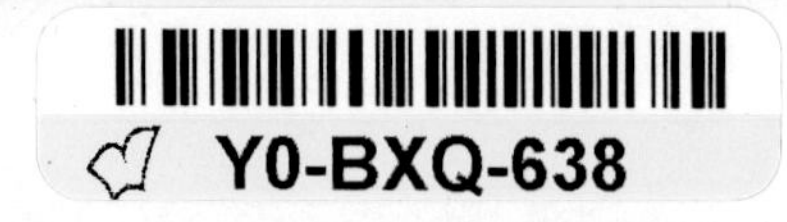
Y0-BXQ-638

NATURAL CELL-MEDIATED IMMUNITY AGAINST TUMORS

Academic Press Rapid Manuscript Reproduction

NATURAL CELL-MEDIATED IMMUNITY AGAINST TUMORS

Edited by

Ronald B. Herberman

Laboratory of Immunodiagnosis
National Cancer Institute
National Institutes of Health
Bethesda, Maryland

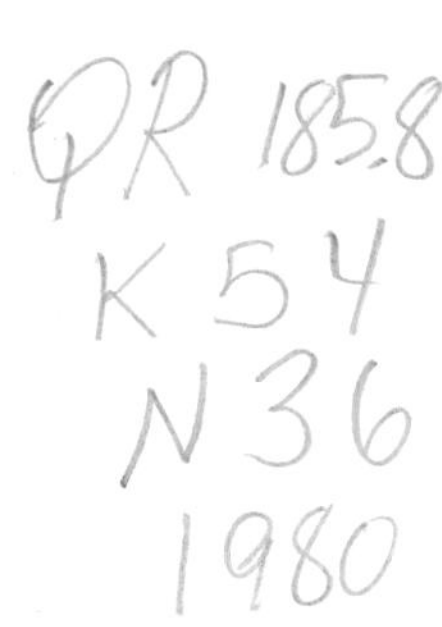

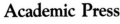

Academic Press

A Subsidiary of Harcourt Brace Jovanovich, Publishers
New York London Toronto Sydney San Francisco 1980

ACADEMIC PRESS, INC.
111 Fifth Avenue, New York, New York 10003

United Kingdom Edition published by
ACADEMIC PRESS, INC. (LONDON) LTD.
24/28 Oval Road, London NW1 7DX

Library of Congress Cataloging in Publication Data
Main entry under title:

Natural cell-mediated immunity against tumors.

Includes index.
1. Killer cells. 2. Tumors—Immunological aspects.
3. Cellular immunity. I. Herberman, Ronald B.,
Date. [DNLM: 1. Neoplasms—Immunology. QA200
N321]
QR185.8.K54N36 616.99′20795 80-15103
ISBN 0-12-341350-8

PRINTED IN THE UNITED STATES OF AMERICA

80 81 82 83 9 8 7 6 5 4 3 2 1

CONTENTS

PARTICIPANTS

Susanne Becker, Department of Obstetrics and Gynecology, University of North Carolina Medical Center, Chapel Hill, North Carolina 27514

Phyllis B. Blair, Department of Bacteriology and Immunology, University of California, Berkeley, California 94720

Barry Bloom, Department of Microbiology and Immunology, Albert Einstein College of Medicine, Bronx, New York 10461

Reinder L. H. Bolhuis, Radiobiological Institute TNO, 151 Lange Kleiweg, Rijswijk, The Netherlands

Michael J. Brunda, Laboratory of Immunodiagnosis, National Cancer Institute, National Institutes of Health, Bethesda, Maryland 20205

Robert C. Burton, Transplantation Unit, Massachusetts General Hospital, Boston, Massachusetts

Denis M. Callewaert, Department of Chemistry, Oakland University, Rochester, Michigan 48053

Edward A. Clark, Regional Primate Research Center, University of Washington, Seattle, Washington 98195

Gustavo Cudkowicz, Department of Pathology School of Medicine, 232 Farber Hall, State University of New York at Buffalo, Buffalo, New York 14214

Jeannine M. Durkik, Fred Hutchinson Cancer Research Center, 1124 Columbia Street, Seattle, Washington 98104

Rachel Ehrlich, Department of Microbiology, The George S. Wise Faculty of Life Sciences, Tel Aviv University, Tel Aviv, Israel

Stefan Einhorn, Karolinska Hospital, Stockholm, Sweden

Oleg Eremin, Division of Immunology, Department of Pathology, University of Cambridge, Cambridge CB2 2QQ, England

James T. Forbes, Division of Oncology, Department of Medicine, Vanderbilt University Hospital, Nashville, Tennessee 37232

James M. Gerson, Department of Pediatrics, The Milton S. Hershey Medical Center, Hershey, Pennsylvania 17033

Magnus Gidlund, Department of Immunology, University of Uppsala Biomedical Center, Biomedicum, Box 582, S-751 23 Uppsala, Sweden

Jerome Mark Greenberg, The Center for the Health Sciences, University of California, School of Medicine, Los Angeles, California 90024

Otto Haller, Institute of Medical Microbiology, University of Zurich, POB 8028, Zurich, Switzerland

Mona Hansson, Department of Tumor Biology, Karolinska Institutet, Stockholm 60, Sweden

Ronald B. Herberman, Laboratory of Immunodiagnosis, National Cancer Institute, National Institutes of Health, Bethesda, Maryland 20205

Pamela J. Jensen, Division of Immunology, Department of Microbiology and Immunology, Duke University Medical Center, Durham, North Carolina 27710

Tsuneo Kamiyama, Department of Surgery, The Center for Health Sciences, School of Medicine, University of California, Los Angeles, California 90024

Joseph Kaplan, Department of Pediatrics, Wayne State University School of Medicine, Detroit, Michigan 48201

H. David Kay, Division of Rheumatology, Department of Internal Medicine, Box 412, The University of Virginia School of Medicine, Charlottesville, Virginia

Robert Keller, Immunobiology Research Group, University of Zurich, Schonleinstrasse 22, CH-8032 Zurich, Switzerland

Holger Kirchner, Deutsches Krebsforschungszentrum Heidelberg, Institut für Virusforschung, 69 Heidelberg, Im Neuenheimer Feld 280, West Germany

Eva Klein, Department of Tumor Biology, Karolinska Institutet, Stockholm 60, Sweden

Yukio Koide, Second Department of Internal Medicine, Nagoya City University Medical School, Kawasumi, Mitzuko-ku Nagoya 467, Japan

Stefan Korec, Laboratory of Immunodiagnosis, National Cancer Institute, National Institutes of Health, Bethesda, Maryland 20205

Hillel S. Koren, Division of Immunology, Department of Microbiology and Immunology, Duke University Medical Center, Durham, North Carolina 27710

Gloria C. Koo, Sloan Kettering Institute for Cancer Research, New York, New York 10021

Santo Landolfo, Università degli Studi di Torino, Istituto di Microbiologia, Via Santena 9, 10126 Torino, Italy

Mary-Ann Lane, Sidney Farber Cancer Center, 35 Binney Street, Boston, Massachusetts 02115

Wolfgang Leibold, Institute of Pathology, Hannover Veterinary School, Hannover, West Germany

Maria-Luise Lohmann-Matthes, Max-Planck-Institut für Immunobiologie, 78 Freigurg-Zahringer, Stubeweg 51, Postfach 1169, West Germany

Eva Lotzová, Department of Developmental Therapeutics, M.D. Anderson Hospital & Tumor Institute, Texas Medical Center, Houston, Texas 77030

Alberto Mantovani, Istituto di Recerche Farmacologiche "Mario Negri," Via Eritrea, 62, 20157 Milano, Italy

Michael Moore, Division of Immunology, Paterson Laboratories, Christie Hospital & Holt Radium Institute, Manchester Area Health Authority (South), Manchester M20 9BX, England

Anders Örn, Department of Immunology, University of Uppsala Biomedical Center, Biomedicum, Box 582, S-751 23 Uppsala, Sweden

John R. Ortaldo, Laboratory of Immunodiagnosis, National Cancer Institute, National Institutes of Health, Bethesda, Maryland 20205

Bice Perussia, Wistar Institute, 36th and Spruce, Philadelphia, Pennsylvania 19101

Hans H. Peter, Dept. Innere Medizin, Med. Hochschule, D-3000 Hannover, West Germany

Sylvia B. Pollack, Department of Biology and Immunology, ZD-08, University of Washington, Seattle, Washington 98185

Hugh F. Pross, Department of Pathology, The Ontario Cancer Foundation, Kingston Clinic, Kingston, Ontario, Canada K7L 2V7

Carlo Riccardi, Universita̓ degli Studi di Perugia, Istituto di Farmacologia, Via Del Giochetto, 06100 Perugia, Italy

Gert Riethmüller, Eberhard-Karls-Universität Tübingen, Chirurgische Klinik, Abteilung für Exp. Chirugie u. Immunologie, D 7400 Tübingen 1, Den Calwer Strasse 7, West Germany

John C. Roder, Department of Microbiology and Immunology, Queen's University, Kingston, Ontario, Canada K7L 3N6

Eero Saksela, Department of Pathology, University of Helsinki, Haartmaninkatu 3, SF-00290 Helsinki 29, Finland

Daniela Santoli, Wistar Institute, 36th and Spruce, Philadelphia, Pennsylvania 19101

Angela Santoni, Laboratoria di Immunologia e Chemotherapia, Universita̓ di Perugia, Via Del Giochetto, 06100 Perugia, Italy

William E. Seaman, Immunology & Arthritis Section (151T), Veterans Administration Hospital, 4150 Clement Street, San Francisco, California 94121

Janet K. Seeley, Laboratory of Immunodiagnosis, National Cancer Institute, National Institutes of Health, Bethesda, Maryland 20205

Osias Stutman, Cellular Immunology Section, Sloan Kettering Institute for Cancer Research, New York, New York 10021

Anna Tai, Departments of Pathology and Medicine, School of Medicine, University of New Mexico, Albuquerque, New Mexico 87131

Aldo Tagliabue, Istituto di Ricerche Farmacologiche, M. Nigri Via Eritrea, 62, 20157 Milano, Italy

Milton R. Tam, Fred Hutchinson Cancer Research Center, 1124 Columbia Street, Seattle, Washington 19804

Giorgio Trinchieri, Wistar Institute, 36th and Spruce, Philadelphia, Pennsylvania 19101

Brent M. Vose, Patterson Laboratories, Christie Hospital and Holt Radium Institute, Manchester M20 9BX, England

Raymond M. Welsh, Jr., Department of Immunopathology, Scripps Clinic and Research Foundation, 10666 North Torrey Pines Road, La Jolla, California 92037

Joyce M. Zarling, Immunology Research Center, 1150 University Avenue, Madison, Wisconsin 53706

PREFACE

Most immunologists have long tended to regard natural or spontaneous immunity as an amorphous subject of rather dubious import. In part, this view was due to traditional training and approaches to immunologic problems. By comparison with acquired immunity, and the extensive information on its characteristics, poorly understood observations of natural immunity met with much skepticism about their biologic significance. Furthermore, immune responses are generally considered to be induced by a particular, known antigen. There is almost an instinctive belief of immunologists that all immune phenomena must be in response to an immunogen. Thus, uninduced reactivity, not under the control of the investigator and directed against ill-defined structures, is suspect. The prevailing view has been that natural immunity differs from acquired immunity only in the nature of the inducing antigen or in some quantitative aspects, but that the mechanisms involved are the same. Efforts were often directed toward identification of an environmental or endogenous antigenic stimulus and, if none were found, the reactivity would be judged nonspecific or even nonimmunologic.

Changes in this attitude have been slow to develop and a beginning appreciation of the potential of this spontaneously arising state of immune reactivity has only recently come to the fore. As the extensive investigations on NK cells attest, this traditional view was based on a tacit assumption rather than a coherent analysis and was unwarranted, for it is now clear that in many ways the cellular basis and regulatory factors for natural immunity differ strikingly from those involved in "classical" acquired immunity. Indeed, in certain key biologic situations such as the germ-free state, and in nude or thymectomized mice, natural immunity remains quite unimpaired. Moreover, in neoplasia this noninduced cellular system may in some situations make a more effective contribution to host resistance and survival than the highly vaunted T cell-based immune cytotoxicity.

We are entering a new era in which the mechanism and operational basis for the host's innate capability to cope with threats of the environment are undergoing far-reaching reassessment. Investigators in this neglected sector of modern immunobiology now proceed apace, being limited mostly by the need for development of requisite techniques, reagents, and approaches, a new awareness of the implications of noninduced resistance and its possible complementary role or even primary role in host defenses, and the abandonment of past bias.

Natural killer (NK) cells were discovered only about eight years ago. Thereafter, a small number of investigators became interested in this subpopulation of lymphoid cells and began to explore their characteristic ability to lyse a wide variety of tumor cells and their possible role *in vivo.* More recently, with the marked burgeoning of interest in natural cell-mediated immunity, experienced investigators worldwide have turned to this field. NK cells are now known to be present in a variety of animal species and their characteristics have been extensively studied. Although the reactivity of NK cells against tumors continues to attract most of the effort, the field has diversified in a number of important aspects: It has become evident that the reactivity of NK cells is by no means restricted to tumor cells as these cells also recognize and lyse certain normal cells, including subpopulation of thymocytes, macrophages, and bone marrow cells. The reactivity against bone marrow cells has provided a major new insight into the mechanisms that could account for natural resistance to engraftment of allogeneic and xenogeneic bone marrow. Thus, the NK cell may well be involved in regulation of differentiation of normal hematopoietic cells, as well as in resistance against tumors. Moreover, NK cells may also have a role in resistance to viral diseases as they have been found to be quite active against cells infected with a variety of viruses.

Research on NK cells has extended into other fields of investigation and has contributed new knowledge on problems in these areas. The accumulating evidence for a close relationship of NK cells to K cells [effector cells for antibody-dependent cell-mediated cytotoxicity (ADCC) against tumors] has helped in the characterization of K cells. Similarly, the discovery that interferon plays a central role in augmentation of NK activity reveals an appealing new interpretation for the antitumor effects of this agent.

Research on natural cell-mediated immunity has identified other categories of natural effector cells, particularly macrophages and granulocytes. It is especially noteworthy that other cytotoxic effector cells have also been discerned, which have a number of differences from, as well as some similarities with, NK cells. Moreover, natural cell-mediated immune functions apart from cytotoxicity are now perceived, such as the natural production of lymphokines in response to tumor cells and other stimuli.

Much of the research covered in this volume got underway at the very time major changes were taking place in the prevailing views regarding tumor immunology. Much of the deep-seated belief that immonology was destined to play a major role in understanding and coping with cancer centered around three concepts that enjoyed wide acceptance: (a) the presence of tumor-specific or tumor-associated antigens on most or all tumors; T cell-mediated immunity against these antigens, especially cytotoxic T cells, was considered to play a central role in resistance against tumor growth; (b) immune surveillance against tumors, again with T cell-mediated immunity assigned paramount importance; (c) implicit faith that immunotherapy represented a major advance in dealing with the realities of clinical cancer. Here, too, the role of T cells, especially cytotoxic T cells, was the major focus. Considerable efforts have been made to account for the effects of immunotherapy by the induction or increase in T cell-mediated immunity or by the elimination of factors interfering with this arm of the immune response. Extensive immunological monitoring of cancer patients receiving immunotherapy focused on the levels of T cells and their functions and on specific T cell-mediated immunity against tumor-associated antigens.

Each of these components of the foundation of faith in, and enthusiasm for, tumor immunology has now been seriously challenged, and painstaking efforts are directed toward separating reality from unrealistic expectations. This questioning of the importance of the immune system in resistance against cancer results from findings that spontaneous tumors are often nonimmunogenic, the absence of specific cytotoxic T cells reactive against many human tumors (indeed, much if not most of what had been previously described is likely due to NK cells or other naturally cytotoxic cells), apparent contradictions to some major predictions of the immune surveillance hypothesis (e.g., lack of a major increase in tumor incidence in nude, athymic mice, or in neonatally thymectomized mice), and failure to demonstrate convincingly efficacy in most of the clinical trials of immunotherapy (accompanied by the frustrating failure to detect clear effects on the immunologic parameters that were monitored, even in those trials where immunotherapy was actually providing clinical benefits).

The discovery and understanding of NK cells and other natural effector cells have revealed new vistas for coping with some of these problems and have given a new perspective to the concept of immune surveillance and a distinctive role for the immune system in resistance against tumor growth, even in T cell-deficient individuals and against nonimmunogenic tumors. These developments suggest new possibilities for immunotherapy and alternative explanations for some of the beneficial effects of immunotherapeutic agents in current use.

This volume is designed to provide the first comprehensive treatment of the subject of natural cell-mediated immunity against tumors. Up to now, only selected aspects of NK cell research has been dealt with in review articles. With the rapid proliferation of information on NK and other natural effector cells, it has become progressively more difficult for most experimentalists and clinicians to sort through and assimilate this complex literature. The nature of the NK cell and its relationship to the known categories of lymphoid and other hematopoietic cells has proved to be especially confusing. There has been a shift from the earlier consideration of the NK cell as having no distinguishing characteristics, and consequently described as a null cell, to the present where the cell has been reported to have, in fact, a variety of positive features, some suggestive of a relationship to T cells and others of a possible link to macrophages or even to B cells. With the identification of other forms of natural cell-mediated immunity, it has become increasingly difficult to determine which effects are due solely to NK cells and to other effector cells, or even to distinguish adequately between these various cell types. It therefore became essential to sift through this accumulated information and to systematize and assess the data and identify the current problems, issues, and delineate the needs, opportunities, and prospects for this research area.

This volume brings together contributions from the leading laboratories presently conducting research in this field. Each was invited to summarize one or more main aspects of their research, in a brief but relatively comprehensive fashion, and was encouraged to emphasize current information, including unpublished data. In view of the immediate character of these contributions, the editor and the publisher had committed themselves to seeing this volume to completion within six months of submission of manuscripts. The brevity of the processing period necessitated the utilization of "camera ready" format. Hopefully, the benefits of speedy publication will outweigh any inconveniences such as inconsistency in style, typeface, and typographical errors. Regrettably, a few of the important contributors to the field were unable to meet the short deadline and, hence, the omission of their contributions. However, the overall response and cooperation in this plan has been excellent and each area appears amply documented. Since the planned schedule has been realized, the overall product reflects a truly current exposition of the state of knowledge in the field.

The main topics to be covered were selected in the planning and organization of this volume. Rather than having contributors prepare a review on all aspects of their investigations on natural immunity, they were asked to segregate their information into segments relevant to the main topics that make up the structure of this volume. This made for the integration of information on each major topic, avoiding the diffuse quality that would otherwise result. To further assist the reader in evaluating and comprehending the diverse range of complex data, the editor has prepared descriptive, critical synopses for each section, highlighting the main points.

This volume seeks to provide a better perspective of how these natural mechanisms fit in with and relate to the traditional, more extensively studied components of the immune system. It is now apparent that many unexplained phenomena that have been noted during the course of immunologic research, e.g., increased baseline response or unexpectedly rapid or "nonspecific" responses to immunization, may well involve NK cells or other natural effector mechanisms. It therefore becomes mandatory to consider and control for the possible contributions of NK cells in studies of "immune" T cell reactivities. Similarly, those concerned with macrophages and granulocytes must also consider the natural activity of these effector cells. Indeed, as investigators proceed apace, it becomes compellingly evident that these natural, noninduced effectors constitute a very broad spectrum of cell types, primarily perceived by their distinct activities, their membrane characteristics, susceptibility to modulation, genetics, etc. They transcend the few neatly categorized cell types that heretofore have dominated immunobiologic investigation.

INTRODUCTION

Ronald B. Herberman

National Cancer Institute
Bethesda, Maryland

The chapters in this book are mainly summaries of current information regarding natural killer (NK) cells and other aspects of natural cell-mediated immunity. To put this large amount of data into perspective, it is worthwhile to briefly review the chronology of developments in this rapidly advancing field of research.

Cell-mediated cytotoxicity against tumors first began to be extensively examined about 13 years ago, when Hellström (1967) developed the colony inhibition assay. Cytotoxicity against a variety of experimental tumors in rodents and against cultured cells from some human tumors was observed with lymphoid cells from tumor-bearing or tumor-immune individuals. Shortly thereafter, the technically simpler microcytotoxicity assay was developed (Takasugi and Klein, 1970) and with this many laboratories began studies on cell-mediated immunity against tumors. During the next two to three years, there were many reports on cell-mediated cytotoxicity against tumors in rodents and other experimental species. There was even a more rapid and extensive proliferation of reports on reactivity of cancer patients, with a wide assortment of tumor types (for review of these assays and findings, see Herberman, 1974). Both the colony inhibition and microcytotoxicity assays required the rather tedious visual counting of large numbers of cells. Shortly after Brunner *et al.* (1968) developed the ^{51}chromium release cytotoxicity assay, this and other radioisotopic release techniques began to be applied to tumor systems (Oren *et al.*, 1971; Lavrin *et al.*, 1972, 1973; Leclerc *et al.*; 1972, Jagarlamoody *et al.*, 1971; Cohen *et al.*, 1973). Particularly for studies with leukemia or lymphoma target cells, it was possible to perform ^{51}Cr release assays in 4 hours and this rapid and quantitative

ISBN 0-12-341350-8

assay has become the method of choice for most studies of lymphocyte cell-mediated cytotoxicity.

During this early period of research, the focus was on specific cell-mediated cytotoxicity against tumor-associated antigens. Tumor-bearing or tumor-immune individuals were found to react against their own or related tumors but usually not against skin fibroblasts or unrelated tumors. Since normal individuals were assumed to be unreactive, the effects of normal lymphocytes were taken as the baseline control or zero point and results were expressed as the activity above that of the normal control. In studies with neuroblastoma, Hellström *et al*. (1968) noted that some normal relatives of patients reacted but suggested that this was due to some contact-induced sensitization against the disease.

Although this concept of almost ubiquitous, specific tumor associated cell-mediated cytotoxic reactivity against tumors became generally accepted, some exceptions to the expected specificity in clinical testing began to be noted by a few investigators. This led to a Conference and Workshop on Cellular Immune Reactions to Human Tumor-Associated Antigens, held in June 1972 (for proceedings and discussion, see Herberman and Gaylord, 1973). Many problems with the cytotoxicity tests with human tumor cells were apparent, but the majority of participants considered these to be due to technical difficulties with the target cells and/or with the preparation of the effector cells. However, a few reports were discussed which indicated that normal individuals, including those unrelated or unexposed to cancer patients, could react against leukemic cells (Rosenberg *et al*., 1972) or against cell lines derived from tumors (McCoy *et al*., 1973; Oldham *et al*., 1973). Because of this, the following comments were included in the concluding remarks at the Conference: "Most of us have seen a variety of effects produced by the lymphocytes of normal individuals. Does this represent real immunologic activity against tumor-associated antigens, or is this just noise or problems with setting the baseline in the assays?... It is certainly possible that some or all normal individuals have immune reactivity against tumor cells or cell lines derived from tumors...These reactions could play an important role in immune surveillance" (Herberman, 1973).

The discussion at this Conference stimulated much reevaluation of disease-related specificity by many of the participants and in fact, by the time of submission of their manuscript for the Monograph, Skurzak *et al*. (1973) included a description of reactivity by non-malignant controls against glioma target cells. Within the next 1-2 years, many investigators, including some of those initially obtaining good specificity, reported on cytotoxic reactivity by normal individuals and a lack of complete histologic type-specific reactivity by cancer patients (Takasugi *et al*., 1973; Heppner *et al*., 1975; Peter *et al*., 1975; Kay *et al*., 1976; Canevari *et al*., 1976).

In the midst of this transition period, in November 1974, there was a Workshop on Cell-Mediated Cytotoxicity for Bladder Carcinoma (see Bean *et al*., 1975 for report) at the Sloan-Kettering Institute in New York. The focus was on human bladder cancer and secondarily on malignant melanoma, since these were thought to be the main types of cancer for which specific, disease-related cell-mediated cytotoxicity still could be demonstrated. From comparative tests by several groups on a limited number of blood specimens, it was clear that differences in preparation of effector cells did affect the results. However, the most impressive outcome was that, despite these differences, there was rather good correlation in results among investigators. Since at the Workshop and in most of the investigators' own laboratories, effector cells frequently showed reactivity restricted to some of the target cell lines, Dr. Eva Klein suggested the new operational term, selective cytotoxicity, to denote cytotoxicity for some target cells, including, for the cancer patients tested, those of unrelated histological types, but not for all test target cells. In retrospect, and as illustrated by some of the chapters in this book, this appears to be a good description for the reactivity pattern of NK cells and related natural effector cells. However, it is noteworthy that, at the time of the Workshop, just five years ago, there was very little direct discussion of natural cell-mediated cytotoxicity.

Concurrent with the initial recognition of cytotoxic reactivity by normal human donors were similar observations in rodent systems. When spleen cells from young, 6-8 week old normal rats were tested as controls for studies of immunity to a Gross virus-induced leukemia, they were found to frequently give substantial levels of lysis above the medium control and often as high as those from tumor-immune rats. After this natural reactivity was found to be a consistent phenomenon (Nunn *et al*., 1973), similar observations were made with normal mice and initially reported at the Second International Immunology Congress, July 1973 (Herberman *et al*., 1974). Within the next two years, the initial characterization of mouse and rat NK cells was completed (e.g., Kiessling *et al*., 1975a,b; Herberman, 1975a,b; Nunn *et al*., 1976).

As a result of the above reports, another international conference on immunity to human tumors (Stevenson and Laurence, 1975), and two editorials in J. Natl. Cancer Inst. (Baldwin, 1975; Herberman and Oldham, 1975), during 1975 awareness of the limitations in the search for specific disease-related cell-mediated cytotoxicity and of the possible role of natural effector cells became widespread. Thus began a rapid expansion of research activity on natural cell-mediated immunity, with particular emphasis on characterization of the effector cells and on determination of the possible *in vivo* role of these cells (reviewed by Baldwin, 1977; Herberman and Holden, 1978; Kiessling and Haller, 1978; Möller, 1979).

The field has moved more rapidly with mice and rats than with humans, probably because of the availability of many markers for characterization of lymphocyte subpopulations and of inbred strains for analysis of genetic factors and because of the ability to readily perform in vivo manipulations. A major advance in our understanding of the regulation of NK activity began with the observations that inoculation with a variety of stimuli (Herberman *et al*., 1976, 1977; Wolfe 1976) led to a rapid augmentation of NK activity. When poly I:C, a well-known inducer of interferon was found to have this activity in rats (Oehler *et al*., 1978), the possible mediation of the augmentation by interferon was suggested. This possibility was soon thereafter confirmed for mouse (Gidlund et al., 1978; Djeu *et al*., 1979) and human (Trinchieri and Santoli, 1978; Herberman *et al*., 1979) NK cells.

The progress in this field has been remarkable during the approximately eight years of its existence. Cytotoxicity by cells from normal individuals has evolved from an overlooked or maligned, undesirable effect (thought to be an artifact) to a well-studied area of research. It is rather ironic how great the shift has been, from an almost exclusive emphasis on specific cell mediated immunity against tumor associated antigens to a predominance now, at least for human studies, of reports on NK and other natural effector cells and very few continuing reports of disease-related cytotoxic effector cells.

The current status of the field is well summarized by the contributions in this book. However, it should be clear that there are still more unresolved problems than there are clear answers. Perhaps this book will provide another milestone in this field, and stimulate more extensive efforts to definitively characterize the effector cells and determine their biological roles.

REFERENCES

Baldwin, R. W. (1975). *J. Natl. Cancer Inst. 55,* 745.

Baldwin, R. W. (1977). *Nature 270,* 557.

Bean, M. A., Bloom, B. R., Herberman, R. B., Old, L. J., Oettgen, H. F., Klein, G., and Terry, W. D. (1975). *Cancer Res. 35,* 2902.

Brunner, K. T., Mavel, J., Cerottini, J. C., and Chapuis, B. (1968). *Immunol. 14,* 181.

Canevari, S., Fossati, G., and DellaPorta, G. (1976). *J. Natl. Cancer Inst. 56,* 705.

Cohen, A. M. (1973). *Cancer 31,* 81.

Djeu, J. Y., Heinbaugh, J. A., Holden, H. T., and Herberman, R. B. (1979). *J. Immunol. 122,* 175.

Gidlund, M., Orn, A., Wigzell, H., Senik, A., and Gresser, I. (1978). *Nature 223,* 259.

Hellström, I. (1967). *Int. J. Cancer 2,* 65.

Hellström, I., Hellström, K. E., Pierce, G. E., and Bill, A. H. (1968). *Proc. Nat. Acad. Sci. USA 60,* 1231.

Heppner, G., Henry, E., Stolbach, L., Cummings, S. F., McDonough, E., and Calabresi, P. (1975). *Cancer Res. 35,* 1931.

Herberman, R. B. (1973). *Nat'l. Cancer Inst. Monogr. 37,* 217.

Herberman, R. B. (1974). *In* "Advances in Cancer Research," Vol. 19, (G. Klein and S. Weinhouse, eds.) p. 207. Academic Press, New York.

Herberman, R. B., and Gaylord, C. E. (eds.), (1973). *Nat'l. Cancer Inst. Monogr. 37,*.

Herberman, R. B., and Holden, H. T. (1978). *Adv. Cancer Res. 27,* 305.

Herberman, R. B., and Oldham, R. K. (1975). *J. Nat'l Cancer Inst. 55,* 749.

Herberman, R. B., Ting, C. C., Kirchner, H., Holden, H., Glaser, M., and Lavrin, D. (1974). *In* "Progress in Immunology, II" (L. Brent and J. Holborow, eds.) p. 285. North-Holland Publishing Co., Amsterdam 285.

Herberman, R. B., Nunn, M. E., and Lavrin, D. H. (1975a). *Int. J. Cancer 16,* 216.

Herberman, R. B., Nunn, M. E., Holden, H. T., and Lavrin, D. H. (1975a). *Int. J. Cancer 16,* 230.

Herberman, R. B., Campbell, D. A. Jr., Oldham, R. K., Bonnard, G. D., Ting, C. C., Holden, H. T., Glaser, M., Djeu, J., and Oehler, R. (1976). *Ann. N. Y. Acad. Sci. 276,* 26.

Herberman, R. B., Nunn, M. E., Holden, H. T., Staal, S., and Djeu, J. Y. (1977). *Int. J. Cancer 19,* 5.

Jagarlamoody, S. M., Aust, J. C., Tew, R. H., and McKhann, C. F. (1971). *Proc. Nat'l. Acad. Sci. 68,* 1346.
Kay, H. D., Thota, H., and Sinkovics, J. G. (1976). *Clin. Immunol. Immunopathol. 5,* 218.
Kiessling, R., and Haller, O. (1978). *In* "Contemporary Topics in Immunology" (N.L. Warner, ed.) 8, 171.
Kiessling, R., Klein, E., and Wigzell, H. (1975a). *Europ. J. Immunol. 5,* 112.
Kiessling, R., Klein, E., Pross, H., and Wigzell, H. (1975a). *Europ. J. Immunol. 5,* 117.
Lavrin, D., Nunn, M., and Herberman, R. B. (1972). *Proc. Amer. Assoc. Cancer Res. 13,* 66.
Lavrin, D. H., Herberman, R. B., Nunn, M., and Soares, N. (1973). *J. Nat'l. Cancer Inst. 51,* 1497.
Leclerc, J. C., Gomard, E., and Levy, J. P. (1972). *Int. J. Cancer 10,* 589.
McCoy, J. L., Herberman, R. B., Rosenberg, E. B., Donnelly, F. C., Levine, P. H., and Alford, C. (1973). *Nat'l. Cancer Inst. Monogr. 37,* 59.
Möller, G. (1979). *Immunol. Rev. 44,* 1.
Nunn, M., Djeu, J., Lavrin, D., and Herberman, R. (1973). *Proc. Amer. Assoc. Cancer Res. 14,* 87.
Nunn, M. E., Djeu, J. Y., Glaser, M., Lavrin, D. H., and Herberman, R. B. (1976). *J. Nat'l. Cancer Inst. 56,* 393.
Oehler, J. R., Lindsay, L. R., Nunn, M. E., Holden, H. T., and Herberman, R. B. (1978). *Int. J. Cancer 21,* 210.
Oldham, R. K., Siwarski, D., McCoy, J. L., Plata, E. J., and Herberman, R. B. (1973). *Nat'l. Cancer Inst. Monogr. 37,* 49.
Oren, M. E., Herberman, R. B., and Canty, T. G. (1971). *J. Nat'l. Cancer Inst. 46,* 621.
Peter, H. H., Pavie-Fischer, J., Fridman, W. H., Aubert, C., Cesarini, J. P., Roubin, R., and Kourilsky, F. M. (1975). *J. Immunol. 115,* 539.
Rosenberg, E. B., Herberman, R. B., Levine, P. H., Halterman, R. H., McCoy, J. L., and Wunderlich, J. R. (1972). *Int. J. Cancer 9,* 648.
Skurzak, H. M., Steiner, D., Klein, E., and Lamon, E. W. (1973). *Nat'l. Cancer Int. Monogr. 39,* 93.
Stevenson, G. T., and Laurence, D. J. R. (1975). *Int. J. Cancer 16,* 887.
Takasugi, M., and Klein, E. (1970). *Transplant. 9,* 219.
Takasugi, M., Mickey, M. R., and Terasaki, P. I. (1973). *Cancer Res. 33,* 2898.
Trinchieri, G., and Santoli, D. (1978). *J. Exp. Med. 147,* 1314.
Wolfe, S. A., Tracey, D. E., and Henney, C. S. (1976). *Nature 262,* 584.

CHARACTERISTICS OF NK AND RELATED CELLS

Reinder Bolhuis

Rotterdam Radio-Therapy Institute,
Rotterdam;
and
Radiobiological Institute TNO,
P.O. Box 5815
2280 HV Rijswijk
The Netherlands

A. Characteristics of NK Cells and Related Cells

1. General

Many reports have eventuated demonstrating disease-related anti-tumor cytotoxic activity of lymphocytes of tumor patients (1-4). Documentation of NK cytotoxicity against a wide variety of cell lines of lymphocytes derived from both normal donors and cancer patients seriously questioned the validity of determination of disease-related cytotoxicity of cancer patients' lymphocytes (5-7).

Although these spontaneous cytotoxic reactivities were initially considered as "undesired background", it was then suggested that this NK cytotoxicity, taking place without deliberate sensitization against notably malignant cells, may serve as an alternative immune surveillance mechanism.

Antibody dependent and/or antibody independent cell-mediated cytotoxicity operate in healthy donors and, for instance, in cancer patients. The former effector cells, which are involved in antibody dependent cell-mediated cytotoxicity (ADCC) against IgG-coated mouse mastocytoma cells (K-cell cytotoxicity), express receptors for the Fc portion of IgG (IgG-FcR). Monocytes have also been show to bear these FcR. A

The work presented here was supported by grant X-67 of the Dutch National Cancer League, the "Koningin Wilhelmina Fonds"

ISBN 0-12-341350-8

number of cell types have been determined to exert the "spontaneous" or NK cytotoxicity in man, such as IgG-FcR bearing cells (8, 9), complement receptor bearing cells (10), carry ing FcR as well as complement receptors (11), and activated T-cells (12).

Thus, substantial information is available in the literature to favor the following possibilities:
1. IgG-FcR are present on both NK-cells cytotoxic against monolayer target cells (8, 12) or K-562 cells (13) and K-cells (8, 14-17);
2. soluble factors or antibodies are involved in NK cell killing (18, 19);
3) (a proportion of) NK cells belong to the T-cell lineage of lymphocytes (13, 20, 21). The suggested involvement of antibodies would implicate that the NK cytotoxic cell mechanism is of an ADCC type.

The experiments described here aimed to address the following questions: 1) are the characteristics of the cells exerting NK cytotoxicity against the K-562 erythroleukemic cells growing in suspension (as measured in a short term ^{51}Chromium release assay), the same as those active against human tumor derived cell lines growing in monolayers (as measured in a longterm cytotoxic assay)?; 2) are NK and K reactivities both antibody dependent and possibly displayed by identical cells?

METHODS

1. Purification of mononuclear cells.

Lymphocyte purification: Mononuclear cells were obtained from healthy donors by Ficoll-Isopaque centrifugal sedimentation of heparinized blood. Contaminating phagocytic cells in the isolated lymphoid cells were removed by treating the cells with carbonyl iron plus magnetism. Table I shows the percentage cell yield of the cell separations.

Isolation of sheep red blood cell (SRBC) rosette forming cells: E-RFC enriched and E-RFC depleted populations were obtained. The technique has been described in detail (13, 20, 21).

Separation of cells lacking the IgG-Fc receptor (IgG-FcR) and recovery of cells with IgG-FcR: IgG coated SRBC (EA-RFC) were eliminated by adsorbing these IgG-FcR positive cells to antibody-antigen immune complex monolayers. The technique described by Kedar et al. (22) with some modifications (21,

TABLE I

CELL YIELD EXPRESSED AS PERCENTAGE OF THE INITIAL LYMPHOCYTE NUMBER (% total yield) ± SE AND PERCENTAGE OF THE LYMPHOCYTE NUMBER USED FOR A PARTICULAR SEPARATION STEP (% step-wise yield) ± SE

Lymphocyte fractions	% total yield ± SE	% step-wise yield ± SE	no. of experiments
Ficoll-Isopaque purified lymphocytes	100	100	7
Lymphocytes plus iron and magnetism treatment	80 ± 3.1	80 ± 3.1	10
E-RFC enriched fraction (T cell fraction)	55 ± 7.0	68 ± 4.8	6
E-RFC depleted fraction (non-T cell fraction)	7 ± 1.3	8 ± 1.4	6
Direct EA-RFC depleted fraction	63 ± 6.3	64 ± 9.3	12
Direct EA-RFC recovered fraction	21 ± 4.3	23 ± 6.8	1

23) was used. The principal of the technique is depicted in Scheme 1.

Preparation of pure lymphocytes: Ficoll-Isopaque separated lymphocytes were further purified by passing the cells over a nylon column. The procedure used has been described (7). In short, the cells were placed onto a column of unstained spun nylon with a length of 5 cm and a diameter of 15 mm, which had been prewashed with medium supplemented with 5% fetal calf serum. The column was then incubated for 30 min at 37° C. The lymphocytes were eluted with RPMI-1640 plus 5% fetal calf serum, and the eluted cells were washed in medium.

Preparation of monocyte enriched fraction: Monocytes were prepared from Ficoll-Isopaque purified mononuclear cells. One milliliter leukocyte suspension (30×10^6/ml) in RPMI-1640 1640 plus 20% fetal calf serum was added to a Falcon petri dish (60 x 15 mm) and cells were allowed to adhere to the

Scheme 1

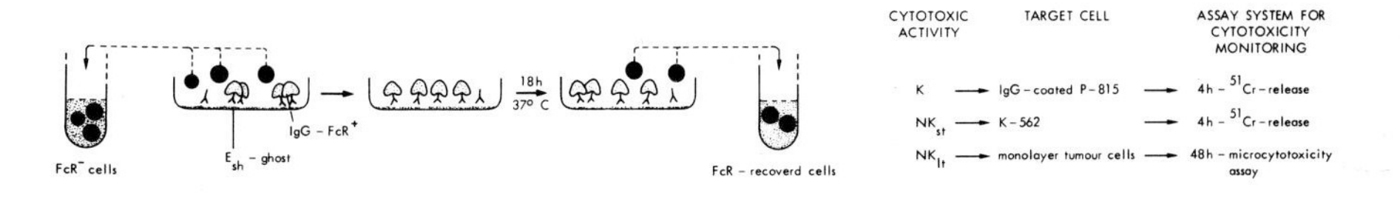

surface by incubating the cells for 1 h at 37° C. After washing the plates thoroughly to remove nonadherent cells, the adherent cells were collected by gently scraping the plates with a rubber policeman. The percentage monocytes present in this recovered fraction was 50-60% as judged by electronic sizing (24) and counting of non-specific esterase positive cells (25).

Target cells: P-815-X2 mouse mastocytoma cells and K-562 erythroid leukemic cells were maintained as suspension cultures and used as target cells in a 4 h ^{51}Cr release assay assay (20, 21,26). Colon carcinoma cells and two melanoma cells (Mel-I and NKI-4) were cultured as monolayers and used as target cells in the Takasugi-Klein cytotoxicity assay (26).

It should be noted that the data presented in this section were obtained using cryopreserved lymphoid cells as effector cells. This was due to the fact that for the simultaneous analysis of functional and morphological (i.e. cell surface markers) of unfractionated and fractionated populations, 500 x 10^6 lymphocytes per donor were needed. After the cells were thawed they were incubated overnight before they were used (20, 21).

Determination of T cells by rosette formation with SRBC and anti-T-cell serum, of EA-RFC and of B cells by immunofluorescence after staining the cells with FITC-labelled goat anti-human Fab (Ga/Hu/Fab, Nordic, Tilburg, The Netherlands) has been described in detail (27).

NK_{st} and killer (K) cell antibody dependent cell-mediated cytotoxicity (ADCC): NK_{st} (short-term) and K cytotoxicity were measured in a 4 h ^{51}Cr-release assay using K-562 and P-815 sensitized with anti-P-815-IgG, as target cells (20, 21).

The 48-h microcytotoxicity test has been described by Takasugi and Klein (26). This assay was used to determine the cytotoxic effect of NK cells against monolayer target cells. These effector cells were operationally defined as NK_{lt} (long-term) cells.

RESULTS

1. NK and K (ADCC) activities of unseparated mononuclear lymphoid cells and IgG-FcR negative lymphoid cells:

The results of EA-RFC-separation studies (20,21) are presented in Table II. The aim was to resolve the question

TABLE II

PER CENT CYTOTOXICITY OF VARIOUS LYMPHOCYTE FRACTIONS

Lymphocyte donor	per cent reduction of target cells					% E-RFC	immunofluorescence				% EA-RFC
	NKI-4	NK_{lt}[1] Mel-1	colon	NK_{st}[2] K-562	K[3] P-815		% T^+	% Ig^+	% T^+/Ig^+	% T^-/Ig^-	
Donor A											
1) unfractionated lymphocytes	37*[4]	25*		20*	14*	71[5]	73	8	1	18	12
2) EA-RFC depleted fraction	33*	11		4	0	76	89	1	5	5	1
Donor B											
1) unfractionated lymphocytes	64*		44*	35*	39*	82					22
2) EA-RFC depleted fraction	18		28*	4	5	87	93	1	0	6	0
Donor C											
1) unfractionated lymphocytes		22*	44*	24*		76					20
2) EA-RFC depleted fraction	19*			2	0	93					1
Donor D											
1) unfractionated lymphocytes	35*		31*	47*		74	80	8	2	10	17
2) EA-RFC depleted fraction			35*	0	0	77	98	1	0	1	0
Donor E											
1) unfractionated lymphocytes	15		48*	14*	23*	80	87	6	1	6	20
2) EA-RFC depleted fraction	- 3		4	4	0	96	96	0	0	4	0

1 NK_{lt}: NK cell cytotoxicity against monolayer cultures (48 h MCT)
2 NK_{st}: NK cell cytotoxicity against K-562 (4 h ^{51}Cr-release assay)
3 K: K cell cytotoxicity against IgG-coated P-815 (4 h ^{51}Cr-release assay)
4 * p value $\leq$ 0.05
5 lymphocytes were not treated. The average yield of 2, 43 % of 1.

whether all NK cells carried FcR on their surface, irrespective of their target cell type. The unfractionated mononuclear cells were cytotoxic against all monolayer tumor target cells and K-562 target cells and displayed K-cell (ADCC) activity. When the EA-RFC were eliminated from the mononuclear cells, no NK_{st} cytotoxicity against K-562 target cells or K (ADCC) cytotoxicity against IgG-P-815 target cells was observed in a 4 h ^{51}Cr-release assay.

The EA-RFC depleted fraction of a number of individuals still displayed cytotoxicity against monolayer target cells in the long-term microcytotoxicity assay (Table II). These results indicate that NK cells in human peropheral blood represent a heterogeneous population of effector cells (20, 21, 28).

The NK_{lt} effector cells are heterogeneous among themselves since elimination of the EA-RFC from the mononuclear cells may a) reduce the level of cytotoxicity against one monolayer target cell but not against the other (Table II, donor A); b) reduce the level of cytotoxicity against both monolayer target cells (Table II, donor B). Apparently, the NK_{lt} consists of both IgG-FcR positive and IgG-FcR negative cells and, moreover, there appears to be selectivity in the recognition and killing of mononuclear cells, also after elimination of IgG-FcR positive effector cells.

The efficacy of EA-RFC depletion is demonstrated by our data showing that no ADCC and no EA-RFC (Table II) are observed after elimination of IgG-FcR positive cells.

One possibility to explain the cytotoxicity of IgG-FcR negative cells against monolayer target cells would be that IgG-FcR are regenerated during the 48 h time period which is needed in the NK_{lt} assays. Regeneration of FcR under certain conditions has been reported (29). This possibility could be excluded since EA-RFC effector cells, being cytotoxic against monolayer target cells in a 48 h microcytotoxicity assay were not able to lyse monolayer target cells or IgG-P-815 target cells in a 4 h ^{51}Cr release assay after prior incubation for 48 h of these effector cells on monolayer target cells (unpublished results).

As for the presence of IgG-FcR on most NK cells, especially those cytotoxic against K-562 this finding is in agreeagreement with data reported by others (8, 9, 11, 30, 31, 32).

2. NK and K (ADCC) activities of E-RFC enriched and E-RFC depleted cell fractions:

The majority of reports indicated that NK cells belong to a so-called non-T "null" cell fraction. This was concluded on the basis of cell separation studies and subsequent determination of percentages T and non-T cells in the isolated fractions. Table III gives NK_{lt}, NK_{st} and K cytotoxicity data of such cell separation studies and the simultaneous analysis of the cellular composition of these isolated fractions. The isolation of the E-enriched fraction was performed under optimal conditions (13, 20, 21, 33). Both T and non-T cell fractions appeared to be cytotoxic against monolayer cell lines as well as K-562 cells (our data; 13). The per cent lysis of unfractionated cells is given in Table II.

Analysis of the lymphocyte subpopulations by means of E-rosette formation indicated that the T-cell fraction was highly enriched in T-cells and the E-RFC depleted fraction contained virtually no T-cells. When, however, an anti-T cell antiserum (21, 34) was used for the identification of T-cells the following results were obtained:

1) the E-RFC enriched fraction contained virtually pure T-cells (Table III);

2) the E-RFC depleted fraction contained a significant percentage of T-cells as shown by the anti T-cell antiserum (Table III).

That this is not due to non-specific binding of TRITC labelled anti-T-cell serum to the FcR of the cells is illustrated by analysis of individual lymphocytes for the presence of (SIg) and T-cell specific antigen using the two wavelength immunofluorescence method (35). This analysis revealed that virtually no double staining is observed in the unfractionated lymphocytes, containing T-cells and B-cells (SIg bearing cells) and the non-T-cell fraction, containing a high percentage of B-cells as would be expected in case of non-specific staining (Table III; % T^+/Ig^+). Our observation indicates that after rosette formation and separation, T-cells do not form E-rosettes as readily as before the E-RFC depletion. This conclusion is supported by the good correlation between the per cent T-cells as determined by E-rosette formation and by immunofluorescence, when performed before fractionated of these cells on Ficoll (Table III, % E-RFC and % T^+). The implications of this finding are important and may explain a number of the apparent contradicting results in the literature. Kiuchi and Takasugi (9) defined the NK-cell as a null cell, i.e. without T and/or B cell characteristics except the presence of IgG-FcR. These authors used E-rosette formation and separation and subsequently checked the purity of the separated fractions by E-rosette formation. West et al. (13) concluded that the T-cells showing the NK-cell activity belong to a subpopulation of T-cells bearing low affinity receptors of E_{sh}. Apparently, the optimal conditions employed for E-rosette formation and separation do not completely prevent the dissociation of low avidity E-RFC, resulting in the

TABLE III

PER CENT CYTOTOXICITY OF VARIOUS LYMPHOCYTE FRACTIONS

Lymphocyte donor	per cent reduction of target cells						immunofluorescence				
	NKI-4	NK_{lt}[1] Mel-1	colon	NK_{st}[2] K-562	K[3] P-815	% E-RFC	% T^+	% Ig^+	% T^+/Ig^+	% T^-/Ig^-	% EA-RFC
Donor A											
3) T-cell fraction: E-RFC	15*[4]	- 5		34*		89[5]	93	1	0	6	7
4) E-RFC depleted fraction	43*	38*		32*		5[5]	16	30	1	54	39
Donor B											
3) T-cell fraction: E-RFC	15		9	46*	25*	95	90	1	2	9	14
4) E-RFC depleted fraction	55*		33*	35*	19*	3	6	30	0	62	61
Donor C											
3) T-cell fraction: E-RFC		20*	19*	13*		85	96	0	0	4	3
4) E-RFC depleted fraction		13	40*	24*		3	19	45	1	36	50
Donor D											
3) T-cell fraction: E-RFC	17*		40*	21*		84	97	2	0	1	3
4) E-RFC depleted fraction	- 9		38*	34*		3	17	36	0	47	73

1 NK_{lt}: NK cell cytotoxicity against monolayer cultures (48 h MCT)
2 NK_{st}: NK cell cytotoxicity against K-562 (4 h ^{51}Cr-release assay)
3 K : K cell cytotoxicity against IgG-coated P-815 (4 h ^{51}Cr-release assay)
4 * p value $\leqslant 0.05$
5 lymphocytes were not treated. The average yield of 3, 55 % of 1; of 4, 7% of 1.

appearance of T-cells with low affinity receptors for E_{sh} after this separation procedure in the interface (21, 36). Since these low-affinity E-RFC have been shown to exhibit the strongest NK-cell activity (13) this could explain the fact that lymphocytes in the non-T-cell fraction, containing only 6-17% T-cells, show a similar level of NK-cell activity as the T-cell fraction (containing virtually pure T-cells, see above) at the same lymphocyte target cell ratio: the latter is relatively depleted and the former relatively enriched for T-cells (NK cells) which bear low-affinity receptors for E_{sh} (our data, 20, 21).

Hersey et al. (12) showed T-cells, bearing FcR, to be cytotoxic. Our data clearly demonstrate that other techniques than the one used for the separation of a cell subpopulation in order to demonstrate the purity of that isolated subpopulation. Thus not all T-cells form E-rosettes after E-RFC separation on Ficoll (36) and a proportion of these T-cells may bear FcR (33, 37). Hence, the cells from the interface, showing NK-cell activity would be characterized as non-T, non-B, IgG-FcR bearing cells on the basis of their E-, EA- and SIg markers. Analysis of cells in this interface fraction with the anti-T cell antiserum, however, proved the presence of T-cells. The simultaneous analysis of cell surface markers and cytotoxicity testing also demonstrated that T-cells (E-RFC, anti-T cell serum positive) can form EA-rosettes and exert K-cell activity (ADCC) confirming data of others (23,37).

The T cell nature of the NK cells was further confirmed by Kaplan and Callewaert (38). These authors succeeded to abrogate NK cell activity by pre-treating the effector cells with anti-T cell antiserum plus complement. Furthermore, significant fraction of NK cells express a receptor for helix pomatia and this receptor is considered to be a T cell marker (39).

The E-RFC depleted fractions are strongly enriched for SIg positive cells (B) (Table III) (7, 21) without a concomittant rise in NK activity, confirming reports by others that human NK cells lack SIg (20, 21, 32). The data presented in Table IV demonstrates that monocytes do not display cytotoxicity themselves i.e. the monocyte enriched fraction exerting the lowest per cent lysis of target cells. Furthermore, human NK cells lack adherent and phagocytic properties (12, 13, 21, 40) and the majority of NK cells do not carry complement receptors (13, 41).

From the data discussed so far it can be concluded that the various NK cell reactivities can be observed and that these NK cells may differ with respect to their characteristics:

1) NK cells displaying cytotoxicity against monolayer target cells and against K-562 suspension target cells as tested in

TABLE IV

PER CENT NK-CELL ACTIVITY OF PURE LYMPHOCYTES WITH AND WITHOUT THE ADDITION OF MONOCYTES, AND/OR A MONOCYTE ENRICHED FRACTION AGAINST NKI-4, Mel-I AND K-562.

Effector cells	Target cells		
	NKI-4[1]	Mel-I[1]	K-562[2]
Nylon purified lymphocytes	39*	83*	47*
Nylon purified lymphocytes + 1% monocytes	49*	78*	50*
Nylon purified lymphocytes + 5% monocytes	58*	83*	48*
Monocytes enriched fraction[3]	27*	69*	19*

1 NK_{lt} : NK cell cytotoxicity against monolayer cultures (48 h MCT)
2 NK_{st} : NK cell cytotoxicity against K-562 (4 h ^{51}Cr-release assay)
3 The monocyte enriched fraction contained 60% monocytes
* p value 0.05

long-term and short-term cytotoxicity assays respectively. These NK cells express IgG-FcR (NK_{lt} and NK_{st}, IgG-FcR positive);
2) NK cells displaying NK cytotoxicity against monolayer cultured target cells exclusively tested in a microcytotoxicity assay, with no demonstrable membrane IgG-FcR: EA-RFC and ADCC negative;
3) NK cells belong, at least in part, to the T cell lineage.

The investigation reported here and by others illustrate that human NK cells are heterogenous and cannot easily be distinguished from K-cells which are present in the same cell fractions as NK_{lt} and NK_{st} cells. One exception was described here, i.e. the IgG-FcR negative cell fraction comprising the IgG-FcR negative NK_{lt}. Thus, NK cell lysis may be of an ADCC type of reaction. Our data concerning the mechanism of NK cytotoxicity in relation to ADCC will be presented in section I.B (this issue).

ACKNOWLEDGEMENTS

The author wishes to thank Mr. C.P.M. Ronteltap, Mrs. A.M. Nooyen, Mrs. R. de Rooy for superb technical assistance. Mrs. M. van der Sman for inventive secretarial help.

REFERENCES

1. Bubenik, J., Perlmann, P., Helmstein, K. and Moberger, G. Int. J. Cancer 5, 1970, 310.
2. Hellström, I., Hellström, J.E., Sjögren, H.O. and Warner, G.A. Int. J. Cancer 7, 1971, 1.
3. Fossati, G., Canevaki, S., Della Porta, G., Balzarini, G.P. and Veronesi, U. Int. J. Cancer 10, 1972, 391.
4. O'Toole, C., Stejskal, V. and Perlmann, P. J. exp. Med. 139, 1974, 457.
5. Takasugi, M., Mickey, M.R. and Terasaki, P.I. Cancer Res. 33, 1973, 2898.
6. Oldham, R.K., Djeu, J.Y., Cannon, G.B., Siwarski, D. and Herberman, R.B. J. Nat. Cancer Inst. 55, 1975, 1309.
7. Bolhuis, R.L.H. Cancer Immunol. Immunother 2, 1977, 245.
8. Peter, H.H., Pavie-Fischer, J., Fridman, W.H., Aubert, C., Cesarini, J.P., Roubin, R. and Kourilsky, F.M. J. Immunol. 115, 1975, 539.
9. Kiuchi, M. and Takasugi, M. J. Nat. Cancer Inst. 56, 1976, 575.
10. De Vries, J.E., Cornain, S. and Rumke, P. Int. J. Cancer 14, 1974, 427.
11. Jondal, M. and Pross, H. Int. J. Cancer 15, 1975, 596.
12. Hersey, P., Edwards, A., Edwards, J., Adams, E., Milton, G.W. and Nelson, D.S. Int. J. Cancer 16, 1975, 173.
13. West, W.H., Cannon, G.B., Kay, H.D., Bonnard, G.D. and Herberman, R.B. J. Immunol. 118, 1976, 355.
14. McLennan, I.C.M. Transplant. Rev. 13, 1972, 67.
15. Perlmann, I.C.M., Perlmann, H. and Wigzell, H. Transplant. Rev. 13, 1972, 91.
16. Dickler, H.B. J. Exp. Med. 140, 1974, 508.
17. Pape, G.R., Troye, M. and Perlmann, P. J. Immunol. 118, 1977, 1919.
18. Saal, J.G., Rieber, E.P., Hadam, M. and Riethmüller, G. Nature 265, 1977, 158.
19. Akira, D. and Takasugi, M. Int. J. Cancer 19, 1977, 747.
20. Bolhuis, R.L.H., Thesis Erasmus University Rotterdam, 1977.
21. Bolhuis, R.L.H., Schuit, H.R.E., Nooyen, A.M. and Ronteltap, C.P.M. Eur. J. Immunol. 8, 1978, 731.
22. Kedar, E., de Landazuri, M.O. and Bonavida, B.J. J. Immunol. 112, 1974, 1231.
23. Van Oers, M.H.J., Zeylemaker, W.P. and Schellekens, P.Th. A. Eur. J. Immunol. 7, 1977, 143.
24. Loos, J.A., Blok-Schut, B., Kipp, B., Van Doorn, R. and Meerhof, L. Blood 48, 1976, 743.
25. Yam, L.T., Li, C.Y. and Crosby, W.H. Am. J. Clin. Pathol. 55, 1971, 283.

26. Takasugi, M. and Klein, E. Transplantation 9, 1970, 219.
27. Bolhuis, R.L.H. and Nooyen, A.J.M. Immunol. 33, 1977, 679.
28. Eremin, O., Ashby, J. and Stephens, J.P. Int. J. Cancer 21, 1978, 35.
29. Ortaldo, J.R., Bonard, G.D. and Herbermann, R.B. J. Immunol. 119, 1977, 1351.
30. Pross, H.F. and Baines, M.G. Int. J. Cancer 18, 1976, 593
31. Kay, H.D., Bonnard, G.D., West, W.H. and Herbermann, R.B. J. Immunol. 118, 1977, 2058.
32. Bakacs, T., Gergely, P., Cornain, S. and Klein, E. Int.J. Cancer, in the press.
33. West, W.H., Payne, S.M., Weeze, J.L. and Herbermann, R.B. J. Immunol. 119, 1978, 548.
34. Asma, G., Schuit, H.R.E. and Hijmans, W. Clin. Exp. Immunol. 29, 1977, 286.
35. Knapp, W., Bolhuis, R.L.H., Radl, J. and Hijmans, W. J. Immunol. 111, 1973, 1295.
36. Bolhuis, R.L.H. and Schuit, H.R.E., Clin. Exp. Immunol. 35, 1979, 317.
37. Samarut, C., Brochier, J. and Revilland, J.P. J. Immunol. 5, 1976, 221.
38. Kaplan, J. and Callewaert, D.M. J. nat. Cancer Inst. 60, 1978, 961.
39. Pape, G.R., Troye, M. and Perlmann, P. Scand. J. Immunol. 10, 1979, 109.
40. Levin, A., Marsey, R., Deinhardt, F., Schauf, U. and Wolter, J. In: Neoplasm Immunity Therapy and Application. (ed. R.G. Crispen), p. 107, 1975. ITR, Chicago.
41. Pross, H.G., Bains, M.G. and Jondal, M. Int. J. Cancer 20, 1977, 353.

ALLOANTISERA SELECTIVELY REACTIVE WITH NK CELLS: CHARACTERIZATION AND USE IN DEFINING NK CELL CLASSES

Robert C. Burton[1]

Transplantation Unit
General Surgical Services and Department of Surgery
Harvard Medical School
Massachusetts General Hospital
Boston, Massachusetts

I. INTRODUCTION

The phenomenon whereby lymphoid cells derived from the lympho-hemapoietic organs of non-immune laboratory animals and human subjects lyse normal and neoplastic cells *in vitro* has been termed natural killing, and the effector cells natural killer or NK cells (Herberman et al., 1979, Kiessling and Wigzell, 1979). The broad range of susceptible targets and the associated variations in the conditions under which optimal degrees of *in vitro* lysis have been observed have suggested a heterogeneity among the effector cells, and, indeed, recent observations from a number of laboratories have provided evidence for such a heterogeneity. The purpose of this review is to summarize investigations performed in this laboratory on the development of NK specific alloantisera and their use with other antisera which has shown a heterogeneity of NK cells (Burton and Winn, 1980a; 1980b), and to relate these findings to those of others.

[1]*The author is the John Mitchell Crouch Fellow of the Royal Australasian College of Surgeons, and the studies were supported by Grants CA-17800 and CA-20044 awarded by the National Cancer Institute, Bethesda, Maryland, and by Grants AM-07055 and HL-18646 from the National Institutes of Health, Bethesda, Maryland.*

ISBN 0-12-341350-8

II. METHODOLOGY

The mice used in the studies reported herein were purchased from Jackson Laboratories, Bar Harbor, Maine, and the antisera and methodology used in the experiments have been reported in detail elsewhere (Burton et al., 1978a, Burton and Winn, 1980a; 1980b). The tumor cell lines employed were as follows: YAC, an A/Sn strain Moloney virus induced T lymphoma; EL-4, a C57BL/6 carcinogen induced T lymphoma (T-LYM), P-815, a carcinogen induced mast cell tumor (MST) and WEHI-164, a carcinogen induced BALB/c fibrosarcoma (FSA). Their origins have been dealt with elsewhere (Burton et al., 1977; Burton and Winn, 1980a). Monoclonal anti-Thy 1.2 IgM antibody was purchased from New England Nuclear, Boston, Massachusetts.

III. ALLOANTISERA WITH ANTI-NK ACTIVITY

A. Definition of NK Specificity

In 1977 Glimcher et al. reported that a C3H anti-CE alloantiserum contained specific anti-NK activity in addition to anti-Ly 1.2 activity. This NK specific alloantigen has subsequently been designated NK 1.1 (Cantor et al., 1979). Two further NK specific alloantisera have been defined in this laboratory using the following criteria.

1. Backcross Genetic Analysis. The anti-NK alloantiserum must contain anti-NK activity that segregates separately to any cytotoxicity as detected by the trypan blue test in a backcross analysis of spleen cells from (NK susceptible x NK resistant) F1 x NK resistant mice. Alloantisera made between H-2 compatible mice of different strains potentially contain many different antibodies, and can probably never be regarded as monospecific. NK cells are so small a subpopulation of the spleen (1-2%) that they should not be detected in the trypan blue test (Kiessling and Wigzell, 1979; Dr. N. L. Warner, personal communication). Therefore, the analysis should contain individual mice whose spleen cells are not killed above the complement (C) background, and yet NK activity is removed by treatment with anti-NK serum and C.

2. *Functional Tests.* In addition to the above, functional tests which indicate that an anti-NK alloantiserum and C does not remove T and B cell activity from a spleen cell suspension for which it does abolish NK activity are also employed.

3. *Strain surveys.* Strain surveys may provide supplementary evidence to the backcross analysis if strains can be found against whose spleen cells the alloantiserum has anti-NK activity, but for which there is little or no cytotoxic activity in the trypan blue test.

Although all these tests may indicate that an alloantiserum contains only anti-NK activity against a particular strain, it is still possible, and, indeed, even likely, that other antibodies which are non-cytotoxic with rabbit C and/or are directed at other subpopulations, both defined (e.g. macrophages) and as yet undefined, are present in the serum. The usefulness of these alloantisera is not, however, necessarily impaired by the presence of other antibodies, so long as the experimental conditions under which they are used take account of this.

B. *Analysis of Three Anti-NK Alloantisera*

1. *Titrations of Three Anti-NK Alloantisera.* Three anti-NK alloantisera produced in this laboratory are shown in Figure 1. Spleen cells of susceptible strains have been treated first with various concentrations of antiserum, and then with pretested rabbit C to produce titration curves of residual NK activity against YAC. As can be seen, the CE anti-CBA serum has by far the highest titer, and, indeed, the anti-NK activity of this pool was 1:1024. The reverse immunization, CBA anti-CE, gave a much weaker anti-NK serum which also contained modest amounts of auto-antibody, and thus required absorption prior to use. This serum is probably an anti-NK 1.1 serum (Table I), and low anti-NK activity plus autoreactivity have been encountered by others using anti-NK 1.1 sera (Dr. G. Koo, personal communication). The C3H anti-ST serum was intermediate in activity against NK cells. The four pools of this serum produced to date have had anti-NK titers in the range 1:8 - 1:32, while the four CE anti-CBA pools have titered in the range 1:32 - 1:1024.

2. *Backcross Analysis of Two Anti-NK Alloantisera.* All pools of CE anti-CBA and C3H anti-ST alloantisera produced to date have mediated high levels of C dependent lysis of spleen cells of the immunizing strain in the trypan blue test, and

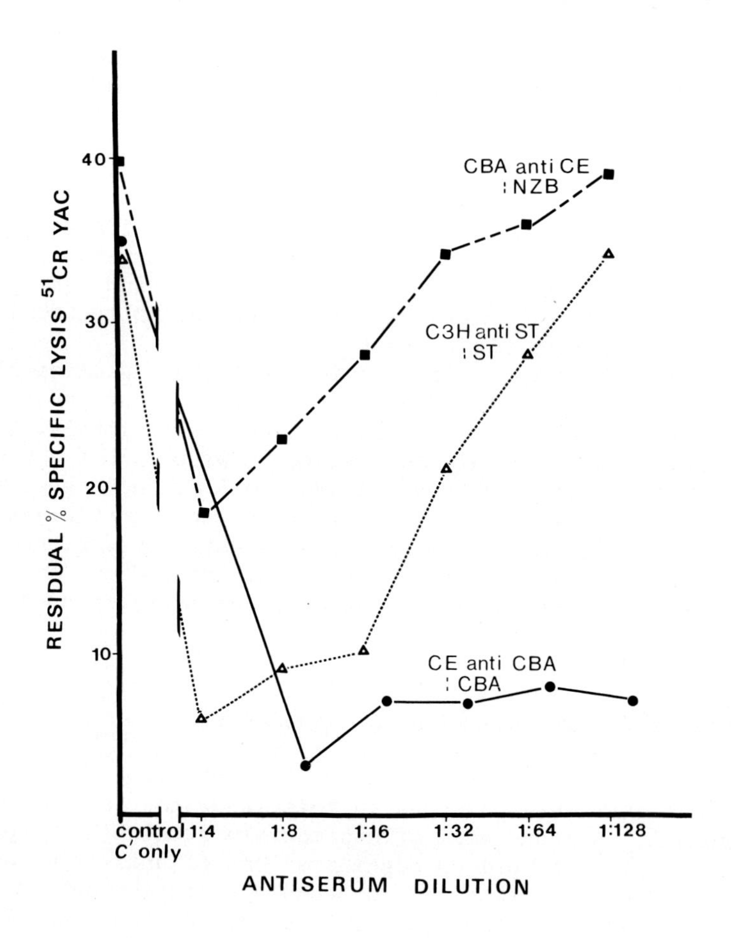

FIGURE 1. Titration of three anti-NK alloantisera.

so clearly contain antibodies in addition to those directed at NK cells. The backcross analyses, however, clearly show that anti-NK activity is separate to the major cytotoxic activity of these antisera (Table II).

a. CE anti-CBA. As can be seen, the cytotoxicity of the CE anti-CBA serum for spleen cells in the trypan blue test segregated quite separately to its anti-NK activity against YAC (Table II - A). These backcross results also indicate that CE anti-CBA serum probably contains two anti-NK antibodies directed against NK specific alloantigens, and that these alloantigens are probably determined by two loosely

TABLE I. *Strain Distribution of NK Alloantigens Detected by Specific Alloantisera*

	Mouse strains[a]								
Anti-NK alloantisera	CBA	C3H	C57BL	ST	NZB	Ma/My	BALB/c	DBA/2	DBA/1
CE anti-CBA	+	+	+	+	-	-	+	+	-
(NZB x CE)F1 anti-CBA[b]	+	+	+	+	-	-	+	n.d.	-
C3H anti-ST[c]	-	-	+	+	+	+	+	+	+
C3H anti-ST	-	-	+	+	+	+	-	-	n.d.
(C3H x DBA/2)F1 anti-ST	-	-	+	+	+	n.d.	-	-	n.d.
CBA anti-CE	-	n.d.	+	+	+	n.d.	-	-	n.d.
(BALB/c x C3H)F1 anti-CE[d]	-	n.d.	n.d.	+	+	+	n.d.	n.d.	-
Anti-NK 1.1[e]	-	-	+	n.d.	+	n.d.	-	-	n.d.

[a]Murine spleen cells treated with anti-NK alloantiserum and C. Positive if NK activity against YAC was reduced by 50% or more; n.d., not done.

[b](NZB x CE)F1 anti-CBA antiserum from Dr. N. L. Warner

[c]Some pools of C3H anti-ST serum contain additional anti-NK activity against BALB/c and DBA/2.

[d](BALB/c x C3H)F1 anti-CE antiserum from Dr. G. Koo.

[e]From Cantor et al. (1979).

linked genes. Functional tests have indicated that at least some of the cytotoxic activity of CE anti-CBA serum in the trypan blue test is probably anti-Ly 1.1.

b. C3H anti-ST. The other backcross analysis (Table II - B) indicated that the C3H anti-ST serum (#36) contained NK specific activity, as defined, because four of the backcross mice were negative in the trypan blue test, yet NK activity was removed from their spleen cells by treatment with C3H anti-ST serum and C. These four mice have subsequently been backcrossed to C3H in order to begin the development of an NK congenic line on the C3H (high NK) background. To date, the fourth backcross mice have been tested with C3H anti-ST serum and C and the NK alloantigen is present, while there is no detectable cytotoxicity in the trypan blue test. The results

TABLE II. Backcross Analysis of Anti-NK Alloantisera

NK alloantigens[a]	*Trypan blue cytotoxicity test*[b]		
	Positive	*Negative*	*Total*
A. CE anti-CBA: (CExCBA)F1 x CE[c]			
Positive	*20*	*15*	*35*
Negative	*15*	*5*	*20*
Total	*35*	*20*	*55*
B. C3H anti-ST: (C3HxST)F1 x C3H[c]			
Positive	*11*	*4*	*15*
Negative	*16*	*2*	*18*
Total	*27*	*6*	*33*

[a]*Spleen cells from individual mice treated with anti-NK + C. Positive if NK activity against YAC was reduced by 50% or more.*

[b]*Spleen cells from individual mice treated with anti-NK + C. Positive if killing of spleen cells above C background.*

[c]*Backcross mice of both sexes individually splenectomized.*

of the backcross analysis also indicate that the NK alloantigen detected by pool #36 C3H anti-ST serum is probably determined by a single segregating locus. Some pools of C3H anti-ST serum, however, contain an additional anti-NK specificity, and there is, as yet, no evidence that this extra specificity is NK specific (Table I).

C. *Anti-NK Alloantisera Made in F1 Recipients*

On the basis of the findings of Cantor et al. (1979), and of strain surveys performed with the CE anti-CBA and C3H anti-ST defined anti-NK alloantisera, a number of other anti-NK alloantisera have been produced by immunization of appropriate F1 mice. The use of F1 recipients reduces the number of alloantigens by which the strains differ, and thus may reduce the number of antibodies in addition to anti-NK that a serum contains. This is well shown with the (BALB/c x C3H)F1 anti-CE anti-NK 1.1 alloantiserum which, unlike the C3H serum, does not have anti-Ly 1.2 activity (Glimcher et al., 1977). This serum was provided for study here by Dr. G. Koo, and the (CE x NZB)F1 anti-CBA serum was made by Dr. N. L. Warner in a collaborative study. This latter serum appears to sort only NK cells of strain C3H when studied by fluorescence activated cell sorter analysis (Tai et al., 1980), and so may be truly NK cell specific in this strain.

D. *Strain Surveys with Anti-NK Alloantisera*

The results of strain surveys performed with the NK specific alloantisera in this laboratory have been summarized in Table I. Further genetic analysis of what seems to be a polymorphic system of NK specific alloantigens is currently in progress, and will be the subject of a future review (in preparation). However, it has become apparent that, although NK cells are a very minor subpopulation in lymphoid organs such as spleen, high titer anti-NK alloantisera can be raised when mice are immunized with spleen cells. Thus far, genetic analysis of these sera has indicated that at least two loci which determine NK specific alloantigens are present in NK cells which kill lymphoid tumors such as YAC.

IV. HETEROGENEITY OF NK CELLS

A. *The NK_L Cell and the NK_S Cell*

When fresh murine spleen cell suspensions are treated with either of the two anti-NK specific alloantisera CE anti-CBA or C3H anti-ST and rabbit C, *in vitro* lysis of lymphoma targets is abolished, while lysis of a solid tumor target is not (Table III); thereby defining two different NK cell populations within the one spleen cell suspension: NK_L cells which lyse lymphoid tumor targets and NK_S cells which lyse solid tumor targets (Burton and Winn, 1980b). Based largely on studies of the differential sensitivity to incubation at 37°C of NK cells which lysed solid or lymphoid targets Stutman et al., (1978) and Paige et al., (1978) had suggested that two subpopulations of NK might exist in fresh spleen cell suspensions. The above serological studies now provide definitive evidence for two NK cell types in fresh spleen, NK_L and NK_S cells. Additional experiments with beige mice, which have a near absolute defect in NK activity against YAC (Roder, 1979), have provided further evidence for the two NK cell types (Table III). As can be seen, NK_L activity is virtually absent in beige mice (C57BL/6-bg/bg Jackson Laboratories, Bar Harbor, Maine), while NK_S activity is present.

B. *Do Subclasses of NK_L Cells Exist?*

Although the anti-NK alloantisera have defined NK_L cells as a separate NK cell class, studies on the natural killing of lymphoma targets in other laboratories have suggested that further heterogeneity might exist within NK_L cells.

1. NK_L Cells which Kill EL-4 or YAC. Kumar et al. (1979a; 1979b) have reported that mice treated with the bone seeking radioisotope ^{89}Sr lose NK activity against YAC but retain NK activity against EL-4, and that NK activity against EL-4 appears earlier after adoptive transfer of spleen and bone marrow cells. These studies suggest that two different effector cells are involved at the lytic stage, but do not exclude the possibility that they are both in the same cell lineage. Since both NK cells are sensitive to the CE anti-CBA anti-NK alloantiserum plus C (Table III), it is possible that the EL_4 NK_L cell is a precursor, while the YAC NK_L cell is a more mature cell which is dependent upon an intact bone marrow for its function (Kumar et al., 1979a, 1979b).

TABLE III. *Differentiation of NK_L Cells from NK_S Cells*

Spleen cell treatment[a]	Percent specific lysis[b] EL-4 (T-LYM)	YAC (T-LYM)	WEHI-164 (FSA)
CBA[c]			
C	28 ± 1	44 ± 1	53 ± 2
CE anti-CBA + C	0	1 ± 0	53 ± 2
NZB			
C		21 ± 1	62 ± 1
C3H anti-ST + C		2 ± 1	64 ± 2
BALB/c			
C		59 ± 1	53 ± 1
CE anti-CBA + C		4 ± 1	49 ± 1
B6AF1 anti-B10.D2 + C		6 ± 1	44 ± 1
Rat anti-mouse + C		4 ± 1	29 ± 1
C57BL/6-bg/bg			
Nil		1 ± 0	46 ± 3

[a]Antisera used at 1:4 B6AF1 anti-B10.D2 and rat anti-mouse, 1:10 C3H anti-ST, 1:50 CE anti-CBA; rabbit C at 1:4.

[b]Mean ± s.e.m., 1:2 effector dilution after treatment, 16 hour assay, 10^4 target cells.

[c]Mouse strain of origin of spleen cells.

2. *Thy-1.2 Negative and Positive NK_L Cells.* The question as to whether NK cells which lyse lymphoid targets (NK_L cells) express Thy 1.2 has been a source of controversy for nearly five years, and the advent of monoclonal anti-Thy 1 antibodies has not, as yet, resolved the issue. To date, the controversy has largely revolved around the question of the sensitivity of NK_L cells to anti-Thy 1.2 serum, or monoclonal anti-Thy 1 antibodies, and C, with different laboratories reporting positive and negative results, even when the same monoclonal antibodies were used (Herberman et al., 1979; Kiessling and Wigzell, 1979; Karre and Seeley, 1979; Kumar et al., 1979a; Matthes et al., 1979; Lake et al., 1979). Recent studies using monoclonal anti-Thy 1.2 and the fluorescence activated cell sorter have contributed significantly to this question (Matthes et al., 1979). Their studies indicated that NK_L cells included both Thy 1.2 negative and Thy 1.2 positive subpopulations, and that the relative frequency of each subpopulation was different in nude and normal mice. Thy 1.2

positive NK_L cells predominated in nudes, while the converse was true of normal mice. Since most of the studies referred to above were performed in normal mice, a minor subpopulation of Thy 1.2 positive NK_L cells might not have been detected, especially if C with less than optimal activity was used.

Taken together, these findings suggest that at least three subpopulations of NK cells may exist within the NK_L cell class that lyses lymphoma targets.

C. *Other Alloantigens of NK_L Cells*

A number of studies have been reported in which alloantisera containing antibodies directed against subpopulations of cells of the lymphohemapoietic system have been used to study NK cells which lyse lymphoma targets *in vitro*. Although the alloantigens which these reagents identify are *not* NK specific these studies have been useful in the investigation of the function and possible cell differentiation pathway of NK_L cells.

1. Ly-5. Ly-5 is an alloantigen which is expressed on most cells of the lymphohemapoietic system (Scheid and Triglia, 1979), including NK_L cells (Cantor et al., 1979; Pollack et al., 1979). In addition, it also appears to be involved in the *in vitro* effector function of NK_L cells, as Cantor et al. (1979) observed that NK activity against a lymphoma target was blocked by an alloantiserum containing anti-Ly 5.1 antibodies. This suggests that antibodies in this serum were binding to structures on the NK_L cell surface very close to or actually involved in target cell recognition and/or lysis. Studies with monospecific anti-Ly 5 reagents might, therefore, provide further insights into the mechanism of NK_L cell recognition of target cell structures.

2. Mph-1. I/st anti-B10.M alloantisera contain antibodies which react with 60% of PEC but not with lymph node cells (Archer and Davies, 1974). This serum, designated anti-Mph 1.2, was used to study promonocyte enriched cultures of mouse bone marrow cells, which are able to lyse YAC *in vitro* (Lohmann-Matthes et al., 1979). It was shown that these cultured cells lost their ability to kill YAC after treatment with anti-Mph 1.2 and C. Although these results suggest that promonocytes might be involved in natural killing, additional studies are clearly necessary. It is possible that anti-Mph 1.2 serum also contains anti-NK_L activity as a separate specificity, and the tissue distribution of Mph 1 itself has not been sufficiently characterized to be certain that it is restricted to cells of the macrophage/monocyte lineage (Archer and Davies, 1974). The promonocyte enriched effector populations tested also contained about 20% granulocytes (Lohmann-Matthes et al., 1979), and so it is possible that the modest levels of NK activity detected were mediated by granulocytic cells or a minor subpopulation of NK_L cells present in cultured bone marrow.

D. *Is NK_S Activity Cell Mediated?*

Paige et al., (1978) found that natural cytotoxic activity (NC) against solid tumor targets (NK_S activity) was *not* abolished by treatment of spleen cells with a variety of alloantisera and C. Investigations performed in this laboratory confirm those findings (Burton and Winn, 1980b), but, in addition, show that NK_S activity can be reduced by treatment of spleen cells with high titer rat anti-mouse serum and C (Table III). Of particular interest has been the finding that NK_S activity survives treatment of a spleen cell suspension with anti-H-2 alloantiserum and C, which usually kills all but 1-3% of the cells, including all NK_L cells (Table IV).

In order to be certain that NK_S activity was cell mediated, these 1-3% of live cells were separated from the dead cells by density gradient centrifugation. When tested, the small number of live cells did contain all the NK_S activity. In addition, culture supernatants of fresh spleen cells were tested and, although they had some activity against solid tumor targets, this was very much less than that of cells assayed for the same period of time. Therefore, the NK_S cell seems to be a non-adherent cell, to be deficient in the expression of a number of cell surface antigens and/or resistant to C, to be more resistant to *in vitro* culture than the NK_L cell, and to lyse only solid tumor targets.

E. *The NK_C Cell*

1. *Killer Cells Develop in Unstimulated Spleen Cell Cultures.* *In vitro* studies of the weak cytotoxic T cell (Tc) response to syngeneic tumor cells have focused attention on the generation of cytotoxic effector cells (CL) in unstimulated spleen cell cultures (Burton et al., 1978b). It has been observed that, while the effector cells recovered from stimulated cultures are highly sensitive to anti-Thy 1.2 serum and C treatment, those CL recovered from unstimulated cultures of the same spleen cell pool may show only partial sensitivity to the same treatment (Burton et al., 1977). Furthermore, the tumor target used in the ^{51}Cr release assay

TABLE IV. Properties of NK_S Cells[a]

Effector cells	Treatment	% VCR[b]	Percent specific lysis	
			YAC (T-LYM)	WEHI-164 (FSA)
BALB/c	Nil		51 ± 1	54 ± 1
	Adherent cell depletion[c]	50	54 ± 1	50 ± 1
	CE anti-CBA + C	35	6 ± 1	54 ± 2
	B6AF1 anti-B10.D2 + C	2	0	51 ± 2
	B6AF1 anti-B10.D2 + C	3	n.d.	41 ± 0
	B6AF1 anti-B10.D2 + C[d]		n.d.	37 ± 1
BALB/c	5 x 10^5 spleen cells + 10^4 target cells in 200 ul			41 ± 0
Culture Supernatant	from 2.5 x 10^6 spleen cells in 1 ml			6 ± 0
	from 5 x 10^6 spleen cells in 1 ml			10 ± 0
	from 10 x 10^6 spleen cells in 1 ml			11 ± 0
	from 40 x 10^6 spleen cells in 1 ml			10 ± 0

[a] Antiserum + C treatment and assay conditions as for Table III.
[b] Percent viable cell recovery after treatment.
[c] Adherent cell depletion by 3 passages of 1 hour at 37°C in plastic petri dishes.
[d] Dead cell removal by density gradient centrifugation.

appears to be an important factor in this phenomenon. For some tumor targets the CL activity is totally abolished by treatment with anti-Thy 1.2 serum and C, while for others it is largely unaffected (Burton et al., 1977, Ching et al., 1978).

2. *Studies with Anti-NK and Other Antisera.* The serological characteristics of the cultured CL which lyse lymphoid and solid tumor targets are shown in Table V. These CL were totally resistant to treatment with CE anti-CBA serum or anti-Thy 1.2 serum and C under conditions in which all NK_L activity of fresh spleen cells and alloreactive Tc activity induced in culture was abolished. In a previous study these CL were defined as cultured natural killer cells or NK_C (Burton and Winn, 1980b). The additional studies shown here with monoclonal anti-Thy 1.2 antibody, however, indicate that two effector populations can be distinguished. Lysis of the YAC and P-815 tumor cells was mediated largely or totally by CL which were sensitive to anti-Thy 1.2 monoclonal antibody and C, while lysis of the solid tumor target was mediated largely by CL which were resistant to this treatment. The former population are probably Tc, although their resistance to treatment with anti-Thy 1.2 serum and C under conditions which kill all alloreactive Tc induced *in vitro* suggests that their surface density of Thy 1.2 and/or their sensitivity to C mediated lysis must be different.

On the basis of these results, NK_C cells should probably be re-defined as those Thy 1.2 negative CL which mediated most of the lysis of the FSA WEHI-164 and some of the lysis of the T lymphoma YAC.

3. *Other Killer Cells which Develop in Culture.* Four days of spleen cell culture are required before NK_C activity, as defined above, can be detected, and peak activity is on day 6 (Burton et al., 1977). Under a variety of circumstances, however, cytotoxic effector cells can be detected in 1-3 day cultures. Spleen cells which were cultured with tumor necrosis serum developed two peaks of cytotoxic activity, one at 1-2 days, and a second at 6 days (Chun et al., 1979). The 6 day peak effectors were resistant to monoclonal anti-Qa 5 antibody and C and partially sensitive to monoclonal anti-Thy 1.2 antibody and C, and were probably a mixture of Tc and NK_C as described above. The 1-2 day peak effectors, however, were totally resistant to anti-Thy 1.2 monoclonal antibody and C, and very sensitive to anti-Qa 5 monoclonal antibody and C. Since NK cells which lyse lymphoid targets also express Qa 5 (Dr. G. Koo, personal communication) these effector cells may well have been NK_L cells. Experiments with anti-NK alloantisera could settle this question.

TABLE V. Properties of NK_C Cells[a]

Effector cells	Treatment	Percent specific lysis		
		YAC (T-LYM)	P-815 (MST)	WEHI-164 (FSA)
BALB/c anti-CBA[b] 6 day culture	C	47 ± 2		
	Anti-Thy 1.2 + C	6 ± 2		
	Monoclonal anti-Thy 1.2 + C	2 ± 1		
BALB/c[c] Fresh spleen	C	51 ± 1		
	CE anti-CBA + C	6 ± 1		
BALB/c 6 day culture	C	45 ± 1	37 ± 1	54 ± 3
	Anti-Thy 1.2 + C	45 ± 2	36 ± 2	42 ± 2
	Monoclonal anti-Thy 1.2 + C	13 ± 1	0	35 ± 2
	CE anti-CBA + C	47 ± 1	31 ± 2	50 ± 2
	B6AF1 anti-B10.D2 + C	n.d.	n.d.	11 ± 1
	Rat anti-mouse + C	n.d.	n.d.	7 ± 1
	Pretreat CE anti-CBA + C[d]	37 ± 3	23 ± 5	41 ± 1
	Pretreat B6AF1 anti-B10.D2 + C[d]	7 ± 3	n.d.	36 ± 1

[a] Antiserum + C treatment and assay conditions as for Table III.
[b] Alloreactive Tc induced in vitro as positive control for anti-Thy 1.2 serum.
[c] Fresh spleen (NK_L) cells as positive control for CE anti-CBA anti-NK serum.
[d] Same spleen cell pool treated as shown before culture; controls showed abolition of NK_L activity and preservation of NK_S activity after treatment (day 0).

CL with a spectrum of target activity like that of NK cells in fresh spleen have been detected early in the course (1-3 days) of mixed lymphocyte cultures (Karre and Seeley, 1979). These effector cells, unlike NK_L or NK_S cells, were relatively sensitive to treatment with monoclonal anti-Thy 1.2 antibodies and C, suggesting that they were Tc rather than NK cells.

F. *The Relationship Between NK_L, NK_S and NK_C Cells*

The NK_C cells are clearly differentiated from NK_L cells by their target preference and resistance to CE anti-CBA allo-antiserum and C; however, their relationship to NK_S cells is less clear. They were highly susceptible to treatment with anti-H-2 or rat anti-mouse serum and C, but this could represent a development of C sensitivity by culture of NK_S cells. However, the NK_C cells, in contrast to the NK_S cells, also killed the lymphoma target. When spleen cells were cultured following treatment with CE anti-CBA serum and C, normal levels of cultured CL activity against both lymphoma and solid tumor targets were observed (Table V), indicating that Tc and NK_C do not arise directly from NK_L. When the 1-3% of spleen cells which survived treatment with anti-H-2 serum and C were cultured, it appeared that only NK_C developed (Table V). The results suggest, but do not prove, that NK_C develop from NK_S.

G. *Comments and Conclusions*

On the basis of the studies reviewed herein it seems certain that the phenomenon of natural killing is mediated by more than one NK cell type. A minimum of three NK cells (NK_L, NK_S and NK_C) can be differentiated from each other on the basis of target preference, the expression of cell surface antigens and the effects of culture. The effect of culturing spleen cells seems quite variable. Short term culture (24 hours) destroys NK_L cells but not NK_S cells, and long term culture (6 days) generates at least two effector populations, NK_C cells and Tc. Culture in the presence of tumor necrosis serum generates a new NK cell type in 1-3 days, which can be clearly differentiated from the NK_C cell on the basis of the expression of Qa 5. Its relationship to the NK_L cell or NK_S cell is not yet known.

Further studies of the cell lineage(s) to which NK cell(s) belong, other possible *in vitro* functions such as ADCC against lymphoid targets, and their possible *in vivo* relevance should take account of this heterogeneity of the effectors of natural killing. For example, studies in this laboratory have shown that the effectors of ADCC against chicken red blood cells do not express NK specific alloantigens, while those that mediate ADCC against lymphoid targets do, suggesting that they are NK_L cells (Hamilton, et al., manuscript in preparation). The discovery of specific alloantigens of NK cells of a particular class should enable further dissection of the phenomenon of natural killing to proceed both rapidly and with precision.

ACKNOWLEDGMENTS

The author wishes to acknowledge the excellent technical assistance of Mrs. Joanne Fortin and the constructive and helpful discussions with Dr. Henry J. Winn.

REFERENCES

Archer, J. R., and Davies, D. A. L. (1974). *J. Immunogenetics 1,* 113.
Burton, R. C., Chism, S. E., and Warner, N. L. (1977). *J. Immunol. 119,* 1329.
Burton, R. C., Grail, D., and Warner, N. L. (1978a). *Br. J. Cancer 37,* 806.
Burton, R. C., Chism, S. E., and Warner, N. L. (1978b). *Contemp. Topics Immunobiol. 8,* 69.
Burton, R. C., and Winn, H. J. (1980a). Submitted for publication.
Burton, R. C., and Winn, H. J. (1980b). Submitted for publication.
Cantor, H., Kasai, M., Shen, F. W., Leclerc, J. C., and Glimcher, L. (1979). *Immunol. Rev. 44,* 3.
Ching, L. M., Marbrook, J., and Walker, K. Z. (1977). *Cell Immunol. 31,* 284.
Chun, M., Pasanen, V., Hammerling, U., Hammerling, G. F., and Hoffman, M. K. (1979). *J. Exp. Med. 150,* 426.
Glimcher, L., Shen, F. W., and Cantor, H. (1977). *J. Exp. Med. 145,* 1.
Herberman, R. B., Djeu, J. Y., Kay, H. D., Ortaldo, J. R., Riccardi, C., Bonnard, G. D., Holden, H. T., Fagnani, R., Santoni, A., and Puccetti, P. (1979). *Immunol. Rev. 44,* 43.
Karre, K., and Seeley, J. (1979). *J. Immunol. 123,* 1511.
Kiessling, R., and Wigzell, H. (1979). *Immunol. Rev. 44,* 165.

Kumar, V., Luevano, E., and Bennett. (1979a). *J. Exp. Med. 150*, 531.
Kumar, V., Ben-Ezra, J., Bennett, M., and Sonnenfeld, G. (1979b). *J. Immunol. 123*, 1832.
Lake, P., Clark, E. A., Khorshidi, M., and Sunshine, G., (1979). *Eur. J. Immunol.*, in press.
Lohmann-Matthes, M. L., Domzig, W., and Roder, J. (1979). *J. Immunol. 123*, 1883.
Matthes, M. J., Sharrow, S. O., Herberman, R. B., and Holden, H. T. (1979). *J. Immunol. 123*, 2851.
Paige, C. J., Figarella, E. F., Cuttito, M., Cahan, A., and Stutman, O. (1978). *J. Immunol. 121*, 1827.
Pollack, S. B., Tam, M. R., Nowinski, R. C., and Emmons, S. L. (1979). *J. Immunol. 123*, 1818.
Roder, J. C. (1979). *J. Immunol. 123*, 2168.
Scheid, M. P., and Triglia, D. (1979). *Immunogenetics*, in press.
Stutman, O., Paige, C. J., and Figarella, E. F. (1978). *J. Immunol. 121*, 1819.
Tai, A., Burton, R. C., Winn, H. J., and Warner, N. L. (1980). Submitted for publication.

ASIALO GM1 AND THY 1 AS CELL SURFACE MARKERS OF MURINE NK CELLS

Jeannine M. Durdik
Barbara N. Beck
Christopher S. Henney

Basic Immunology Program
Fred Hutchinson Cancer Research Center
Seattle, Washington

Natural killer (NK) cells were originally defined as a distinctive cell type because they lacked those surface markers characteristic of mature T cells, B cells and macrophages (1). In the six years since this definition, there have been intensive efforts to define the cell surface characteristics of NK cells. These efforts have had two principal goals: (i) documentation of the lymphoid lineage of NK cells and (ii) characterization of a membrane marker confined to NK cells. The latter would have obvious usefulness in the isolation of homogeneous NK cell populations and in determining the identity and contribution of NK cells to the activity of heterogeneous cytotoxic cell populations.

The question of the lineage of NK cells has stimulated considerable interest, and there have been several suggestions that NK cells represent a pre-T cell population. Such proposals have been based principally on the ability of some anti-Thy 1 sera to reduce NK reactivity (2, 3). The validity of this argument has been undermined by the failure of several investigators to affect NK cell activity with anti Thy 1 sera (4). Whether such discrepancies reflect differences in the specificity of the antisera employed or differences in the NK cell populations used has not been satisfactorily resolved. We have addressed this issue by testing the sensitivity of BCG-induced NK cell populations of C57BL/6 mice to treatment with a number of anti Thy 1 reagents. The antibody preparations included conventional AKR anti C3H thymocyte serum and the products of two hybridomas with anti-Thy 1 reactivity.

In search of a membrane marker whose display was confined to NK cells, we have focused on a characterization of the neutral glycolipids and gangliosides of murine NK cells. We have done so because different lymphoid cell subpopulations appear to display characteristic glycolipid profiles (5, 6). We thus asked whether NK cells could be differentiated from other cytotoxic cells on the basis of membrane glycolipid display.

ISBN 0-12-341350-8

I. EFFECT OF ANTI THY I ANTIBODIES ON NK CELL ACTIVITY

Three antibody preparations with anti Thy 1.2 specificity were used in these experiments to explore effects on BCG induced C57BL/6 NK cells (7). Each antibody was tested, in the presence of either guinea pig or rabbit complement, for its ability to reduce, in parallel, the lytic activities of NK cells and of cytotoxic T cells. In each case, reduction of BCG induced NK activity was observed (Table I). This reduction was dependent upon the presence of complement, since no change in lytic activity was seen in the presence of antibody alone. It was clear however that the reduction in NK activity was much less than that seen when cytotoxic T cells were treated with the same reagents. Comparison of the titration data (Table I) clearly revealed that the cytotoxic T cells were more sensitive to the two mouse antibody preparations. Interestingly, studies with the rat monoclonal antibody showed less distinction between T and NK effector cell populations. In all cases, at the highest antibody concentrations tested, NK cell activity was reduced, (82, 45, and 59% respectively) but, at the same concentrations, inhibition of T cell activity was considerably greater (100, 84 and 88% (Table I)).

Interpretation of these results requires analysis of the specificity of the reagents employed. Employing a 51-Cr release assay with rabbit serum as a complement source, the conventional serum, raised in AKR mice by injection with C3H thymocytes by the method of Reif and Allen (8), showed no reactivity with AKR or C3H bone marrow or with AKR thymus and spleen, when used at a 1:10 dilution. At a 1:50 dilution, the serum lysed greater than 90% of C3H thymocytes and 35-45% of C3H and C57BL/6 spleen cells.

A lyophilized preparation of a mouse monoclonal IgM antibody (F7D5) was the gift of Dr. E. A. Clark (Regional Primate Center at the University of Washington). The antibody was the product of a cell hybrid derived from the fusion of NS-1/1-Ag4-1 cells of the BALB/c P3 (MOPC 21) plasmacytoma and spleen cells of AKR mice responding to immunization with CBA thymus cells. The anti Thy 1.2 specificity of the antibody produced by this hybridoma was demonstrated using Thy 1 congenic mice, in tests of function and tissue distribution (9). Thus, the antibody abolished T helper cell activity for IgM and IgG responses in vivo and in vitro, ablated suppressor T cell activity, and suppressed proliferative responses to the T cell mitogens PHA and Con A. The antibody had no effect on spleen cell responsiveness to LPS. When its cytotoxic activity towards spleen cells was assessed, fifty per cent of the maximal cytotoxicity was observed at a dilution of 1:1000 in the presence of a guinea pig complement source.

The third reagent used in these studies was a concentrated supernatant from an in vitro culture of a rat-mouse hybridoma (Jlj, a gift of Dr. F. Symington). The hybridoma was produced by the fusion of rat spleen cells (immune to C3H thymus) with cells of the mouse myeloma SP2/0. The resulting hybrids were cloned and the Jlj

TABLE I. Effect of anti-Thy I antibodies on NK cell activity

Source of anti-Thy I antibody	Source of effector cells	% specific cytolysis of L5178Y target cells by cytotoxic cells after treatment with complement and anti-Thy I antibody at the following dilutions					
		1:20	1:40	1:80	1:160	1:320	C alone
AKR anti C_3H	alloimmune T[a]	0	0	0	7	15	45[e]
	NK[b]	5	5	15	18	25	28
Mouse monoclonal anti-Thy 1.2	alloimmune T[c]	7	4	5	7		44[f]
	NK[b]	40	47	54	55		71
Rat monoclonal anti-Thy 1.2	alloimmune T[d]	6	30		50		50[g]
	NK[d]	15	25		33		37

Effector cells (2-3 X 10^7/ml) were pretreated with the indicated dilutions of anti Thy I antibody at 4^oC for 30 minutes followed by the addition of C for 45 minutes at 37^oC. After washing, these cells were tested for residual cytotoxic activity against L5178Y cl 27v. This target cell is Thy 1.2 negative and was selected for its NK sensitivity. NK cell populations were BCG induced pec from C57BL/6 mice given 10^8 viable BCG organisms 4-5 days earlier. Alloimmune T cells were generated either in vivo (expt. I) or in vitro (expts. II & III) against 10^7 L5178Y cl 27 ascites cells (NK resistant). E:T ratios: [a]100:1, [b]50:1, [c]25:1, [d]30:1. C: [e]normal rabbit serum 1:16 final dilution, [f]1:12 guinea pig serum, [g]1:24 guinea pig serum.

hybridoma was selected for its high toxicity towards (C57BL/6 x C3H)F1 thymocytes at dilutions where no toxicity towards AKR thymocytes occurred.

On the basis of the strain distribution of lymphocyte alloantigens, the possible additional specificities which could be present in AKR anti C3H anti Thy 1.2 serum include Ly 1.1, Ly 3.2, Ly 6.1, Ly 7.1, Ly 8.1 and Ala 1.1. Other investigators have identified antibodies to the predicted Ly 1, 3, and 8 alloantigens in conventional sera raised in an identical manner to that employed here (10). With the exception of Ly 3.2, C57BL/6 mice do not carry the appropriate alleles for these loci. NK cell populations have been tested with anti Ly 3.2 serum plus C and found to be negative for this marker (11, and unpublished results). It is therefore unlikely that the reactivity of the AKR anti C3H thymocyte serum towards C57BL/6 NK cells is due to any known contaminant in this serum.

The studies with monoclonal antibodies with documented specificity for Thy 1.2 further substantiate that BCG-induced NK cells bear an antigenic structure resembling Thy 1.2. The reduction of BCG induced NK activity with the mouse anti Thy 1.2 monoclonal antibody, F7D5, is of interest, as this reagent has been previously employed by Clark et al. (12) and by Mattes et al. (3) with conflicting results. In their studies of NK activity present in nude and normal mice, Clark et al. concluded that neither of these sources had NK cells which bore Thy 1. In contrast, Mattes et al. concluded that Thy 1 was present on the major portion of NK cells present in unstimulated BALB/c nude spleen and upon a more limited fraction of cells from CBA spleen. One hypothesis, which would reconcile these conflicting results and would be consistent with our observations, would be that expression of Thy 1 may be correlated with the "activated" state of NK cells. The nude mice which Clark et al. employed demonstrated a much lower activity than those employed by Mattes et al., which suggests the mice differed in their levels of endogenous stimulation. Our own findings with BCG induced NK cells taken together with the findings of Mattes, imply that "activated" NK cells display a higher density of Thy 1 on their surface than do unstimulated NK cells.

The sensitivity of C57BL/6 BCG-induced NK cells to treatment with anti Thy 1.2 antibodies demonstrates either that these cells express a low density of Thy 1.2 (compared to cytotoxic T cells), or that they express a structure antigenically cross-reactive with Thy 1.2. If the macromolecule on the surface of NK cells is not indeed Thy 1, then it must be closely related to it both antigenically and in its expression, for BCG induced NK cell populations from AKR mice (Thy 1.1) were not susceptible to the anti Thy 1.2 reagents used (data not shown). If this structure is not identical with Thy 1.2, eventually a discordance should be observed when comparing T cell and NK cell sensititivity to several monoclonal anti Thy 1.2 antibodies. With the two anti Thy 1.2 monoclonal antibodies we have used, such differences were not apparent. The presence of Thy I on NK cells is compatible with earlier suggestions that these cells are of the T cell lineage.

II. GLYCOLIPID MARKERS OF NK CELLS

Experiments by Marcus and his colleagues (5, 6) have indicated that lymphocyte subpopulations have distinctive glycolipid profiles. By immunofluorescence, they noted that rabbit antisera raised against ganglioside GMI reacted with peripheral T cells and thymocytes. On the other hand, antiserum against the unsialated derivative, asialo GMI, reacted with only 30% of peripheral T cells and not with thymocytes. The reactivities of both antisera were independent of the Thy I phenotype of the cells.

These observations encouraged us to examine whether NK cells, both endogenous and BCG-induced, might express a particular glycolipid, which would then be useful as an identifying marker. We have assessed the sensitivity of NK cell mediated lytic activity to treatment with a series of rabbit anti glycolipid antisera (13). These experiments were carried out in collaboration with Drs. W. Young, L. Patt and S-I. Hakomori, who kindly provided us with the antisera which they had raised (14).

Pretreatment of peritoneal exudate cells from BCG stimulated mice with anti asialo GM2 or with anti globoside, with or without C, did not alter NK activity (Table II). In striking contrast, however, pretreatment of the effector population with anti asialo GMI (or with affinity-purified anti asialo GMI), in the presence of C completely eliminated NK activity. This elimination of cytotoxic activity was accompanied by lysis of approximately 15% of the cells in the effector population. Anti ganglioside GMI reduced NK activity by approximately 25%. Analysis of the specificity of this reagent suggested that this could be explained entirely by cross reactivity with anti asialo GMI (as previously noted, 6).

Comparative studies were undertaken to define the difference, if any, in membrane antigen display between the uninduced NK cell and the BCG induced NK cell. Figure I illustrates that similar reduction patterns are seen in both activities after treatment with anti asialo GMI and complement. Kasai et al. (15) have also identified asialo GMI as a marker for uninduced NK cells.

It is important to note that although asialo GMI was described initially as a marker for cells lacking surface immunoglobulin, and thus presumably for T cells, we and others have found that alloimmune T killer cells were unaffected by treatment with anti-asialo GMI and C (Figure I; see also (15)). Thus, anti-asialo GMI serum appears to be a useful tool in defining a cytotoxic cell as an NK cell. Additionally, it can be used for both positively and negatively selecting for NK cells, since unlike Ly 5 serum (11, 16), anti asialo GMI serum does not block NK activity in the absence of C (data not shown).

TABLE II. Effect of Anti-Glycolipid Antibodies on NK Activity

Effector cell pre-treatment		NK activity % specific cytolysis at effector to target ratios of:			% cells killed by antiserum
Antiserum directed to:	Complement	45:1	15:1	5:1	
-	-	37.0	20.4	12.0	-
-	+	40.2	22.6	12.4	0
asialo GM_1	-	27.8	14.3	4.0	0
	+	1.0	-1.4	-2.4	18
asialo GM_1 (affinity purified)	-	30.7	16.2	-	5
	+	1.0	-2.7	-3.0	13
GM_1	-	38.6	15.5	9.5	5
	+	28.2	15.1	7.2	1
globoside	-	37.4	20.2	9.3	-2
	+	30.5	19.7	9.6	4
asialo GM_2	-	42.8	17.9	7.0	0
	+	35.6	18.6	8.6	0

BCG induced peritonal exudate cells (4×10^6/ml) were incubated for 30 min. at 4° with the indicated antisera (1:10 final dilution) followed by addition of native guinea pig serum as complement source (final 1:24 dilution). Incubation was continued for 45 min. at 37°, after which the cells were washed three times and brought to a constant volume (0.4 ml). The microcytotoxicity assay was performed with 10^4 51Cr-labeled target cells at the indicated effector:target cell ratio in a final volume of 0.2 ml. After 4 hours incubation at 37°, 0.1 ml of the cell-free supernatant was assayed for 51Cr content. The percentage of the effector cell population killed by antiserum treatment was determined by vital dye exclusion.

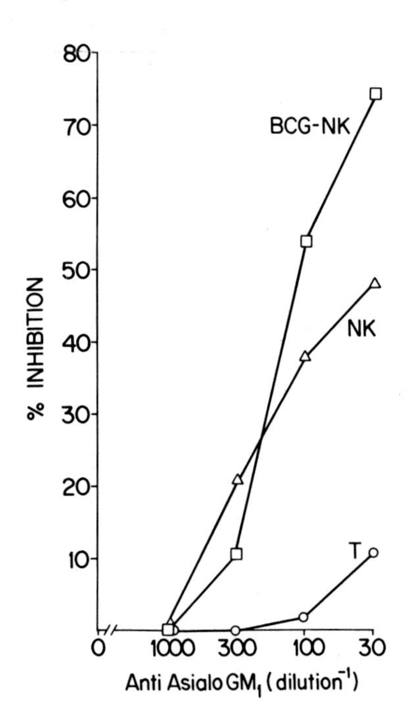

FIGURE 1. Effect of anti asialo GM1 serum on NK cell, BCG induced NK cell and cytotoxic T cell activity. Various effectors were pretreated with anti asialo GM1 at 4°C for 30 minutes followed by incubation at 37°C for 45 minutes with or without the addition of C (guinea pig serum final dilution 1/24). The values shown are relative to lysis after C treatment alone at an effector:target ratio of 25:1. The target is L5178Y clone 27v. The values for specific lysis for untreated, C treatment alone, and anti asialo GM1 (1/30) treatment alone are: 35.8, 33.9, and 35.3 for BCG induced pec of C57BL/6 origin ( ), 14.6, 12.6, and 13.2 for spleen cells from normal CBA mice ( ), and 37.9, 36.6, and 39.3 for alloimmune T cells ( ). BCG pec were harvested 4 days after inoculation i.p. with 10^8 BCG. Alloimmune T cells were generated in 5 day cultures utilizing the NK resistant ascites line as antigen (L5178Y clone 27a).

In our studies comparing the cell surface display of asialo GM1 on endogenous and BCG-induced NK cell populations, we became interested in examining the status of induced NK cell populations from C57BL/6 bgJ/bgJ (beige) mice. Homozygous beige mice are reported to have a lysosomal defect resembling Chediak-Higashi syndrome in man (17) and recently have been reported to lack NK activity (18). Attempts to induce activity with interferon, or the interferon inducers tilorone and poly I:C, were reportedly unsuccessful (18). However, we have found that peritoneal exudate cells harvested from beige mice given BCG i.p. have significant lytic activity (Table III), although no activity was demonstrable in normal peritoneal exudate cells or in normal spleen cell populations from beige mice. This BCG induced activity has been found to reside in the nylon wool non-adherent population and to be resistant to concentrations of anti Thy 1.2 antiserum which eliminated cytotoxic T cell activity but not NK activity (data not shown). In keeping with the data presented in Table I, when using higher concentrations of anti Thy 1.2 serum we ablated the NK activity of beige mice. Additionally, we demonstrated that the cytotoxic activity of beige mice was sensitive to treatment with anti asialo GM1 serum plus complement (Table IV). Thus, although no (or very little) endogenous NK activity could be measured in beige mutant mice, it appeared that the activity which arose upon stimulation with BCG was identical with that in normal mice.

In sum, BCG induced NK cell populations from C57BL/6 mice bear either Thy 1.2 alloantigen, or a macromolecule which antigenically cross-reacts with it to a considerable degree. The density of Thy 1 display on NK cells appeared to be considerably less than on cytotoxic T cells, since all of the antibodies used ablated cytotoxic T cell activity at greater dilutions than those at which they inhibited NK cell function.

The neutral glycolipid asialo GM1 was readily demonstrable on murine NK cells. This was true both for NK cell populations from normal CBA spleen and for BCG-induced NK cell populations from CBA, C57BL/6 and beige mutant mice. In contrast, although 30% of peripheral murine T cells are reported to display asialo GM1, this glycolipid could not be demonstrated on cytotoxic T cells. These findings suggest that asialo GM1 may prove to be a useful marker for the identification and isolation of NK cell populations. Furthermore, investigation of the display of this marker during NK cell ontogeny may prove to be useful in delineating the cellular origin of these cells.

TABLE III. NK activity in *beige* mutant mice and normal littermates.

PEC Effector cell Source	% specific lysis of YAC-1 cells at E:T 40:1	20:1	10:1
Homozygous *beige*			
BCG-induced	28.0 ± 0.4	18.1 ± 1.2	11.6 ± 0.2
Uninduced	--	0.7 ± 0.5	--
Littermates			
BCG-induced	77.9 ± 1.3	69.4 ± 0.5	58.5 ± 1.4
Uninduced	--	4.0 ± 0.2	--

Specific lysis was measured in a 4 hr 51-Cr-release assay with BCG-induced and normal PEC as effector cells.

TABLE IV. Effect of anti-asialo GM_1 plus complement on *beige* NK cell activity.

Treatment	% specific lysis of YAC-1 cells by BCG induced PEC from: Homozygous *beige*	Littermates
Guinea pig serum (C)	13.0 ± 1.1	70.1 ± 0.5
anti-asialo GM_1	14.1 ± 0.2	67.7 ± 1.8
anti-asialo GM_1 + C	-3.0 ± 0.2	20.0 ± 2.0

Specific lysis was measured in a 7 hour 51-Cr-release assay at an effector:target cell ratio of 20:1. The effector cells were pretreated with the antiserum (1:10) and/or C (1:12) and washed before readjustment to equal cell numbers and use in the assay.

REFERENCES

1. Kiessling, R., Petranyi, G., Karre, K., Jondal, M., Tracey, D. and Wigzell, H. J. Exp. Med. 143, 772 (1976).
2. Herberman, R. B., Nunn, M. E. and Holden, H. T. J. Immunol. 121, 304 (1978).
3. Mattes, M., Sharrow, S. O., Herberman, R. B. and Holden, H. T. J. Immunol. 123, 2851 (1979).
4. Kiessling, R. and Wigzell, H. Immunologic Rev. 44, 165 (1979).
5. Stein-Douglas, K. E., Schwarting, G. A., Naiki, M. and Marcus, D. M. J. Exp. Med. 143, 822 (1976).
6. Stein, K. E., Schwarting, G. A. and Marcus, D. M. J. Immunol. 120, 676 (1978).
7. Tracey, D. E., Wolfe, S. A., Durdik, J. M. and Henney, C. S. J. Immunol. 119, 1145 (1977).
8. Reif, A. E. and Allen, J. M. V. J. Exp. Med. 120, 413 (1964).
9. Lake, P., Clark, E. A., Khorshidi, M. and Sunshine, G. Eur. J. Immunol. (in press).
10. Davidson, W. F., Betel, I., Sharrow, S. O. and Mathieson, B. J. Journal of Supramolecular Structure, Supplement 3, 247 (1978).
11. Pollack, S. B., Tam, M. R., Nowinski, R. C. and Emmons, S. L. J. Immunol. 123, 1818 (1979).
12. Clark, E. A., Russell, P. H., Egghart, M. and Horton, M. A. Int. J. Cancer (in press).
13. Young, W. W., Hakomori, S-I., Durdik, J. M. and Henney, C. S. J. Immunol. (in press, January 1980).
14. Hakomori, S-I., in "Methods in Enzymology" 28, 232. Academic Press, New York, (1972).
15. Kasai, M., Iwamori, M., Nagai, Y., Okumura, K. and Tada, T. Eur. J. Immunol. (in press).
16. Kasai, M., LeClerc, J. C., Shen, F. W. and Cantor, H. Immunogenetics 8, 153 (1979).
17. Lutzner, M. A., Lowrie, C. T. and Jordan, H. W. J. Heredity 58, 299 (1967).
18. Roder, J. and Duwe, A. Nature 278, 451 (1979).

CHARACTERISTICS OF NATURAL CYTOSTATIC EFFECTOR CELLS

Rachel Ehrlich
Margalit Efrati
Isaac P. Witz[1]

Department of Microbiology
George S. Wise Faculty of Life Sciences
Tel-Aviv University
Tel-Aviv, Israel

I. INTRODUCTION

Anti-tumor activities mediated by immunocytes of normal individuals (i.e. those without clinical evidence of a malignant growth) raised the interest of numerous investigators since it is not unlikely that such cells are involved, inter alia, in surveillance of nascent tumor cells.

Whereas cytotoxicity mediated by effector immunocytes from normal individuals is being studied rather thoroughly, (Herberman and Holden, 1978) the study of cytostasis and of the naturally occuring cells mediating it is, with a few exceptions (Jerrels et al, 1979)somewhat neglected. With this in mind, and in view of the possibility that cytostasis may be a mechanism by which dormant but potentially malignant cells (Haran-Ghera, 1978) are somehow under check and inhibited from extensive proliferation, we studied the cytostatic abilities of normal mouse splenocytes against adherent B-16 melanoma cells.

[1]*This investigation was supported by Contract NO1-CB-74134 awarded by the National Cancer Institute DHEW and by a grant from The United States-Israel Binational Science Foundation (BSF) Jerusalem, Israel.*

ISBN 0-12-341350-8

II. EXPERIMENTAL

A. *Cytostatic Activity of Normal Splenocytes*

An ^{125}IUDR incorporation inhibition (^{125}IUDR I-I) assay was utilized. The assay was performed according to Fish et al,(1974) with some modifications (Ehrlich et al, submitted for publication). A brief description of the assay is given below. B16-F10 (F10) melanoma cells were used as targets. These cells were readapted to adherent stationary culture conditions following several in-vivo passages in syngeneic C57BL/6 mice as solid subcutaneous tumors. The original tumor line was selected by Fidler for its ability to form a high number of experimental pulmonary colonies (Fidler, 1973).

Cultured F10 cells were kindly sent to us by Dr. I. Fidler Frederick Cancer Research Center, Frederick M.d. The target cells were distributed to flat bottom sterile microculture plates and incubated for 5-6 hours at 37°C to allow their adherence to the bottom of the plates. Normal effector cells, usually splenocytes were added to the plates and the incubation continued for 4 or 16-18 hours. The effector cells were then washed away and ^{125}IUDR prepared in our laboratory (Fish et al, 1974)was added. The incubation with ^{125}IUDR was for 8-16 hours. The microplates were then washed, dried and cut by an electrically heated chrome-nickel wire. Cell associated ^{125}IUDR was determined by an Auto-Gamma Spectrometer.

Inhibition of ^{125}IUDR incorporation into F10 target cells could be detected already after a 2 hour exposure of target cells to effectors (Ehrlich et al, submitted for publication). The inhibition reached maximal levels following an incubation period of 4-6 hours, and cytostatic activity was not significantly increased by further incubation.

All the strains and hybrids tested (C57BL, BALB/C, C3HeB, A, AxA.BY, AxC57BL/6 had cytostatic activity against the melanoma line and there was no evidence for an H-2 restriction in this system. Allogeneic splenocytes exhibited as good an effector function or better than syngeneic cells. In the experiments to be described below we either used C57BL/6 or BALB/C effector cells.

B. *Cytostatic Activity of Splenocytes, Peritoneal Exudate Cells and Thymocytes*

Figure 1 shows that both splenocytes as well as thioglycolate-induced peritoneal exudate cells (PEC) express cyto-

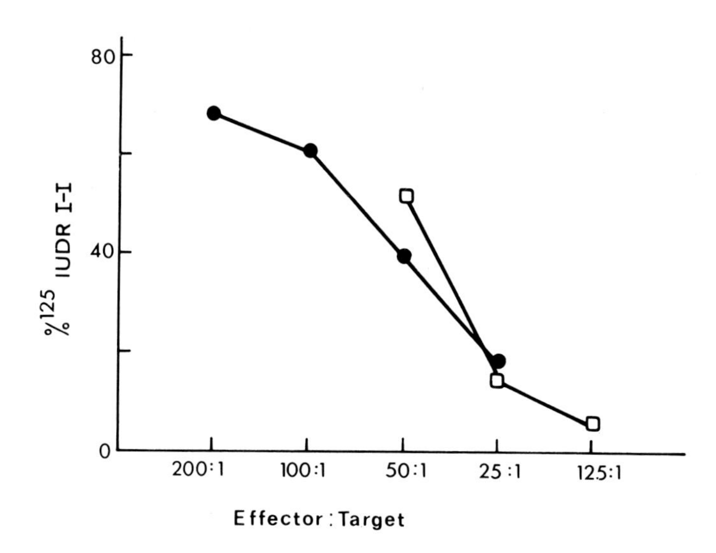

FIGURE 1. Inhibition of ^{125}IUDR incorporation into F10 targets mediated by splenocytes (●——●) and by peritoneal exudate cells (□——□).

stasis of B16-F10 (F10) melanoma cells. The fact that thymocytes were inactive fits a characteristic of NK cells (Herberman and Holden, 1978) but not that of NC cells (Stutman et al, 1978). In order to find out whether or not soluble factors released from the splenocytes or from the PEC were responsible for the cytostatic activity by competing against labeled IUDR or by degrading it, we assayed the cytostatic activity of effector cell supernatants. Supernatants of splenocytes or PEC alone or supernatants of mixed cultures of effector and target cells have no cytostatic activity whatsoever (results not shown). These experiments show that the effector cells per se rather than soluble factors released from such cells caused the cytostasis of the target cells. Furthermore, we demonstrated previously that high concentrations of thymidine (20μg/ml) inhibited ^{125}IUDR incorporation into target cells (Ehrlich et al, submitted for publication). The lack of activity of the culture supernatants in cytostasis shows that they did not contain degradation products of DNA such as thymidine which could compete against the ^{125}IUDR.

TABLE I: *Cytostasis and NK Activity Mediated by Splenocytes from 3 Month and 12 Month Old C57BL/6 Mice After 4 or 18 Hours Incubation with Target Cells*

E/T Cell Ratio	Age (months)	^{125}IUDR I-I[a] (Mean±S.D.)[b]		%^{51}Cr Release[c] (Mean±S.D.)	
		Time of Incubation			
		4 hrs(3)[d]	18 hrs(3)	4 hrs(4)	18 hrs(4)
200 :1	3	53.0± 2.6	61.7±13.6		
100 :1		36.7±12.4	34.0±14.7	22.3± 9.4	35.3±12.0
50 :1		22.7±17.5	21.0±14.7	15.0±10.2	35.8± 6.3
25 :1		10.0±11.8	6.0± 5.6	11.3± 5.7	28.3± 6.2
12.5:1				7.3± 5.4	19.3± 8.7
200 :1	12	34.5± 0.7	59.0± 1.4		
100 :1		28.0±15.6	42.5± 7.8	12.0± 3.6	29.3±13.8
50 :1		22.5±20.5	24.5± 9.2	9.5± 4.7	26.5± 8.2
25 :1		16.5±12.0	10.5± 0.7	6.3± 3.5	18.0± 7.1
12.5:1				4.0± 2.9	13.8± 6.8

a ^{125}IUDR incorporation inhibition (^{125}IUDR I-I) was performed with cultured B16-F10 (F10) cells as targets.

b S.D. = Standard deviation

c The ^{51}Cr release assay was performed with cultured YAC-1 lymphoma cells as targets.

d Numbers in parenthesis indicate the number of experiments performed. A pool of three spleens was used in each experiment.

C. Effects of Aging on Cytostatic Activity

In view of the fact that older mice have a low NK activity (Herberman et al, 1975a, Kiessling et al, 1975) we asked the question whether or not aging mice also express a declined cytostatic activity. The results indicated that cytostatic activity of splenocytes from aging mice is not reduced at all (Table I). In fact, the cytostatic activity of splenocytes from aging mice was sometimes moderately enhanced.

The results of parallel comparative experiments indicated that the difference in NK activity between young and aging mice was evident mainly in a 4 hour assay but much less in an 18 hour assay (Table I). During the 18 hour assay, the aging NK cells became apparently activated. The in-vivo activation occuring spontaneously in young mice have been somehow prevented in the older ones. In light of these results we compared the degree of cytostasis mediated by splenocytes from 3 and 12 month-old mice in a 4 and an 18 hour assay. As shown in Table I the splenocytes from the aging mice were capable to exert almost a maximal cytostatic effect even in the 4 hour assay.

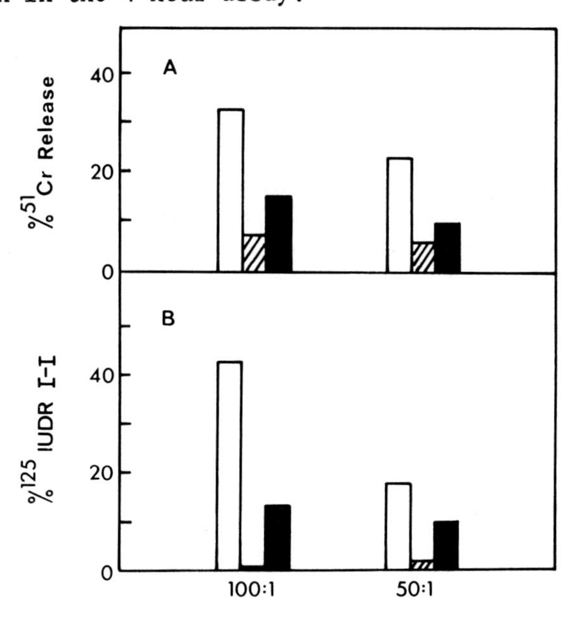

FIGURE 2. A. Cold target inhibition of NK activity (□) by YAC-1 (▨) and F10 (■) tumor cells.
B. Cold target inhibition of ^{125}IUDR I-I (□) by mitomycin-c treated YAC-1 (▨) and F10 (■) tumor cells.

This indicates that unlike NK activity of old splenocytes which can be spontaneously boosted at least 3 fold during the prolonged in-vitro assay, cytostatic cells of old mice are almost fully activated and the duration of the assay can not be held responsible for the lack of demonstrable differences in cytostatic activity between young and aging mice.

D. *The Target Specificity of NK and Cytostatic Cells*

In a previous study (Ehrlich et al, submitted for publication) we demonstrated that B16-F10 (F10) cells were resistant to NK-mediated lysis even in an 18 hour ^{51}Cr release assay. Fig. 2A which summarizes a cold-target inhibition assay shows that F10 cells are able, nontheless, to compete against labeled YAC-1 cells for NK cells. In the reciprocal cold-target inhibition assay both mitomycin-c treated YAC-1 cells as well as F10 cells competed successfully against target F10 cells for cytostatic splenocytes (Fig. 2B). These experiments suggest that NK cells and cytostatic splenocytes recognise similar or possible even cross-reactive determinants on the target cells.

E. *A Partial Characterization of Cytostatic Splenocytes*

1. *Adherence*. ^{125}IUDR I-I mediated by splenocytes from 3 month and 12 month-old C57BL/6 mice was tested with effector populations which were non-adherent to plastic surfaces or to G-10 sephadex columns (TableII).

The results show that non-adherent splenocytes from the young mice expressed constantly a lower cytostatic activity than the unfractionated population. Splenocytes from aging mice which did not adhere to the plastic surface had a cytostatic activity which was comparable to the unfractionated population. However, the cytostatic activity of splenocytes from aging mice decreased significantly after passage through G-10 sephadex columns.

These results suggest that cytostasis is mediated by at least 2 effector populations differing in their adherence properties. Moreover, it seems that some of the properties of the cytostasis-mediating effector cells may be different in young and aging mice.

2. *Phagocytosis*. Phagocytic macrophages were depleted from splenocyte populations by iron and magnetism (Lundgren et al, 1968). The results summarized in TableIII show that phagocyte-depleted splenocytes from the young but not from the aging mice expressed a slight decrease in cytostatic activity.

TABLE II: Cytostasis Mediated by Non-Adherent Splenocytes from 3 Month and 12 Month-Old C57BL/6 Mice

E/T Cell Ratio	Treatment	% ^{125}IUDR I-I[a] (Mean±S.D.)[b]			
		3 months		12 months	
		Unfractionated	Non-Adherent	Unfractionated	Non-Adherent
200 :1	Adherence	61.7±17.7	37.8±16.6	69.8±19.2	64.3±24.4
100 :1	to plastic	43.0±23.0	31.5±19.6	49.0±16.8	55.2±17.9
50 :1	surfaces(6)[c,d]	31.8±21.3	15.0±14.3	44.0± 9.0	35.8±25.5
25 :1		22.1±20.7	12.0±15.8	11.0±15.8	23.6±19.1
200 :1		44.5± 9.2	23.0±12.7	62.5± 3.5	21.0± 7.1
100 :1	retention on	33.0±17.0	18.0±14.1	41.0± 5.7	14.5± 9.2
50 :1	sephadex G-10	11.5± 5.0	16.0± 1.4	26.5±12.0	3.0± 4.2
25 :1	columns(2)[c,e]	4.0± 5.7	0.0± 0.0	12.0± 1.4	6.5± 6.4
12.5:1		3.0± 4.2	0.0± 0.0	1.5± 2.1	0.0± 0.0

a,b,c See footnotes a,b,d of Table 1.

d Spleen cells were incubated for 1 hour at 37°C on plastic petri dishes. The non-adherent cells were used for the tests.

e Spleen cells were eluted from G-10 sephadex columns (Ly and Mishell, 1974). The cell population that was not retained on the column was used for the tests.

TABLE III: *Cytostasis Mediated by Phagocyte-Depleted Splenocytes from 3 and 12 Month-Old C57BL/6 Mice*

	% ^{125}IUDR I-I[a] (Mean±S.D.)[b]			
E/T Cell Ratio	3 month		12 month	
	Unfractionated(5)[c]	Phagocyte[d] Depleted(4)	Unfractionated(7)	Phagocyte Depleted(7)
200:1	69.8±17.9	51.0±15.0	77.1±15.7	69.0±28.2
100:1	59.0±21.7	43.7±14.8	67.4±14.9	67.1±23.8
50:1	45.2±25.6	27.5±21.7	40.8±23.7	46.8±24.5
25:1	23.4± 8.7	14.3±15.3	15.8±16.0	25.1±24.9

a,b,c See footnotes a,b,d of Table 1.

d Depletion of phagocytes was performed by iron and magnet.

TABLE IV: Cytostasis Mediated by Fc-receptor-depleted splenocytes

Treatment	*E/T Cell Ratio*	*% ^{125}IUDR I-I[a][b] (Mean±S.D.)*
	200:1	*32.0± 8.5*
E[c]	*100:1*	*20.0± 7.1*
Monolayer	*50:1*	*13.5± 3.5*
	25:1	*8.5±12.0*
	200:1	*16.5± 2.1*
EA[c]	*100:1*	*10.5± 5.0*
Monolayer	*50:1*	*2.0± 1.4*
	25:1	*4.0±12.0*
	200:1	*30.5± 2.1*
Untreated	*100:1*	*28.0± 2.8*
Control	*50:1*	*18.0±15.6*
	25:1	*14.0± 2.8*

a,b *See footnotes a,b of Table 1.*

c *Monolayers of sheep-erythrocytes (E) or of antibody-coated E (EA) were prepared according to Herberman et al. (1977).*

3. Fc-Receptors. Herberman et al (1977) suggested that mouse NK-cells have Fc-receptors as surface markers although they are not required for the killing activity. Depletion of Fc-receptor positive cells by binding to sheep erythorcytes (SRBC) coated with rabbit antibodies against SRBC (EA) did not decrease, in our hands, NK mediated cytotoxicity while the recovery of non-binding cells was 25-40%. Under the same conditions depletion of EA-binding cells caused a significant reduction in the cytostatic ability of the non-binding population (TableIV). Depletion of E-binding cells did not cause any significant decrease in cytostasis activity. The results show that the effector cells mediating the cytostasis of melanoma cells express avid Fc-receptors. This stresses again that the cytostasis-mediating cells differ from the cells mediating NK cytotoxicity.

4. Incubation at 37^oC. Herberman et al (1975b) demonstrated that NK activity is very much decreased after effector cells had been incubated for 24 hours at 37^oC. We tested whether or not incubation at 37^oC had a similar effect on cytostatic activity. Table V shows that there is no decrease

TABLE V: *Cytostasis and NK Activity Mediated by Splenocytes from 3 and 12 Month-Old C57BL/6 Mice Preincubated for 24 hours at 37°C*

E/T Cell Ratio	Age (Months)	% ^{125}IUDR I-I[a] (Mean±S.D.)[b] 37°C Incubation[e] (3)[d]	Control (3)	% ^{51}Cr Release[c] (Mean±S.D.) 37°C Incubation (3)	Control (3)
200 :1		57.6±26.2	70.3±23.5		
100 :1		36.3±19.8	61.3±18.2	11.0±6.2	34.3± 8.1
50 :1	3	33.0±17.1	41.0±24.5	10.0±3.0	26.7± 6.7
25 :1		17.6±16.6	36.3±17.5	8.7±3.8	21.0± 7.2
12.5:1		20.3±18.8	20.5±21.9	7.0±5.3	17.0± 5.3
200 :1		75.3±10.1	75.7± 7.0		
100 :1		62.6± 9.0	50.3±22.3	2.0±2.7	26.0±17.4
50 :1	12	50.3± 5.8	37.0±21.5	3.7±2.5	27.3±11.4
25 :1		22.7± 8.1	18.0±18.5	4.0±1.0	19.7± 8.1
12.5:1		15.7±13.8	21.5±14.9	4.7±0.6	17.0± 6.8

a,b,c,d See footnotes a,b,c,d of Table I.

e Preincubation of splenocytes at 37°C was performed in tubes so as to minimize depletion of adherent cells.

in ^{125}IUDR I-I in young or in old mice while there was a sharp decrease in the NK activity of the same splenocytes confirming thus the results of the abovementioned investigators.

This data provides support for the tentative conclusion that most of the cytostasis and of the NK activity is mediated by 2 different cell populations.

III. CONCLUDING REMARKS

The results of this study indicated that adherent B-16 melanoma cells expressing determinants recognized by NK cells, are resistant to cytoxicity mediated by such effectors. These tumor cells are however rather sensitive to cytostasis mediated by normal splenocytes. This finding by itself accentuates the biological importance of naturally occuring cytostatic effectors.

One of the main difficulties in attempting to characterize natural cytostatic effector splenocytes is the probable heterogeneity of the cytostatic cell population. All the conventional cell depletion methods used could at best remove only partially the cytostatic activity indicating the involvement of more than one cell population in this activity. The results of the reported experiments are compatible with the possibility that both "classical" NK cells as well as non-phagocytic cells belonging possibly to the monocyte-macrophage series participate in the cytostasis reactivity. This cell population differs in some important characteristics from NK cells. The activity of the former population does not decrease by incubation at 37°C whereas NK cells do. Some of the cells inhibiting ^{125}IUDR incorporation adhere to plastic surfaces or to G-10 sephadex columns whereas, NK cells don't and the Fc-receptors of the former cells seem to bind more avidly to EA than those of NK cells. In order to sort out the nature of the effector cells it will become necessary to deplete NK cells from the splenocyte populations. Attempts to follow this approach are being performed at present.

Whatever the exact nature of cytostatic cell populations, it seems that their activity may be of some importance in the resistance against the development of tumors from apparent potentially malignant cells. The existance of long-term survival of "dormant" NK-resistant tumor cells, for example preleukemic cells, without a formation of a malignant tumor can be attributed, at least partially, to the activity of cytostatic effector cells.

REFERENCES

Fidler, I.J. (1973). Nature New Biol. 242, 148-149.

Fish, F., Yaacubovicz, M. and Witz, I.P. (1974) J.Natl.Cancer Inst. 53, 1743-1747.

Haran-Ghera, N. (1978). J. Natl.Cancer Inst. 60, 707-710.

Herberman, R.B., Nunn, M.E. and Lavrin, D.H. (1975a). Int. J. Cancer 16, 216-229.

Herberman, R.B., Nunn, M.E., Holden, H.T. and Lavrin, D.H. (1975b). Int. J. Cancer 16, 230-239.

Herberman, R.B., Bartram, S., Haskill, J.S., Nunn, M., Holden, H.T. and West, W.H. (1977). J. Immunol. 119, 322-326.

Herberman, R.B. and Holden, H.T. (1978). Adv. Cancer Res. 27, 305-375.

Jerrels, T.R., Dean, J.H., Richardson, G., Cannon, G.B. and Herberman, R.B. (1979). Int. J. Cancer 23, 768-776.

Kiessling, R., Klein, E. and Wigzell, H. (1975). Eur. J. Immunol. 5, 112-117.

Lundgren, G., Zukoski, Ch. F. and Möller, G. (1962). Clin. Exp. Immunol. 3, 817-836.

Ly, I.A. and Mishell, R.I. (1974). J. Immunol. Meth. 5, 239-247.

Stutman, O., Paige, C.T. and Figarella, E.F. (1978). J. Immunol. 121, 1819-1826.

CHARACTERIZATION OF THE NK CELL IN MAN AND RODENTS

Oleg Eremin

Division of Immunology
Department of Pathology
University of Cambridge
Cambridge

I. INTRODUCTION

Natural cell-mediated immunity or natural cytotoxicity has been extensively documented in man and certain rodents (for review see Herberman and Holden, 1978). The precise nature and biological function of the effector cell, the natural killer (NK) cell, on the other hand, has not been satisfactorily resolved.

Sporadic accounts in the literature have described the NK cell as a phagocytic cell (Gomard et al., 1974; Takasugi et al., 1975). The consensus of opinion, however, is that the NK cell is a lymphocyte, both in man (Hersey et al., 1975; Jondal and Pross, 1975; Cooper et al., 1977; Nelson et al., 1977; Ono et al., 1977; West et al., 1977; Kall and Koren; 1978; Kristensen and Langvad, 1978) and in mice and rats (Herberman et al., 1975; Kiessling et al., 1976; Nunn et al., 1976; Shellam, 1977).

Numerous attempts have been made by various workers, often using different techniques, to characterize further the natural killer cells into defined lymphocyte subsets. The findings from such studies have often been contradictory and the surface marker characteristics, in both man and rodents, have still to be unequivocally determined.

The aim of this article is to summarize our attempts at elucidiating the surface marker profile of natural killer cells in the different lymphoid compartments of man, rabbit and rat. The findings suggest a heterogeneity of NK cells in

ISBN 0-12-341350-8

the various lymphoid compartments of man and offer an explanation for the low level of NK cell activity in the rabbit.

II. CHARACTERIZATION OF THE HUMAN NK CELL

A. *Blood*

1. *Methodological Considerations.* The human NK cell in blood was characterized by carrying out various selective lymphocyte subpopulation depletion and enrichment procedures, using rosetting techniques and Ficoll-Hypaque gradients (SG 1.077).

Lymphocytes were isolated from heparinised venous blood of healthy adults on Ficoll-Hypaque gradients and the phagocytic cells removed by a magnet following pretreatment with carbonyl iron. The resultant lymphocytes were 98% viable and free of contaminating cells (≤3%) (Eremin et al., 1976).

Lymphocyte membrane markers were determined by various rosetting techniques. Thymus-derived lymphocytes were detected by their ability to adhere to sheep red blood cells (T^+). The Fc receptor-bearing (Fc^+) lymphocyte subset was determined by rosette formation with ox red blood cells (ORBC) coated with a subagglutinating dose (but in the plateau range) of rabbit IgG anti-ORBC antiserum. The C3 receptor-bearing ($C3^+$) lymphocyte subpopulation was estimated by the numbers of lymphocytes rosetting with ORBC coated with a subagglutinating dose (but in the plateau range) of rabbit IgM anti-ORBC antiserum and C5 deficient mouse complement.

The B lymphocyte subpopulation with surface immunoglobulin (sIg^+) was estimated by the direct antiglobulin rosetting (DAR) assay (Coombs et al., 1977). Rabbit anti-human Fab was coupled by chromic chloride to the surface of trypsin-treated ORBC. Following coupling, the Fc portion of the rabbit Ig was masked by chromic chloride, and was not detected by the Fc receptors on the lymphocyte surface. Normal rabbit IgG, coupled with chromic chloride to trypsin-treated ORBC, was the control for chromic chloride masking of the Fc portion of IgG and always failed to rosette with the different lymphocyte preparations.

Suspensions of rosettes, lymphocytes and red blood cells were layered onto Ficoll-Hypaque gradients and spun in a stepwise manner with an increasing interphase force (250 to 450 g). lymphocytes depleted of a particular subpopulation were recovered from the interphase layer. Rosetted lymphocytes and contaminating unrosetted cells were isolated from the pellet by vigorous mechanical disruption and lysis of red blood cells with distilled water. Pretreatment with distilled water, in contrast to ammonium chloride, has been shown not to be detrimental to the lytic capacity of the NK cell (Eremin et al., 1978c).

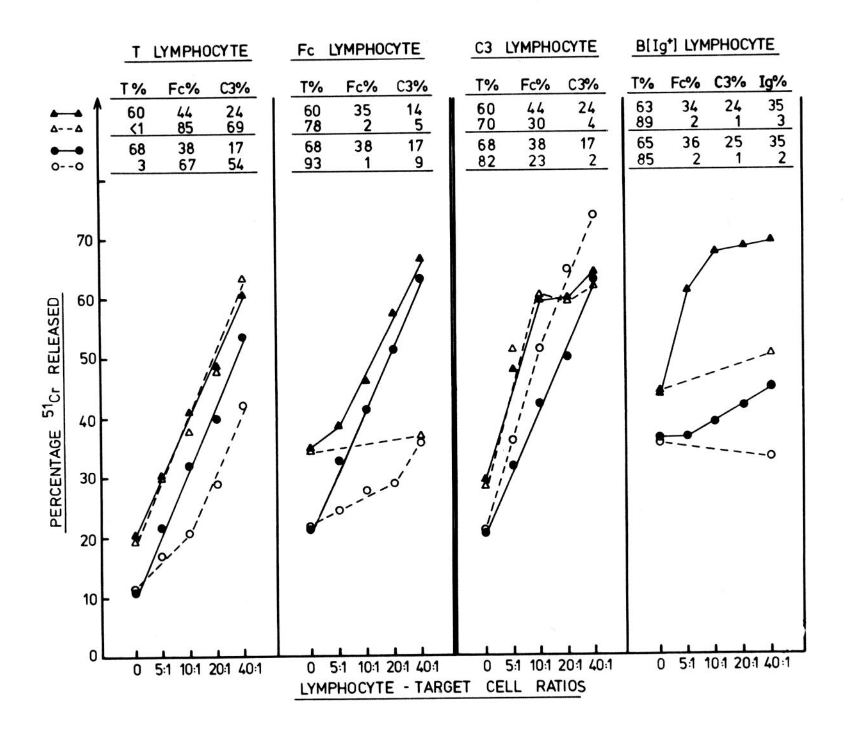

FIGURE 1. Natural cytotoxicity of selectively depleted blood lymphocyte preparations. Lymphocyte suspensions [untreated (▲,●) or depleted of a particular lymphocyte subpopulation (T, Fc, C_3, B(Ig+) : Δ,o)] were added to ^{51}Cr labelled CLA4 target cells at various lymphocyte to target cell ratios (0 to 40:1) and the mixture incubated at 37°C for 24 hrs. Statistical analysis : significant reduction ($p<0.05$) of natural cytotoxicity after depletion of T (o), Fc receptor-bearing (Δ,o) and B(Ig+) (Δ,o) lymphocyte subpopulations. Significant augmentation ($p<0.05$) of natural cytotoxicity after depletion of C3 receptor-bearing (o) lymphocyte subpopulation. No significant change in natural cytotoxicity after depletion of T(Δ) and C3 receptor-bearing (Δ) lymphocyte subpopulations.

In the *in vitro* assays used to measure NK cell activity, the different lymphocyte preparations were added, at varying lymphocyte to target cell ratios (5:1 to 50:1) to ^{51}Cr-labelled CLA4 target cells (Epstein-Barr virus positive lymphoblastoid cell line growing as a suspension culture) and the cell mixtures incubated at 37°C for 18 to 24 hrs (Eremin et al., 1978a).

2. *Surface Marker Characteristics of the Blood NK Cell.* Our findings (see Figures 1 and 2) indicate that the human NK cell in blood is a non-thymus-derived, ($Fc^{\pm}$ $C3^-$), immunoglobulin-bearing lymphocyte (Eremin et al., 1978b).

Substantial evidence has accumulated in the literature showing that the predominant, if not the sole, killer cell in natural cytotoxicity is a non-SRBC-rosetting cell or non-T lymphocyte (De Vries et al., 1974; Matthews and MacLaurin, 1975; Peter et al., 1975; Pross and Jondal, 1975; Kiuchi and Takasugi, 1976; Parkman and Rosen, 1976; Bakacs et al., 1977; Cooper et al., 1977; Mackler et al., 1977; Ono et al., 1977; Pross et al., 1977; Takasugi et al., 1977; Gupta et al., 1978; Kall and Koren, 1978; Ozer et al., 1979).

Kay et al. (1977) and West et al. (1977), on the other hand, found that the NK cell was a T lymphocyte subset, possessing low affinity receptors for SRBC (detected when the rosetting assay was carried out at 4°C). Other workers, using anti-T lymphocyte antiserum, have claimed that the killer cell, although failing to rosette with SRBC possessed the T lymphocyte surface antigen (Bolhuis et al., 1978; Kaplan and Callewaert, 1978). Gupta et al. (1978) even found that some SRBC rosetting (standard assay) T lymphocytes were cytotoxic.

Evidence has been presented by some workers that the thymus-derived cytolytic lymphocyte also has receptors for the Fc portion of IgG (T^+ Fc^+) (Bakacs et al., 1977; Saal et al., 1977; Gupta et al., 1978; Kall and Koren, 1978; Kristensen and Langvad, 1978). At least two groups of workers have shown that the $T\mu$ lymphocytes (with receptors for Fc IgM) lacked any killer cell activity, whilst the $T\gamma$ lymphocyte subset (with receptors for Fc IgG) were cytolytic in the *in vitro* assays used (Gupta et al., 1978; Kall and Koren, 1978).

Our own evidence (Figures 1 and 2; Eremin et al., 1978b), suggests that the predominant natural killer cell in the *in vitro* killer assays was not a thymus-derived lymphocyte and that the SRBC rosetting blood lymphocyte (T^+) was a non-lytic cell. We were unable to isolate selectively the (T^+ Fc^+) subpopulation, due to concomitant contamination by the (Fc^{+} $C3^{-}$) lymphocytes (the lymphocyte subset in which the NK cells reside). Mixed rosetting assays confirmed the presence of both subsets in the T lymphocyte enriched pellets. Our studies therefore cannot exclude the lytic role of (T^{+} Fc^{+}) lymphocyte subset, which from the data of others appears to possess NK cell activity.

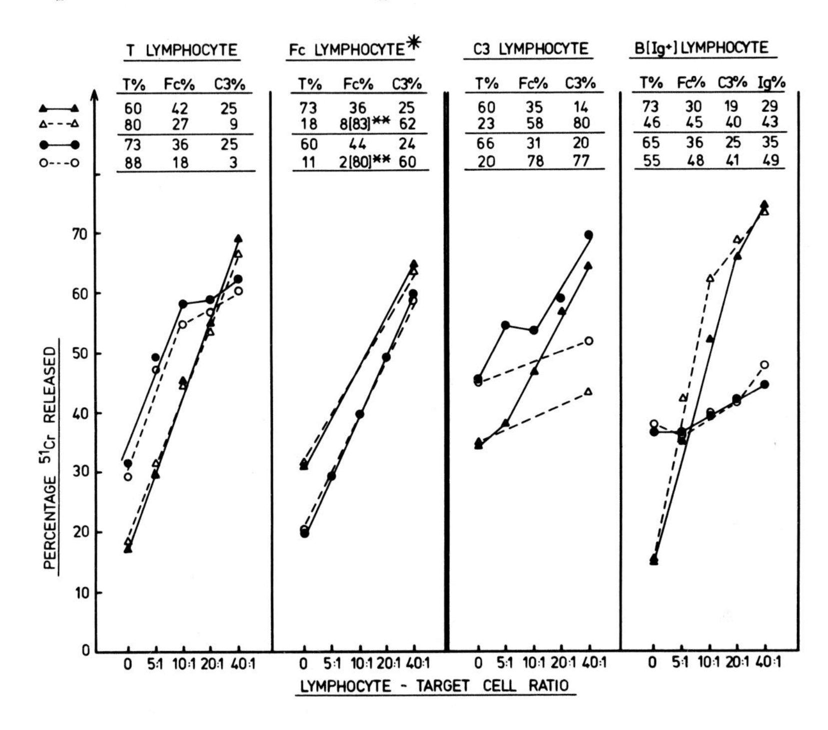

FIGURE 2. Natural cytotoxicity of selectively enriched blood lymphocyte preparations. Lymphocyte suspensions [untreated (▲,●) or enriched for various lymphocyte subpopulations (T, Fc, C3, B(Ig^{+}): Δ,o) from the pellet fractions] were added to ^{51}Cr labelled CLA4 target cells at various lymphocyte to target cell ratios (0 to 40:1) and the mixture incubated at 37°C for 24 hrs. Lymphocytes recovered from Fc rosettes had their Fc receptors blocked. ** Percentage of Fc rosetted lymphocytes in pellet prior to disruption. Statistical analysis : significant reduction ($p<0.05$) of natural cytotoxicity after enrichment for C3 receptor-bearing (Δ,o) lymphocyte subpopulation. Significant augmentation ($p<0.05$) of natural cytotoxicity after enrichment for B(Ig^{+}) (Δ -5:1, 10:1) lymphocyte subpopulation. No significant change in natural cytotoxicity after enrichment for T (Δ,o), Fc receptor-bearing (Δ,o) and B(Ig^{+}) (Δ -20:1, 40:1; o) lymphocyte subpopulations.*

Although several workers have found the non Fc receptor-bearing lymphocyte (Fc^-) to show minor natural lytic activity (Ono et al., 1977; Bolhuis et al., 1978; Kristensen and Langvad, 1978), the majority of workers accept that, whatever other surface markers it may or may not have, the NK cell in the blood of man is an Fc receptor-bearing lymphocyte (Fc^+) (Hersey et al., 1975; Jondal and Pross, 1975; Peter et al., 1975; Bakacs et al., 1977; Cooper et al., 1977; Nelson et al., 1977; Ono et al., 1977; Pape et al., 1977; Pross et al., 1977; Saal et al., 1977; West et al., 1977; Bolhuis et al., 1978; Kristensen and Langvad, 1978; Vierling et al., 1978).

The importance of the Fc receptor for the lytic process is contentious, some authors claiming that the NK cell was only a K cell (responsible for antibody-dependent cellular-cytotoxicity) which had been pre-armed with the appropriate IgG anti-target antibody *in vivo* (for a discussion of this topic see Herberman and Holden, 1978). Blocking of the Fc receptor with Fc fragments, aggregated IgG or immune complexes has produced a variable but often incomplete reduction of NK cell activity, in contrast to the complete abolition of K cell activity detected following such pre-treatments (Peter et al., 1975; Parkman and Rosen, 1976; Timonen and Saksela, 1977; Bolhuis et al., 1978; Kristensen and Langvad, 1978).

We found that blocking of the Fc receptor, which occurred following mechanical disruption and red blood cell lysis of the Ficoll-Hypaque column pelleted Fc rosettes, did not affect NK cell activity, whilst it totally abolished K cell activity (Eremin et al., 1977b; Eremin et al., 1978b). Similarly, Kay et al. (1977) and Gupta et al. (1978) reported no detrimental effect on natural cytotoxicity following blocking of the Fc receptor, although the K cell activity was significantly reduced.

The presence or absence of the receptor for the third component of complement on the blood natural killer cell has not been satisfactorily resolved. Many authors find that some or all of the killer cells are ($C3^+$) (De Vries et al., 1974; Jondal and Pross, 1975; Peter et al., 1975; Parkman and Rosen, 1976; Pross et al., 1977; Jondal and Targan, 1978). Many other workers, however, report that the killer cell lacks a C3 receptor on its cell surface (Hersey et al., 1975; Kiuchi and Takasugi, 1976; Takasugi et al., 1977; West et al., 1977; Vierling et al., 1978).

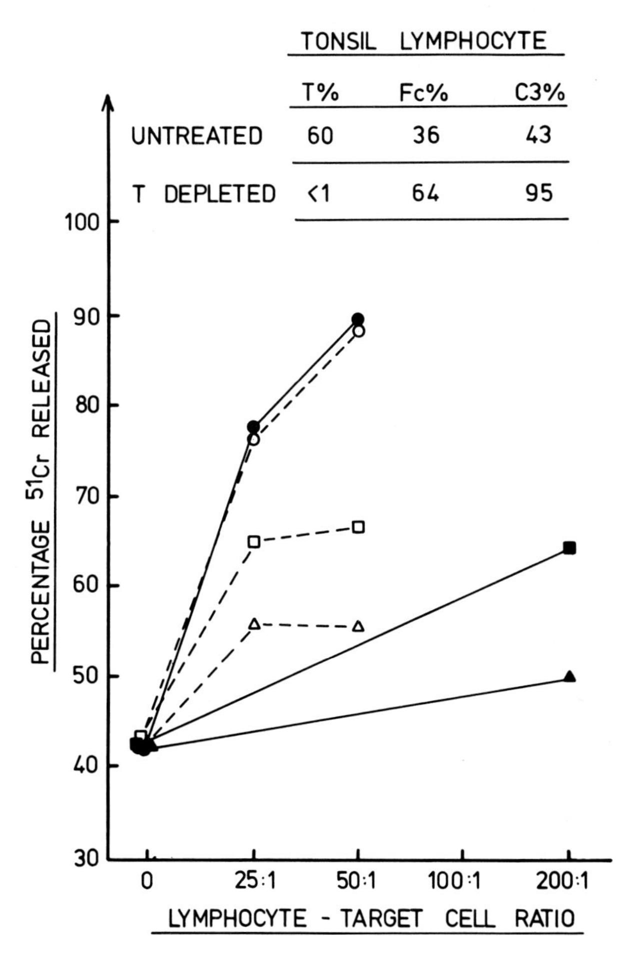

FIGURE 3. Reduction of blood NK cell activity by (Fc^+ $C3^+$) lymphocytes. Lymphocyte suspensions [untreated blood lymphocytes (●), untreated tonsillar lymphocytes (■), tonsillar lymphocytes enriched for (Fc^+ $C3^+$) cells (▲), untreated blood lymphocytes mixed (1:4) with ox red blood cells (o), untreated blood lymphocytes mixed (1:4) with untreated tonsillar lymphocytes (□), untreated blood lymphocytes mixed (1:4) with tonsillar lymphocytes enriched for (Fc^+ $C3^+$) cells (Δ)] were added to ^{51}Cr labelled CLA4 target cells and incubated at 37°C for 24 hrs. Statistical analysis: significant reduction ($p<0.05$) of blood natural cytotoxicity by untreated tonsil (□) lymphocytes and (Fc^+ $C3^+$) enriched tonsil (Δ) lymphocytes; tonsil suspension (▲) depleted of T lymphocytes. No significant change in natural blood cytotoxicity by ox red blood cells (o).

We found the natural killer cell to lack receptors for the third component of complement (Fc^+ $C3^-$), but the (Fc^+ $C3^+$) subpopulation was able to regulate the *in vitro* cytotoxicity of the (Fc^+ $C3^-$) NK cell (Figure 3), either by competitive inhibition for the available target cell surface antigens or by a "suppressor type" mechanism (Eremin et al., 1978b). Suppressor or autoregulatory cells modifying NK cell activity have been recently described in human blood (Parkman and Rosen, 1976; Osband and Parkman, 1978; Ozer et al., 1979). This suggests that the lytic capacity of a lymphocyte preparation, depends on both the absolute and relative numbers of natural killer and suppressor cells present in the preparation. This probably explains why the level of cytotoxicity in cell suspensions depleted of T lymphocytes or enriched for Fc receptor-bearing lymphocytes (see Figures 1 and 2) was not greater, there being a concomitant increase of both the (Fc^+ $C3^-$) and (Fc^+ $C3^+$) subpopulations.

Many workers, using nylon wool columns or anti-human Ig coated Degalan beads or Sephadex G200 columns (whole Ig or $F(ab')_2$ preparations), have found the human blood NK cell to lack demonstrable surface immunoglobulin (sIg^-) as measured by the direct immunofluorescence (DIF) technique (Parkman and Rosen, 1976; Bakacs et al., 1977; Cooper et al., 1977; Kalden et al., 1977; Nelson et al., 1977; Pape et al., 1977). Kaplan and Callewaert (1978) found the NK cell to lack B cell antigens and Ozer et al. (1979) found no evidence of an Ia like antigen on its cell surface. A few authors, however, have found evidence of sIg on the NK cell (Peter et al., 1975; Kiuchi and Takasugi, 1976; Takasugi et al., 1977; Koide et al., 1977).

We have used a rosetting technique to specifically deplete (sIg^+) lymphocytes on Ficoll-Hypaque columns. This rosetting assay specifically detects immunoglobulin-bearing lymphocytes, the percentage of sIg^+ cells is not diminished by prolonged incubation and washing at 37°C and the indicator cells do not interact through the lymphocyte Fc receptor (Coombs et al., 1977; Haegert et al., 1978).

The direct antiglobulin rosetting reaction, when compared with direct immunofluorescence, detects a significantly higher percentage of (sIg^+) lymphocytes both in man (Haegert et al., 1978) and in various domestic animals (Binns et al., 1979). With the DAR assay the number of "null" cells (lacking demonstrable T lymphocyte markers and detectable sIg) in the peripheral blood lymphocyte preparations is very low (1 to 3%) and in many instances none can be detected (Eremin et al., 1978b and unpublished findings; Haegert et al., 1978; Haegert and Coombs, 1979). This very sensitive assay does not discriminate between lymphocytes with significant amounts and those with small amounts of surface immunoglobulin.

Although some "null" cells presumably belong to the non-lymphoid series of cells, others appear to be precursors of the lymphocyte lineage. Chess et al. (1975) isolated a "null" cell population and found that in *in vitro* culture approximately 50% of these "null" cells acquired detectable sIg. They also found, using an I^{125}-labelled $F(ab')_2$ anti-Fab preparation, that some "null" cells possessed sIg^+ but at a very much reduced concentration - 1% that of ordinary B cells (DIF positive). Warr et al. (1978) similarly found that in the athymic mouse, splenic "null" cells possessed typical B cell surface immunoglobulins, but between 10 and 30% of the amount found on typical B cells. Great variation in the surface density of sIg has also been found on B cells at varying stages of maturation (Nossal and Lewis, 1972; Melchers and Andersson, 1973). It is possible that the DIF technique does not detect the mature B cell with its low density of sIg.

Most typical B lymphocytes (sIg^+ by DIF) are found to be Fc receptor-bearing and to have C3 receptors, that is are (Fc^+ $C3^+$) (Chess et al., 1974; Horwitz and Lobo, 1975; Ehlenberger et al., 1976). Such a lymphocyte subpopulation has been shown by us to lack NK cell activity (Eremin et al., 1978b). Many, if not most, "null" cells express high-affinity receptors for the Fc portion of IgG (Froland and Natvig, 1973; Lobo and Horwitz, 1976; Horwitz et al., 1978) and a substantial number lack C3 receptors (Fc^+ $C3^-$) (Horwitz and Lobo, 1975; Horwitz et al., 1978). Some of these "null" cells also had low levels of Ia antigen on the cell surface (Horwitz et al., 1978).

Our findings with the DAR assay, in conjunction with the data presented above suggest that the natural killer cell is an (Fc^+ $C3^-$) lymphocyte with probably low density sIg, which is not detected by DIF. This could either be an immature precursor of the B cell lineage or conversely a more mature type of B lymphocyte.

B. *Tonsil : Lymph Node*

In man, natural cytotoxicity has been documented and the NK cell characterized primarily in blood; studies of NK cell activity in other lymphoid compartments are scanty. Natural killer cell activity has been found in cell preparations from the spleen (Lotzová and McCredie, 1978; Eremin, unpublished findings) and bone-marrow (Lotzová and McCredie,

1978). We have previously described natural cytotoxicity in cell preparations from the tonsil and lymph node (Eremin et al., 1978a), although some authors have failed to detect NK cell activity in both lymphoid compartments (Nelson et al., 1977; Herberman and Holden, 1978).

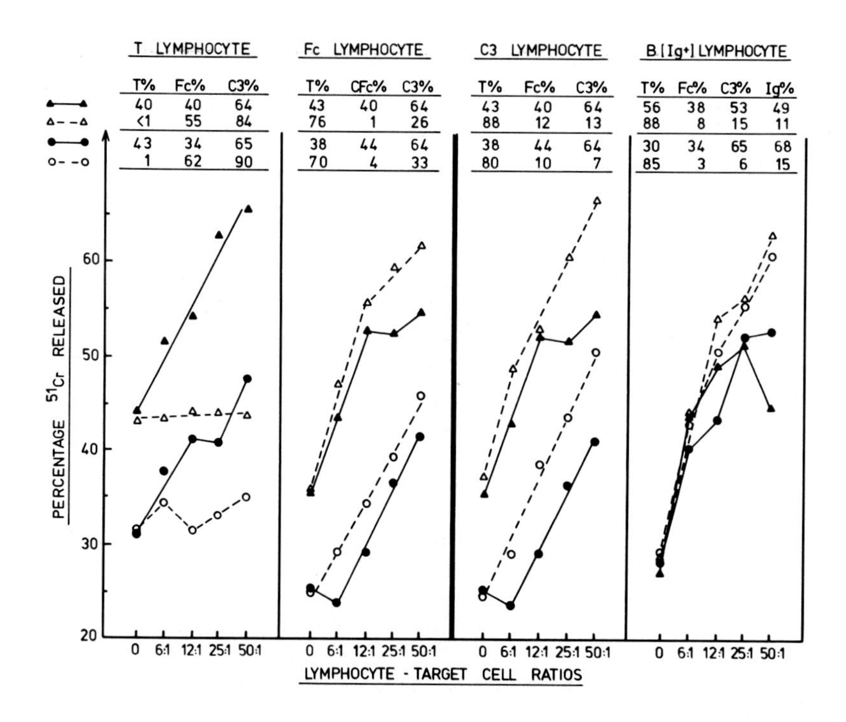

FIGURE 4. Natural cytotoxicity of selectively depleted tonsil lymphocyte preparations. Lymphocyte suspensions [untreated (▲,●) or depleted of a particular lymphocyte subpopulation (T, Fc, C3, B(Ig+) : △,o)] were added to ^{51}Cr labelled CLA4 target cells at various lymphocyte to target cell ratios (0 to 50:1) and the mixture incubated at 37°C for 24 hrs. Statistical analysis : significant reduction ($p < 0.05$) of natural cytotoxicity after depletion of T(△,o) lymphocyte subpopulation. Significant augmentation ($p < 0.05$) of natural cytotoxicity after depletion of Fc receptor-bearing (△ - 25:1, 50:1; O), C3 receptor-bearing (△ - 6:1, 25:1, 50:1; O) and B(Ig+) (△ - 12:1, 25:1, 50:1; O) lymphocyte subpopulations.

Lymphocytes, isolated from tonsils and lymph nodes (Eremin et al., 1976), were selectively depleted or enriched for various subpopulations by rosetting and centrifuging on Ficoll-Hypaque gradients, and set up in *in vitro* NK cell assays (Eremin et al., 1978a, 1978b). As the results from both tonsil and lymph node preparations were very similar, only the findings for tonsil lymphocytes are presented here (Figures 4 and 5).

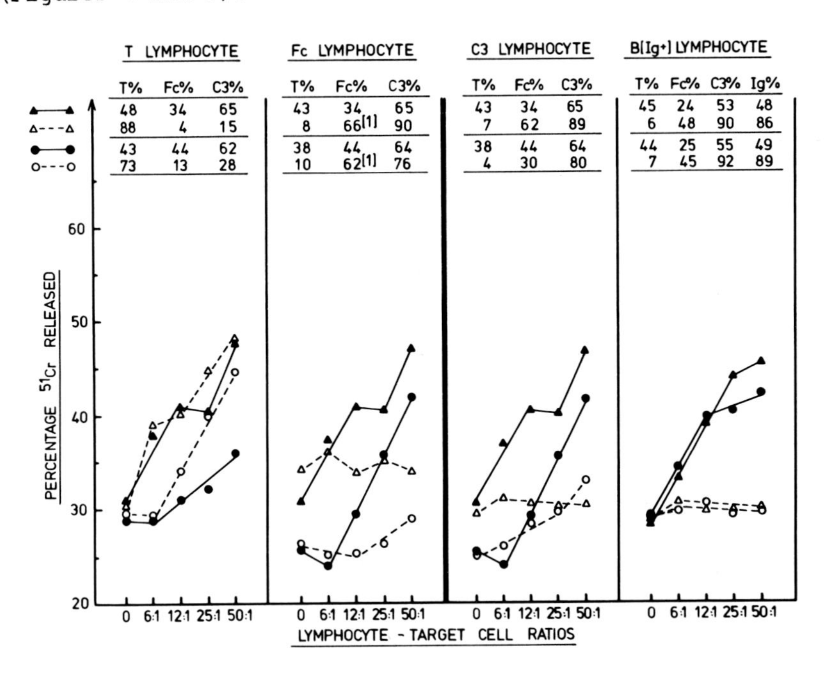

FIGURE 5. Natural cytotoxicity of selectively enriched tonsil lymphocyte preparations. Lymphocyte suspensions [untreated (▲,●) or enriched for various lymphocyte subpopulations (T, Fc, C3, B(Ig⁺) :Δ,o) from the pellet fractions] were added to ^{51}Cr labelled CLA4 target cells at various lymphocyte to target cell ratios (0 to 50:1) and the mixture incubated at 37°C for 24 hrs. (1) lymphocytes recovered from Fc rosettes had some of their Fc receptors blocked. Statistical analysis : significant reduction ($p<0.05$) of natural cytotoxicity after enrichment for Fc receptor-bearing (Δ; 0 - 12:1, 25:1, 50:1), C3 receptor-bearing (Δ,0 - 25:1, 50:1) and B(Ig±) (Δ,o) lymphocyte subpopulations. Significant augmentation ($p<0.05$) of natural cytotoxicity after enrichment for T (0 - 12:1, 25:1, 50:1) lymphocyte subpopulation. No significant change in natural cytotoxicity after enrichment for T (Δ) lymphocyte subpopulation.

In contrast to the findings in blood, our studies revealed (Figures 4 and 5) that the NK cell in tonsil and lymph node was a non-sIg-bearing, thymus-derived (T^+) lymphocyte, lacking both the Fc and C3 receptors (Eremin et al., 1978b).

TABLE 1. Mixed Rosetting (Fc, C3) Populations in Various Lymphoid Compartments of Man[a]

Lymphocyte donor	Percentage of total rosettes counted[b]		
	Fc rosettes (Fc^+ $C3^-$)	Mixed rosettes (Fc^+ $C3^+$)	C3 rosettes (Fc^- $C3^+$)
Blood (n = 6)	43 ± 13	49 ± 11	8 ± 3
Tonsil[c] (n = 6)	3 ± 1	44 ± 10	53 ± 10
Lymph node[d] (n = 6)	6 ± 2	44 ± 9	50 ± 11

[a]*Mixed rosetting reactions were carried out with fluorescein isothiocyanate-labelled indicator cells as outlined previously (Eremin et al., 1976).*

[b]*Values expressed as a mean ± standard deviation.*

[c]*Tonsils obtained at tonsillectomy from patients who had had recurrent bouts of tonsillitis but were in a quiescent phase.*

[d]*Lymph nodes obtained from inguinal area or abdomen and which were not draining a site of inflammation or tumour growth.*

This heterogeneity of NK cell activity in the different lymphoid compartments of man was suggested by the very low numbers of (Fc^+ $C3^-$) lymphocytes found in tonsils and lymph nodes (Table 1), and by the differential lytic responses elicited from these lymphoid compartments following pretreatments with trypsin and ammonium chloride. Trypsin treatment of tonsil and lymph node lymphocytes had no effect on NK cell activity, in contrast to the significant reduction of blood lymphocyte cytotoxicity following such enzyme treatment (Eremin et al., 1978a). The susceptibility of the blood NK cell to trypsin treatment is well documented in the literature (Peter et al., 1975; Pross and Jondal, 1975; Kay et al., 1977; Nelson et al., 1977). Pretreatment of blood and tonsil lymphocytes with ammonium chloride reduced NK cell activity. Recovery of blood lymphocyte cytotoxicity occurred after 24 hrs of incubation at 37°C, but the lytic capacity of the tonsillar NK cell was still reduced following this period of incubation (Eremin et al., 1978c).

C. *Summary and Conclusions*

1. In summary, our findings (based on selective lymphocyte subpopulation depletion and enrichment procedures) suggest that in man there is a heterogeneity of natural killer cells present in the different lymphoid compartments examined - blood, tonsil and lymph node.

2. In the blood, the predominant cell mediating natural cytotoxicity is a non-thymus-derived, (Fc^+ $C3^-$), immunoglobulin-bearing lymphocyte. The sIg on the killer cell appears to be only detectable by the DAR assay and is not picked up by the DIF technique, and is probably present in reduced amounts on the cell surface. The NK cell therefore could possibly be either an immature precursor or a fully mature cell of the B lymphocyte lineage, which by conventional immunofluorescence techniques is classified as a "null" cell. Our procedures did not allow us to specifically isolated the (T^+ Fc^+) subset from blood, which may also have a lytic capacity *in vitro*.

3. The sIg-bearing, (Fc^+ $C3^+$) lymphocyte subset (which is probably the B lymphocyte population detected by DIF) appears not only to lack natural killer cell activity *in vitro* but to be able to suppress the *in vitro* cytotoxicity of the (Fc^+ $C3^-$) blood NK cell. The level of natural

cytotoxicity detected in lymphocyte preparations is therefore governed by the absolute and relative numbers of the NK and its "suppressor" cell.

4. In human tonsils and lymph nodes, the NK cell is a thymus-derived (T^+) lymphocyte, lacking both Fc and C3 receptors. The (Fc^+ $C3^-$) lymphocyte subset (the blood NK cell) is present in very low numbers. Various treatments of this tonsillar (T^+) natural killer cell with trypsin and ammonium chloride further confirms this heterogeneity.

III. NK CELL ACTIVITY IN THE RAT AND RABBIT

Lymphocytes were isolated from the blood, lymph nodes and spleens of the rat and rabbit as previously described (Eremin et al., 1979). Figures 6 and 7 show the variable

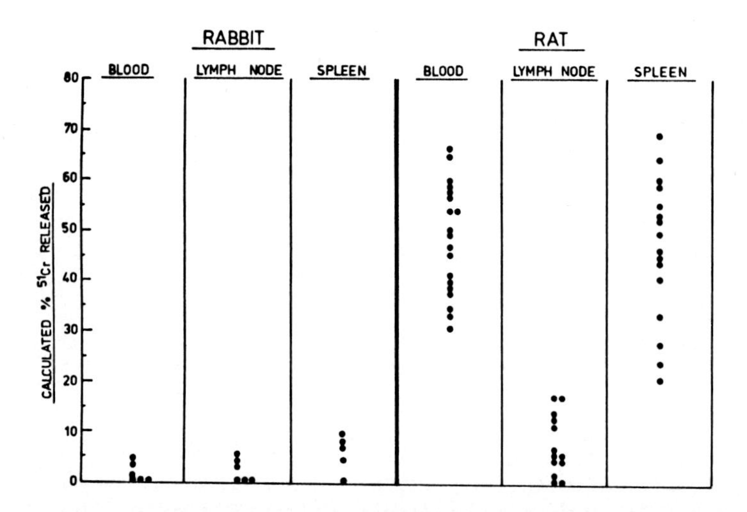

FIGURE 6. Natural cytotoxicity of rabbit and rat lymphocytes against CLA4. Rabbit and rat lymphocyte suspensions, prepared from blood, lymph node and spleen, were added to ^{51}Cr labelled CLA4 target cells and the mixture incubated at 37°C for 24 hrs. ^{51}Cr release was calculated by subtracting the background release (in the absence of lymphocytes) from the obtained experimental release. Maximal lymphocyte to target cell ratios only shown (50:1).

levels of NK cell activity detected in the different lymphocyte preparations from the rat and rabbit against ^{51}Cr labelled CLA4 and Detroit 6 (D6) (Hela subline growing as a monolayer) target cells respectively.

Variable but prominent levels of NK cell activity were found in lymphocyte preparations from the blood and spleen of the rat against both target cells. The NK cell activity of lymph node preparations from the rat, on the other hand, was substantially lower against both target cells (Figures 6 and 7).

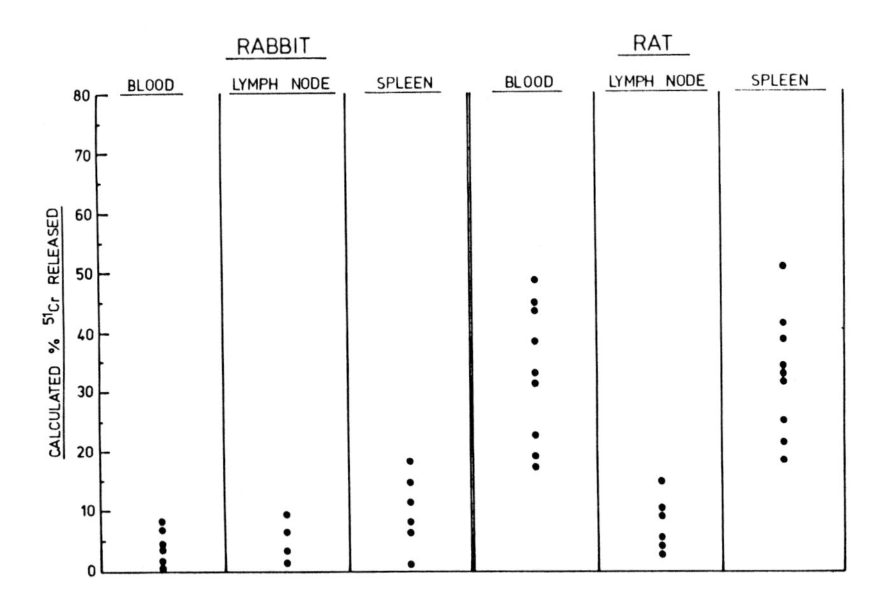

FIGURE 7. Natural cytotoxicity of rabbit and rat lymphocytes against D6. Rabbit and rat lymphocyte suspensions, prepared from blood, lymph node and spleen, were added to ^{51}Cr labelled Detroit 6 (D6) target cells and the mixture incubated at 37°C for 24 hrs. ^{51}Cr release was calculated by subtracting the background release (in the absence of lymphocytes) from the obtained experimental release. Maximal lymphocyte to target cell ratios only shown (50:1).

TABLE 2. *Mixed Rosetting (Fc, C3) Populations in Various Lymphoid Compartments of the Rabbit and Rat*[a]

Lymphocyte Donor	Percentage of total rosettes counted								
	Blood[b]			Lymph Node			Spleen		
	Fc rosettes (Fc^+C3^-)	Mixed rosettes (Fc^+C3^+)	C3 rosettes (Fc^-C3^+)	Fc rosettes (Fc^+C3^-)	Mixed rosettes (Fc^+C3^+)	C3 rosettes (Fc^-C3^+)	Fc rosettes (Fc^+C3^-)	Mixed rosettes (Fc^+C3^+)	C3 rosettes (Fc^-C3^+)
Rabbit 1	4	46	50	1	43	56	2	58	40
Rabbit 2	3	42	55	1	32	67	3	67	30
Rat 1	38	57	5	8	80	12	19	65	16
Rat 2	33	63	4	6	67	27	20	70	10

[a] *Mixed rosetting reactions were carried out with fluorescein isothiocyanate-labelled indicator cells as outlined previously (Eremin et al., 1976).*

[b] *Rabbits were bled from a marginal ear vein into a receptacle containing ACD (1 part ACD to 3 parts blood), as the citrate inhibited complement activation which occurred in vitro during the isolation of lymphocytes from heparinized or defibrinated blood. Centrifugation on Ficoll-Hypaque was also avoided as this leads to a selective loss of T lymphocytes (Eremin et al., 1979).*

Rabbit lymphocyte preparations, however, irrespective of the origin of the lymphoid compartment (blood, lymph node and spleen), showed very low or absent levels of natural cytotoxicity (Figures 6 and 7).

Mice (Nunn and Herberman, 1979), rats (see above; Nunn and Herberman, 1979) and guinea pigs (unpublished findings) can lyse heterologous target cells *in vitro*. To exclude the possibility that rabbits are unable to do so, cytotoxicity against homologous rabbit cell lines needs to be evaluated further. It does appear, however, from the data presented that the rabbit, not only lacks K cells (responsible for antibody-dependent cellular-cytotoxicity) (Eremin et al., 1979) but seems to have very few, if any, NK cells.

It can be seen from Table 2 that the (Fc^+ $C3^-$) lymphocytes (the NK cell subset in man) are present in very low numbers in the blood and spleen of the rabbit and in the lymph nodes of both the rabbit and rat. The (Fc^+ $C3^+$) lymphocytes (the NK suppressor cell subset in man) are prominent in all of the lymphoid compartments of the rabbit and rat.

These subpopulation findings, in association with the *in vitro* lytic assays suggest that the surface marker profile of the NK cell in the rabbit and rat is (Fc^+ $C3^-$), similar to that of the natural killer cell in human blood. The data also indicates that the (Fc^+ $C3^+$) lymphocyte lacks cytolytic capacity and offers an explanation for the very low levels of NK cell activity detected in the rabbit.

Selective lymphocyte subpopulation depletion studies, carried out in the rat to date, confirm this postulate. Rat lymph nodes, in contrast to the findings in man, appear to lack a second (thymus-derived) NK cell (unpublished findings).

ACKNOWLEDGMENTS

The data presented was obtained in collaboration with Professor R.R.A. Coombs, J. Ashby and D. Plumb. The work was supported by the Cancer Research Campaign (UK). Figures 1, 2, 3, 4 and 5 are reproduced, by kind permission, from the International Journal of Cancer, 21, 42-50, 1978. Table 1 is reproduced in part, by kind permission, from the International Archives of Allergy and Applied Immunology, 52, 277-290, 1976. Table 2 is reproduced in part, by kind permission, from Cellular Immunology, 47, 332-346, 1979. I gratefully acknowledge the encouragement and help provided by Professor R.R.A. Coombs, Head of the Division of Immunology, Department of Pathology, University of Cambridge.

REFERENCES

Bakacs, T., Gergely, P. and Klein, E. *Cell. Immunol. 32,* 317 (1977).

Binns, R.M., Licence, S.T., Symons, D.B.A., Gurner, B.W., Coombs, R.R.A. and Walters, D.E. *Immunology 36,* 549 (1979)

Bolhuis, R.L.H., Schuit, H.R.E., Nooyen, A.M. and Ronteltap, C.P.M. *Eur. J. Immunol. 8,* 731 (1978).

Chess, L., MacDermott, R.P., Sondel, P.M. and Schlossman, S.F. *Prog. in Immunol. II, 3,* 125 (1974).

Chess, L., Levine, H., MacDermott, R.P. and Schlossman, S.F. *J. Immunol. 115,* 1483.

Coombs, R.R.A., Wilson, A.B., Eremin, O., Gurner, B.W., Haegert, D.G., Lawson, Y., Bright, S. and Munro, A.J. *J. Immunol. Methods 18,* 45 (1977).

Cooper, S.M., Husen, D.J. and Friou, G.J. *Cell. Immunol. 32,* 135 (1977).

De Vries, J.E., Cornain, S. and Rümke, Ph. *Int. J. Cancer 14,* 427 (1974).

Ehlenberger, A.G., McWilliams, M., Phillips-Quagliata, J.M., Lam, M.E. and Nussenzweig, V. *J. Clin. Invest. 57,* 53 (1976).

Eremin, O., Plumb, D. and Coombs, R.R.A. *Int. Arch. Allergy appl. Immunol. 52,* 277 (1976).

Eremin, O., Kraft, D., Coombs, R.R.A., Franks, D., Ashby, J. and Plumb, D. *Int. Arch. Allergy appl. Immunol. 55,* 112 (1977).

Eremin, O., Ashby, J. and Stevens, J.P. *Int. J. Cancer 21,* 35 (1978a).

Eremin, O., Coombs, R.R.A., Plumb, D. and Ashby, J. *Int. J. Cancer, 21,* 42 (1978b).

Eremin, O., Ashby, J. and Plumb, D. *J. Immunol. Methods 24,* 257 (1978b).

Eremin, O., Wilson, A.B., Coombs, R.R.A., Plumb, D. and Ashby, J. *Cell. Immunol. 47,* 332 (1979).

Froland, S.S. and Natvig, J.B. *Transp. Rev. 16,* 114 (ed. G. Moller), Munksgaard, Copenhagen.

Gupta, S., Fernandes, G., Nair, M. and Good, R. *Proc. Natl. Acad. Sci. 75,* 5137 (1978).

Haegert, D.G., Hurd, C. and Coombs, R.R.A. *Immunology 34,* 5 (1978).

Haegert, D.G. and Coombs, R.R.A. *Lancet ii,* 1051, (1979).

Hersey, P., Edwards, A., Edwards, J., Adams, E., Milton, G.W. and Nelson, D.S. *Int. J. Cancer 16,* 173 (1975).

Horwitz, D.A., Lobo, P.I. *J. Clin. Invest 56,* 1464 (1975).

Horwitz, D.A., Niaudet, P., Greaves, M.F., Dorling, J. and Deteix, P. *J. Immunol. 121,* 678 (1978).

Jondal, M. and Targan, S. *Clin. exp. Immunol. 33,* 121 (1978).
Kalden, J.R., Peter, H.H., Roubin, R. and Césarini, J.P. *Eur. J. Immunol. 7,* 537 (1977).
Kall, M.A. and Koren, H.S. *Cell. Immunol. 40,* 58 (1978).
Kaplan, J. and Callewaert, D.M. *J. Natl. Cancer. Inst. 60,* 961 (1978).
Kay, H.D., Bonnard, G.D., West, W.H. and Herberman, R.B. *J. Immunol. 118,* 2058 (1977).
Kiuchi, U. and Takasugi, M. *J. Nat. Canc. Inst. 56,* 575 (1976).
Koide, Y., Takasugi, M. and Billing, R. *Transpl. Proc. 7,* 731 (1977).
Kristensen, E. and Langvad, E. *Cancer Immunol. Immunoth. 5,* 71 (1978).
Lobo, P.I. and Horwitz, D.A. *J. Immunol. 117,* 939 (1976).
Lotzová, E. and McCredie, K.B. *Cancer Immunol. Immunoth. 4,* 215 (1978).
Mackler, B.F., O'Neill, P.A. and Merstrich, M. *Eur. J. Immunol. 7,* 55 (1977).
Matthews, N. and MacLaurin, B.P. *Lancet i,* 581 (1975).
Melchers, F. and Andersson, J. *Transplant. Rev. 14,* 76, (ed. G. Moller), Munksgaard, Copenhagen.
Muchmore, A.V., Decker, J.M. and Blaese, R.M. *J. Immunol. 119,* 1680 (1977).
Nelson, D.L., Strober, W., Abelson, L.D., Bundy, B.M. and Massin, D.L. *J. Immunol. 118,* 943 (1977).
Nossal, G.S.U. and Lewis, H. *J. exp. Med. 135,* 1416 (1972).
Nunn, M.E., Djeu, J.Y., Glaser, M., Lavrin, D.H. and Herberman, R.B. *J. nat. Cancer Inst. 56,* 393 (1976).
Nunn, M.E. and Herberman, R.B. *J. nat. Cancer Inst. 62,* 765 (1979).
Oehler, J.R., Lindsay, L.R., Nunn, M.E. and Herberman, R.B. *Int. J. Cancer 21,* 204 (1978).
Oldham, R.K., Ortaldo, J.R. and Herberman, R.B. *Cancer Res. 37,* 4467 (1977).
Oldham, R.K., Forbes, J.T., Niblach, G.D. *Proc. Am. Assoc. Cancer Res. 19,* 161 (1978).
Ono, A., Amos, D.B. and Koren, H.S. *Nature 266,* 546 (1977).
Osband, M. and Parkman, R. *J. Immunol. 121,* 179 (1978).
Ozer, H., Strelkauskas, A.J., Callery, R.T. and Schlossman, S.F. *Eur. J. Immunol. 9,* 112 (1979).
Pape, G.R., Troye, M. and Perlmann, P. *J. Immunol. 118,* 1925 (1977).
Parkman, R. and Rosen, F.S. *J. exp. Med. 144,* 1520 (1976).
Peter, H.H., Pavie-Fischer, J., Fridman, W.H., Aubert, Ch., Césarini, J.P., Roubin, R. and Kourilsky, F.J. *J. Immunol. 115,* 539 (1975).

Pollack, S.B. and Emmons, S.L. *J. Immunol. 122,* 719 (1979).
Potter, M.R. and Moore, M. *Clin. exp. Immunol. 34,* 78 (1978).
Pross, H.F. and Jondal, M. *Clin. exp. Immunol. 21,* 226 (1975).
Pross, H.F., Baines, M.G. and Jondal, M. *Int. J. Cancer 20,* 353 (1977).
Saal, J.G., Rieber, E.P., Hadam, M. and Rietmüller, G. *Nature 265,* 158 (1977).
Shellam, G.R. *Int. J. Cancer 19,* 225 (1977).
Shellam, G.R. and Hogg, N. *Int. J. Cancer 19,* 212 (1977).
Takasugi, M., Kiuchi, M. and Opelz, G. *Transpl. Proc. 9,* 789 (1977).
Timonen, T. and Saksela, E. *Cell. Immunol. 33,* 340 (1977).
Vierling, J.M., Steer, C.J., Bundy, B.M., Strober, W., Jones, E.A., Hague, N.E. and Nelson, D.L. *Cell. Immunol. 35,* 405 (1978).
Warr, G.W., Lee, J.C. and Marchiolonis, J.J. *J. Immunol. 121,* 1767 (1978).
West, W.H., Cannon, G.B., Kay, H.D., Bonnard, G.D. and Herberman, R.B. *J. Immunol. 118,* 355 (1977).

CHARACTERISTICS OF MURINE NK CELLS IN RELATION TO T LYMPHOCYTES AND K CELLS

Magnus Gidlund
Otto Haller [1]
Anders Örn
Emmanuel Ojo [2]
Peter Stern
Hans Wigzell

Department of Immunology, Biomedical Center
University of Uppsala
Uppsala, Sweden

INTRODUCTION

Progress in cellular immunology has to a marked degree been dependant upon development of technology allowing the physical and functional separation and analysis of the various cells in the immune system. In the present article we will describe and discuss the murine NK cells in relation to two other cell types with potential lytic abilities, namely T lymphocytes and the heterogeneous group of killer cells or K cells that participate in antibody-dependant cell-mediated cytolysis (ADCC). The article will, as requested, be biased to predominantly contain and discuss our own results in this area considering that other workers in the same area in this volume will put forward their results and views.

[1] *Present adress: University of Zürich, Switzerland.*

[2] *Present adress: University of Ife, Ife, Benin, Nigeria.*

ISBN 0-12-341350-8

SURFACE MARKERS ON NK CELLS IN COMPARISON TO T AND B CELLS AND MACROPHAGES.

Several groups of investigators have contributed to our present understanding of the surface markers on murine NK cells in relation to other cells involved in immune reactions. Our own studies in this regard representing a mixture of original discoveries and confirmations are summarized in table 1.We have in these comparisons been excluding cell types such as granulocytes which for morphological reasons can be excluded to constitute NK cells(1).

Table 1.A comparative analysis of surface markers on murine NK cells in relation to other relevant immune cells.

Markers	*NK cells*	*T cells*	*B cells*	*Macrophages*
H-2K/D	+(-?)	+	+	+
Ia	−	−(+)	+	+
Lyt-1,2,3	−	+	−	−
Thy-1	−(+)	+	−	−
Mph	−	−	−	+(−)
Asialo-GM$_1$	+	−(+)	−	?
Ig	−	−	+	−
Fc-receptors	±	−(+)	+	+
C3-receptors	−	−	+	+
Helix pomatia A	+	+	−(+)	−(+?)
Vicia villosa	−	−(+)	−	−

+ or − =majority of cells positive or negative for the marker.
± =weak reactions indicating low avidity or few receptors.
( )=signs within brackets denote that a minority subgroup within a major group has the marker.
Mph=an alloantigen in the mouse for macrophages (2)
Asialo-GM$_1$=rabbit antisera against the asialo-GM$_1$ ganglioside, provided for by Drs S.I.Hakomori and M.Kasai resp.(3,4).
Helix pomatia A=a lectin from the snail with the same name with specificity for the N-acetylgalactoseamine as dominant group (5,6).
Vicia villosa=the N-acetylgalactoseamine specific lectin from seeds of the plant.
?=not properly studied by us.

The results as depicted in table 1 requires comments.The H-2 antigens were originally considered to be present in"normal" amounts on murine NK cells (1).More recent data have indicated that a fraction of mouse natural killer cells may have a quite low amount of such antigenic determinants (unpublished data) as judged by sensitivity to cytotoxic antibodies.Whether this indeed represents heterogeneity with regard to density of antigen or sensitivity to cytoxic antibodies with complement would require availability of pure NK cells.A marker of debate over the years with regard to mouse NK cells has been the Thy-1 antigen (1,7,8,9).Our own results using either monoclonal or polyclonal anti-theta reagents in presence of complement have by and large failed to wipe out more than a fraction of NK lytic ability (in the range of 20-40% in the positive cases).However,we have also noted that the Thy-1 constitution of the target cell in some situations constituted an unexpected contributing factor to the outcome of such tests (not published results).We would thus at present still be somewhat reluctant to accept this marker as a "safe" one for murine NK cells.The last allo-antigen of interest is the Mph-1 antigen known to constitute a marker for monocytes/macrophages (2) and antisera against this marker in presence of complement will not eliminate NK activity (10).

Reports have been forthcoming as to the possible relatively select representation of asialo-GM_1 gangliosides on murine NK cells in relation to other lymphoid cells (3,4).Using antisera kindly provided to us from these investigators we have been able to confirm that not only mouse but also rat NK cells have a high density of asialo-GM_1 like sites whereas human NK cells fail to express such markers.However,using these antisera at tenfold-higher concencentrations it was possible to also quite efficiently eliminate cytotoxic murine T cells in the presence of complement.We would thus at present consider this marker to be a useful one but of limited discriminatory power with regard to cytolytic cell types in the mouse.

Lectins have been found of usefulness in the characterization of mouse lymphoid cells.Helix pomatia A agglutinin can thus be shown to react with NK cells after removal of sialic acid from the cells but the reactivity of the lectin to killer T cells is even higher (6).Yet,this lectin shows quite a select reactivity with regard to other cell types from the immune system.A second lectin with even more narrow specificity is the N-acetylgalactoseamine-reactive one derived from Vicia villosa seeds (11).This lectin would seem to have a quite distinct reactivity for mouse killer T cells with little or no measurable reactivity for NK or ADCC-reactive cells (12).

From the surface markers delineated in table 1 it would seem clear that NK cells do not classify as cells belonging to the "classical" sets of B or T lymphocytes and macrophages or monocytes.Other approaches using organ distribution patterns, effects of organ-deprivation and selective immune deficiencies have yielded similar conclusions (13,14,15).

Notes of caution should,however,be taken as to the actual placing of NK cells as being a cell type outside any of the classical pathways of differentiation.Likewise,it is necessary to explore each "new" cell type for possible activities in "old" functional assays.For this reason we have further tested the possibilities that NK cells may a)be on the way to develop into another cell type,e.g. a cytolytic T cell and b)may be able to exert lytic functions beyond the defined NK area such as K cell activity in antibody-dependant cell-mediated cytototixicity.Finally,although we have in our comparison as presented in table 1 so far found no major difference between the surface markers present on normal versus "activated" NK cells it is evident from other articles in this volume that such differences do surely exist at some levels.

THE RELATIONSHIP BETWEEN NK CELLS AND T LYMPHOCYTES.

No doubts exist that NK cells can functionally develop and appear in the physical absence of the thymus (16,17).Yet,when comparisons are made between previously known subgroups in the immune cellular system and the newly found NK cells as to surface markers there certainly exist some suggestive evidence for a T-like behaviour of NK cells.In the mouse we have already mentioned the Thy-1 marker (7) and the Helix pomatia A binding abilities (6).In the human a substantial fraction of NK cells do express sheep erythrocyte-binding ability (18),a marker considered a quite select T cell marker (19).On the other hand certain "typical" T markers such as Lyt-1,2 and 3 antigens are not demonstrable on the murine NK cells (20).Still one can certainly make a forceful argument that NK cells may be of pre-T nature (21),with a possibility to differentiate into mature T lymphocytes under given conditions .

There exist a well known antagonistic relationship between the presence of a thymus and the levels of NK cells in the individual animal (16,17).Three possibilities exist that can explain these results:a)The thymus has a direct negative impact on NK cells via some presumably hormonal action which may induce NK cells to become non-active as NK cells(mature to T cells?).Against this one may argue that experiments in vivo as well as in vitro using purified thymic hormones from many sources have so far failed to have any significant positive or negative impact on NK activities in the mouse (own data as well as Dr.R.B.Herberman´s).b)The thymus is generating cells of suppressor type for NK cells.Strong arguments for such a possibility come from data showing that autologous thymocytes can function as natural target for the individual´s own NK cells with high numbers of NK-susceptible thymocytes being present in animals with low NK levels (22).One could thus put forward the reasoning that the known organ distribution so typical for NK cells may in fact merely be an inverse picture of the distribution pattern of such suppressor cells.(7). c)The third possibility is based on the knowledge that interferon is a major regulator of NK levels in vivo and in vitro (24,25).As an intact T cell system is instrumental in an efficient defense towards infections a deficiency in that part of the immune system may automatically lead to increases in endogenous interferon levels due to infections.This may then in a secondary manner lead to the known variations in NK levels known to exist between T-deficient and normal mice.If the claim is confirmed that mice reared under patogen free conditions are virtually zero with regard to NK activity with recovery to normal levels within a week after placing the animals under normal conditions (26) we would favour the last of these three alternatives.Analysis of potential differentiation of NK cells into T cells under controlled conditions in vitro and/or assays of such a sensitivity that they could measure the normal endogenous serum levels of interferon in mice would allow more definite conclusions as to these alternatives.

A consideration of NK cells being like a more primitive form of cytotoxic T lymphocytes,CTL:s,is also worth discussing. We already know that one "typical" CTL marker in the mouse,the T145 glycoprotein,is lacking on the surface of the NK cells (12),but this marker may be associated with a late,mature T cell activity.Killing by contact between cells is an old mechanism of pre-T nature and NK cells could thus be viewed as a deviant form of CTL:s.In this regard specificity tests may be of interest.CTL:s are well known to express a close to complete restriction as to concommitant MHC recognition in order to be able to exert their lytic activities (27). In contrast,the specificity of NK cells is still very much under debate (see other articles in this volume) and views of clonal specificity a la sophisticated immunocompetent T and B lymphocytes exist in parallel to results suggesting a more general,group-restricted selectivity being the same for all NK cells of the species.It is already known that NK cells fail to express MHC restriction in their lytic actions (28).Here we include data to show that MHC determinants at the target cell level plays no detectable role whatsoever for the murine NK cells in contrast for the CTL:s.

Table II. MHC determinants on the target cell surface play no role for NK cells but are essential for CTL:s.

A. NK cells but not T cells can kill murine teratocarcinoma cells lacking MHC determinants.

Effector cells	*Target cells (% specific lysis)* Nulli	YAC
CBA spleen	14%	24%
" -, *Tilorone*	43%	46%
AKR spleen	3%	5%
- " -, *Tilorone*	12%	13%
"Immune T anti-Nulli"	0%	0%

B. F(ab)$_1$ rabbit-anti-H-2 fragments block CTL:s but not NKcells

Effector cells	*Blocking reagent*	*Target cell=Yac*
A.BY-anti-A CTL	*Normal F(ab), 400ug/ml*	67,1%
- " -	*Anti-H-2-"- - " -*	37,6%
C57BL spleen NK	*Normal F(ab) - " -*	53,8%
- " -	*Anti-H-2 -"- - " -*	57,9%

Immune anti-nulli were raised by in vivo immunization with Nulli teratocarcinoma cells or normal spleen cells of 129 genotype across an H-2 barrier followed by in vitro restim. for 5 days before testing(33).
ABY-anti-A CTL were derived from a 5 days MLC.
CBA is a "high" NK and AKR a "low" NK strain (1). Tilorone is an interferon inducer secondarily in vivo activating NK cells (23).

These results would thus clearly distinguish CTL:s from NK cells at yet another level, that of target structure requirements with regard to MHC. Assumptions of clonal specificity being present on NK cells in a T-like manner would thus have to require a different set of receptor specificities than are present on ordinary T cells endowed with cytolytic potential.

THE RELATIONSHIP BETWEEN NK CELLS AND K CELLS.

Several cell types are known to be able to function as killer cells against IgG-coated target cells (29). It is clear that the target cell can contribute in a decisive manner as to what effector cell types can function in such K cell lysis. When NK cells were discovered it was thus natural to explore the possible ability of such cells to also function as K cells well realizing that NK cells do exert their spontaneous selective lytic ability via own, actively synthesized receptors (30).We (31) and others(32) have in the murine system been able to demonstrate that NK cells may exert a dual activity,that is function both as NK cells against certain targets and as K cells against other,select target cells.These conclusions were drawn from sets of experiments exploring in parallel the lytic abilities against IgG-coated NK-resistant tumor targets or erytrocytes in parallel to conventional NK assays.Experiments were also carried out including blocking experiments where the results indicated that the very same NK cells reactive against YAC Moloney lymphoma cells could be selectively inhibited in their lytic action by adding competing IgG-coated NK-resistant tumor targets (31).However,NK cells seemed select in their lytic function as K cells against IgG-coated targets in the sense that they did not seem able in the murine system to lyse IgG-coated chicken red blood cells.Table III depicts experiments of such a nature showing the select,T-independent linkage between NK cells and K cell activity against IgG-coated NK-resistant tumor cells with no linkage to K cell activity against the IgG-coated erythrocytes.

Table III.In vitro lytic activities of spleen cells derived from normal or thymectomized bone-marrow chimeras.

Effector cells	NK-YAC	NK-P8I5	ADCC-P8I5	ADCC-CRBC
A/C,0	9,2%	0%	0%	22,6%
A/C,NDV	I6,6%	0,5%	I,2%	I6,5%
A/A,0	7,2%	0,2%	0,5%	2I,4%
C/C,0	27,3%	0%	4,4%	36,3%
C/A,0	32,4%	0,3%	3,4%	24,6%
C/A,NDV	53,3%	8,I%	I8,6%	27,0%
C/A-X,0	29,2%	0,I%	7,4%	26,I%
C/A-X,IF	52,5%	I3,7%	28,4%	28,2%

Effector cells:A=AKR.C=CBA.First letter=marrow donor.Second letter=lethally irradiated recipient.0=untreated.NDV=donors treated with Newcastle disease virus 24 hrs previously.IF= donors treated with 5xI0^4 units of type I interferon 24 hrs previously.X=thymectomized recipient.Effector cells were spleen cells from mice more than 3 weeks after transfer of bone marrow cells to irradiated recipients.Results expressed in % specific lysisYAC=an A/Sn highly susceptible Moloney lymphoma whereas P8I5=a DBA/2 mastocytoma relatively resistant to NK cells unless in activated form.CRBC=chicken red blood cells.Effector:target ratio 50:I.

The results in table III do also illustrate the relative term of NK sensitivity versus resistance.The P8I5 tumor is using normal NK cells a resistant target.However,when NK cells are being activated there is a significant increase in their lytic capacity in the sense that previously resistant targets may now become relatively susceptible to NK attacks.In our hands,however,we have never noticed any significant changes in specificity subsequent to such activations.Another finding worth mentioning is the fact that trypsin treatment of the NK cells will remove the lytic ability of the NK cells but will still allow the same cells to function as efficient K cells in ADCC against certain targets (32).

From the above findings we would thus conclude that NK cells can exert K cell activity against some but not all IgG-coated target cells.However ,the activity in the NK effector systems is using additional or completely different receptor structures compared to those used by the NK cells when functioning as K cells in ADCC systems.

SUMMARY

Murine NK cells exist as a distinct cell type but with some surface markers similar and maybe identical to other already classified cells of the immune system.Judged by surface markers one may consider NK cells to possibly belong to a pre-T lineage but further studies are required to establish this possibility.Several distinct differences exist between NK and CTL:s involving both surface structures and specificity requirements.This would mean that NK cells if using receptors of a clonally distributed type endowing specificity to these cells must have receptor structures distinctly different from those present on CTL:s.Finally,NK cells can certainly be shown to also express K cell activity in ADCC systems against some but not against all IgG-coated target types.This dual activity would thus further emphasize the potential importance of the NK cells in several in vivo situations.

ACKNOWLEDGMENTS

This work was supported by the Swedish Cancer Society,by NIH contract NOI-CB-64033,by the Swiss National Science Foundation (No.3.I39-0.77) and by an EMBO fellowship (P.S.).

REFERENCES

1. Kiessling, R., Petrányi, G., Kärre, K., Jondal, M., Tracey, D., and Wigzell, H., *J.Exp.Med. 143,* 112 (1976).
2. Archer, R., *Genet.Res. (Camb.) 26,* 213 (1975).
3. Young, W.W., and Hakomori, S-I, *J.Immunol. in press.*
4. Kasai, M., Iwamori, M., Nagai, Y., Okumura, K., and Tada, T., *J.Immunol. in press.*
5. Hammarström, S., and Kabat, E.A., *Biochemistry 8,* 2929 (1969).
6. Haller, O., Gidlund. M., Hellström, U., Hammarström, S., and Wigzell, H., *Eur.J.Immunol. 8,* 765 (1978).
7. Kiessling, R., and Wigzell, H., *Immunol.Rev. 44,* 165 (1979).
8. Herberman, R.B., Nunn, M.E., and Holden, H.T., *J.Immunol. 121,* 304 (1978).
9. Clark, E.A., Russel, P.H., Egghart, M., and Horton, M.A., *Int.J.Cancer in press.*
10. Ojo, E., Haller, O., and Wigzell, H., *Scand.J.Immunol. 8,* 215 (1978).
11. Kimura, A., Wigzell, H., Holmquist, G., Ersson, B , and Carlsson, P., *J.Exp.Med. 149,* (1979).
12. Kimura, A., Örn, A., Holmquist, G., Wigzell, H., and Ersson, B., *Eur.J.Immunol. 9,* 575 (1979).
13. Kiessling, R., Klein, E., Pross, H., and Wigzell, H., *Eur.J.Immunol. 5,* 117 (1975).
14. Haller, O., Gidlund, M., Kurnick, J., and Wigzell, H., *Scand.J.Immunol. 8,* 207 (1978).
15. Roder, J., and Duwe, A., *Nature 278*, 451 (1979).
16. Kiessling, R., Klein, E., and Wigzell, H., *Eur.J. Immunol. 5,* 112 (1975).
17. Herberman, R.B., Nunn, M.E., Holden, H.T., and Lavrin, D.H., *Int.J.Cancer 26,* 230 (1975).
18. West, W.H., Cannon, G.B., Kay, H.D., Bonnard, G.D., and Herberman, R.B., *J.Immunol. 118,* 335 (1977).
19. Jondal, M., Holm. G., and Wigzell, H., *J.Exp.Med. 136,* 207 (1973).
20. Glimcher, L., Shen, F., and Cantor, H., *J.Exp.Med. 145,* 1 (1977).
21. Herberman, R.B., and Holden, H.T., *Adv.Cancer Res. 27,* 305 (1978).
22. Hansson, M., Kiessling, R., Andersson, B., Kärre, K., and Roder, J., *Nature 278,* 174 (1979).
23. Gidlund, M., Örn, A., Wigzell, H., Senik, A., and Gresser, I., *Nature 273,* 759 (1978).
24. Trinchieri, G., and Santoli, D., *J.Exp.Med. 147,* 1314 (1978).

25. Djeu, J.Y., Heinbaugh, J.A., Holden, H.T., and Herberman, R.B., *J.Immunol. 122,* 175 (1979).
26. Clark, E.A., and Harmon, R.C., *Adv.Cancer Res. in press.*
27. Zinkernagel, R.M., Solter, D., and Knowles, B.B., *Nature 266,* 361 (1977).
28. Becker, S., Fenyö, E.M., and Klein, E., *Eur.J.Immunol. 6,* 882 (1976).
29. Perlman, P., and Cerottini, J.C., *Adv.Cancer Res. in press.*
30. Kärre, K., Haller, O., Becker, S., Kiessling, R., Ranki, A.M., Andersson, L.C., and Häyry, P., *submitted for publication.*
31. Ojo, E., and Wigzell, H., *Scand.J.Immunol. 7,* 297 (1978).
32. Santoli, A., Herberman, R.B., and Holden, H.T., *J.Natl. Cancer Inst. 62,* 109 (1979).
33. Stern, P.L., Gidlund, M., and Wigzell, H., *submitted for publication.*

CHARACTERISTICS OF NK CELLS

Ronald B. Herberman
Tuomo Timonen
Craig Reynolds
John R. Ortaldo

Laboratory of Immunodiagnosis
National Cancer Institute
Bethesda, Maryland

I. INTRODUCTION

Our laboratory has been interested in the comparative characterization of natural killer (NK) cells in mice, rats and humans. We have been quite impressed with the many similarities in the effector cells among the three species. Repeatedly, observations have been first made for a particular characteristic of NK cells in one species and when the analogous characteristic was examined in the others, parallel or at least consistent results were obtained. However, there have been a few features that have varied considerably among the species and understanding of the mechanisms underlying those differences might provide important clues to some of the basic factors involved in the development and regulation of NK cells. In this chapter, we will briefly summarize some of the main similarities and differences in rodent and human NK cells.

II. CELL SURFACE CHARACTERISTICS

A. T Cell Markers

The possibility of NK cells being in the T cell lineage remains a point of considerable controversy. None of the supporting evidence, taken separately, can be considered

ISBN 0-12-341350-8

conclusive. However, the total amount of information, with the similarities among the species (summarized in Table I), makes the association of NK cells with the T cell lineage more compelling.

In the mouse, expression of Thy 1 on lymphoid cells appears to be mainly, if not exclusively, associated with T cells and precursors of T cells. Treatment of spleen cells,

TABLE I. Similarities in Cell Surface Characteristics of Mouse, Rat, and Human NK Cells

Characteristic	*Mouse*	*Rat*	*Human*
T cell markers	*Low density of Thy 1 on portion of NK cells; reactivity with variety of anti-thymocyte alloanti-sera, (e.g., Ly 5, Ly 9)*	*At least partial depletion of activity by heterologous anti-T and by antibody in anti-thymocyte alloanti-serum (ART-1^a)*	*Elimination of activity by hetero-logous anti-T sera; low affinity receptors for E on majority of NK cells*
Fcγ receptors	*Low affinity receptors on at least majority of NK cells*	*Low affinity receptors on at least majority of NK cells*	*Easily de-tectable on all NK cells reactive with K562*
C3 receptors	*Undetectable*	*Undetectable*	*Undetectable on at least most NK cells*
Surface membrane immunoglobulin	*Undetectable*	*Undetectable*	*Undetectable*
Adherence	*Nonadherent, but after boosting, a portion adherent*	*Mainly but not com-pletely nonadherent*	*Nonadherent, but after* in vitro *generation, a portion adherent*

TABLE II. Expression of Thy 1 Antigen on NK Cells of Nude and Conventional Mice, and Detected by Monoclonal Anti-Thy 1.2 (from Mattes et al., *1979)*

Fractionation procedure	*BALB/c nude mice*	*CBA euthymic mice*
Cytotoxicity by antibody + C	*75-90% activity Thy 1+*	*33-67% activity Thy 1+*
Fluorescence-activated cell sorter	*30-60% activity Thy 1+*	

particularly those from nude mice, with anti-Thy 1.2 allo-antiserum plus complement was found to cause a partial depletion of NK activity (Herberman *et al.*, 1978). By use of mice congenic for Thy 1, it appeared likely that the observed effects were due to antibodies to Thy 1, rather than to any contaminating antibodies. This conclusion has recently been confirmed by use of monoclonal antibodies to Thy 1 (Mattes *et al.*, 1979). These results are summarized in Table II. Several points about these findings should be noted, since they may account for apparent discrepancies from results of other investigators: 1) Treatment with antibody plus complement never resulted in complete elimination of activity, as is typically seen when cytotoxic T cells are similarly treated. Thus, it seems clear that a portion of splenic NK cells have no detectable expression of Thy 1. 2) It has been consistently difficult to detect the effects of anti-Thy 1 plus C on spontaneous activity of conventional, euthymic mice. Partial depletion of activity has only become apparent by some calculation of total residual activity, taking into account the large proportion of cells lysed by this treatment. In contrast, the effects of treatment on nude spleen cells or on spleen cells after *in vivo* boosting have been more apparent, indicating that a higher proportion of these NK cells have detectable Thy 1. This may be due to variation in expression of this antigen, depending on the state of differentiation or activation of the cells. 3) The Thy 1+ NK cells appear to have a lower density of antigen on their cell surface than do most typical, mature T cells. With both the alloantiserum and the monoclonal antibodies, it has been necessary to perform the depletion studies with substantially higher concentrations than those needed for complete

TABLE III. Expression of Receptors for Helix pomatia *on NK Cells and on Cytotoxic or Mitogen-Responsive T Cells (from Mattes and Holden, 1980)*

Fractionation procedure	*NK cells*	*Cytotoxic T-cells*	*Mitogen-responsive T-cells*
Rosetting	*Most of activity in non-rosetting fraction*	*50-70% of activity in non-rosetting fraction*	*No activity in non-rosetting fraction*
Sepharose affinity column	*>90% activity specifically bound and elutable*	*About 50% activity specifically bound and elutable*	*All activity specifically bound and elutable*

elimination of cytotoxic T cells or of proliferative responses to T cell mitogens. The low density of Thy 1 was confirmed in the studies done with the fluorescence activated cell sorter (FACS). The Thy 1+ cells in nude spleen cells had low fluorescence intensity. The lower estimate of the proportion of Thy 1+ cells from the FACS analysis is probably related to this, since it was difficult to set the optimal level of fluorescence intensity to sort the weakly positive from negative cells.

Mouse NK cells have also been examined in our laboratory (Mattes and Holden, 1980) for expression of receptors for *Helix pomatia* lectin, which have been largely associated with T cells. These results, as summarized in Table III, varied with the fractionation procedure that was used. Receptor-bearing cells were removed by passage over a solid-phase affinity column, as previously described by Haller *et al.*, (1978), or by rosetting with human erythrocytes. Both procedures were effective in removing most mature T cells, as reflected by the elimination of lymphoproliferative responses to T cell mitogens. As previously reported (Haller *et al.*, 1978), most NK cells appeared to have receptors for the lectin, but these appeared to have insufficient affinity to allow their separation by rosetting. Low affinity receptors were also found in some non-T cells and therefore this lectin does not appear to help in the determination of the lineage of NK cells. These studies also appeared to indicate that some cytotoxic T cells were heterogeneous in their expression of receptors for the Helix lectin. Only about half of the cytotoxic activity of spleen cells immune to murine sarcoma virus was removed on the affinity column, and the receptor-positive immune effector cells also appeared to have low affinity for binding.

Rat NK cells have also been examined for their expression of T cell associated antigens. Treatment of spleen cells with a high concentration of a heterologous burro anti-rat T cell serum (Djeu *et al.*, 1974) plus complement caused a partial depletion of NK activity. (R. Oehler and J. Djeu, unpublished observations). To examine this issue in more detail, we have recently treated nylon wool nonadherent spleen cells with a variety of other anti-T cell antibodies and then tested for residual NK activity (Table IV). Rat T cells have

TABLE IV. Effects of Anti-T Cell Antibodies on Rat NK Activity

		Antibody pretreatment[1]						
Strain	ART phenotype	NRtS	ART-1a	Thy 1.1[2]	W3/13[2]	W3/25[2]	BC-84	OX-1[2]
M520	1a	23.2[3]	3.1	--[4]	--	19.3	--	--
COP	1a	18.2	6.2	16.7	--	--	15.5	--
LEW	1a	36.1	6.3	--	--	--	--	12.6
W/Fu	1b	49.3	10.2	--	41.1	37.5	52.0	--
W/Fu	1b	43.2	5.6	--	33.1	32.2	--	18.1
NBR	1b	56.7	56.6	--	--	--	--	--

[1]Nylon-passed spleen cells treated with antibody and rabbit complement and then tested against ^{51}Cr-labelled W/Fu Gl lymphoma target cells, at 100:1 effector:target cell ratio, in a 4 hour assay.

[2]These antibodies not directly cytotoxic but became cytotoxic when goat anti-mouse immunoglobulin reagent was added.

[3]% cytotoxicity above autologous control.

[4]Not tested.

been shown to express specific alloantigens, antigens of rat thymus (ART), detectable by appropriately absorbed, antithymocyte alloantisera (Lubaroff, 1977). One such antiserum, anti-ART-1^a, produced in NBR rats against Lewis thymocytes, was found to cause substantial complement-dependent depletion of NK activity. However, the antibody responsible for this effect does not appear to be directed against the 1^a allo-antigen, since it had similar effects on 1^b rat strains. Furthermore, BC-84, a monoclonal antibody that appears to be specific for ART-1^a (D. Lubaroff and C. Reynolds, unpublished data), did not affect NK activity in either ART-1^a or 1^b rats. It does not appear to be an autoantibody since it had no effect on NK activity of NBR spleen cells. It seems likely that it is a contaminating alloantibody, perhaps analogous to the anti-NK 1 antibody that was initially found in mouse alloantisera to Ly 1 (Glimcher *et al.*, 1977).

Recently it was reported that NBR anti-Lewis alloantisera contain antibody against LC, a leukocyte-common antigen, expressed on thymocytes, bone marrow cells, and macrophages as well as on some peripheral lymphocytes (Fabre and Williams, 1977). Experiments with OX-1, a monoclonal antibody to LC antigen (Sunderland *et al.*, 1979) have indicated that the majority of NK cells express this antigen. Whether reactivity against this specificity is completely responsible for the effects observed with the anti-ART-1^a alloantisera remains to be determined. If all of the effects of anti-ART-1^a sera are due to antibodies to LC, no conclusions regarding the cell lineage of rat NK cells could be drawn.

We have also examined a number of other monoclonal antibodies to rat T cells and found some to be effective in removing NK activity (Table IV). Because of the finding of Thy 1 on a portion of mouse NK cells, it was of interest to study the effect of anti-Thy 1.1 on rat NK cells. This antiserum reacts with precursors of T and B lymphocytes and with thymocytes in the rat, but with very few peripheral T cells (Ritter *et al.*, 1979). The W3/13 and W3/25 antibodies have been shown to bind to most mature T cells (Williams *et al.*, 1977) and depleted 40% and 25% of spleen cells, respectively, but these had little if any effect on NK activity.

In studies on human NK activity, the majority of effector cells were found to rosette with sheep erythrocytes, when the rosetting was done under optimal conditions (Kay *et al.*, 1977; West *et al.*, 1977). These results are different from those of several other groups, but the failure to detect rosette-forming NK cells appeared to be due in part to the usual use of ammonium chloride solutions to remove E (sheep erythrocytes) from the pelleted cells. In addition, the rosette-forming NK cells appeared to be mainly in a subpopulation of cells with low affinity receptors for E (West *et al.*, 1978). Thus, if

TABLE V. E Receptors on Human NK Cells

Cell Fraction[a]	*Lytic units/ 10^7 cells*	*Total lytic units/ fraction*	*Percent unfractionated activity*
Unfractionated	*70*	*70*	*100*
Total E-RFC	*75*	*60*	*86*
high affinity	*28*	*16*	*23*
low affinity	*210*	*40*	*57*
Non-E-RFC	*66*	*13*	*19*

[a]*Total E-rosette forming cells (E-RFC), and high- and low-affinity E-RFC subsets, and an E-RFC depleted cell fraction were separated from peripheral blood mononuclear cells of a normal donor and then, without lysis of E in E-RFC fractions, tested in 4 hour ^{51}Cr release assay against K562.*

the rosetting procedure was performed under suboptimal conditions, only high affinity rosette-forming cells, with low NK activity, would be isolated. An example of the distribution of NK activity into various fractions by E-rosetting is shown in Table V. It should be noted that although 80-90% of the total activity was in rosette-forming fractions, a consistent small subpopulation of receptor negative NK cells was found.

Virtually all human NK cells, including those not forming rosettes with E, have been reported to be eliminated by a specific anti-T cell serum (Kaplan and Callewaert, 1978, and chapter in this book). Using this antiserum, we have been able to confirm their results (Ortaldo *et al.*, 1979). We have obtained essentially the same results with another anti-human T cell serum, produced by immunization of rabbits with cultured T cells of a normal donor and absorbed with an autologous B cell line (Bonnard *et al.*, 1978, and in preparation). This reagent, in the presence of complement, appears to be quite selective for T cells, eliminating all E-RFC and T cell associated functions but having no detectable effect on B cells or monocytes. However, this antiserum, as that of Kaplan and Callewaert, does react with a portion of "null" cells. It remains to be determined whether this reflects the presence of some non-E-rosetting T cells or reactivity against a differentiation antigen, present on immature cells of non-T as well as T cell lineage.

B. Fc Receptors

Another feature which appears to be characteristic of most NK cells from each of the species studied is their expression of receptors for the Fc portion of IgG (Pross and Jondal, 1975; Peter *et al.*, 1975; Hersey *et al.*, 1975; Herberman *et al.*, 1977; West *et al.*, 1977; Oehler *et al.*, 1978). These were quite difficult to detect on mouse and rat NK cells and this may reflect low affinity binding of IgG to the Fc receptors (FcR) on these cells. Adequacy of depletion of FcR+ cells on immune complex monolayers has been best monitored by parallel testing for antibody-dependent cell-mediated cytotoxicity (ADCC) against tumor target cells. This is consistent with substantial evience that NK and ADCC activities are associated with the same subpopulation of lymphocytes (Ojo and Wigzell, 1978; Santoni *et al.*, 1979a,b). Although FcR have been readily detected on human NK cells which react with the K562 myeloid cell line and some other targets, there have been some recent indications of another subpopulation of NK cells, lacking detectable FcR, that react against some monolayer target cells (Bolhuis, 1977, and chapter in this book; Eremin *et al.*, 1978, and chapter in this book). During the course of a study in our laboratory designed to look for disease-related cytotoxicity by cells from breast cancer patients, similar observations were made (W. West, G. D. Bonnard, K. Pfifner and R. B. Herberman, unpublished). NK activity against K562 was eliminated by adsorption on immune complex monolayers and residual activity by the FcR- cells against 3 monolayer cell lines derived from breast cancer was evaluated (Table VI). With some donors, not only breast cancer patients but also some normal adults or patients with benign breast disease, the FcR- subpopulation was found to make a significant contribuiton to the activity against these monolayer cell lines. However, detectable reactivity by FcR- cells was not seen with the majority of donors. It is difficult at this time to determine what the interrelationships are among the NK cells with somewhat divergent properties. It is quite possible that they are all within the same subpopulation of cells, with some variation in the subsets of NK cells reactive with different specificities on target cells (see our chapter on specificity, section ID).

C. Other Characteristics

Other similar features of NK cells in the various species are summarized in Table I. All studies have shown that NK cells lack surface membrane immunoglobulins and are

TABLE VI. Cytotoxicity Against Human Breast Cancer-Derived Monolayer Cell Lines by FcR- Lymphocytes

		Number with significant residual activity after depletion of FcR+ cells (range residual activity)[a]				
Donors	No. tested	K562	Ab-Chang	MCF7	MDA231	G11
Normal adults	15	0	0	3(10-60%)	4(15-70%)	5(13-65%)
Breast cancer	8	0	0	1(30%)	1(40%)	1(28%)
Benign breast disease	16	0	0	4(15-61%)	4(22-75%)	6(18-90%)

[a]PBL of donors were incubated on EA monolayers, as previously described (West et al., 1977), and nonadherent cells were tested against K562, antibody-coated Chang cells (as measure of residual K cell activity), and against three monolayer cell lines derived from patients with breast cancer, all in a four hour ^{51}Cr release assay. In tests with significant levels of cytotoxicity by FcR- cells, lytic units/10^7 cells were calculated. The numbers in parentheses are the ranges of lytic units remaining/lytic units in unfractionated population.

nonphagocytic. Most studies have indicated that spontaneous NK cells are nonadherent to plastic or various adherence columns. However, as with Warner and his associates (see chapter in section IA), we have found that a portion of augmented NK cells obtained from virus or poly I:C-inoculated mice bound to nylon or Sephadex G-10 columns. In the rat, we have noted that a significant portion of even spontaneous NK cells adhere to nylon wool, rayon or G-10 columns. In contrast to the mouse or human, NK activity is never enriched by column passage of lymphoid cells. A portion of human NK cells generated during *in vitro* culture in medium with fetal bovine serum has been found to adhere to nylon columns

(Ortaldo *et al.*, 1979). Increased adherence properties may be associated in a particular state of differentiation or activation of NK cells.

III. SIZE OF NK CELLS

At various times in our laboratory, attempts were made to determine the size of NK cells by fractionation of lymphoid cells by velocity sedimentation. In most experiments, both mouse and human NK cells were found in fractions with the bulk of small to medium lymphocytes (Herberman *et al.*, 1977; A. Levin, J. Gerson, J. Ortaldo and R. B. Herberman, unpublished observations). However, recently Timonen *et al.*, 1979,

TABLE VII. Frequency of Lymphoid Cell/K562 Conjugates in Lymphoid Cell Fractions Obtained from Discontinuous Density Gradients[a]

Population[b]	% Lymphoid[c] cells in conjugates	% LGL among conjugate-forming cells	% Cells per fraction	NK activity[d]
Input	18	33		18
0	42	83	10	44
1	50	83	14	49
2	12	25	20	22
3	9	20	25	3
4	6	0	20	0
5	12	0	11	0

[a]*Median of five experiments.*

[b]*Peripheral blood lymphocytes, depleted of adherent cells by incubation on plastic and filtration through nylon wool, were separated into six fractions (0-5) in discontinuous Percoll density gradients as described in chapter by Saksela and Timonen.*

[c]*Contacts analysed from lymphoid cell/K562 mixtures (1/1 ratio, incubation time 2 hr), cytocentrifuged on microscope slides, fixed in methanol and stained with Giemsa. Minimum 100 cells counted.*

[d]*% ^{51}Cr release during 4 hour cytotoxicity assay with K562, effector/target ratio of 25:1.*

found that the majority of human lymphocytes forming conjugates with NK-sensitive target cells were large cells with prominent granules (large granular lymphocytes, LGL). As described elsewhere in this book (Saksela and Timonen, section IA), it has been possible to enrich for LGL on discontinuous Percoll density gradients. We have recently used this procedure in an attempt to enrich for, and thereby better characterize, NK cells. The results indicated, as shown in a representative experiment in Table VII, that most of the NK activity resided in fractions 0 and 1 from the gradients. Since only about one-fourth of the cells were in these fractions, this provided a substantial enrichment step. LGL were also concentrated in these fractions. While some cells in other fractions formed conjugates with K562, they did not have the morphology of LGL. Treatment with interferon augmented activity in the fractions 0 and 1, but did not induce activity in the other fractions. Thus, it seems likely that NK cells are included among the subpopulation of conjugate-forming LGL and that the other lymphocytes forming conjugates (about two-thirds of conjugate-forming cells in the input population) are unrelated to active NK cells or their immediate precursors. To further

TABLE VIII. The Effect of Depletion of Fc Receptor Positive Cells on the Frequency of Lymphocyte-K562 Conjugates

Fraction	*% LGL in conjugates/ % LGL*[a]	*% other lymphocytes in conjugates/ % other lymphyocytes*	*Lysis ($LU/10^7$ Cells)*[b] *NK*	*ADCC*
Exp. 1				
0/1	*60/72*	*12/28*	*706*	*1369*
0/1, FcR-	*1/2*	*10/98*	*<1*	*<1*
Exp. 2				
0/1	*63/85*	*4/15*	*321*	*250*
0/1, FcR-	*1/2*	*8/98*	*<1*	*<1*

[a]*Denominator for each percentage is total lymphoid cells counted, out of a minimum of 100 cells counted; lymphocyte/ K562 ratio in conjugate analyses 1:1, incubation time 2 hr.*
[b]*NK activity tested against K562, ADCC against RL♂1 coated with rabbit anti-mouse brain serum.*

analyze the relationship between LGL and NK cells, the effects of depletion of FcR+ cells from the 0/1 Percoll fractions were examined (Table VIII). The results indicated that almost all LGL as well as all NK and ADCC activity, were removed by this procedure. Furthermore, treatment of the FcR- cells with interferon did not induce cytotoxic activity. These data thus strengthen the association of LGL with NK cells. Other lymphocytes that formed conjugates with K562 were unaffected by depletion of FcR+ cells, indicating that, even within the NK-enriched 0/1 fractions, a portion of the conjugate-forming cells are unrelated to NK activity. It would appear that the FcR+ cells in Percoll fractions 0 and 1 represent a highly enriched population of NK cells and studies with this population should lead to more insights into the characteristics of human NK and K cells.

IV. EFFECTS OF OVERNIGHT INCUBATION ON NK ACTIVITY

The kinetics of development and maintenance of NK activity *in vivo* differ substantially between the rodents and humans. With both mice and rats, activity first becomes detectable at 3-4 weeks of age, reaches peak levels at 5-8 weeks of age, and then declines to low levels after 10-12 weeks of age (Herberman, 1975b; Kiessling *et al.*, 1975; Nunn *et al.*, 1976). In contrast, human NK activity appears to remain stable for years, is similar in young and elderly individuals, and some NK activity can be detected in most individuals at birth (see Herberman and Holden, 1978). Another major difference among the species, which bear at least some superficial similarities to these differences in *in vivo* kinetics, is in the maintenance of NK activity after overnight incubation at 37°C (see Herberman and Holden, 1978). Human PBL, maintained in media with either fetal bovine or human serum, either show no change or actually increase in activity. In contrast, mouse NK activity has tended to be quite labile, often decreasing markedly or disappearing after overnight incubation. In the rat, yet another pattern has been seen, with activity usually increasing substantially during culture at 37°C. Even spleen cells from older rats that have very low immediate activity usually become quite reactive after overnight incubation. This may account for the lack of variation in activity with age that has been seen in long term cytotoxicity assays with rat spleen cells (Oldham *et al.*, 1977).

Some recent studies may provide clues to the differences seen after overnight incubation. X-irradiation (2000R) of human mononuclear cells had no immediate effect on NK activity but after overnight incubation, most activity was lost. However, treatment of the irradiated cultured cells with interferon caused a strong increase in activity, to levels similar to those of unirradiated cells. This could be interpreted as a differential effect of irradiation on NK cells and pre-NK cells, with pre-NK cells being resistant to irradiation. This would be similar to differences in effects of *in vivo* irradiation that have been observed in rats and mice (Oehler and Herberman, 1978; *Djeu et al.*, 1979c). Alternatively, the NK cells themselves may be radioresistant but maintenance of their activity may depend on a radiosensistive precursor population, perhaps needed to produce interferon.

Mouse NK cells have been found not to be invariably labile *in vitro* at 37°. By adjustments in cell density and

TABLE IX. Effect of Overnight Incubation and Role of Nylon Wool Adherent Cells on Rat NK Activity[a]

Incubation conditions	*Removal of nylon-adherent cells*	In vitro *culture with:*		*% Cytotoxicity*
		C. Parvum	*Poly I:C*	
Exp. 1				
None	–			*4.7*
	+			*1.0*
4°C	–			*14.9*
	+			*5.5*
37°C	–	–		*51.4*
	+	–		*10.6*
	–	+		*56.9*
	+	+		*47.9*
Exp. 2				
4°C	–	–	–	*13.8*
37°C	–	–	–	*29.5*
	–	+	–	*32.0*
	–	–	+	*31.1*
	+	–	–	*11.7*
	+	+	–	*30.4*
	+	–	+	*14.8*

[a]*Spleen cells from >12 week-old W/Fu rats, unseparated or after passage over nylon wool column, were incubated for 18 hr, in medium alone or in the presence of* C. parvum, *450 μg/ml, or poly I:C, 100 μg/ml, and then tested for cytotoxicity against W/Fu Gl in 4 hr* ^{51}Cr *release assay at 100:1 effector:target cell ratio.*

other modifications in environmental conditions, it has been possible to get substantial persistence in activity (e.g., Djeu *et al.*, 1979a). However, even with the improved conditions, there has been considerable experiment-to experiment variability in the proportion of activity maintained. As with the human studies, treatment with interferon has yielded some interesting data on this issue. Incubation overnight of spleen cells with interferon or poly I:C added at time 0 has uniformly resulted in persistence and usually augmentation of activity. In contrast, after overnight incubation, treatment with interferon has been unable to restore a loss of activity. Thus, the *in vitro* lability of mouse NK cells may be due, at least in part, to a loss in responsiveness to interferon which, as suggested above for human cells, may need to be produced by accessory cells in order to maintain reactivity.

Recent studies with overnight incubation of rat spleen cells have also pointed to a complex situation, with probable involvement of accessory cells (Table IX). The NK activity of older rats was found to increase after incubation at 4°C, although not to the high levels seen after incubation at 37°C. The augmentation did not seem to require the presence of fetal bovine serum or endotoxin in the medium, but did require the presence of nylon wool adherent cells. The required accessory cells appear to be macrophages, being also adherent to rayon and G10, removed by carbonyl iron and magnet treatment, and surface membrane immunoglobulin negative. Boosting by poly I:C was almost abrogated by removal of nylon adherent cells. In contrast, the NK activity of nylon wool passaged cells could still be boosted well by incubation with *C. parvum*. These results could be explained by a role of interferon in the *in vitro* augmentation of activity by interferon, with macrophages being the cells producing interferon spontaneously or, as previously shown in mice (Djeu *et al.*, 1979b), in response to poly I:C, but with nonadherent cells producing interferon in response to *C. parvum*.

From the available results from the above studies that are in progress, it is not yet possible to clearly define the factors involved in maintenance of NK activity *in vitro*. However, most of the data are consistent with an important role of interferon production. Further studies in this area may provide insight into the factors involved in *in vivo* regulation of spontaneous NK activity.

REFERENCES

Bolhuis, R. L. H. (1977). "Cell-mediated immunity to carcinoma of the urinary bladder. Specificty of the reaction and the nature of the effector cells." Radiobiological Institute of the Organization for Health Research TNO, Rijswijk, The Netherlands.

Bonnard, G. D., Schendel, D. J., West, W. H., Alvarez, J. M., Maca R. D., Yasaka, K., Fine, R. L., Herberman, R. B., de Landazuri, M. O., and Morgan, D. A. (1978). *In* "Human Lymphocyte Differentiation: Its Application to Human Cancer." (B. Serrou and C. Rosenfeld, eds.), p. 319. Elsevier/North-Holland Biomedical Press, Amsterdam.

Djeu, J. Y., Glaser, M., Kirchner, H., Huang, K. Y., and Herberman, R. B. (1974). *Cell. Immunol. 12,* 164.

Djeu, J. Y., Heinbaugh, J. A., Holden, H. T., and Herberman, R. B. (1979a). *J. Immunol. 122,* 178.

Djeu, J. Y., Heinbaugh, J. A., Holden, H. T., and Herberman, R. B. (1979b). *J. Immunol. 122,* 182.

Djeu, J. Y., Heinbaugh, J., Vieira, W. D., Holden, H. T., and Herberman, R. B. (1979c). *Immunopharmacology 1,* 231.

Eremin, O., Coombs, R. R. A., Plumb, D., and Ashby, J. (1978). *Int. J. Cancer 21,* 42.

Fabre, J. W. and Williams, A. F. (1977). *Transplantation 23,* 349.

Glimcher, L., Shen, F. W., and Cantor, H. (1977). *J. Exp. Med. 145,* 1.

Haller, O., Gidlund, M., Hellström, U., Hammarström, S., and Wigzell, H. (1978) *Eur. J. Immunol. 8,* 765.

Herberman, R. B. and Holden, H. T. (1978). *Adv. Cancer Res. 27,* 305.

Herberman, R. B., Nunn, M. E., Holden, H. T., and Lavrin, D. H. (1975a). *Int. J. Cancer 16,* 230.

Herberman, R. B., Nunn, M. E., and Lavrin, D. H. (1975b). *Int. J. Cancer 16,* 216.

Herberman, R. B., Bartram, S., Haskill, J. S., Nunn, M., Holden, H. T., and West, W. H. (1977). *J. Immunol. 119,* 322.

Herberman, R. B., Nunn, M. E., and Holden, H. T. (1978). *J. Immunol. 121,* 304.

Hersey, P., Edwards, A., Edwards, J., Adams, E., Milton, G. W., and Nelson, D. S. (1975). *Int. J. Cancer 16,* 173.

Kaplan, J., and Callewaert, D. M. (1978). *J. Natl. Cancer Inst. 60,* 961.

Kay, H. D., Bonnard, G. D., West, W. H., and Herberman, R. B. (1977). *J. Immunol. 118,* 2058.

Kiessling, R., Klein, E., Pross, H. and Wigzell, H. (1975a). *Eur. J. Immunol., 5,* 117.

Lubaroff, D. M. (1977). *Cell. Immunol. 29,* 147.

Mattes, M. J., and Holden, H. T. (1980). Submitted for publication.

Mattes, M. J., Sharrow, S. O., Herberman, R. B., and Holden, H. T. (1979). *J. Immunol. 123,* 2851.

Nunn, M. E., Djeu, J. Y. , Glaser, M., Lavrin, D. H., and Herberman, R. B. (1976). *J. Natl. Cancer Inst. 56,* 393.

Oehler, J. R., and Herberman, R. B. (1978). *Int. J. Cancer,* 204.

Oehler, J. R., Lindsay, L. R., Nunn, M. E., and Herberman, R. B. (1978). *Int. J. Cancer 21,* 204.

Ojo, E., and Wigzell, H. (1978). *J. Immunol. 7,* 297.

Oldham, R. K., Ortaldo, J. R., and Herberman, R. B. (1977). *Cancer Research 37,* 4457.

Ortaldo, J. R., Bonnard, G. D., Kind, P. D., and Herberman, R. B. (1979). *J. Immunol. 122,* 1489.

Peter, H. H., Pavie-Fischer, J., Fridman, W. H. Aubert, C., Cesarini, J. P., Roubin, R., and Kourlisky, F. M. (1975). *J. Immunol. 115,* 539.

Pross, H. F., and Jondal, M. (1975). *Clin. Exp. Immunol. 21,* 226.

Ritter, M. A., Gordon, L. K. and Goldschneider, I. (1978). *J. Immunol. 121,* 2463.

Santoni, A., Herberman, R. B., and Holden, H. T. (1979a). *J. Natl. Cancer Inst. 62,* 109.

Santoni, A., Herberman, R. B., and Holden, H. T. (1979b) *J. Natl. Cancer Inst. 63,* 995.

Sunderland, C. A., McMaster, W. R. and Williams, A. F. (1979). *Eur. J. Immunol. 9,* 155.

Timonen, T., Saksela, E., Ranki, A., and Hayry, P. (1979). *Cell Immunol. 48,* 113.

West, W. H., Cannon, G. B., Kay, H. D., Bonnard, G. D., and Herberman, R. B. (1977). *J. Immunol. 118,* 335.

West, W. H., Boozer, R. B., and Herberman, R. B. (1978). *J. Immunol. 120,* 90.

Williams, A. F., Galfre, G., and Milstein, C. (1977). *Cell 12,* 663.

ANTIGENIC PHENOTYPE OF MOUSE NATURAL KILLER CELLS[1]

Gloria C. Koo

Memorial Sloan-Kettering Cancer Center
New York, New York

Antoinette Hatzfeld[2]

Institut de Pathologie Moleculaire
Paris, France

I. INTRODUCTION

The term Natural Killer (NK) cell is used, in this article, in reference to cells which have the surface phenotype Nk-1$^+$, and are cytolytic for cultured cells of the radiation induced leukemia cells, BALB RL. male 1 (RL.1), in a short term (5 hours) chromium-release assay. The discovery of the Nk-1 alloantigen system, which distinguished the natural killer cell population we are studying, occurred when Glimcher et al., (1977) found that the antiserum, anti-Lyt-1.2, could eliminate NK activity against RL.1 cells. This at first implied that NK cells are Lyt-1$^+$, but control tests showed that elimination of NK cells with anti-Lyt-1.2 serum occurred equally with effector populations from C57BL/6(B6) mice (Lyt-1.2) and from congenic strain, B6-Lyt-1.1. This indicated a previously unrecognized antibody, present in the anti-Lyt-1.2 serum (C3H vs. CE), that reacted with NK cells.

Accordingly, a second antiserum was prepared: (C3H x BALB) v. CE. This antiserum exhibited no Lyt-1.2 activity (because of the introduction of the BALB genotype into the immunized recipient), but was as effective as the original serum in

[1]*Supported in Part by Grants from NIH: CA-08748 CA-254 1 6, ACS:FRA-167, NSF and NATO*

[2]*Present address: Memorial Sloan-Kettering Cancer Center, New York, New York*

ISBN 0-12-341350-8

eliminating NK cells. The alloantigen system thus identified will be referred to as Nk-1, and the alloantigen present on CE and other positive strains as Nk-1.1.

NK activity of the unfractionated B6 spleen population is relatively low (< 10% lysis). We found it more effective to enrich NK cells by discontinuous BSA gradient centrifugation (Scheid et al., 1978). We used BSA concentrations of 10%, 23%, 26%, 29%, and 35% giving interfaces A,B,C, and D. Layers A and B provide cells for both lytic and serological assays, layers C and D contain few NK cells as shown in Table I. Nk-1.1$^+$ cells were enumerated by Protein-A-sheep red blood cell (PA-SRBC) rosette assay (Koo, et al., 1978). There exists a very good correlation between the specific % lysis and the proportion of Nk-1.1 cells in each layer, confirming the previous data that Nk-1 antigen is a marker for NK cells.

Therefore, we routinely used layers A and B for both serological and lytic assays. This enrichment is necessary especially for definitive serotyping. We also used B6 mice throughout our study because of the possibility of anti-Lyb-2.3 and other undefined contaminants in the Nk-1.1 antiserum.

By serological absorptions with a wide range of tissues, we found that spleen, lymph node cells, and bone marrow cells

TABLE I. BSA Density Gradient for Enrichment of NK Cells[a]

Splenic effector cells	*% Cell recovery*	*% Lysis*	*% Nk-1.1 Cells*[b]
Unfractionated		*10 ± 2*	*15 ± 2*
Layer A	*18 ± 6*	*26 ± 4*	*24 ± 1*
Layer B	*45 ± 2*	*15 ± 5*	*15 ± 4*
Layer C	*30 ± 4*	*4 ± 2*	*8 ± 1*
Layer D	*8 ± 4*	*2 ± 4*	*7 ± 3*
A + B + C + D	*100*	*12 ± 1*	*12 ± 6*

[a] *Mean (± SD) values of 3 separate tests*

[b] *% Nk-1.1 cells - assessed by PA-SRBC rosette assay*

are the only tissues from B6 mice that can absorb Nk-1.1 antibody. Thus, the Nk-1.1$^+$ cells were confined to tissues known to contain NK cells. We have also serotyped 50 backcross mice-(B6 x BALB) F_1 backcrossed to BALB - and determined that there was one spcificity detected in the Nk-1.1 antiserum, using B6 as the source of NK cells.

Having established Nk-1 antigen as the surface marker for NK cells, we attempted to define this lymphoid subpopulation more precisely by studying the antigenic profile of NK cells. To achieve this, we used a panel of conventional as well as some newly discovered monoclonal antisera to lymphocytic alloantigens.

II. PROCEDURES USED TO DETERMINE ANTIGENIC PHENOTYPE OF NK CELLS

As NK activity and Nk-1.1 antigen are both criteria for measuring NK cells, we could determine the antigenic phenotype of NK cells by monitoring both the change in NK activity and Nk-1.1$^+$ cells after elimination of NK cells with various antisera. Table II lists the antisera applied to serotype NK cells. We have used two elimination procedures depending on the antiserum and antigenic system: Elimination by complement (C) mediated cytoxicity was used whenever there was IgM class antibody (e.g., Lyt-1.1, Qa-4, and Qa-5 antisera). C mediated elimination was also more efficient when the antigen positive cells constituted a high (50-60%) proportion of the A and B layers of fractionated spleen population (e.g., Qa-2, 3). Another elimination procedure was to deplete PA-SRBC rosetted cells by Ficoll-isopaque gradient centrifugation (Parish and Hayward, 1974). Effector cells were sensitized with serum and reacted with PA-SRBC. They were then layered on a Ficoll-isopaque (specific gravity 1.10) layer and centrifuged in the cold at 600g for 7 minutes (Koo, et al., 1980). Non-rosetted cells were situated at the interface and rosettes in the pellet. The Ficoll elimination procedures were most effective when the antigen positive cells constituted about 30-40% of the total population (e.g., Nk-1.1$^+$ and Thy-1 $^+$ cells). Furthermore, when Nk-1 antiserum was used in Ficoll elimination, both Nk-1$^+$ cells and NK activity were enriched in the pellet.

TABLE II. Antisera

Specificity	Antisera Description	Marker for T or B cell	References
Nk-1.1	(C3H x BALB) anti-CE	NK	Glimcher et al., 1977
Thy-1.2	Monoclonal	T	Hammerling et al., 1978
Qa-1	B6 x A.Tla^b anti-A strain leukemia	T	Stanton et al., 1977
Qa-2.3	B6-Kl anti-B6	T + B	Flaherty et al., 1978
Qa-3	B6-Kl anti-B6 absorbed with leukemia cell EL_4	T + B	Hammerling et al., 1978
Qa-4	Monoclonal	T + non-T	Hammerling et al., 1979
Qa-5	Monoclonal	T + non-T	Hammerling et al., 1979
Lyt-1.1	Monoclonal	T	U. Hammerling, unpublished data
Lyt-2.2	Monoclonal	T	Hammerling et al., 1979
Lyb-2.2	SJL/J x CE anti-A.SW	B	Shen et al., 1977

III. ANTIGENIC PHENOTYPE OF NK CELLS

A. *NK Cells are Positive for Nk-1, Thy-1, Qa-2, Qa-4, Qa-5, Ly-5 and Lyt-1 antigens (Figure 1).*

1. Nk-1. Nk-1.1 antiserum routinely eliminated 75-80% of Nk-1.1$^+$ cells and NK activity detected in A and B layers of the BSA fractionated spleen (Figure I and Table III). Since technical problems in elimination procedures could have prevented us to eliminate 100% of Nk-1.1$^+$ cells, all NK cells are interpreted to express Nk-1.1 antigen. Treatment of plaque - forming cells with anti-Nk-1.1 serum does not affect their activities (Glimcher et al., 1977) and anti-Nk-1.1$^+$ serum does not eliminate cytotoxic T cells in T-cell mediated cytotoxicity (Glimcher et al., 1977, and Pollack et al., 1979). Nk-1 is very likely the surface marker for all NK cells directed against various lymphoma target cells, since Nk-1.1 antigen is also detected on NK cells responsible for lysing YAC (Pollack et al., 1979, and our unpublished data) EL_4 and Meth A infected with Rauscher MuLV (unpublished data).

2. Thy-1. Thy-1 antigen was detected on 50% of NK cells. This is reflected by the decrease of Nk-1.1$^+$ cells in the BSA fractionated spleen cells (Table III) and the concommitant decrease of NK activity, (Figure 1). Specificity of anti-Thy-1.2 reactivity was assured by using congenic mouse strains, A and A-Thy-1.1 mice: elimination of NK activity was obtained only in A mice, but no elimination was obtained in A-Thy-1.1 mice. The reduction of NK cells was achieved by both conven-

TABLE III. Proportion of Nk-1$^+$ and Thy-1$^+$ Cells After Ficoll Elimination of B6 Effector Cells with Anti-Nk-1.1 and Anti-Thy-1.2 Antisera

Eliminated with	*% PASRBC-rosettes after elimination*[a]	
	Nk-1.1$^+$ cells	*Thy-1.2$^+$ cells*
NMS	*21 ± 4*	*21 ± 1*
Anti-Nk-1.1	*7 ± 3*	*14 ± 1*
Anti-Thy-1.2	*12 ± 5*	*4 ± 1*

[a] *Mean (± S.D.) values of 5-10 separate tests*

$$\% \text{ Rosettes} = \frac{\text{rosetted cells}}{\text{rosetted + non-rosetted cells}} \times 100$$

tional and monoclonal Thy-1.2 antisera. This is in agreement with earlier findings (Herberman et al., 1978) and more recent findings of Mattes et al., (1979) and Minato et al., (1979). The fact that we observed an efficient elimination of NK cells with anti-Thy-1.2 antiserum is probably due to the elimination procedures and the enrichment of NK cells by BSA density gradient. Thy-1$^+$ cells in A and B layers constitute 50-60% of all Thy-1$^+$ cells in spleen and a subpopulation (about 30%) of these are Nk-1$^+$ (Table III).

To test the possibility of adsorption of Thy-1 antigen on NK cells, we performed elimination tests on irradiated A-mice reconstituted with A-Thy-1.1 bone marrow and spleen cells. In this case, the NK cells were not eliminated by anti-Thy-1.2 antiserum, proving that there was no nonspecific adsorption of Thy-1.2 antigen on Thy-1.1 cells.

Thy-1 has generally been used as a T-cell marker in the lymphoid system, even though it is also expressed on brain and epidermal cells (Williams, 1977). Detection of Thy-1 antigen on NK cells suggests that NK cells may derive from the T-cell lineage.

3. Qa-2. Qa-2 antigen was detected on 50% of NK cells. The polyvalent Qa-2,3 antiserum (B6-K.1 anti-B6) detects both Qa-2 and Qa-3 determinants. Additional experiments suggest that Qa-2, and not Qa-3, is present on NK cells: (1) The observation that effector cells of DBA/1 mice (phenotype: Qa-2$^+$, Qa-3$^-$) are also partially eliminated (50% reduction of lytic activity) points to Qa-2 as the responsible antigen. (2) When anti-Qa-2, 3 antiserum rendered specific for Qa-3 by exhaustive absorption with EL_4 leukemia cells (Qa-2$^+$, Qa-3$^-$) was used for elimination, only marginal reduction (11%) was produced.

Qa-2 antigen is found on thymus, spleen and bone marrow, and it is predominantly expressed on T cells, but also on B cells and granulocytes - macrophage progenitor cells (Kincade, P., and L. Flaherty - personal communications). Therefore, expression of Qa-2 antigen on NK cells does not provide evidence for T-cell lineage for NK cells.

4. Qa-4 and Qa-5. Qa-4 and Qa-5 antigens were detected on all NK cells. These two antigenic systems were recently defined by Hammerling et al., (1979) using two monoclonal antisera. They are closely linked to Qa-2, 3 locus and it is not clear if they are allelic to Qa-2, 3 antigens. Qa-4 antigen is found on 75% of Thy-1$^+$ cells, and Qa-5 antigen is found on 35% of Thy-1^+ cells. Both are absent on thymocytes. They were originally defined as T-cell antigens, however, in nude mice, there is a population of Qa-4^+, Thy-1^- cells, suggesting that non-T cells as well express Qa-4, 5 antigens, probably similar to those cells expressing Qa-2 antigen. At the present moment, NK cells are the only immunologically functional cells expressing Qa-4, 5 antigens. No significant effect was observed on plaque-forming cells or cytotoxic T-cells when spleen cells were treated with Qa-4, 5 antisera. (U. Hammerling, personal communication).

5. Ly-5. Two laboratories have independently demonstrated Ly-5 antigens on NK cells (Cantor et al., 1979, and Pollack et al, 1979). We have also obtained similar results (data not shown). Again, Ly-5 is not an exclusive T-cell marker. In fact, it is expressed on B cells, and other hemopoeitic stem cells, as well (Scheid and Triglia, 1979).

6. Lyt-1. Lyt-1 was detected on 28% of NK cells. Of the six antigens listed here, only Lyt-1 is considered a T cell restricted surface marker. It is found on T-helper cells (Cantor et al., 1975), and cytotoxic T-cells (Nakayama et al., 1979). It may have been overlooked previously because anti-Nk-1.1 specificity was a contaminant in the Lyt-1.2 antiserum (Glimcher et al., 1977).

B. NK Cells are Negative for Qa-1, Qa-3, Lyt-2, Lyb-2, Ly-6 and Ly-10 Antigens (Figure 1).

Antisera to Qa-1 and Lyt-2 and Lyb-2 antigens did not eliminate NK activity. Qa-1 and Lyt-2 are both T-cell specific alloantigens (Stanton et al., 1978, and Cantor et al., 1975). Lyb-2 is a B-cell marker, detectable on all B cells, even prior to expression of surface immunoglobulins. (U. Hammerling, personal communications). Therefore, the absence of these antigens on NK cells indicates that NK cells are not typical T cells nor are they B cells. Ly-10 antigen was recently described by Kimura et al., (1980) to be a marker for T cells, B cells, and progenitor cells, including prothymocytes. Monoclonal antiserum to Ly-10, kindly provided by S. Kimura and N. Tada in our laboratory, also did not affect NK activity (data not shown), suggesting that NK cells are not prothymocytes. We also did not observe significant effect on NK activity when NK cells were treated with monoclonal Ly-6 antibody (data not shown).

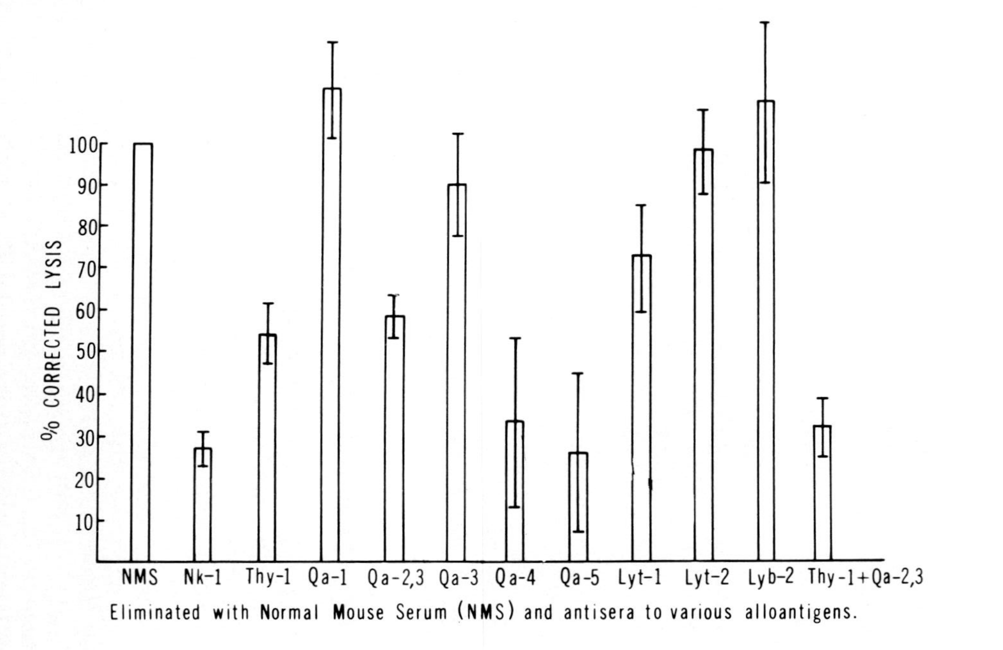

FIGURE 1. Percent corrected lysis obtained after elimination of B6 effector cells with various antisera. Effector cells are pooled from A and B layers of the BSA gradient. B6-Lyt-1.1 mice were used for the Lyt-1.1 elimination experiments. Ficoll elimination was used with Nk-1, Thy-1, Qa-1, Qa-3, and Lyt-2 antisera. C'elimination was used with Qa-2,3, Qa-4, Qa-5, Lyt-1, and Lyb-2 antisera. E:T ratio is 100:1. Each bar represents mean values (± S.D.) from 5-10 experiments

$$\% \text{ corrected lysis} = \frac{\% \text{ specific lysis obtained after elimination by antisera}}{\% \text{ specific lysis obtained after elimination by NMS}} \times 100$$

IV. CONCLUDING REMARKS

Our results clearly show that NK cells share some surface antigens with T cells. Nearly all NK activity resides in a population of cells expressing Nk-1, Qa-4, Qa-5, and Ly-5 antigens. Because of the partial elimination achieved with monoclonal anti-Thy-1.2 and anti-Qa-2, 3 antisera and to some extent with anti-Lyt-1.1 antiserum, we surmise that this population can be divided into distinct subpopulations. Whether or not Thy-1.2 and Qa-2 reside on the same cells is undecided. Experiments in which spleen cells were exposed to a mixture of anti-Thy-1.2 and anti-Qa-2,3 sera resulted in a 70% reduction of NK activity (see Figure 1). This may be due to a low density of both antigens on NK cells, requiring the synergistic effect of both antibodies for complete elimination. Alternatively, Thy-1^+ NK cells may be qualitatively different from Qa-2^+ NK cells.

The present knowledge of the antigenic profile of NK cells does not allow us to assign NK cells to any particular hemopoietic lineage. It is, however, clear from our studies as well as those of others, that NK cells are not B cells because they lack universal B cell markers IgM, and Lyb-2. They are most likely also not prothymocytes, because by definition prothymocytes are Thy-1^- and thymopoeitin does not induce Nk-1^+ cells nor NK activity (unpublished results). Furthermore, Ly-10, expressed on prothymocytes, is not present on NK cells. The identification of the Qa and Ly-5 antigens on NK cells does not contribute toward a solution on the question of NK cell derivation. These antigens have been demonstrated on B and T cell subpopulations, and occur on non-lymphoid cells as well (Scheid and Triglia, 1979, P. Kincade and L. Flaherty, personal communication).

The presence of Thy-1 antigen on NK cells could not justify the assignment of NK cells to the T-cell lineage. By definition, T cells are dependent on thymus for their differentiation and clearly the development of NK cells in nude mice is independent of thymus. The presence of Lyt-1 on NK cells, however, would substantiate the derivation of NK cells from the T-cell lineage (it is not known if nude mice have Lyt-1 cells in their spleen). The enigma presented by NK activity in nude mice is worth discussing here: Despite the absence of thymus, nude mice do have some Thy-1^+ cells in their spleen (Raff, 1973; Loor and Roelants, 1974). These Thy-1^+ cells are assumed to have differentiated from environmental induction. The nude mice, however, do not have mature T cell functions, yet their

NK activity appears normal and the Thy-1$^+$ cells seem to constitute the majority of NK activity (Mattes et al., 1979, and our own observation). It is interesting to note that Thy-1$^+$ cells from nude mice reside mostly in A and B layers when spleen cells from nude mice are separated on a BSA density gradient (personal observation). This suggests that the majority of the Thy-1$^+$ cells in nude mice have similar physical property to Nk-1$^+$, Thy-1$^+$ cells of normal mice. Thus, the nude mice have nature's enriched NK population. It is possible that NK cells in nude mice as well as normal mice belong to the alternate route of maturation of the Thy-1$^+$ cells, that could differentiate independent of thymus.

Regardless of the eventual assignment of NK cells to T cells, promonocytes or a new lineage of hemopoietic cells, we have furnished evidence of heterogeneity among the family of NK cells that have lytic activity to RL.1 cells. The Thy-1 and Qa-2 markers distinguish two functionally similar subpopulations. This heterogeneity may be the same as the one described by Mattes et al., (1979) that there are Thy-1$^+$ and Thy-1$^-$ NK cells, and may also relate to the finding reported earlier (Chun et al., 1979) that antigenically distinct NK population can be induced in tissue culture. The NK cells induced by TNS or interferon in spleen population within 24 hours do not require the presence of T cells for their production (phenotype: Qa-5$^+$, Thy-1$^-$), whereas the NK cells produced in 4 days without addition of any inducer appear to depend on T cells for their production (phenotype: Qa-5$^-$, Thy-1$^+$). The authors remarked, however, cultured cells are more resistant to treatment with Thy-1 antibody so the expression of Thy-1 antigen on the TNS induced NK cells may be equivocal. Therefore, the TNS induced NK cells are similar to the spontaneous NK cells in their surface antigen expression, but the tissue culture induced NK cells are apparently different from the spontaneous NK cells.

In summary, the antigenic profile of the family of NK cells with lytic activity to RL.1 can be presented as follows:

Percentage of NK Cells Expressing the Surface Markers:

100%	*50%*	*25%*	*<10%*
Nk-1	*Thy-1*	*Lyt-1*	*Qa-1*
Qa-4	*Qa-2*		*Lyt-2*
Qa-5			*Lyb-2*
Ly-5			*Ly-6*
			Ly-10

Our study shows that BSA enrichment makes it possible to serotype NK cells. In addition to functional definition of NK cells, we could identify NK cells by their surface marker, Nk-1. This allows us to follow the differentiation and development of $Nk\text{-}1^+$ cells that are not yet functional NK cells. Thus, the establishment of antigenic profile of NK cells provides a means to define and analyze the ontogeny of NK cells.

ACKNOWLEDGMENTS

We thank Janet Jacobson and Lillian Mittl for excellent technical assistance, Drs. U. Hammerling and F. W. Shen for helpful discussions and generous supply of antisera, and Barbara LoFaso for preparation of the manuscript.

REFERENCES

Cantor, H., and Boyse, E.A., (1975). *J. Exp. Med., 141, 1376.*

Cantor, H., Kasai, M., Shen, F.W., Leclerc, J.C., and Glimcher, L., (1979). *In* "Imm. Rev." (G. Moller ed.) Vol. 44, p. 3 Munksgaard, Copenhagen.

Chun, M., Vilo, P., Hammerling, U., Hammerling, G.J., and Hoffman, M.K., (1979). *J. Exp. Med., 150, 426.*

Flaherty, L., Zimmerman, D., and Hansen, T.H., (1978). *Immunogenetics, 6, 245.*

Glimcher, L., Shen, F.W., and Cantor, H., (1977). *J. Exp. Med. 145, 1.*

Hammerling, G.J., Lemke, H., Hammerling, U., Hohmann, C., Wallich, R., and Rajewsky, J., (1978). *In* "Current Topics in Microbiology" (F. Felchers, M. Potter and N. Warner eds.) Vol. 81., p. 100. Springer-Verlag, Berlin.

Hammerling, G.J., Hammerling, U., Flaherty, L., (1979). *J. Exp. Med., 150, 108.*

Herberman, R.B., Nunn, M.E., and Holden, H.T., (1978). *J. Immunol., 121, 304.*

Kimura, S., Tada, N., and Hammerling, U., (1980). *Immunogenetics, In press.*

Koo, G.C., and Goldberg, C.L.,(1978). *J. Imm. Methods, 23, 197.*

Koo, G.C., Jacobson, J.B., Hammerling, G.J., and Hammerling, U., (1980). Manuscript submitted for publication.

Loor, F., and Roelants, G.E., (1974). *Nature (London), 251, 229.*

Minato, N., Bloom, B.R., Jones, C., Holland, J., and Reid, L. M., (1979). *J. Exp. Med. 149, 1117.*

Mattes, M.J., Sharrow, S.O., Herberman, R.B., and Holden, H.T. (1979). *J. Immunol., 123, 2851.*

Nakayama E., Shiku, H., Stockert, E., Oettgen, H.F., and Old, L.J., (1979). *Proc. Natl. Acad. Sci., U.S.A., 76, 1977.*

Parish, C.R., and Hayward, J.A., (1974). *Proc. R. Soc. Lond. B., 187, 65.*

Pollack, S.B., Tam, M.R., Nowinski, R.C., and Emmons, S.L., (1979). *J. Immunol., 123, 1818.*

Raff, M.C., (1973). *Nature, (London), 246, 350.*

Scheid, M.P., Goldstein, G., and Boyse, E.A., (1978). *J. Exp. Med., 147, 1727.*

Scheid, M.P., and Triglia, D., (1979). *Immunogenetics, In press.*

Shen, F.W., Spanondis, M., and Boyse, E.A., (1977). *Immunogenetics 5, 481.*

Stanton, T.H., and Boyse, E.A., (1976). *Immunogenetics 3, 525.*

Williams, A.F., (1977). *Contemp. Top. Mol. Immunol. 6, 83.*

NATURAL CYTOTOXICITY OF MACROPHAGE PRECURSOR CELLS AND OF MATURE MACROPHAGES

Maria-Luise Lohmann-Matthes[1]
Wolfgang Domzig[1]

Max-Planck-Institute for
Immunbiology Freiburg, Germany

I. INTRODUCTION

Cells of the macrophage series at different stages of their maturation can act as cytotoxic effector cells by several independent mechanisms. Mature macrophages are activated by lymphokines to cytotoxicity (1,2,3), and this cytotoxicity shows a certain preference for tumor targets, although also normal proliferating cells are lysed to a significant degree (4,5). The young bone marrow-derived monocyte, but not the resting peritoneal macrophage, has the capacity to lyse antibody-coated tumor target cells in a K-cell-like manner (6,7).

A nonadherent and nonphagocytic precursor cell of the macrophage series, the promonocyte, has been shown recently to possess two strongly cytotoxic properties: it kills antibody-coated targets in a K-cell-like manner (8), like the young monocyte, and, in addition, it kills certain susceptible tumor cells like the YAC-1 in an NK-like manner (9). This latter NK-like cytotoxic mechanism is significantly enhanced in vitro when interferon is added to the test (9).

Two of these cytotoxic mechanisms occur as "natural cytotoxicity": promonocytes obtained from in vitro cultures of mouse bone marrow spontaneously perform strong NK-like cytotoxicity against YAC-1 target cells, whereas P815 targets remain unaffected. This spontaneous promonocyte cytotoxicity seems to take part in the in vivo natural killing capacity of mouse spleen cells and induced peritoneal exudate cells.

Present address: Max-Planck-Inst. f. Immunbiol.
Stübeweg 51, D-7800 Freiburg, Germany

ISBN 0-12-341350-8

The second type of natural macrophage mediated cytotoxicity shows the lymphokine-induced type of cytotoxicity. This type of cytotoxicity in our hands occurs only in conventionally kept mice. Conventionally kept mice have a high incidence of peritoneal macrophages which are nonspecifically cytotoxic to tumor targets without any apparent prior infection or stimulation of the mice. Whether these two types of natural macrophage-mediated cytotoxicity are in fact truly natural or whether the observed cytotoxic effects are a result of inapparent in vivo stimulation or immune reactions and resulting in the production of small amounts of interferon lymphokines, remains so far an open question. Both types of natural cytotoxicity can be enhanced by the appropriate stimulus, i.e. either by interferon or lymphokines.

A third type of natural macrophage-mediated resistance, the more or less pronounced cytostatic effect, which is performed by all mature macrophages (10), will not be included in this contribution.

II. MATURATION STAGES OF MACROPHAGES OBTAINED IN AN IN VITRO LIQUID CULTURE SYSTEM OF MOUSE BONE MARROW.

We have cultivated mouse bone marrow in the presence of L-fibroblast-conditioned medium, fetal calf serum and horse serum (11) which is a slight modification of the technique of Goud (12) and Sumner (13). The L-fibroblast-conditioned medium supports proliferation of cells of the macrophage and granulocytic series only. The latter cell type is functionally inactive in our test systems, and also the peak of granulocyte proliferation occurs earlier than the peak of macrophage proliferation. From these cultures we collect macrophage precursor cells which can be highly enriched by methods described elsewhere (8). The earliest identifiable cell is the monoblast, a round cell of a 10 μm diameter with a small rim of dark blue basophilic cytoplasma.

The next stage is a cell with a diameter of 10-15 μm which has completely lost the basophilia of the cytoplasma and has more cytoplasma than the monoblast. The nucleus is slightly indented and bean-shaped (Figure 1).

This cell still lacks the typical criteria of a mature monocyte: it is nonadherent, nonphagocytic and stains negative or only slightly positive for nonspecific esterase depending on the staining technique applied. We called this cell promonocyte, although it definitely represents a younger, more immature stage than the cell which in the van Furth nomenclature is called promonocyte (16). This cell matures within 24 to 48 h to an adherent and phagocytic cell, at least in the mouse system. In the human system, this maturation takes much longer (15). These monoblasts and promonocytes mature in the bone marrow cultures within 5-12 days into monocytes and macrophages which form confluent monolayers.

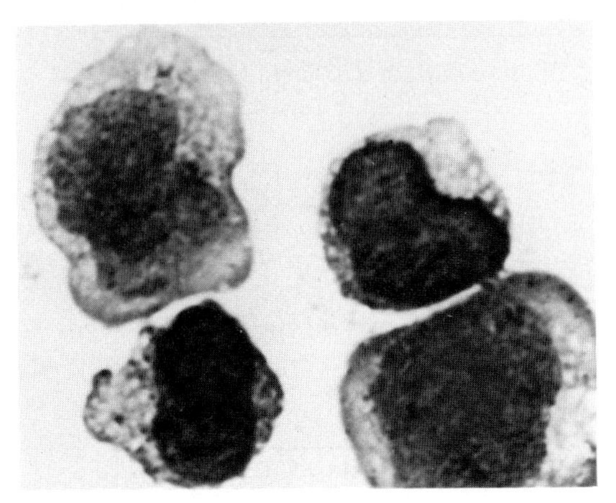

FIGURE 1. Promonocytes isolated from a 5 day old bone marrow culture.

III. THE PROMONOCYTE AS NATURAL KILLER CELL

A) Natural cytotoxicity of promonocytes from bone marrow cultures

We have reported recently that promonocytes, which are collected from liquid bone marrow cultures and separated from mature monocytes, perform a cytotoxic activity which resembles the activity of natural killer cells (9). Promonocytes spontaneously kill a variety of susceptible tumor lines in a short-term ^{51}Cr or $^{125}IdUrd$ release assay, whereas other tumor lines remain unaffected (Fig. 2).

This activity has been shown to be enhanced by interferon added to the test (9).

B) In vivo presence of promonocytes and promonocyte natural killer activity.

The effector promonocytes which we used were always taken from bone marrow cultures. Therefore, it was necessary to test whether this cell type occurs outside the bone marrow under in vivo conditions.

To clarify this, we used three different populations of cells with high natural killer activity and tested for the presence of promonocytes, namely 1) the peritoneal exudates of mice, which had been injected 3 days before i.p. with corynebacterium parvum (CP) (16), 2) the spleen of nude mice (17) and 3) the human peripheral blood of healthy volunteers (18).

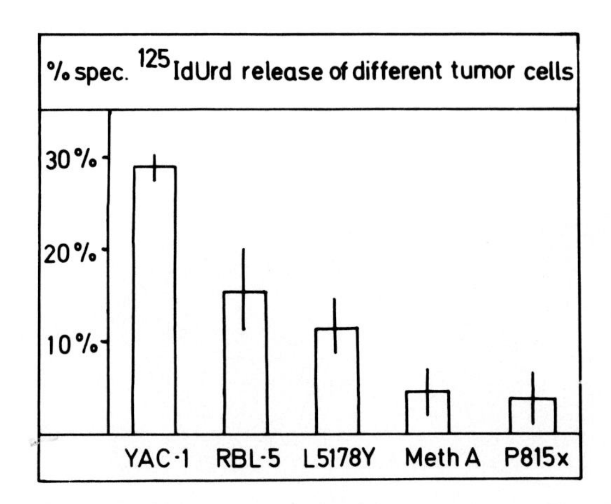

Figure 2. Natural killer activity of promonocytes against different tumor cells. A 5 day old bone-marrow culture was passed through nylon wool columns. The effluent cells (mostly promonocytes) were tested against various targets at a ratio of 20:1 in a 6 h test.

1) Peritoneal exudates of mice, previously injected i.p. with CP according to Ojo et al. (16), were passed through columns of nylon wool and glass beads. The effluent cells were depleted of adherent cells and of cells staining strongly positive for nonspecific esterase. When these cells were cultivated for 3 days, a monolayer of mature macrophages developed indicating that a high proportion of precursor cells of macrophages must have been present in the cell population. The column effluent cells were also treated with the alloanti-macrophage serum Mph 1.2 + C' and then tested for natural killer activity. Table 1 shows that the treatment of corynebacterium parvum-induced peritoneal exudate cells with Mph 1.2 + C' resulted in about 70% inhibition of the NK activity as compared to untreated controls.

The alloanti-macrophage serum Mph 1.2 was raised according to Archer in two congenic mouse strains (19) which only differ in a surface antigen present on macrophages. This antiserum kills bone marrow macrophages completely, whereas T- and B-lymphocytes are unaffected. The choice of the complement batch which works with this antiserum turned out to be very critical. None of the guinea pig complements we used produced any lytic effect, and out of 30 rabbits tested, only 3 had a suitable complement which lysed macrophages in the presence of Mph 1.2 alloantiserum.

2) Spleen cells of nude mice were treated similarly with the alloanti-macrophage serum Mph 1.2 + C' and were then either tested

against YAC-1 target cells for natural killing or were further cultured for 3 days for macrophages to spread or to mature from precursor cells.

Table 1: Natural killer activity of column passed corynebacterium parvum induced peritoneal cells. Inhibition by treatment with anti Mph 1.2 serum + C'.

Effector cells	% total release from ^{51}Cr labeles YAC-1	% inhibition of cytotoxicity
CP induced column passed peritoneal exudate	59 ± 4	—
CP induced column passed peritoneal exudate treated with C'	61 ± 3	—
CP induced column passed peritoneal exudate treated with Mph 1.2 + C'	27 ± 2	72
Mature 12 day old bone marrow macrophages	15 ± 2	feeder effect
Medium	19 ± 2	

CP induced column passed exudates were first incubated for 30' with Mph 1.2 (1:20) and then for 90' with a selected nontoxic batch of rabbit C' (1:6). After this two-step treatment cells were washed and target cells were added. Effector/target ratio was 20:1. Assay time was 4 h.

Table 2 shows, that also with these effector cells, NK activity was abolished after treatment with Mph 1.2 + C'. When growth and spreading of macrophages was controlled for 72 h, we observed that in the untreated wells, a confluent monolayer had developed, whereas in the treated wells hardly any macrophages were present. This indicates that in the treated wells nearly all mature macrophages and also the precursor cells had been eliminated by the antiserum treatment.

Table 2: NK-killing of nu/nu spleen cells against YAC-1 inhibited by Mph 1.2 antiserum + C' treatment.

	% total lysis	% spec. lysis
	of ^{51}Cr labeled YAC-1	
Spleen cells untreated	48 ± 4	30 ± 4
Spleen cells treated with C'	48 ± 3	30 ± 4
Spleen cells treated with anti Mph 1.2 + C'	21 ± 5	3 ± 5
Spleen cells treated with anti Mph 1.2	48 ± 2	30 ± 4
Spont. lysis of YAC-1	18 ± 4	

Spleen cells were incubated 30' with Mph 1.2 (1:20) and then for another 90' with a selected nontoxic batch of rabbit C' (1:6). The effector to target cell ratio was 50:1. The test was done for 4 h.

3) Human peripheral blood leukocytes were first separated on Ficoll hypaque, and the cells of the interphase were passed through adherence columns. The effluent cells were tested for nonspecific esterase staining. In contrast to the monocyte-rich interphase fraction which stains strongly positive for nonspecific esterase, the column-passed cells contained no or only slightly esterase positive cells. However, when these cells were plated and allowed to mature for 3-5 days, monolayers of macrophages which showed strongly positive nonspecific esterase staining, developed indicating that macrophage precursors must have been present in the column-passed fraction. This human system, however, shows tremendous variability in terms of the quantitiy of precursor cells which mature into macrophages, even within the same individual tested several times. These data indicate that precursor cells of monocytes and not only the mature monocytes are released into the periphery, where they actively participate in natural resistance (Zähringer, Domzig, Lohmann-Matthes, in preparation).

C) Inhibition of natural promonocyte killing

The natural killing effect in our bone marrow cultures was only detectable when the precursor cells had been separated from the mature monocytes by passage through adherence columns. Therefore, we tested whether the adherent, mature bone marrow macrophages had in fact an inhibitory function on natural killing of promonocytes. Table 3 demonstrates that indeed the addition of mature macrophages inhibits the natural killing of promonocytes. This finding is similar to experiments performed with mouse spleen cells as natural killer cells, which were inhibited in their natural killing function by the addition of "macrophage like" cells (20). The data of Droller and Perlmann (21) provide an explanation for the inhibitory effect of macrophages, since these authors have shown that prostaglandins inhibit natural killing of mouse spleen cells. In the system described here, this explanation would indicate that the mature bone marrow macrophage which synthesizes and secretes high amounts of prostaglandins (22) inhibits the natural NK killer activity of its precursor cell. A similar negative feedback mechanism in the macrophage system has been described by Sachs and Pluznik (23), who have shown that mature macrophages secrete an inhibitor which blocks macrophage proliferation in the bone marrow.

Table 3: Inhibition of NK activity of promonocytes by the addition of mature bone marrow macrophages to the test

Effector cells	% lysis of ^{51}Cr labeled YAC-1
$1x10^6$ promonocytes	65 $\pm$ 4
$1x10^6$ promonocytes + $5x10^4$ mature macrophages	50 $\pm$ 3
$1x10^6$ promonocytes + $2,5x10^5$ mature macrophages	43 $\pm$ 2
$1x10^6$ promonocytes + $5x10^5$ mature macrophages	25 $\pm$ 2
$5x10^5$ mature macrophages	26 $\pm$ 3
Medium	29 $\pm$ 3

Ratio promonocytes/target cells: 20:1. Assay time : 18 h.

NK activity of column-passed bone marrow cells is also absent when the bone marrow cells have been pretreated for 24 h with the lymphokine MCF (= MAF). This lymphokine activates macrophages and accelerates the maturation process (Lohmann-Matthes unpublished observation). In fact, from such MCF-pretreated bone marrow cultures no promonocytes could be collected, since they all mature under the influence of MCF into macrophages. This effect may also explain why spleen cells, which were treated overnight with MCF, lost all NK activity, whereas the untreated controls retained a good deal of their activity (24). Under these experimental conditions, abolishment of the natural killing, which is performed by promonocytes in the spleen, must have occurred, since promonocytes mature into macrophages under the influence of MCF.

D) Relationship between promonocytes and the "natural killer cell"

1. Surface markers. In the last few months we have been working on surface markers of promonocytes. However, the results are not yet completely clearcut due to problems with antisera and complement batches. Looking at the published evidence of surface markers of NK-cells, a broad variety is obvious. Several T-cell markers have been reported such as Thy 1.2 (25), Ly 5 and Ly 6 (26,27). When monoclonal antibodies were used, they were applied at exceedingly high concentrations. Such high concentrations may cause cross-reactions with other surface markers, when the antibody was prepared from ascites. Those antibodies which are not monoclonal may always have some cross-reactions with surface components of macrophage precursors. Since the surface markers of promonocytes have not yet been analyzed in a sufficient way, there is no possibility to know whether promonocytes have anything in common with NK cells.

2. Morphology of NK cells and promonocytes. The morphology of the promonocyte is easy to define (see Sect.1). The morphology of the natural killer cell seems to be somewhat controversial in mouse and human systems, although it is not very likely that the same activity is performed by two completely different effector cells in both species. J. Roder in his target binding cell (TBC) test described the NK cell as a typical small "resting" lymphocyte (28). In contrast Saksela and Timonen (29), using a rather similar technique, described that in the human situation, the participation of small lymphocytes can be excluded, and the effector cell is a medium-sized lymphocyte or a "large granular lymphocyte" (29). Morphologically, these two cells very much resemble what we call a promonocyte. The only reason why Saksela regards them as lymphocytes is based on the observation that the positive staining for nonspecific esterase, which these cells show, cannot be inhibited by natriumfluoride (NaF). The inhibition of the nonspecific esterase by NaF is assumed to be specific for cells of the

monocytic series, whereas lymphocytic, nonspecific esterase is suppo sed not to be inhibited. However, Löffler (30) and Leder (31) have shown that this inhibition is very unreliable and unstable, and often monocytic cells lack this inhibition phenomenon. Our data confirm their observation. This inhibition can only be taken for granted when for every uninhibited preparation and inhibited control preparation is done, since the degree of inhibition varies with the batch of the substrates and also with the maturation stage of the cells (Zähringer and Lohmann-Matthes, unpublished observation). Thus, the fact that medium sized lymphocytes (MSL) and large granular lymphocytes (LGL) are not inhibited by NaF is probably not sufficient evidence to exclude their possible monocyte origin.

3. NK and promonocyte activity in NK low responder mice. We have described that in contrast to the NK activity of spleen cells of low responder A/J mice, the promonocytes cultured from the bone marrow show completely normal levels of natural killing. The same has been described with beige mice (32). This discrepancy seems to indicate that the promonocyte does not contribute to the actual natural killing activity in vivo; this assumption is unlikely because of the data with the alloanti-macrophages serum + C' treatment reported in section IIIB. Another explanation would be that either promonocytes are inhibited in vivo in the low responder mice or that in low responder mice the maturation from promonocytes to macrophages is very much accelerated. The normal amount of effector cells binding to target cells in the TBC test (33) in low responder mice seems to favour the first explanation. However, the fact that based on target cell binding in one lab the small lymphocyte was characterized as effector cell, whereas in another lab this same cell was excluded using a similar technique, may indicate that a considerable amount of nonspecific binding makes this test comparatively unsensitive with regard to number of binding cells. Probably many of the binding cells have, in fact, nothing to do with the actual killing. Such an effect would also explain data where normal amounts of TBC were reported although no killing occurred (34).

E) Promonocyte natural killing is enhanced by anti-target cell antibody

Promonocytes obtained from bone marrow cultures have strong K-cell-like activity (8). This K-cell-like activity can enhance the natural killing of promonocytes in a similar fashion as has been described for K and NK cells (35,36).

IV. COMMENTS TO THE NATURAL KILLING OF PROMONOCYTES

The data presented, show that an immature macrophage precursor cell the promonocyte has the property to kill spontaneously susceptible target cells in an NK like manner.

This precursor cell is Fc-receptor positive but has not yet developed the typical criteria of a mature macrophage, since it is nonadherent, nonphagocytic and stains negative or only slightly positive for non-specific esterase. This cell develops into a mature macrophages within 24-48 h. It has also been shown that such promonocytes are present in vivo in the peripheral blood, in the induced peritoneal cavity and in the spleen. The characterization of this cell and its relation to the macrophage lineage is based on the following facts: it develops in tissue culture under conditions, which favour the proliferation of macrophage precursor cells. It matures into an adherent typical macrophage and it is killed by the alloanti-macrophage serum Mph 1.2 + C'.

This antiserum which is raised in two congenic strains differing in a macrophage surface antigen, was obtained from Searle laboratory. It was tested in our lab for activity against peritoneal cells, bone marrow macrophages, T- and B-lymphocytes. The T- and B-lymphocytes were neither functionally nor morphologically damaged by treatment with this antiserum + C'. Peritoneal macrophages and also bone marrow macrophages were killed (as already mentioned, the choice of the suitable complement batch is very critical with this antiserum). Thus there is no doubt that this antiserum has a strong and specific activity against macrophages and macrophage precursors. Whether however, this antiserum is probably cross-reacting with NK cells cannot be excluded, since it is not a monoclonal antibody.

To characterize further the specificity of the Mph 1.2 antiserum, we absorbed the antiserum with mature adherent bone marrow macrophages of a 12 day old culture. In such a culture no other cell type than mature macrophages are present. Thus the absorption effect would be exclusively due to the elimination of anti-macrophage antibodies. Effector cells from CP induced peritoneal exudates as well as spleen cells which had been treated with such absorbed Mph 1.2 antiserum + C' retained NK activity, whereas those treated with unabsorbed Mph 1.2 + C' lost their most of their activity (unpublished observation). The fact that not all activity was abolished by treatment with Mph 1.2 + C' can either be explained by the presence of two effector cell-populations, pre-T-cells (25) and promonocytes, or by insufficient antiserum concentrations. In any case, experiments with such antisera will only provide clearcut results when they are repeated with a monoclonal antibody against macrophages and macrophage precursor cells. Similar problems may be relevant for the antisera used for characterization of the surface markers of NK cells like antisera against Thy 1.2, Ly 5 and Ly 6. Although it is known that mature macrophages lack these surface markers it remains to be estabilshed whether promonocytes may probably crossreact with such surface antigenic structures. The experiments showing T-lymphocyte markers on the surface of NK cells as well as our experiments suggest, that natural killing activity is a property of immature precursor cells. It is very likely that precursor cells of different cell lineages like macrophages and lymphocytes contribute to the natural killing activity in vivo.

V. NATURAL MACROPHAGE MEDIATED CYTOTOXICITY

Our lab had been working for years on cytotoxicity of macrophages induced to cytotoxicity by the activation with lymphokines (37). Our experiments always deal with the problem that a certain percentage of the mice which are used had nonspecifically cytotoxic macrophages in their noninduced peritoneal cavity. Therefore we could not test our lymphokine preparations on the peritoneal macrophages of these mice. This was the primary reasion for us, to establish the liquid culture system of mouse bone marrow described in Section II. This system provided us with macrophages in large numbers which were never preactivated, at least not in terms of cytotoxicity against tumor cells and measured in a 24 h ^{51}Cr release assay. However, for certain experiments we kept using the peritoneal macrophages of untreated mice. We thus compared the quality of the peritoneal macrophages of conventionally kept mice with those of mice which had been kept under SPF conditions until the day of use.

Our experience with these two groups of mice was quite clear cut. Whereas the macrophages obtained from SPF mice showed never any cytotoxicity the macrophages from conventionally kept mice showed a large variability ranging from strong nonspecific cytotoxicity to absence of any cytotoxicity. The type of the cytotoxicity was of the lymphokine type: it was nonspecifically directed against all tumor targets tested and was performed by a mature non-induced peritoneal macrophage. We deduced from these findings that the conventionally kept mice passed frequently inapparent infections, which resulted in lymphokine production although the animals looked perfectly healthy. No other parameter tested in such mice showed any sign of such an passed infection: T-cell cytotoxicity, in vitro antibody presentation, and MLR were perfectly normal with these mice. The only parameter which demonstrated in a very sensitive way the health-conditions of the animal was the degree of nonspecific cytotoxicity of their peritoneal macrophages. Since the human population resembles a conventionally kept mouse colony more than an SPF colony, this type of cytotoxicity may be called natural macrophage mediated cytotoxicity. Keller (38) and Montovani (39) have reported a similar type of cytotoxicity also with SPF mice. The reason, why we so far never detected such an effect in SPF mice, may be that Keller and

Montovani have much more sensitive assays. Both authors prelabel their targets with ^{3}H thymidine, which has a particularly low spontaneous release. Therefore they can extend their assay time much longer and detect cytotoxicity effects which do not come up in an 24 h assay. In addition the sensitivity of such an assay depends totally on the target cell used.

In conclusion cells of the macrophage lineage contribute with two mechanisms to natural resistance of the organism: the macrophage precursor cell promonocyte performs an NK like activity. When the cell matures to a monocyte or macrophage this activity is lost. Under conventional breeding conditions, a natural cytotoxicity occurs which is of the lymphokine-induced type of macrophage cytotoxicity.

Acknowledgements

This work was supported by a grant of the Volkswagenwerk foundation.

REFERENCES

1. Evans, R., Grant, C.K., Cox, H., Steele, K. and Alexander P., J. Exp. Med. 136, 1318 (1972).
2. Lohmann-Matthes, M.-L., Ziegler, F.G. and Fischer, H., Eur. J. Immunol. 3, 56 (1973).
3. David, J.R. and Renold, H.G. in: "Biology of the lymphokines" Academic press p. 121 (1979).
4. Keller, R., J. Natl. Cancer Inst. 56, 369 (1976).
5. Lohmann-Matthes, M.-L., Kolb, B. and Meerpohl, H., Cell. Immunol. 41, 231 (1978).
6. Haskill, J.S. and Fett, J.W., J. Immunol. 117, 1992 (1976).
7. Lohmann-Matthes, M.-L., and Domzig, W., Eur. J. Immunol. 9, 261 (1979).
8. Domzig, W., and Lohmann-Matthes, M.-L., Eur. J. Immunol. 9, 267 (1979).
9. Lohmann-Matthes, M.-L., and Domzig, W., J. Immunol. 123, 1883 (1979).
10. Keller, R., Cell. Immunol. 17, 542 (1975).
11. Meerpohl, H.G., Lohmann-Matthes, M.-L., and Fischer, H., Eur. J. Immunol. 6, 213 (1976).
12. Goud, T.J.L.M., Schotte, C., and van Furth, R., in: "Mononuclear Phagocytes" (R van Furth, ed.), p. 189. Blackwell Scient, Publ., Oxford (1975).
13. Sumner, M.A., Bradley, T.A., Hodgson, G.S., and Cline, M.J., Brit. Journ. Haemat. 23, 221 (1972).
14. van Furth, R. and Diesselhoff den Dulk, M., J. Exp. Med. 132, 794 (1970).

15. Zähringer, M. and Lohmann-Matthes, M.-L., in preparation.
16. Ojo, E., and Wigzell, H., J. Immunol. 8, 215 (1978).
17. Herberman, R.B., in "The nude mouse in experimental and clinical research" (J. Fogh and B.C. Giovanella, eds.), p. 135. Acad. Press N.Y. (1978).
18. Ortaldo, J.R., Oldham, R.K., Cannon, G.C. and Herberman, R.B., J. Natl. Cancer Inst. 59, 77 (1977).
19. Archer, J.R. and Davies, D.A.L., J. Immunol., 1, 113 (1974).
20. Cudkowicz, G. and Hochman, P., Immunological Reviews, 44, 13 (1979).
21. Droller, M.J., Schneider, M.V. and Perlmann, P., Cell. Immunol., 39, 165 (1978).
22. Rietschel, E., Schade, U., Lüderitz, O., Fischer, H., Peskar, B.: "Microbiology 1980", Americ. Soc. Microbiol. Wash. D.C. in press.
23. Ichikawa, Y., Pluznik, D.H. and Sachs, L., Proc. Nat. Acad. Science. 58, 1480 (1967).
24. Roder, J.C., Lohmann-Matthes, M.-L., Domzig, W., Kiessling, R. and Haller, O., Eur. J. Immunol., 9, 263 (1979).
25. Herbermann, R.B., Nunn, M.E. and Holden, H., J. Immunol. 121, 304 (1978).
26. Cantor, H.M., Kasai, F.W., Shen, J.C., Leclerc, J.C. and Glimcher, P., Immunol. Rev. 44, 1 (1979).
27. Pollack, S.B., Tam, M.R., Nowinski, R.C. and Emmons, S.L., J. Immunol. 123, 1818 (1979).
28. Roder, J.C., Kiessling, R., Biberfeld, P. and Andersson, B., J. Immunol. 121, 2509 (1978).
29. Saksela, E., Timonen, T., Ranki, A. and Häyry, P., Immunol. Rev. 44, 71 (1979).
30. Löffler pers. commun.
31. Leder, L.D., Experimentelle Medizin, Pathologie und Klinik, 23, 16 (1967).
32. Roder, J.C., Lohmann-Matthes, M.-L., Domzig, W. and Wigzell, H., J. Immunol. 123, 2174 (1979).
33. Roder, J.C., J. Immunol. 123, 2168 (1979).
34. Kumar, V., Ben-Ezra, J., Bennett, M. and Sonnenfeld, G., J. Immunol. 123, 1832 (1979).
35. Herbermann, R.B., Djeu, J.Y., David, K.H., Ortaldo, J.R., Riccardi, C., Bonnard, G.D., Holden, H.T., Fagnani, R., Santoni, A. and Puccetti, P., Immunol. Rev. 44, 43 (1979).
36. Troye, M., Perlmann, P., Pape, G.R., Spiegelberg, H.L., Näslund, I. and Gidlöf, A., J. Immunol. 119, 1061 (1977).
37. Lohmann-Matthes, L.-M. in "Immunobiology of the macrophage (D.S. Nelson, eds.), p. 463 (1976).
38. Keller, R., Br. J. Cancer, 37, 732 (1978).
39. Montovani, A., Jerrells, T.R., Dean, J.H. and Herberman, R.B., Int. J. Cancer, 23, 18 (1979).

CENTRIFUGAL ELUTRIATION ALLOWS ENRICHMENT OF NATURAL KILLING AND SEPARATES XENOGENEIC AND ALLOGENEIC REACTIVITY

Eva Lotzová

Department of Developmental Therapeutics
The University of Texas System Cancer Center
M.D. Anderson Hospital and Tumor Institute
Houston, Texas

We have reported previously that centrifugal elutriation augments significantly murine NK cell activities to YAC-1 (1). Moreover, in contrast to other separation techniques, it represents a rapid and highly reproducible method,achieving high cell recovery and not exposing the cells to frequently harmful changes in pH, osmolarity, ion concentration, electrical changes etc.. Hence, it appears that this technique could be a useful step on the path to NK cell purification and perhaps, to separation of heterogeneous NK cell clones.

In this series of experiments we have employed centrifugal elutriation (2-3), to study murine splenic and human peripheral blood NK cell activities. Spleens of $B6DF_1$ mice were tested against allogeneic tumor targets, YAC-1 and EL-4 and xenogeneic target, BL (human, EBV-negative Burkitt's lymphoma line). Human peripheral blood NK cell reactivity was similarly examined against xenogeneic target, YAC-1 and allogeneic target, CEM (human T lymphoblastoid cell line).Short-term (4 hrs) ^{51}chromium release cytotoxicity test, as described previously was used in these studies (4-5). All experiments were done in a 1:50 target-to-effector cell ratio.

Human peripheral blood mononuclear cells were isolated by Ficoll-Hypaque gradient procedure before processing by elutriation. Approximately $1x10^8$ to $2x10^8$ murine splenocytes or human

This work was supported by Grant CA 21062 from NCI.

ISBN 0-12-341350-8

peripheral blood cells were introduced into a JE-6 elutriator rotor, (Beckman Instruments) at 4°C, spinning at 3260 rpm, at a flow rate of 16.7 ml/min. Nine different fractions of cells were collected after elutriation from both, murine and human samples. Fractions 1 to 8 were collected at the flow rates of 16.7, 20.0, 26.5, 33.0, 39.5, 46.0, 59.0 and 72.0 ml/min, respectively at a constant rotor speed. Fraction 9, collected after the rotor decelerated and at a maximum flow rate, represented the wash fraction. The recovery of cells after elutriation was 75 to 80%.

I. MURINE STUDIES

As can be seen from Fig.I (that represents a pool of 5 experiments) a signficiant increase in NK cell cytotoxicity in comparison to unfractionated B6DF$_1$ murine splenocytes was achieved after centrifugal elutriation fractionation. This increase in NK cell cytotoxicity was expressed against all three types of target cells, i.e. against YAC-1 and BL,to which B6DF$_1$ mice are good responders and also against EL-4, to which the same mice are poor responders. Highest cytotoxicity was consistently seen in fraction 3 where the enrichment was 2-fold to YAC-1 and BL ($P<0.01$) and 5-fold to EL-4 ($P<0.01$). Lower,although significant increase in NK cell activity was seen in fraction 4 to YAC-1 and BL ($P<0.02$) in which,fraction NK reactivity against EL-4 maintained the same level as in fraction 3. Slight increase in NK cell cytotoxicity was still evident in fraction 2 to BL and YAC-1, but not to EL-4. No significant increase in fraction 5-6 was seen to any of the target cells tested. Fractions 7-9 were either comparable, or lower than unseparated controls. From these experiments it appears that the reactivity of B6DF$_1$ splenocytes to all three type of target cells show the same pattern,an observation indicating that killing of xenogeneic and allogeneic targets is mediated by the same NK cell populations, or at least by subpopulation, expressing similar physical characteristics, such as size, density and cell shape

II. HUMAN STUDIES

As illustrated in Fig. II, substantial enrichment of human peripheral blood NK cell activity was also achieved by centrifugal elutriation (the results represent a pool of two experiments). However, in contrast to murine studies, human NK cells showed different pattern of reactivity to allogeneic

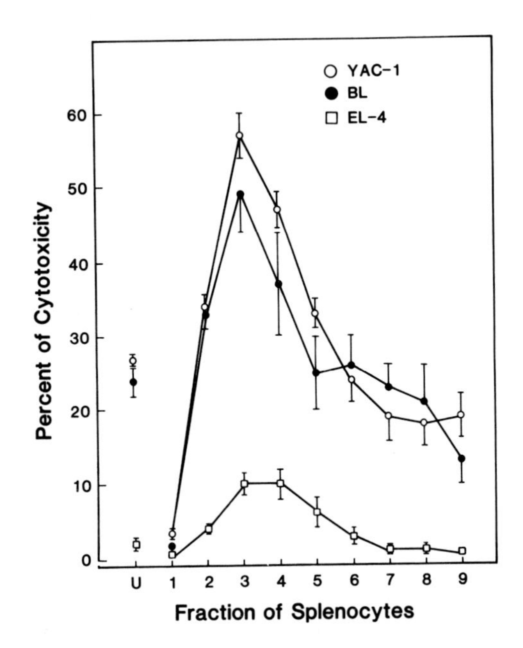

FIGURE I. NK Cell Activities of Unseparated and Centrifugal Elutriation Fractionated B6DF$_1$ Splenocytes Against Allogeneic and Xenogeneic Tumors. U-unseparated; 1 to 9 -various fractions after centrifugal elutriation.

and xenogeneic tumor target. Specifically, fraction 3 and 4 consistently showed enrichment of NK cell cytotoxicity to CEM target (increase in fraction 3 was 2.5-fold, $P<0.01$, and in fraction 4, 1.6-fold, $P<0.02$) but no enrichment to xenogeneic target, YAC-1. On the contrary, fractions 5 and 6 were enriched significantly for anti YAC-1 NK cell activities (3.2 times

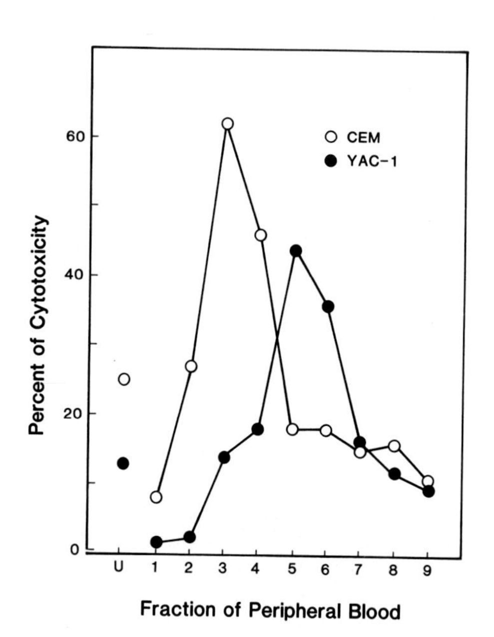

FIGURE II. NK Cell Activity of Unseparated and Centrifugal Elutriation Fractionated Human Peripheral Blood to Allogeneic and Xenogeneic Tumor Cells. U-unseparated; 1 to 9-various fractions after centrifugal elutriation.

and 2.8 times, respectively; P values <0.005), but were appreciably lower than unseparated controls with regard to anti CEM activity. Fractions 1,2,7 and 8 were either lower or comparable to unseparated controls with regard to both types of target cells. These results suggest that human peripheral blood NK cells reacting to xenogeneic targets are distinguishable from those reacting to allogeneic targets on the basis of their physical properties.

III. MEAN SEDIMENTATION VELOCITY AND CELL SIZE DISTRIBUTION OF HUMAN PERIPHERAL BLOOD CELLS AND MURINE SPLENOCYTES

To obtain information on the physical properties of the cells expressing NK cytotoxicity, the mean sedimentation velocity and percentage of cells in specific size ranges in each fraction was calculated and correlated with cytotoxicity (Table I). Fraction 3 and 4, which showed greatest enrichment in murine NK cell activities to both, allogeneic and xenogeneic targets and fraction 2 that showed some enrichment had average sedimentation velocity of 4.2, 5.4 and 3.3 mm/h/g, respectively, and contained predominantly (65-81%) cells of sizes 100-160 μm^3. However, these fractions also contained relatively high number of the cells of sizes greater than 160 μm^3, and very small number of the cells with sizes smaller than 100 μm^3 Fractions 5-8, which did not show enriched NK cell activity, were collected at sedimentation rates of 6.6, 7.8, 9.5 and 11.9 mm/h/g, respectively and the cells sedimenting in these fractions were of heterogenous sizes with approximately 6-19% of the cells ranging from 60-100 μm^3, 40-50% of the cells in the range of 100-160 μm^3 and 35-50% of the cells of sizes larger than 160 μm^3. Fraction 9 contained cells of all sizes, as expected, since it was a pellet fraction, which also included some cells entrapped within debris.

These data suggest that cells of sizes 100-160 μm^3 may be relevant for NK cytotoxicity, however, participation of cells >160 μm^3 could not be eliminated. This is suggested, especially in the view of cell size distribution in fraction 2, which has high numbers of cells of 100-160 μm^3 sizes and even though still enriched expresses lower NK cell cytotoxicity than fraction 3 and 4.

In human peripheral blood, high allogeneic NK cell activity coincided with high percent of cells of average sedimentation velocity 4.2 and 5.4 mm/h/g and cell sizes of 100-195 μm^3. However, this fraction was also contaminated with 14-17% of cells of higher sizes (195-293 μm^3) that could have effected NK cell activity. Contrary to murine NK cell profiles, a gap in the sedimentation velocities and sizes was evident between the cells reacting to allogeneic and those reacting to xenogeneic tumors, since the latter expressed average sedimentation velocity 6.6 and 7.8 mm/h/g and coincided with cells of sizes >293 μm^3 (fractions 5 and 6). However, again some contamina-

TABLE I. Mean Sedimentation Velocity and Cell Size Distributions of Human Peripheral Blood Cells and Murine Splenocytes Separated by Centrifugal Elutriation

Elutriation Fraction	Mean Sedimentation Velocity in mm/h/g (range)[a]	Cell Size Distributions in μm^3 (%)[b]					
		Murine			Human		
		60–100	100–160	>160	100–195	195–293	>293
1	1.5(0.0– 3.0)	48	45	7	86	10	4
2	3.3(3.0– 3.6)	8	81	11	86	10	4
3	4.2(3.6– 4.8)	5	75	20	81	14	5
4	5.4(4.8– 6.0)	5	65	30	58	17	25
5	6.6(6.0– 7.2)	6	50	44	23	12	65
6	7.8(7.2– 8.3)	10	40	50	20	12	68
7	9.5(8.3–10.7)	14	45	41	25	9	66
8	11.9(10.7–13.1)	19	46	35	24	12	64
9	max.(13.1– ∞)	30	46	24	40	15	45

[a]Mean sedimentation velocity was determined using the equation 1.93x flow rate: $(rpm/1000)^2$.

[b]Cells in each fraction were counted with a Coulter Counter and the cell size distribution was determined using a multichannel pulse height analyzer connected to the counter. The percentage of cells in each size range was compared by measurement of the areas under the curve.

tion of the fractions with cells of smaller and larger sizes was observed (see Table I).

It is not possible to determine from these studies, either the type of the cells involved in natural killing or the nature of other cell populations present in individual fractions; however, we are currently in the progress in evaluating individual fractions with regard to the cell surface and functional characteristics and specific NK-target binding properties. We believe, that despite this impermanent obscurity regarding the qualitative composition of individual fractions, centrifugal elutriation presents a useful technique for NK cell enrichment and, as indicated by our studies, may be instrumental in separating various clones of NK cells.

REFERENCES

1. Phillips, J.H., Lotzová, E.,and Mesitrich, M.L.,*Fed. Proc. 38*, 915 (1979).
2. Meistrich, M.L., Nell, L.J., Richie, E.S., Mackler, B.F., and O'Neill, P.A., *Fed. Proc. 38 (Abstract)*, 1014 (1979).
3. Mackler, B.F., O'Neill, P.A., and Meistrich, M.L., *Eur. J. Immunol. 7*, 55 (1977).
4. Lotzová, E., *"Experimental Hematology Today, 1979" (S.J. Baum, G. David Ledney, Eds)*, p.207. Springer-Verlag, New York, (1979).
5. Savary, C.A., and Lotzová, E., *J. Immunol. 120*, 239, (1978).

EFFECTS OF ALLOANTISERA ON MURINE K AND NK CELL ACTIVITY[1]

Sylvia B. Pollack

Division of Tumor Immunology
The Fred Hutchinson Cancer Research Center
Department of Microbiology and Immunology
University of Washington, Seattle, Washington

Sandra L. Emmons
Linda A. Hallenbeck
Milton R. Tam

Divisions of Tumor Immunology and Tumor Virology
The Fred Hutchinson Cancer Research Center
Seattle, Washington

I. INTRODUCTION

We recently evaluated the expression of T cell-associated antigens on natural killer (NK) cells of C57Bl/6 (B6) mice by cytotoxic depletion experiments using alloantisera to Thy 1, Ly 1, Ly 2, Ly 5, Ly 6 and NK 1 antigens (Pollack *et al.*, 1979). The NK activity of B6 spleen cells (SC) was markedly reduced after treatment of the cells with complement (C) and antisera to the NK 1.1 and Ly 5.1 antigens. Some pools of anti-Ly 6.2 serum also depleted NK activity. In contrast, NK activity was not affected by antisera to Thy 1.2, Ly 1.2 or Ly 2.2.

[1]*These studies supported by grant CA 18647 from the National Cancer Institute, DHEW.*

ISBN 0-12-341350-8

In this report, we use those antisera to evaluate the phenotype of B6 killer (K) lymphocytes which mediate antibody-dependent cellular cytotoxicity (ADCC) to tumor targets. Experiments are included to determine whether the effects of antiserum on K cell activity are in fact due to depletion of K cells or to nonspecific inhibition of K cell activity by free or cell-bound antibodies.

II. MATERIALS AND METHODS

A. *Mice*

B6 mice were purchased from The Jackson Laboratory or were bred in this laboratory. Breeding stock for the semicongenic strain C3H/CE and for the congenic strains B6.Ly 1.1 and B6.Ly 2.1/3.1 were kindly provided by Dr. E. A. Boyse (Sloan-Kettering Institute). Mice of the C3H/He, SJL/J, A.SW, BALB/c, CXBD, A, AKR, and 129 strains were purchased from The Jackson Laboratory. F_1 hybrids were bred in our laboratory. AKR/Cu mice were purchased from Cumberland Farms.

B. *Antisera*

Alloantisera used for these experiments have been described previously (Pollack *et al.*, 1979). The general protocol used to raise the antisera was as follows: mice were immunized every 2 weeks beginning with the equivalent of one thymus (and/or spleen) per 10 recipient mice. The amount of immunizing tissue was gradually increased so that at the fifth immunization, one thymus (and/or spleen) per 1 to 2 recipients was used. Mice were bled at days 4 and 7 after the fifth immunization and screened individually for specific antibody and autoantibodies. Nonresponders and mice producing high titers of autoantibody were discarded. Immunizations of the remaining mice were continued every 10-14 days. Mice were bled and sera pooled at days 4 and 7 after each booster immunization. Sera used in these studies were generally from the 7-10th immunization. Specificity was determined by titration of the antisera on thymocytes or SC from mice bearing appropriate or inappropriate alleles.

Monoclonal IgM anti-Thy 1.2 serum was kindly provided by Dr. Edward Clark (University of Washington). Monoclonal IgG_{2a} anti-Thy 1.1 serum, used to induce ADCC to SL-2 target cells, was provided by Dr. Irwin Bernstein (FHCRC).

C. *Complement-Dependent Antibody Cytolysis of Spleen Cells*

Spleens were removed from normal B6 mice and single cell suspensions of SC were prepared as described previously (Pollack *et al.*, 1979). For depletion of SC bearing particular alloantigens, the cells were mixed with equal volumes of antiserum and C in a one step-procedure as described (Pollack *et al.*, 1979). A single pool of newborn rabbit sera, screened for low cytotoxicity to mouse lymphoid cells, was used as a source of C at an optimal final dilution of 1:36. Controls consisted of SC and C incubated with no antiserum or of SC and antiserum without C.

After incubation at 37° for 45 min, SC mixtures treated with both antiserum and C were placed on ice for 10 min and then were underlayered with 5 ml cold Ficoll-hypaque (d=1.090). The cells were centrifuged at 1200 g for 15 min at 4° C to pellet dead cells. Viable cells were collected from the interface, washed three times in cold PBS, counted, and resuspended in RPMI 1640 medium containing 5% fetal calf serum (5% RPMI). The resulting SC were greater than 95% viable.

Control SC which were treated with antiserum in the absence of C, and which consequently were not lysed during the 45 min incubation were washed three times in PBS, counted and resuspended in 5% RPMI. The viability of these cells was also greater than 95%.

D. *^{51}Cr-Release NK and ADCC Assays*

The A/Sn Moloney sarcoma virus-induced lymphoma, YAC-1, was used as the target to detect NK activity of the SC. The spontaneous AKR T cell lymphoma, SL-2, was used as a target for ADCC. The target cells were labeled with ^{51}Cr and washed as described previously (Pollack *et al.*, 1979). After labeling, SL-2 cells were resuspended in a 10^{-4} dilution of monoclonal IgG_{2a} anti-Thy 1.1 serum and were held on ice for 45 min. The antibody-coated SL-2 cells were then spun through 2 ml FCS to remove unbound antibody before use in the ADCC assay.

10^4 ^{51}Cr-labeled YAC-1 or antibody-coated SL-2 target cells were mixed with normal B6 SC at various effector: target (E:T) ratios in Cooke round bottom microtest plates. After incubation for 4 hr at 37° C, an aliquot was removed from each well for the assessment of ^{51}Cr-release as described (Pollack *et al.*, 1979).

III. INTERACTIONS OF K AND NK CELLS WITH ALLOANTISERA

A. C-Dependent Lysis of B6 SC

All antisera were first titered to determine the lowest concentration at which each antiserum produced maximal cytotoxicity to B6 SC in a C-dependent assay. Trypan blue dye exclusion was used to assess the recovery of viable cells after treatment with C and each of the antisera except for anti-NK 1.1. This serum bound to less than 10% of B6 SC and did not lyse enough SC to be detectable with the dye exclusion assay (Tam *et al.*, 1980). To titer the anti-NK 1.1 serum, SC were treated with dilutions of the antiserum and C and then tested for NK effector activity. The endpoint was determined as the last serum dilution at which significant depletion of NK activity was observed. The mean titers for the antisera are listed in Table I.

B. K and NK Effector Activity of SC Treated with Various Concentrations of Antisera plus C

C-dependent depletion assays were also used to determine the effects of various dilutions of the antisera on K cell-mediated killing of antibody-coated SL-2, and to compare those with the effects on NK cell-mediated killing of YAC-1. Three different patterns of antiserum effects were observed.

1. Antisera to Ly 6.2 and to NK 1.1. SC treated with low dilutions of these antisera and C were markedly depleted of both K and NK activity (Fig. 1). The effect on K cell activity was particularly striking with the anti-NK 1.1 serum. At higher antiserum dilutions neither K nor NK cell activity was affected.

TABLE I. Highest Initial Antisera Dilutions Producing Maximal C Dependent Lysis[a]

Thy 1.2	*Ly 1.2*	*Ly 2.2*	*Ly 3.2*	*Ly 5.1*	*Ly 6.2*	*NK 1.1*
1:5x10^5	1:50	1:100	1:200	1:400	1:100	1:30

[a]*Antisera were titered in a one-step C-dependent assay as described in Materials and Methods to determine the highest dilution producing maximal lysis of SC, or, for anti-NK 1.1, maximal depletion of NK effector activity.*

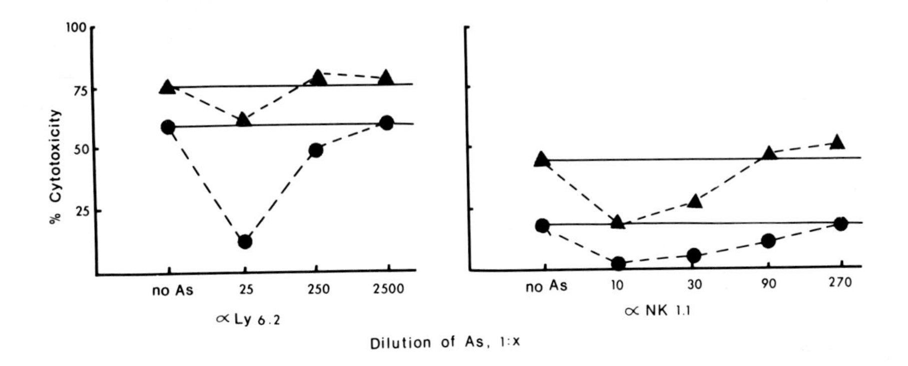

FIG. 1. Cytotoxicity of B6 SC treated with varying dilutions of anti-Ly 6.2 or anti-NK 1.1 and C (broken lines) or with C alone (no As; solid line). ▲--▲, NK to YAC-1 (E:T=50:1) ●--●, ADCC to SL-2 (E:T=100:1)

2. *Antisera to Ly 1.2, 2.2, and 3.2.* As shown in Fig. 2, antisera to Ly 1.2, 2.2 and 3.2 did not significantly decrease either K or NK cell activity at any dilution tested. In some cases K and NK cell activity was significantly enhanced.

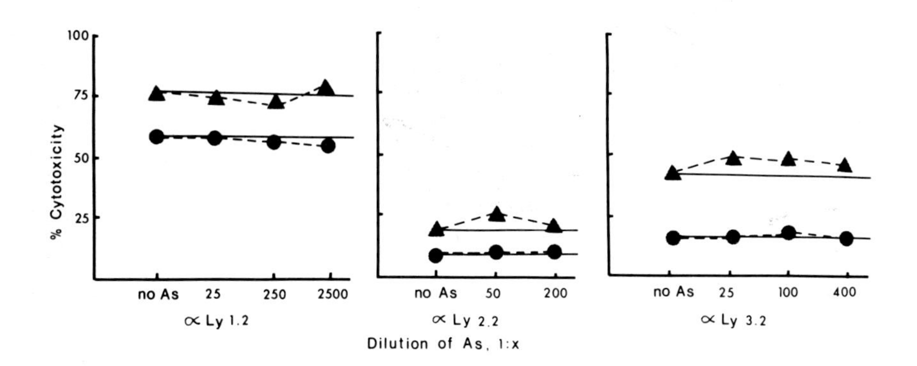

FIG. 2. Cytotoxicity of B6 SC treated with anti-Ly 1.2, 2.2 or 3.2 and C. Symbols and conditions as in Fig. 1.

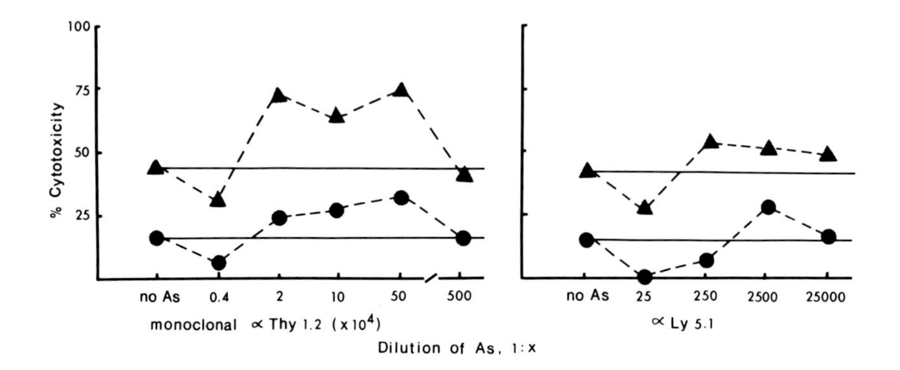

FIG. 3. Cytotoxicity of B6 SC treated with anti-Thy 1.2 or Ly 5.1 and C. Symbols and conditions as in Fig. 1.

3. *Antisera to Thy 1.2 and Ly 5.1.* A third pattern was observed when the SC were treated with C and antiserum to Thy 1.2 or Ly 5.1 (Fig. 3). Both K and NK cell activity were reduced when the antisera were used at low dilutions. However, at higher dilutions, at which maximal lysis of B6 SC was still obtained, enhancement of both K and NK cell-mediated cytotoxicity was observed (Table II).

TABLE II. Effect of Antiserum Dilution on Number of SC Lysed and on K and NK Cell Activity[a]

	Thy 1.2 + C		*Ly 5.1 + C*	
	1:5x10^3	*1:5x10*^{5}	*1:50*	*1:400*
% SC killed	*49 ± 3*	*53 ± 1*	*64 ± 11*	*65 ± 10*
% change[b] *in*				
ADCC	*-33 ± 13*	*+51 ± 25*	*-83 ± 8*	*+82 ± 14*
NK	*-7 ± 9*	*+32 ± 15*	*-24 ± 4*	*+46 ± 7*

[a]*Summarized data from 4 experiments presented as means ± S.E.M.*

[b]*% change calculated from 100x (% lysis with control SC - % lysis with exptl. SC) ÷ (% lysis with control SC).*

Such results were consistently observed with two different pools of Ly 5.1 antiserum. The results with the monoclonal anti-Thy 1.2 were somewhat more variable. In 2 of 4 experiments, K and NK cell activity were markedly enhanced after treatment of SC with C and $5x10^{-5}$ anti-Thy 1.2, but in 2 other experiments (e.g. Fig. 4), the cytotoxic activity of the treated SC was not significantly different from that of control SC.

At the highest dilutions tested, where the antisera were no longer cytolytic to SC, K and NK cell activities returned to baseline.

C. *C-Dependency of the Effects of Antisera on K and NK Effector Activity*

Once the sera had been titered for their C-dependent effects on both cytotoxicity to SC and depletion (or enrichment) of K and NK effector function, optimal serum dilutions were tested to determine whether the effects on K and NK cells were, in fact, C-dependent. This was, of course, of primary concern in the case of K cells which rely on Fc receptors (FcR) for their activity. Nonspecific blocking of FcR by free or cell-bound antibody could inhibit ADCC whether or not the antibody was directed towards an alloantigen on the K cells themselves.

The results of one of a series of experiments comparing the effects of antisera in the presence or absence of C are shown in Fig. 4. All antisera except anti-Thy 1.2 and anti-Ly 5.1 were tested at the highest dilution which, in the C-dependent assays, showed maximal effect on K or NK function. K cell results are shown in the upper panels, NK in the lower panels. Thy 1.2 and anti-Ly 5.1 were each tested at two optimal dilutions which, in the C-dependent titrations, produced two opposing effects.

1. Monoclonal Anti Thy 1.2 Antibody. In the experiment presented in Fig. 4, monoclonal anti-Thy 1.2 did not produce increased activity when used at a dilution of $1{:}5x10^{5}$. Both K and NK cell activity were decreased when the antibody was used at 1:5000. This decrease was clearly C-dependent.

2. Antisera to Ly 1.2, 2.2 or 3.2. In the absence of C, these antisera had no significant effect on either K or NK cell activity. A significant enrichment for K cell activity was observed with SC treated with anti-Ly 2.2 and C. Increases in both K and NK occurred after treatment with anti-Ly 3.2 and C. K cell activity was increased more than NK cell activity.

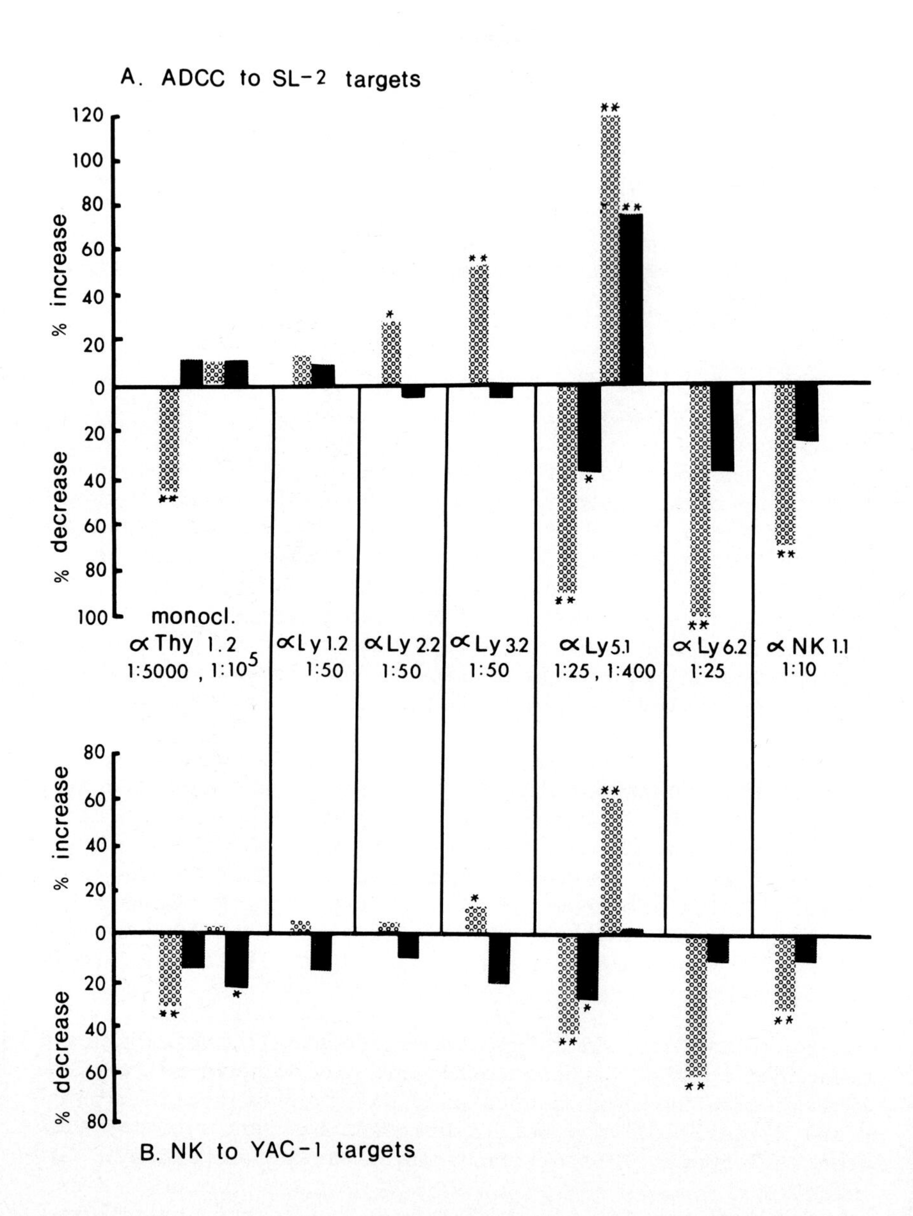

FIG. 4. The effect of antiserum plus C (open bars) or antiserum alone (hatched bars) on the K (panel A) and NK (panel B) activity of B6 SC. % change calculated as shown in the legend for Table II.

3. Antiserum to Ly 5.1. Results with the 1:25 initial dilution of Ly 5.1 confirmed the observation that this antiserum can decrease NK cell activity in the absence of C (Cantor *et al.*, 1979; Pollack *et al.*, 1979). The present experiments showed that K cells were similarly affected. However, in the samples treated with a 1:400 dilution of anti-Ly 5.1 and no C, K cells were consistently highly increased in activity whereas NK cells were unaffected.

The C-dependent effects of anti-Ly 5.1 serum paralleled the effects of serum alone. SC treated with a 1:25 initial dilution of anti-Ly 5.1 and C displayed markedly reduced levels of both K and NK activity. However, when the initial dilution of anti-Ly 5.1 was 1:400, K cell activity was more than doubled in the C-treated cells. NK cell activity was also significantly increased, although less so than K cell activity.

4. Antisera to Ly 6.2 and NK 1.1. Results with anti-Ly 6.2 and NK 1.1 showed that the maximal effects of these antisera on both K and NK cell activity were C-dependent. K cell activity, however, was also reduced in each of three experiments by anti-Ly 6.2 and by anti-NK 1.1 alone, although the decrease in effector activity was substantially less than when the antisera were used with C to lyse alloantigen bearing cells.

IV. CONCLUSIONS AND DISCUSSION

The reactions of murine K and NK cells with antisera to cell surface alloantigens are generally similar. Both activities are depleted from SC treated with anti-NK 1.1 serum and C. Thus K cells bear the NK cell-associated antigen, NK-1. This conclusion is bolstered by a comparison between the results with antiserum to NK 1.1 and, *e.g.*, anti-Ly 1.2. Whereas anti-NK 1.1 does not lyse detectable numbers of SC, it does deplete K cells. In contrast, antiserum to Ly 1.2 lyses a significant percentage of SC, presumably releasing antigen-antibody complexes in the process, but does not affect K cell activity. Thus it cannot be argued that lysis of irrelevant (non-K) cells within the SC population is sufficient to inhibit ADCC under the conditions used in these experiments. It should be noted that dead SC are removed after treatment with antiserum and C and the remaining viable cells washed extensively before use in the cytotoxicity assays.

Our results with anti-Ly 6.2 are similar to those with anti-NK 1.1, suggesting that NK and K cells also bear Ly 6.

However, this conclusion is tempered by the fact that in previous experiments not all pools of anti-Ly 6.2 serum decreased NK activity (Pollack *et al.*, 1979). Clark *et al.* (1979) have suggested that anti-NK 1.1 may appear as a contaminant specificity in some pools of anti-Ly 6.2 serum.

The results with antisera to Ly 1.2, Ly 2.2 and Ly 3.2 demonstrate that neither K cells nor NK cells bear those alloantigens. SC treated with these antisera in either the presence or absence of C had control or greater levels of cytotoxicity in the NK and ADCC assays.

The question of whether murine NK cells express Thy 1 has been controversial (Herberman *et al.*, 1975; Kiessling *et al.*, 1975; Pollack *et al.*, 1979; Santoni *et al.*, 1979b; Mattes *et al.*, 1979). Using a conventional alloantiserum to Thy 1.2, we found no significant depletion of NK activity at any of the dilutions tested (Pollack *et al.*, 1979). In the experiments reported here, we have used a high-titered monoclonal IgM anti-Thy 1.2 antibody from Dr. Edward Clark. Low dilutions of this antibody plus C deplete both NK and K cell activity. However, when the antiserum is used at an additional 100-fold dilution, the same percentage of SC are lysed as at the lower antibody dilution, but both NK and K cell activities are enhanced.

These data can be interpreted in several ways. If NK and K cells lack the Thy-1 alloantigen, then lysis of Thy-1 bearing cells at high antibody dilutions (10^{-5} to 5×10^{-5}) would enrich for NK and K cells. The decreased NK and K cell activity observed at low antibody dilutions might be due to nonspecific blocking by excess antibody (free or complexed) bound to the effector cells.

Alternatively, if NK and K cells do bear the Thy 1 antigen, the decreased activity in SC treated with the low dilution of anti-Thy 1.2 and C would be due to depletion of those cells. The increased activity in cells treated with C and high dilutions of antibody can be explained if the Thy 1 antigens on K and NK cells are so sparse that at low concentrations of anti-Thy 1.2 antibody, not enough antibody binds to effect C-dependent lysis. Since K and NK cells represent only a small proportion of a normal SC population, their lysis would not be detected by dye exclusion (cf. Table II). Discriminatory effects of C and low or high dilutions of anti-Thy 1.2 could, therefore, produce lysis of or passive enrichment for K and NK cells. Unanalyzed mechanisms of crosslinking or activation of effector cells cannot, of course, be excluded.

It is important to emphasize that the SL-2 cells used as targets in the K cell assay are Thy 1.1 positive. Thus the increased ADCC observed with SC treated at some concentrations of anti-Thy 1.2 cannot be ascribed to an interaction of the anti-Thy 1.2 serum with the target cells.

Recent evidence from Mattes *et al.* (1979) indicates that some NK cells do bear a low density of Thy 1.2 antigen. SC were separated with the fluorescence activated cell sorter into Thy 1.2 positive and Thy 1.2 negative populations. NK activity was found in both populations. The variability in our results with anti-Thy 1.2 may reflect this heterogeneity of NK cells and suggests a similar heterogeneity of K cells.

The effects of low dilutions of anti-Ly 5.1 are largely C-independent. Decreased NK activity in the presence of low dilutions of anti-Ly 5.1 has been reported previously (Cantor *et al.*, 1979; Pollack *et al.*, 1979). This observation is now extended to K cells. High dilutions of anti-Ly 5.1 greatly enhanced both K and NK activity. The same sort of discriminatory serum dilution effect suggested for anti-Thy 1.2 may be responsible for this enhancement. Of all the antisera tested, the only one which distinguished between K and NK cells was anti-Ly 5.1 at high dilutions (1:400-600) in the absence of C. This treatment greatly enhanced K but not NK activity and is being investigated further. It should be noted that both targets, YAC-1 and SL-2, are Ly 5.1 positive cells, but, in our hands, YAC-1 is resistant to ADCC in a short term assay.

In general, the patterns of reactivity of K and NK cells with the various antisera are very similar. We conclude that murine K cells are NK 1 positive cells which do not bear Ly 1, Ly 2 or Ly 3. They also interact with antiserum to Ly 5 and Ly 6. The results with Thy 1 remain equivocal but suggest that some K cells are Thy 1 positive and/or that K cells express only low amounts of the Thy 1 antigen.

Other similarities between the cells mediating K and NK activities have been reported (see Herberman *et al.*, 1979, for review). NK and K cells have comparable tissue distribution (Santoni *et al.*, 1979a) and appear to be small to medium sized lymphocytes (Herberman *et al.*, 1979) which do not adhere to nylon wool and do not bear surface immunoglobulin (Herberman *et al.*, 1975; Kiessling *et al.*, 1975). Both activities are relatively resistant to X-irradiation (Santoni *et al.*, 1979b) and are boosted by either *in vivo* or *in vitro* treatment with interferon or interferon-inducing agents such as virus and *C. parvum* (Ojo and Wigzell, 1978; Santoni *et al.*, 1979a).

The questions of whether NK cells require antibody for their function and the role and/or presence of FcR have not been clearly resolved (Herberman *et al.*, 1975, 1977; Kiessling, *et al.*, 1975; Santoni *et al.*, 1979b). In our hands, SC depleted of FcR-bearing cells by adherence to 7s antibody-coated sheep erythrocytes are depleted of K cell activity but enriched for NK cell activity (unpublished observations, using the assays reported here). The difference between K and NK is apparent even when the data are expressed in terms of lytic units. Herberman *et al.* (1977; Santoni *et al.*, 1979a) have reported depletion of both K and NK cell activity after removal of FcR-bearing cells. However, in their experiments, ADCC was measured with an NK sensitive target in an overnight assay.

Functional differences between the K and NK cells have been observed (Santoni *et al.*, 1979b). Whereas NK activity is decreased by treatment of the lymphocytes with trypsin, K cells are unaffected or even enhanced in activity. Murine NK activity is also reduced after *in vivo* treatment of mice with hydrocortisone while K cell activity is unaffected.

Although K and NK cells are phenotypically indistinguishable in our experiments with alloantisera, it is still unclear whether the two activities reside in different populations of cells or are physiologically separable functions of one cell type. Several investigators favor the latter hypothesis (Ojo and Wigzell, 1978; Mattes *et al.*, 1979). However, it is also plausible that K and NK cells are developmentally related but functionally discrete cells. Precedent for phenotypically similar but functionally separate lymphocyte subclasses exists within the T cell system. The precise nature of the relationship between K and NK cells remains unresolved.

REFERENCES

Cantor, H., Kasai, M., Shen, F.W., LeClerc, J.C., and Glimcher, L. (1979). *Immunol. Rev. 44*, 1.

Clark, E.A., Russell, P.H., Egghart, M., Horton, M.A. (1979). *Int. J. Cancer 24*, 688.

Herberman, R.B., Nunn, M.E., Holden, H.T., and Lavrin, D.H. (1975). *Int. J. Cancer 16*, 230.

Herberman, R.B., Bartram, S., Haskill, J.S., Nunn, M., Holden, H.T., and West, W.H. (1977). *J. Immunol. 119*, 322.

Herberman, R.B., Djeu, J.Y., Kay, H.D., Ortaldo, J.R., Riccardi, C., Bonnard, G.D., Holden, H.T., Fagnani, R., Santoni, A., and Puccetti, P. (1979). *Immunol. Rev. 44*,43.

Kiessling, R., Klein, E., Pross, H., and Wigzell, H. (1975). *Eur. J. Immunol. 5*, 117.

Mattes, M.J., Sharrow, S.O., Herberman, R.B., and Holden, H.T. (1979). *J. Immunol. 123*, 2851.

Ojo, E., and Wigzell, H. (1978). *Scand. J. Immunol. 7*, 297.

Pollack, S.B., Tam, M.R., Nowinski, R.C., and Emmons, S.L. (1978) *J. Immunol. 123*, 1818.

Santoni, A., Herberman, R.B., and Holden, H.T. (1979a). *J. Natl. Cancer Inst. 62*, 109.

Santoni, A., Herberman, R.B., and Holden, H.T. (1979b). *J. Natl. Cancer Inst. 63*, 995.

Tam, M.R., Emmons, S.L., and Pollack, S.B. (1980). *J. Immunol.* in press.

CHARACTERISTICS OF HUMAN NATURAL KILLER CELLS[1]

Hugh F. Pross[2]

Departments of
Radiation Oncology and Microbiology & Immunology
Queen's University
Kingston, Ontario, Canada

Malcolm G. Baines

Departments of
Obstetrics & Gynecology and Microbiology & Immunology
Queen's University
Kingston, Ontario, Canada

I. INTRODUCTION

It is now almost a decade since natural killer (NK) cells first appeared to haunt cell-mediated cytotoxicologists (1-3). During this interval there has been a gradual but relentless evolution in our concept of the role and importance of these cells, to the point where, in human systems at least, a lymphoid cell capable of lysing tumour targets *in vitro* is an NK cell until proven otherwise. To a large extent this situation has been brought about by the demonstration that spontaneous lymphocyte-mediated cytotoxicity (SLMC) (4) against tumour target cells could be attributed to an identifiable lymphocyte subpopulation with characteristic, albeit not unique, surface markers (4-8),

[1] *Support for this work was received from the Ontario Cancer Treatment and Research Foundation (HFP) and the Medical Research Council of Canada (MGB).*

[2] *Research Associate of the Ontario Cancer Treatment and Research Foundation.*

ISBN 0-12-341350-8

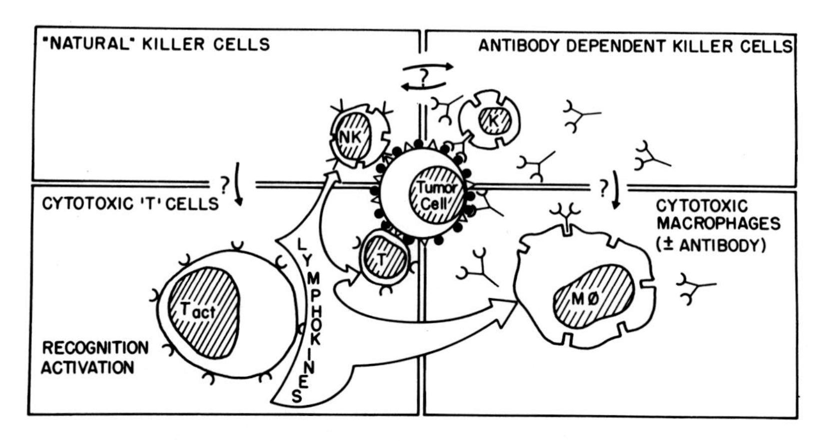

FIGURE 1. Four mechanisms of cell-mediated cytotoxicity.

and which was presumably distinguishable from other cell types capable of cell-mediated lysis (Fig 1). The numerous surface marker studies which have been done on NK cells have led to considerable debate as to the inter-relationship between the NK cell and other cell types, especially with respect to whether or not NK cells are pre-T cells, identical to K cells, or promonocytes (9-15). Most publications on this subject have addressed the question of the characteristics of NK cells by systematically fractionating normal human lymphocytes using various rosette depletion and column separation techniques. Much of this work has been reviewed in this volume and elsewhere (16,17), and will not be dealt with here. Instead, we would like to treat the subject of the "characteristics of human NK cells" from a somewhat different point of view, and attempt to answer the question, "When can a lymphocyte capable of cell-mediated cytotoxicity be called an NK cell?" The problem of defining killer cells has arisen recently in several situations, both clinical (e.g. the killer cell activity seen in the blood of immunodeficient or cancer patients) and experimental (e.g. interferon-induced killer cells in mice), although perhaps the best example of this problem is that of culture-induced killer cells, which have been labelled with such names as NK-like cells (18) and anomalous killer (AK) cells (19).

II. NK CELLS DEFINED -- SOURCE, SURFACE RECEPTORS, SELECTIVITY

Obviously the source of the cells used in *in vitro* cytotoxicity assays may define whether or not the effects seen are due to NK cells. Cytotoxic cells in the monocyte/granulocyte-depleted blood of disease-free, unimmunized normal donors are NK lymphocytes, *by definition*. These cells are therefore the standard by which similarly treated patients' lymphocytes must be compared. Because of the lack of a specific anti-human NK cell antiserum, at the moment, this comparison between "unknown" and normal lymphocytes must be based on the surface characteristics and the target selectivity of the cytotoxic cells.

The surface markers of NK cells can be divided into those markers present on virtually all NK cells and those markers which are present on only a certain proportion. Table I summarizes our attempts to identify these markers by assessing the effect of depleting various rosette-forming cell types on cytotoxicity. It can be seen from Table I that virtually all NK cells are Fc receptor positive, a large proportion of which are E rosette-forming T cells. As stated by West *et al.* (9), the T NK cells are low affinity E rosette-forming cells, and this is shown in Table I by the large difference in the effect caused by total ERFC depletion compared with the minimal effect of "high affinity" ERFC depletion. None of these conclusions with respect to T cells are incompatible with our earlier work or that of others, the difference being in the interpretation of the enhancing effects of depleting the largely inert ERFC population. The intriguing question at the moment concerns the nature of the non-E rosetting NK cells. The most simple explanation is that all NK lymphocytes are of the same lineage, and therefore that the non-E rosetting cells are pre-T in nature. To some extent this is supported by the results of Kaplan *et al.* (20), who obliterated NK activity with an anti-T cell antiserum.

Table I also illustrates a problem which is common to these types of experiments. First, as noted in the Figure legend, the data is derived from an experiment using the blood of only one donor. This is necessary because of the variation between different normal donors, both in rosette proportions and cytotoxicity, which makes the data much less clear cut when the results are pooled. A more serious problem lies in the fact that it is virtually impossible to totally deplete for a particular cell type, leaving open the possibility that the last remaining rosette-forming cells are in fact the killer cells. To some extent we have overcome this problem by measuring the proportions of the different RFC types found in all the various depleted and control preparations, and then performing linear regression

TABLE I. Surface Receptors on NK Cells

Rosette type depleted	% RFC[a] Pre-	Post- depletion	Relative cytotoxicity[b] Observed	Expected[c]	% NK cells with receptor
19S EAC	21	4	0.64	1.2	36
7S EA	20	3	0.002	1.2	95
E (total)	68	7	1.3	2.6	49
E ("high affinity")[d]	68	18	1.8	2.0	11

[a]Percent rosettes pre- and post-depletion from the iron plus magnetism treated, Ficoll-Isopaque purified peripheral blood of a single donor. Ficoll-Isopaque was also used for RFC depletion as described previously (21).

[b]Ratio of k_2(test)/k_1(control) using the equation for the dose response curve $R = A(1-e^{-kc})$ where R = percent chromium release, A = maximum attainable lysis, c = cell number, and k = slope, which is directly proportional to cytotoxic activity (22).

[c]Relative (enhanced) cytotoxicity expected if none of the killer cells have the receptor being depleted (a = 0), calculated according to the formula

$$K_2 = \frac{K_1 - aK_1}{1 - b}$$

where K_1 and K_2 are the cytotoxic activities before and after rosette depletion, a = the proportion of NK cells with the receptor under study, and b = the proportion of cells in the original lymphocyte sample removed by RFC depletion. If RFC depletion is complete, b is the proportion of RFC in the unfractionated sample, assuming non-specific cell loss due to the procedure is uniformly distributed among the other cell types. It should be noted that $K_1/K_2 = k_1/k_2$ in the equation described above, and that when all NK cells have the receptor being depleted, a = 1 and $K_2 = 0$, as expected.

[d]In the case of "high affinity" E rosette depletion, the pre- and post-depletion proportion of total E rosettes is indicated.

analysis on the data to determine the relationship between RFC and NK. By extrapolating the data back to the y intercept (i.e. RFC = 0), it was possible to estimate the level of cytotoxicity in preparations completely lacking a particular rosette-forming cell type (21). Using this method, we determined that all NK cells in fresh peripheral blood have the Fc receptor, and that the C3 receptor is present on some but not all NK cells. The latter data also proved that the C3 receptor was not necessary for NK cell-mediated lysis to occur. Although the Fc receptor may be present on all the NK cells, this does not mean that it is necessary for lysis to occur, however, and, in fact, it has recently been shown that NK activity is still detectable after the Fc receptor has been removed from the NK cell (11,23).

In conclusion, human NK cells in fresh peripheral blood appear to be heterogeneous with respect to E and EAC RFC formation (21,24). They may be identified, however, by the fact that their activity is removed by EA rosette depletion and enhanced by routine, predominantly high affinity, E rosette depletion.

Unfortunately, it is not possible to unequivocally state that a lymphocyte is, or is not, an NK cell on the basis of standard surface markers. A specific cytotoxic T cell may well have Fc receptors and conversely, as shown by Kay *et al.* (23), Fc receptor negative NK cells can be produced under certain conditions. For this reason the most reliable marker of NK activity at present is the target cell *selectivity* of the cytotoxic effect. For some reason, which is as yet unknown, certain target cells are lysed much more readily than others (Table II). This hierarchy of target susceptibility is more or less the same with all normal donor lymphocytes, and we have yet to find a normal donor who does not have at least some NK activity against K562. In view of this fact, we selected the K562 target cell assay as the method of choice for the detection of NK cells (5). Aside from the extreme sensitivity of this target cell, there were a number of other compelling reasons for its choice, and these are indicated in Table III and in the accompanying chapter on NK in tumour-bearing patients. One of the most interesting characteristics of K562 is the fact that it is HLA-A, B and C negative (25), ruling out these antigens as targets of the NK cells. Other target surface antigens which have been studied with respect to NK sensitivity are shown in Table III, derived from experimental data and the list of known sensitive targets shown in Table II. The fact that autologous B cell lines are also sensitive

TABLE II. Human NK Target Selectivity[a]

---

1. *K562 (chronic myeloid leukemia-derived (26), erythroleukemia (27))*
2. *T cell lines (e.g. Molt-4)*
3. *PHA-stimulated thymocytes (28)*
4. *B cell lines (autologous and allogeneic) (5)*
5. *Well-established lines from solid tumours*
6. *Some xenogeneic lines (e.g., P815, a murine mastocytoma (4))*
7. *Fibroblast lines (29)*
8. *Fresh tumour cells*
9. *Fresh normal cells*

---

[a]*Target cells are listed in approximate decreasing order of susceptibility, ranging from very susceptible (K562) to negligibly susceptible (normal cells) based on our own experience (4,5, unpublished observations). The position of PHA-stimulated thymocytes on this list was suggested by Dr. H. Koren (personal communication). Some lines are only sensitive in overnight assays. Discrepancies within this list may be found from lab to lab.*

to NK lysis indicates that effector-target HLA differences are not responsible for the triggering of NK cytotoxicity and, conversely, the broad range of sensitive allogeneic targets from many donors indicates that HLA similarity is not essential either. Several years ago we began culturing K562 in human serum, including serum autologous to the potential lymphocyte donor, in order to investigate the role of serum-derived antigens as the target of the NK cell (30). These lines are still NK-sensitive, ruling out fetal calf serum and allogeneic serum-derived antigens as necessary target structures (31). Our lines were also checked and found negative for mycoplasma contamination by both culture and DNA staining. In addition, Tylocine (GIBCO, New York) has been routinely added to the medium used for longterm culture of the cell lines in order to ensure that the lines remain mycoplasma-free (32). In line with our earlier observations and those of others (4,33), the use of mycoplasma-free cultures has not affected our results.

Thus, the nature of the target antigen remains a mystery. Although it has been reported (34) that malignant cells, including fresh pleural effusion cells, are better than

TABLE III. Target Cell Antigens Which Are Not Necessary for NK Sensitivity[a]

1. *Fetal calf serum-derived antigens*
2. *Allogeneic serum antigens*
3. *EBV-derived antigens*
4. *HLA-A,B,C (differences or similarities)*
5. *T and B lymphocyte antigens*
6. *Mycoplasma-derived antigens*
7. *Tumour-specific antigens*

[a]*Although these antigens are not necessary for NK sensitivity, it has not been proven whether or not they are sufficient for this effect to occur. The presence of some of these antigens (e.g. mycoplasma) may enhance cytotoxicity (35), but this is not always the case (4,33).*

normal cells at competitively inhibiting NK against K562 (and hence presumably display a greater amount of the NK target "antigen"), the comparative insensitivity to lysis of fresh tumour cells, combined with the sensitivity of fibroblast cell lines, suggest that tumour-specific or associated antigens are neither sufficient nor necessary for the NK effect to occur. This does not negate the potential importance of NK cells as a mechanism of defense against tumour development *in vivo*, but it does suggest that NK cells may have a broader function than simply surveillance against malignancy.

III. CONCLUSION

Human NK cells may be identified on the basis of source, surface receptors and target cell selectivity. The "standard" NK lymphocyte is detected in the monocyte/granulocyte depleted peripheral blood of virtually all normal donors, is removed by depletion of Fc-receptor-bearing cells while being enriched by depletion of "high affinity" E rosette-forming cells, and is characterized by the selective nature of the target cells which are susceptible to lysis. Using the K562 assay, almost 100% of NK cells can be shown to be Fc receptor-positive, of which at least 50% are low affinity E rosette-forming, and about one-third are complement receptor positive. The nature of the NK target antigen has not been established, but several artefactual and genuine surface antigens have been ruled out as the universal cause of the NK phenomenon.

ACKNOWLEDGMENTS

We are grateful to Mrs. M. Chau, Mrs. J. Tremblay, Mrs. V. Masters and Mrs. B. Milgrom for excellent technical assistance, to Miss Helen Roughton for drawing bloods for us, and to Mrs. Nancy Wainman for typing the manuscript.

REFERENCES

1. Oldham, R.K., Siwarski, O., McCoy, J.L., Plata, E.J., and Herberman, R.B., *Natl. Cancer Inst. Monogr. 37*, 49 (1973).
2. Takasugi, M., Mickey, M.R., and Terasaki, P.I, *Cancer Res. 33*, 2898 (1973).
3. Hellstrom, K.E., and Hellstrom, I., *Adv. Immunol. 18*, 209 (1974).
4. Pross, H.F., and Jondal, M., *Clin. Exp. Immunol. 21*, 226 (1975).
5. Jondal, M., and Pross, H.F., *Int. J. Cancer 15*, 596 (1975).
6. De Vries, J.E., Cornain, S., and Rumke, P., *Int. J. Cancer 14*, 427 (1974).
7. Peter, H.H., Pavie-Fischer, J., Fridman, W.H., Aubert, C., Cesarini, J.P., Rougin, R., and Kourilsky, K.M., *J. Immunol. 115*, 539 (1975).
8. Hersey, P., Edwards, A., Edwards, J., Adams, E., Milton, G.W., and Nelson, D.S., *Int. J. Cancer 16*, 1973 (1975).
9. West, W.H., Cannon, G.B., Kay, H.K., Bonnard, G.D., and Herberman, R.B., *J. Immunol. 118*, 355 (1977).
10. Pape, G.R., Troye, M., Axelsson, B., and Perlmann, P., *J. Immunol. 122*, 2251 (1979).
11. Bolhuis, R.L., Schuit, H.R.E., Nooy, A.M., and Ront-elap, C.P.M., *Eur. J. Immunol. 8*, 732 (1978).
12. Kay, H.D., Bonnard, G.D., and Herberman, R.B., *J. Immunol. 122*, 675 (1979).
13. Pross, H.F., Gupta, S., Good, R.A., and Baines, M.B., *Cell. Immunol. 43*, 160 (1979).
14. Koren, H.S., Amos, D.B., and Buckley, R.H., *J. Immunol. 120*, 796 (1978).

15. Lohmann-Mathes, M.L., Domzig, W., and Roder, J., *J. Immunol. 123*, 1883 (1979).
16. Herberman, R.B., Djeu, J.Y., Kay, H.D., Ortaldo, J.R., Riccardi, C., Bonnard, G.D., Holden, H.T., Fagnani, R., Santoni, A., and Puccetti, P., *Immunol. Rev. 44*, 33 (1979).
17. Pross, H.F., and Baines, M.G., *Cancer Immunol. Immunother. 3*, 75 (1977).
18. Golub, S.H., Golightly, M.G., Zielske, J.V., *Int. J. Cancer 24*, 273 (1979).
19. Seeley, J.K., Masucci, G., Poros, A., Klein, E., and Golub, S.H., *J. Immunol. 123*, 1303 (1979).
20. Kaplan, J., Callewaert, D.M., and Peterson, W.D., *J. Immunol. 121*, 1366 (1978).
21. Pross, H.F., Baines, M.G., and Jondal, M., *Int. J. Cancer 20*, 353 (1977).
22. Dunkley, M., Miller, R.G., and Shortman, K., *J. Immunol. Methods 6*, 39 (1974).
23. Kay, H.D., Fagnani, R., Bonnard, G.D., *Int. J. Cancer 24*, 141 (1979).
24. Vessela, R.L., Gormus, B.M., Lange, P.H., and Kaplan, M.E., *Int. J. Cancer 21*, 594 (1978).
25. Klein, E., Ben Bassat, H., Neumann, H., Ralph, P., Zeuthen, J., Polliack, A., Vanky, F., *Int. J. Cancer 18*, 421 (1976).
26. Lozzio, C.B., and Lozzio, B.B., *J. Natl. Cancer Inst. 50*, 535 (1973).
27. Andersson, L.C., Jokinen, M., and Gahmberg, C.G., *Nature 278*, 364 (1979).
28. Ono, A., Amos, D.B., and Koren, H.S., *Nature 266*, 546 (1977).
29. Saksela, E., Timonen, T., Ranki, A., and Hayry, P., *Immunol. Rev. 44*, (1979).
30. Irie, R.F., Irie, K., and Morton, D.L., *J. Natl. Cancer Inst. 52*, 1051 (1974).
31. Pross, H.F., Luk, S., and Baines, M.G., *Int. J. Cancer 21*, 291 (1978).
32. Friend, C., Patuleia, M.C., Nelson, J.B., *Proc. Soc. Exp. Biol. and Med. 121*, 1009 (1966).
33. DeVries, J.E., Meyerling, M., Van Dongen, A., and Rumke, P., *Int. J. Cancer 15*, 391 (1975).
34. Ortaldo, J.R., Oldham, R.K., Cannon, G.C., and Herberman, R.B., *J. Natl. Cancer Inst. 59*, 77 (1977).
35. Brooks, C.G., Rees, R.C., and Leach, R.H., *Eur. J. Immunol. 9*, 159 (1979).

PHENOTYPIC CHARACTERISTICS OF NK CELLS IN THE MOUSE[1]

John C. Roder

Department of Microbiology and Immunology
Queen's University
Kingston, Ontario
Canada K7L 3N6

I. INTRODUCTION

One of the current enigmas in the study of NK cells relates to their origin and cell lineage within the immunological network. Although we are far from a definitive answer to this difficult question a picture is emerging regarding the nature of the NK cell itself. In this paper I discuss the ontological development of NK cells and recent data concerning their surface antigens, morphology, ultrastructure, cytochemistry and physical characteristics.

II. DEVELOPMENT

One of the characteristic features of the NK system in rats and mice, but not in man, is the rapid rise and fall in NK activity with age. NK mediated cytolysis is low or absent in fetal liver and spleens of newborn mice, appears at 3-4 weeks of age (which is later than immunocompetent T cells appear) and shows a peak at 5-8 weeks followed by a slow decline to low levels in mice 6-12 months of age (1,2). This age distribution of *in vitro* activity is well correlated with resistance to growth of the same tumors *in vivo* (3) and appears to reflect an intrinsic, pre-programmed developmental pathway in NK cell ontogeny. Hence, bone marrow transfer experiments between young and old donors and recipients revealed that recipients always expressed the level of NK activity found in the bone marrow donors (4). With the development of a sensitive technique for assessing the frequency of NK cells by their capacity to selectively adhere

[1] *Supported by the M.R.C. and N.C.I. of Canada.*

ISBN 0-12-341350-8

to target cells, we found that very young (2 week) and very old (1 year) mice possessed only one half the total number of NK cells present in 6 week old mice (5). Therefore the rise and fall of NK activity with age was due to a decline in the numbers of NK cells generated rather than functional deficiencies in those NK cells which did arise. Confirmation of this conclusion awaits the development of NK markers which are independent of the recognition structure.

Several lines of evidence suggest that NK cells are marrow derived. As alluded to above, radiation chimeras repopulated with small numbers of bone marrow or fetal liver cells generate NK activity (4). In addition NK function is markedly suppressed in mice treated with (i) the bone-seeking isotope, ^{89}Sr, (6), (ii) chronic B-estradiol administration (7) or (iii) in congenitally osteopetrotic mice (8). In ^{89}Sr treated mice however the frequency of NK cells was normal as judged by target-effector binding (9). The absence of suppressor cells and the failure to restore NK cytolytic function in ^{89}Sr treated mice with bone marrow infusions indicates that NK cells are not only bone marrow derived but also marrow-dependent (9).

NK cells do not require an intact thymus for development and may in fact be somewhat inhibited by the presence of a thymus and/or thymic hormones as discussed previously (10). Hence, congenitally athymic nude mice (12) or thymectomized mice (10, 11) develop normal or elevated levels of NK activity. In addition splenectomized (11) or congenitally asplenic mice (10) also fall within normal limits. In summary it would appear that NK cells arise in the bone marrow and develop independently of thymic or splenic influence.

III. SURFACE MARKERS

New and exciting work by Kasai et al (12) has revealed an unusual glycolipid on the surface of NK cells, namely gangliotetraosyl ceramide or asialo-GM1. Rabbit antisera against purified asialo-GM1 was highly cytotoxic to NK cells in the presence of complement as recently confirmed in our laboratory. Cytotoxic T cells, thymocytes, bone marrow cells, carrier specific helper T cells and conA reactive T cells were not susceptible to anti-asialo GM1 and complement which indicates that this antigen may be largely restricted to NK cells (12). By using fluorescent antibody techniques to stain individual NK cells in target-effector conjugates we found that the majority of splenic lymphocytes stained were indeed NK cells (Beaumont and Roder, unpublished). It cannot be concluded however that asialo-GML is specific for NK cells since it has been reported that some peripheral T cells react weakly (12, 13). The results suggest rather that asialo-GM1, or a cross-reacting determinant, is preferentially expressed in high concentration on NK cells relative to other cell types.

NK cells have been traditionally classified as "null" cells, lacking the surface characteristics of mature B cells, T cells or macrophages. There is universal agreement that NK cells do not express surface Ig (14, 16) as indicated by lack of depletion on anti-Ig columns or after anti-Ig plus complement treatment. Furthermore, NK cells do not stain with fluoresceinated anti-Ig at the single cell level (Roder, unpublished) in a target binding cell (TBC) assay, nor do they express Ia antigens (Kiessling, R., Hogg, N., personal communication). NK cells do however express serologically detected antigens of the H-2K and H-2D ends of the MHC locus. NK cells do not possess C3 receptors as shown in rosette depletion assays using C3 coated erythrocytes (15, 17). Finally NK function is normal in mice chronically depleted of B cells by anti-IgM treatment since birth (18). These results strongly suggest that NK cells are not B cells and may not lie on the B cell lineage. The one possible exception is the observation that cell fractionation with the B cell selective lectin, soybean agglutinin (19), removes approximately 50% of the splenic NK activity (Reisner, Y., and Karre, K., unpublished observation). Therefore it cannot be ruled out at this time that some NK cells are very early B cells which lack surface or cytoplasmic Ig but express terminal N-acetyl-D-galactosamine residues.

Fc receptors on murine NK cells proved difficult to detect. Initial attempts to remove NK cells on Ig-anti-Ig columns (14) or to block NK activity with immune complexes were unsuccessful (17). Later however low avidity Fc receptors were detected by NK depletion on IgG coated monolayers, a process which could be blocked by the Fc binding protein A (20). These findings together with the observations that NK cells can kill antibody coated tumor targets (21, 23) suggest that murine NK cells like human NK cells possess FcR, albeit of lower avidity.

NK cells resemble small lymphocytes morphologically (16) and with the exception of one report (24) it is generally agreed that they are non-adherent and non-phagocytic, since they pass through columns of nylon wool, sephadex G-10 or glass beads are not removed by treatment with carbonyl iron and a magnet (14, 15, 25, 26). It is unlikely therefore that NK cells are mature macrophages. In support of this view a detailed comparative study revealed that NK cells and activated macrophages had a distinct range of target selectivities and a different genotype pattern of high and low responders (27). In addition it has been shown that (i) NK cells are peroxidase negative (16) whereas promonocytes and macrophages are peroxidase positive (28), (ii) mouse NK cells possess receptors for Helix pomatia lectin (29) whereas cells of the monocyte-macrophage lineage lack this receptor (30), (iii) macrophage and NK cytolysis differ with respect to organ distribution and age dependence (31). NK cells therefore are not mature macrophages but a modifying role for macrophages in the development of NK cells cannot be excluded (discussed in ref. 27).

It is somewhat more controversial whether NK cells represent an earlier stage in monocyte differentiation, namely the promonocyte, as suggested by Marie-Luise Lohmann-Matthes and her colleagues. Both NK cells and promonocytes are non-adherent, non-phagocytic cells with a nucleus/cytoplasm ratio greater than one and both cell types stain negatively or very slightly positive for esterase (16, 32). Functionally both cell types exhibit spontaneous killing of YAC but not P815 cells and are capable of antibody-dependent cell-mediated cytotoxicity (ADCC) (21, 23, 32 - 34). Furthermore cytolytic activities of both cell types are enhanced by interferon (33, 35). In spite of these striking parallels we believe that NK cells and promonocytes belong to separate cell lineages which have evolved convergent effector functions. First, each cell type responds differently to macrophage cytotoxicity factor (MCF) which induces promonocytes (36) but not NK cells (27) to become adherent, phagocytic, activated macrophages with a change in the selectivity pattern of targets sensitive to cytolysis. Both YAC and P815 are lysed by activated macrophages (27) whereas promonocytes lyse only YAC (33). Secondly, promoncytes but not NK cells (33, 37) express a macrophage alloantigen (mph-1) (38).

Thirdly, a detailed analysis of NK cells and a new promonocyte permanent cell line revealed distinct target selectivity patterns, kinetics of lysis and cell properties (39). Fourthly, the level of cytolysis by promonocytes and NK cells follows a different genotype pattern (33) and finally perhaps the strongest argument comes from observations in the beige mouse. This mutant strain has a selective impairment of NK cytolysis with no apparent effect on promonocyte or macrophage effector functions (23,40). Therefore one must conclude at present that promonocytes represent a class of cells distinct from NK cells although a partial convergence of effector mechanisms has occurred.

Perhaps the most controversial area in the characterization of NK cells lies in their phenotypic properties which are shared with T cells. At least two independent groups have now confirmed that NK cells bear the Ly 5 alloantigen (41, 42) which is also present on thymocytes and mature T cells but not on B cells or macrophages (43). Both the Ly 5.1 and Ly 5.2 alleles (42) were expressed in the appropriate congenic strains. It is interesting to note that pre-treatment of NK cells with anti-Ly 5 antisera in the absence of complement also blocks NK cytolysis which suggested that Ly 5 or some closely related structure may be directly involved in target cell recognition or lysis (41, 42). Another presumptive alloantigen, NK-1, has also been found on NK cells of some strains (41, 42, 44) but is not present on mature T cells, B cells, kidney cells or brain cells (44). NK-1 is not expressed on cytotoxic T lymphocytes(CTI) and could serve to distinguish NK and CTL in mixed populations (44).

Most groups have been unable to detect thy 1 on NK cells from conventional strains using antibody plus complement cytotoxicity techniques (14, 15, 17, 25, 41, 44, 45, 46) or monoclonal anti-thy 1 (47). One group, using thy 1 congenic mice or nude mice in particular were able to demonstrate a subpopulation of thy 1 positive cells which exhibited "NK-like" activity (48). In contrast to the negative cytotoxicity results reported by others (47, 49) Matthes et al (50) could successfully separate some but not all NK cells on a fluorescence activated cell sorter using the same monoclonal reagent. The results re-emphasize that NK cells, like NK cell investigators, are a heterogeneous population.

The expression of some T cell antigens on NK cells does not in itself warrent the conclusion that NK cells belong to the T cell lineage. Thy 1, for example, is found not only on all T cells and some NK cells but also on cells far removed from the T cell lineage such as brain cells, epithelial cells and fibroblasts (51). In addition NK cells do not express receptors for peanut agglutinin, a marker for pre-T cells (see below), nor do they express T145, a unique glycoprotein which appears on the surface of cytotoxic T cell precursors upon alloantigenic stimulation (Kimura and Wigzell, personal communication). In summary it would be premature at this stage to place NK cells on the T cell lineage.

Lectins with diverse carbohydrate specificities have also been used to analyze NK cells. Receptors for Helix pomatia lectin, analogous to human blood group A, are uncovered on neuraminidase treated T cells and NK cells but not on B cells or macrophages (52). Since NK cells possess low affinity HP receptors compared to high affinity receptors on T cells, affinity chromatography on sepharose coupled HP has allowed a relative degree of enrichment for NK cells. Others (50) have reported that not all NK cells are HP+, in particular that subpopulation which is thy 1+. If true, these two reagents could provide a useful tool for dissecting the heterogeneous NK pool into HP+ thy 1- and HP- thy 1+ cells.

Vicia villosa lectin has been found to bind strongly to CTL but not NK cells (Kimura et al, unpublished observation). Peanut agglutinin binds to non-reducing terminal D-galactosyl residues on immature, hydrocortisone sensitive murine thymocytes, fetal liver lymphocytes and stem cells in the spleen and bone marrow whereas these residues are masked by sialic acid on mature lymphocyte subpopulations (53). NK cells were not agglutinated by PNA and therefore it is unlikely that they belong to the majority of early, immature T cells (Reisner and Karre, unpublished observations). Soybean agglutinin on the other hand binds to splenic B cells but not T cells (19). Using agglutination techniques coupled with gravity sedimentation it was found that approximately 50% of splenic NK cells had receptors for SBA (Reisner and Karre, unpublished observations). These results suggest that NK cells are heterogeneous regarding expression of the SBA receptor and imply that splenic NK cells are more similar to B cells than T cells regarding the expression of surface glycoproteins.

IV. MORPHOLOGY, CYTOCHEMISTRY AND ULTRASTRUCTURE

NK cells resemble small, metabolically inactive lymphocytes in the mouse as revealed by electron microscopy of target-effector conjugates (16). The majority of effector cells comprising such conjugates have previously been shown to consist of functional NK cells (5, 16, 54). NK cells detected in such a manner had a high N/C ratio, scanty cytoplasm, relatively numerous large mitochondria, inconspicuous Golgi zones, a lack of endoplasmic reticulum or polyribosomes and a predominantly heterchromatic nucleous with a crescent nucleolus. In scanning E.M. the surface was moderately villous. Point contacts were established between target and effector villi and NK cells could often be seen actively engulfing processes on the target. Although most target were eventually lysed by the attached NK cell, no regions of specialized membrane structures or local cytopathogenic changes were noted.

Cytochemical staining of TBC revealed that NK cells were negative for alphanaphthyl acid esterase (ANAE) which was previously shown to stain T cells but not B cells in the mouse (55). NK cells were negative for peroxidase and only weakly stained by acid phosphatase, two chemicals which normally stain cells of the monocyte-macrophage lineage (56). On the basis of cytochemical staining it can be tentatively concluded that NK cells are lymphoid in nature and distinct from B cells, T cells or monocytes.

V. PHYSICAL PROPERTIES

Free flow electrophoresis indicated that NK cells and cells mediating ADCC had a unique electrophoretic mobility midway between that of splenic CTL (high net negative charge) and B cells (low net negative charge) (57). At unit gravity NK cells sedimented with a velocity (4-5mm/hr) comparable to that of small to medium sized lymphocytes. The sedimentation profile was broad however which suggests some heterogeneity in the size of NK cells. Fractionation on linear iso-osmotic density gradients revealed that NK cells were somewhat higher in density (1.082-1.070 g/mm^2) than the median value for the whole spleen cell population. Similar results were obtained in the rat using countercurrent distribution in an aqueous two phase-system (58). Three peaks of cells were partitioned and the peak of NK and ADCC activity was distinct from immunized cells mediating specific cytolysis, cells responding to ConA or PHA and cells bearing sIg. In summary then, physical separation techniques also reveal that NK cells are distinct from the majority of classical B cells, T cells and macrophages.

VI. CONCLUSIONS

As shown in the summary table, NK cells in the mouse possess their own unique spectrum of surface antigens and physiological properties. The available evidence does not firmly place the NK lymphocyte on any known developmental pathway within the lymphoreticular system but rather supports the existence of a separate and unique lineage. The point at which NK cells diverge from T and B cells during development remains an avenue for future research. It is encouraging that several surface markers, some unique, are finally available to allow the unequivocal identification of NK cells. Future work in this area will undoubtedly involve further attempts to subdivide NK cells into subpopulations.

TABLE I. Characteristics of Murine NK cells

Marker	NK	B	T	Promono-cyte	Macro-phage
sIg	-	+	-	-	-
C_3R	-	+	-	+	++
FcR	-/+wk.	+	-/+	+	+
Ly 1	-	-	+	nt	-
Ly 2	-	-	+	nt	-
Ly 3	-	-	+	nt	-
Ly 5	+	-	+	nt	-
Ly 6	?	+act.	+	nt	nt
Thy 1	-/+wk.	-	+	nt	-
NK-1	+	-	-	nt	nt
mph-1	-	-	-	+	+
H-2K,D	+	+	+	+	+
Ia	-	+	-	nt	+/-
asiaol-GM1	++	-	-/+wk.	nt	nt
GM1	-/+wk.	+	++	nt	nt
HP lectin	+	-	++	nt	-
PNA	-	-	+pre-T	nt	nt
SBA	-/+	+	-	nt	nt
V. villosa	-	-	+	nt	nt
ANAE	-	-	+	-	-
esterase	-	-	-	-/+wk.	+
acid phos.	-/+wk.	-	-	+	+
peroxidase	-	-	-	+	+
adherence	-	-/+wk.	-	-	++
Phagocytosis	-	-	-	-	++
Thymus dep.	-	-	+	-	-
B.M. dep.	++	+	+	-	-
Spleen dep.	-	-	-	-	-
cortisone sens.	+	-	+	-	-
89 Sr. sens.	++	-	-	-	-
silica sens.	-/+	-	-	nt	++

Symbols denote the presence (+) or absence (-) of a given marker or property. Subpopulations which are both positive and negative are designated -/+; ?, uncertain data; wk, the marker is weak and difficult to detect; act., present on activated cells only; nt, not tested to the best of our knowledge. References are given in text except for in vivo cortisone (59) and silica sensitivity (60).

REFERENCES

1. Kiessling, R., Klein, E., and Wigzell, H., *Eur. J. Immunol.* 5, 112 (1975).
2. Herberman, R.B., Nunn, M.E., and Lavrin, D.H., *Int. J. Cancer* 16, 216 (1975).
3. Haller, O., Hannson, M., Kiessling, R., and Wigzell, H., Nature 270, 609 (1977).
4. Haller, O., Kiessling, R., Orn, A., and Wigzell, H., *J. Exp. Med.* 145, 1141 (1977).
5. Roder, J., and Kiessling, R., *Scand. J. Immunol.* 8, 135 (1978)
6. Haller, O., and Wigzell, H., *J. Immunol.* 118, 1503 (1977).
7. Seaman, W.E., Blackman, M.A., Gindhart, T.D., Roubinian, J.R., Loeb, J.M. and Talal, N., *J. Immunol.* 121, 2193 (1978).
8. Seaman, W.E., Gindhart, T.D., Greenspan, J.S., Blackman, M.A., and Talal, N. *J. Immunol.* 122, 2541 (1979).
9. Kumar, V., Ben-Ezra, J., Bennett, M., and Sonnenfeld, G., *J. Immunol.* 123, 1832 (1979).
10. Herberman, R.B., and Holden, H.T., *In* "Advances in Cancer Research" (ed. Klein, G., and Weinhouse, S.) 27, 305 (1978). Academic Press, N.Y.
11. Haller, O., Gidlund, M., Kurneck, J.T., and Wigzell, H., *Scand. J. Immunol.* 8, 207 (1978).
12. Kasai, M., Iwamori, M., Nagai, Y., Okumura, K., and Tada, T., *Eur. J. Immunol.* (in press).
13. Stein, K.E., Schwarting, G.A., and Marcus, D.M., *J. Immunol.* 120, 676 (1978).
14. Kiessling, R., Klein, E., Pross, H., and Wigzell, H., *Eur. J. Immunol.* 5,117 (1975).
15. Herberman, R.B., Nunn, M.E., Holden, H., and Lavrin,D.H., *Int. J. Cancer* 16, 230 (1975).
16. Roder, J.C., Kiessling, R., Biberfeld, P., and Anderson, B., *J. Immunol.* 121, 2509 (1978).
17. Kiessling, R., Petranyi, G., Karre, K., Jondal, M., Tracey, D., and Wigzell, H., *J. Exp. Med.* 143, 112 (1976).
18. Gidlund, M., Ojo, E., Orn, A., Wigzell, H., and Murgita, R., *Scand. J. Immunol.* 9, 167 (1979).
19. Reisner, Y., Ravid, A., and Sharon, N., *Bioch. Biophys. Res. Commun.* 72, 1585 (1976).
20. Herberman, R.B., Bartram, S., Haskill, S., Nunn, M.E., Holden, H.T., and West, W.H., *J. Immunol.* 119, 322 (1977).
21. Ojo, E., and Wigzell, H., *Scand. J. Immunol.* 7,297 (1978).
22. Santoni, A., Herberman, R.B., and Holden, H.T., *J. Natl. Cancer Inst.* 62, 109 (1979).

23. Roder, J.C., and Duwe, A.K., Nature, *278*, 451 (1979).
24. Paige, C., Figarella, E., Cuttito, M., Cahan, A., and Stutman, O., *J. Immunol.* *121*, 1827 (1978).
25. Sendo, F., Aoki, T., Boyse, E.A., and Buofo, C.K., *J. Natl. Cancer Inst.* *55*, 603 (1975).
26. Zarling, J.M. Nowinski, R.C., and Bach, F.H., *Proc. Natl. Acad. Sci.* *72*, 2780 (1975).
27. Roder, J.C., Lohmann-Matthes, M.L. Domzig, W., Kiessling, R., and Haller, O., *Eur. J. Immunol.* *9*, 276 (1979).
28. van Furth, R., Hirsch, J., and Fedorko, E., *J.Exp. Med.* *132*, 794 (1970).
29. Haller, O., Gidlund, M., Hellstrom, U., Hammarstrom, S., and Wigzell, H., *Eur. J. Immunol.* *8*, 765 (1978).
30. Hellstrom, U., Hammarstrom, S., Diliner, M., Perlmann, H. and Perlmann, P., *Scand. J. Immunol.* *5*, 45 suppl.5, (1976).
31. Keller, R., *Br. J. Cancer* *37*, 732 (1978).
32. Domzig, W., and Lohmann-Matthes, M. L., *Eur.J. Immunol.* *9*, 267 (1979).
33. Lohmann-Matthes, M. L., Domzig, W., and Roder, J., *J. Immunol.* *123*, 1883 (1979).
34. Herbermann, R.B., Djeu, J.Y., Kay, H.D., Ortaldo, J.R., Riccardi, C., Bonnard, G.D., Holden, H.T., Fagnani, R., Santoni, A., and Puccetti, P., *Immunol. Rev.* *44*, 43 (1979).
35. Gidlund, M., Orn, A., Wigzell, H., Senik, A. and Gresser, I., Nature *273*, 759 (1978).
36. Meerpohl, H. B., Lohmann-Matthes, M.L. and Fisher, H., *Eur. J. Immunol.* *6*, 213 (1976).
37. Ojo, E., Haller, O., and Wigzell, H., *Scand. J. Immunol.* *8*, 215 (1978).
38. Archer, R. *Genet. Res. (Camb.)* *26*, 213 (1975).
39. Kerbel, R.S., Roder, J. and Pross H. submitted.
40. Roder, J., Lohmann-Matthes, M.L., Domzig, W., and Wigzell, H., *J. Immunol.* *123*, 2174 (1979).
41. Pollack, S.B., Tam, M.R., Nowinski, R., and Emmons, S.L. *J. Immunol.* *123*, 1818 (1979).
42. Cantor, H., Kasai, M., Shen, F.W., Leclerc, J., and Glimcher, L., *Immunol. Rev.* *44*, 3 (1979).
43. Komuro, K., Itakura, K., Boyse, E.A., John M., Immunogenetics *1*, 452 (1975).
44. Glimcher, L., Shen, F.W., and Cantor, H., *J. Exp. Med.* *145*, 1 (1977).
45. Greenberg, A.H., and Playfair, J.H.L., *Clin. Exp. Immunol.* *16*, 99 (1974).
46. Gomard, E., Leclerc, J.C. and Levy, J. Nature *250*, 671 (1974).

47. Karre, K., and Seeley, J.K., *J. Immunol.* *123*, 1511 (1979).
48. Herberman, R.B., Nunn, M.E., and Holden, H.T., *J. Immunol.* *121*, 304 (1978).
49. Clark, E.A., Russell, P., Egghart, M., and Horton M., *Int. J. Cancer* (in press).
50. Mattes, M. J. Sharrow, S., Herberman, R. B. and Holden H.T., *J. Immunol.* *123*, 2851 (1979).
51. Williams, A.F., *Contemp. Top.Mol. Immunol.* *6*,83 (1977).
52. Haller, O., Gidlund, M., Hellstrom, U., Hammarstrom S., and Wigzell, H., *Eur. J. Immunol.* *8*, 765 (1978).
53. Reisner, Y., Linker-Israeli, I., and Sharon, N. *Cell Immunol.* *25*, 129 (1976).
54. Roder, J.C., Rosen, A., Fenyo, E.M., and Troy, F.A. *Proc. Natl. Acad. Sci.* *76*, 1405 (1979).
55. Mueller, J., Brundel, R., Buerki, H., Keller, H., Hess, O.W., and Gottier, H., *Eur. J. Immunol.* *5*, 270 (1974).
56. Goud, T.J., Schotte, C., and vanFurth, R., *J.Exp. Med.* *142*, 1180 (1975).
57. Karre, K., Haller, O., Becker, S., Orn, A., Andersson, L., Ranki, A.M., Kiessling, R., and Hayry, P., submitted.
58. Nelson, K., Malmstrom, P., Jonsson, A., and Sjogren, H.O., *Cell. Immunol.* *37*, 422 (1978).
59. Hochman, P.S., and Cudkowicz, G., *J. Immunol.* *119*, 2013 (1977).
60. Kiessling, R., Hochman, P.S., Haller, O. Shearer, G.M., Wigzell, H., and Cudcowicz, G., *Eur. J. Immunol.* *7*, 655 (1977).

MORPHOLOGY AND SURFACE PROPERTIES OF HUMAN NK CELLS

Eero Saksela[1]
Tuomo Timonen

Department of Pathology
University of Helsinki
Finland

I. INTRODUCTION

The basic requirement for the killer action of natural killer cells (NK cells) is their ability to establish close contacts with the representative target cells (1,2). We have taken advantage of this fact and developed methods for enrichment of human NK cells by allowing them to form conjugates with the target cells and then separating the conjugates from the unbound cells by suitable gradient centrifugations (3). The adsorbed effector cells can be dissociated from the targets by agitation and separated from them by subsequent velocity gradients. The method is suitable for adsorption-elution of the NK cells attacking suspension-grown targets, such as K-562 (an erythroleukemia cell line), but it can also be adapted to anchorage-dependent target cells, such as fetal fibroblasts, by the use of microcarrier cultures, which can be treated analogously with the suspension-grown targets (4).

The advantage of the techniques outlined above is that they allow a direct morphological observation of the cell populations selected for the main

[1]*Supported by grant No. 1 RO 1 CA 23809-01 from the National Cancer Institute, NIH, Bethesda, Md.*

ISBN 0-12-341350-8

parameter under study, i.e. the natural killer function. By applying in situ surface marker analyses one may obtain information of the surface characteristics and other properties of this selected population and use morphology as a marker in fractionation studies of human NK cells.

II. MORPHOLOGY OF HUMAN NK CELLS

By using the adsorption-elution techniques outlined above and reported in detail elsewhere (3,5) the natural killer activity of human lymphocytes can be greatly enriched in the adsorbed eluted fractions. This can be accomplished either by using anchorage--dependent or suspension-grown target cells as summarized in Figure 1. Differential analyses of cells on Giemsa stained cytocentrifuge preparations showed that a particular cell type, termed large granular lymphocyte, was particularly enriched in the adsorbed eluted fractions as compared to the input populations (Table I).

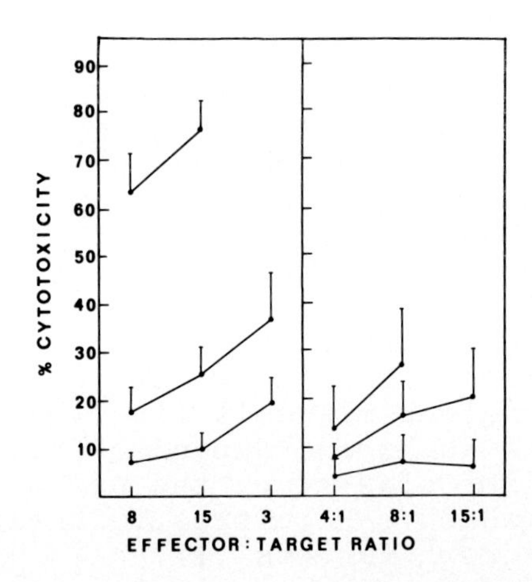

FIGURE 1. Cytotoxicity of target-cell adsorbed-eluted (upper curve), input (middle) and target-cell non-adherent effector cells on K-562 (left) and fetal fibroblast (right) target cells. Means of five experiments (± SD), 18h chromium release assays.

TABLE I. Pattern of Enrichment by Adsorption-elution (AE) of Various Mononuclear Cell Types Using Fetal Fibroblasts or K-562 Cells as Adsorbants

Differential	Adsorbant cells			
	Fetal fibroblasts[z]		K-562[a]	
	Input (%)	AE (%)[d]	Input (%)	AE (%)[d]
Lymphoid cells[c]				
LGL	20 ± 3	52 ± 8[xxx]	20 ± 7	65 ± 8[xxx]
MSL	51 ± 5	40 ± 8[xx]	43 ± 7	24 ± 6[xx]
SL	23 ± 6	5 ± 3[xxx]	32 ± 5	8 ± 5[xxx]
Unclassified	4 ± 2	1 ± 1	2 ± 1	1 ± 1
Monocytes	2 ± 1	1 ± 1	3 ± 2	2 ± 1
Other WBC	1 ± 1	1 ± 1	1 ± 1	1 ± 1
Cytotoxicity	15 ± 6	39 ± 25	25 ± 11	76 ± 22

[a]Mean ± SD of six experiments; ^{51}Cr release test, 18 h, E:T ratio 8:1, FF as targets

[b]Mean ± SD of six esperiments; ^{51}Cr release test, 18 h, E:T ratio 15:1, K-562 as targets

[c]LGL = large granular lymphocytes; MSL = medium-sized lymphocytes; SL = small lymphocytes

[d]Student's t-test, [xxx]$P < .0005$; [xx]$P < .005$ from input

In contrast, other lymphocyte types were significantly reduced in numbers. As already pointed out above, conjugate formation with the target cells is a prerequisite for the killing to occur. Therefore, the relative proportion of the various lymphocyte types making contact with K-562 cells was correlated with the level of NK activity in nine individuals. As seen in Figure 2 the number of LGL making contact with the target cells was linearly correlated to the level of cytotoxicity obtained, whereas no such correlation existed concerning the other lymphocyte classes. The data thus strongly suggested that the human NK activity resided in a lymphocyte population characterized by the LGL morphology.

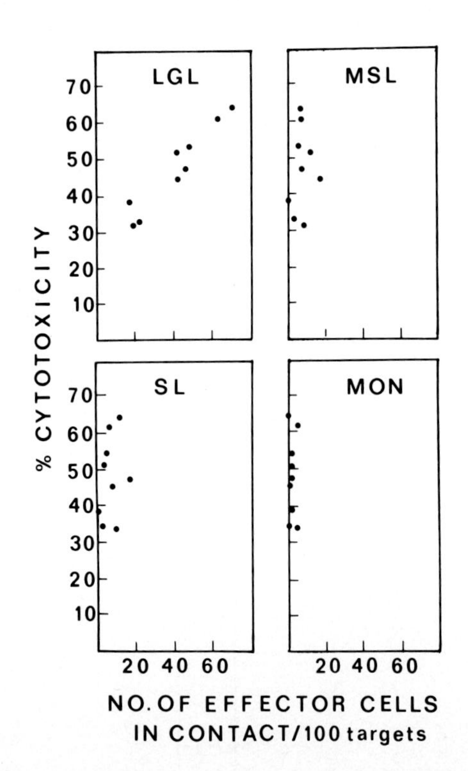

FIGURE 2. The number of various mononuclear cell types making conjugates with K-562 cells correlated to NK activity against the same targets in nine individuals. LGL = large granular lymphocyte; MSL = medium-sized lymphocyte; SL = small lymphocyte; MON = monocyte.

Using the morphological criteria of LGL, which were easy to discern on Giemsa stained cytocentrifuge preparations we screened a number of different fractionation methods to enable a more practical way of enriching human NK cells in large numbers. Percoll gradients (Pharmacia, Uppsala, Sweden) proved to have high resolution power in this respect (6). When discontinuous Percoll gradients were used starting from 37.5% (V/V) with 2.5% steps up to 47.5%, five distinct fractions could be obtained with the NK activity peaking on one single fraction. As shown in Figure 3 the cytotoxicity obtained peaked at a fraction containing over 80% of large granular lymphocytes and followed in intesity the percentual proportion of LGL in each fraction. The bottom

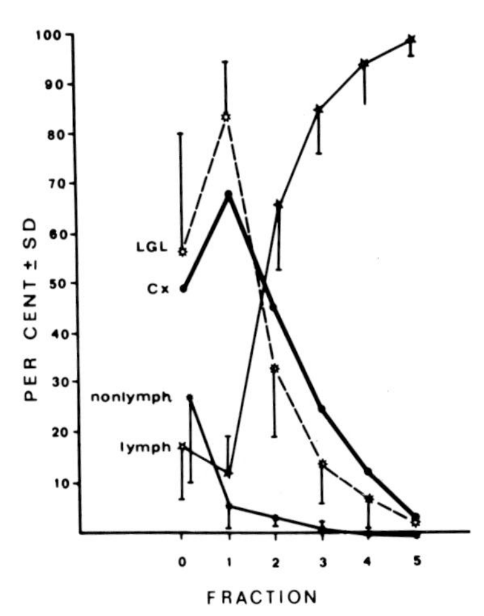

FIGURE 3. Percoll fractionation of Ficoll-Isopaque separated, adherent-cell depleted human buffy coat lymphocytes. Fractions start from 37.5% (v/v) with 2.5% steps, 300g, 45 min. Cx = cytotoxicity against K-562 cells in 4h chromium release assay; LGL = large granular lymphocytes.

fraction contained almost exclusively medium sized and small lymphocytes and had no cytotoxic activity. The fractionation studies thus corroborated the conclusion above that LGL are the mediators of human NK activity. It is also possible to delete specifically the human lymphoid cell populations of LGL by incubating the cells in the presence of 4mM sodium butyrate which leaves other specialized functions, such as MLC response and PHA blastogenesis intact (7). In such LGL depleted populations the NK activity is also lost adding further evidence to the conclusion.

Large granular lymphocytes represent in the average 20% of all lymphocytes in the peripheral blood, ie. about 4-6% of all white blood cells. We do not know whether every LGL is endowed with the capacity to NK activity, although such a conclusion would perhaps not be unreasonable considering the potential importance of the system. Morphologically the LGL are larger and less dense than the lymphocytes in general as shown by velocity and density fractionations (5). They have a larger nucleocytoplasmic ratio and the nuclei are slightly eccentric with an often reniform outline and inconspicuous chromatin. The cytoplasm is weakly basophilic and contains small azurophilic granules best discerned in Giemsa stained cytocentrifuge preparations (4,5,8). The cytoplasm shows a strong granular or sometimes diffuse staining pattern in a modified alpha-naphtyl--acetate-esterase (ANAE) staining (9). This activity is not inhibited by fluoride in contrast to the monocyte esterase activity which is in line with the proposed T-cell lineage of the cells as discussed below (11). In transmission electron microscopy (Fig. 4) the LGL showed relatively abundant cytoplasm containing mitochondria and sparse endoplasmic reticulum. Distinct membrane-coated granules could be detected as a characteristic feature. The nuclei were slightly irregular, often reniform in contour and the chromatin peripherally denser. In time--lapse cinematographic analyses the LGL are highly mobile cells forming polar pseudopodia and changing their appearance rapidly from round to irregular, mobile forms. The cells make short (10-15 min) contacts with the target cells and move from one target to another apparently not suffering damage at the lysis of the target cells.

III. SURFACE MARKERS OF HUMAN NK CELLS

Human NK cells are non-phagocytic and non-adherent cells. Removal of the phagocytosing cells by iron magnetism and removal of the glass-adherent and/or nylon-wool adherent cells increases the NK

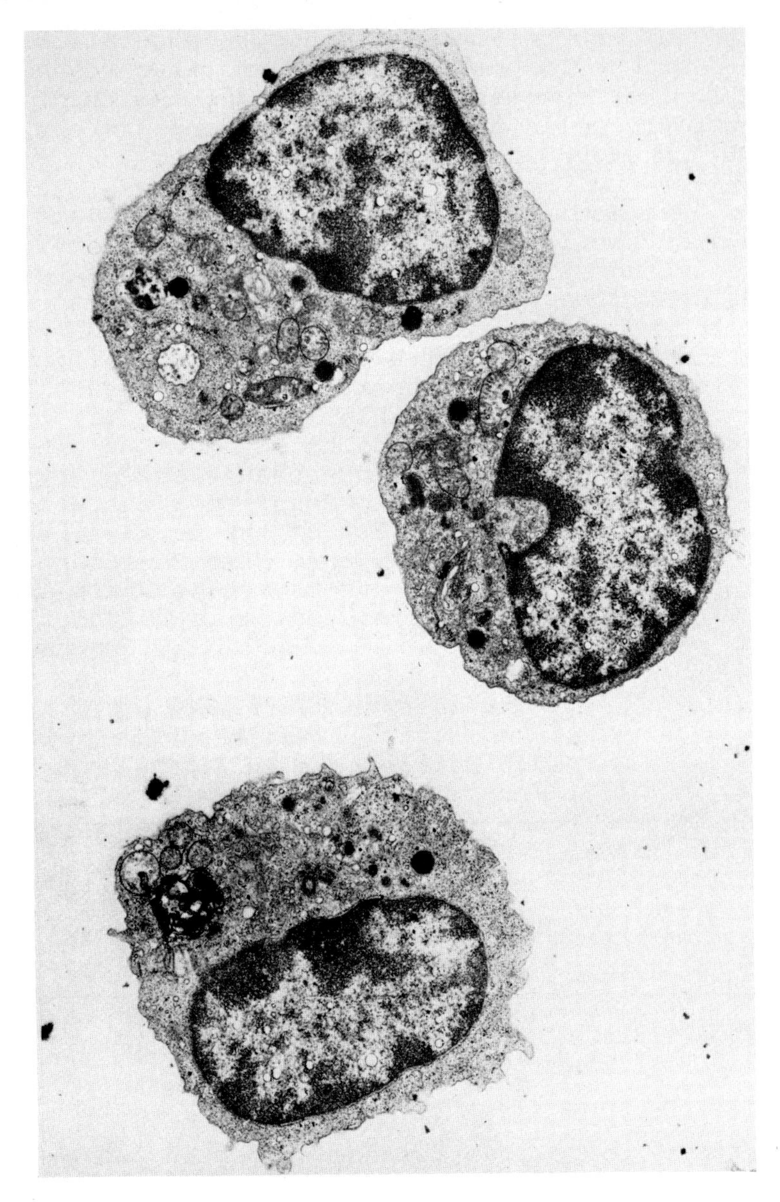

FIGURE 4. Transmission electron micrograph of Percoll purified large granular lymphocytes. Note the relative abundance of mitochondria, sparce endoplasmic reticulum and the characteristic electron dense granules. Nuclei are slightly reniform with inconspicuous chromatin structure (courtesy of Dr. Olli Carpen).

activity of the remaining lymphocyte populations (10). Surface Ig positive cells are also regularly a small minority (less than 5%) among the fractions of cytotoxic cells described above, and are not obviously involved in the NK activity.

We have applied the direct rosette analysis of large granular lymphocyte utilizing Giemsa stained cytocentrifuge preparations according to the techniques described previously (5,8). These procedures allow the morphological identification of LGL on the preparations together with the assignment of the same cells either to the rosetting or non-rosetting categories. As seen in Table II, a large majority of both fetal fibroblast and K-562 adsorbed eluted LGL form E-rosettes (bind more than 4 sheep erythrocytes per cell) and thus express T-cell characteristics. A large majority (76%) of the fetal fibroblast adsorbed-eluted cells form also EA-rosettes (bind IgG opsonized human erythrocytes) whereas only 32% of the K-562 adsorbed eluted cells do this.

TABLE II. Rosetting Characteristics of the Adsorbed-Eluted Human NK Cells Using Fetal Fibroblasts or K-562 Cells as Adsorbants

Adsorbant cells	*E-RFC (%)*	*EA-RFC (%)*
Fetal fibroblasts[a]	65	76
K-562[b]	81	32

[a] *Mean of two experiments*
[b] *Mean of three experiments*

There seems to be a difference either in the avidity or expression of Fc-IgG receptors on the surface of the human NK cells obtained by adsorption elution with these different cell types. As is shown elsewhere in this volume K-562 cells in contact with human lymphocytes augment their NK activity whereas fetal fibroblast do not. The augmentation seems to occur via recruitment of an initially inactive, "pre-NK" cell population to cytotoxic activity. The rosette analysis data are compatible with the interpretation that such augmentable "pre-NK" cells enriched by K-562 adsorption elution but not by fibroblast adsorption are Fc-IgG negative cells.

The above argument on the different expression of Fc-IgG receptors among human NK cells is also reflected in the blocking experiments with aggregated IgG which inhibits the NK activity of Fc-IgG positive cells apparently by steric hindrance. Aggregated IgG blocked significantly the NK activity of human lymphocytes against K-562 cells in a 4 hour assay (Fig. 5). However, preincubation of the lymphocytes with K-562 made the NK activity increasingly insensitive to aggregated IgG blockade indicating that most of the augmented activity was due to Fc-IgG negative cells as the rosetting data above suggested. The data apparently also suggest that the augmented "pre-NK" cells do not acquire the capacity to express high avidity Fc-IgG receptors at least during an 18 h incubation with the augmenting target cells. Morphologically, however, also the augmented "pre-NK" cells have the characteristics of LGL cells, since target cell effector cell conjugates analysed using augmented effector cell populations show the same predominance of LGL cells in contact with the targets (5).

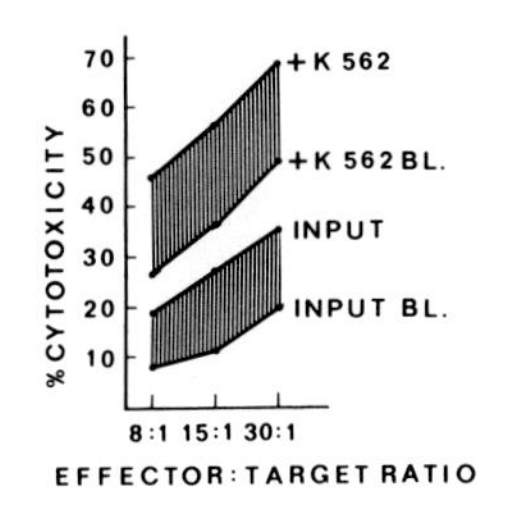

FIGURE 5. Blocking of target-cell augmented and non-augmented human NK activity by aggregated human IgG. Input = cells incubated in medium only for 18h prior to an 18h chromium release assay on fetal fibroblast targets; Input bl. = as above but 160µg/ml aggr IgG added during the assay; +K-562 = effector cells co-cultured with K-562 cells for 18h prior to assay; +K-562 = as above but aggr IgG added to assay.

IV. SURFACE LABELLING PATTERN OF HUMAN NK CELLS

The availability of enriched LGL fractions made it possible to analyse these cells by surface labelling techniques. The LGL fractions were run twice through the density gradients described above and the few remaining cells of the monocyte-macrophage series were removed with iron phagocytosis and magnetism. The fractions contained over 90% of cells with LGL morphology. Their surface labelling pattern was compared to the bottom fractions of practically pure small and medium-sized lymphocytes. The surface labelling was performed by Dr. C.G. Gahmberg (Department of Serobacteriology, University of Helsinki) using galactoseoxidase followed by tritiated borohydride reduction. The homogenized cells were subsequently run on polyacrylamide gels according to methods described in detail earlier (12) and the pattern of radioactive proteins analysed on autoradiographs. The patterns of surface labelling of the above two cell fractions are shown in Figure 6. The LGL cells had a characteristic banding pattern which was different from other lymphocyte patterns in human peripheral blood (13). The cells had a strong

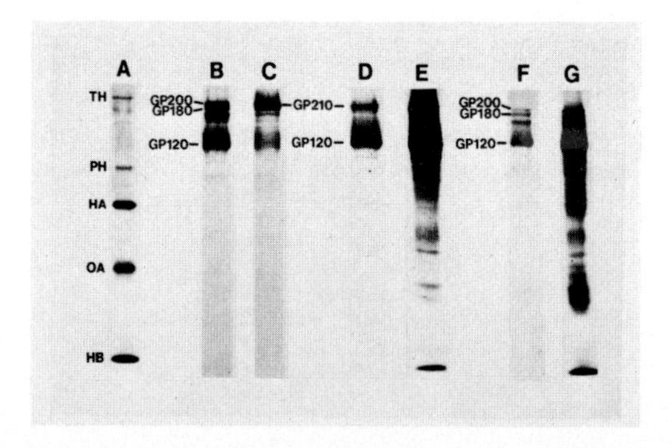

FIGURE 6. Banding pattern of LGL enriched and depleted Percoll fractions using surface labelling techniques outlined in the text. B = reference T-cells; C = reference null cells; D = Percoll fraction no 1 containing 90% LGL; E = the same but with long exposure to show minor bands; F = fraction 5 containing 100% medium-sized and small lymphocytes. G = as E. A = marker protein bands.

band (GP 120) which mature T-cells have but lacked the two distinct bands (GP 200 and 180) of these cells. Instead, the LGL had a strong band (GP 120) characterizing null-cells lacking typical T or B cell markers. The bottom fraction consisted of cells with pure T-cell banding pattern. On the basis of these data the human NK cells resembled T-cells to a certain extent but they had also a typical band of null--cells, and in this sense fell between null-cells and mature T-cells in banding characteristics. Whether one can assign this type of pattern to "pre-T" cells is uncertain but would tentatively be an appealing suggestion.

V. CONCLUDING REMARKS

We feel safe to conclude that human NK cells are morphologically large granular lymphocytes. This cell type represents a sizable population of human peripheral blood lymphocytes, but its characteristic morphologic features are not as readily detected on regular hematological smear preparations as they are on Giemsa stained cytocentrifuge slides. However, Grossi et al. (14) have described human Fc-IgG receptor positive T cells with similar morphology and Ault and Weiner (15) have identified cells with LGL morphology as effectors of human ADCC activity. We have also shown previously that the fetal fibroblast adsorbed eluted LGL are excellent effector cells of ADCC (16). We do not know, however, what proportion of the LGL population is involved in the human NK activity. Thorough adsorption with target cells utilizing the methods described above fail to remove all cells with LGL morphology from the starting population. On the other hand, density gradient fractions devoid of cells with LGL morphology are effectively depleted of NK activity suggesting that functionally the human peripheral blood NK system is confined to the LGL category of cells.

The nature of LGL was studied using known subclass-specific surface markers. Practically all cells with LGL morphology were sheep-erythrocyte binding. The ANAE distribution varied from granular to diffuse positive and the activity could not be inhibited by sodium fluoride. The LGL cells obtained from density gradient fractionations were good responders for PHA and Con-A mitogenesis and our data thus support the findings of Hersey et al. (17), West et al. (18) and Kaplan & Callewaert (19) that human NK cells belong to the T cell lineage of lymphocytes. On surface labelling experiments they also expressed certain T-cell characteristics but had also features of 0-cells suggesting a less well differentiated, perhaps a "pre-T" cell.

Our data indicated that "mature" human NK cells adsorbed-eluted with non-augmenting target cells, such as fetal fibroblasts, were Fc-IgG receptor positive cells whereas "pre-NK" cells, augmentable to NK activity by contact with cell line target cells, such as K-562, were mostly Fc-IgG negative. The functional interrelationships of these NK cell populations will be discussed in a separate chapter of this volume.

ACKNOWLEDGEMENTS

The technical assistance of Ms. Maija-Liisa Mäntylä and Pirkko Kalliomäki is gratefully acknowledged.

REFERENCES

1. Haller, O., Kiessling, R., Örn, A., and Wigzell, H., *J. Exp. Med.* 145, 1411 (1977).
2. Roder, J. C., Kiessling, R., Biberfeld, P., and Andersson, B., *J. Immunol.* 121, 2509 (1978).
3. Timonen, T., and Saksela, E., *Cell. Immunol.* 40, 69 (1978).
4. Saksela, E., Timonen, T., Ranki, A-M., and Häyry, P., *Immunol. Rev.* 44, 71 (1979).
5. Timonen, T., Saksela, E., Ranki, A-M., and Häyry, P., *Cell. Immunol.* 48, 133 (1979).
6. Timonen, T., and Saksela, E., *J. Immunol. Methods* (1979) (submitted).
7. Timonen, T., and Saksela, E., (1979) (in preparation).
8. Timonen, T., Ranki, A., Häyry, P., and Saksela, E., *Cell. Immunol.* 48, 121 (1979).

9. Ranki, A., Tötterman, T. H., and Häyry, P., *Scand. J. Immunol.* 5, 1129 (1976).
10. Timonen, T. (Thesis) University of Helsinki (1979).
11. Ranki, A., and Häyry, P., *J. Clin. Lab. Immunol.* 1, 333 (1979).
12. Gahmberg, C. G., and Hakomori, S., *J. biol. Chem.* 248, 4311 (1973).
13. Andersson, L. C., Nilsson, K., and Gahmberg, C. G., *Int. J. Cancer* 23, 143 (1979).
14. Grossi, C. E., Webb, S. R., Zicca, A., Lydyard, P. M., Moretta, L., Mingari, M. C., and Cooper, M. D., *J. Exp. Med.* 147, 1405 (1978).
15. Ault, K. A., and Weiner, H. L., *Clin. Immunol. Immunopath.* 11, 60, (1978).
16. Timonen, T., *Scand. J. Immunol.* 9, 239 (1979).
17. Hersey, P., Edwards, A., Edwards, J., Adams, E., Milton, G. W., and Nelson, D. S., *Int. J. Cancer* 16, 173 (1975).
18. West, W. H., Cannon, G. B., Kay, H. D., Bonnard, G. D., and Herberman, R. B., *J. Immunol.* 118, 355 (1977).
19. Kaplan, J., and Callewaert, D. M., *J. Nat. Cancer Inst.* 60, 961 (1978).

NATURAL CYTOTOXIC (NC) CELLS AGAINST SOLID TUMORS IN MICE: GENERAL CHARACTERISTICS AND COMPARISON TO NATURAL KILLER (NK) CELLS[1]

Osias Stutman
Elizabeth Feo Figarella
Christopher J. Paige
Edmund C. Lattime

Cellular Immunobiology Section
Memorial Sloan-Kettering Cancer Center
New York, New York

I. INTRODUCTION

The natural occurrence of cell-mediated cytotoxicity (CMC) against tumor cells in vitro has been established in mice (1-8) and other species, including man (1,3). The effector cells of this CMC are collectively known as "natural killer" (NK) cells (1-5). We have used the term "natural cytotoxic" (NC) cells to describe an effector cell closely related to the NK system (7,8). The term "natural" designates the appearance of such reactions in the absence of overt experimental stimulation (1-8). Most of the studies on natural CMC agree that these responses may represent a novel mechanism mediated by lymphoid cells, not sharing some of the established properties of the more conventional immunologically mediated CMC reactions (1-4). Among the unique features of NK and NC cells we could mention (1-8): a) no major histocompatibility com-

[1]*Supported by National Institute of Health Grants CA-08748, CA-15988 and CA-17818 and American Cancer Society Grant IM-188. Elizabeth Feo Figarella was supported by a grant from the "Consejo de Desarrollo Cientifico y Humanistico" and the "Centro Nacional de Referencia en Inmunologia Clinica" from the Universidad Central de Venezuela.*

ISBN 0-12-341350-8

plex restriction of killing; b) no defined "specificity", since these cells kill a wide range of tumor and non-tumor targets; c) no classical immunological memory; d) pre-existence at high levels in the host, in contrast to other immunologic effector mechanisms, which require priming and need time for development; e) their levels and activity are strongly influenced by interferon and e) appear not to belong to any of the well-defined cellular lineages (T, B, macrophage) since the conventional markers used to define such lineages are either absent or difficult to detect on NK and NC cells. Furthermore, it is possible that these natural cytotoxic reactions may be part of a complex defense mechanism directed against a variety of tumoral, viral, parasitic or bacterial aggressions (6), or even against normal non-tumor tissues (1-4). Although some well defined patterns concerning characteristics of the effector cells, regulatory mechanisms, inducibility by interferon, genetic control, etc. have emerged for NK cells (1-4), it is also becoming apparent that a high level of heterogeneity is also part of the system, as indeed the *in vivo* and *in vitro* studies in mice seem to indicate (1-4, 7,8).

During our studies on the *in vitro* measurement of specific CMC against solid tumors in mice, we observed that normal lymphoid cells showed in many instances, high levels of CMC against these adherent targets (7-9). In some instances, as was the case for virus-induced mammary tumors, most of the spontaneous CMC appearing late in life in these mice was mediated by conventional T cells (9), and will not be further discussed in this paper. However, a non-T CMC was also observed, especially using chemically induced fibrosarcomas (7, 8). Although such natural cytotoxicity shared a large number of properties with the CMC mediated by NK cells (tested in short term assays and mostly against lymphomas in suspension), some distinct qualities were observed in this model, using longer cytotoxicity assays with 3H-proline pre-labelled adherent cells derived from solid tumors as targets (7,8). Thus we used the term"natural cytotoxic"(NC) cells to describe the effectors of the observed cytotoxic responses *in vitro* (7,8). The results from comparisons between the properties and qualities of NC and NK cells prompted the interpretation that, although showing some important differences, both lymphoid cell types shared enough similarities to warrant the hypothesis that they belong to a group of "functionally related effector cells" that may be involved in some form of anti-tumor surveillance *in vivo*, as well as having other defense and regulatory functions (7,8). In the same context, and based on the apparent thymus-independency of NK and NC cells (1-8), we also postulated that the "normal" incidence of spontaneous and induced tumors observed in athymic nude mice (10-14), was probably mediated by "alternate pathways" (i.e. non-thymus dependent) of surveillance (10-12), of which NC and NK cells, as well as other mechanisms (11), would be prime candidates (10-14).

In this review we will discuss and summarize some of the properties of NC cells and compare them with NK cells, as well as present some new studies currently under way in our laboratory. Among these new studies, and due mostly to space limitations, we will discuss preferential experiments showing differences in behavior between NC and NK cells, such as the observation that mice receiving chronic estrogen or treated with 89Sr, although having low levels of NK activity measured against YAC-1 targets (as was observed by others, 15-18), have normal levels of NC activity in spleen, when tested against NC-sensitive adherent targets.

However, it should be stressed that, at present writing, it is impossible to clearly decide if NC and NK cells actually belong to different cellular lineages or if they represent different subsets of a functionally related effector population (7,8).

II. THE MURINE NC SYSTEM

A. *Some General Characteristics.*

1. *Assay.* Adherent target cells from solid tumors, prelabelled with 3H-proline in a 24 hr assay, in the presence of variable numbers of effector cells derived from normal animals, were used in most of our experiments (see references 7, 8 and 19 for detailed description of methods). Based on our results with T cell-mediated cytotoxicity, we could show that while the early component of the assay was quite comparable with the short term 51Cr cultures, the later components revealed complex cellular interactions which amplify the T response (19). For the NC system, the time course of cytotoxicity shows low but detectable levels within the first 6 hrs, with a progressive increase and completion of most of the cytotoxicity by 18 hrs, with a slow rising plateau thereafter (8). Figure 1 depicts such a time course of NC-mediated cytotoxicity. Variations of the effector:target (E:T) ratio from 10 to 100:1 showed a good linear relationship (7,8). However, with higher E:T ratios, either no further increase in CMC or an actual prozone-type decrease in CMC was consistently observed (unpublished results). Thus, most of the "standard" experiments were done testing the different target cells at

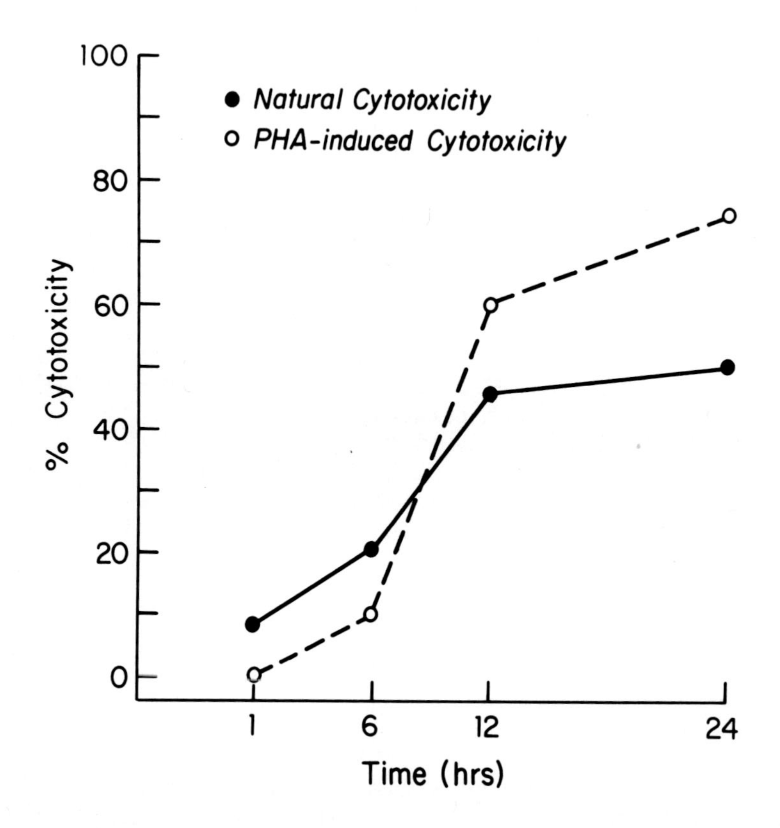

FIGURE 1. Time course of NC-mediated cytotoxicity of normal BALB/c spleen cells against syngeneic 3H-proline pre-labelled adherent Meth A targets, with (•) and without (o) the addition of 2 µg PHA/well, at an effector: target ratio of 100:1.

10, 50 and 100:1 E:T ratios in 24 hr assays (7,8). An NC-like activity against Moloney sarcoma virus-induced adherent sarcoma targets, using a quite similar 3H-proline pre-labelling method and 24-48 hr assays, has been recently described (20).

2. *Target Cells.* Most of our studies have been done with Meth A, a chemically induced fibrosarcoma of BALB/c origin (7,8). This cell line serves as the "prototype" susceptible target for NC cells, in a manner similar to YAC-1 for the NK system (1-5). We also used Meth 113, which is a BALB/c chemically-induced fibrosarcoma (7), which is resistant to NC

cells from syngeneic BALB/c sources, although it is killed by NC cells from certain allogeneic mouse strains (7 and our Chapter in the Immunogenetics Section).

Target cells in the NC system can fall into two categories: a) cells like Meth A which are highly susceptible and killed by NC cells from all the mouse strains tested and b) targets like Meth 113 which show a restricted pattern of susceptibility and are killed by NC cells from only some mouse strains, which may or may not include the same syngeneic strain as the tumor (7). In general, normal adherent target cells such as fetal or adult fibroblasts, are not affected by NC cells (7). Mammary tumor virus-induced breast adenocarcinomas of C3H origin, tested in 3H-proline assays, were consistently resistant to NC-mediated cytotoxicity (7,9), although the generality of this observation needs detailed study. However, it is interesting to point out that of 14 such tumors studied, only one showed high susceptibility to NC killing (9). A mammary tumor established cell-line also was resistant to NC mediated cytotoxicity (7). Some Moloney sarcoma virus-induced tumors appear to be quite susceptible to NC-like cytotoxicity (20).

TABLE I. Susceptibility of Meth A and YAC-1 Adherent or Suspension Target Cells to Natural Cyto-Toxicity Measured in 3H-proline and 51Cr Long and Short In Vitro Assays.

Target cells[a]	*Effector cells*[b]	*Assay*[c]	*Percent CMC at Diff.Ratios*		
			100:1	*50:1*	*10:1*
1.Meth A	*SP*	*3H-P (24)*	*52*	*33*	*24*
2.Meth A	*SP*	*51Cr (4)*	*6*	*3*	*0*
3.Meth A	*SP*	*51Cr (18)*	*20*	*13*	*9*
4.YAC-1	*SP*	*3H-P (24)*	*12*	*8*	*4*
5.YAC-1	*SP*	*51Cr (4)*	*43*	*29*	*16*
6.Meth A	*CTL*	*3H-P (12)*	*89*	*68*	*59*
7.YAC-1	*CTL*	*3H-P (12)*	*86*	*63*	*46*

[a] *Targets were grown in suspension for 51Cr assays and as monolayers for the 3H-proline (3H-P) tests. Artificial monolayers with poly-L-lysine (21) were made with YAC-1 cells.*

[b] *Effector cells were either normal spleen (SP) from 4-8 week old CBA/H donors or immune cytotoxic T cells (CTL) obtained in mixed lymphocyte cultures using CBA/H responder cells and either BALB/c or A/Sn irradiated cells as stimulators.*

[c] *51Cr or 3H-proline (3H-P). Incubation times in hrs in parentheses. For details on tests see refs. 7 and 8.*

However, susceptibility or resistance to NC activity is influenced by many factors. One important factor is whether the target cells grow in suspension or monolayer cultures. Table I shows susceptibility of Meth A and YAC-1 to CMC by normal spleen cells, when grown in suspension or adherent cultures (in the case of YAC-1, artificial monolayers were made using poly-L-lysine, as in 21). Cytotoxicity was measured with a 51Cr assay for the cells in suspension and with 3H-proline for the adherent targets. Meth A, while highly susceptible to CMC by normal CBA/H spleen cells when measured with 3H-proline (Table I, line 1), was resistant to CMC by the same cells when grown in suspension and measured in a 4 hr 51Cr release assay (Table I, line 2). However, higher CMC was observed with the same Meth A targets in suspension tested in an 18 hr 51Cr release assay (Table I, line 3). Conversely, YAC-1 cells were resistant when tested as monolayers with a 3H-proline assay (Table I, line 4) while showing the well known susceptibility to CMC when tested in a 4 hr 51Cr release assay (Table I, line 5). However, both targets grown as monolayers were equally destroyed in a 12 hr 3H-proline assay by specific alloreactive T cells (Table I lines 6 & 7). Thus, the resistance of YAC-1 when grown as an artificial monolayer to natural CMC, cannot be ascribed to technical factors. In addition, we have shown that Meth A and Meth 113 can produce competitive inhibition for NK-killing of YAC-1 cells in a 4 hr 51Cr assay (see our Chapter in the "Specificity" Section).

Nevertheless, these differences in susceptibility to lysis whether the targets are grown in suspension and monolayers are not absolute. For example, RBL-5 and EL4 are quite susceptible to natural CMC when measured either in suspension or as artificial monolayers; P815 is resistant to natural CMC by BALB/c cells when tested in both assays, while Meth E4 (a chemically induced fibrosarcoma of C57Bl/6 origin, see 7), is susceptible to natural CMC when tested in suspension or as adherent target, in a 51Cr or 3H-proline assay, respectively (unpublished observations).

Another important factor determining the magnitude of the cytotoxicity of NC cells against adherent solid tumor targets is mycoplasma infection of the cultures. With mycoplasma infected targets, cytotoxicity indices are markedly increased, reaching at least 70 to 80% at 100:1 E:T ratios, a level of cytotoxicity which is maintained at lower E:T ratios. The presence of the effector cells is necessary to show this effect, since the spontaneous target loss of mycoplasma free or infected target cells alone, within 24 hrs, is comparable (usually less than 10%). This spurious natural cytotoxicity is probably related to nutrient depletion from the culture medium or some form of "activation" of the effector cells by the mycoplasma, since it can be partially prevented by re-feeding the cultures every 6 hrs or by addition of anti-mycoplasmal antibiotic (such as kanamycin) to the medium. We have not made a detailed analysis of this problem, but a similar observation with rat tumors has been described (22). However, this seems to be an important source of a possible in vitro artifact which may mimic as some form of natural cytotoxicity. In our studies, the mycoplasma-related CMC appears to be mediated by a macrophage-like cell, quite different from the NC cell (unpublished observations). All our reported studies using 3H-proline assays have been done with mycoplasma free tumor targets (periodically tested by Dr. J. Fogh, Sloan-Kettering Institute). We have not tested the possible effect of mycoplasma infected targets in the NK system. We have obtained YAC-1 cells from Dr. G. Cudkowicz (State Univ of New York at Buffalo) and from Dr. P. Ralph (Sloan-Kettering Institute), which are mycoplasma free. For other details on growth of the targets, media selection, screening of fetal calf serum, prevention of mycoplasma contamination and other technical aspects of the in vitro assays, see references 7, 8, 9 and 19.

B. *The NC Effector Cell.*

Many of the properties of NC cells (and the comparisons with NK cells) have been presented in some detail in our publications (7,8). We will discuss briefly some of the main features of NC cells, including some additional unpublished information. Other aspects such as ontogeny, genetic influences, "specificity,", etc. will be discussed on other Chapters.

1. *Tissue Distribution.* In our studies with cells from normal BALB/c mice tested for NC activity against syngeneic Meth A target cells in a 24 hr 3H-proline assay, we found a rank of NC activity with different organs at 100:1 E:T ratios (7). The highest activity was observed in spleen and marrow, followed by thymus, peritoneal washings and nodes (7). Table II shows a summary of these rankings, expressed as percent NC activity of the different tissues if spleen activity is considered 100. Our unpublished data with white blood cells gave consistent values of approximately 40-50% of spleen activity. Table III shows some results when marrow and spleen cells from mice of different strains were tested for NC activity against Meth 113 targets (7). Marrow and spleen were concordantly high or low reactors, following the patterns of strain distribution of NC reactivity against this target (7, see also our Chapter in the Immunogenetics Section). However, BALB/c and B10.D2n strains showed higher activity in marrow than in spleen (Table III).

TABLE II. NC and NK Activity in Different Tissues Expressed as Percent of Spleen Cytotoxic Activity

Strain	Target	Assay	Percent Activ. Compared to Spleen[a]						Ref.
			LN(P)	LN(M)	PC	BL	BM	T	
BALB/c	Meth A	NC	32	39	49	40	108	63	7
BALB/c nude	RBL-5	NK	115	207	27	96	15	-	23
C57Bl/6	RBL-5	NK	116	67	50	39	58	0	23
CBA	RBL-5	NK	47		106	-	44	2	24
CBA	YAC-1	NK	36		-	-	40	2	25
BALB/c nude	WEHI-7	NK	48		12	48	12	-	26
BALB/c	WEHI-7	NK	43		86	43	31	0	26
CBA	YAC-1	NK	18		-	142	25	0	39
CBA	YAC-1	NK*	36		-	98	36	0	39

[a]Activity of different tissues expressed as percent of activity in spleen (spleen=100). The abbreviations used are: LN(P), peripheral lymph nodes; LN (M), mesenteric lymph nodes (note that the last 4 experiments used pooled P and M lymph nodes); PC, peritoneal cells; BL, blood white cells; BM, bone marrow and T, thymus.

NC cells were tested in 24 hr assays, using 3H-proline prelabelled targets; NK cells were tested in 4-5 hr assays using 51Cr labelled lymphoma targets. The fourth experiment (ref. 24) used an 18 hr 51Cr-release assay. The last experiment compared normal and tilorone-induced (*) NK cells.

TABLE III. NC Activity in Marrow and Spleens of Different Mouse Strains against Meth 113 Targets.

Strain	No. of exper.	Percent Cytotoxicity[a] Bone Marrow	Spleen
BALB/c	12	10 ± 3.0	5 ± 2.1
BALB/c nu/nu	3	6,11,22 (13)	7,7,20 (11)
NZB	3	33,38,46 (39)	36,39,47 (41)
A/J	3	26,29,35 (30)	33,37,41 (37)
C57Bl/6	3	6,12,23 (14)	8,11,14 (11)
C57Bl/10	2	3,14 (8)	7,11 (9)
B10.D2n	2	15,27 (21)	7,13 (10)
B10.A	2	10,14 (12)	9,13 (11)
I/St	2	12,20 (16)	14-21 (17)

The tissue distribution of murine NK activity shows some similarities and some differences with NC cells: a) there is general agreement that spleen cells are good sources of NK cells, and indeed most of the published work in mice uses spleen cells (1-8); b) with the exception of the thymus, which is consistently negative for NK activity in 4 and 18 hr 51Cr assays (23-26), activity in nodes, marrow, blood and unstimulated peritoneal washings is present, but the magnitude of the response is quite variable (23-27). A summary of some of these experiments is presented in Table II (which also includes data on NC cells), with the results expressed as percent NK activity in different organs, if spleen is considered 100. The variability of the NK levels in normal and nude mice for the different tissues studied (with the exception of the thymus) is quite apparent.

Studies of tissue distribution of NK activity in rats, have also shown variability, although blood and spleen have shown consistently high NK levels (28-30). One study showed that thymus had approximately 50% of the NK activity of spleen (28), while others have shown either low (29) or no activity (30). In humans, most studies have used blood lymphocytes (1), however bone marrow (31) as well as lymph nodes (32) have shown substantial NK-like activity.

In the murine NC system we have found that activity in lymph nodes may be quite variable, and influenced by a variety of environmental factors (i.e. animals obtained from "dirty" animal rooms had consistently higher activity in nodes than animals in clean facilities; tumor bearing animals had very high levels of NC activity in nodes, see our Chapter in the "Tumor-bearers" Section).

The NC-like activity in thymus is presently under study and our results indicate that 90% of the activity is detected on a nylon-wool adherent population and that 50% of the cytotoxic activity of such adherent population can be eliminated after treatment with the appropriate anti-Thy 1 reagent and C. On the other hand, the NC activity in marrow is mediated by cells which share all the properties described for NC cells in spleen (unpublished results).

In summary, the tissue distribution of NK and NC activity

Footnote: Table III.

[a]*Values given for percent cytotoxicity at 100:1 E:T ratios, tested against 3H-proline pre-labelled Meth 113 target cells in a 24 hr assay as described in ref. 7. For all strains except BALB/c the actual paired values for marrow and spleen are given from each experiment, mean values in parentheses. For BALB/c the values are means* $\pm$ *SEM.*

in mice is quite comparable, with one exception: NC shows a consistently high activity in bone marrow which is not observed with NK cells (7, 23-26). The NK-like activity that we reported earlier in the thymus (7) appears to be due to a different cell population. Thus, the "presence of activity in thymus" reported in our earlier publications as one of the differences between NK and NC (7) can presently be dismissed.

2. *Augmentation of NC activity.* In our published work we have shown that NC activity in the peritoneal cavity could be markedly increased within a few days after local administration of BCG or complete Freund's adjuvant (7,8). We also showed that such cytotoxicity was mediated by NC cells, with the same features as those found in normal spleens (7,8). A similar augmentation of NK activity in the peritoneal cavity after administration of BCG (33) and Corynebacterium parvum (34) has been reported. In addition, BCG and C. parvum produced increased NK activity in the spleens of BALB/c mice, with lesser effects on BALB/c nudes (35). Another report, however, indicates that intraperitoneal C. parvum, although increasing NK activity locally, had only marginal effect on spleen NK activity (36). In addition, NK activity can be augmented by interferon inducers such as Tilorone or Poly I:C (37-39) as well as interferon itself (27-39). The role of interferon as a critical regulatory factor of NK activity is well accepted (1-4).

Our own additional studies on augmentation of NC activity in spleen or peritoneal cavity with BCG, C.Parvum and Poly I:C show patterns comparable to those described with the murine NK system (33-39). Experiment 1 in Table VI extends our observations with BCG, showing a marked augmentation of NC activity in the peritoneal cavity against Meth A and Meth 113 targets, either 2 or 7 days after BCG. Normal BALB/c mice show low NC activity against Meth 113 (7), that can be enhanced by BCG (as well as C.parvum and Poly I:C). However, the effect of BCG on spleen NC activity was minimal, against both targets. Table IV also shows that the BCG effect on the peritoneal cavity is not due to mobilization of NC cells from spleen, since the augmentation was also observed in animals that had been splenectomized (Spx) 2 weeks before the BCG administration. Experiment 2 in Table IV shows the effect of two dosages of C.parvum administered intraperitoneally on NC activity in spleen and peritoneal cavity. A marked augmentation of NC activity against Meth A and Meth 113 was observed at both C.parvum dosages. On the other hand, only the high dose of C.parvum produced augmentation of NC activity in spleen, against both targets. Thus, these results with NC cells, follow the same pattern as those observed with NK cells (34, 35). The differences in effect, of intraperitoneal

TABLE IV. Augmentation of NC Activity in Spleen and Peritoneal Cavity by BCG, C. parvum and Poly I:C

Treatment[a]	Percent Cytotoxicity[b]			
	Spleen Cells		Peritoneal cells	
	A	113	A	113
1. None	43	5	26	7
BCG (day 2)	49	13	77	36
BCG (day 7)	56	12	80	53
Spx. None	-	-	32	5
Spx. BCG (day 7)	-	-	78	73
2. None	53	6	18	4
C.parvum (0.7mg)	55	7	84	79
C.parvum (7mg)	83	65	80	77
3. None	46	5	-	-
Poly I:C (1µg)	50	12	-	-
Poly I:C (10µg)	82	71	-	-

[a]All the agents were injected intraperitoneally. BCG (Pasteur) as 10^7 live bacteria (from Trudeau Institute, Saranac Lake, N.Y.); C. parvum at 0.7 or 7 mg per mouse (C. parvum without preservative at a concentration of 7 mg/ml, Batch PX383, CN 6134, from Burroughs Wellcome Co., Triangle Park, N.C.) and Poly I:C and 1 and 10 µg/mouse (Sigma Chemicals, St. Louis, Mo.) Spleen and peritoneal cells from the treated animals were obtained at 2 and 7 days after treatment in the BCG experiments; 7 days in the C.parvum (comparable data, not presented, with cells obtained 3 days after C. parvum) and 3 days after treatment for Poly I:C. Six week old BALB/c mice were used in all the experiments. "Spx" indicates splenectomy performed at 4 weeks of age (i.e. 2 weeks before BCG treatment).

[b]Cytotoxicity at 100:1 effector: target ratios in 24 hr assays, using Meth A (A) or Meth 113 (113) BALB/c fibrosarcoma adherent target cells, pre-labelled with 3H-proline as in references 7 and 8.

C.parvum on spleen NK activity, may be explained by dosage, i.e. the dose showing an effect of C. parvum on spleen was 2.1 mg/mouse (35), while the dose showing no effect on spleen was 0.1 mg/mouse (36). Experiment 3 in Table IV shows the augmentation of NC activity in spleen by Poly I:C. Again, a dose effect was observed, since only the higher dose produced augmentation of NC activity of spleen cells from BALB/c mice against Meth A and Meth 113 targets.

In summary, our preliminary results with agents that augment NK activity, such as BCG, C.parvum and Poly I:C, indicate that comparable augmentation is observed for NC cells, in spleen and peritoneal cavity. This again points to possible relationships between these two systems of natural cytotoxicity in mice.

3. No H2 Restriction. The phenomenon of H2 restriction of T cell-mediated cytotoxicity is well established (40). Thus, homology at the H2 region between effector and target cells is required for optimal lysis, especially in short term assays (40). Niether NC (7, 8) nor NK (1-4) cells show H2 restriction for lysis, and high cytotoxicity levels can be detected using either syngeneic, allogeneic or even xenogeneic targets (1-8). Since most of the H2 restriction work has been done using short term 51Cr release assays (40), and H2 restriction appears to be less strict in longer assays (20, 41), it should be noted that H2 restriction can be detected under the appropriate culture and timing conditions, using the 3H-proline assay with adherent target cells (41).

4. Effect of Pre-incubation. One remarkable property of murine NK cells is their lability after short-term incubation at 37°C (1-4, 42-44), with marked decrease in activity after a few hours in culture. This phenomenon is still unexplained and contrasts with NK cells in rats (29) and humans (1,3) which do not show such in vitro lability. As a matter of fact, both in rats (29) and humans (1), NK activity is increased after pre-incubation, either as a consequence of activation by factors in the culture (such as fetal calf serum, 45) or loss of regulatory cells (46). On the other hand, if murine NK cells are so labile in culture, it is difficult to explain their activity in 18 hr 51Cr assays (24) or that the decreased activity after trypsin treatment may show recovery after 18 hr incubation (44). However, the in vitro lability of murine NK cells may show some strain variation (i.e. spleen NK cells from Swiss nude mice being more labile than NK cells from CBA mice, 44). It is also possible that re-induction of NK activity may take place in the longer assays. As a matter of fact, an increase in NK-like activity has been observed after 6 days of culture (47) or after 3 days in mixed-lymphocyte cultures (48).

Whatever the cause and explanation for this in vitro lability, murine NC cells are stable and not affected by either short or long-term incubation at 37°C (8). NC activity in spleens from normal or nude BALB/c mice was not affected by incubation periods that ranged from 6 hrs to 6 days (8).

NK activity of BALB/c spleen cells declined after 6 hr incubation (8). None of these cultures included 2-mercaptoethanol (8). The addition of different concentrations of 2-mercaptoethanol (2ME) did not affect the decline of BALB/c spleen NK cells (unpublished). With NC cells, the addition of $5x10^{-5}$ M 2ME to the media in which the spleen cells were incubated for 12 or 18 hrs before testing produced a 25% reduction of cytotoxic activity, compared to the activity of the cultures without 2ME (unpublished).

Some recent studies with NK cells have generated ideas that NK and K cells which are effectors in antibody-dependent cellular-cytotoxicity (ADCC) against tumor targets may be identical (1-4, 24, 44, 49-51). This is not the place to discuss whether such assumption is justified or not. However, our own studies have shown that after 6 days of incubation, ADCC effector cells are depleted, while NC activity is still present (8), suggesting that some procedures may be able to dissociate between these effector cells (8). ADCC was measured using 3H-proline adherent mammary tumor cells as targets (8).

In summary, the differences in the effects of pre-incubation on NK and NC activity are supportive of the idea of heterogeneity of these effector cells.

5. *Physical Properties*. A wide variety of procedures for cell separation have been used in the characterization of NK and NC cells (1-8). In this section we will discuss the use of ammonium chloride treatment, nylon wool columns, Sephadex-G10 columns, adherence to plastic surfaces, velocity sedimention at unit gravity and treatment with carbonyl iron and magnetism. All these techniques have been used for the study of NC cells (8).

Ammonium chloride pre-treatment of the effector cells at 4°C, room temperature or 37°C had no effect on murine NK activity (5, 52-54). Similarly, ammonium chloride pre-treatment had no effect on NC activity in normal or nude spleen cells (8). On the other hand, human NK cells are sensitive to inhibition by ammonium chloride buffer treatment (55, 56), although such inhibition is reversible and returns to normal values after 24 hr incubation (56). In guinea pigs' spleen, NK-like cells were not affected by ammonium chloride treatment, while NK activity in blood lymphocytes was markedly depressed (57).

On the other hand, the effector cell in human ADCC against tumor targets is also inhibited by ammonium chloride treatment, although such inhibition is reversible (56, 58, 59). In our own studies we have confirmed this observation using mouse spleen cells as effector cells in an ADCC model that uses murine mammary tumor cells as targets: ammonium chloride produced a profound inhibition of ADCC activity (8), which recovered after 12-24 hrs in culture (unpublished). In those same experiments we had shown that ammonium chloride had no effect on NC cells in spleen (8). Thus, it seems that ammonium chloride treatment is a procedure that may differentiate between NC cells and ADCC effector cells against tumor targets (8). As was mentioned in the previous section, there is a current hypothesis which considers NK and ADCC cytotoxicity against tumor targets in suspension as mediated by the same effector cells, via different mechanisms, in mice (1-4, 24, 44, 49-51) as well as in man (1, 3, 56).

Nylon wool columns have been extensively used for the fractionation of NK (see 1-4 for reviews) and NC cells (8, 20). It is well accepted that nylon wool filtration does not affect NK activity of mouse lymphoid cells (1-4, 35, 39, 42-44, 60-62). On the other hand, although somewhat variable, a 20 to 40% reduction of NC activity was observed after nylon wool filtration of spleen cells from normal or nude mice (8). In addition, cytotoxicity was also observed in the nylon adherent fraction in the NC studies (8). On the other hand, when tested, NK activity has usually been found in the nylon adherent population, although at lower levels than in the non-adherent fractions (43, 60-64). A detailed study on nylon-adherent and non-adherent NK activity in different tissues shows that, although the non-adherent cells have consistently higher activity, a substantial amount of NK cytotoxicity is detected in the nylon-adherent population (64). For example, if the non-adherent spleen value is considered 100, the non-adherent cells in other tissues had values of 112 for blood, 87 for nodes and 44 for marrow (compare also with values in Table II). On the other hand, the values for the nylon-adherent fraction (considering, again, non-adherent spleen as 100) were 48 for blood, 46 for spleen and 22 for nodes and marrow (64). This nylon-adherent NK fraction is consistently eliminated in many studies of NK activity which use nylon wool columns as a routine separation procedure (1-4, 64-66). Furthermore, virus-activated NK cells appear to be more nylon adherent (R.M. Welsh & R. Kiessling, Scientific Report, 78-79, Scripps Clinic and Research Foundation, p. 109). Another feature of the nylon wool filtration studies with NK cells was that, although activity was not affected, only rarely was a true enrichment of NK activity observed (60). In addition, one report indicates that nylon adherence of NK activity may be variable depending on the lymphoma target used for the assay (61). In our own studies with NC cells, we observed that the mild reduction of cytotoxicity after removal of the nylon-adherent cells could be restored by addition of the adherent cells to the effector population (8).

We suggested that such effects could be due to the "...regulatory interaction between cells that differ in nylon adhesiveness" (8), required for proper NC (and NK?) function. Supporting this view is the fact that an adherent macrophage population is required for the augmentation of NK activity by Poly I:C (63). It is possible that some form of in vitro activation may take place in the long-term assays that measure NC activity (and perhaps even in the short term assays, as suggested by the rapid effects of interferon, see 3). Such in vitro activation may explain, among other things, the time course for cytotoxicity (Fig. 1), and the need for nylon-adherent cells, which may be required for adequate in vitro function or activation of NC cells. However, the cytotoxic activity detected in the nylon-adherent fractions, both in NK (43, 60-64) and NC (8) systems, deserves further study.

A good correlation between "target-binding cells" (TBC) and NK activity has been described (64, 65). However, two types of TBC were found, one which was non-adherent to nylon wool and which correlates well with NK activity and a second TBC population which was retained by nylon wool and did not correlate with NK activity, based especially on target binding preference to NK-susceptible or resistant targets (64, 65). Although there is no doubt that the nylon-non-adherent TBC correlates well with NK activity in the YAC-1 system (65), and that binding and lysis may be independent events (50, 65, 167), the relatively high frequency of TBC, even considering only the nylon non-adherent fraction, does not agree with the actual estimates of total NK cells per spleen (25, 62). In addition, the role of the nylon-adherent TBC requires further study. Especially, if the NK-NC systems will turn out to be heterogeneous. For example, the genetic control patterns established for NK cells and non-adherent TBC in the YAC-1 model (2,4) do not seem to apply to NC cells (7, see also our Chapter in Immunogenetics Section) or even to NK cells tested against other targets (18).

Sephadex G10 columns have also been used to separate NC (8) and NK cells (18, 34, 36, 43, 49, 61), showing good agreement with the nylon wool results: NK activity was not decreased after such filtration, whether from normal lymphoid tissues (18, 49, 61) or from peritoneal exudates induced with BCG (43) or C. parvum (34, 36). On the other hand, some reduction (20-35%) of NC activity was observed after G10 with normal spleen cells, as well as with BCG-induced peritoneal exudates (8). G10 filtration completely abrogated cytotoxicity produced by BCG-activated macrophages (8). One interesting feature of the effects of G10 filtration on NC activity was that the reduction was higher (in some experiments reaching 70%) at lower effector:target ratios (8), suggesting that the limiting factor may be an adherent "accessory" cell and not

TABLE V. Effect of Pre-treatment with Anti-Thy 1 and C on NC Activity

Reagent[a]	Strain	Cells[b]	% CMC[c]	% Inhibition[d]	
				C alone	Thy 1+C
Allogeneic	BALB	SP	54	12	7
Allogeneic	BALB-nude	SP	60	14	8
Congenic	BALB	SP	39	13	0
Congenic	BALB/nude	SP	49	19	0
Congenic x 2	BALB	SP	66	10	5
Congenic x 2	BALB-nude	SP	59	6	2
Hybridoma	BALB	SP	56	6	0
Hybridoma[e]	BALB	SP	43	10	0
Hybridoma	BALB-nude	SP	67	16	0
Hybridoma x2	BALB	SP	54	8	0
Hybridoma x2	BALB-nude	SP	63	12	1
Hybridoma	CBA/H	SP	44	10	0
Hybridoma	CBA/H-nude	SP	66	11	2
Hybridoma	A/J(Meth 113)	SP	43	7	0
Hybridoma	NZB(Meth 113)	SP	57	12	0
Hybridoma	BALB	BM	37	17	0
Hybridoma	BALB-nude	BM	48	17	0
Hybridoma	BALB	Thy	36	21	47
Congenic Thy.1.1	BALB	SP	52	8	0
Congenic Thy.1.1 x 2	BALB	SP	44	8	2

[a]"Allogeneic" anti-Thy 1.2 was obtained commercially (Litton Bionetics, Kensington, MD) and used at 1:2 dilutions after absortion with AKR thymocytes as in ref. 79; the "congenic" reagent was obtained from Dr. F.W. Shen (Sloan-Kettering Inst) and was used at 1:50 dilution; the "hybridoma" reagent was provided by Dr. U. Hammerling (Sloan-Kettering Inst) and used at 1:50 dilutions. Noncytotoxic rabbit serum at 1:10 dilutions was used as source of complement. The two step mass cytolysis procedure was described in ref. 8. Effector cells were treated before using them in the CMC assay. "x2" means that the procedure was repeated two times.

[b]Spleen (SP), bone marrow (BM) or thymocytes (Thy) from the indicated strains were obtained from 5-8 week donors.

[c]Percent CMC was calculated for untreated cells as in ref. 7 and 8 for effector:target ratios of 100:1, tested against 3H-proline pre-labelled Meth A target cells of BALB/c origin in a 24 hr assay. A/J and NZB spleen cells were tested against Meth 113 targets (see 7 and 8).

the NC cell proper.

Adherence to plastic surfaces does not affect NC activity (8) nor NK activity of normal lymphoid tissues (18, 60, 61) or of BCG or C.parvum-induced peritoneal exudates (34, 43). One study tested the adherent cells for NK activity, finding most of the activity in the non-adherent fraction (34). However, the plastic adherent cells showed some cytotoxicity against YAC-1 targets (34), which were comparable to those observed by others with non-adherent cells tested against other lymphoma targets (23, 35).

In summary, the studies with nylon wool columns and adherence to plastic suggest that, although the bulk of NK and NC cytotoxic activity is in the non-adherent fractions, some activity is associated to the adherent cells.

Velocity sedimentation at unit gravity. The separation of effector cells by this procedure shows that most of the activity is on fractions that migrate between 4.0 to 5.0 mm/hr, both for NK (34, 44, 50, 65, 68) and NC cells (8), indicating a cell of medium to small volume. The effector cells of ADCC against tumor cells in suspension also fall within that range (44), while the effector cells in ADCC against adherent targets were slightly larger, with a mean migration of 5.7 mm/hr (8).

Carbonyl iron and magnetism. There is also agreement that treatment of the effector cells with carbonyl iron and magnetism does not affect NK (25, 27, 38, 42, 44, 69-71) nor NC cells (8, 20). This procedure, provided that care is taken to avoid non-specific binding of the carbonyl iron (72), removes phagocytic cells. One single report on a late appearing NK-like activity in AKR mice, described marked reduction after carbonyl iron (73). However, a late appearing NK-like cell in BALB/c mice, somewhat similar to that in ref. 73, was not affected by carbonyl iron treatment (71). It should be kept in mind that promonocytes, which may show natural cytotoxicity in vitro, are non-phagocytic cells (74). Thus, the fact that NK and NC cells are not affected by carbonyl iron is presented here only as functional evidence for being non-phagocytic, and not as an absolute property of the macrophage lineage.

Footnotes for Table V, continuted.

[d]*Results expressed as percent inhibition from CMC values of untreated cells.*

[e]*One step treatment with anti-Thy 1. and C.*

6. *Surface antigens*. Our studies with a variety of antisera that recognize surface alloantigens on T, NK and other lymphoid and macrophage cells have shown that murine NC cells in spleen are Thy 1, Lyt 1, Lyt 2, Lyt 3, Ala 1.2, NK 1.1 and Mph 1.2 negative (8 and Tables V and VI). For details on the characteristics of these antigenic systems see 75 for Thy 1 and Lyt, 76 for Ala 1, 66 and 77 for NK 1 and 78 for Mph. Table V shows a summary of our studies with different types of Thy 1 reagents that include antisera produced in congenic mice and monoclonal antibodies (kindly provided by Drs. F.W. Shen and U. Hammerling, Sloan-Kettering Institute). No major effects of the treatment with Thy 1 and C on NC activity were observed. A certain toxicity of C alone was observed in most experiments (ranging from 6 to 19% inhibition). Commercial anti-Thy 1 (marked "allogeneic" in Table V) produced 7-8% reduction of NC activity in BALB normal and nude spleen cells. No such effects were observed with the other reagents, and neither spleen nor marrow NC activity from BALB/c or CBA/H normal or nude mice tested against Meth A targets, were affected by the treatment, even if the treatment was repeated 2 times (8, 79) or whether the treatment was done using a two step (8 and Table V) or a one step procedure (80). In addition, NC activity in spleens from A/J and NZB mice against Meth 113 targets was also not effected by anti-Thy 1 and C. The only exception being the NC-like activity of thymus cells against Meth A, which showed a marked susceptibility to Thy 1 and C, as well as C alone (see Sections II. B.1 and II.B.5 for further discussion of thymus cells). All the results in Table V are with 100:1 E:T ratios, however the same results were obtained with 50 and 10:1 ratios, with or without adjustment for cell numbers after the cytolysis procedures (8, 51). Similarly, not shown in the Table, the same type of results were obtained with different dilutions of the Thy 1 antisera. In summary, NC cells appear to be Thy 1 negative (8, 20). Results, showing no effect of treatment with anti-Thy 1 and C, were found using the type of analysis applied to the NK data (1,44, 51, 79). Then the NC cytotoxic activity was expressed in "lytic units" obtained from the linear part of the dose-response curve in 6 or 12 hr assays (see Fig. 1), no effect of anti-Thy 1 was observed, beyond the effects of C alone (unpublished), whether the lytic units were defined as the number of effector cells needed for production of 25 (79), 15 (51) or 1 (44) percent cytotoxicity above baseline.

Small amounts of Thy 1 on NK cells have been reported (1, 3, 35, 42, 51, 79) and this fact is generally accepted, as judged from review articles (1-4). However, the issue of the presence of Thy 1 on NK cells is not completely settled: a) with the usual cytolysis procedures that will eliminate Thy 1 positive cells or other types, many laboratories have shown no effect of the treatment on NK activity, in a variety of natural or augmented murine models (15, 18, 25, 34, 39, 43, 61,

62, 66, 69, 71, 73, 80-83); b) some effects on NK cells (1, 3, 35, 42, 51, 60, 79), especially after two consecutive treatments (79), as well as partial enrichment after fluorescent cell-sorting (51), have been reported, suggesting that some NK cells have low but detectable amounts of surface Thy 1 (1, 3, 51, 79); c) however, studies from the same laboratory as those discussed in (b) have shown that the issue is not simple and that Thy 1+ as well as Thy 1- NK cells may coexist (38, 44, 51) depending on strain and whether the cells were from normal or nude mice (44); d) in addition, when tested in 18 hr 51Cr assays, treatment of the effector cells could either increase NK activity or show no effect, depending on whether the cells were from normal or nude mice (44); e) similarly, Poly I:C augmented NK activity was also not affected by treatment with anti-Thy 1 (38); f) the NK-like activity appearing 3 days after mixed lymphocyte culture is mediated by a Thy 1 positive blast cell, termed "anomalous killer" (48): and g)on the other hand, the NK cells which appear after 6 days of culture (47) or after 4 days in Mishell-Dutton cultures (83), are Thy 1 negative. Thus, it is tempting to postulate that the NK compartment comprises cells with a range of surface Thy 1 expression, which goes from the undetectable to the clearly positive. On the other hand, NC cells are Thy 1 negative. Whether these cells represent the true lineage of the NK system or the heterogeneity is indicative of different effector cells all capable of exerting an NK-like cytotoxicity, deserves further analysis. A third, less attractive possibility, is that cross-reactive contaminants in the biological reagents may be involved in some of those results. It is obvious, on the other hand, that the presence of Thy 1 on some NK cells, does not necessarily mark them as belonging to the T cell lineage, since Thy 1 is expressed on other tissues as well (75).

Table VI shows that NC cells from mice of the appropriate "positive" (+) strains for the different alleles of several serological reagents that recognize antigenic systems on T cells (Lyt 1, 2, 3), NK cells (NK 1), T and B cells (Ala 1) and macrophages (Mph 1) are not affected by such treatments. Only occasional marginal effects are observed, sometimes in cells of mice of the inappropriate phenotype, suggesting contaminants or other technical reasons. Thus, one can postulate that NC cells do not express Lyt 1, 2 or 3, Ala 1, NK 1 or Mph 1 antigens on their surface. In addition, we have shown that treatment with rabbit anti-mouse brain and C had no effect on NC activity (8).

Ala 1 recognizes an antigen on "activated" lymphoid cells, including T and B cells (76). Genetic studies have suggested a close relationship between Ly 6, Ly 8 and Ala 1, to the point that either these loci are "extremely closely linked or

TABLE VI. *Effect of Pre-treatment with Anti-Lyt, NK and Mph and C on NC Activity in Spleen*

Reagent[a]	Source of cells[b]	Percent CMC[c]	Percent inhibition[d] C alone	Percent inhibition[d] Ab+C
Ala 1.2[e]	DBA/2 (+)	48	5	0
	C57Bl/6 (+)	56	3	0
	BALB/c (-)	60	5	0
Lyt 2.1	DBA/2 (+)	53	16	3
	CBA/H (+)	49	9	2
	B6.Ly 2.1 (+)	46	14	0
	BALB/c (-)	56	11	2
Lyt 2.2	C57Bl/6 (+)	48	7	7
	A/J (+)	53	6	2
	BALB/c (+)	60	14	4
	CBA/H (-)	51	10	0
Lyt 1.1	CBA/H (+)	77	8	0
	DBA/2 (+)	49	13	5
	B6.Ly 1.1 (+)	43	7	0
	BALB/c (-)	71	5	8 (?)
	C57Bl/6 (-)	63	8	0
Lyt 1.2	C57Bl/6 (+)	49	3	3
	BALB/c (+)	45	18	0
	CBA/H (-)	52	8	2
Lyt 3.2	CBA/H (+)	63	7	2
	BALB/c (+)	42	8	0
NK 1.1 (1:10)	C57Bl/6 (+)	73	7	3
	NZB (+)	60	9	2
	BALB/c (-)	59	7	0
NK 1.1 (1:2)	C57Bl/6 (+)	56	11	2
	BALB/c (-)	68	6	0
NK 1.1 (1:2)[e]	C57Bl/6 (+)	54	10	3
Mph 1.2[e]	BALB/c (+)	66	5	0
	I/St (-)	59	6	0
	BALB/c (+)[f]	70	6	2
	BALB/c (+)[g]	89	4	45

[a]Ala 1.2 was obtained from Dr. A. Feeney (Univ. California at San Diego, CA), Lyt reagents and NK 1.1 were obtained from Dr. F.W. Shen (Sloan-Kettering Inst.) and Mph 1.2 from Searle Laboratories (High Wycombe, England). For further details on these reagents see 76, 75, 77 and 78 respectively. For details on two step or one step cytolysis procedures see ref. 8. With the exception of the Lyt 2.1 reagent which was used at 1:100 dilutions, all other antisera were used at 1:10 dilutions, unless otherwise stated. In two step procedures cells were incubated for 30 min with antibody and subsequently another 30 min with C. The one step assay used 45 min incubations.

that the sera recognize different antigenic sites on a single gene product" (84). Ly 6 has been reported as present on NK cells (80). The *Lyt 1, 2 and 3* antigens are well accepted markers for T cells (75). However, NK 1 was defined, from studies on a contaminant of Lyt 1.2 antisera (66). With this proviso, NK cells have been found negative for Lyt 2 (66, 77, 80) as well as Lyt 1 (66, 80). *Mph 1* is an antigen present on a subpopulation of macrophages (78). One study reports that C. parvum induced NK cells in peritoneal cavity are Mph negative (34), while another study shows approximately 40% reduction of NK-like activity mediated by promonocytes (74). Our own studies show that Mph 1 is absent from BCG-induced peritoneal NC cells, while the antiserum produced a 45% reduction of the cytotoxicity mediated by peritoneal activated macrophages (last line, Table VI).

NK 1 was the first antigenic marker which appears to be exclusive for NK cells, tested against RL♂1 targets (66, 77). Table VI shows that treatment with anti-NK 1.1 and C in a one or two step cytolysis procedure had no effect on NC activity of spleen cells from mice of the appropriate strains (8). On the other hand, the same treatment produced a 40% reduction of NK activity of spleen cells from C57Bl/6 mice tested against RBL-5 targets (8) and 65 to 79% reduction against YAC-1 targets (unpublished). A recent publication also shows reduction of NK activity against YAC-1 targets by an anti-NK 1.1

Footnotes for Table VI, continued.

Mph 1.2 used a one step incubation assay of 90 min. Rabbit serum pre-screened for low toxicity at 1:12 dilutions was used for all assays except Ala 1.2 which used 1:8 dilution of guinea pig serum and Mph 1.2 which used 1:2 dilutions of guinea pig serum.

[b] *Spleen cells were derived from the indicated strains from 5-8 week donors. In parentheses, whether the strains are "positive" or "negative" for the antigens detected by the different alloantisera.*

[c] *Cell-mediated cytotoxicity (CM) calculated as in ref. 7, 8 for 100:1 effector target ratios, tested against Meth A targets in a 24 hr assay.*

[d] *Percent inhibition after treatment with C alone or antibody + C, compared to the control values of untreated spleen.*

[e] *Indicates a one-step cytolysis assay.*

[f] *Peritoneal cells, 5 days after BCG administration.*

[g] *Peritoneal cells, 15 days after BCG, tested in a 48 hr CMC assay.*

(80). Some of our preliminary results with anti-NK 1.1 antiserum (obtained from Dr. F.W. Shen, Sloan-Kettering Inst.), deserve comment. As mentioned before, NC cells from adult spleens appear as NK 1 negative, however, we have found a 34 and 41% reduction of NC activity by pretreatment with anti-NK 1.1 and C in two experiments in which newborn C57Bl/6 spleen cells were studied against Meth A targets (see also our Chapter in the "Ontogeny" Section). If this observation is further documented, it may represent an interesting link between the NC and NK system, since the only apparent discrepancy between presence of NK 1 positive cells and NK cytotoxic activity, happens to be the newborn and infant spleen (G. Koo, Sloan-Kettering Inst., personal communication).

Other antisera that react against NK cells (among other cell types which include T cells) have been described, such as Ly 5 (77, 80), Ly 6 (80) and Qa 5 (83). None of these reagents have been tested against NC cells, although we have tested Ala 1, which is closely related to Ly 6 (84), with negative results (Table VI). Using a CE anti-CBA reagent which appears to recognize the other allele of NK.1, Drs. R.C. Burton and H.J. Winn from the Massachusetts General Hospital, Boston, MA, have demonstrated an interesting heterogeneity among NK cells (personal communication, manuscript submitted to J. Immunology). NK_L which lyse lymphoma cells in 4 hr 51Cr assays are destroyed by treatment with the anti-NK reagent and anti H-2 antisera, while NK_S cells which lyse solid tumors in a 16 hr 51Cr assay, were resistant to treatment with the anti-NK as well as H-2 antibodies and C. The correlation between NK_S and NC cells deserves further study.

7. *Surface Ig, Fc Receptors, etc.* As the nylon wool, and especially the Sephadex G10 columns data suggested, neither NK (1-4, 25, 36, 39, 42, 43, 61, 62, 73, 81, 85) nor NC cells (8) have detectable *surface Ig*, demonstrated by several separation procedures including Ig-anti Ig columns. In addition B-cell deprived mice, obtained by treatment with heterologous anti-IgM serum showed normal levels of NK activity (85). Similarly, good NK (1, 23) and NC (7) activity were observed in CBA/HN mice, which have a B cell defect. As part of a study to define the resistance to polyoma tumor development observed in 4-5 month old CBA/H nude mice (11), we studied a small number of nude CBA/H animals with a marked B cell deficiency and low or undetectable Ig levels, produced by administration of a heterologous anti-mouse mu chain since birth (as described in 85), for NK and NC activity in spleen tested against YAC-1 and Meth A target cells, respectively, at 5-8 weeks of age. In 6 anti-mu treated nudes and 6 control nudes (treated with normal rabbit Ig), no major differences in NK or NC activity were observed, and in some animals

of the anti-mu group, an actual increase in NK and NC activity was observed (approximately 10 to 15% increase versus the controls). For example, at 100:1 E:T ratios, the NC levels were 42, 47, 46, 50, 57, 60 for the controls and 50, 54, 66, 67, 58 and 60 for the paired anti-mu-treated nudes.

The presence of *Fc receptors* on murine NK cells is still open to some debate (1-4). The enrichment of NK activity after passage through Ig-anti-Ig columns (25, 62), as well as the lack of depletion when passed through antigen-antibody complex columns (42), enrichment after removal of Fc positive cells by a rosette technique (39) or the lack of effect after absortion onto antigen-IgG antibody complex monolayers (18, 42), suggest that either NK cells do not display Fc receptors or that such receptors, if present, are of low avidity. However, when antigen-IgG antibody monolayers were used and the calculation was done taking into account the cell recovery in the fractions and the cytotoxicity values were expressed in lytic units capable of 25 (68) or 10% (44) target lysis, a 70% reduction in NK lytic units after such absortions was observed and the depletion could be blocked by treatment of the monolayers with Protein A (44, 68). It is well accepted that human NK cells display readily detectable Fc receptors (1,3).

There is some evidence that NK and K cells which mediate ADCC against tumor targets may be quite similar (1-4, 24, 44, 49, 50, 69). On the otherhand, aggregated IgG does not block NK-mediated cytotoxicity (42, 43, 62) while it blocks ADCC against tumor targets (49). Thus, whatever the avidity of the Fc receptors on some NK cells, such receptors do not seem to be involved in the NK-lytic event (42, 43, 62) while they still may be sufficiently functional for some of those cells to act as effectors in ADCC against tumor targets (24, 44, 49). In summary, it is generally accepted that either "in the mouse, NK cells do not display high avidity receptors for IgG" (49); that the Fc receptors are "detected with difficulty" and the avidity may be "quite heterogeneous" (1) or that one should be "reluctant to accept the presence of Fc receptors for IgG on murine NK cells from binding data alone" (4). The functional data on ADCC, on the other hand, suggests that Fc positive cells may represent another subpopulation within the NK compartment (44, 49).

Our own data with NC cells showed that NC-mediated cytotoxicity, as was the case with NK cells, was not affected by aggregated Ig (8), indicating that, if present, the Fc receptor was not involved in the lytic event.

Table VII shows some of our unpublished results on depletion of Fc positive cells and their effects on NC and ADCC activity. It is apparent that, absortion of cells to the antigen-antibody monolayers produced an enrichment of NC ac-

TABLE VII. Effect of Removal of Fc Positive Cells on NC and ADCC Activity of BALB/c Spleen Cells

Treatment[a]	Percent recovery[b]	Percent cytotoxicity[c] NC (Meth A)	ADCC (MT)
Unfractioned	100	49	53
E-monolayers	60	45 (9%)	50 (6%)
EA-monolayers	26	76 (0%)	12 (78%)
EA-Prot. A monolayers	54	46 (7%)	47 (12%)
Unfractioned	100	38	44
FcR depletion	16	91 (0%)	5 (89%)

[a]Spleen cells from 5-8 week old BALB/c mice were fractioned using sheep-red blood cell monolayers (E), SRBC-anti-SRBC monolayers (EA), or Protein A treated EA-monolayers, produced as described in refs. 44 and 68; FcR depletion was produced by formation of rosettes with anti-Forssman IgG coated SRBC, and the rosettes removed by velocity sedimentation in Ficoll, as described in ref. 39.

[b]Recoveries after absortion or fractionation, as percent of unfractioned spleen.

[c]Percent cytotoxicity calculated as in ref.7, 8, using 100:1 effector: target ratios (data, with comparable results for 50 and 10:1, not shown). Percent reduction of activity after fractionation in parentheses. NC cells were tested against 3H-proline pre-labelled Meth A targets in a 24 hr assay (as in ref. 7, 8). ADCC, tested against a C3H mammary tumor target, pre-labelled with 3H-proline, in the presence of rabbit anti-whole-disrupted mammary tumor virus, in a 12 hr assay as described in 8.

tivity which was also observed after removal of the Fc positive cells by a rosette technique. Conversely, both procedures produced a 78 and 89% reduction, respectively, of ADCC activity against an adherent mammary tumor target. The same type of results were obtained if the values were expressed as activity per recovered fraction (68). Thus, NC cells appear to have undetectable Fc receptors and this property can differentiate them from the K cells which act as effector cells in ADCC responses against tumor targets. When we tested the NK activity of similarly separated spleen cells (against YAC-1 cells in a 4 hr 51Cr assay), using the FcR depletion procedure, the percent cytotoxicity for the unfractioned population was 33, 21 and 10 (at 100, 50 and 10:1 effector:target ratios) and 72, 55 and 39 for the FcR-depleted population, showing a substantial enrichment of anti-YAC NK activity, as was observed by others using a similar technique (39). With the EA monolayers, the percent recovery of lytic units (LU_{25}) after absorption ranged from 50 to 79% (unpublished) which is much higher than the approximately 20% recovery described by Herberman et al. (68), using RL♂1 targets. Whether these differences are due to subpopulations of NK cells or of different requirements for Fc-positive NK cells, depending on targets, awaits further study.

The treatment of NC (8) or NK cells (43, 44, 62) with *trypsin* produced a reversible decrease in cytotoxic activity. Thus, a "trypsin-sensitive" structure appears important for cytotoxicity mediated by NC and NK cells. On the other hand, although a relationship between NK and ADCC effectors against tumor targets has been proposed (see above), trypsin treatment of the effector cells had no effect on the ADCC system (44). NC cells could recover after trypsin treatment within 4-8 hrs, even when cultured in serum free medium or after depletion of B cells and adherent cells (unpublished), suggesting that, as appears to be the case for NK cells (4, 44), cytotoxic activity is not mediated via arming by antibodies or serum components, as has been suggested by some human (86 and murine studies (87).

In summary: a) both NC and NK cells do not display surface Ig; b) some NK cells may have low avidity Fc receptors, while NC appear as having no Fc receptors; c) some NK cells may act as effector cells in ADCC systems against tumor targets, while with our ADCC tumor target model, NC cells can be separated from the ADCC effectors (8); d) both NC and NK cytoxicity is not affected by aggregated Ig or similar treatments, suggesting that, if present, the Fc receptor is not involved in the lytic event; e) both NC and NK cells have trypsin-sensitive structures and trypsin treatment produces reversible inhibition of cytotoxicity and finally, f) both NC and NK activity is not mediated by some "arming" mechanism.

8. Nude versus Normals. NC activity is detected both in nude as well as in normal mice (7, 8). However, we could not find consistent differences in NC activity in spleen, marrow or other tissues between nude and normal animals (7, 8). In the NK system, several studies have shown higher activity in nudes (23, 25, 29, 35, 88), while others have shown only modest differences (24, 33), and in some cases, especially after augmentation of NK activity by different agents, no differences between nudes and normal were observed (18, 39, 81). Therefore, the "high" NK levels in nudes has been considered to be indicative of some form of T cell regulation of NK activity (1). Indeed, a decrease in NK activity after thymus grafting has been described in nudes (1).

However, in view of the interferon-dependent augmentability of the NK system (35, 37-39, 81, 89) it is also possible that the high NK activity in nudes may be secondary to the increased susceptibility to infections which arises as a consequence of the thymus deficiency in nudes (10, 12). Thus, the correction of the defect by thymus grafting, would bring down the NK levels not through a direct T cell regulation but as the secondary consequence of a better handling of infections by the restored animals. In addition, in radiation chimeras made between cell donors and hosts that differ in NK levels, the addition of T cells had no effect on the NK levels produced by the donor marrow (90). Thus, T cells from a low NK strain did not affect the high NK levels produced by marrow from a high NK strain in a low NK recipient (90).

As part of our studies on the genetic control of NC activity against Meth 113 targets (see our Chapter in the Immunogenetics Section), we made radiation chimeras of low NC-C57Bl/6 mice (B6) and high NC-B6.Tla^a bone marrow donors and found that the chimeras, tested 8 weeks after reconstitution, showed that high NC activity of the marrow donor, as was observed in the NK system (2, 4, 90). In these studies we also included thymectomized hosts, which were restored with high NC-marrow plus T cells from the high (B6.Tla^a) or the low (B6) NC strains. No differences in the high NC levels in spleen or other tissues, were observed between these chimeras, suggesting that neither the thymus nor T cells play a major role in regulating NC levels of activity (unpublished, see our Chapter in the Immunogenetics Section).

C. *Other Properties of the NC System*

In this section we will mainly discuss the effects of irradiation, cyclophosphamide (and other drugs including chemical carcinogens), hydrocortisone, ^{89}Sr and estrogen on NC activity and compare the results with the effects of such treatments on NK cells. It is obvious that all the procedures described above, whether or not they affect NC or NK levels, may be doing so by very different mechanisms. Accepting a minimal, four compartment model for NK or NC differentiation these agents may be acting at any of all levels which may affect NC-NK activity in a given organ. Our simple model includes: a) a precursor compartment (pre-NC or NK); b) an accessory-cell compartment (63), which contains the cell/s that either present the "interferon signal" to the pre-NC cell or actually produce interferon by themselves; c) the effector cell compartment that contains the "mature" NC or NK cells and d) a regulatory compartment (92-94), probably acting on the other three. The actual NC or NK levels measured in the cytotoxicity assays with cells from a given organ are just the summation of the possible interactions between compartments. One important characteristic that will emerge from the brief description of our unpublished results with these procedures is that NC cells are more resistant to these treatments than NK cells, and in some cases not affected at all by treatments that produce almost total abrogation of NK activity.

1. Irradiation. From the available literature on murine NK cells, the effects of irradiation are still open to analysis. In reviews, murine NK cells have been called "moderately resistant" (1) or showing "relative insensitivity" (2) to whole body irradiation. As a matter of fact, the possible association of NK activity and resistance to hemopoietic grafts, is centered on the radioresistance of both functions in mice (2, 17, 91). However, the information on NK is contradictory: a) no decline of NK activity in spleen, or even enrichment, was observed 1 day after 100 to 1100 R of whole body irradiation (17, 91, 92, 93, 94); b) one report indicates approximately 70-75% reduction of NK activity in spleen only after 2200 or 4400 R (91); c) on the other hand, while NK cells in spleen were quite resistant to in vitro irradiation, activity was totally abrogated 1 or 2 days after 800 R of whole body irradiation (44), while another study showed only a 42% reduction of NK activity in spleen 1 day after 800 R (95), both these studies using nude mice; and d) finally, after a single dose of 700 R in vivo, increased activity above controls was observed from day 1 to approximately day 12, with a sharp decrease thereafter, with recovery of splenic NK activity beginning on day 28 and reaching control values at approximately 40-60 days (93, 94). This last study showed "suppressor cells" detectable during the period of lowest NK activity (day 17-19), suggesting that regulatory mechanisms of NK activity are also influenced by irradiation. Thus, one may summarize these somewhat heterogeneous results by saying: a) the "mature" effector NK cells in spleen are relatively radioresistant cells with a probable life-span (based on 93) of approximately 2 weeks; b) the progenitors, probably of bone marrow origin (2, 4, 15-18, 90), are radiosensitive and c) the kinetics of decline and recovery of NK cell activity in spleen may be influenced by regulatory cells as proposed in 93 and 94.

Table VIII summarizes our studies on the effects of different irradiation dosages and schedules on NC activity in spleen and marrow (the results being expressed as percent activity of control response at 100:1 effector:target ratios). One day after a single dose of whole body irradiation, NC activity in spleen showed only a modest reduction (ranging

TABLE VIII. *Effect of Different Dosages and Schedules of Whole Body Irradiation on NC Activity in Spleen and Marrow*

Treatment[a]	Cells[b]	% of Control Response at Different Days[c] 1	2	3	5	7	8	12	14	16	19	30
A. 400 R	SP	96	-	-	-	-	99	-	-	-	-	-
500 R	SP	80	-	-	-	-	108	129	104	80	115	99
600 R	SP	78	-	-	-	-	94	105	131	65	80	96
700 R	SP	97	98	98	97	100	95	95	103	60	-	90
700 R	BM	100	95	68	7	10	3	6	4	5	7	35
800 R	SP	94	96	96	90	-	-	-	-	-	-	-
B. 400 + 600 R	SP	-	-	-	-	-	96	-	-	-	-	-
600 + 600 R	SP	-	-	-	-	-	75	-	-	-	-	-
700 + 700 R	SP	-	-	-	-	-	50	-	-	-	-	-
700 + 700 R	BM	-	-	-	-	-	9	-	-	-	-	-
C. 900 R	SP	87	-	-	-	-	-	-	-	-	-	-
1100 R	SP	96	-	-	-	-	-	-	-	-	-	-
1100 R	BM	12	-	-	-	-	-	-	-	-	-	-
2500 R	SP	98	-	-	-	-	-	-	-	-	-	-
4000 R	SP	87	-	-	-	-	-	-	-	-	-	-
5000 R	SP	80	-	-	-	-	-	-	-	-	-	-

[a]In Exp. A and C, a single dose of whole body irradiation; in Exp. B, two doses, one week apart, and testing 1 day after 2nd dose.

[b]SP: spleen; BM: bone marrow.

[c]Results expressed as percent response compared to non-irradiated controls. All animals were BALB/c mice and their spleen or marrow cells were tested at 100:1 effector-target ratios against pre-labelled Meth A targets in a 24 hr assay. The mean cytotoxicity for the control spleen cells in 25 experiments was 55.4% ± 2.4; and for bone marrow controls it was 55.7 (48, 50, 56, and 69). The percent reduction in spleen cellularity one day after a single dose of irradiation was approximately 70% for 400-600 R; 85 % for 700 and 98% for 900 or higher dosages.

from 2 to 22%), at dosages ranging from 400 to 5000R. On the other hand, bone marrow NC activity, although not affected by 700R was markedly reduced by 1100 R. Later after irradiation,

NC activity in spleen was not affected (or increased), up to 14 days, with a moderate decline (approximately 40% reduction) on day 16, especially at the 600-700 R dose range, with recovery to control levels by day 30. With bone marrow NC activity the picture was quite different: marked decline on day 5 onwards, after 700 R, with impaired recovery still present on day 30. With a double dose of irradiation one week apart (Exp. 2 in Table VIII), one day after the second dose (day 8 in the Table), 700 + 700R produced a 50% reduction of NC activity in spleen and a marked reduction in marrow. In summary, NC activity in spleen and marrow show a marked difference in radiation sensitivity, rate of decline and recovery rates after irradiation. In addition, NC activity in spleen appears more resistant to irradiation than NK, and also shows a more rapid rate of recovery after 700 R. Determination of the site of action of irradiation on NC or NK activity needs additional work.

2. *Cyclophosphamide (CY) and Other Drugs.* Due to space limitations and the lack of effect on NC levels, we will just list the drugs and protocols of administration used, without presentation of the results, which are being prepared for publication elsewhere. No inhibition of NC activity in spleen was observed for *any* of the agents tested, and increase activity above controls ranging from 15 to 25% was observed in some instances. The following drugs were tested: a) *Cy* at 100, 200 and 300 mg/kg, IP or 20 mg/kg daily x 5, IP, and the NC activity was tested at 24 or 48 hrs (the single 100 mg dose or the 20 mg x 5, produced consistent increase in activity); b) *Vinblastine* at 100 µg/mouse, IV; c) *Carrageenan* (a mixture of 80% kappa and 20% lambda, Sigma Chemicals, St. Louis, MO) at a dose of 1.0 or 2.5 mg/mouse, IV and spleen cells tested 18, 24 and 48 hr later; d) *Silica* (Min-U-Sil, from Whittaker, Clark and Daniels Inc., So. Plainfield, NJ) at 2.5 and 5.0 mg/mouse, IV and spleen cells tested 1 day later or at 15.0 mg/mouse, IP and spleen cells tested at 2, 4 and 6 days after the drug (increase activity observed on day 4, after IP silica, ranging between 5 to 25% of controls); e) *Trypan blue* at 4 mg/mouse, SC in a single or a two dose, one week apart; and f) *3-methylcholanthrene* at a 1.0 mg/mouse, SC dose, and NC activity in spleen tested 4, 6 and 12 days later. As was indicated before, none of these drugs nor schedules of administration produced any inhibition of NC activity in spleen. All these studies were done with BALB/c, as well as some other mouse strains, and NC activity was tested against Meth A targets in 24 hr proline assays.

NK cells have been reported to be susceptible to inhibition by CY (17, 18, 91, 96) as well as other cytotoxic drugs used in chemotherapy (96). Treatment with silica was inhibitory for NK cells against YAC-1 targets (17, 91) but not against EL4 targets (18). Carrageenans also depress NK activity (17, 91, 93) and probably act by inducing a regulatory supressive cell population (93). Thus, as was the case for the irradiation studies, NC cells seem more resistant to CY, silica and carrageenans than the NK cells. The other agents such as trypan blue or hydrocarbon carcinogens have not been tested for their effects on NK cells.

3. Hydrocortisone (HC). Table IX shows the effect of HC on NC activity in spleen, tested against Meth A targets. While no effect was observed at 24 hr with either 5 or 10 mg/mouse doses, a significant decline of NC activity of approximately 60% inhibition was observed 48 hr after HC. However, such effect was transient and NC activity returned to normal (or showed an over-shoot after 10 mg HC) at 72 hrs. Somewhat similar results have been observed with NK cells (18, 44, 92, 94). HC treatment affects NK cells by the induction of a suppressive population (94). In addition, although an association between the NK and ADCC effector cells against tumor targets has been postulated (1, 3, 24, 44, 49), HC treatment does not seem to affect ADCC effector cells (44, 92, 94). On the other hand, HC decreases NK activity tested against YAC-1 (44, 92) as well as against EL4 (18). NK cells against these two targets differ in their sensitivity to treatment with ^{89}Sr (16, 17, 18).

Table IX. Effect of Hydrocortisone (HC) on NC Activity in Spleen

HC dose (mg)	*Time after HC*	*Percent of control activity[a]* 100:1	50:1	10:1
5 mg	24 hr	81	100	116
5 mg	48 hr	43*	43*	37*
5 mg	72 hr	94	103	133
10 mg	24 hr	88	105	111
10 mg	48 hr	43*	41*	16*
10 mg	72 hr	145*	134*	211*

[a]BALB/c mice were injected IP with 5 or 10 mg of HC and NC activity in their spleens tested at 24, 48 and 72 hr after HC. Meth A targets pre-labelled with 3H-proline were used in 24 hr assays. The control cytotoxicity for the 3 E:T ratios were 41, 32, and 22 respectively. (*) indicates significant difference using Student T test.

4. *^{89}Sr and estrogen.* Both ^{89}Sr (16-18, 67, 81, 94) and chronic estrogen administration (15, 97) produce a marked decrease of NK activity in spleen, when tested against YAC-1 targets. ^{89}Sr also depresses other "natural" defense mechanisms which are probably related to the NK-NC systems (6, 98). On the other hand, NK cells tested against EL4 targets are not affected by treatment with ^{89}Sr, as evidence of marrow-dependence, may be considered as the main characteristic defining these natural defense mechanisms mediated by non-conventional NK or similar cells (6, 98). The actual mechanism of the depression of NK activity by these procedures is still undefined, and it may involve elimination of marrow precursors (16, 17, 18) or some other form of marrow dependency, since although inactive NK cells capable of binding to the target are found in the ^{89}Sr-treated animals (67), interference with augmenting mechanisms (81, 97) or development of suppressor cells (94), may also depress NK activity.

TABLE X. Effect of ^{89}Sr or Beta-estradiol on NC and NK Activity in Spleen Tested Against Meth A, YAC-1 and EL4 Targets

Experimental group[a]	Percent cytotoxicity at 100:1 ratios[b]								
	Meth A			YAC-1			EL4		
	1	2	3	1	2	3	1	2	3
Control	43	40	37	25	43	52	14	16	15
^{89}Sr	67	49	31	3	11	16	6	19	12
Control	50	42	33	24	21	19	10	10	10
Estradiol	51	44	37	6	2	1	10	7	2

[a]C57Bl/6J mice were used in all the experiments. The ^{89}Sr mice and the untreated age-matched controls were kindly provided by Dr. M. Bennett (Boston Univ. School Med., Boston, Mass). These mice received two doses of 100 μCi of ^{89}Sr and were tested 4-6 weeks after the last injection as in ref. 18. The estradiol mice and their sham implanted controls were kindly provided by Dr. W.E. Seaman (Ft. Miley Vet. Hosp, San Francisco, CA) and were implanted with beta-estradiol containing plastic tubing as in ref. 15, at 4 weeks of age, and tested 8 weeks after implantation.

[b]Percent cytotoxicity for three pairs of individual mice per treatment type (marked 1, 2, 3) at 100:1 effector spleen cells to target, tested against Meth A (in a 24 hr proline assay) and against YAC-1 and EL4 in a 4 hr ^{51}Cr release assay.

Our preliminary studies on the effects of ^{89}Sr and estrogen (beta-estradiol) on NC activity show that neither treatment produced inhibition, while marked inhibition of anti-YAC-NK activity, with only modest effects on anti-EL4-NK activity were observed in those same animals. Table X shows the results with three representative pairs of animals treated with either ^{89}Sr as in ref. 16-18 or with beta-estradiol as in ref. 15. Such animals were kindly provided by Drs. Michael Bennett and William E. Seaman, respectively. NC activity was either not affected or enriched in the spleens of the treated animals. The same results were obtained with 50 and 10:1 effector:target ratios (data not shown). On the other hand, those same animals showed a marked inhibition of NK activity tested against YAC-1 targets, as was observed by others with both treatments (15-18). In all three animals, higher NK levels were observed at 10:1 ratios in the ^{89}Sr group (data not shown), suggesting dilution of a suppressor population (94). No significant effect of the ^{89}Sr-treatment was observed when the NK cells were tested against EL4 targets, as was observed by Kumar et al. (18). In addition, estradiol did not affect NK activity against EL4 in 2 of the three animals.

In summary, NC cells in spleen are not affected by treatment of the animals with ^{89}Sr or beta-estradiol, procedures which produce a decline in NK activity tested against YAC-1 targets. At first glance, this seems to represent a major difference between NC and NK cells. However, the recent description of ^{89}Sr-resistant NK cells (18) and our confirmation of such results, supports our views that NC and NK, including the slowly emerging NK sub-types, may represent a family of related effector cells.

D. *Possible In Vivo Activity of NC Cells*

The ability of NK cells to recognize and lyse tumor cells preferentially has suggested the hypothesis that they are involved in anti-tumor surveillance (1-4, 7, 10-14, 99, 100). As a matter of fact, based on studies with nude mice, we proposed some form of thymus-independent surveillance (10-14) of which NK and NC may represent one of the effector mechanisms (7). Especially, since in vivo activity of NK cells, exemplified as resistance to small tumor inocula, is well documented in normal and nude mice (1-4, 82, 95, 99, 101, 102).

In the original description of the chemically-induced Meth A fibrosarcoma, Old and collaborators (103) showed a remarkable cell dose dependency for tumor growth, where either trocar pieces or large cell inocula would grow progressively, while lower cell dosages would fail to grow. Thus, it was reasonable to try to correlate in vivo growth patterns, especially the actual cell dosage to establish a tumor transplant, and susceptibility in vitro to NC cytotoxicity. The prediction being that, NC-susceptible targets would require high cell dosages, while NC-resistant ones would require small cell inocula for establishment of local tumor growth after transplantation to syngeneic hosts. Table XI shows our studies with 29 newly arisen chemically-induced fibrosarcomas in CBA/H mice, and also shows that the prediction was correct. A good correlation between cell dosage to establish tumor takes and in vitro susceptibility to NC kill is clearly observed. Of 15 tumors that required cell dosages of 10^5 or higher for implantation, 11 (73%) were highly susceptible to NC killing. Conversely, of 14 tumors that grew with the smaller inocula of 10^4 or less cells, 13 (93%) were resistant to NC killing. Thus, it appears that NC cells may be operative at local subcutaneous sites, controlling tumor development, as the good correlation between local growth and susceptibility-resistance to NC killing in vitro, seems to indicate. It is obvious,

TABLE XI. Correlation of Susceptibility to NC Killing and Cell Numbers Required to Establish Tumor Growth

Cell Dose for 50% Tumors[a]	*No. of Tumors Tested for Susceptibility to NC Killing*		
	High	*Intermediate*	*Low*[b]
10^6 *or more*	8	1	0
10^5	3	2	1
10^4	0	0	4
10^3	0	1	9

[a]*All tumors were fibrosarcomas induced by methylcholanthrene in CBA/H mice, tested in syngeneic hosts. All tumors were in their 2nd-3rd transplant generation, and also grown as secondary cultures in vitro. Cells were injected SC. A total of 29 tumors tested.* LD_{50} *for tumor development up to 4 weeks after tumor inoculation.*

[b]*"High, intermediate and low" levels of NC susceptibility were defined by the percent lysis produced by CBA/H spleen cells at 100:1 ratios in a 24 hr proline assay: 50% cytotoxicity or more (High), 30-40% (Intermediate) and 20% or less (Low).*

that these results may represent only circumstantial evidence in favor of an in vivo role for NC (and NK) cells as a defense mechanism against tumor development. Other important factors for the effectiveness of these natural defense systems, besides target cell susceptibility, may include local delivery of NC-NK cells to the appropriate sites, interference with amplification or renewal of NC-NK cells, masking of recognition units on the effector cells, etc. If one accepts a putative surveillance role for NC (and NK) cells, all tumors that appear clinically, had, by definition, escaped the surveillance mechanism, and thus should be resistant to NC-NK cytotoxicity. The fact that chemically induced fibrosarcomas in mice are polyclonal (104) would suggest that complex in vivo selections may take place (105). On the other hand, in vitro transformed cells, not exposed to such selective pressures by NC-NK cells, should be susceptible. We tested 6 in vitro chemically transformed lines and found that, indeed, all were quite susceptible to NC killing (unpublished). Thus, it may well be that "susceptibility" to NC-NK lysis may be a property of the transformed phenotype, but a property that can be readily modulated by surface rearrangement. As a matter of fact, the increased resistance to lysis by NC-NK produced by in vivo passage (7, 53) would support this view.

III. CONCLUDING REMARKS ON NC AND NK CELLS AND ON HETEROGENEITY OF NATURAL CYTOTOXICITY

After re-reading the previous Sections in this Chapter, it appears that agreement as well as dissent dominate the views on characteristics of natural cytotoxic or killer cells. One of the reasons for some of the disagreements is that several "facts" concerning NK cells have reached the levels of accepted truths, especially after being included in review articles, and have established some "absolute"properties of the NK cell, properties, which, after further study appear to be quite variable. Suffice it to cite the example of the effects of ^{89}Sr on NK activity (1-4, 6, 16-18, 67, 81, 89, 91, 94, 98), which has been considered as the litmus test for defining the "natural resistance" mechanisms, including NK (6, 98). It now seems that ^{89}Sr-resistant NK cells do exist, depending on the target used for testing (18). We have confirmed this observation and also showed that NC cells are not affected by ^{89}Sr treatment of the cell donors (see Section II. C.4). In addition, other cytotoxic mechanisms such as macrophages are also abrogated by ^{89}Sr treatment (106). Similar comments can be made concerning the effects of pre-culture versus in vitro activation; nylon-wool adherence; presence of

Thy 1, NK 1 or FcR, etc. (see Section II. B. 4, 5 & 6).

Our interpretation of these apparent discrepancies was proposed when we described a population of natural killer cells which, although sharing many properties with NK cells, also had enough unique qualities to be considered a different, albeit related, cell population which we termed NC cells (7, 8). We even proposed a "family" of functionally related effector cells mediating these natural responses (7). We think that the "natural defense" system (6) of which NK and NC are examples, is heterogeneous. And even if it be a "single lineage" of cells distinct from T, B and macrophages, it may represent different levels of development within that lineage, as well as sub-sets of effector cells with different functional properties, which are detected as functional heterogeneity.

Functional heterogeneity mediated by sub-sets of cells is well accepted for the T system (75, 77). With NK-NC cells, it is probable that functional sub-sets with different properties and different specificities will be clearly defined in the future. It is apparent that the separation of a subset of cells capable of cytotoxicity against adherent targets (NC) which differ from NK cells by its genetic control and some properties of the effector cell, is a step in that direction. It is also apparent that a workable model for NK-NC development, renewal and regulation is necessary, before statements such as whether NK or NC cells, or any other subclass, belong to the same lineage or are in separate lineages, can be made. Even with the simplest model proposed in Section II. C (two compartments of Pre-NC (NK) $\longrightarrow$ NC (NK), i.e. precursor and effector, which are affected by an "accessory" cell compartment that gives the "interferon" signal, and a "regulatory" cell compartment that affects any of the other cells, either directly or indirectly), it is impossible, at present writing to talk seriously of lineages. Especially, since most of the procedures or reagents that appear to influence NC-NK activity, may be doing so at single or multiple levels, and may represent "markers" of the "mature" effector cell, as well as of the precursor, accessory or regulatory compartments*.

However, an important caution should be kept in mind. Functional heterogeneity may be due to two non-exclusive mechanisms: a) real heterogeneity in which different sub-sets of

**For evidence of the accessory and regulatory compartments being distinct, compare adherence and macrophage-like properteis of cells required for NK activation (63, 107), with some of the non-adherent suppressor cells described in reference 94.*

effector cells within the NC-NK lineage are capable of killing different tumor or other targets (as discussed above) and b) spurious heterogeneity, in the sense that "natural" in vitro cytotoxicity may be a final common pathway for a variety of different effector cells and mechanisms, which may include NC-NK, as well as putative T cells (48, 71), promonocytes (74), macrophages (6, 73, 107) or armed ADCC-like mechanisms (44, 49, 86, 87). One example of this is the description of promonocytes with the "functional characteristics of NK cells" (74). However, when tested against YAC targets the promonocytes showed a strain distribution of activity quite different from NK cells (C57Bl/6 and A mice had comparably high levels of promonocyte-mediated cytotoxicity) and in addition, mice homozygous for the beige trait have good levels of promonocyte-mediated cytotoxicity (69) while NK activity is low or absent (50, 69).

Thus, it is reasonable to assume that the apparently contradictory results between different laboratories concerning some of the properties of NK cells described in Sections II.B and II.C, may be due to heterogeneity of the NK compartment, especially since different target cells (besides YAC-1) have been used in these experiments.

A brief listing of some discrepancies suggesting heterogeneity of the NK-NC cell system could be attempted, as a Summary of this Chapter.

Preincubation versus in vitro induction (see Section II.B. 4). The effects of short-term pre-incubation can clearly differentiate between NC and NK cells (1, 8). On the other hand, longer incubations, as well as different procedures of in vitro activation of NK activity, seem to indicate that different NK populations can be generated in culture, with differential expression of Thy 1 and other surface markers (47, 48, 83, 88).

Nylon-wool adherence (see Section II.B.5). Non-adherent as well as nylon-adherent subfractions of NK (61, 64) and NC cells (8) have been described. However, most of the work is focused on the non-adherent fractions. Similarly, with the "target-binding cells" described by Roder et al. (64, 65), it appears that the nylon-non-adherent binding cells conform with anti-YAC NK cells, however, it will be interesting to determine the role and function of the nylon-adherent target-binding cells, which are presently being dismissed from those studies, because they do not fit with the expected properties of anti-YAC NK cells (4, 64, 65).

Presence or absence of Thy 1 (see section II.B). This property may also serve to define NK subpopulations, as well as spurious NC-NK like responses, such as the NC activity present in thymus (7 and see Section II.B.1). The coexistence of Thy 1+ and Thy 1- NK cells appears to be dependent on mouse strain, whether the animals are nude or normal and the type of assay used for testing the activity (1, 3, 38, 44, 51, 79). Are these differences reflecting different sub-sets of NK cells or different stages in NK development, or just affecting regulatory cells? These questions are still unanswered. In addition, the "activated" NK cells appear to be different from the "resting" NK cells, especially by the absence of Thy 1 (38) and by being nylon-wool adherent (see Section II B. 5). The same comments apply to the *presence or absence of NK 1* antigens (see Section II. B. 6), since it appears that both NK 1+ and NK 1- cells have been described (Burton and Winn, personnal communication). To some extent, the same type of comment can be made concerning *presence or absence of Fc receptors* (see Section II. B. 7) and effector activity in ADCC against tumor targets (44, 49, 50). The discrepancies between laboratories could be due to coexistence of FcR+ and FcR- NK cells (as well as due to the low affinity of the receptors).

Radiation sensitivity (see Section II.C. 1) As discussed above, the discrepancy between high sensitivity (44) or apparent resistance (17, 91-94) to a single dose of 800R, may be explained by coexistance of NK cells (or precursors or other cells) with differences in radiation sensitivity. NC cells are radioresistant.

Hydrocortisone and other drugs (see Section II. C. 2 & 3). While NC cells are also resistant to procedures that depress NK activity (such as cyclophosphamide, carrageenan and silica), they are affected in a similar way by high dosages of hydrocortisone. Further studies are needed to determine if the hydrocortisone effect on NC cells has a similar mechanism (i.e. mediated by suppressor cells) as in the NK system (94). It should be noted that hydrocortisone depresses NK activity without affecting the effectors for ADCC against solid tumors (44, 92, 94), which some authors consider mediated by the same effector cells (1, 3, 44, 49).

^{89}Sr treatment (or estrogen, see Section II. C. 4). NC (Table X) and NK cells tested against EL4 targets (18) are resistant to ^{89}Sr, while NK-cells tested against YAC (16, 17, 91) or activated by LCM virus (81) are susceptible to depression by ^{89}Sr treatment. The EL4 NK data (18) was confirmed by our studies (Table X). Thus, even within the NK system, differences in susceptibility to procedures such as ^{89}Sr suggest sub-classes of effector cells depending on the targets used for testing. In addition, the strain distribution of NC activity (7 and our Chapter in the Immunogenetics Section) is quite different from that of anti-YAC NK cells (4), which is also different from the strain distribution of activity of the anti-EL4 NK activity (18) or when other targets or activation procedures are used for measuring NK activity (26,

81, 88). These results suggest a complex genetic pattern of control of NC-NK subclasses, which is supported by the in vivo genetic studies (108).

In summary, from our definition of the NC cell as a cell closely related to the NK system (7, 8), but showing enough differences to warrant the sub-division, we are now proposing an intrinsic heterogeneity of precursor, effector and regulatory cells within the "natural defense" system that is tested by measuring cell-mediated cytotoxicity against certain tumor (and other targets). Quoting Alexander Pope seems appropriate to support this working hypothesis: "Not chaos-like, together crushed and bruised,/But as the world harmoniously confused:/Where order in variety we see,/And where, though all things differ, all agree." (Windsor Forest, 13). Thus, although at first glance we all may seem "together crushed and bruised," especially if comparing the murine NK-NC systems with similar systems in other species including man, it is also becoming apparent that "order in variety we see," and from a possible in vitro artifact, NK cells have become an important compartment in our systems of natural defense. However, we feel that through analysis of the systems as intrinsically heterogeneous, we may reach the level at which, "though all things differ, all agree."

ACKNOWLEDGMENTS

We wish to thank Michael J. Cuttito, Roberta Wisun, Gene Pecoraro and Robert Bohnenberger for their assistance in this work and Linda Stevenson for preparing this manuscript. We would also like to thank Drs. Henry J. Winn and Robert C. Burton for sharing their unpublished results.

REFERENCES

1. Herberman, R.B. and Holden, H.T., Adv. Cancer Res. 27, 305 (1978).
2. Kiessling, R. and Haller, O., Contemp. Top. Immunobiol. 8, 171 (1978).
3. Herberman, R.B., Djeu, J.Y., Kay, H.D., Ortaldo, J.R., Riccardi, C., Bonnard, G.D., Holden, H.T., Fagnani, R., Santoli, A. and Puccetti, P., Immunological Rev. 44, 43 (1979).
4. Kiessling, R. and Wigzell, H., Immunological Rev. 44, 165 (1979).
5. Kiessling, R., Klein, E. and Wigzell, H. Eur. J. Immunol.

5, 112 (1975).
6. Cudkowicz, G., Landy, M. and Shearer, G.M. (eds)., "Natural resistance systems against foreign cells, tumors and microbes," Academic Press, New York (1978).
7. Stutman, O., Paige, C.J. and FeoFigarella, E., J. Immunol. 121, 1819 (1978).
8. Paige, C.J., FeoFigarella, E., Cuttito, M.J., Cahan, A., and Stutman, O., J. Immunol. 121, 1827 (1978).
9. Stutman, O.,Cancer Res. 36: 737 (1976).
10. Stutman, O., Adv. Cancer Res., 22, 261 (1975).
11. Stutman, O., J. Immunol. 253, 142 (1975).
12. Stutman, O., in "The Nude Mouse in Experimental and Clinical Research" (J. Fogh and B. Giovanella, eds.), p. 411, Academic Press, New York (1978).
13. Stutman, O., Exp. Cell. Biol. 74, 129 (1979).
14. Stutman, O., J. Natl. Cancer Inst. 62, 353 (1979).
15. Seaman, W.E., Blackman, M.A., Gindhart, T.D., Roubinian, J.R., Loeb, J.M., and Talal, N., J. Immunol. 121, 2193 (1978).
16. Haller, O. and Wigzell, H., J. Immunol. 118, 1503 (1977).
17. Kiessling, R., Hochman, P.S., Haller, O., Shearer, G.M., Wigzell, H. and Cudkowicz, G., Eur. J. Immunol. 7, 655 (1977).
18. Kumar, V., Luevano, E. and Bennett, M., J. Exp. Med. 150, 531 (1979).
19. Stutman, O., Shen F.W. and Boyse E.A., Proc. Natl. Acad. Sci. USA. 74, 5667 (1977).
20. Henin, Y., Gomard, E., Gisselbrecht, S., and Levy, J.P. Brit. J. Cancer 39, 51 (1979).
21. Stulting, R.D. and Berke, G., J. Exp. Med. 137, 932 (1973).
22. Brooks, C.G., Rees, R.C. and Leach, R.H., Eur. J. Immunol. 9, 159 (1979).
23. Herberman, R.B., Nunn, M.E. and Lavrin, D.H., Int. J. Cancer 16, 216 (1975).
24. Santoni, A., Herberman, R.B. and Holden, H.T., J. Natl. Cancer Inst. 62, 109 (1979).
25. Kiessling, R., Klein, E., Pross, H. and Wigzell, H., Eur. J. Immunol. 5, 117 (1975).
26. Burton, R.C., Grail, D. and Warner, N.L., Br. J. Cancer 37, 806 (1978).
27. Greenberg, A.H. and Playfair, J.H.L., Clin. Exp. Immunol. 16, 99 (1974).
28. Nunn, M.E., Djeu, J.Y., Glaser, M., Lavrin, D.H. and Herberman, R.B., J. Natl. Cancer Inst. 56, 393 (1976).
29. Shellam, G.R. and Hogg, N., Int. J. Cancer 19, 212 (1977).
30. Potter, M.R. and Moore, M., Clin. Exp. Immunol. 34, 78 (1978).

31. Targan, S., Brown, D., Gale, R. and Jondal, M., J. Clin. Lab. Immunol. 2, 139 (1979).
32. Vose, B.M., Vanky, F., Agrov, S. and Klein, E., Eur. J. Immunol. 7, 753 (1977).
33. Tracey, D.E., Wolfe, A.A., Durdik, J.M and Henney, C.S., J. Immunol. 119, 1145 (1977).
34. Ojo, E., Haller, O. and Wigzell, H., Scand. J. Immunol. 8, 215 (1978).
35. Herberman, R.B., Nunn, M.E., Holden, H.T., Staal, S. Djeu, J.Y., Int. J. Cancer 19, 555 (1977).
36. Ojo, E., Haller, O., Kimura, A. and Wigzell, H., Int. J. Cancer 21, 444 (1978).
37. Gidlund, M., Orn, A., Wigzell, H., Senik, A., and Gresser, I., Nature 273, 759 (1978).
38. Djeu, J.Y., Heinbaugh, J.A., Holden, H.T. and Herberman, R.B., J. Immunol. 122, 175 (1979).
39. Senik, A., Gresser, I., Maury, C., Gidlund, M., Orn, A., and Wigzell, H., Cell. Immunol. 44, 186 (1979).
40. Zinkernagel, R.M. and Doherty, P.C., Contempt. Topics, Immunobiol. 7, 179 (1977).
41. Stutman, O. and Shen, F.W., Nature 276, 181 (1978).
42. Herberman, R.B., Nunn, M.E., Holden, H.T. and Lavrin, D.H., Int. J. Cancer 16, 230 (1975).
43. Wolfe, S.A., Tracey, D.E. and Henney, C.S., J. Immunol. 119, 1152 (1977).
44. Santoni, A., Herberman, R.B. and Holden, H.T., J. Natl. Cancer Inst. 63, 995 (1979).
45. Zielske, T.V. and Golub, S.H., Cancer Res. 36, 3842 (1976).
46. Muchmore, A.V., Decker, J.M. and Blaese, R.M., J. Immunol. 119, 1686 (1977).
47. Burton, R.C., Chism, S.E. and Warner, N.L., J. Immunol. 119, 1329 (1977).
48. Karre, K. and Seeley, J.K., J. Immunol. 123, 1511 (1979).
49. Ojo, E. and Wigzell, H., Scand. J. Immunol. 7, 297 (1978).
50. Roder, J.C., J. Immunol. 123, 2168 (1979).
51. Mattes, M.J., Sharrow, S.O., Herberman, R.B. and Holden, H.T., J. Immunol. 123, 2851 (1979).
52. Haller, O., J. Natl. Cancer Inst. 60, 1433 (1978).
53. Becker, S., Kiessling, R., Lee, N., and Klein, G., J. Natl. Cancer Inst. 61, 1495 (1978).
54. Haller, O., Gidlund, M., Hellstrom, U., Hammarstrom, S., and Wigzell, H., Eur. J. Immunol. 8, 765 (1978).
55. Bean, M.A., Bloom, B.R., Herberman, R.B., Old, L.J., Oettgen, H.F., Klein, G. and Terry, W.D., Cancer Res. 35, 2902 (1975).
56. Kay, D.H., Bonnard, G.D., West, W.H. and Herberman, R.B., J. Immunol. 118, 2058 (1977).
57. Altman, A. and Rapp, H.J., J. Immunol. 121, 2244 (1978).

58. Kodera, Y. and Bean, M.A., Int. J. Cancer 16, 579 (1975).
59. Yust, I., Smith, R.W., Wunderlich, J.R. and Mann, D.L., J. Immunol. 116, 1170 (1976).
60. Sendo, F., Aoki, T., Boyse, E.A. and Buafo, C.K., J. Natl. Cancer Inst. 55, 603 (1975).
61. Tufveson, G., Riesenfeld, I., Ronnblom, L., Hedman, A. and Alm, G.V., J. Natl. Cancer Inst. 59, 1491 (1977).
62. Kiessling, R., Petranyi, G., Karre, K., Jondal, M., Tracey, D. and Wigzell, H., J. Exp. Med. 143, 772 (1976).
63. Djeu, J. Y., Heinbaugh, J.A., Holden, H.T. and Herberman, R.B., J. Immunol. 122, 182 (1979).
64. Roder, J.C. and Kiessling, R., Scand. J. Immunol. 8, 135 (1978).
65. Roder, J.C., Kiessling, R., Biberfeld, P. and Andersson, B., J. Immunol. 121, 2509 (1978).
66. Glimcher, L., Shen, F.W. and Cantor, H., J. Exp. Med. 145, 1 (1977).
67. Kumar, V., Ben-Ezra, J., Bennett, M. and Sonnenfeld, G., J. Immunol. 123, 1832 (1979).
68. Herberman, R.B., Bartram, S., Haskill, J.S., Nunn, M., Holden, H.T. and West, W.H. J., Immunol. 119, 322 (1977).
69. Roder, J.C., Lohmann-Matthes, M.L., Domzig, W. and Wigzell, H., J. Immunol. 123, 2174 (1979).
70. Zarling, J., M., Nowinski, R.C. and Bach, F.H., Proc. Natl. Acad. Sci. USA 72, 2780 (1975).
71. Kende, M.,Hill, R., Dinowitz, M., Stephenson, J.R. and Kelloff, G.J., J. Exp. Med. 149, 358 (1979).
72. Sanderson, C.J., Clark, I.A. and Taylor, G.A., Nature 253, 376 (1975).
73. Gomard, E., Leclerc, J.C. and Levy, J.P., Nature 250, 671 (1974).
74. Lohmann-Matthes, M.L., Domzig, W. and Roder, J., J. Immunol., 123, 1883 (1979).
75. Boyse, E.A. & Old, L.J., Harvey Lectures 71, 32 (1978).
76. Feeney, A.J. and Hammerling, U., Immunogenetics 3, 369 (1976).
77. Cantor, H., Kasai, M., Shen, F.W., Leclerc, J.C. and Glimcher, L., Immunological Rev. 44, 3 (1979).
78. Archer, J.R. and Davies, D.A.L., J. Immunogenet. 1, 113 (1974).
79. Herberman, R.B., Nunn, M.E. and Holden, H.T., J. Immunol. 121, 304 (1978).
80. Pollack, S.B., Tam, M.R., Nowinski, R.C. and Emmons, S.L, J. Immunol. 123, 1818 (1979).
81. Welsh, R.M., J. Exp. Med. 148, 163 (1978).
82. Minato, N., Bloom, B .R., Jones, C., Holland, J. and Reid, L.M., J. Exp. Med. 149, 117 (1979).
83. Chun, M., Pasanen, V., Hammerling, U., Hammerling, G.F., and Hoffmann, M.K., J. Exp. Med. 150, 426 (1979).

84. Horton, M.A., Beverly, P.C.L. and Simpson, E., Immunogenetics 7, 173 (1978).
85. Gidlund, M., Oho, E.A., Orn, A., Wigzell, H. and Murgita, R.A., Scand. J. Immunol. 9, 167 (1979).
86. Koide, Y. and Takasugi, J., J. Natl. Cancer Inst. 59, 1099 (1977).
87. Blair, P.B. and Lane, M.A., J. Immunol. 115, 184 (1976).
88. Croker, B.P., Zinkernagel, R.M. and Dixon, F.J., Clin. Immunol. Immunopathol. 12, 410 (1979).
89. Welsh, R.M., J. Immunol. 121, 1631 (1978).
90. Haller, O. A., Gidlund, M., Kurnick, J.T. and Wigzell, H., Scand. J. Immunol. 8, 207 (1978).
91. Trentin, J.J., Kiessling, R., Wigzell, H., Gallagher, M. T., Datta, S.K. and Kulkarni, S.S., in "Experimental Hematology Today" (S.J. Baum & G.D. Ledney, eds.), p. 179. Springer-Verlag, New York (1977).
92. Hockman, P.S. and Cudkowicz, G., J. Immunol. 119, 2013 (1977).
93. Hochman, P.S., Cudkowicz, G. and Dausset, J., J. Natl. Cancer Inst. 61, 265 (1978).
94. Cudkowicz, G. and Hochman, P.S., Immunol. Rev. 44, 13 (1979).
95. Warner, N.L., Woodruff, M.F.A. and Burton, R.C., Int. J. Cancer 20, 146 (1977).
96. Mantovani, A., Luini, W., Peri, G., Vecchi, A. and Spreafico, F., J. Natl. Cancer Inst. 61, 1255 (1978).
97. Seaman, W.E., Merigan, T.C. and Talal, N. J. Immunol. 123, 2541 (1979).
98. Bennett, M., Baker, E.E., Eastcott, J.W., Kumar, V. and Yonkosky, D., J. Reticuloendothel. Soc. 20, 7 (1976).
99. Haller, O., Hanson, M., Kiessling, R. and Wigzell, H. Nature 270, 609 (1977).
100. Klein, G. and Klein, E., Transplant Proc. 9, 1095 (1977).
101. Riccardi, C., Pucetti, P., Santoni, A. and Herberman, R.B., J. Natl. Cancer Inst. 63, 1041 (1979).
102. Ojo, E., Cell. Immunol. 45, 182 (1979).
103. Old, L.J., Boyse, E.A., Carswell, E. and Clarke, D.A., Ann. N.Y. Acad. Sci. 101, 80 (1962).
104. Reddy, A.L. and Fialkow, P.J., J. Exp. Med. 150, 878 (1979).
105. Patek, P.Q., Collins, J.L. and Cohn, M., Nature 276, 510 (1978).
106. Keller, R., Immunology 37, 333 (1979).
107. Tracey, D.E., J. Immunol. 123, 840 (1979).
108. Klein, G., Klein, G.O., Karre, K. and Kiessling, R. Immunogenetics 7, 391 (1978).

Addendum

For further discussion on NK cell heterogeneity, see the Chapters by R.C. Burton and by G.C. Koo and A. Hatzfeld in the present Volume. Also see Clark et al. (Int. J. Cancer 24, 688, 1979) and Macfarlan et al. (Infect. Immun. 26, 832, 1979). These papers were not available to us at the time of completion of the present manuscript.

ONTOGENY AND OTHER AGE-RELATED EFFECTS OF NATURAL CYTOTOXIC (NC) CELLS IN MICE[1]

Osias Stutman

Cellular Immunobiology Section
Memorial Sloan-Kettering Cancer Center
New York, New York

I. EFFECTS OF AGE ON NK AND NC ACTIVITY

A. Introduction

As was discussed in our original description of the NC cell (natural cytotoxic cell, tested against adherent tumor targets in long-term in vitro assays), one major difference between NC and NK cells was the age-related effect on activity (1). NC activity was detected in the spleens of BALB/c and NZB mice from birth, showed no clear patterns of age-related changes and was present (and high), at the oldest ages studied, such as 52 and 104 weeks (1). On the other hand, there is agreement that NK cells in mice are not detected in spleens until 3-5 weeks of age, usually reach peak activity at approximately 8 weeks and show a subsequent decline to low levels thereafter (2-8). Thus, NC activity appears earlier in life and remains functional for longer periods than NK cells in mice (1). However, as will be discussed in the following sections, these statements should be handled with caution, since activity levels, both for NC and NK cells, may be the result of complex inductive and regulatory events, still not

[1]*This work was supported by grants CA-08748, CA-15988, and CA-17818 of the National Institutes of Health and grant IM-188 from the American Cancer Society.*

ISBN 0-12-341350-8

properly defined (1-8). For example, while there is good agreement on the age of appearance of NK activity in spleen (2-8), the actual age-dependent decline is less well defined (9-12). And, while it is stated that no detectable NK activity could be detected in mice older than 12 weeks (5), other studies have shown peak activity in mice that were 20 weeks or older (9, 10) or even in 36-week old mice (11). One study shows that in CBA mice "over 1 year old," NK activity was present in the spleen, although at lower levels than younger controls, however the values were of approximately 30 and 50% cytotoxicity against YAC-1 target cells at 50:1 ratios (12). This study also showed that young into old (or vice versa) bone marrow radiation chimeras expressed the NK pattern of reactivity of the age of the marrow donor, suggesting that these age-related changes are expressed at the "bone marrow precursor level" (12), although activity levels may also be related to regulatory cells (7, 8). Cells capable of suppressing young adult NK activity in vitro have been described in the spleens of infant mice (7,8). Supporting this view is the observation by Dr. G. Koo (Sloan-Kettering Institute, personal communication) that mouse newborn spleens contain detectable levels of $NK.1^+$ cells which do not show NK cytotoxic activity. NK.1 is an antigen which is probably expressed exclusively on NK cell populations (13, 14).

Studies with NK-like cells in other species than mice also suggest a complex picture for the effects of age on activity levels (15-27). In rats, there is agreement from all laboratories that activity is detected from 2-3 weeks of age and peaks at 5-8 weeks (15-19). On the other hand, some laboratories find a decline by 10 weeks of age (15,17) while others find activity for much longer periods of time, from 36 (16,18) to 88 weeks (19). One report suggests that using long-term assays (and probably as a consequence of in vitro activation of cytotoxic activity), NK-like activity can be detected in the older rats (16). On the other hand, the low activity in infant rats seems not related to some form of suppressor cells (19), as may be the case in mice (7,8). In hamsters, an NK-like activity has been described which appears at 4-7 days of age and shows no age-related decline (20). No clear age variation was observed in guinea pigs for an NK-like activity at ages ranging from 3 to 40 weeks (21). In pigs, newborn animals showed no NK-like activity, however such function was detected in 8 week old animals or older, with no evidence of decline in animals tested at 8 and 42 months of age (22). In humans there are no clear effects of age on NK levels of activity (23-27), and the situation can be aptly summarized by a statement from a review by Herberman & Holden (5),"... age has not been found to have a major effect on human NK activity." In addition, NK activity has been detected in cord blood, indicating an early appearance of this function in ontogeny (25).

B. *Ontogeny of NC Function in Mice*

Our published work showed that spleen cells from newborn, as well as infant BALB/c mice from 4 to 21 days of age, had levels of NC activity comparable to those observed in the adult controls, when tested against Meth A, a syngeneic chemically induced fibrosarcoma adherent target (1). NC activity of newborn or infant spleen cells against Meth A targets was also observed with NZB, CBA/H, A/J and I/StUmc strains (1). Table I shows some additional studies on the ontogeny of NC cells in BALB/c mice, tested against Meth A targets, as described in ref. 1. It can be seen that the hemopoietic embryonic liver from animals at 14-17 or 18-19 days of gestation

TABLE I. Ontogeny of NC Activity in BALB/c Mice Against Syngeneic Meth A Adherent Target Cells

Age (days)[a]	*Cells*[b]	*Percent cytotoxicity*[c] *100:1*	*50:1*	*10:1*
14-17 (*)	*Liver*	2	0	3
18-19 (*)	*Liver*	6	7	0
17-19 (*)	*Spleen*	12	9	4
17-19 (*)	*Spleen (NA)*	12	11	6
Birth	*Spleen*	29	19	10
Birth	*Spleen (NA)*	28	12	7
4	*Spleen*	44	36	22
8	*Spleen*	33	25	14
60	*Spleen*	49	37	29

[a] *(*) means days of gestation*
[b] *(NA) means nylon non-adherent, for details on nylon wool columns see ref. 28.*
[c] *Percent cytotoxicity at different effector:target ratios, measured against 3H-proline pre-labelled target cells in a 24 hr assay, as described in ref. 1.*

showed no significant cytotoxicity (higher effector:target ratios, not shown in the Table, were also negative). Some marginal NC activity was detected in embryonic spleen (17-19 days of gestation) and was apparent at birth. Both the marginal activity in the embryonic spleen as well as the NC activity observed in newborn spleen were mediated by nylon-wool, non-adherent cells, suggesting a property in common with the adult type NC-cell (28). The lack of enrichment after nylon wool filtration was also observed with adult NC cells (28). NC levels at 4 and 8 days of age in spleen were comparable to those observed in 60-day-old animals, as was observed in our previous publication (1). The particular experiment in Table I shows the lowest level of activity of newborn BALB/c spleen (in relation to the "adult" 60-day old control) observed in a series of 14 experiments. Thus, development of NC activity in spleen of BALB/c mice, measured against Meth A syngeneic targets in a 24 hr proline assay, is absent in embryonic hemopoietic liver and spleen and appears in spleen since birth (note that, based on our mouse colony procedures, "birth" means less than 18 to 24 hrs old). On the other hand, no detectable NK activity was observed in such embryonic, newborn or infant tissues, when tested against YAC-1 target cells in a 4 or an 18 hr 51Cr assay (data not shown). The 60-day old controls showed NK cytotoxicity indices of 20 to 43% at 100:1 effector: target ratios in 4 hr assays against YAC-1, comparable to the values observed by others (3).

Table II shows that this pattern of NC reactivity since birth may be variable, depending on the target used for the assay. Newborn or 14 and 28 day-old BALB/c, A/J and (BALB x A)F1 mice were tested for NC activity against Meth A and Meth 113 targets (see 1 for details on these BALB/c fibrosarcomas), as well as NK activity against YAC-1 targets. It is apparent that, while all newborn animals showed good NC activity against Meth A, a progressive maturation of NC activity was observed against Meth 113. NC reactivity against this tumor is strain dependent (BALB being a low and A/J a high reactor, with high reactivity being dominant in the F1 hybrids, see ref. 1), thus low NC reactivity was observed with BALB cells of any age, while a pattern of NC "maturation" or progressive increase of activity with age was observed with spleen cells from the high reactors A/J and the F1 hybrid. The 28 day-old animals showed "adult" levels of activity, compared to those observed in older animals (1). A comparable age and strain dependency for maturation was observed for spleen NK cells tested against YAC-1 targets: BALB and the F1 hybrids are intermediate reactors in this system, while A/J is a prototype low reactor. A recent report has shown NK activity at 2 weeks of age in C3H mice tested against RBL-5 targets, while activity in CBA mice appeared at 4-5 weeks (29).

TABLE II. Effect of Age on NC Activity Against Meth A and Meth 113 BALB/c Fibrosarcomas (and on NK Activity Against YAC-1 Targets)

Strain	Age (days)	Percent cytotoxicity on different targets[a]		
		Meth A	Meth 113	YAC-1
BALB/c	newborn	56	2	2
BALB/c	14	49	12	12
BALB/c	28	53	5	38
A/J	newborn	40	4	7
A/J	14	52	22	3
A/J	28	50	43	6
(BALBxA)F1	newborn	59	10	4
(BALBxA)F1	14	63	21	16
(BALBxA)F1	28	67	36	24

[a]*Spleen cells from mice of the different ages and strains were tested against Meth A or Meth 113 adherent target cells prelabelled with 3H-proline in a 24 hr assay, using effector:target ratios of 100:1 (as well as low ratios not shown). For YAC-1 targets, NK cytotoxicity of spleen cells measured in a 4 hr 51Cr release assay and the cytotoxicity is presented for 100:1 effector:target ratios. For further technical details see ref. 1.*

Whatever the hypothesis used to explain the low NK reactivity of newborn or infant mice (i.e. suppressor cells, 7,8; environmental factors such as infections that affect interferon levels, 5; genetic influences regulating maturation, 6, 12, etc.), it appears that "age of appearance" as one of the major differences between the NK and NC system, as proposed earlier (1), is not absolute. From the present results, such age effects appear to depend on the target used for NC detection: with Meth A targets NC activity is detected since birth in all mouse strains tested (1), while for Meth 113 NC activity is low at birth and reaches adult levels at 4 weeks of age (Table II), a pattern quite comparable to the one observed in the NK system (2-8). In addition, age-dependent NC development against Meth 113 targets followed the strain patterns of reactivity, whether high or low reactors (1, see also our Chapter on Immunogenetics).

The possible role of environmental factors (such as infections) to explain the NC activity observed in newborns, is ruled out by the present results, since both patterns of reactivity, the newborn and the late appearing, were observed with animals reared in the same housing facilities.

The target dependency for detection of these differences suggests that some targets (like Meth 113) may require additional steps of NC cell "activation" for cytotoxicity to occur, steps which are not provided by the long-term incubation used in these assays (16).

In addition, the observed differences of age-related effects on NC cells could not be explained by in vitro factors such as: a) mycoplasma infection of the targets, which increases target cell susceptibility to lysis (30), since both Meth A and Meth 113 used in the experiments are free of mycoplasma (however, this is an important factor which increases target cell susceptibility due to depletion of the culture medium, see Sections I.A and I.B); b) differences in target cell susceptibility to be lysed, since both targets are equally sensitive to lysis by other cell-mediated mechanisms (1); and c) reactivity to fetal calf serum components (31, 32), since the same age-patterns of reactivity were observed whether using serum free conditions (as described in ref. 33) or horse serum (unpublished results).

In summary, the ontogeny of NC effector cells has two main characteristics: a) it is absent in lympho-hemopoietic tissues of embryonic mice and b) may be present from birth in spleen or show age-dependent "maturation" reaching peak activity at 4 weeks, depending on the target used for the assay. This last pattern of reactivity is somewhat comparable to that observed for NK cells (2-8). Both newborn as well as the later appearing cytotoxicity are mediated by cells which share the same properties as adult spleen NC cells (1, 28), supporting our views of heterogeneity of these natural cytotoxicity systems (1, 28).

C. Aging and NC Activity

In our previous studies on NC cells in BALB/c mice (1), we could show that activity levels were comparable between 4 and 8-week old animals and animals tested at older ages (12, 17, 25,52 and 104 weeks of age). Thus, NC cells in mice do not show the age-dependent decline observed with murine NK cells, and show somewhat, a pattern comparable to that observed for NK cells in rats and humans (5, 18, 19, 23-27). Table III shows an example of these results testing spleen cells from mice of different strains and ages against Meth A targets. Although there are some scattered results showing somewhat lower NC reactivity in some of the older animals

TABLE III. NC Activity of Spleen Cells from Different Mouse Strains and Different Ages Against Meth A Targets

Age (days)	Percent cytotoxicity at 100:1 ratios[a]							
	BALB/c	CBA/H	NZB	I/St	A/J	C57Bl/6	dw/+	dw/dw
90	66	66	60	72	50	53	47	40
120	60	67	ND	72	60	59	ND	ND
180	53	50	67	70	59	50	45	46
365	70	63	44	70	55	48	31	30
450	55	53	50	73	42	ND	ND	ND
730	72	70	ND	66	70	ND	ND	ND

[a]*Spleen cells from mice of the indicated strains and ages were tested as described in ref. 1 against 3H-proline prelabelled Meth A target cells of BALB/c origin, in a 24 hr assay. Percent cytotoxicity calculated as in ref. 1.*

(i.e. 365-day old NZB, dw/+ and dw/dw; 450-day old A/J), it is apparent that NC activity is well preserved in aging mice of different strains, and certainly well beyond the 8-12 week (56-84 days of age) limit observed by several laboratories for detectability of NK activity in spleens (2-8). As it was indicated in the Introduction to this paper, the age for decline of NK activity in mice is not too well defined, since NK activity has been observed in older animals (9-12). Our own studies, with some of the animals described in Table III, showed that NK activity tested against YAC-1 targets is usually present in the spleens of older animals, although we studied only a few age groups. For example, the cytotoxic index at 100:1 effector to target ratios in 4 hr 51Cr release assays using YAC-1 as targets was 29,33 and 48% respectively for spleen cells from 365, 450 and 730-day old CBA/H mice, while the 30-day old control had 57% cytotoxicity. Similarly, 365-day old CBA/H nu/nu showed 63% cytotoxicity against YAC-1, while the 30-day old controls showed 69%. Similar results were observed with C57Bl/6 and BALB/c animals. Whether these results show a real "reappearance" of NK activity in aging animals due to environmental activation or loss of suppressive controls, deserves further study.

In summary, NC activity seems to remain well preserved during the life-span of most mouse strains tested, as was observed in our initial publication (1). Although there is substantial evidence for a decline of NK activity with age (2-8), I feel that such decline needs further definition, based on some of the published work (9-12) as well as our own preliminary results.

II. CONCLUSIONS

The following conclusions can be drawn from the present paper: a) NC activity in mice appears earlier than NK activity, and depending on the type of target used, can be detected in spleens since birth; b) with other targets, "adult" levels of NC activity are reached by 4 weeks of age and c) NC activity in spleen is well preserved throughout life in several mouse strains, and does not show age-dependent decline, even in aging mice. Thus, the ontogeny as well as the affects of advancing age, suggest some differences between NK and NC cells. However, it is still possible to support the view that they may belong to a group of functionally related effector cells.

ACKNOWLEDGMENTS

I wish to thank Michael Cuttito and Roberta Wisun for their able technical assistance and Linda Stevenson for preparation of this manuscript.

REFERENCES

1. Stutman, O., Paige, C.J. and FeoFigarella, E., J. Immunol. 121, 1819 (1978).
2. Herberman, R.B., Nunn, M.E. and Lavrin, D.H., Int. J. Cancer 16, 216 (1975).
3. Kiessling, R., Klein, E., Pross, H. and Wigzell, H., Eur. J. Immunol. 5, 117 (1975).
4. Kiessling, R., Hochman, P.S., Haller, O., Shearer, G.M., Wigzell, H. and Cudkowicz, G., Eur. J. Immunol. 7, 655 (1977).
5. Herberman, R.B. and Holden, H.T., Adv. Cancer Res. 27, 305 (1978).
6. Kiessling, R. and Haller, O., Contemp. Topics Immunobiol. 8, 171 (1978).
7. Savary, C.C. and Lotzova, E., J. Immunol. 120, 239 (1978).
8. Cudkowicz, G. and Hochman, P.S., Immunol. Rev. 44, 13 (1979).
9. Gomard, E., Leclerc, J.C. and Levy, J.P., Nature 250, 671 (1974).

10. Zarling, J., Nowinski, R.C. and Bach, F.H., Proc. Natl. Acad. Sci. USA, 72, 2780 (1975).
11. Greenberg, A.H. and Playfair, J.H.L., Clin. Exp. Immunol. 10, 99 (1974).
12. Haller, O., Kiessling, R., Orn, A. and Wigzell, H., J. Exp. Med. 145, 1411 (1977).
13. Glimcher, L., Shen, F.W. and Cantor, H., J. Exp. Med. 145, 1 (1977).
14. Cantor, H., Kasai, M., Shen, F.W., Leclerc, J.C. and Glimcher, L., Immunol. Rev. 44, 3 (1979).
15. Nunn, M.E., Djeu, J., Glaser, M., Lavrin, D.H. and Herberman, R.B. J. Natl. Cancer Inst. 56, 393 (1976).
16. Oldham, R.K., Ortaldo, J.R. and Herberman, R.B., Cancer Res. 37, 4467 (1977).
17. Oehler, J.R., Lindsay, L.R., Nunn, M.E. and Herberman, R.B., Int. J. Cancer 21, 204 (1978).
18. Shellam, G.R. and Hogg, N., Int. J. Cancer 19, 212 (1977).
19. Brooks, G.C. and Flannergy, R.G., Immunology, in press (1980).
20. Datta, S.K., Gallagher, M.T. and Trentin, J.J., Int. J. Cancer 23, 728 (1979).
21. Altman, A. and Rapp, H.J., J. Immunol. 121, 2244 (1978).
22. Koren, H.S., Amos, D.B. and Kim, Y.B., Proc. Natl. Acad. Sci. USA, 75, 5127 (1978).
23. Takasugi, M., Mickey, M.R. and Terasaki, P.I., Cancer Res. 33, 2898 (1973).
24. Rosemberg, E.B., McCoy, J.L., Green, S.S., Donnelly, F.C., Siwarski, D., Levine, P.H. and Herberman, R.B., J. Natl. Cancer Inst. 52, 345 (1974).
25. Jondal, M. and Pross, H., Int. J. Cancer 15, 596 (1975).
26. Oldham, R.K., Djeu, J.Y., Cannon, G.B., Siwarski, D. and Herberman, R.B., J. Natl. Cancer Inst. 55, 1305 (1975).
27. Takasugi, M., Akira, D., Takasugi, J. and Mickey, M.R. J. Natl. Cancer Inst. 59, 69 (1977).
28. Paige, C.J., FeoFigarella, E., Cuttito, M.J., Cahan, A. and Stutman, O., J. Immunol. 121, 1827 (1978).
29. Santoni, A., Herberman, R.B. and Holden, H.T., J. Natl. Cancer Inst. 62, 109 (1979).
30. Brooks, C.G., Rees, R.C. and Leach, R.H., Eur. J. Immun Immunol. 9, 159 (1979).
31. Zielske, J.V. and Golub, S.H., Cancer Res. 36, 3842 (1976).
32. Golstein, P., Luciani, M.F., Wagner, H. and Rollinghoff, M., J. Immunol. 121, 2533 (1978).
33. Peck, A.B. and Bach, F.H., J. Immunol. Methods 3, 147 (1973).

Addendum

After this manuscript was completed we became aware of the paper by Kende et al. (Kende, M., Hill, R., Dinowitz, M., Stephenson, J.R. and Kelloff, G.J., J. Exp. Med. 149, 358, 1979) describing an NK-like activity which appeared at approximately 18 months of age in BALB/c spleens, and showed a striking virus specificity against targets productively infected with either an endogenous ecotropic BALB virus or R-MuLV. Cytotoxicity was mediated by a nylon non-adherent, non-phagocytic, Thy 1 negative cell with no detectable receptors for Ig or C. Activity was measured in an 18 hr 51Cr assay with target cells in suspension. It would be of interest to determine with Lyt reagents if these effectors are T cells with low Thy 1 surface antigen or if they truly belong to a unique type of NK cell with "specific" antiviral reactivity.

BIOPHYSICAL AND SEROLOGICAL CHARACTERIZATION OF MURINE NK CELLS

Anna Tai
Noel L. Warner

Immunobiology Laboratories
University of New Mexico
School of Medicine
Albuquerque, New Mexico

I. BIOPHYSICAL CHARACTERIZATION OF NK CELLS FROM NORMAL AND AUGMENTED MICE BY ADHERENCE AND SEDIMENTATION PROPERTIES

Previous investigation from several groups have indicated that endogenous NK cells from normal untreated mice are non-phagocytic and of low adherence (Herberman et al. 1975a; Kiessling et al. 1975a, b; Sendo et al. 1975; Zarling 1975). Thus the passage of reactive spleen cell suspensions over nylon wool columns has been used as a means of enrichment for NK cell activity. In addition, in morphological studies performed by Kiessling et al. (1975b), Roder et al. (1978) and Herberman and Holden, (1978), in which T, B and phagocytic cells were first depleted and the remaining cells examined under the microscope, the endogenous NK effector cells were visualized as being small to medium in size.

Augmentation of NK activity *in vitro* and *in vivo* by a variety of chemical, cellular and viral agents has been well documented (see Section C this volume). The augmented population of NK cells appears to show generally similar target specificities as the endogenous effectors (however see Tai and Warner Section D this volume), and to be nonphagocytic, and non-adherent to rayon wool (Djeu et al. 1979) and to plastic (Welsh and Zinkernagel 1977).

Although this evidence suggested that endogenous and augmented NK cells share generally similar characteristics, it was felt that a more rigorous examination of the two populations was warranted. Thus the goals of these studies were to

ISBN 0-12-341350-8

compare endogenous and augmented NK cells in terms of adherance and sedimentation properties, and to extablish whether these procedures could lead to enrichment of NK effector cells.

A. *Velocity Sedimentation*

The size distribution of spleen cells from normal, polyriboinosinic-polycytidilic acid (Poly I-C) and lymphocytic choriomeningitis virus (LCMV) treated BALB/c mice was examined by 1xg sedimentation in a "staput" apparatus. The sedimentation profiles of total viable cells from the 3 different sources were quite similar indicating that the overall sizes of the majority of the spleen cells are not affected by the various treatments of the host. Pooled fractions were tested for NK reactivity using ^{51}Cr labeled YAC-1 (T lymphoma) and WEHI-164 (fibrosarcoma), (Fig. 1, A-F) in the standard 4 hour chromium release assay.

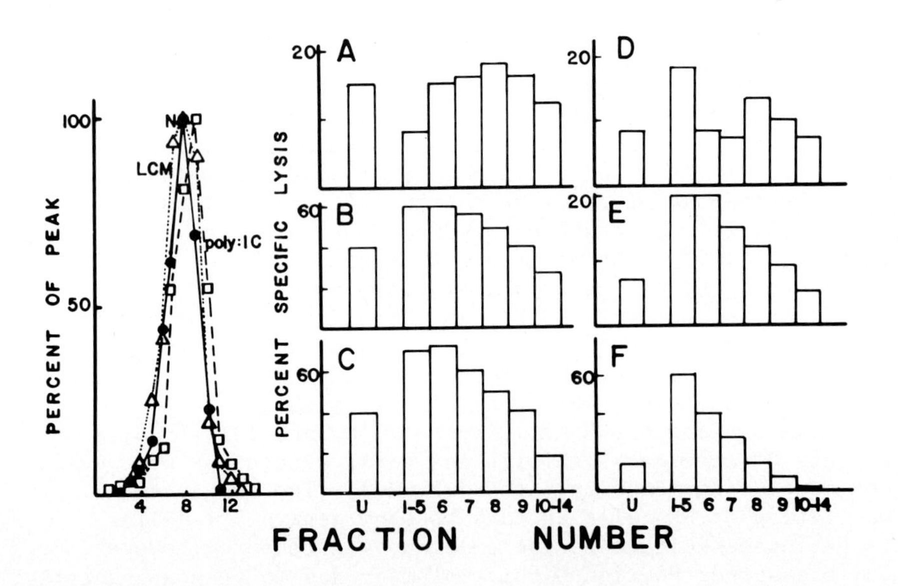

FIGURE 1. Velocity sedimentation separation of NK effector cells from spleens of normal (A, D) poly-I-C (B, E) and LCMV treated BALB/c mice (C, F). Fractions were pooled from the separation procedure at various intervals (largest cells at low fraction numbers), and assayed for lytic activity on YAC-1 (A-C) and WEHI-164 (D-F).

The cytotoxicity profiles of the untreated NK cells using YAC-1 as target cells indicate activity to reside in small to medium size cells. However the activity against WEHI-164 seems to reside in two separate populations, one of large size and the other small-medium size. With the poly I-C population, NK activity against both targets was resident to a greater degree in large cells. The same shift in the profile of cytotoxic activity occurred to an even greater extent with LCMV induced effector cells for both targets. Thus although size heterogeneity was evident for cells with NK activity in all situations, there was also a most distinct shift in NK activity following augmentation of NK levels with both poly I-C and LCMV.

B. *Nylon Wool Separation*

The adherence of the different populations of NK cells to nylon wool was also examined. In view of the functional lability of the NK effector cells at 37°C, fractionation was performed at room temperature, using a modified procedure of Julius et al. (1973). The cytotoxicity of fractionated poly I-C and LCMV induced spleen cells on YAC-1 (Fig. 2A) indicates

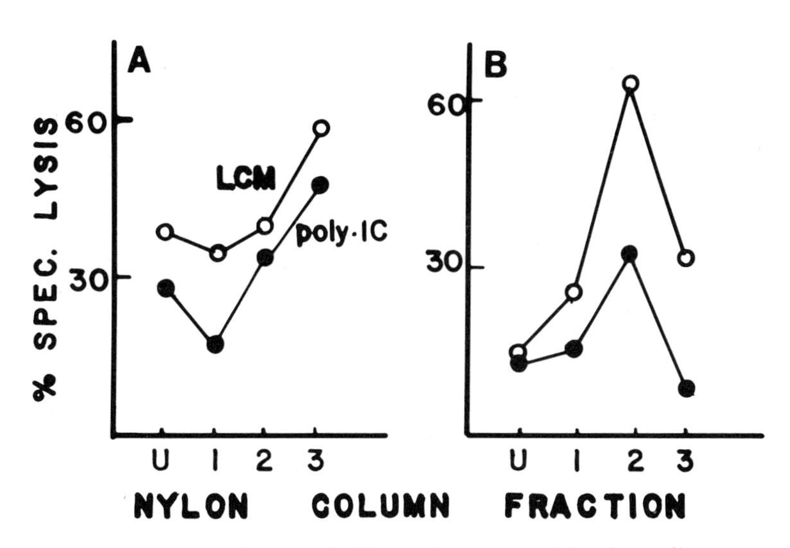

FIGURE 2. Separation of NK effector cells by adherence to nylon wool columns at room temperature (A) or 37°C (B). Fractions represent immediate run through (1), second 50 ml wash through (2), and ringette fraction eluted by compression of additional medium (3). Target tumor is YAC-1, and effector spleen cells were obtained from Poly I-C or LCMV treated mice.

that, in contrast to the usual "non-adherent" nature ascribed to NK effector cells, these effector cells are adherent to nylon wool at room temperature. When the fractionation was performed at 37°C, (Fig. 2B) most of the activity was found in the wash through fraction (Fraction 2), indicating a reduced adherence of these cells at higher temperatures. Comparison of the percent specific lysis of fractionated (Fraction 3) cells indicates a 3-4 fold enrichment over the unfractionated cells for the room temperature separation, and a 2-3 fold enrichment for the 37°C separation (Fraction 2).

C. Sephadex G10 Separation

LCMV induced spleen cells were similarly fractionated through sephadex G-10 at room temperature according to the procedure of Ly and Mishell (1974). Non-adherent cells eluted by the first 60 ml of medium showed a marked decrease in their ability to lyse tumor targets. When G-10 adherence and

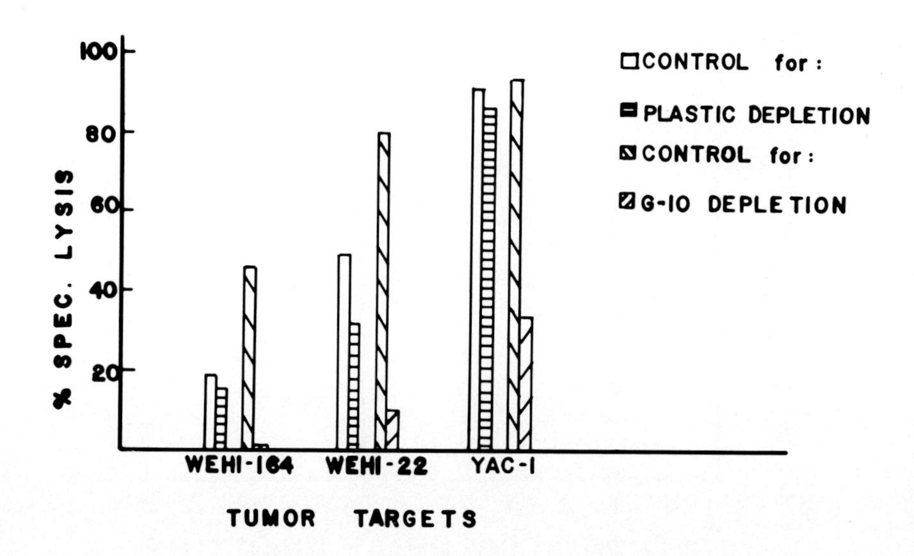

FIGURE 3. Specific lysis of different tumor targets by effector spleen cell preparation from LCMV treated mice, separated by either plastic or G-10 adherence.

plastic adherence properties were compared, the results (Fig. 3), showed that LCMV induced spleen cells were non-adherent to plastic, but were adherent to G-10 sephadex. Similar results were in general obtained with different tumor targets, although some minor quantitative differences were noted in degree of depletion.

D. Conclusions

These studies of the use of biophysical procedures to enrich and characterize populations of NK effector cells have yielded several specific conclusions:

i) NK effector cells from most sources and reactive with several targets, are heterogeneous in volume and adherence properties.

ii) However, a distinct shift in the size distribution of NK effector cells occurs following augmentation of the total level of NK reactivity by various treatments that are associated with elevation of interferon levels (see Section C this volume). The shift is towards larger cells which may represent a blastogenic response of the NK effector population, or alternatively, may represent the emergence of a new distinct NK cell population that is distinct from these in untreated mice. The results to be described later in this section however suggest that these are serologically related cell types.

iii) NK effector cells from poly I-C or LCMV treated mice show considerably greater surface adherence to G-10 and nylon columns than do NK cells from untreated mice. This may also reflect a change in the differentiation status of these cells following interferon induction. It should be noted however, that the demonstration of surface adherence is quite temperature dependant, as has also been noted for other hemopoietic cell types (Shortman et al. 1971).

iv) Both volume and adherence separation procedures can result in some enrichment of NK activity in selected fraction. However in view of the lability of NK cells, this is probably somewhat less than might have been expected, and does not yield a sufficient degree of enrichment to warrant general application for NK cell isolation purposes. As will be discussed in the next section, the cell volume shift can however also be utilized as a parameter for selection in combination with other specific approaches in flow sorting procedures.

II. CHARACTERIZATION OF SURFACE ALLOANTIGENS OF MURINE NK CELLS BY SPECIFIC ALLOANTISERA

Although NK effector cells constitute a cell type that can be clearly distinguished from previously defined cytotoxic cells, relatively few specific surface markers have been identified for the murine NK cell. Unlike cytotoxic T cells, the NK cell does not express Lyt-1, 2 or 3 or T145 (Kimura and Wigzell, 1978), nor does it express surface immunoglobulin, Ia products or C3 receptors (Kiessling et al. 1975b; Kiessling et al. 1976a; Glimcher et al. 1977; Herberman and Holden, 1978). In addition anti-macrophage antibody treatment followed by complement does not eliminate NK activity (Ojo and Wigzell, 1978).

On the other hand, NK cells may share some markers which are common to T or B cells although possibly at different cell surface densities. NK cells exhibit on their surface the appropriate H-2K and D molecules and neuraminidase treated cells like T lymphocyte or immature B lymphocytes, will bind Helix pomatia A (Haller et al. 1978a). Herberman et al. (1977) showed that NK cells have low but detectable amounts of Fc receptors although of low avidity for Ig binding. The detection of Thy-1 (theta) antigen has been a point of considerable debate. NK cells from nude mice and augmented mice, and to a lesser extent from normal mice, have been shown by cytotoxicity assays to possess a low level of Thy-1. However, repeated treatment with anti-Thy-1 sera and rabbit complement, (but not guinea pig complement), were necessary to demonstrate substantial abrogation of NK activity. The issue of Thy-1 expression is considered in more detail elsewhere in this volume, and by those advocates of its expression is considered a strong argument favoring the possible interpretation that NK cells may belong to the T cell lineage - possibly at a stage analogous to the prothymocyte. We would however like to emphasize certain cautions in regard to such an interpretation:

i) The presence of a specific well characterized cell surface marker on a cell type of unknown nature, does not necessarily imply that the particular cell in question synthesized that component. Several cell surface components can be readily shed from a cell that produced that component, and be then picked up by other cells. Such shedding may well be accelerated through antibody induced capping.

ii) Even if NK cells do synthesize Thy-1 of intrinsic origin, this need not imply the cells are in the T cell lineage. Although Thy-1 can indeed be considered a unique marker to distinguish T cells from B cells, other cell types can express Thy-1. For example we have recently detected abundant Thy-1 expression on an unequivocal myelomonocytic leukemia which does not express any other "specific" T cell markers (Warner, N.L., Ledbetter, J., and Herzenberg, L.A., manuscript in preparation).

Another surface marker that has been clearly identified on NK cells is the Ly-5 component. Both normal and athymic mice were shown to express one of 2 allelic forms of the products specified by this locus and antibody specific for Ly-5 was shown to abrogate NK activity even in the absence of complement (Kasai et al. 1979). The Ly-5 component however is not specifically expressed on only T cells, but may be present on most hemopoietic cells. The cell surface density of its expression on NK cells may however be more similar to that of T cells, since antibody and complement does eliminate both cell types. The identification of surface alloantigens specific for NK cells will however be of considerably greater value for their characterization, and has met with some success. One such component, the NK-1.1 antigen, was serologically defined by Glimcher et al. (1977) by the C3H anti-CE thymocyte antiserum, and shown to be distinct by absorption studies from the known anti-Ly-1.2 antibody also present in that serum.

In studies performed in collaboration with R.C. Burton and H. Winn (Harvard Medical School, Mass. General Hospital), several new reagents which serologically define other NK specific surface alloantigens, have been generated (see section by Burton, R.C. and Winn, H. this volume). Two basic methods were used in the study of these antisera. The first involved pretreatment of effector cells with the reagent at $4^{o}C$ for 30 minutes followed by fluorescein-conjugated anti-mouse IgG1 and analysis of staining reaction using the fluorescence activated cell sorter (FACS III, Becton Dickinson). Results on these sorting and analysis studies will be addressed in the next section. The serum we have extensively used was raised by 6-10 weekly injections of CBA spleen cells into $(NZBxCE)F_1$ hybrid mice. The treatment of LCMV augmented BALB/c ByJ splenic cells by an $(NZBxCE)F_1$ anti-CBA antiserum (anti-NK antiserum) at $4^{o}C$ or $37^{o}C$ in the absence of complement, does not affect the lytic capacity of the NK effector cells on the YAC-1 tumor target. The second method used was pretreatment of the effector spleen cell population with the antiserum, followed by complement. The cells were washed after each treatment and readjusted to the original volume and tested for lytic activity.

TABLE 1. Effect of Incubation Temperature and Complement Source on NK Killing by anti-NK Alloantiserum.

Reagent	Temp. of Incubation	C' Source	% specific lysis ± S.E.M. Medium Control	Comp. Control	Serum and Comp.
$(NZBxCE)F_1$ anti-CBA	4°	guinea pig complement	47.3±0.8	52.0±2.2	51.0±2.7
	37°	"	60.6±6.0	52.0±1.4	50.2±2.7
	4°	rabbit complement	48.0±4.9	55.3±0.1	39.7±0.5
	37°	"	50.8±1.4	44.2±4.7	20.4±1.8

As indicated by the results in Table 1, the temperature of incubation and the complement source were both important factors for abrogation of NK activity. As shown by Burton and Winn (this volume) the use of low toxicity rabbit complement is essential for lytic activity to be found using these alloantisera. The importance of incubation temperature is further illustrated by the titration data in Fig. 4. The distribution of the alloantigen on spleen cells of different mouse strains was examined by treating spleen cells from mice of different genetic backgrounds with the anti-NK serum, and assaying for remaining activity. Treatment of BALB/c, CBA, C57Bl/6, and C3H splenic lymphoid cells substantially reduced NK activity. On the other hand spleen cells from NZB mice were not affected by this alloantiserum. A wider strain distribution survey of this surface alloantigen, and those defined by the several alloantisera of Burton and Winn (see this volume) is presently under further investigation. Whether this serum defines an alternate allele to that defined by the NK-1.1 specificity, or another locus (NK-2?) at present remains unknown. We thus provisionally will refer to this as the $(NZBxCE)F_1$ anti-CBA/NK specificity.

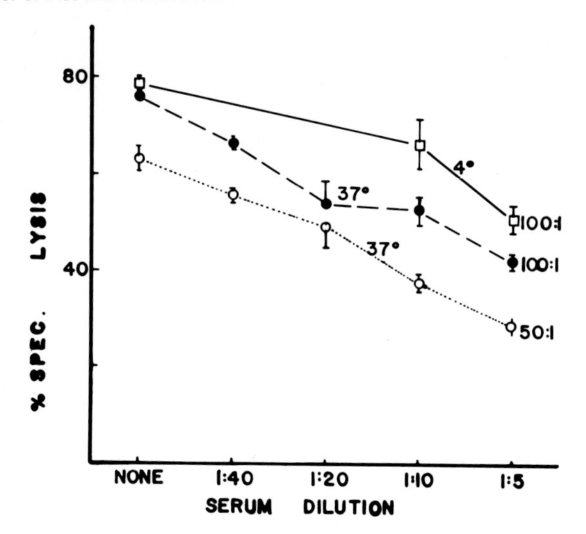

FIGURE 4. Elimination of NK effector cells from spleen cell preparations of LCMV treated mice, using (NZBxCE)F_1 anti-CBA spleen alloantiserum and complement. E/T ratios at 100:1 and 50:1 were used with YAC-1 targets.

III. IDENTIFICATION AND ISOLATION OF NK CELLS BY FLOW CYTOMETRY

The identification of specific cell surface markers on NK effector cells provides a new approach to the positive selection of NK effector cells by varios procedures that involve the application of the specific alloantiserum and a method to identify and isolate such reactive cells. In this reaction we will describe our studies with the (NZBxCE)F_1 anti-CBA/NK serum using the fluorescence activated cell sorter.

In such studies, it is essential that the procedure itself not result in an inactivation of the effector function of the cell. Such potentially could occur through either:

i) binding of the alloantiserum to the cell (as in the case of anti-Ly5 treatment); this fortunately does not occur with the anti-NK sera so far described;

ii) inactivation of the cell by its short pulse with the argon ion laser;

iii) admixture with any of the reagents used in the flow procedure;

iv) the time involved in the procedure

In view of the unusually high lability of the NK cell observed in many studies, it was somewhat unexpected in fact to discover that the flow sorting procedure can be used to achieve selection and enrichment of NK cells. It should be stated at the outset however, that we feel the more appropriate control for comparison of degrees of enrichment of NK cells, is a preparation of effector cells diluted in sheath fluid, and held under similar condition to the sorted cells, but not sorted through the system. The standard preparation procedure for sorting involved the treatment of spleen cells with ammonium chloride to remove erythrocytes, incubation of such cells with either the alloantiserum or control normal mouse serum at 4°C for 30 minutes, washing once, and further incubation with fluorescein iso-thiocyanate (FITC)-conjugated goat anti-mouse IgG_1 at 4°C for 30 minutes. The stained cells were then washed twice, resuspended in phosphate buffered saline (PBS) with 1% fetal falf serum (FCS), filtered to remove cell clumps and then sorted or analyzed in a FACS-III (Becton Dickinson) system.

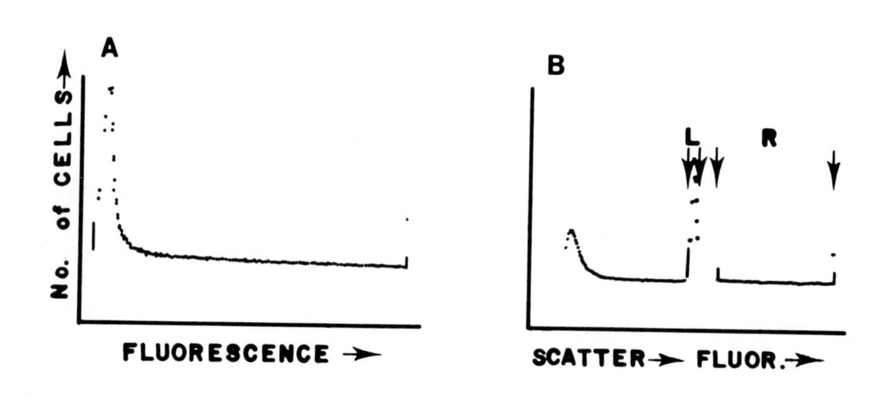

FIGURE 5. (A) Analysis of the staining of C3H spleen cells with (NZBxCE)F_1 anti-CBA/NK alloantiserum (anti-NK) or with normal mouse serum (NMS), followed by FITC-conjugated goat anti-mouse IgG_1. No significant difference in the fluorescence distribution of the two preparation was observed. Panel A is an overlay of the two fluorescence pattern. (B) Criteria for sorting of NK cells. Both preparations from panel A, were sorted on the basis of all scatter, and fluorescence channels of 128-134 (left), or 149-255 (right).

One of the questions encountered in the studies of NK cytotoxicity is the frequency of NK cells in a splenic population. Spleen cells from LCMV treated C3H mice were stained either with normal mouse serum (NMS) or with the alloantiserum followed by the FITC-conjugated goat-anti mouse IgG_1. No significant difference in the staining of these two samples was observed. The overlay of both fluorescence profiles is shown in Fig. 5A which indicates no discernible differences in the two staining patterns. Approximately 8-10% of the cells were in channels above 140, which is close to the inflection point of the curve. This was the case for both profiles, and is primarily due to IgG_1 bearing cells in the spleen. Over numerous such runs, only 1-4% of spleen cells could be concluded to be "stained" by the $(NZBxCE)F_1$ anti CBA/NK reagent. Thus only a very small percentage of the splenic population was "positive" for the surface alloantigen. However when the 2 populations were sorted by FACS into non-fluorescent cells (L) and mid-bright to very bright fluorescent cells (R) (Fig. 5B) and all populations tested for NK cytotoxicity on YAC-1 tumor target (Fig. 6A), the left and

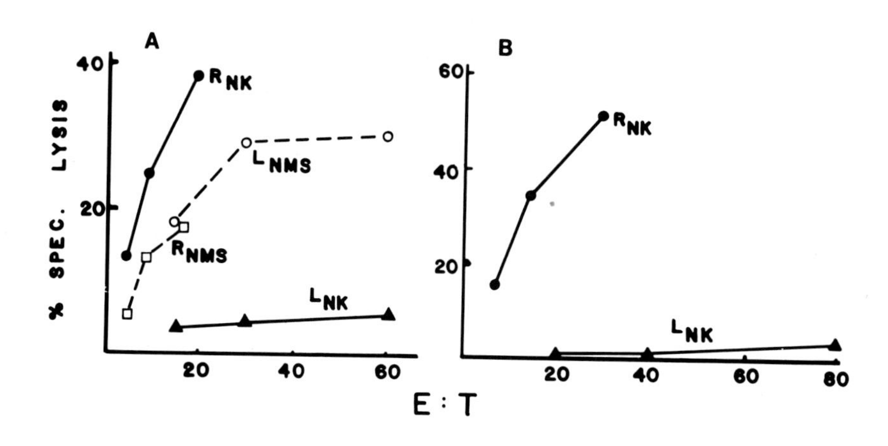

FIGURE 6. NK mediated lytic activity on YAC-1 target cells, of C3H (A) or BALB/c (B) spleen cells from LCMV mice separated by FACS on the basis of staining with $(NZBxCE)F_1$ anti-CBA/NK alloantiserum as defined in Fig. 5.

right population of NMS stained cells (L_{NMS}, R_{NMS}) showed a similar degree of cytotoxicity, while the right population of the alloantiserum stained cells (R_{NK}) was greatly enriched in NK activity when compared to the left population (L_{NK}). Similar results (Fig. 6B) were obtained with spleen cells from LCMV-treated BALB/c ByJ mice. Thus the alloantiserum selected for a very rare population of cells which has virtually all of the NK mediated killing capacity.

To further localize the NK effector population into as restricted a population as possible, spleen cells from LCMV treated C3H mice were sorted into four regions on the basis of fluorescense intensity and tested for NK lytic activity. As shown in Fig. 7, the non-fluorescent population (channels 128-136) which constituted over 90% of the spleen cell population, contained no NK activity. The low-fluorescent population

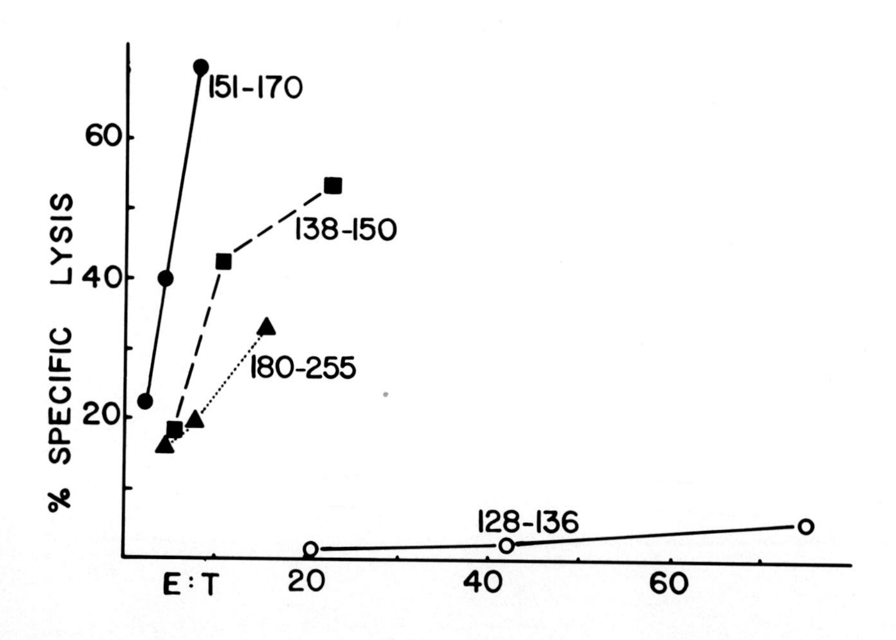

FIGURE 7. NK mediated lytic activity of spleen cells from LCMV treated C3H mice sorted on the basis of staining intensity with an (NZBxCE)F_1 anti-CBA/NK serum. The non fluorescent cells are in channels 128-136 (negative), dim fluorescent (138-150), mid-bright (151-170) and brightest in 180-255.

(ch. 138-150) was enriched in NK activity, and the mid-bright fluorescent cells (ch. 151-170) was greatly enriched in NK cytotoxicity. The brightest cells (ch. 180-255) however, had lower activity than the preceding population. Thus the majority of the NK population and the greatest degree of enrichment was found in the mid-fluorescent intensity region and yielding significant lysis even with an E:T of 2:1.

In addition to sorting on the basis of fluorescence intensity, spleen cells could also be sorted on the basis of light scatter, a parameter closely parallel to the volume of the cells. In prior experiments on velocity sedimentation of mouse spleen cells, we found that in LCMV or poly I:C treated mice, functional NK activity was associated with the larger cell population. Thus LCMV treated C3H spleen cells were sorted into four subpopulations based on light scatter, and the sorted populations were tested for lytic activity on ^{51}Cr labeled YAC-1 (Fig. 8). The highest level of NK activity

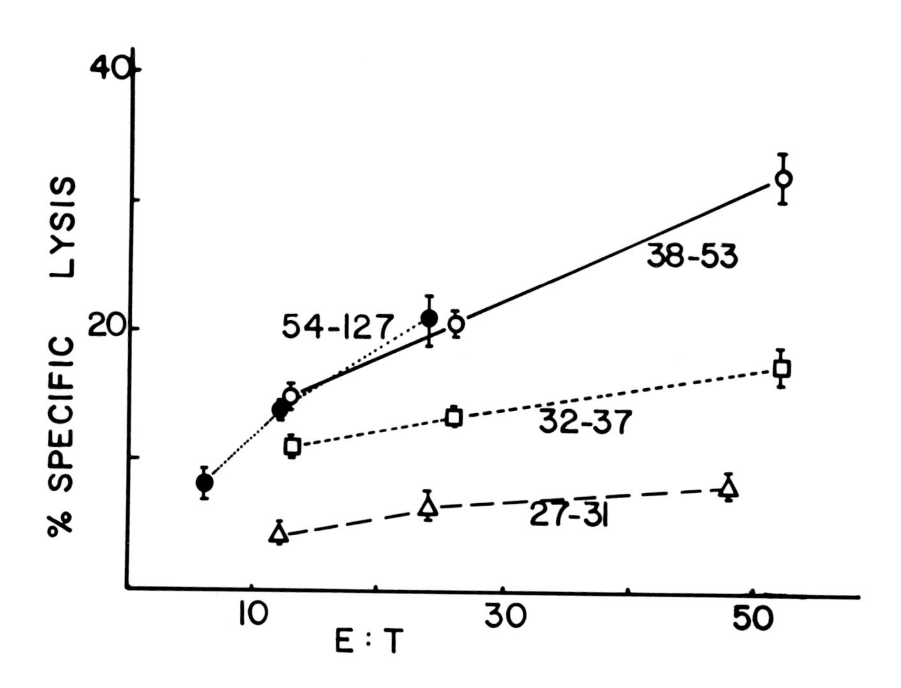

FIGURE 8. NK mediated lytic activity of spleen cells from LCMV treated C3H mice sorted on the basis of light scattering intensity. Smallest cells would be in low channel numbers. Target tumor is YAC-1.

was associated with the cell fractions having the greatest degree of light scattering. Similar results were also found using the fibrosarcoma target WEHI-164, with the only difference being that virtually no lytic activity was found in the cell fraction with low scattering properties (small cells). These results thus closely parallel the observation using velocity sedimentation (Fig. 1) in which the larger cells have more activity with both lymphoma and fibrosarcoma targets, but that the ratio of activity in large to small cell fractions is greater for the fibrosarcoma target than for the lymphoma. This type of result would thus be more compatible with the view that different subsets of NK effector cells exist for the different targets.

Preliminary studies employing a combination of light scatter for larger cells and the mid-fluorescence bright intensity, suggest that further enrichment of NK effector population can be obtained.

A. *Conclusion*

These studies therefore lead to several provisional conclusions concerning the nature of the NK effector population:

i) On the basis of staining with the NK specific alloantiserum, it is concluded that the NK effector population represents a very rare cell type in the spleen. Further studies using directly fluoresceinated IgG fractions of the alloantiserum, or biotin-conjugated fractions followed by FITC avidin (which does not give any background staining as with the FITC goat anti-mouse IgG_1) should provide a more direct and precise assessment of the frequency of NK effector cells in various cell populations - such as comparisons for frequency of effector cells for different targets (on the basis of sorting and assay), and comparisons of cell numbers in normal and augmented mice.

ii) If the resolution of this staining and sorting can be further improved, it may then be possible to isolate the effector population in pure or considerably enriched fashion, and then further stain such cells with other reagents that may more precisely define the nature of the NK effector cell differentiation lineage.

iii) These studies have also demonstrated that the NK effector population from LCMV treated mice which lyse the fibrosarcoma WEHI-164, also bear the NK alloantigen recognized by the (NZBxCE)F_1 alloantiserum. Since the NK effector population from normal mice which lyse tumor cells from carcinomas and sarcomas have been reported to *not* express the NK specific alloantigens (Paige et al. 1978; Burton, R.C. and Winn, H. manuscript submitted), it is perhaps suggestive that the relationship between these NK effector populations may be of a sequential differentiation nature, in that they are both in the same differentiation lineage, with the NK alloantigens being expressed at only one particular stage.

Further analysis of this possibility is in progress.

REFERENCES

Djeu, J.Y., Heinbaugh, J.A., Holden, H.T., and Herberman, R.B. *J. Immunol. 122,* 175 (1979).

Glimcher, L., Shen, F.W. and Cantor, H. *J. Exp. Med. 145,* 1 (1977).

Haller, O., Gidlund, M., Hellstrom, U., Hammerstrom, S., and Wigzell, H. *Eur. J. Immunol. 8,* 765 (1978).

Herberman, R.B., Nunn, M.E., Holden, H.T., and Lavrin, D.H. *Int. J. Cancer 16,* 230 (1975a).

Herberman, R.B., Bartram, S., Haskill, J.S., Nunn, M.E., Holden, H.T. and West, W.H. *J. Immunol. 119,* 322 (1977).

Herberman, R.B., and Holden, H.T. *Advances in Cancer Res. 27,* 305 (1978).

Julius, M.H., Simpson, E., Herzenberg, L.A. *Eur. J. Immunol. 3,* 645 (1973).

Kasai, M., Leclere, J.C., Shen, F.W. and Cantor, H. *Immunogenetics 8,* 153 (1979).

Kiessling, R., Klein, E., and Wigzell, H. *Eur. J. Immuno. 5,* 112 (1975a).

Kiessling, R., Klein, E., Pross, H., and Wigzell, H. *Eur. J. Immunol. 5,* 117 (1975b).

Kiessling, R., Petranyi, G., Karre, K., Jondal, M., Tracy, D., and Wigzell, H. *J. Exp. Med. 143,* 112 (1976).

Kimura, A. and Wigzell, H. *J. Exp. Med. 147,* 1418 (1978).

Ly, I.A. and Mishell, R.J. *J. Immunol. Methods 5,* 239 (1974).

Ojo, E., and Wigzell, H. *Scand. J. Immunol. 8,* 215 (1978).

Paige, C.J., Figarella, E.F., Cutteto, M.J., Cahan, A., and Stutman, O. *J. Innumol. 121,* 1827 (1978).

Roder, J.C., Kiessling, R., Biberfeld, P., and Anderson, B. *J. Immunol. 121,* 2509 (1978).

Sendo, F., Aoki, T., Boyse, E.A., and Buofo, C.K. *J. Natl. Cancer Inst. 55,* 603 (1975).

Shortman, K., Williams, N., Jackson, H., Russell, P., Byrt, R., and Diener, E. *J. Cell Biol. 48,* 566 (1971).

Welsh, Jr., R.M., and Zinkernagel, R. *Nature 268,* 646 (1977).

Zarling, J.M., Nowinsky, R.C., and Bach, F.H. *Proc. Nat. Acad. Sci. U.S.A. 72,* 2780 (1975).

ANALYSIS OF RECOGNITION PATTERNS OF NK CELLS THROUGH USE OF VARYING COMBINATIONS OF MOUSE STRAINS AND TUMOR TARGETS

Anna Tai
Noel L. Warner

Immunobiology Laboratories
University of New Mexico
School of Medicine
Albuquerque, New Mexico

I. INTRODUCTION

One of the major questions concerning the NK system concerns the nature of the recognition event between the NK cell and its tumor target. Involved in this issue is both a consideration of the nature of the effector cells recognition unit - whether it is a V gene based specific recognition system as in T and B cells, or of less specific and unknown nature; and the corresponding nature of the tumor "antigen" that is seen by the NK cell. At the present time, it would be perhaps reasonable to suggest that although there are numerous instances suggesting "specificity", none of these reach the level of the fine recognition of an Ig V gene based system. One approach to determining whether there is positive evidence for specificity in NK effector-target cell recognition is to survey a wide range of both effector cell sources (normal versus augumented, different mouse strains) and of tumor target cell lines.

Since their initial recognition (Oldham et al. 1973; Herberman et al. 1973, 1974; Rosenberg et al. 1974) NK cells have been shown to have a wide range of cytotoxicity. Originally it was thought that killing was restricted to lymphomas (Zarling 1975; Kiessling 1975) but has since been shown to be cytotoxic for many different types of tumors including lymphomas, fibrosarcomas and carcinomas (Kiessling et al. 1975; Herberman et al. 1975, Shellam and Hogg 1977;

ISBN 0-12-341350-8

Nunn et al.1976, 1977; Sutuman et al. 1978; Warner and Li 1979; Tai et al. 1980). In addition, mouse, rat and human NK cells have been reported to exhibit both intra- and inter- species cytotoxicity (Hansson et al. 1978; Haller et al. 1977). Furthermore, other results indicated that NK cells could also lyse normal haemopoietic cells, including allogeneic bone marrow cells and thymus cells (Haller et al. 1977; Ono et al. 1977; Nunn et al. 1977; Hansson et al. 1979). These results in general would seem to infer that NK cells either posses a very broad or nonspecific type of receptor, or that the NK population is composed of many distinct subpopulations each having a quite defined and restricted specificity. Further evidence for this latter thesis came from cold target competition experiments (Herberman et al. 1975) who concluded that NK cells recognized several antigen specificities associated with C-type viruses. Correlation between susceptibility and release of exogenous C-type viral antigens was found by Shellam and Hogg (1977); and Lee and Ihle (1977) were able to block NK lysis of AKR thymomas with the relevant viral gp70. In contrast, studies by Becker et al. (1976) advocated no involvement of viral related antigens, and Kiessling showed the absence of correlation between expression of surface MuLV antigens and sensitivity to lysis (Kiessling et al. 1978). In our hands, tumor cell lines which have been shown to be actively budding virus, for example WEHI-22 a T lymphoma, were not always susceptible to NK lysis. In addition we have purified extracellular virus from 3 different T lymphoma cell lines using the procedure of Ihle et al. (1976), and tested the ability of these viruses to block NK activity from LCMV augmented mice. *No blocking* was observed in any effector-target-virus-combination. Roder et al. (1979) have isolated NK target structures from YAC-1 cell line and found no common determinants between these and gp70, p30 ro MCSA. Thus the subject of possible viral invovlement is still open to question, although present data would tend to negate viral antigen involvement.

II. COLD TARGET BLOCKING

One of the most useful techniques for analyzing the possible nature of effector cell specificities in cytotoxicity systems is the cold target blocking assay (Ortiz de Landazuri and Herberman 1972). Although this is considered in detail elsewhere in this volume, we would like to stress two aspects of the utilization of this system in NK studies.

The first issue concerns the apparent ability of some tumor cell lines to inhibit NK mediated lysis of susceptible tumor targets even though the inhibitory tumor is itself apparently resistant to lysis by the same NK effector cell population. There are two non-specific explanations of such an observation that are in essence "trivial", and must first be eliminated in such an observation, and these are:

a) That the tumor line is inherently resistant to lysis in the particular isotope release system used, and

b) that the tumor produces a substance - such as prostaglandins, that can directly inhibit the lytic process mediated by the effector cell. One example of this phemonenon, in which neither of these "trivial" explanations is feasible, involves the T cell lymphoma line WEHI-22, which is completely resistant to lysis by NK effector cells from BALB/c mice (Burton et al. 1978), however is quite suseptible to lysis by spleen cells from LCMV or poly I:C treated mice (Tai et al. 1980). Furthermore, in other studies not shown, this tumor shows no non-specific inhibitory properties. Thus we provisionally conclude that the WEHI-22 tumor, which is susceptible to lysis with certain NK effector cells, does express NK recognized target structures. However these may be in sufficiently low density to permit effective tumor-NK interaction for lysis to result when using untreated mouse spleen derived NK cells as the effectors.

We might thus suggest that in considering the mechanism of NK killing, one can assume that in NK lysis, as in CTL mediated lysis, a series of steps occur, the first of which is recognition, and the final of which is lysis (Cerrotini and Brunner 1974; Martz 1975). At least two of the events have been dissociated by Roder et al. (1978) who inhibited the lytic event, while allowing the recognition event to occur. One might thus argue, that although all murine tumors possess common target determinants, a rather specific "fit" is required to permit lysis to occur. Thus changes in avidity or hydrophobicity of the effector population, the latter of which has been shown by Becker et al. (1979) to be relevant to susceptibility of tumor cells to NK lysis, can alter the efficiency of the lytic event. Augmentation of the NK effector cell population by various agents has been shown to result in some distinct changes including adherence, volume heterogeneity, and perhaps expression of distinct NK specific alloantigens (see Tai and Warner previous section I). Possibly this might be considered as analogous to an increased maturation as occurs in the cytotoxic T cell lineage from an Lyt-1, 2, 3 positive cytotoxic cell to an Ly-2, 3 cell. The "augmented" NK cell, perhaps through an altered density of surface recognition structures, now shows a higher efficeincy of killing such previously "resistant" tumor targets.

The second aspect we wish to stress is that although there is indeed considerable evidence for heterogeneity in the NK population, there may also be common target structures present on many tumors that are recognized by the one NK subset, but that there are distinct quantitative differences in the expression of these target structures on different cell lines. We again use the T cell lymphomas as an example of this observation. As shown in Figure 1, NK effector cells from the spleen of LCMV treated BALB/c mice, are capable of lysing all three T cell lymphomas to a similar extent. However when this NK population is used with any of the three ^{51}Cr labeled tumors, and the three tumors are compared as cold target inhibitors, YAC-1 tumor is consistently the most efficient inhibitor (Fig. 1, B-D). We would thus conclude that within this triad of T cell lymphomas, there need be only one NK subset and one tumor target structure, but the target component differs quantitatively in amount, and shows greatest expression on YAC-1 cells.

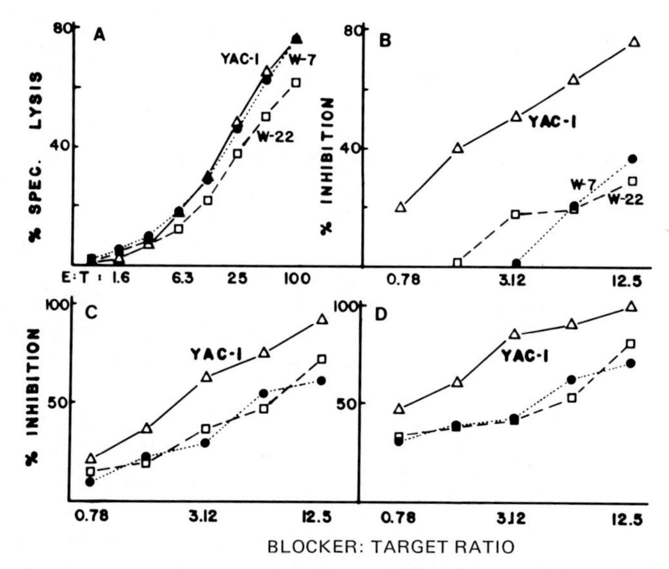

FIGURE 1. A) Lysis of YAC-1, WEHI-7, and WEHI-22 cell lymphomas by spleen cells from LCMV treated BALB/c mice. (B-D) Inhibition of this lysis using the same NK effector population as in A, with either ^{51}Cr labeled YAC-1 (B), WEHI-7 (C) or WEHI-22 (D) as targets, and all three unlabeled tumors as cold target blockers.

III. COMPARISON OF DIFFERENT NK EFFECTOR SOURCES ON DIFFERENT TUMOR TARGETS

Mouse strains have been classified into high-, intermediate and low- NK reactive depending on the cytotoxicity they demonstrate on several tumor targets (Herberman and Holden 1978; Kiessling et al. 1975; Petranyi et al. 1975). In general, targets susceptible to NK mediated lysis by spleen cells of one mouse strain are also susceptible to lysis by other mouse strains. However we would like to point out some *exceptions*, which suggest that target-dependence exists in addition to strain dependence in overall NK reactivities.

When normal spleen cells of various mouse strains were tested on several tumor targets (Table 1), we found that NZB/NIH spleen cells, which were cytotoxic for YAC-1, a T lymphoma, were only minimally cytotoxic for WEHI-22 and WEHI-164, a T lymphoma and a fibrosarcoma. Conversely CBA/J and NZB showed higher cytotoxicity for WEHI-164 than for YAC-1, and none of the mouse strains tested were very cytotoxic for WEHI-22. The differential killing was also demonstrated by spleen cells from LCMV treated mice. The results of Figure 2 indicated that BALB/c ByJ spleen cells were highly cytotoxic for YAC-1, moderately for WEHI-274 a premacrophage tumor, and not at all for ABE-8, a pre-B lymphoma. C3H/HeJ again showed similar NK levels as BALB/c ByJ, but with higher relative killing for WEHI-274 and again no cytotoxicity for ABE-8. On the other hand, C57Bl/6, while showing moderate to low killing of YAC-1 and WEHI-274, was able to kill ABE-8 to a greater extent than BALB/c or C3H spleen cells. Thus the phenomenon of target dependence is operative in both endogenous as well as the augmented situations.

Two previous examples of tumor target differences were also noted in our previous section on characterization of NK cells. Thus in Figure 1 and Figure 3 of section I, we showed that by either velocity sedimentation or adherence depletion, relative differences were observed between different fractions in their lytic capacity of YAC-1 (T lymphoma) versus the fibrosarcoma WEHI-164. Again this indicates heterogeneity at the effector level that differs for different tumor targets.

In this instance we again wish to stress that there have been previous indications of different effector populations that lyse solid tumors versus lymphomas (Stutman et al. 1978; Burton, R.C. and Winn H., manuscript submitted), however our studies were performed with spleen cells from LCMV treated mice, in which the effector cells for *both* targets bear the

TABLE I. Comparison of Endogenous NK Activity for Various Mouse Strains with Several Tumor Targets

Mouse strains	*Assay time*	*% Specific lysis (+S.E.M.) for:*		
		WEHI-22	*WEHI-164*	*YAC-1*
NZB/NIH	*4 hr*	*5.3±0.7*	*4.2±0.5*	*20.5±1.2*
CBA/J	*4 hr*	*1.6±0.9*	*23.5±1.6*	*10.3±0.7*
C57Bl/6	*4 hr*	*1.6±0.9*	*10.0±1.6*	*7.2±0.6*
NZW	*4 hr*	*4.5±0.7*	*7.6±0.5*	*3.9±0.3*
	8 hr	*NT*	*27.0±0.3*	*20.1±0.6*

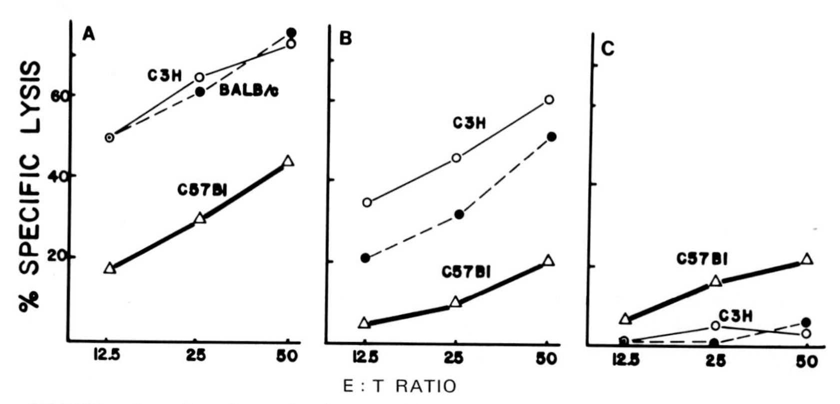

FIGURE 2. Lysis of three different tumor targets by spleen cells from LCMV treated mice of indicated strains (A:YAC-1; B:WEHI-274; C:ABE-8). Although only minimal lysis is observed with ABE-8 the relative effectiveness of C57B1/6 cells versus BALB/c or C3H is clearly different than with the other targets.

alloantigen recognized by the (NZBxCE)F_1 anti-CBA serum.

A further possible example of the selective proliferation of NK subsets comes from studies with the MRL/L mouse strain. This strain of mouse carries a gene (lpr) which determines a massive lymphoproliferation and autoimmune processes (Murphy and Roths 1978). The disease becomes clearly evident in mice of 4-5 months of age. When splenic and mesenteric lymph node cells from young (8 weeks old) MRL/L and MRL/N mice were compared, both strains demonstrate low NK mediated lytic activity on WEHI-22 and YAC-1. Effector cells from older mice (4-5 months) however showed a striking difference in their reactivities (Figure 3), with the MRL/L effector cells, especially the mesenteric lymph node cells, showing a noticeable increase in cytotoxicity compared to the MRL/N spleen cells. This increase was target-dependent, with WEHI-22 being lysed to a greater extent than YAC-1 by both spleen and mesenteric lymph node cells.

This combination thus represents one of the few situations where:

i) lymph node cells have shown more lytic activity than spleen cells, and

ii) where WEHI-22 is *more* susceptible to lysis than YAC-1.

Clearly further studies are necessary to define the exact nature of the cell in the MRL/lpr mouse that is responsible for this lysis, however this again provides further evidence of heterogeneity in natural killer effector cell populations--in this case most clearly distinguished by an unusual target tumor specificity pattern.

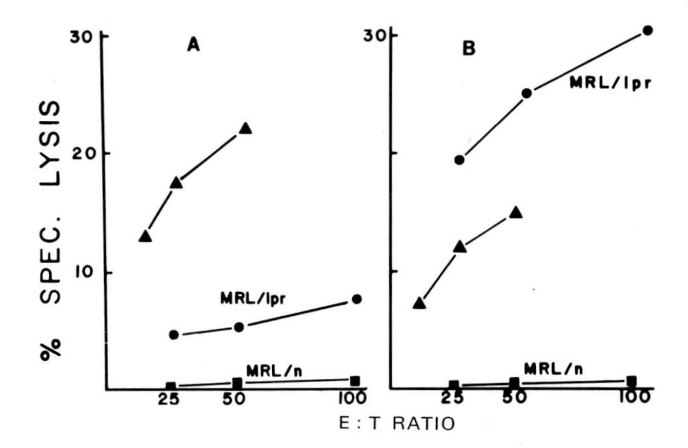

FIGURE 3. Lysis of YAC-1 (A) and WEHI-22 (B) T lymphomas by mesenteric lymph nodes of MRL/n and MRL/L mice. For comparison, lytic activity of spleen cells from MRL/n mice given LCMV is shown (closed triangles).

In conclusion, we would thus emphasize that the use of selective combinations of effector cell populations and different tumor targets, has resulted in clear evidence of multiple NK effector subsets. Superimposed upon this however, is a distinct impression of additional common target structures, which may however differ in amount between tumors. We certainly do *not* have evidence of very restricted NK subsets with fine specificity for single target structures. The issue that must yet be resolved is whether the heterogeneity of NK subsets is related to stages in differentiation of one cell lineage, multiple branches of a common differentiation lineage, or, like T and B cells, members of a common lineage each of which however express a distinct recognition structure.

REFERENCES

Becker, S., Fenyo, E.M., and Klein, E. *Eur. J. Immunol. 6,* 882, (1976).
Becker, S., Stendahl, O., and Magnusson, K. *Immunolog. Comm. 8,*73 (1979).
Burton, R.C., Grail, D., and Warner, N.L. *Brit. J. Cancer, 37,* 806 (1978).
Cerrotini, J.C., and Brunner, K.T. *Advance Immunol. 18,* 67 (1974).
Chism, S.E., Burton, R.C. Grail, D.L., Bell, P.M., and Warner, N.L. *J. Immunol. Methods 16,* 245 (1977).
Haller, O., Kiessling, R., Orn, A., Karre, K., Nilsson, K., and Wigzell, H., *Int. J. Cancer 20,* 93 (1977).
Hansson, M., Karre, K., Bakacs, T., Kiessling, R., and Klein, G. *J. Immunol. 121,* 6 (1978).

Hansson, M., Kiessling, R., Anderson, B., Karre, K., and Roder, J. *Nature 278,* 174 (1979).
Herberman, R.B., Nunn, M.E., Lavrin, D.H., and Asofsky, R. *J. Natl. Cancer Inst. 51,* 1509 (1973).
Herberman, R.B., Ting, C.C., Kirchner, H., Holden, H., Glaser, M., Bonnard, G.D., and Lavrin, D. *Prog. Immunol. Int. Congr. Immunol., 2nd 1974 vol. II.* p. 285 (1974).
Herberman, R.B., Nunn, M.E., and Lavrin, D.H. *Int. J. Cancer 16,* 216 (1975).
Herberman, R.B., and Holden, H.T., *Adv. Cancer Res, 27,* 305 (1978).
Ihle, J.N., Denny, T.P., and Bolognesi, D.P. *J. Virol. 17,* 727 (1976).
Kiessling, R., Klein, E., and Wigzell, H. *Eur. J. Immunol. 5,* 112 (1975).
Kiessling, R., Haller, O., Fenyo, E.M. Steinitz, M., and Klein, G. *Int. J. Cancer 21,* 460 (1978).
Lee, J.C., and Ihle, J.N. *J. Immunol. 118,* 928 (1977).
Martz, E. *J. Immunol. 115,* 261 (1975).
Murphy, E.D., and Roths, J.B. Genetic Control of Autoimmune Disease. Eds. N.R. Rose, P.E. Bigazzi, and N.L. Warner. Elsenvier, North-Holland. p. 207 (1978).
Nunn, M.E., Djeu, J.Y., Glaser, M., Lavrin, D.H., and Herberman, R.B. *J. Natl. Cancer Inst. 56,* 393 (1976).
Nunn, M.E., Herberman, R.B., and Holden, H.T. *Int. J. Cancer 20,* 381 (1977).
Oldham, R.K., Siwarski, D., McCoy, J.L. Plata, E.J., and Herberman, R.B. *Natl. Cancer Inst. Monogr. 37,* 49 (1973).
Ono, A., Amos, D.B., and Koren, H.S. *Nature 266,* 546 (1977).
Ortiz de Landazuri, M., and Herberman, R.B. *Nature New Biol. 238,* 18 (1972a).
Petranyi, G., Kiessling, R., Povey, S., Klein, G., and Wigzell, H. *Immunogenetics 2,* 53 (1975).
Roder, J.C., Kiessling, R., Biberfeld, P., and Anderson, B. *J. Immunol. 121,* 2509 (1978).
Roder, J.C., Rosen, A., Fenyo, E.M., and Troy, F.A. *Proc. Natl. Acad. Sci. 76,* 1405 (1979).
Rosenberg, E.B., McCoy, J.L., Green, S.S., Donnelly, F.C., Siwarski, D.F., Levine, P.H., and Herberman, R.B. *J. Natl. Cancer Inst. 52,* 345 (1974).
Shellam, G.R., and Hogg, N. *Int. J. Cancer 19,* 212 (1977).
Stutman, O., Paige, C.J., and Figarella, E.F. *J. Immunol. 121,* 1819 (1978).
Tai, A., Burton, R.C., and Warner, N.L. *J. Immunol.* in press, (1980).
Warner, N.L., and Li, A.T. Immunobiology and Immunotherapy of Cancer, Eds. W. Terry and Y. Yamamura. Elsevier, North-Holland p. 119 (1979).
Zarling, J.M., Nowinsky, R.C., and BAch, F.H. *Proc. Nat. Acad. Sci. U.S.A. 72,* 280 (1975).

FACS ANALYSIS AND ENRICHMENT OF NK EFFECTOR CELLS[1]

Milton R. Tam
Sandra L. Emmons
Sylvia B. Pollack

Divisions of Tumor Virology and Tumor Immunology
The Fred Hutchinson Cancer Research Center
Seattle, Washington

I. INTRODUCTION

Murine NK cells which lyse certain tumor and normal cells *in vitro* have been characterized as non-adherent, non-phagocytic, non-immunoglobulin-bearing lymphocytes of unknown lineage. Early studies failed to identify characteristic B or T lymphocyte markers on these cells, which led to their designation as "null" lymphocytes. Recently, however, these "null" cells have been shown to possess receptors for the lectin *Helix pomatia A* (Haller *et al.*, 1978), and to react with sera generated against the T cell-associated antigens Ly 5 (Cantor *et al.*, 1979; Pollack *et al.*, 1979; Kasai *et al.*, 1979) and Ly 6 (Pollack *et al.*, 1979). In addition, Herberman *et al.* (1978) and Mattes *et al.* (1979) have reported that NK cells from both normal and nude mice are partially susceptible to complement (C)-mediated lysis with either monoclonal or conventionally raised anti-Thy 1 sera, suggesting that the NK cell may be in the T cell lineage. Glimcher *et al.* (1977) have reported production of an antiserum identifying an NK cell-specific alloantigen. Treatment of normal spleen lymphocytes with this antiserum and C lysed fewer than 5% of the cells, yet depleted NK activity when tested on target tumor cells. Cantor *et al.* (1979) have termed this antigen NK-1 and identified strains of NK 1.1^+ and NK 1.1^- mice.

[1] *This work was supported in part by grants AI 18074 and CA 18647 from the National Cancer Institute and institutional grant IN-26T from the American Cancer Society.*

ISBN 0-12-341350-8

The objectives of studies presented here are to more fully characterize the phenotype of murine NK cells, to enrich for and purify NK effector cells from normal spleen with the aid of the fluorescence activated cell sorter (FACS), and to describe the discrepancy in NK cell phenotype *vs.* NK effector cell function found in old (9 to 13 months of age) C57BL/6 (B6) and C57BL/6-*beige* (B6-*bg*) mutant mice.

II. METHODS AND MATERIALS

A. *Mice and Tumor*

Mice of the C3H/He, SJL, A.SW, BALB/c, CXBD, A, AKR, and 129 strains were purchased from The Jackson Laboratory, Bar Harbor, Maine. B6 and B6-*bg* mice were purchased from the Jackson Laboratory and subsequently bred in our facilities. For the preparation of antisera the special congenic lines B6.Ly 1.1 and B6.Ly 2.1/3.1, and the semi-congenic line C3H/CE were used; breeding stock was kindly provided by Dr. E.A. Boyse (Sloan-Kettering Institute, New York). YAC, an A strain Moloney virus-induced lymphoma, was adapted to *in vitro* growth and maintained in complete RPMI 1640 medium supplemented with 10% heat-inactivated fetal calf serum (FCS).

B. *Preparation of Antisera*

For production of all antisera, a generalized protocol was followed: mice were immunized starting with cells obtained from one spleen or thymus per 10 recipient mice. Increasing numbers of immunizing cells were administered every 10 to 14 days so that by the fifth immunization one thymus or spleen per 1 to 2 mice was used. Four days after the fifth inoculation the mice were bled individually and their sera tested for C-dependent cytotoxic activity on target and appropriate control cells (or depletion of NK activity for anti-NK 1.1 serum). Sera from nonresponders and mice producing autoantibody were removed from the group. Immunizations of selected mice were continued every 10 to 14 days, with bleedings at 4 and 7 days after each booster immunization.

C. *Preparation of Effector Cells*

Spleens were removed from donor mice, the cells teased from the splenic capsule with bent 18 gauge needles, and filtered through a glass wool pad to remove debris. Red cells were removed by hypotonic lysis, the remaining cells washed once with PBS, and resuspended in RPMI containing 5% FCS (5% RPMI). Some effector cell preparations were passed over nylon wool columns (Julius *et al.*, 1973) to remove B cells and adherent cells. To test the effects of antisera on spleen NK effector cells, equal volumes of spleen cells (SC) at 2 x 10^7/ml, dilutions of antiserum, and newborn rabbit serum as a source of C (screened for low toxicity) at an initial dilution of 1:15 were incubated for 45 min at 37°, washed once in PBS, and resuspended in 5% RPMI. Viable cells were counted by trypan blue dye exclusion and the treated cells adjusted to the desired concentrations for use in subsequent assays. ^{51}Cr-release assays were performed as previously described (Pollack *et al.*, 1979).

D. *Fluorescein Labeling of SC*

Nylon wool-passed SC were adjusted to 1.5 x 10^7/ml and anti-NK 1.1 serum added at a final dilution of 1:20 to 1:30. The SC were held on ice for 30 min, centrifuged through a FCS cushion to remove unreacted antibody, and resuspended to 1.5 x 10^7/ml in fluorescein-conjugated goat anti-mouse Ig (F-GAMIG, Hyland Laboratories or Meloy, Inc.) diluted 1:25. After 30 min on ice, the cells were again centrifuged through FCS and resuspended in 5% RPMI for analysis or sorting.

Nylon wool-passed SC often contained as many as 10% contaminating Ig or Fc receptor bearing B cells which reacted directly with the F-GAMIG. To remove this background staining the SC in some experiments were first incubated with a 1:25 dilution of goat anti-mouse Ig (GAMIG, Meloy, Inc.) for 30 min at 37° prior to fluorescein labeling. This pretreatment decreased the interference of B cells with the detection of the small proportion of specifically staining NK 1.1^+ cells.

E. *Analysis and Sorting of SC with the FACS*

SC which had been fluorescein labeled were analyzed or sorted on the FACS-II (Becton-Dickinson, Mountain View, Calif.) at a flow rate of 2500 to 3500 cells/sec. Data were collected as histograms correlating (1) cell size, and (2) fluorescence intensity, against the number of cells analyzed. A FACS-generated dot plot correlating light scatter (cell size) *vs.* the fluorescence intensity was also photographed. From the analytical data generated "gates" were selected to sort the SC into fluorescence-bright (NK-1^+) and fluorescence-dull (NK-1^-) populations. The two cell populations were collected with 5% RPMI on ice until use in subsequent effector NK cell assays.

E. *The Target Binding Cell (TBC) Assay*

The TBC assay of Roder and Kiessling (1978) is thought to quantitate NK cells based on their affinity for appropriate target cells. Briefly, 2 x 10^5 SC were combined with 1 x 10^6 YAC-1 in a final volume of 0.4 ml. Samples were centrifuged at 1000 rpm, held on ice for 30 min, and resuspended with a Pasteur pipette. Wet mounts were made, examined under a Zeiss fluorescence microscope, and at least 250 SC per sample counted. The percentages of bound SC to free SC were calculated, and in experiments using fluorescein-labeled SC, the percentages of fluorescent SC and YAC-1-bound fluorescent SC were also calculated.

III. RESULTS

A. *Effect of Alloantisera on the NK Activity of B6 SC*

To determine their effects on NK cytotoxic activity, several T cell-associated antisera and anti-NK 1.1 were titrated against normal B6 SC and tested on the NK-sensitive YAC-1 target cell. As shown in Table I, antisera to NK 1.1, Ly 5.1, and Ly 6.2 significantly reduced lysis of target cells, even at dilutions of 1:60. In contrast antisera to Thy 1.2, Ly 1.2, and Ly 2.2 did not significantly reduce effector cell activity within the range of dilutions tested.

Whereas pretreatment of SC with either anti-NK 1.1 or Ly 6.2 in the absence of C had no effect on NK activity, treatment with anti-Ly 5.1 *alone* inhibited NK cells (data not shown). We have not determined the mechanism by which anti-Ly 5 serum inhibited NK activity. One possibility is that the antibodies interacted with NK cell surface recognition or binding structures, thus inhibiting later steps involved with lysis of target cells.

B. *Cytolysis of NK Effector Cells With Anti-NK 1.1 Serum*

When normal B6 SC were treated with anti-NK 1.1 (1:20 initial dilution) and C, less than 5% of the SC were lysed, as measured by a trypan blue dye exclusion assay. When treated SC were assayed for effector cell activity with YAC-1 cells, virtually all NK activity was lost (Figure 1), even at an effector to target cell ratio of 100:1.

TABLE I. *Titration of Alloantisera on B6 Spleen Cells: Reduction of NK Activity*

Effector Cell Treatment[a]	% Reduction in Target Cell Lysis at Initial Serum Concentrations of:			
	1:7.5	1:15	1:30	1:60
Anti-NK 1.1	80***[b]	64***	40**	20**
Anti-Thy 1.2	15	15	15	-15*
Anti-Ly 1.2	-4	-4	4	-24*
Anti-Ly 2.2	-12	-16	-16	-20
Anti-Ly 5.1	100***	96***	100***	88***
Anti-Ly 6.2	100***	100***	96***	92***

[a]SC from normal mice were treated with the above initial dilutions of antiserum and a 1:15 initial dilution of C in a one-step lytic assay.

[b]Percent reduction in lysis as calculated in Pollack et al., 1979. The effector:target cell ratio was 50:1 in all instances. Data shown are compiled from two experiments: in one instance control SC produced 25% specific lysis and in the other, 20% specific lysis. ***, $p<0.001$; **, $p<0.01$; *, $p<.05$

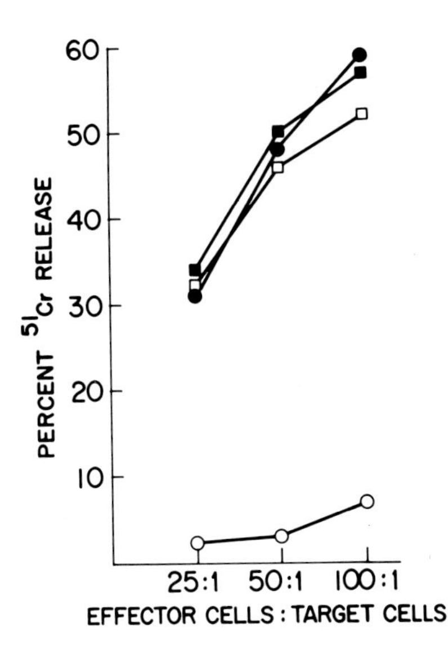

FIGURE 1. Pretreatment of SC with anti-NK 1.1 and C removes natural killer activity against YAC-1 target cells. ^{51}Cr-labeled YAC-1 (1×10^4/well) were combined with 2.5, 5.0, or 10×10^5 pretreated SC in a 4 hr chromium release assay. The SC were treated with: anti-NK 1.1 and C (o), anti-NK 1.1 only (●), C only (□), or medium only (■).

C. *Analysis of Fluorescein-Labeled NK Effector Cells*

As observed by conventional fluorescence microscopy, treatment of GAMIG-blocked, nylon wool passed SC with anti-NK 1.1 and F-GAMIG specifically labeled 10 to 15% of the B6 SC, but less than 1% of 129 strain SC. When stained B6 SC were analysed by flow fluorometry on the FACS, a labeled NK-1^+ subpopulation of small to medium-sized SC could be resolved from the majority of unlabeled cells (Figure 2A). NK-1^+ cells were not observed in control B6 SC preparations reacted with F-GAMIG alone (Figure 2C), or strain 129 SC reacted with anti-NK 1.1 and F-GAMIG (Figure 2B).

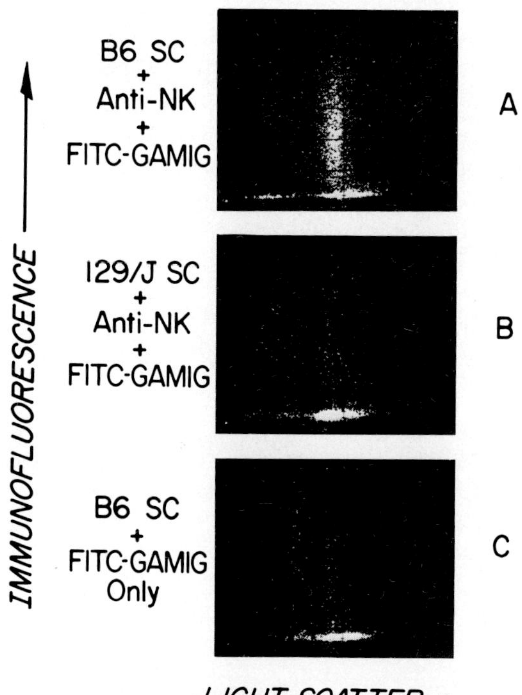

FIGURE 2. FACS-generated dot plots illustrate the specificity of anti-NK 1.1 serum. Dot plots are generated on a FACS cathode ray tube by plotting individual cells for size and fluorescence intensity. Increasing size is plotted on the horizontal axis and increasing fluorescence on the vertical axis. The origin is represented by the dot of light in the lower left hand corner. 2A, B6 (H-2^b, NK 1.1^+) SC labeled with anti-NK 1.1 (1:20 final dilution)+ F-GAMIG; 2B, 129 (H-2^{bc}, NK 1.1^-) SC labeled with anti-NK 1.1 (1:20)+ F-GAMIG; 2C, a control B6 SC preparation labeled with F-GAMIG only. In each dot plot 4000 cells are represented.

D. *Enrichment of NK-1$^+$ Cells with the FACS*

Selected populations of NK-1$^+$ and NK-1$^-$ cells were sorted for and collected with the FACS. Appropriate deflection "gates" were set and a 10 to 20 channel barrier used to ensure the collection of non-overlapping cell populations. A consistent 20 to 30% of the nylon wool-passed SC were sorted as NK-1$^+$. Approximately 60% were sorted as NK-1$^-$ and the remainder, 10 to 20% of the total cells were coincidence analyzed because of the high flow rate, and discarded by the FACS rather than sorted. Reanalysis of the sorted fractions demonstrated that all SC sorted as NK-1$^+$ were labeled, whereas those sorted as NK-1$^-$ were unlabeled. NK-1$^+$ cells did not lose their stain and remained more than 95% viable even though processing of the SC often required more than 6 hr.

E. *Functional Analyses of Sorted SC*

1. *Cytotoxic Assays Using ^{51}Cr-Labeled YAC-1 Target Cells* In a series of 8 experiments sorted NK-1$^+$ cells effected significantly more NK lysis than parallel preparations of unsorted SC. Enrichment in NK activity ranged from 4 to 8-fold compared with the control nylon wool-passed samples, and up to a 13-fold enrichment when compared with an untreated SC preparation. In the experiment illustrated in Figure 3 an 8-fold enrichment was obtained compared with the parallel unsorted SC preparation. In 6 of 8 experiments no NK effector activity was found in the NK-1$^-$ sorted fraction; only very low levels of activity were found at the highest effector:target cell ratios in the remaining 2 assays.

2. *TBC Assays*. In the experiment shown in Table II, the sorted, nylon wool-passed SC were not blocked by incubation with GAMIG prior to the fluorescein labeling. Ten percent of the SC were thus stained with the F-GAMIG alone, but these fluorescent cells did not bind the YAC-1 targets. In contrast all of the complexes formed by the NK-1$^+$ sorted SC and YAC-1 included a fluorescent cell. These NK-1$^+$ cells were enriched for target binding activity approximately 3-fold over control, unsorted SC. The NK-1$^-$ sorted cells neither bound target cells nor killed them in an effector cell assay.

3. *Winn Assay*. In a preliminary assay to test the *in vivo* activity of sorted cells, 1.25 x 10^3 YAC cells and either 1 x 10^4 NK-1$^+$ or NK-1$^-$ sorted SC were mixed and inoculated subcutaneously into groups of 3 A/J mice. The NK-1$^+$ cells completely suppressed outgrowth of the tumor in all 3 mice, whereas the tumor was observed to grow in all 3 mice inoculated with NK-1$^-$ cells (MTD=6.5 mm at 21 days post inoculation).

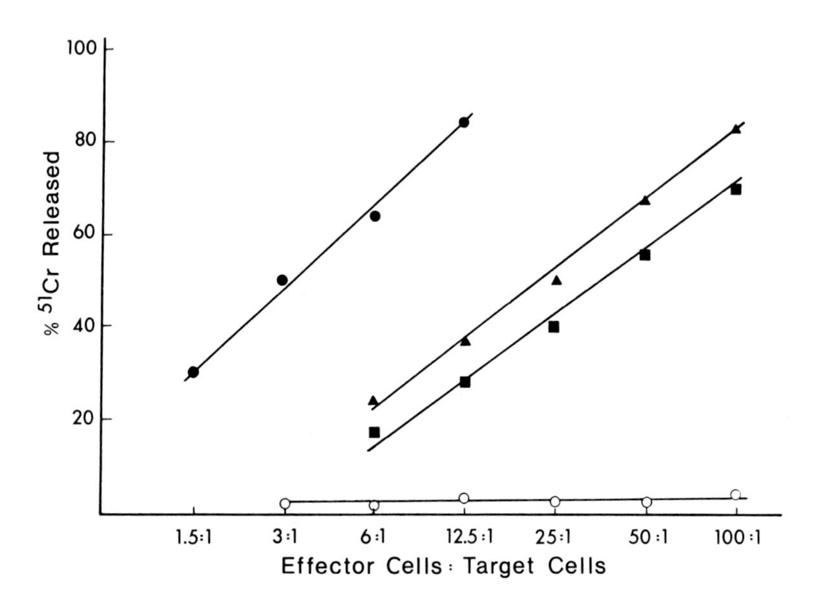

FIGURE 3. Sorting for NK-1+ SC enriches for and isolates effector NK activity. Nylon wool-passed SC were labeled with anti-NK 1.1 and F-GAMIG and separated into NK-1+ and NK-1− populations on the FACS. Sorted NK-1+ cells (●); sorted NK-1− cells (o); unsorted, nylon wool-passed, anti-NK 1.1-labeled SC (▲); unsorted, unlabeled SC (■). Sorted and unsorted SC were tested at SC:YAC-1 ratios of 0.7:1 to 100:1 in a 4 hr ^{51}Cr-release assay. One of eight experiments is illustrated.

TABLE II. Target Binding by Sorted NK-1+ and NK-1− SC

SC Treatment[a]	% Fluor-escent SC	% SC Binding to YAC-1[b]	% Fluorescent SC Binding YAC-1
Anti-NK 1.1, F-GAMIG, NK-1+ sorted	93[c]	17	17
Anti-NK 1.1, F-GAMIG, NK-1− sorted	1	1	0
F-GAMIG, unsorted	10	5	0
Unsorted SC		6	

[a]Nylon wool-passed SC were treated with the reagents listed in sequence, and sorted on the FACS into NK-1+ and NK-1− cells.

[b]As observed by visible light microscopy.

[c]Percentages are based on at least 250 SC counted.

F. *Discordance in NK Phenotype and Function*

1. NK Cells in Old B6 Mice. To determine whether old mice, previously determined to be deficient in NK activity (Kiessling *et al.*, 1975), were lacking in $NK\text{-}1^+$ cells, SC were labeled with anti-NK 1.1 and F-GAMIG and analyzed with the FACS. Fluorescence histograms obtained from six 9 to 13 month old B6 mice were virtually identical to control preparations of young (2 months) B6 mice such as was illustrated in Figure 2. FACS analysis determined the presence of a similar proportion (20 to 25%) of NK 1.1^+ cells in nylon wool-passed SC from young and old mice. However, the SC from the same 6 old mice had less than 50% of the NK effector activity on YAC-1 when compared with SC from young mice.

2. $NK\text{-}1^+$ Cells in B6-bg Mutant Mice. We have confirmed the data of Roder and Duwe (1979) in that B6-*bg* mice are deficient in NK effector activity when compared with normal B6 mice using either normal or nylon wool-passed SC on YAC-1 target cells (Figure 4). Yet, FACS analysis of B-cell depleted SC preparations from B6 and B6-*bg* mice indicated a similar number of $NK\text{-}1^+$ cells present (B6, 31.1% $NK\text{-}1^+$, n=2; B6-*bg*, 33.7% $NK\text{-}1^+$, n=3).

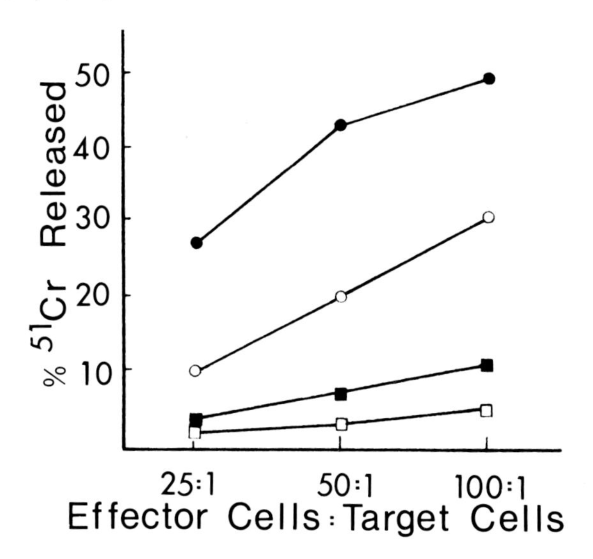

FIGURE 4. B6-bg mice are impaired in NK effector cell function. 1×10^4 labeled YAC-1 cells were combined with 2.5, 5.0, or 10×10^5 normal B6 SC (o), nylon wool-passed B6 SC (●), B6-bg SC (□), or nylon wool-passed B6-bg SC (■) in a 4 hr cytotoxicity assay.

III. DISCUSSION

An important question concerning NK cell lineage is their relationship with T cells. We have assessed the presence of six different T cell-associated alloantigens on NK cells by a cytotoxic depletion assay. Antisera to Thy 1, Ly 1, Ly 2, and Ly 3 (data not shown for Ly 3.2) did not significantly deplete NK activity. However, antisera generated to Ly 5 and Ly 6 were cytotoxic to NK cells in the presence of C, and in addition, anti-Ly 5 inhibited NK activity without C (Pollack *et al.*, 1979). These findings confirm the observation of Cantor *et al.*(1979) who reported that treatment of SC with anti-Ly 5 affects NK activity regardless of whether C is present. Our conclusions regarding the presence of Ly 6 on the surface of NK cells have been tempered by (1) the report of Clark *et al.* (1980) who have shown that certain pools of anti-Ly 6.2 serum may contain antibodies directed to NK cell antigens, and (2), that the treatment of SC with monoclonal anti-Ly 6 serum and C does not deplete SC of NK activity (G. Koo, personal communication).

We have demonstrated that a minor SC population can be labeled with anti-NK 1.1 and fluorescein-conjugated antiglobulin and subsequently enriched for and isolated with the FACS. The sorted cells, characterized as small to medium in size, were shown to be functionally active in target cell lysis, a TBC assay, and *in vivo* in a preliminary Winn assay. When sorted NK-1$^+$ cells were used in a functional lytic assay, as much as an 8-fold enrichment of NK activity was observed over control unsorted SC. In 6 of 8 experiments the NK-1$^-$ cells were inactive; in the remaining 2 assays only low levels of NK effector cell activity were seen at the highest effector: target cell ratios (50:1 to 100:1).

The slopes of the cytotoxicity curves obtained with NK-1$^+$ sorted SC from young adult B6 were always parallel with the slopes of both the normal and the nylon wool-passed control SC preparations. If sorting (or nylon wool passage) removed suppressor type cells, the cytotoxicity curve of the treated cells would be steeper than the control SC. Instead, a simple enrichment was always seen. In the TBC assay 3 times as many NK-1$^+$ sorted cells bound YAC-1 targets when compared with control SC, while no NK-1$^-$ sorted SC were bound to target cells, visually confirming NK cell enrichment. However, only 17% of the NK-1$^+$ sorted cells bound YAC-1 targets. Some NK-1$^+$ sorted cells may have been functionally immature, inactive, or capable of reacting only with a different set of target cells. Alternatively, the binding of some NK-1$^+$ cells to targets may not have been stable enough to withstand resuspension by pipetting.

Despite a similar number of NK-1$^+$ cells in old and young B6 mice, SC from old mice were not as cytolytically active as those from young mice. The disparity between NK 1.1 expression and functional NK activity observed in SC from old mice was even more striking in the case of lymph node cells (LNC). In young mice LNC NK activity was usually 20% of SC NK activity, whereas in old mice LNC had only 0.1% of the NK activity of old SC (unpublished data). One explanation for the apparent discrepancy is that, in maturation of NK cells in old mice, pre-NK cells acquire the NK-1 antigen, but not a lytic capacity. Alternatively, old NK-1$^+$ cells may more rapidly lose their lytic activity. These two possibilities, of course, cannot be distinguished without relevant kinetic data. Also plausible, however, is that the difference between phenotype and function could be explained by the presence of proportionately more inhibitory cells in old mice. Preliminary data from mixing experiments showed that adding LNC from old mice to SC from young mice inhibited NK effector activity significantly more than adding young LNC to SC from young mice. While these preliminary experiments indicate the inhibition is due to an noncompetitive mechanism, this remains to be determined.

The B6-*bg* spontaneous mutation has been shown to impair the function of both K and NK cells, but not any other T cell-mediated functions. The mutation is believed to provide an animal model of the Chediak-Higashi syndrome in man. While the exact mechanisms involved are uncertain, the genetic defect is presumed to be within the lytic mechanism and not with the attachment of effector cells to target cells (Roder and Duwe, 1979). Our results indicate that B6-*bg* mice have normal numbers of effector NK-1$^+$ cells with normal amounts of NK-1 antigen per cell. Thus, a purified population of NK-1$^+$ cells from *beige* mutant mice such as those obtained on the FACS could be used *in vitro* to determine the nature of the genetic defect.

The availability of a potent NK 1.1 antiserum and the consequent ability to obtain purified or enriched NK cells now makes it possible to directly attack some of the lingering questions regarding the biology of NK cells. For example, *in vivo* effects of NK-1$^+$ cells in tumor immunotherapy may now be thoroughly studied. Marrow engraftment and the relationship between NK-1 and hybrid histocompatibility (Hh-1) antigen-bearing cells and their activities (Kiessling *et al.*, 1977) can be studied using purified NK-1$^+$ and NK-1$^-$ sorted preparations. In addition purified NK cells can be studied *in vitro* in an attempt to determine the developmental relationship of NK cells to other cytolytically active lymphocytes, including

K cells. If, as Herberman *et al.* suggest, NK cells are within the T cell lineage, then culture of sorted spleen (or thymus) cells in the presence of mitogens or T cell growth or maturation factors may induce differentiation.

ACKNOWLEDGMENTS

We thank Drs. Robert Nowinski and E. A. Clark for valuable discussions, and Ms. Rosa Mae MacDonald for assistance with cell sorting and analysis. We thank the Williams and Wilkins Co. for the permission to use copyrighted material from the *Journal of Immunology* in the preparation of this manuscript.

REFERENCES

Cantor, H., Kasai, M., Shen, F.W., Leclerc, J.C., and Glimcher, L. (1979). *Immunol. Rev. 44,* 1.

Clark, E.A., Russell, P.H., Egghart, M., and Horton, M.A. (1980). *Int. J. Cancer, in press.*

Glimcher, L., Shen, F.W., and Cantor, H. (1977). *J. Exp. Med. 145,* 1.

Haller, O., Gidlund, M., Hellström, U., Hammarström, S., and Wigzell, H. (1978). *Eur. J. Immunol. 8,* 765.

Herberman, R.B., Nunn, M.E., and Holden, H.T. (1978). *J. Immunol. 121,* 304.

Julius, M.H., Simpson, E., and Herzenberg, L.A. (1973). *Eur. J. Immunol. 3,* 645.

Kasai, M., Leclerc, J.C., Shen, F.W., and Cantor, H. (1979). *Immunogenetics 8,* 153.

Kiessling, R., Klein, E., and Wigzell, H. (1975). *Eur. J. Immunol. 5,* 112.

Mattes, M.J., Sharrow, S.J., Herberman, R.B., and Holden, H.T. (1979). *J. Immunol. 123,* 2851.

Pollack, S.B., Tam, M.R., Nowinski, R.C., and Emmons, S.L. (1979). *J. Immunol. 123,* 1818.

Roder, J.C. and Kiessling, R. (1978). *Scand. J. Immunol. 8,* 135.

Roder, J.C. and Duwe, A. (1979). *Nature 278,* 451.

SUMMARY: CHARACTERISTICS OF NK AND RELATED CELLS

As reflected by the chapters in this section, there has been much recent effort directed towards characterization of NK cells and of other, possibly related, effector cells. On some issues, there has been a convergence of data and opinions, but on other major points, controversy has continued or even intensified. In this summary, I will attempt to identify the main topics that have been discussed, indicate the characteristics that have come to be agreed upon, and point out the controversial issues and weigh the existing evidence.

I. CELL LINEAGE OF NK CELLS

Since the initial placement of NK cells into the category of ill-defined and heterogeneous population of null cells, there have been many efforts to find cell surface markers and/or other characteristics that would indicate the relationship of NK cells to the three main classes of lymphoid cells, i.e. T cells, B cells, and macrophages.

A. Possible Relationship to T Cells

Most of the evidence and consequent debate has focused on whether NK cells belong to the T cell lineage. In rodents, it has been clear that NK cells occur spontaneously in nude mice and neonatally thymectomized mice and rats, and thus, these cells are not thymic dependent and not typical mature T cells. However, in mice and humans, NK cells have been reported to have several markers that suggest some relationship to the T cell lineage, possibly being early, pre-thymic cells of the T lineage. Table I summarizes the evidence that has been presented here on this issue. Each of these markers has been detected on at least a portion of NK cells and appears to be strongly associated with peripheral T cells of the T lineage. Thy 1 is not completely restricted to T cells, being found on some non-lymphoid cells and on one myelomonocytic leukemia

ISBN 0-12-341350-8

TABLE 1. Expression on NK Cells of Markers Associated or Consistent With the T Cell Lineage

Marker	Known Distribution	Expression on NK Cells (authors of chapters)
Mouse Thy1	Lymphoid cells: on normal cells, has been found only on T cells and pre-T cells and not on B cells or macrophages, but has been detected on a myelomonocytic leukemia (Tai and Warner) Non-lymphoid cells: brain and epidermal cells	Low density on potion of spontaneous (Burton, Gidlund et al., Herberman et al., Koo, and Hatzfeld, Pollack et al.) and boosted (Durdick et al., Herberman et al.) NK cells. On a higher proportion of NK cells of nude than euthymic mice (Herberman et al.)
Ly1	Only on mouse thymocytes and peripheral T cells	Usually undetectable (Gidlund et al. Pollack et al.) but with use of monoclonal antibody on enriched population of spleen cells, detected on 28% of NK cells (Koo and Hatzfeld)
asialo GM1	On 30% of peripheral T cells and at high concentration can inhibit cytotoxic T cells (Gidlund et al.); undetected on thymus, bone marrow, B cells	On most or all NK cells (Durdik et al., Gidlund et al.)
Human E receptors	On most or all periperhal T cells and thymus cells; undetected on cells of B or macrophage lineage	Low affinity receptors on a portion (50-80%) but not all NK cells (Bolhuis, Herberman et al., Pross and Baines, Saksela and Timonen)
HTLA	On thymus cells, all peripheral cells with E receptors plus portion of null cells; undetected on surface Ig + cells, macrophages, or bone marrow stem cells (Kaplan and Callewaert)	On all NK cells, including those without E receptors (Bolhuis, Herberman et al., Kaplan and Callewaert); also on precursors of NK cells (Ortaldo and Herberman)
gp 120	On mature T cells (Saksela and Timonen)	On enriched population of large granular lymphocytes containing most or all NK activity (Saksela and Timonen)

(Tai and Warner)[1], but for normal lymphoid cells it has been very widely accepted as a reliable and specific marker for cells of the T lineage.

[1]*In this and subsequent summaries, citation of chapters in this book will be by authors, not followed by year, to allow discrimination from references to papers published elsewhere. Most but not all chapters will be in the section corresponding to the summary. The reader is referred to the chapters for more detailed references.*

The information regarding expression of Thy 1 on mouse NK cells and of receptors for sheep erythrocytes (E receptors) on human NK cells has been somewhat controversial but now many groups, including all of those presenting data on this point in this book, have obtained positive results. Some of the apparent discrepancies may be attributed to expression of these markers on only a portion of NK cells and then only in low density or low affinity relative to to that seen with mature T cells.

In regard to human anti-T cell antisera, several different heteroantibodies, all apparently specific for T cells, have been found to react with NK cells, even those that lack detectable E receptors, and also with precursors of NK cells (see Ortaldo and Herberman in section IC2). However, it should be noted that one group (Reinherz *et al.*, 1980) has failed to detect reactivity of NK cells with monoclonal anti-T cell antibodies (OKT1 and OKT3), but these antibodies did not react with all cells with E receptors and may only be recognizing a major subpopulation, but not all, of T cells.

In addition to information presented in the chapters regarding the possible T cell lineage of NK cells, another recent piece of evidence is that mouse (Orn *et al.*) and human (T. Timonen, G. Bonnard, and R. B. Herberman, unpublished observations) NK cells have receptors for T cell growth factor and can be propogated in culture in the presence of conditioned medium from PHA-stimulated lymphocytes.

Because of the evidence for some relationship of NK cells to T cells, one must reconsider the points of difference between NK cells and cytotoxic T lymphocytes (CTL), and particularly the practical methods for discriminating between these two classes of effector cells. Until recently, elimination of cytotoxic activity of mouse lymphoid cells by treatment with anti-Thyl plus C, or the finding of E receptors on human effector cells, was taken as good evidence for involvement of CTL. However, it is now clear that these criteria are not sufficiently helpful. Mouse CTL appear to have a higher density of Thyl than NK cells and similarly, most human CTL have high affinity E receptors, whereas NK cells have low affinity E receptors. However, the quantitative differences may not be large enough to permit complete separation of these effector populations. Despite these overlapping properties of NK cells and CTL, there does appear to be a number of major differences that could be used for discrimination: 1) The important role of the major histocompatibility complex (MHC) in CTL and the general inability of CTL to react with targets deficient in MHC antigens. In contrast, NK cells do not display any MHC restriction, reacting at least as well against allogeneic targets and further, as shown by some chapters (e.g. Gidlund *et al*.), targets lacking MHC antigens, or having their MHC antigens blocked by antibodies, still react well with NK cells. Also, as discussed further in the section on specificity of NK cells, PHA blasts, which are excellent targets for alloimmune CTL, have been found consistently to be resistant to lysis by NK cells and they don't cold target inhibit the lysis of NK-susceptible target cells. Thus, the specificity of NK cells versus CTL can often be a useful distinction. 2) With mouse NK cells, some of the recent information regarding selective markers would seem to be of considerable value in discriminating them from CTL. Anti-asialo-GM1 at low concentrations, anti-NK 1.1 and related anti-NK antibodies, and anti-Qa4 and anti-Qa5 all appear promising for this purpose. The value of anti-Ly 5 for discrimination is not clear, since no information is reported in the chapters here on expression of Ly5 on CTL. The use of *Viccia villosa* lectin (Gidlund *et al*.) also appears valuable for discrimination, since under the same conditions in which all mouse CTL are positive, NK cells have been found to be negative. 3) With human NK cells, there are fewer clear procedures for discriminating them from CTL. However, the anti-T cell monoclonal antibodies (OKT1, OKT3, and others) referred to above would be expected to adequately discriminate between these two classes of effector cells.

B. Possible Relationship to B Cells

Most investigators have failed to detect an association of NK cells with B cells (Table II). For example, treatment of effector cells with anti-immunoglobulin antibodies plus C has not affected activity. However, there have been sporadic reports of surface immunoglobulin on NK or K cells (e.g. MacDermott *et al*., 1975). However, such results could be attributed to IgG bound to the effector cells through their Fc-IgG receptors. Eremin in his chapter raises this issue again regarding human NK cells, since he found that they formed rosettes in a sensitive procedure said to detect low amounts of surface immunoglobulins, and they remained positive after incubation at 37°C. However, one must carefully examine the evidence and remain cautious regarding the interpretation since it is still possible that small amounts of cytophilic immunoglobulins are involved rather than intrinsic membrane immunoglobulins.

TABLE II. Expression of B Cell Associated Markers on NK Cells

Marker	*Known Distribution*	*Expression on NK Cells*
Surface membrane immunoglobulin	*most B cells*	*undetected by most groups but detected by sensitive rosette method method on human NK cells (Eremin)*
Ia	*most B cells and also some monocytes and activated T cells*	*not detected on mouse or human NK cells*
C3 receptors	*most B cells and monocytes*	*not detected on mouse or rat NK cells; undetectable or detectable on a small portion (Pross and Baines) of human NK cells*
Lyb-2	*all mouse B cells, even before expression of surface immunoglobulin (Koo and Hatzfeld)*	*undetected on mouse NK cells*

The failure of mouse NK cells to react with anti-Lyb-2 (Koo and Hatzfeld) adds new negative data regarding their possible relationship to B cells. The consistent failure to detect Ia antigens on mouse and human NK cells, and the absence of C3 receptors on at least most NK cells also point to important distinctions from most B cells.

C. Possible Relationship to Macrophages

Ever since their initial characterization, NK cells of mice, rats, and humans have been reported to be nonphagocytic and nonadherent, and, therefore, little consideration was given to their possible relationship to macrophages. It seems clear that macrophages, including those from normal individuals, can have cytostatic and cytolytic activity against tumor cells. However, a number of characteristics of macrophage-mediated cytotoxicity, including the range of susceptible targets and strain distribution, has pointed to a class of natural effector cells different from NK cells (see section III). Despite the rather clear distinction between NK cells and typical macrophages, some recent studies have raised the question of NK cells being in the macrophage lineage.

One such series of studies to carefully consider is that of Lohmann-Matthes and Domzig on the relationship of mouse NK cells to cells early in the macrophage lineage. Their basic system has involved cells from the bone marrow that are cultured for several days in L-fibroblast conditioned medium. The majority of the cells are nonadherent and nonphagocytic, and esterase negative, and have a large irregular nucleus and abundant cytoplasm. They have called these cells promonocytes, although in their chapter they point out that such cells would have to precede the stage of cells that van Furth has designated as promonocytes. Cultures with a predominance of this type of cell have been found to have high cytotoxic activity against NK-susceptible target cells.

These observations raise two important questions: 1) Are the effector cells in these bone marrow cultures NK cells? 2) If so, are these NK cells in the macrophage lineage? It would not be surprising for NK cells to grow out from bone marrow cultures, since other studies have provided strong evidence for the origin of mouse NK cells from bone marrow stem cells (see Haller *et al.*). In addition, it is of interest that the morphology of the predominant cell type in the bone marrow cultures bears some resemblance to the human large granular lymphocyte (LGL) which, as discussed below, posses-ses most or all human NK activity. However, it is unclear whether this is more than just a superficial resemblance. It would be of particular interest to know whether the bone marrow-cultured cells have the same type of cytoplasmic granules as the LGL. Despite this possible similarity of some bone marrow-derived cells to human NK cells, the more direct question is whether the cells in culture share phenotypic and functional characteristics of NK cells. In regard to cell surface markers, insufficient data are available. It will be important to determine whether these cells react with some of the antisera described above (e.g. to Thyl, asialo GM1, Qa4 or 5, NK1.1 and other antigens) that have been found to be selective for mouse NK cells. In less conclusive support of these cells being NK cells, they are spontaneously cytolytic in short term assays against NK-susceptible but not NK-resistant target cells. However, against the involvement of NK cells is the major difference in strain distribution of reactivity. Bone marrow cells from low NK strains, such as beige and A, have been found to have similar levels of reactivity as cells from high NK strains. This discrepancy is also not conclusive, since, as pointed out by the authors, the cultured cells from low strains may be released from *in vivo* negative control mechanisms. Overall, it would appear uncertain as to whether the observed cytotoxic activity in the bone marrow cultures is due to NK cells or to another type of cytotoxic effector cell.

If one assumes that NK cells are indeed responsible for the cytotoxicity, it is then essential to carefully weigh the evidence for the effector cells being related to macrophages. Based on available data, this also appears to be difficult to decide. The population of cultured cells is probably heterogeneous and NK cells may only be a small subset. The observation that within a few days all cells have the characteristics of mature macrophages is not conclusive evidence, since one could postulate that NK cells and some other cells in the population died prior to this point. In general, it has been very difficult to settle such issues with activities in a mixed population of many cells. Most of the evidence in support of the macrophage derivation of the bone marrow effector cells comes from the results of treatment with anti-Mph 1 plus C. The antisera used in these studies was prepared by the original procedure of Archer and Davies and is reported to react well with macrophages and not T or B cells. However, since this is a critical issue, the authors detailed data on the specificity of the reagent would have to be thoroughly assessed. Of concern is the conflicting data on this point from Gidlund *et al.* When they treated NK cells with anti-Mph 1 plus C, under conditions in which a high proportion of macrophages were lysed, no effect on cytotoxic reactivity was observed. Thus, taken together, these studies of Lohmann-Matthes and Domzig raise some important and intriguing questions about the lineage of NK cells, but, as yet, do not provide clearcut answers.

A similar question about the relationship of human NK cells to monocytes has been raised very recently by the study of Reinherz *et al.* (1980). They have reported that NK cells and a substantial portion of Tγ cells react with a monoclonal antibody, OKM1, said to be specific for monocytes. As with the data with anti-Mph 1, the central question is the restriction of the detected antigen to cells of the monocyte lineage. This antibody has been found to also react with granulocytes, and it seems possible that it may actually detect an antigen expressed on some cells of various lineages.

For example, an interesting possibility to be examined is whether the OKM1 antibody is directed against the Fc-IgG receptor (FcγR) which is known to be expressed on monocytes, granulocytes, NK cells and Tγ cells.

II. OTHER CELL SURFACE MARKERS ON NK CELLS

A. Markers characteristic of, but not restricted to, NK cells

Most investigators have come to agree that most rodent and human NK cells have FcγR. These receptors are readily detectable on human NK cells reactive with K562, but appear to be of low affinity on mouse and rat NK cells. The presence of FcγR on NK cells is frequently a useful point of distinction from CTL, especially in studies with human lymphocytes. However, it would appear that one can not rely solely on this marker. As discussed below and in section 1B, FcγR do not appear to be invariably associated with NK cells. NK cells in some tissues or reacting with certain target cells appear to lack FcγR, and it has been clearly shown that FcγR can be modulated off NK cells without concomitant loss of cytotoxic activity.

Ly5 antigen appears to be present on most or all mouse NK cells. Antibodies to this cell surface antigen now also appear to be responsible for reports of reactivity of anti-Ly6 sera with NK cells. This marker does not appear to be particularly selective for NK cells, being expressed on some cells of most types with hematopoietic origin (Scheid and Triglia, 1979). Since most investigators have found that anti-Ly5 without C can inhibit NK activity, it seems unlikely that this marker will be of use for positive selection of NK cells. However, this complement-independent inactivation has prompted Burton to raise the intriguing possibility that Ly5 is physically quite close to the recognition structure on NK cells. It is of interest to note that rat NK cells appear to possess an analogous marker, LC antigen (Herberman *et al*.), which is also expressed on a variety of lymphoid cell types. The monoclonal antibody to this antigen has also produced appreciable inhibition of rat NK activity in the absence of complement.

B. Markers Characteristic of, and Possibly Restricted to, NK Cells

It is very encouraging that several markers have been found that appear selective for mouse NK cells. If one or more of these antigens can be documented to be completely restricted to NK cells and their immediate precursors, we would have a powerful tool for enumerating and isolating NK cells and for characterizing them in great detail. NK1.1, the other NK antigens described by Burton, Qa4, and Qa5 have thus far only been demonstrated on NK cells. Treatment of mouse spleen cells with antisera to these markers has been useful for almost complete depletion, or enrichment, of NK cells. In contrast, these reagents have not affected CTL, or the few other functional or morphological cell types examined. However, it still needs to be documented that only NK cells, and IF-inducible pre-NK cells, have these markers. It would be of great interest to study cells positively selected for these markers with and without IF treatment, for the proportion of conjugate-forming cells and in single cell cytotoxicity assays (Grimm and Bonavida, 1979), to determine the frequency of cells capable of recognizing and lysing NK-susceptible target cells. The only data presented here on this important point, from Tam *et al.*, is that 17% of NK 1.1 + cells formed conjugates with YAC-1. It remains to be determined whether the remaining 83% of such cells could, under some circumstances, also react with and lyse NK-susceptible targets. Determination of the degree of association of each of these antigens with NK cells is needed for adequate evaluation of the data presented regarding the incidence of marker-positive cells in various situations. For example, Tam *et al.* report that older mice with low NK activity have the same numbers of NK1.1 + cells as do young, high NK-reactors. These data appear to be at variance with the data of Roder and Haliotis, showing a decrease in conjugate-forming cells with age. Such discrepancies can only be settled by better determination of the specificity of each of the procedures.

III. EVIDENCE FOR SUBPOPULATIONS OF NK CELLS WITH VARYING CELL SURFACE AND OTHER CHARACTERISTICS

Considerable evidence points to heterogeneity of cells that, as a total population, appear sufficiently similar to refer to as NK cells. In addition, some natural effector cells have been described that may be distinct from NK cells. It is currently difficult to clearly assign the various spontaneously cytotoxic cells to one category or another. On the one hand, it would seem very useful to reserve the designation of NK cell for effector cells sharing a number of cell surface and functional characteristics, and to separately categorize natural effector cells with divergent properties. However, it remains quite unclear just where the dividing line should be drawn. Such discrimination probably should await more complete phenotyping of each of the effector cells.

One major indication of heterogeneity of NK cells has come from studies of expression of Thyl on mouse NK cells and of E receptors on human NK cells. As discussed above, only a portion of NK cells have detectable expression of these markers. Qa2 appears to be another cell surface antigen on only about 50% of mouse cells and it is of interest in that it seems to some extent to mark a separate subset of NK cells than does Thyl.

With human NK cells, another indication for heterogeneity has come from studies of expression of FcγR. While this appears to be an excellent marker for NK cells reactive with K562, it does not seem to be expressed on all NK cells reacting with other targets. Also, Eremin has found that NK cells in lymph nodes or tonsils appear to lack FcγR, and those effector cells also differ from NK cells in the peripheral blood in their resistance to inactivation by trypsinization or by ammonium chloride.

Other indications for subsets of effector cells have also been noted when different target cells have been tested. Lotzova has noted differences in the size of effector cells reacting with heterologous rather than syngeneic or allogeneic target cells. Even more dramatic differences have emerged from studies of mouse spleen cells with solid tumor target cells. The NC cells of Stutman *et al*., bear some resemblance to NK cells, but also differ in several major respects (see their chapter for details).

The studies of Burton provide further indication of major differences between effector cells for the usual lymphoma target cells (which he designates NK_L) and those reacting with a fibrosarcoma target (designated as NK_S). Upon initial examination, it would appear that NK_S cells are quite different from typical NK cells, failing to be depleted by anti-NK1.1 plus C. However, the observation that NK_S cells also resist lysis by anti-H2 and other antisera blurs this distinction. It seems possible that NK_S cells are related to NK_L cells, but are at a point in differentiation or in a physiologic state that make them express less cell surface antigens or be resistant to lysis for other reasons. The intermediate phenotype of NK_C cells would tend to support this possibility. It will be important to more extensively determine the phenotype of NC cells, NK_S and NK_C cells relative to NK_L cells and to each other, particularly by complement-independent methods such as separation by the fluorescence activated cell sorter. It is of interest in this regard that Tai and Warner, using this method, found that LCM virus-augmented NK cells reactive with the fibrosarcoma target (and thus NK_S cells) were found to express the NK antigen of Burton.

The relationship to NK cells of the cytostatic effector cells of Ehrlich *et al.* is also difficult to determine. They have some apparent difference from NK cells, but these may be related to the nature of the assay, or the state of activation of the cells. For example, while spontaneous NK cells have been found to be nonadherent, after activation a portion of the effector cells adhere to various fiber columns. Again, we must await more extensive characterization of the cytostatic effector cells.

One interesting possible explanation for some of the observed heterogeneity of NK cells is that within the overall population with some general, common characteristics, the effector cells for each target cell specificity (see discussion in section IB) have varying expression of some markers and possibly even idiotypic determinants. Alternatively, the observed differences in effector cells may just reflect different stages of differentiation or activation. For example, there have been some suggestions for variation in expressions of Thyl, depending on the state of activation of the cells. Similarly, the lack of $Fc_\gamma R$ on some NK cells may be due to *in vivo* modulation of these structures.

IV. MORPHOLOGY OF NK CELLS AND POSSIBLE METHODS TO DIRECTLY ENUMERATE THEM

Various methods have been utilized in attempts to separate NK cells from other lymphoid cells and/or to determine their morphology and frequency: 1) as discussed above in II B, by antisera thought to be specific for NK cells; 2) by formation of conjugates with target cells; and 3) by size or density separation. None of these procedures by themselves have been documented to provide pure populations of NK cells. Each population enriched for NK cells is probably still rather heterogeneous, containing cells unrelated to NK cells. However, some combination of these methods might be quite helpful in enumerating and better characterizing NK cells. For example, the subpopulation of mouse spleen cells that are NK antigen positive and form conjugates may be highly enriched for, or may solely consist of NK cells. In studies with human NK cells, the combination of Percoll density gradient and $Fc\gamma R$ separation, and enumeration by conjugate formation, has been very useful in obtaining strong evidence that human NK cells are within a population of LGL (Saksela and Timonen; Herberman, *et al.*). However, even with this impressive correlation, it is not entirely clear what proportion of LGL are functional NK cells or IF-inducible pre-NK cells. Recent preliminary experiments with the single cell agarose cytotoxicity assay are very encouraging, indicating that almost all of the Percoll-separated conjugate forming LGL are capable of lysing K562 target cells (T. Timonen and R. B. Herberman, unpublished observations). Preliminary data also indicate that rat NK cells have the morphology of LGL and can be separated on Percoll gradients (C. Reynolds, T. Timonen and R.B. Herberman). It is not yet clear whether mouse NK cells have similar morphology or bear some distinctive morphological features. As reported by Roder and Haliotis, the predominant nonadherent cell in mouse spleens that form conjugates has the appearance of a small, "resting" lymphocyte. However, it seems likely that some, or perhaps even the majority of conjugate-forming cells, are not NK cells, and this issue will need to be more closely examined when more highly purified populations of mouse NK cells are available.

REFERENCES

Grimm, E. and Bonavida, B. (1979) *J. Immunol.* *123*, 2861-2869.

Macdermott, R.P., Chess, L. and Schlossman, S.F. (1975) *Clin. Immunol. Immunopathol.* *4*, 415-424

Reinherz, E., and Schlossman, S., *et al.* (1980) *J. Exp. Med.* in press.

Scheid, M.P., and Triglia, D. (1979). *Immunogenetics* *9*, 423-433.

MECHANISM OF CYTOTOXICITY BY NK CELLS AND THEIR RELATIONSHIP TO K CELLS

Reinder Bolhuis

Rotterdam Radio-Therapy Institute,
Rotterdam;
and
Radiobiological Institute TNO,
P.O. Box 5815
2280 HV Rijswijk
The Netherlands

B. Mechanism of Cytotoxicity-Relation to ADCC.

In section I.A we presented evidence that NK cells reactive against monolayer target cells can be either IgG-FcR negative or positive; that they belong to the T cell lineage and that they display selective cytotoxicity against monolayer tumor target cells. Furthermore, NK reactivity against K-562 erythroidleukemic cells, as measured in a 4 h ^{51}Cr release cytotoxicity assay, is displayed by cells expressing IgG-FcR on their surface. K cells (ADCC) also express receptor for the Fc portion of IgG-FcR and their lytic mechanism is antibody dependent. Since these IgG-FcR positive K and NK cells are recovered in the same cell fractions (Section I.A; this issue) this may not only suggest that K and NK cells are identical but also that both lytic reactivities are antibody dependent because some authors reported that:

1) lymphocytes already have naturally occurring antibodies bound to their surface _in vivo_ and with specificity for certain target cells (1-6).
2) antibody is released by lymphocytes and binds to FcR bearing cells during the cytotoxicity assay (7, 8).

However, a number of differences between NK and K cells can be summarized (Table I). It could be argued that corticosteroid treatment inhibited the production and/or release of NK-mediating antibody. Furthermore, the published data regarding the inhibition of NK activity by anti-Ig antibodies

ISBN 0-12-341350-8

TABLE I

DIFFERENTIAL EFFECTS OF SEVERAL TREATMENTS ON HUMAN NK AND K REACTIVITIES

Treatment	NK	K	Reference
Trypsin	reversible loss of activity	no effect	Kay et al., 1977 Koide and Takasugi, 1977 Eremin et al., 1978
Protein A or F(ab)2 anti-IgG in cytotoxicity assay	no effect	inhibition	Kay et al., 1977
Soluble immunocomplexes	decrease	total inhibition	Bolhuis et al., 1978
Cortico steroids	decrease	inhibition	Parillo and Fauci, 1978a; b
Capping of IgG-FcR	no effect or enhancement	total inhibition	Bolhuis, 1977 Bolhuis et al., 1978
Autologous non-T FcR negative cells	no effect	inhibition	Pollack and Emmons, 1979

are conflicting: Inhibition of NK activity by F(ab')2 anti-human IgG was reported by several authors (14).

We have not been able to confirm these data using goat F(ab)2 fragments against human IgG. F(ab)2 was purified by elution from a IgG-immunoadsorbent. Inhibition of K (ADCC) reactivity was observed but NK reactivity was not affected (unpublished observations). Similarly, Kay et al. (15) and Ault and Weiner (16) could not inhibit NK cell activity by use of these antisera.

We have designed experiments to investigate the role of IgG-FcR in NK and K (ADCC) cell lysis of target cells. Soluble IgG-antigen complexes will bind to IgG-FcR and thus are expected to reduce K cell activity (3, 4). We have determined the effects of soluble immune complexes on NK and K reactivity as well as the NK and K reactivity originally IgG-FcR positive cells that have shed their FcR (EA-RFC recovered fraction).

The effect on NK and K reactivity of addition of these antibody-antigen complexes to the cytotoxicity assays is shown in Figure 1. K cell cytotoxicity can be completely inhibited by these complexes whereas inhibition of NK reactivity ranges from 40-65 per cent. Furthermore, no EA-RFC can be detected in the presence of immune complexes in the effector cell preparation (Figure 1). This suggests that at least a subset of NK cells do not need the functional involvement of IgG-FcR for NK cell lysis of target cells.

When IgG-FcR positive cells were isolated by adsorbing these cells to immunocomplex monolayer these cells spontaneously detach upon prolonged incubation on these adsorbents

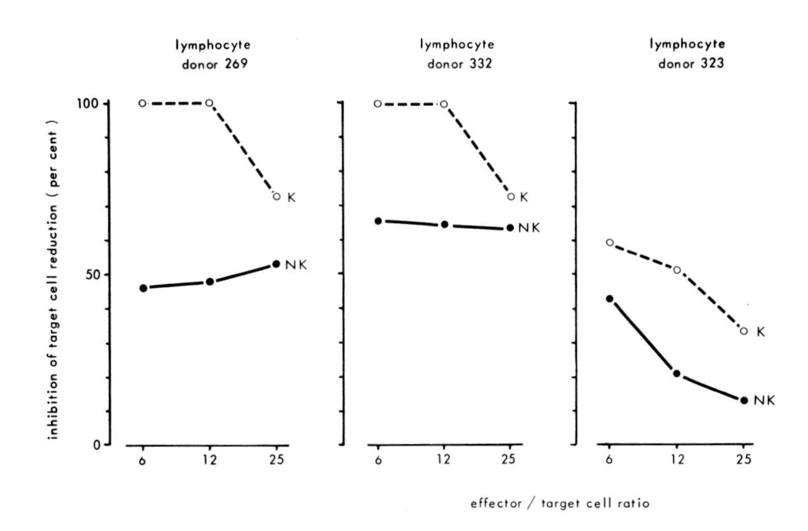

Figure 1:
Per cent reduction by immune complexes of the cytotoxic capacity of NK and K cells (—●—) K-562 (NK) target cell; (--O--) P-815 (K) target cell. Percentage of EA-RFC without complexes: Donor 269, 12%; donor 332, 22%; donor 323, 23%. Percentage of EA-RFC with complexes: donor 269, 1%; donor 332, 4%; donor 323, 1%. Complexes: rabbit anti-ovalbumin (OVA), 1:4 diluted; OVA 17 ug/ml.

(3, 4).

From Figure 2 it can be seen that these EA-RFC recovered lymphocytes have shed their IgG-FcR from their surface: NK cell activity of these cells is not affected or even increased whereas NK reactivity is almost completely reduced. When immune complexes are added to this system when for the unseparated effector cells one sees about 50 per cent and 100 per cent inhibition of NK cell and K cell activity respectively (Figure 3) as shown before in Figure 1.

Addition of immune complexes to recovered EA-RFC cells which have shed their IgG-FcR has no effect on NK reactivity (Figure 3). Since these recovered EA-RFC, lacking IgG-FcR as a result of the isolation procedure, i.e. shedding of the receptor, have no K reactivity, addition of immune complexes is not expected to have an effect. These data clearly indicate the NK reactivity cannot be functionally equated with K (ADCC) reactivity since the NK reactivity does not require the functional involvement of IgG-FcR whereas K reactivity does (Figures 2 and 3). Although the two types of effector cells are always demonstrated to be simultaneously present in cell fractions regardless the fractionation procedure employed, our results indicate that although the NK and K cells

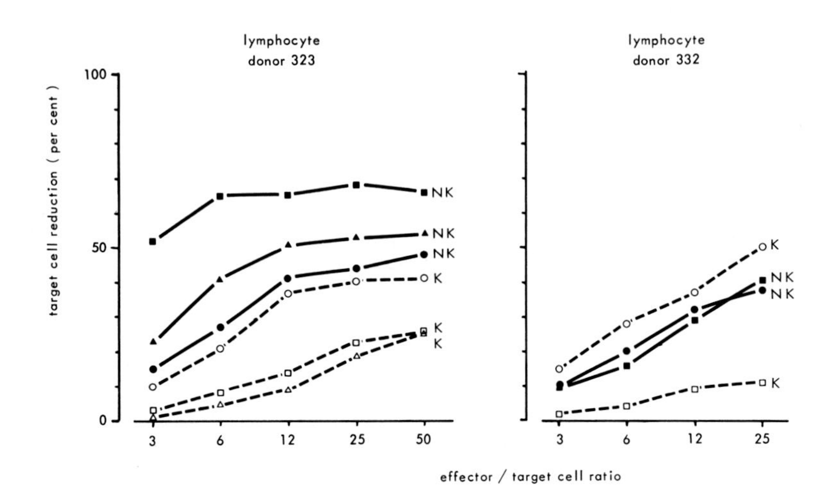

Figure 2:
Separation of NK and K cell activity by means of EA-RFC recovery followed by EA-RFC depletion.
K-562 (NK cell) target cells; IgG-coated P-815 (K cell) target cells:
●, NK cell and ○, K cell cytotoxicity of unfractioned lymphocytes (EA-RFC donor 323) 23% and 20% respectively; ▲, NK cell and △, K cell cytotoxicity of EA-RFC-recovered lymphocytes (EA-RFC donor 323) 5% and 0%, respectively; ■, NK cell and □, K cell cytotoxicity of EA-RFC-recovered lymphocytes depleted for possible EA-RFC (EA-RFC donor 323) both values 0%.

may be identical then the reactivities develop along different pathways. This is also suggested by the observation that lymphocytes of some patients with agammaglobulinemia still display NK cell activity (17).

In conclusion, it can be stated that either a) NK and K cells are distinct cell types; or b) that part of the NK cells may also display K reactivity and that these NK and K cell reactivities are distinct functions of that individual lymphocyte. Although it was demonstrated in our experiments described above that NK cell lysis is independent of IgG-FcR i.e., no antibody is involved, these finding do not exclude such a mechanism of lysis.

ACKNOWLEDGEMENTS

The author wishes to thank Mr. C.P.M. Ronteltap, Mrs. A.M. Nooyen, Mrs. R. de Rooy for superb technical assistance. Miss H. Schuit is greatly acknowledged for the immunofluorescence studies. Mrs. M. van der Sman for inventive secretarial help.

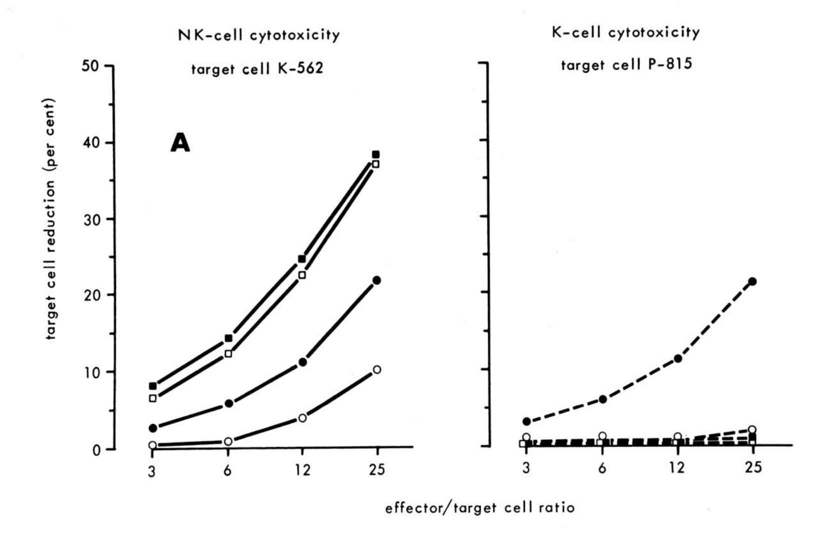

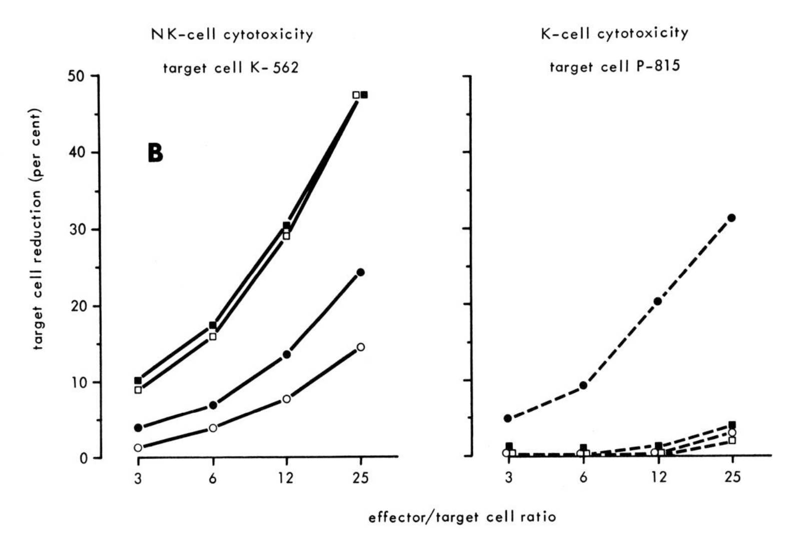

Figure 3:
The influence of immune complexes on NK and K cell activities of ●, unfractionated and ■, EA-RFC-recovered lymphocytes; separation of NK and K cell activities. (a) donor 332; (b) donor 336 (open symbols: cells in the presence of immune complexes).

	donor 332	donor 336
	(% EA-RFC)	
Unfractionated lymphocytes	20	15
Unfractionated lymphocytes + rabbit anti-OVA-OVA complexes	0	1
EA-RFC-recovered lymphocytes	0	0
EA-RFC-recovered lymphocytes + rabbit anti-OVA-OVA complexes	0	0

REFERENCES

1. Pross. H. and Jondal, M. Clin. exp. Immunol. 21, 1975, 226.
2. Akira, D. and Takasugi, M., Int. J. Cancer 19, 1977, 747.
3. Bolhuis, R.L.H., Thesis, Erasmus University Rotterdam, 1977.
4. Bolhuis, R.L.H., Schuit, H.R.E., Nooyen, A.M. and Ronteltap, C.P.M. Eur. J. Immunol. 8, 1978, 731.
5. Kay, H.D., Bonnard, G.D., West, W.H. and Herbermann, R.B. J. Immunol. 118, 1977, 2058.
6. Takasugi, M. and Akira, D., J. nat. Cancer Inst. 82, 1979, 1361.
7. Blair, P.B. and Lane, M.A. J. Immunol. 115, 1975, 184.
8. Pape, G.R., Troye, M. and Perlmann, P. J. Immunol. 118, 1977, 1919.
9. Koide, Y. and Takasugi, M. J. nat. Cancer Inst. 59, 1979, 1099.
10. Eremin, O., Ashby, J. and Stephens, J.P. Int. J. Cancer 21, 1978, 35.
11. Parillo, J.E. and Fauci, A.S. Clin. exp. Immunol. 31, 1978, 1.
12. Parillo, J.E. and Fauci, A.S. Scand. J. Immunol. 8, 1978, 99.
13. Pollack, S.B. and Emmens, S. J. Immunol. 122, 1979, 719.
14. Troye, M., Perlmann, P., Pape, G.R., Spiegelberg, H.L., Näslund, A. and Gidlöv, A. J. Immunol. 119, 1977, 1061.
15. Kay, H.D., Bonnard, G.D. and Herbermann, R.B. J. Immunol. 122, 1979, 675.
16. Ault, K.A. and Weiner, H.L. J. Immunol. 122, 1979, 2611.
17. Koren, H.S., Amos, D.B. and Buckley, R.H. J. Immunol. 120, 1978, 796.

QUANTITATION OF HUMAN NATURAL AND ANTIBODY-DEPENDENT CYTOTOXICITY[1]

Denis M. Callewaert

Department of Chemistry
Oakland University
Rochester, Michigan

I. INTRODUCTION

The ^{51}Cr release microcytotoxicity assay was originally developed as a sensitive assay for cytotoxic T lymphocytes (Brunner *et al.*, 1968), and adapted for the study of antibody-dependent cell-mediated cytotoxicity (Perlmann and Perlmann, 1970). When cultured cell lines were used as target cells in these assay systems, relatively low levels of lysis were occasionally observed in control experiments using unstimulated peripheral blood lymphocytes in the absence of antibody. This "background" lysis was soon recognized as natural cytotoxicity (Rosenberg *et al.*, 1974).

Although a wide range of variations have been reported, the four hour short-term radiochromium release assay, with an effector cell to target cell ratio of 100:1 has been widely used to measure cytotoxicity by activated T cells as well as antibody-dependent and natural cytotoxicity, and may be termed the "standard" assay conditions for measurement of cytotoxicity. The high effector cell to target cell ratio employed in this standard assay allow for high sensitivity in the detection of cytotoxicity. However, the percentage of cytotoxicity values determined under these conditions are not always quantitative measures of cytotoxicity. Thus, several

[1]*This work was supported in part by United States Public Health Service Grant AI-12766 from the National Institutes of Health.*

ISBN 0-12-341350-8

laboratories have recently suggested modifications in the ^{51}Cr release assay which allow for improved quantitation of cytotoxicity. In the following pages we shall briefly review three methods that are currently being used for the quantitation of natural cytotoxicity, along with the advantages and limitations of each method. In a final section we shall then discuss the results of some quantitative studies of the relationship between natural cytotoxicity and antibody-dependent cytotoxicity.

II. THE STANDARD SHORT-TERM RADIOCHROMIUM RELEASE ASSAY

While a wide variety of assay procedures for the measurement of cytotoxicity have been published, the four hour ^{51}Cr release microcytotoxicity assay appears to be the one most frequently employed. This assay is generally performed in microtiter plates or small test tubes at effector cell to target cell ratios of 100:1, with the results expressed as a percentage of cytotoxicity (%C) according to the formula

$$\%C = \frac{\bar{E} - \bar{S}}{\bar{M} - \bar{S}} \qquad (1)$$

where $\bar{E}$, $\bar{S}$, and $\bar{M}$ are, respectively the means of the replicate determinations of experimental (E) assays containing effector cells and target cells, spontaneous (S) release from target cells cultured alone, and the maximum (M) radioisotope released when target cells are subjected to sonication or other mechanical means are used to disrupt their membranes.

These standard assay conditions provide for a high degree of sensitivity in the detection of cytotoxicity, and have proven invaluable in the study of cytotoxicity mediated by sensitized T lymphocytes and of antibody-dependent cell-mediated cytotoxicity. These standard assay conditions are also ideal for many studies of natural cytotoxicity. For example, they can be used to determine if a particular cell line is susceptible to natural cytotoxicity and can be used in quantitative studies which involve target cells that are only moderately susceptible to natural cytotoxicity. However, several laboratories now routinely use cell lines which are highly susceptible to natural cytotoxicity, such as the Myeloid cell line designated K-562. When highly susceptible cell lines are used as targets, and in experiments where precise quantitation is necessary, standard assay conditions may give misleading results. This is illustrated in figure 1, which presents the results of a typical experiment employing K-562 as the target cell. Note that there is not a linear increase in the percent-

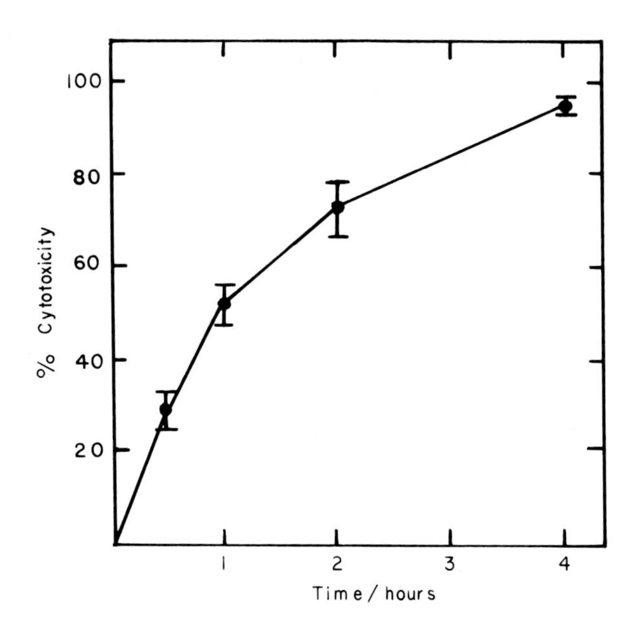

FIGURE 1. Cytotoxicity of K-562 target cells by human peripheral blood lymphocytes as a function of time. The standard 100:1 effector cell to target cell ratio was used and parallel reactions terminated at the indicated intervals. All assays and controls were run in triplicate, and standard deviations were calculated as described by Callewaert et al. (1977)

age of cytotoxicity of K-562 over the four hour assay interval, with the rate of lysis decreasing as the number of remaining target cells diminishes. While deviation from linearity is most severe for effector cell-target cell combinations that produce very high values for percentage of cytotoxicity, a number of factors, including assay conditions, and the source and treatment of effector cells, appear to be involved, so that experiments with relatively low cytotoxicity values may or may not have a linear rate of lysis over the entire assay.

III. VARIATION OF EFFECTOR CELL TO TARGET CELL RATIO AND LYTIC UNITS

The observed nonlinear rate of ^{51}Cr release under standard assay conditions can be attributed, among other things, to a decrease in the probability of effector cells "finding" the remaining target cells after a large number of target cells have been lysed. In order to avoid this impediment to the quantitation of natural cytotoxicity, many investigators now determine the percentage of cytotoxicity at several effector cell to target cell ratios. In these experiments, the target cell concentration is generally held constant while the number of effector cells is varied. A typical example would involve 10^4 target cells and from 10^5 to 10^6 effector cells in a total volume of 0.2ml, giving effector cell to target cell ratios of 10:1 to 100:1. The observed cytotoxicity in a four hour assay is then plotted vs the effector cell to target cell ratio. In order to allow for comparison of the cytotoxicity obtained under different conditions or with different effector cell and target cell combinations, the concept of lytic units has been introduced (Cerottini and Brunner, 1971; Kay *et al.*, 1977). One lytic unit is the number of effector cells required to give a certain percentage of cytotoxicity as determined from a plot of percentage of cytotoxicity vs effector cell to target cell ratio. For example, one may define one lytic unit as the number of effector cells required to achieve 33% cytotoxicity, 50% cytotoxicity, or some other value. Now, since lytic units are inversely related to the cytotoxic potential of a given effector cell population, data is frequently reported as lytic units per 10^7 effector cells, which is directly related to cytotoxic potential.

This technique should, in theory, overcome the problems inherent in the standard assay described above. In our hands, however, plots of percentage of cytotoxicity vs effector cell to target cell ratio are also generally nonlinear. Figure 2 shows the results of a typical experiment of this type. Note that the observed percentage of cytotoxicity of K-562 target cells is not directly proportional to the effector cell to target cell ratio except at the two lowest ratios. However, the error associated with using only these two ratios to calculate lytic units is quite high (*see* Table I). Standard error for lytic units is generally not reported, however, as shown in table I, it may be considerable.

TABLE I. Lytic Units Calculated for the Data in Figure 2

E:T ratios used for the calculation of lytic units	*Lytic units per 10^7 effectors ± S.E.*	
	1 LU = 33% C	*1 LU = 50% C*
1:5, 1:10, 1:20, 1:50, 1:100	*23 ± 7*	*13 ± 4*
1:5, 1:10, 1:20, 1:50	*28 ± 11*	*16 ± 6*
1:5, 1:10	*64 ± 53*	*42 ± 33*

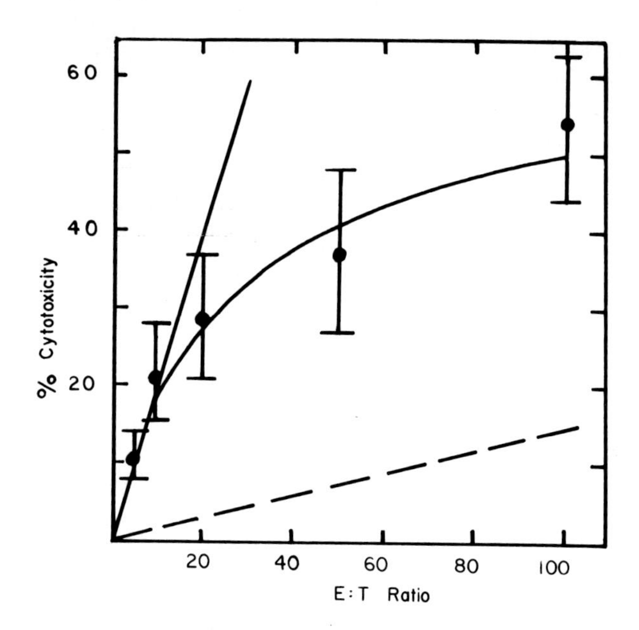

FIGURE 2. Cytotoxicity of K-562 target cells by human peripheral blood lymphocytes as a function of effector cell to target cell (E:T) ratio. All assays and controls were run in triplicate and terminated after four hours. The curved line represents the best fit using all five data points, with the straight solid line generated by using only the two lowest effector cell to target cell ratios. The dashed line represents typical results for a target of low susceptibility to natural cytotoxicity.

Another potential difficulty with the use of lytic units arises when using target cell lines that exhibit low susceptibility to natural cytotoxicity. With these target cells it may not be possible to achieve 33% cytotoxicity - even at an effector cell to target cell ratio of 100:1 (*see* figure 2). If one desires to maintain a standard lytic unit of, say, 33% cytotoxicity, then one must extrapolate from available experimental data. In at least one recent publication, results comparable to those represented in figure 2, about 10% cytotoxicity at a 100:1 ratio, were reported as zero lytic units since the authors were unable to achieve a value of one lytic unit, even at very high effector cell to target cell ratios. Since the majority of cell lines that are susceptible to natural cytotoxicity yield results in this range, it is important to avoid errors such as this.

In spite of these potential difficulties, the use of lytic units allows for generally improved quantitation of cytotoxicity experiments, provided that lytic units are calculated from experiments in which cytotoxicity is reasonably proportional to the effector cell to target cell ratio. In this regard, it is strongly recommended that standard deviations be reported when lytic units are calculated, as experimental results may be misleading when deviation values are omitted.

IV. VARIATION OF TARGET CELL CONCENTRATION AND THE ENZYME-SUBSTRATE ANALOGY

If one draws an analogy between a cytotoxicity reaction and a simple enzyme-catalyzed reaction, then effector cells are analogous to enzyme molecules, target cells are analogous to the substrate, and the kinetic models developed for enzyme-catalyzed reactions can be tested for their applicability to cytotoxicity reactions. Following this analogy, the simplest general model for a cytotoxicity reaction can be symbolized as

$$E + T \underset{k_{-1}}{\overset{k_1}{\rightleftharpoons}} ET \xrightarrow{k_2} E + T_L \qquad (2)$$

where E is an effector cell, T is a target cell, T_L is a lysed target cell analogous to the product of an enzyme-catalyzed reaction, and k_1, k_{-1}, and k_2 are rate constants. According to Michaelis and Menten, the rate of lysis, v, is then

$$v = \frac{V_{max}\ [T]}{K_M\ [T]} \qquad (3)$$

where V_{max} is the maximum possible rate of lysis as the target cell concentration approaches infinity, and $K_M = k_{-1} / k_1$.

This simple model has been tested and found applicable to the study of antibody-dependent cell-mediated cytotoxicity by Zeijlemaker *et al.* (1977), for cytotoxicity mediated by sensitized T lymphocytes (Thorn and Henney, 1976), and for natural cytotoxicity (Callewaert *et al.*, 1978). In these types of experiments, the values of V_{max} and K_M are obtained by measuring the percentage of cytotoxicity at various target cell concentrations with the concentration of effector cells held constant. Since cytotoxicity is generally measured after a fixed time period, conditions must be used for which the rate of lysis does not vary appreciably over the course of the assay. For the effector cell to target cell ratio used in the experiment illustrated in figure 1 this was not the case. However, with higher target cell concentrations and/or short assays one can achieve linearity for virtually all effector cell-target cell combinations. The values of V_{max} and K_M are generally determined graphically, either by plotting $1/v$ vs $1/[T]$ or by plotting $v/[T]$ vs v. For experiments in which the rate of lysis is constant over the entire assay period, either method will yield a straight line. The double-reciprocal method has the advantage of allowing for easy visual comparison of the V_{max} and K_M values obtained under different experimental conditions. However, the second method is preferable from a statistical viewpoint since it weighs all points equally. The results of a typical experiment are plotted using the second method in figure 3.

The value of V_{max} obtained in experiments of this type is a quantitative measure of cytotoxic efficiency that allows for quantitative comparisons of cytotoxicity under different reac-

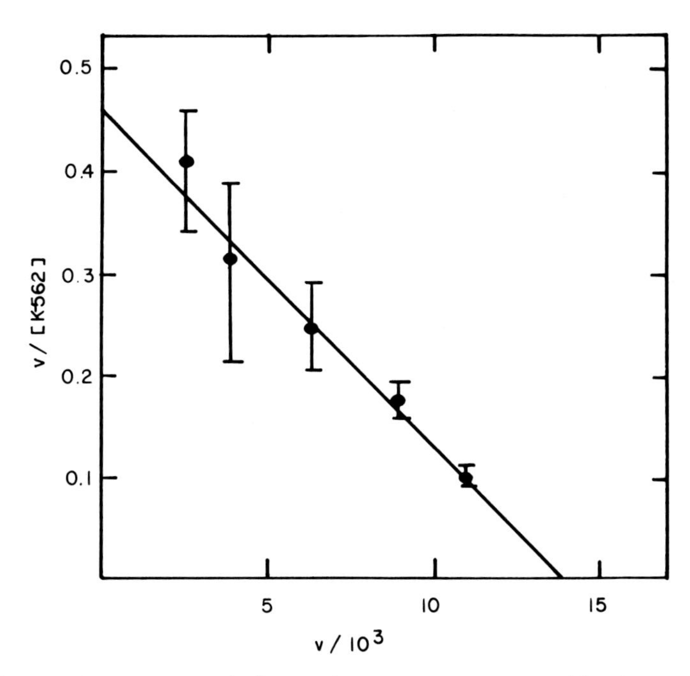

FIGURE 3. Cytotoxicity of K-562 target cells by effector cells obtained from the same donor, and run in parallel with the experiment illustrated in figure 2. The effector cell concentration was held at 5×10^5 per well and the target cell concentration was varied from 6.3×10^3 to 1×10^5 per well. The V_{max} value calculated from this data (the x intercept) is $1.38 \times 10^4 \pm 9.1 \times 10^2$ targets/4 hours, and the K_M value obtained (-1/slope) is $2.94 \times 10^4 \pm 3.4 \times 10^3$.

tion conditions or for different effector-target combinations. Experiments of this type also yield a K_M value which, according to our *simple* model (reaction 2) is equal to k_{-1}/k_1, which is the dissociation constant for effector-target cell complexes if we assume that k_2 is much smaller than k_1 and k_{-1}. However, the studies that have been conducted on T cell mediated cytotoxicity suggest that the model (Grimm *et al.* 1979):

$$E + T \underset{k_{-1}}{\overset{k_{+1}}{\rightleftharpoons}} ET \underset{k_{-2}}{\overset{k_{+2}}{\rightleftharpoons}} ET^* \xrightarrow{k_3} E + T^* \xrightarrow{k_4} T_L \tag{4}$$

effector cell recycling

is more appropriate for cytotoxicity reactions in general. Here T represents a target cell that is "programmed for lysis" in a step with rate constant k_{+2}. T then dissociates from the effector cell (k_3) and releases radiochromium in an effector cell independent step (k_4). According to this model, under steady-state conditions (Dixon and Webb, 1964):

$$V_{max} = k_4 \, [T^*] = \frac{(k_{+2}k_{+3}) \, [E]}{k_{+2} + k_{-2} + k_3} \tag{5}$$

and

$$K_M = \frac{(k_{-1}k_{-2}) + (k_{-1}k_3) + (k_{+2}k_3)}{k_{+1} \, (k_{+2} + k_{-2} + k_3)} \tag{6}$$

These mathematical expressions can be simplified by introducing various assumptions. For example, if k_{+2} is much smaller than k_{+1} and k_3, and if the rates of the reverse reactions are negligible, then $V_{max} = k_{+2}$ E and $K_M = k_{+2}/k_{+1}$. While these assumptions are reasonable for natural cytotoxicity, they remain to be tested. It is clear, however, that the K_M values obtained in cytotoxicity experiments are not simply dissociation constants for effector cell-target cell complexes. More intensive study of cytotoxicity reactions is needed to test the validity and utility of this model.

V. KINETIC CONSTANTS FOR NATURAL AND ANTIBODY-DEPENDENT CYTOTOXICITY REACTIONS

Only a few published reports have appeared to date on the application of enzyme-kinetic models to the study of natural and antibody-dependent cytotoxicity. In general, these studies support the use of models such as those given in reactions (2) and (4), although the reaction conditions used in different laboratories are somewhat different.

For antibody-dependent cytotoxicity, kinetic methods were used to demonstrate that K cell can be recycled (Zeijlemaker *et al.* 1977), and that lymphoid cells autologous to effector cells produce noncompetitive inhibition of target cell lysis (Herrick and Pollack, 1978).

For natural cytotoxicity, kinetic methods revealed identical K_M values for a given effector when tested on various target cell lines (Callewaert *et al.*, 1978), although the K_M values for different effectors against a common target cell line were often substantially different. Recently, Pollack and Emmons (1979) have reported the results of a similar experiment in which the K_M values obtained for a single donor with two different target cells were different. The apparent discrepancy in the results reported by these two laboratories may be due to the different target cells employed or to variations in assay conditions. It should also be noted that both groups used the double reciprocal method for plotting data, and ignored variations between replicate assays when calculating the values of the kinetic constants. In the past several months we have therefore performed a large number of experiments in order to critically compare the kinetic constants obtained in natural cytotoxicity by individual donors against a variety of target cell lines. The K_M values were determined by the preferred graphical method illustrated in figure 3, and deviations between replicate experiments were included in the calculation of the standard deviation for K_M values. The results of these (unpublished) experiments can be summarized as follows: In general, there was no *statistically significant* difference between the K_M values obtained when an individual donor's lymphocytes were tested against several target cell lines susceptible to natural cytotoxicity. However, the calculated standard deviations for K_M values were frequently quite large - even when the reactions were run in sextuplicate and a large number of target cell concentrations were used to generate kinetic constants. The significance of these findings is discussed below.

In one series of experiments, kintic methods have been used to compare the natural and antibody-dependent cytotoxic activity of individual donors (Callewaert *et al.*, 1978). Using the double-reciprocal method for plotting data, similar or identical K_M values were obtained for natural and antibody-dependent cytotoxicity. These findings have also been subjected to more critical experimental testing in recent months. Again, we have found that the K_M values for natural and antibody-dependent cytotoxicity mediated by a single donor's peripheral lymphocytes were not significantly different.

Given the findings that the K_M values obtained for a given donor's lymphocytes in natural cytotoxicity against a number of different target cell lines, and in antibody-dependent cytotoxicity reactions, are *at most* identical, and *at least* of comparible magnitude, what can we conclude? Using the simple model given in reaction (2) and the assumption that k_2 is very small, one might conclude that the K_M for natural cytotoxicity is a measure of the affinity of adsorbed antibody molecules for the antigens on the target cells. Mechanisms have, in fact, been proposed in which natural cytotoxicity results from the *in vivo* (Koide and Takasugi, 1977) or *in vitro* (Troy *et al.*, 1977) adsorption of antibody to F_c receptors on K cells. On the other hand, experiments with cytotoxic T cells suggest that the model given in reaction (4) is a more appropriate representation for cytotoxicity reactions in general (Grimm *et al.*, 1979). Using this model, and without imposing any further assumptions, we can conclude that the comparable magnitude (and perhaps identity) of the K_M values obtained for natural and antibody-dependent cytotoxicity reactions reflect a similar, perhaps common, lytic mechanism. The recognition mechanism employed by these two different phenomena may be, and probably are, not identical, as has been suggested by several lines of evidence presented elsewhere in this volume.

The use of a common lytic mechanism, but distinct recognition mechanisms in natural and antibody-dependent cytotoxicity reactions is compatible with the mounting evidence for these two phenomena being mediated by the same, or overlapping sets, of lymphocytes. The details of the lytic mechanism may be investigated by further application of the enzyme-substrate analogy.

REFERENCES

Brunner, K. T., Manel, J., Cerottini, J. C., and Chapius, B. (1968). *Immunology 14*, 181.

Callewaert, D. M., Kaplan, J., Peterson, W. D., and Lightbody, J. J. (1977). *Cell. Immunol. 33*, 11-19.

Callewaert, D. M., Johnson, D. F., and Kearney, J. (1978). *J. Immunol. 121*, 710-717.

Cerottini, J. C., and Brunner, K. T. (1971). *In "IN Vitro* Methods in Cell-Mediated Immunity" (B. R. Bloom and P. R. Glade, eds.), Academic Press, New York.

Dixon, M., and Webb, E. C. (1964). "Enzymes." Academic Press, New York.

Grimm, E. A., Thoma, J. A., and Bonavida, B. (1979). *J. Immunol. 123*, 2870-2877.

Herrick, M. V., and Pollack, S. B. (1978). *J. Immunol. 121*, 1348-1352.

Kay, H. D., Bonnard, G. D., West, W. H., and Heberman, R. B. (1977). *J. Immunol. 118*, 2058-2066.

Koide, Y., and Takasugi, M. (1977). *J. Nat. Cancer Inst. 59*, 1099-1105.

Perlmann, P., and Perlmann, H. (1970). *Cell. Immonol. 1*, 300.

Pollack, S. B., and Emmons, S. L. (1979). *J. Immunol. 123*, 160-165.

Rosenberg, E. B., McCoy, J. L., Green, S. S., Donnelly, F. C., Siwarski, D. F., Levine, P. H., and Herberman, R. B. (1974). *J. Nat. Cancer Inst. 52*, 345-352.

Thorn, R. M., and Henney, C. S. (1976). *J. Immunol. 117*, 2213-2219.

Troye, M., Perlmann, P., Pape, G. R., Spiegelberg, H. L., Naslund, I., and Gidlof, A. (1977). *J. Immunol. 119*, 1061-1067.

Zeiljlemaker, W. P., van Oers, R. H. J., deGoede, R. E. Y., and Schellekens, P. Th. A. (1977). *J. Immonol. 119*, 1507-1514.

THE RELATIONSHIP BETWEEN NATURAL AND ANTIBODY-DEPENDENT CELL-MEDIATED CYTOTOXICITY[1]

Tsuneo Kamiyama
Mitsuo Takasugi

Department of Surgery
UCLA School of Medicine
Los Angeles, California

I. INTRODUCTION

Since the early 1970's when natural or spontaneous cell-mediated cytotoxicity (NCMC) was first distinguished from specific immune cytotoxicity (1-3), it has received considerable attention because of its potential role in host resistance to malignancy and infection. Many investigators have contributed to the development of our present understanding of the mechanism of NCMC and to the demonstration of its biological significance. However, studies of a related phenomenon, antibody dependent cell-mediated cytotoxicity (ADCC) slightly preceded the discovery of NCMC (4-6) and also contributed to the advancement of our knowledge of NCMC.

Both natural and antibody dependent cell-mediated cytotoxicity have been observed in humans and in most mammals which have been examined. Since the earliest detection of these cellular reactions, controversy has played a major role in their study. Disagreements have arisen over the effector class mediating both reactions and the involvement of antibodies in NCMC as well as ADCC. In this chapter comparing NCMC and ADCC, we will describe some characteristics of the effector cells, the effect of various inhibitors, and an approach to differentiating ADCC from NCMC.

[1]*This work was supported in part by contracts N01-CB 74133 from the Tumor Immunology Section and N01-CP43211 from the Biological Carcinogenesis Branch, Division of Cancer Cause and Prevention, National Cancer Institute.*

ISBN 0-12-341350-8

II. CHARACTERISTICS OF EFFECTOR CELLS

Most investigators agree that effector cells for NCMC or NK cells are nonphagocytic, nonadherent lymphocytes. We have described these cells earlier as N-cells (7). Whether these cells belong to T-, B-cells or an unidentified class of lymphocytes has not been definitely decided. In early studies, they were considered to be neither T- nor B-cells because of the failure to detect characteristic markers on their cell surfaces. Recently, the possibility that NK cells belong to the T-cell lineage has drawn support from several laboratories (8,9) but further study is needed to establish this relationship.

Although several types of effector cells including adherent phagocytic monocytes and granulocytes have been reported to mediate ADCC, this reaction is mediated primarily by a nonadherent, nonphagocytic lymphocyte (K cells) with the same characteristics as NK cells. Whether the same or a different subclass of cells mediates both reactions is currently controversial (10-13).

A. Surface Markers

Markers on human cells which are used most frequently in identifying lymphocyte subsets are surface immunoglobulins (14) and complement receptors (15) on B-cells and receptors for sheep red blood cells (SRBC) on T-cells (10). Several lymphocyte subsets also carry Fc receptors (FcR) for IgG which appear to have a special functional relationship to NCMC-ADCC but are not exclusive to a major lymphocyte subclass. Table I summarizes these results.

1. Surface Immunoglobulins (SIg). In early studies, a class of cells with IgG molecules loosely attached to FcR on the cell surface were included among B-cells (16,17). More recently the B-cell class has been limited to those cells where immunoglobulin is an integral part of the membrane. By this definition, effector cells for NCMC and ADCC are not B-cells. Nevertheless, several groups have now recognized the set of cells with loosely-bound IgG antibodies as one of the more important effector cells which function in NCMC and ADCC (7,18).

2. Receptor for complement (C'). Early studies (19) on effector cells for NCMC suggested that NCMC activity could be eliminated by removal of cells forming rosettes with SRBC, anti-SRBC and C' (EAC-rosettes). Later studies in a number of

TABLE I. Summary of the Activity of Lymphocyte Subsets in NCMC and ADCC

Lymphocyte surface markers	Cytotoxic activity NCMC	ADCC
1. Surface immunoglobulin[a]	Low	Low
2. Complement receptors	Low	Low
3. E rosettes		
a. High affinity	Low	Low
b. Low affinity	High	High
4. EA rosettes (FcR^+)		
a. IgG	High	High
b. IgM	Low	Low

[a]Ig is firmly bound to membrane

laboratories using IgM anti-SRBC and C' indicated that most effector cells for NCMC-ADCC lacked complement receptors, suggesting that previous studies may have included rosettes with SRBC and IgG anti-SRBC (EA-rosettes). If cells with C'_3 receptors are involved in NCMC-ADCC reactions, they represent only a small part of the total effector population (20).

3. *Receptor for Sheep Red Blood Cells (E).* When the effector suspension is separated by formation of spontaneous E-rosettes and centrifugation on Ficoll-Hypaque, NCMC-ADCC activity was observed to be enriched in the interface or nonrosetting fraction (7,21-23). However, a significant part of the activity was still observed in the pellet or rosetting fraction. With a more sensitive rosetting technique, cytotoxic activity was observed to shift toward the rosetting population. Up to 80% of the NCMC and ADCC activity in the original suspension was recovered in the rosetting fraction leading West *et al.* (8,24) to conclude that a cell forming low-affinity E-rosettes mediated NCMC and ADCC. On the other hand, Potter and Moore using several optimal and suboptimal rosette forming procedures demonstrated that both fractions had NCMC activity irrespective of the technique (25). Similar results have been obtained by other laboratories including our own. From these observations, it may be concluded that NK or K cells do not form a distinct subpopulation in relation to the

receptor for SRBC. However, at least a portion of the effector cell population appears to form spontaneous rosettes with SRBC suggesting a T-cell involvement.

4. Receptor for the Fc portion of Immunoglobulin (FcR). The results from most studies indicate that a major part of effector cells mediating both NCMC and ADCC bear FcR (7,22,23, 26,27). When we tested cells separated by EA-rosetting and Ficoll-Hypaque centrifugation for NCMC, activity was greater in the rosetting fraction. However, cytotoxicity was lower than for the original cell suspension indicating that the formation of antigen-antibody (Ag-Ab) complexes during EA-rosette formation may have inhibited the reaction. Ag-Ab complexes and aggregated IgG inhibit NCMC and ADCC by combining with the FcR on the effector cell. Kay *et al.* (28) showed that both NK and K cells bind to monolayers of Ag-Ab complex and the binding was inhibited by the treatment of the monolayer with Staphylococcal protein A. Pape *et al.* (29) using an EA rosette technique also demonstrated that effector fractions containing mostly B-cells but depleted of FcR^+ cells displayed a strong reduction in NCMC and ADCC. A subset of effector cells for NCMC which lacked FcR and was therefore immunoglobulin independent has also been described. No information is available at present whether these cells mediate ADCC.

Recently, T-cell populations have been further divided according to their ability to form EA-rosettes with IgG or IgM-coated ox red blood cells (30,3]). These results indicate that T-cells bearing the receptor for IgG (T_γ) mediated both NCMC and ADCC, while T-cells with the receptor for IgM (T_μ) did not.

B. Separation of Effector Cells for NCMC and ADCC

A subclass of lymphocytes without T- and B-cell markers was discovered in the study of effector cells for ADCC and described as null cells. Many of these cells are now known not to be true null cells since they bear Fc receptors. Recently a set of cells lacking even FcR has been reported (26,]8). Because there are no characteristic surface markers for null cells, they have been isolated by negative selection procedures. A two step isolation technique involving nylon wool or anti-Ig column chromatography for removal of B-cells and E rosette formation followed by centrifugation over Ficoll-Hypaque to remove T-cells has been useful. Recently, Ozer *et al.* reported a rapid isolation method for human null cells involving a single step, double rosette technique using SRBC rosettes to remove T-cells and anti-Ig coated SRBC for B-cells. The isolated null cell population represented less than 5% of the total peripheral mononuclear cells.

The characteristics of effector cells described thus far, do not differentiate between effector cells for NCMC and ADCC and, in fact, may be used to support the proposal that the same subset of cells mediates both reactions. No reports have appeared describing successful separation of effector cells for NCMC and ADCC. The argument against this proposal is based on observations that patients with some immunodeficiencies react in NCMC but not in ADCC (10). However, the conclusion derived from a study of patients with X-linked agammaglobulinemia did not take into consideration the differences in sensitivity between the NCMC and ADCC systems. Healthy controls tested in these systems also showed stronger reactivity in NCMC than in ADCC. This same relationship was observed with effector cells from patients who had generally weaker reactivity allowing detection of cytotoxicity only in the more sensitive system. In another study, *in vivo* and *in vitro* treatment with dexamethasone reduced NCMC but not ADCC (33). In a study where NCMC was tested against Chang cells and ADCC against antibody-coated Chang cells, the absence of an effect by dexamethasone solely in the ADCC system is difficult to understand since the quantification of ADCC includes measurement of an NCMC component.

III. CYTOLYTIC MECHANISMS OF NCMC AND ADCC

Because of the strong similarity between effector cells in NCMC and ADCC, our attention was drawn to the mechanism of cytolysis for the reactions. Even if effector cells could not be separated by physical means, we felt that changing the conditions of the test or the addition of inhibitors might affect the two reactions differentially to emphasize putatively separate mechanisms. These attempts are summarized on Table II.

A. Modulation of NCMC and ADCC

NCMC-ADCC reactions are affected by several inhibitors as well as being influenced by various changes in the test conditions. We will emphasize those factors which are related to a role for immunoglobulins in the reaction in the next section. Here we will discuss physical and chemical factors which influence cellular metabolism.

1. The Effect of Temperature. To obtain optimal cytolysis, the tests should be performed at 37°C. When the tests were carried out at room temperature or at 4°C., both NCMC and ADCC were significantly reduced. Since binding of NK or K cells to

TABLE II. Summary of Modulation in NCMC and ADCC by Different Reagents

	Reagent	Site of effect	Effect NCMC	Effect ADCC
1.	*Aggregated IgG*	*FcR*	*Inhibition*	*Inhibition*
2.	*Ag-Ab complex*	*FcR*	*Inhibition*	*Inhibition*
3.	*Protein A*	*Fc*	*No effect*	*Inhibition*
4.	*Fab anti-Fab*	*Antibody*	*Conflicting results*	*No effect*
5.	*Trypsin*	*Antibody*	*Inhibition*	*Slight enhancement*
6.	*Interferon (NAF)*	*EC*[a]	*Enhancement*	*Enhancement*
7.	*NIF*	*EC*	*Inhibition*	*Inhibition*[e]
8.	*Incubation (1 wk)*	*EC*		
	37°			
	4°		*Reduced*	*Reduced*
9.	*Puromycin*	*PS*[b]	*Inhibition*	*Inhibition*
10.	*Actinomycin D*	*NAS*[c], *PS*	*Inhibition*	*Inhibition*
11.	*Mitomycin C*	*NAS*[c]	*Inhibition*	*Inhibition*
12.	NaN_3	*Respiration*	*Reversible inhibition*	*Reversible inhibition*
13.	*EDTA*	*CDC*[d]	*Inhibition*	*Inhibition*
	+ Ca^{++}		*Recovery*	*Recovery*
	+ Mg^{++}		*Partial recovery*	*Partial recovery*
	+ Ca^{++} and Mg^{++}		*Recovery*	*Recovery*

[a]*EC : effector cells*

[b]*PS : protein synthesis*

[c]*NAS : nucleic acid synthesis*

[d]*CDC : chelation of divalent cations*

[e]*See chapter by Koide and Takasugi*

target cells can take place at low temperature as well as at 37°C., the reduction in temperature affects a stage in NCMC and ADCC which occurs after the initial effector-target recognition step. The temperature-dependent step in the cytolytic process may be an event which requires membrane fluidity and/or active metabolism.

2. *The effect of puromycin, actinomycin D and mitomycin C.* Both NCMC and ADCC were strongly reduced by puromycin, an irreversible inhibitor of protein synthesis. The degree of

TABLE III. Pretreatment of Effector Cells with Mitomycin C, Actinomycin D or Puromycin

Antibiotics[a] *(ug/ml)*	*Percent Inhibition*	
	NCMC NC37	*ADCC IgG-SRBC*
Mitomycin C		
125	*0*	*-2*
250	*79*	*59*
500	*104*	*103*
Actinomycin D		
3.1	*5*	*23*
6.3	*26*	*49*
12.5	*69*	*77*
25.0	*97*	*87*
Puromycin		
200	*7*	*26*
400	*22*	*35*
800	*44*	*48*
1600	*96*	*70*

[a]*Effector cells were treated for 1 hour at 37° C.*

inhibition paralleled the degree of *de novo* protein synthesis assessed by the incorporation of a labeled amino acid, indicating that both NCMC and ADCC were highly dependent on active protein metabolism. Similar results have been reported by others (34). It is unclear, however, what protein is required to mediate cytotoxicity. One possibility is a lymphokine such as lymphotoxin which is capable of killing target cells and another is that the protein produced is a factor like interferon which activates NK and K cells (35). Table III presents the effect of inhibition of nucleic acid and protein synthesis on NCMC and ADCC. A dose-dependent inhibition of the two reactions was observed for the three antimetabolites investigated.

3. *The effect of NaN_3.* The dependency of NCMC and ADCC on an active metabolic process or on temperature suggests that these reactions are also energy-dependent. To test this further, NaN_3, an inhibitor of respiratory enzymes, was added to the test or was used to pretreat effector cells (Table IV). The inhibitor blocked both NCMC and ADCC when present in the test mixture while exhibiting only a weak temporary effect

TABLE IV. The Effect of NaN_3 on NCMC and ADCC

	Percent Inhibition	
NaN_3 (mM)	NCMC NC37	ADCC IgG-SRBC
Added to the test[a]		
3	15	45
10	69	90
30	76	95
100	87	104
Pre-treated[b]		
3	0	4
10	11	3
30	11	11
100	20	25

[a]*NaN_3 was added to the test*
[b]*Effector cells were incubated in NaN_3 for 1 hour at 37°C.*

when effector cells were pretreated. Viability of the effector cells after treatment was greater than 90% at the highest concentration of NaN_3 and more than 95% at the lower concentrations. Thus it is clear that the inhibiting effect of NaN_3 on the effector cell was readily reversible and not due to cell destruction. NaN_3 is also known to inhibit cap formation or catabolism of the capped anti-Ig-Ig complex. Therefore, the study with the inhibitor, NaN_3, supported conclusions from temperature effects that NCMC and ADCC require active respiratory metabolism and/or membrane fluidity of effector cells for completion of the cytotoxic reaction. Other respiratory inhibitors such as dinitrophenol and cyanide also inhibit both cell-mediated cytotoxicity and cap formation by lymphocytes (36-38).

4. The Effect of Ethylenediamine Tetraacetic Acid (EDTA). To assess the role of divalent cations on NCMC and ADCC, EDTA was introduced to the test as a chelating agent. Table V shows the effect of removing divalent cations on NCMC-ADCC by the addition of EDTA and the recovery from this effect through restoration of Ca, Mg, or both. The following conclusions were derived from the study:

(a) Chelation of divalent cations resulted in significant reduction of NCMC and ADCC with a relatively greater loss of NCMC activity. With some effector suspensions, considerable

TABLE V. Effect of EDTA, and Restoration of Cytotoxicity by Addition of Ca^{++} and Mg^{++}

Lymphocyte donor	Reagents[a]	Percent Cytotoxicity NCMC NC37	ADCC IgG-SRBC
197456	control	30.7	18.5
	EDTA	5.5	1.6
	EDTA + Mg^{++}	0.9	4.2
	EDTA + Ca^{++}	23.6	12.2
	EDTA + Mg^{++} & Ca^{++}	4.9	15.6
197457	control	60.8	75.1
	EDTA	4.4	6.8
	EDTA + Mg^{++}	18.6	63.9
	EDTA + Ca^{++}	41.6	70.5
	EDTA + Mg^{++} & Ca^{++}	39.5	71.8

[a] Concentration of the reagents: EDTA = 5 mM; Mg^{++} = 10 mM $MgCl_2$; Ca^{++} = 10 mM $CaCl_2$; Mg^{++} & Ca^{++} = each 5 mM of $MgCl_2$ and $CaCl_2$

ADCC activity was observed in the absence of free divalent cations indicating an additional mechanism for ADCC. In its simplest form, these results might be explained by one set of effector cells dependent on divalent cations and active in NCMC and ADCC and a second set of cells which functions mostly in ADCC and is less dependent on divalent cations.

(b) Supplementation with Ca and Mg after chelation of divalent cations restored most of the cytotoxic activity. Ca was more efficient in the restoration of cytotoxicity. It nearly restored activity to the levels observed with supplementation of both Ca and Mg. Recovery of activity with Mg was only partial and in the case of NCMC depended on the effector cell as well as the target cell. Recovery of ADCC with Mg was always greater than recovery of NCMC. Restoration of Ca and Mg further supported the existence of a heterogeneous effector population with at least two important subsets. These include a subset which is Ca dependent and active in NCMC and ADCC and another which is Mg dependent and more active in ADCC. The Mg dependent cell from some individuals may also be active in NCMC. The combination of cells active in ADCC makes it less sensitive to the withdrawal of divalent cations and more responsive to recovery with restoration of Ca and Mg.

(c) Finally, the pattern of divalent cation dependency in ADCC to antibody coated fresh target cells such as SRBC or peripheral blood lymphocytes (PBL) was quite similar to the pattern for NCMC. This observation suggests that ADCC against noncultured target cells is mediated by an effector subset shared with NCMC.

When effector cells isolated from donors who had previously exhibited Mg dependent recovery in NCMC were further treated with carbonyl iron, the ability to recover activity with Mg supplementation was lost indicating that monocytes might be important in this activity. Effector cells enriched for monocytes were tested for cytotoxicity and although they were active in ADCC, they were ineffective in NCMC. The inability of monocytes to mediate NCMC while influencing recovery of cytotoxicity with Mg suggests an indirect role in NCMC.

B. Participation of Immunoglobulin in NCMC and ADCC

NCMC against adherent or lymphoblastoid cell lines was significantly decreased by treatments which removed immunoglobulins from the lymphocyte surface such as incubation with trypsin or lowering of pH. Moreover, these cells partially regained their cytotoxic activity when incubated in autologous or allogeneic sera. The specificity of the recovered NCMC was consistent with the specificity of the antibodies used for incubation. Serum specifically inactive against a target cell was prepared by absorbing serum from a healthy individual with different target cells. When effector cells were reconstituted with the absorbed serum and tested for cytotoxicity against the same target cells, a selectively lower effect was observed (12). Reconstitution of the effector cells was also performed with eluates from the absorbing target cells producing effector cells which reacted selectively with the target cell. Effector cells armed with monospecific anti-HLA sera were also tested and showed specificity for HLA antigens on target cells (39). From these observations, we postulated that NK cells are "armed" *in vivo* with circulating natural or other antibodies through Fc-FcR interaction at the cell surface.

If the effector cells are armed with IgG antibodies and the antibodies could be detected, the cells should be considered SIg^+. It is generally accepted that B-cells are SIg^+ and can be distinguished from another subset with IgG molecules loosely attached to the cell through Fc-FcR interaction. The immunoglobulins on such cells may be removed by treatment with trypsin and a variety of other techniques. Indeed, Kumagai *et al.* (40) have shown that the antibodies may be removed through elution at low pH and incubation at 37°C. They were also able to detect the recovery of cell surface antibodies when the cells were incubated in serum. Warr *et al.* (41) showed that null cells from athymic mice were SIg^- by immunofluorescence using rabbit antisera to mouse heavy or light chains, but SIg^+ by fluorescence with chicken antibody to the $F(ab')_2$ portion of mouse IgG. The amount of SIg was about 10-30% of that on B-cells. These results suggest that human NK cells may be SIg^+ if tested by a sensitive method.

The proposal that NK cells were armed with antibodies was also supported by Trejdosiewicz *et al.* (42) using statistical analysis of serum antibody titer and NCMC activity against a colon adenocarcinoma cell line in cancer patients and again recently by Kall and Koren (43) who observed both immunoglobulin dependent and independent mechanisms in NCMC. In animal experiments, Prather *et al.* (44) were also able to demonstrate *in vivo* arming. They found NCMC activity against SV40 transformed target cells in normal hamsters passively given anti-SV40 serum. These results suggest that NCMC can be mediated by cells armed *in vivo* with natural antibodies. Thus, the mechanisms of immunoglobulin dependent NCMC and ADCC are quite similar and the primary difference is that an effector cell-antibody complex recognizes the target cells in NCMC while effector cells recognize the antibody-target cell complex in ADCC.

In contrast to the immunoglobulin-dependent mechanisms we have just described, a failure to detect a functional role for antibodies has also been reported. Kay *et al.*(45) and Perussia *et al.* (46) could not demonstrate recovery of cytotoxic activity against K562 cells after trypsin-treatment by incubation with autologous or allogeneic sera. The cells were, however, still active in ADCC. Also according to several investigators, Fab or $F(ab')_2$ fragments against human immunoglobulins did not inhibit NCMC against K562 or adherent target cell lines. NCMC activity by trypsin-treated effector cells against K562 was also observed to recover in culture despite the presence of $F(ab')_2$ fragments against human $F(ab')_2$ in the culture throughout the test. These reports were in contrast to Pape *et al.* who found inhibition of NCMC with Fab anti-human $F(ab')_2$ (18). Pape warns that not all preparations are sufficiently pure and specific to inhibit NCMC and that further processing of reagents with immunoadsorbents may be needed. Even with highly purified Fab, inhibition of NCMC was not complete, further indicating that part of NCMC may be immunoglobulin dependent.

Although we cannot satisfactorily explain the contradictory results without comparative studies, there were distinct differences between our approach and those employed by other laboratories. In reconstituting NCMC, we did not depend solely on the level of activity to show the effect of antibody. Antibodies for reconstitution were selected for specificity to HLA and by absorption and elution. The specificity was demonstrated by testing the reconstituted effector cells against several target cells and differentiating selective cytotoxicity. Moreover, it appears from the results presented (45,46), that our trypsin-treatment was considerably less severe than others and NCMC was only slightly reduced. We felt that treating lymphocytes until a complete loss of activity was observed would result in irreversible damage to the cell.

Despite the conflicting reports, there are encouraging results emerging from several laboratories which might reconcile the differences. The involvement of a heterogeneous population of effector cells has been reported for both NCMC and ADCC with indications that immunoglobulin dependent and independent mechanisms occur simultaneously. Troye *et al.* (47) reported inhibition of NCMC against a transitional cell carcinoma cell line, T24, by Fab fragments specific for either $F(ab')_2$ or Fc fragments of human IgG, but not by immunologically unrelated Fab to ovalbumin. These results indicated that a large part, but not all, of NCMC was induced by antibodies. Further work from the same laboratory (18) on NCMC to K562 and ADCC to T24 indicated that a significant part of NCMC against K562 reflected K cell reactions induced by natural antibodies. However, part of the NCMC also appeared to be immunoglobulin-independent. The relative importance of these two simultaneously occurring mechanisms varied for different lymphocyte donors. Kall and Koren (43) reported that NCMC depended on arming with natural antibodies as well as independently of serum factors. According to their study, NCMC against K562 was independent of serum factors with one exception. This observation might explain why some investigators using only this target system had encountered difficulty in detecting an immunoglobulin dependent mechanism for NCMC. Kay *et al.* showed that NCMC against K562 was partially but significantly inhibited when FcR on effector lymphocytes were modulated by overnight incubation with Ag-Ab complexes (45). The remaining NCMC was strong and not significantly inhibited by additional Ag-Ab complexes or removed by absorption on Ag-Ab monolayers.

In our studies, NCMC against K562 as well as other lymphoblastoid cell lines was strongly inhibited by pretreatment of effector cells with heat-aggregated IgG and Ag-Ab complexes or by the presence of these reagents in the test. The results are in close agreement with those obtained by others (46,18). These observations indicate that the inhibition of NCMC by IgG reagents is determined by the Fc portion of IgG, strongly supporting the functional participation of the FcR and immunoglobulin in NCMC as well as ADCC against most lymphoblastoid cell lines including K562.

As summarized in Table II, most inhibitors and reagents have the same effect on NCMC and ADCC with the exception of trypsin, protein A and possibly divalent cations. The inhibition of only NCMC by trypsin and of ADCC alone by protein A is consistent with our model of one effector cell with Fc receptors mediating both NCMC and ADCC. In NCMC, IgG antibodies react initially with the effector cell while in ADCC, the antibody reacts first with the target cell (See Chapter, Greenberg and Takasugi). The results described in this chapter on the role of divalent cations might seem contradictory to the model of one effector cell for NCMC and ADCC by prescribing an explanation of cytotoxicity through a heterogeneous population of effector cells for both reactions. However, it does not rule out the possibility of sharing one important effector cell subset.

IV. CONCURRENT EXAMINATION OF NCMC AND ADCC TO EPSTEIN-BARR VIRUS (EBV) ASSOCIATED SPECIFICITIES

Determination of ADCC and NCMC differs only by the addition of antiserum to the ADCC test. Thus, tests of ADCC to cultured target cells include an NCMC component as well as ADCC. Since NCMC and ADCC both involve selective as well as nonselective effects and the two reactions interrelate, it is difficult to isolate each effect from the total cytotoxic reaction. ADCC basically involves a relationship between sera and target cells but this relationship is influenced by the effector cells employed which introduce a third variable and NCMC to the test.

ADCC to an EBV-specific system will be used as a model to illustrate how we have approached some of the problems. Raji and Daudi cells were selected as target cells because they can be readily superinfected with the P3Hrl strain of the virus and target antigens associated with EBV are induced on the cell surface. That these antigens are associated with EBV will be shown later through selective cytotoxicity against infected cells only with sera which were known to be seropositive for EBV.

The assessment of precise, specific ADCC to EBV-associated antigens requires differentiation of specific ADCC to EBV-associated antigens from other specificities on target cells and a further discrimination between ADCC and NCMC. The distinction between specific ADCC to EBV target antigens and to other specificities is made by testing several sera versus EBV infected and uninfected target cells in a two dimensional array. Selective cytotoxicity is then derived by application of the interaction analysis and association of selectivity is made with sera positive for EBV or with infected target cells. Since NCMC can also be specific for EBV associated antigens and influences specific ADCC to EBV target antigens, the specificity of the effector cell for the EBV infected target cells should also be discerned by two-dimensional testing. Finally, the relationship between specific ADCC and an underlying specific NCMC requires examination.

A. *Three Dimensional Testing*

The requirement for concurrent testing of ADCC and NCMC to EBV infected target cells calls for testing on a three-dimensional basis. A cubic experimental design is employed. Sera known to be positive or negative for EBV antigens by other serological tests were varied along the Y axis, EBV infected and uninfected target cells along the X axis, and at least 3 effector cells from different individuals along the Z axis. By examining the results achieved through different planes with the two-way interaction analysis, selectivity is investigated for two of the three variables. Selective ADCC is examined through the YX planes, testing sera versus target cells with each of the effector cells. The horizontal planes, XZ, describe the NCMC effect with different sera added to each plane. Finally, the YZ planes measure selective interactions between the effector cell and sera for each target cell, providing information on the relationship between NCMC and ADCC. The complete results may also be examined by the three-way interaction analysis to investigate selective effects on a three-dimensional basis. It provides information on the modulation of NCMC by different sera or the efficiency of ADCC with different effector cells depending on ones point of view.

The tests were conducted in three microtiter U plates with a different effector suspension used on each plate. Within each plate, target cells were tested in triplicate columns and consisted of the original Raji and Daudi cells plus subcultures which had been infected with EBV on the previous day. For the eight rows of the test, lymphocytes were tested by themselves and with five different sera. A spontaneous and a maximum release were also included to determine the range of the test. The percent cytotoxicity was calculated from the results as in Eq. (1).

$$\% \text{ cytotoxicity} = \frac{\text{test release (cpm)} - \text{spontaneous release (cpm)}}{\text{maximum release (cpm)} - \text{spontaneous release (cpm)}} \tag{1}$$

1. *Application of the Two-Way Interaction Analysis*. The two-way analysis of variance was applied to the set of results from each plane of the three-dimensional test to examine selectivity in the interaction between two of the three variables; it assumes that no special relationship existed. The difference between the nonselective score and the observed score was the selective effect reflecting a special interaction. When applied to tests of sera versus target cells as in ADCC (the YX plane) it is represented by the following formulas, (Eq. 2,3):

$$\text{Nonselective reactivity} = \overline{X}_S + \overline{X}_T - \overline{X} \quad (2)$$

$$\text{Selective reactivity} = X_{ST} - \overline{X}_S - \overline{X}_T + \overline{X} \quad \text{(or)} \quad (3)$$

$$= \text{Observed reactivity} - \text{Nonselective reactivity}$$

(notations are described in the next section).

2. *Application of the Three-Way Interaction Analysis*. The three-way interaction analysis is applied to the results from tests employing a three dimensional design and selectivity is differentiated on that basis. An example will be introduced later to improve understanding of its application. The three-way analysis uses the same basic approach as the two-way interaction analysis with the exception that three variables are assayed. Nonselectivity is calculated according to the mean reactivity of each variable and selectivity is calculated as the difference between this nonselective score and the observed test result, (Eq. 4,5):

$$\text{Nonselective reactivity} = \quad (4)$$

$$\overline{X}_{ST} + \overline{X}_{ET} + \overline{X}_{SE} - \overline{X}_S - \overline{X}_T - \overline{X}_E + \overline{X}$$

$$\text{Selective reactivity} = \quad (5)$$

$$X_{SET} - \overline{X}_{ST} - \overline{X}_{ET} - \overline{X}_{SE} + \overline{X}_S + \overline{X}_T + \overline{X}_E - \overline{X}$$

Where:

$\overline{X}$ = mean score for all tests

$\overline{X}_E$ = mean score for all tests with the effector

$\overline{X}_T$ = mean score for all tests with the target

$\overline{X}_S$ = mean score for all tests with the sera

$\bar{X}_{ET}$ = mean score for all tests with the effector and target

$\bar{X}_{ST}$ = mean score for all tests with the serum and target

$\bar{X}_{SE}$ = mean score for all tests with the serum and effector

$X_{ST,SET}$ = observed score for the two- and three-dimensional tests

3. *Sample Results*. Table VI presents the results in percent cytotoxicity. Each section represents the scores from one plate testing one effector cell by itself, with two sera negative for EBV viral caspid antigen (VCA) testing (A and B), and

TABLE VI. Direct Results of Three-Dimensional Testing Against EBV-Infected and Uninfected Target Cells

Effector cell	*Serum*	*Percent cytotoxicity[a] on target cells*			
		Raji	*Raji^{EBV}*	*Daudi*	*Daudi^{EBV}*
1	-	*13.3*	*30.4*	*5.2*	*34.6*
	A	*24.8*	*58.9*	*6.0*	*75.8*
	B	*24.2*	*64.2*	*6.6*	*72.2*
	C	*25.5*	*82.7*	*9.6*	*86.0*
	D	*23.4*	*90.4*	*9.9*	*89.0*
	E	*21.3*	*90.4*	*8.1*	*88.1*
2	-	*0.0*	*8.2*	*1.3*	*13.5*
	A	*17.8*	*38.3*	*2.2*	*39.3*
	B	*17.4*	*29.8*	*3.3*	*10.0*
	C	*16.8*	*79.9*	*3.5*	*76.7*
	D	*15.2*	*72.2*	*2.6*	*84.0*
	E	*2.7*	*81.9*	*1.8*	*64.0*
3	-	*3.7*	*19.3*	*4.0*	*17.3*
	A	*11.7*	*36.8*	*7.8*	*50.4*
	B	*9.6*	*32.4*	*7.0*	*46.2*
	C	*8.4*	*78.3*	*6.9*	*72.0*
	D	*11.2*	*73.1*	*6.1*	*91.5*
	E	*9.6*	*71.5*	*6.9*	*74.2*

[a]*Percent cytotoxocity was calculated from equation (1) of text*

TABLE VII. Two-way Analysis of Results from the Serum versus Target (YX) Plane

Effector cell	Serum	Membrane Fluorescence	Selective Scores on Target cells			
			Raji	Raji^{EBV}	Daudi	Daudi^{EBV}
1	A	–[a]	7.4	-11.9	4.4	0.1
	B	–	6.4	-7.1	4.6	-4.0
	C	+	-1.4	2.3	-1.5	0.7
	D	+	-5.8	7.8	-3.5	1.5
	E	+	-6.7	9.0	-4.1	1.8
2	A		12.4	-13.6	8.1	-6.9
	B		21.3	-12.8	18.5	-27.0
	C		-8.4	8.2	-10.4	10.6
	D		-9.3	1.3	-10.6	18.7
	E		-15.9	16.8	-5.5	4.6
3	A		10.5	-12.7	9.8	-7.6
	B		11.3	-14.2	11.8	-8.9
	C		-7.5	14.1	-5.9	-0.7
	D		-8.8	4.8	-10.7	14.7
	E		-5.5	8.1	-5.0	2.4

[a]negative and positive membrane fluorescence

three sera positive for EBV (C,D, and E) against infected and uninfected Raji and Daudi target cells. Even from the original scores, increased cytotoxicity is observed with positive sera against infected cells.

Tables VII-IX show the selective scores obtained by applying the two-way interaction analysis to the results in Table VI. The Tables from VII-IX show the selective results through planes at right angles to each other. Table VII presents the selective ADCC results assessing sera versus target cells through the YX plane. Sera C, D, and E show selectively positive cytotoxicity for Raji and Daudi infected with EBV. This is selective ADCC. In the same experiment, selective NCMC is detected in another plane (XZ) testing effector cells versus target cells. Table VIII shows these results with effector 1 reacting selectively against infected cells in the absence of sera and with negative sera. With positive sera C, D, and E, this selective effect for infected cells is lost as other effector cells also express selective ADCC to EBV infected target cells. The selective results from the third plane (YZ) are shown in Table IX testing the relationship be-

TABLE VIII. Two-way Analysis of Results from Effector versus Target (XZ) Plane

Serum	Effector cell	Selective Scores on Target cells			
		Raji	$Raji^{EBV}$	Daudi	$Daudi^{EBV}$
---	1	-0.7	2.8	-6.6	4.5
	2	1.2	-4.3	4.6	-1.5
	3	-0.5	1.5	2.0	-3.0
A (-)[a]	1	-5.4	4.2	-9.4	10.6
	2	6.9	-0.2	3.0	-9.7
	3	-1.5	-4.0	6.4	-0.9
B (-)	1	-7.8	7.2	-13.9	14.5
	2	12.1	-0.6	9.4	-21.0
	3	-4.4	-6.6	4.5	6.5
C (+)	1	4.7	-1.5	-0.7	-2.6
	2	2.8	2.5	0.0	-5.2
	3	-7.5	-0.1	0.7	7.8
D (+)	1	1.0	6.0	-2.1	-5.0
	2	2.5	-2.5	0.3	-0.3
	3	-3.5	-3.6	1.8	5.2
E(+)	1	1.5	0.5	-6.1	4.1
	2	-2.7	6.4	2.0	-5.7
	3	1.2	-6.9	4.1	1.6

[a]*negative and positive membrane fluorescence*

tween effector cells and sera. The results on the infected target cells show that effector 1 which is selectively positive to begin with in negative sera, is not increased to the same extent in the presence of EBV-positive sera as are effectors 2 and 3. Selective ADCC for EBV target antigens is more readily demonstrated with effector cells weaker in selective NCMC.

Selective reactivity from the three-way analysis (Table X) includes a third variable but basically supports the conclusions from the two-way analysis. If all effector cells are equally efficient in ADCC with a positive serum, the results would be nonselective. A positive selective score in this

TABLE IX. Two-way Analysis of results from Effector versus Serum (YZ) Plane

Target	Effector	Selective scores Serum				
		A(-)	B(-)	C(+)	D(+)	E(+)
Raji	1	-2.8	-0.3	1.1	-0.7	2.6
	2	2.5	2.1	1.7	0.4	-6.7
	3	0.3	-1.8	-2.8	0.3	4.1
$Raji^{EBV}$	1	2.3	10.1	-9.5	-0.1	-2.8
	2	-1.4	-7.4	4.6	-1.4	5.6
	3	-0.9	-2.8	5.0	1.5	-2.8
Daudi	1	-1.5	-1.2	0.8	1.5	0.3
	2	0.1	0.9	0.0	-0.4	-0.6
	3	1.4	0.3	-0.8	-1.2	0.2
$Daudi^{EBV}$	1	6.4	15.1	-6.5	-13.4	-1.6
	2	-2.7	-19.6	11.6	9.0	1.7
	3	-3.7	4.5	-5.1	4.4	-0.1

TABLE X. Three-way Analysis of Results varying Effector Cells, Serum and Target Cells

Effector	Serum	Selective scores on target cells			
		Raji	$Raji^{EBV}$	Daudi	$Daudi^{EBV}$
1	A	-2.7	0.8	-3.0	4.9
	B	-6.6	4.3	-7.0	9.3
	C	4.4	-5.9	4.4	-2.9
	D	2.2	3.2	4.8	-10.2
	E	2.7	-2.3	0.8	-1.1
2	A	2.3	-0.8	0.7	-2.1
	B	8.3	-1.4	6.8	-13.7
	C	-2.6	0.0	-4.5	7.1
	D	-1.4	-3.3	-2.3	7.0
	E	-6.6	5.5	-0.7	1.7
3	A	0.4	0.0	2.3	-2.7
	B	-1.7	-2.9	0.2	4.4
	C	-1.7	5.9	0.1	-4.2
	D	-0.8	0.2	-2.5	3.1
	E	3.9	-3.2	-0.1	-0.5

analysis describes an especially strong interaction between the serum and effector cell on a given target cell. Effector cell 1 which is selectively positive to infected cells in the presence of negative serum loses this selectivity in positive serum. On the other hand, effector 2 which was weakest in selective NCMC for EBV antigens shows the greatest increase in selective activity for these antigens (ADCC) in the presence of positive sera. The relationship of antibodies to NCMC can then be perceived and the interaction between NCMC and ADCC is clarified.

In summary the similarities in the mechanisms between NCMC and ADCC are greater than the differences. Treatment of the effector cells or changing of the conditions of the tests influence the results in a parallel manner with the exception of trypsin (protease), protein A and divalent cations. The differential effect of trypsin and protein A is compatible with the model that a single class of Fc receptor bearing effector cells mediates both reactions. In NCMC, IgG antibodies arm the effector cells through Fc-FcR interaction and the multispecificity of natural antibodies gives NCMC its polyspecificity for the detection of antigens on most cultured cells. In ADCC specific antibody is reacted with the target cell before it combines with the effector cell through Fc-FcR contact to initiate the cytotoxic reaction. The study with divalent cations indicates that the mechanisms of NCMC and ADCC are actually more complex than the model and involve a heterogeneous effector cell population. It does appear, however, that at least one major subclass of effector cells is shared while others may vary.

In order to detect specific ADCC to a given antigen on cultured cells, it is necessary to differentiate selective ADCC to target cells carrying this antigen. Since the total reaction also includes an NCMC component by the effector cell, ADCC must also be distinguished from NCMC. A three-dimensional test design varying sera, target cells, and effector cells was employed to test ADCC and NCMC concurrently and to visualize the relationship between them. Application of the two-way interaction analysis to different planes and the three-way analysis to the complete results allowed identification of selective ADCC, NCMC and the interrelationships between the two related reactions. Three-dimensional testing and the interaction analysis were quite useful for distinguishing the different effects. This permitted recognition of individual reactions and relationships which are normally obscured in the total cytotoxic effect.

REFERENCES

1. Takasugi, M., Mickey, M. R., and Terasaki, P. I., *Cancer Res. 33,* 2898 (1973).
2. Kay, D. H., and Sinkovics, J. G., *Lancet 2,* 296 (1974).
3. Oldham, R. K., Siwarski, D., McCoy, J. L., Plata, E. J., and Herberman, R. B., *Natl. Cancer Inst. Monogr. 37,* 49 (1973).
4. Moller, E., *Science 147,* 873 (1965).
5. Perlman, P., and Holm, G., *Adv. Immunol. 11,* 117 (1969).
6. Maclennan, I. C. M., and Loewi, G., *Nature (Lond.) 219,* 1069 (1968).
7. Kiuchi, M., and Takasugi, M., *J. Natl. Cancer Inst. 54,* 575 (1976).
8. West, W. H., Cannon, G. B., Kay, H. D., and Herberman, R. B., *J. Immunol. 118,* 355 (1977).
9. Bolhuis, R. L. H., Schuit, H. R. E., Nooyen, A. M. and Ronteltap, C. P. M., *Eur. J. Immunol. 8,* 731 (1978).
10. Koren, H. S., Amos, D. B., and Buckley, R. H., *J. Immunol. 120,* 796 (1978).
11. Koide, Y., and Takasugi, M., *J. Natl. Cancer Inst. 59,* 1099 (1977).
12. Akira, D., and Takasugi, M., *Int. J. Cancer 19,* 747 (1977).
13. deLandazuri, M. O., Silva, A., Alvarez, J., and Herberman, R. B., *J. Immunol. 123,* 252 (1979).
14. Pernis, B., Forni, L., and Amante, L., *J. Exp. Med. 132,* 1001 (1970).
15. Golstein, P., Wigzell, H., and Blomgren, H., *J. Exp. Med. 132,* 890 (1972).
16. Chess, L., Levine, H., MacDermott, R. P., and Schlossman, S. F., *J. Immunol. 115,* 1483 (1975).
17. Lobo, P. I., and Horwitz, D. A., *J. Immunol. 117,* 939 (1976).
18. Pape, R. R., Troye, M., Axelsson, B., and Perlman, P., *J. Immunol. 122,* 2251 (1979).
19. Jondal, M., and Pross, H., *Int. J. Cancer 15,* 596 (1975).
20. Pross, H., Baines, M. G., and Jondal, M., *Int. J. Cancer 20,* 253 (1977).
21. O'Toole, C., Stejskal, V., and Perlman, P., *J. Exp. Med. 139,* 457 (1974).
22. Hersey, P., Edwards, A., Edwards, J., Adams, E., Milton, G. W., and Nelson, D. S., *Int. J. Cancer 16,* 173 (1975).
23. Peter, H. H., Pavie Fisher, J., and Fridman, W. H., *J. Immunol. 115,* 539 (1975).
24. West, W. H., Boozer, R. B., and Herberman, R. B., *J. Immunol. 120,* 90 (1978).
25. Potter, M. R., and Moore, M., *Immunology 37,* 187 (1979).

26. Bakacs, T., Gergely, P., Cornain, S., and Klein, E., *Int. J. Cancer 19*, 441 (1977).
27. Pross, H., and Jondal, M., *Clin. Exp. Immunol. 21*, 226 (1975).
28. Kay, D. H., Bonnard, G. D., West, W. H., and Herberman, R. B., *J. Immunol. 118*, 2058 (1977).
29. Pape, G. R., Troye, M., and Perlman, P., *J. Immunol. 118*, 1925 (1977).
30. Gupta, S., Fernandes, G., Nair, M., and Good, R. A., *Proc. Natl. Acad. Sci. 75*, 5137 (1978).
31. Kall, M. A., and Koren, H. S., *Cell. Immunol. 40*, 58 (1978).
32. Ozer, H., Strelkauskas, A. J., Callery, R. T. and Schlossman, S. F., *Cell. Immunol. 45*, 334 (1979).
33. Parillo, J. E., and Fauci, A. S., *Scand. J. Immunol. 8*, 99 (1978).
34. Strom, T. B., Garavoy, M. R., Bear, R. A., Gribik, M., and Carpenter, C. B., *Cell. Immunol. 20*, 247 (1975).
35. Trinchieri, G., Santoli, D., and Koprowski, H., *J. Immunol. 120*, 1849 (1978).
36. Loar, F., Forni, L., and Pernis, B., *Eur. J. Immunol. 2*, 203 (1972).
37. Roder, J. C., Kiessling, R., Biberfield, P., and Anderson, B., *J. Immunol. 121*, 1849 (1978).
38. Unanue, E. R., Karnovsky, M. J., and Engers, H. D., *J. Exp. Med. 137*, 675 (1973).
39. Takasugi, J. E., Koide, Y., and Takasugi, M., *Eur. J. Immunol. 7*, 887 (1977).
40. Kumagai, K., Abo, T., Sekizawa, T., and Sasaki, M., *J. Immunol. 115*, 982 (1975).
41. Warr, G. W., Lee, J. C., and Marchalonis, J. J., *J. Immunol. 121*, 1767 (1978).
42. Trejdosiewicz, L. K., Trejdosiewicz, A. K., and Dykes, P. W., *Cell. Immunol. 45*, 49 (1979).
43. Kall, M. A., and Koren, H. S., *Cell. Immunol. 47*, 57 (1979).
44. Prather, S. O., Geller, R. W., and Lausch, R. N., *J. Natl. Cancer Inst. 62*, 1273 (1979).
45. Kay, H. D., Bonnard, G. D., and Herberman, R. B., *J. Immunol. 122*, 675 (1979).
46. Perussia, B., Trinchieri, G., and Cerottini, J. C., *J. Immunol. 123*, 681 (1979).
47. Troye, M., Perlman, P., Pape, G. R., Spiegelberg, H. L., Naslund, I., and Gidlof, A., *J. Immunol. 119*, 1061 (1977).

DIFFERENTIAL EFFECTS OF IMMUNE COMPLEXES ON HUMAN NATURAL AND ANTIBODY-DEPENDENT CELL-MEDIATED CYTOTOXICITY

H. David Kay[1]

Laboratory of Immunodiagnosis
National Cancer Institute
National Institutes of Health
Bethesda, Maryland

I. INTRODUCTION

During the past decade, significant advances have been made in our understanding of the importance of an originally "unwanted" *in vitro* phenomenon called "natural" or "spontaneous" cell-mediated cytotoxicity. First reported during the years when "histologic specificity" was being demonstrated in microcytotoxicity assays against cultured tumor cell lines by blood lymphocytes from cancer patients, it soon became apparent that unwanted, high "background" killing of tumor cells by lymphocytes from normal, healthy donors was frequently encountered and had to be investigated more rigorously as a phenomenon in itself. Information derived from a number of studies in mouse as well as in man has since suggested that, contrary to prevailing dogma, natural cytotoxicity (NC) might, in fact, be a critically important cellular defense mechanism against developing neoplastic disease *in vivo* (Kay *et al.*, 1976; Kiessling and Haller, 1977; Pross and Baines, 1977; Herberman and Holden, 1978; Hersey, 1979).

Although early studies emphasized characterization of the effector cells active in NC (Jondal and Pross, 1975; Herberman *et al.*, 1975; Kiessling *et al.*, 1975; West *et al.*, 1977), considerable interest has now been focused on relating NC to

[1]*Present address: Department of Medicine, Division of Rheumatology, University of Virginia School of Medicine, Charlottesville, Virginia 22908*

ISBN 0-12-341350-8

another cytotoxic phenomenon which had been described several years earlier, namely, antibody-dependent cell-mediated cytotoxicity (ADCC), mediated by a subset of peripheral blood lymphocytes called "killer lymphocytes", or K cells (MacLennan, 1972; Perlmann *et al.*, 1972). Since the cytotoxic capacity of K cells was not expressed in the absence of a "coating" of IgG antibody on the surface of an appropriate target cell line; or, since ADCC could be abrogated either by including extraneous immune complexes in the reaction, or by stripping away Fc receptors (FcR) from the surface of effector cells by modulation procedures, it became obvious that FcR for IgG were a necessary means by which these K cells initiated cytolytic reactions against antibody-coated ("sensitized") target cells.

It proved intriguing, therefore, to find that, in experiments in which K cells were removed from effector cell suspensions by adsorption to column- or plastic-immobilized immune complexes containing IgG antibody, both ADCC reactivity, as well as the majority of the natural killer (NK) activity, was removed. Subsequently, it has become clear that FcR expression is not only a hallmark of the K cell, but is equally a characteristic of freshly isolated NK cells, from man (West *et al.*, 1977; Hersey *et al.*, 1975; Peter *et al.*, 1975; Kiuchi and Takasugi, 1976), mouse (Herberman *et al.*, 1977), rat (Oehler *et al.*, 1978), and guinea pig (Arnaud-Battandier *et al.*, 1978).

It has now been shown in several studies that NK and K cells have similar surface markers (Herberman and Holden, 1978; Kiuchi and Takasugi, 1976; Kay *et al.*, 1977; Nelson *et al.*, 1977; Bolhuis *et al.*, 1978), that they migrate together in various procedures designed to separate human blood mononuclear cells (Kay *et al.*, 1977; Nelson *et al.*, 1977; Bolhuis *et al.*, 1978; Parrillo and Fauci, 1978), and that they both appear to derive from the same (or similar) precursors in culture (Ortaldo *et al.*, 1980). It therefore seemed important to determine if, in fact, ADCC and NC were different cytotoxic expression of the same cell (Kay *et al.*, 1977; Ojo and Wigzell, 1978; deLandazuri *et al.*, 1979). Accordingly, during the past several years, we have been simultaneously monitoring human NC on the erythroleukemia cell line K562, and ADCC on antibody-sensitized human Chang liver cells, in a 4-hr ^{51}chromium release assay (CRA). Investigation of NC and ADCC in parallel assays had thus provided us a straightforward means to determine whether various treatments and modifications of effector cells have similar or dissimilar effects on NK and K cell activities. Further, since NC and ADCC are found in the same subpopulations of lymphocytes which bear Fc receptors for IgG, we also investigated whether NC might be a form of ADCC; i.e., were the FcR on the NK cell required for its cytolytic activity?

II. METHODS AND MATERIALS

The methods described below are necessarily brief. For more details, the reader is referred to the original papers cited.

A. *Effector Lymphocytes*

Mononuclear leukocytes were isolated from heparinized peripheral blood of normal laboratory donors, on Ficoll-Hypaque (F/H) gradients, and depleted of adherent cells by incubation on plastic surfaces (West *et al.*, 1977; Kay *et al.*, 1977). Although low levels of NC and ADCC by monocytes is now being reported (Shore *et al.*, 1977; Shaw *et al.*, 1978; Barada and Horwitz, 1978; Horwitz *et al.*, 1979), it was not investigated in the studies being reported here.

B. *Target Cells*

As indicator target cells for the determination of NC activity, cultured cells from the erythroleukemia cell line K562 (Lozzio and Lozzio, 1975) were used in a 4-hr ^{51}chromium release assay (Jondal and Pross, 1975; West *et al.*, 1977). Being one of the most sensitive cell lines for the determination of human NC, K562 cells were maintained in stationary suspension culture in RPMI 1640 tissue culture medium containing 10% fetal calf serum (FCS), as previously described (West *et al.*, 1977; Kay *et al.*, 1977). As to its histology, K562 cells are clearly erythroid in derivation, since they express an exclusively erythroid enzyme, glycophorin, in their membrane (Andersson *et al.*, 1979a), fail to react with antimyeloid antisera (Roberts and Greaves, 1978), and can, upon stimulation *in vitro* with appropriate concentrations of sodium butyrate, synthesize hemoglobin and produce erythrocyte-like particles (Andersson *et al.*, 1979b).

ADCC activity was simultaneously monitored in parallel assays using, as targets, antibody-sensitized human Chang liver cells. Maintained in culture as an adherent cell line, Chang cells were not significantly lysed by effector lymphocytes in the absence of sensitizing antibody, and have therefore proved to be useful targets for ADCC unencumbered by a simultaneously high component of natural cytotoxicity. Procedures for sensitization of Chang cells with rabbit antiserum, and for the ^{51}chromium labeling of target cells, were as previously described (Kay *et al.*, 1979a). In some experiments, Chang cells were also sensitized with potent, human anti-HLA antisera obtained from patients who had been frequently transfused (Kay *et al.*, 1979a).

C. *Cytotoxicity Assay*

The ^{51}chromium release assay (CRA) was performed as previously described (Kay *et al.*, 1979a), except that, in some experiments, the CRA was modified for performance in wells of microtiter plates (Kay *et al.*, 1979b). In most studies, effectors were mixed with radiolabeled targets at multiple effector to target (E/T) ratios, and incubated for 4-6 hr at 37°C. Suspensions were then centrifuged, and the supernatants were collected and counted in a gamma spectrometer. All experiments included media controls and "autologous" (cold target) controls, to measure minimum (background) release. Also included were a set of maximum release controls, in which radiolabeled target cells were incubated in wells containing distilled water mixed with Tween 80 detergent.

D. *Lytic Units*

The percentage of specific ^{51}chromium release was calculated as [(A - B / C) x 100], where A = mean counts per minute (cpm) released in test combinations, B = mean cpm of "autologous" controls, and C = mean cpm of maximum release. When the percentage of chromium release was plotted versus the log of the various E/T ratios, cytotoxicity curves were generated from which could be extrapolated the number of effector lymphocytes required to release 30% of the ^{51}chromium incorporated into the target cells. This number of effector cells represented one lytic unit (LU) in that experiment (Kay *et al.*, 1977, 1979a).

III. RESULTS AND DISCUSSION

A. *Procedures Which Had Similar Effects on NK and K Cell Cytotoxicity*

1. Removal of adherent monocytes from effector cell suspensions. Among the early results of our experiments comparing NC and ADCC was the demonstration that neither function required accessory cell help by adherent monocytes (West *et al.*, 1977; Kay *et al.*, 1977). Removal of monocytes by a variety of procedures, which included adsorption on plastic, adsorption on nylon wool, or treatment with carbonyl iron + magnet, had little or no effect on levels of NC and ADCC by the remaining lymphocytes, and, sometimes, even augmented both activities slightly.

2. Depletion of cells bearing Fc receptors (FcR). The presence of FcR on freshly isolated NK cells was confirmed in a number of experiments by several different procedures, as described below. In one series of studies, when lymphocytes, depleted of adherent monocytes, were incubated on "monolayers" of plastic immobilized antigen-antibody complexes (Kay *et al.*, 1977), effector cells exhibiting NK and K cell activity were simultaneously adsorbed onto the monolayers; i.e., very little of either activity was expressed by the nonadherent cells recovered from the complexes (Table I). When, however, just prior to adding lymphocytes, the monolayers of immobilized complexes were coated with Staphylococcal protein A (SpA), which binds the Fc portion of IgG, the complexes could no longer bind the effector cell suspensions, and all of the original NK and K cell activity was recovered in the nonadherent cell suspensions (Kay *et al.* 1977). Further, as shown by Ortaldo *et al.* (1979), when effector cell suspensions which had been depleted of cells bearing FcR (by the adsorption procedures just described) were placed in culture for up to seven days in medium containing FCS, expression of NC and ADCC activities by the cultured cells reappeared simultaneously, and was correlated with the reexpression of FcR on the surface of the cultured cells.

In another series of experiments, when large, insoluble antigen-antibody complexes, such as IgG-sensitized chicken or bovine erythrocytes (cEA or bEA, respectively), were added to the cytotoxicity assays, both NK and K cell functions were simultaneously and equally inhibited, in direct proportion to the amount of inhibiting complexes added (West *et al.*, 1977; Kay *et al.*, 1977, 1979b). Maximum inhibition occurred at the highest inhibitor to effector ratio of 200 EA per effector lymphocyte (Kay *et al.*, 1979b). Thus, the points clearly emphasized by these types of experiments were 1) both freshly isolated NK and K cells bear easily detectable FcR on their cell membranes; and 2) NK and K cells cannot be distinguished using the adsorption or blocking experiments just described.

B. Procedures With Dissimilar Effects on NK and K Cells

Clear distinction could be made, however, between the effector mechanisms of NK and K cells when several other techniques were used. For example, one or the other, but not both, of the effector mechanisms was abrogated when 1) small,

TABLE I. Both NC and ADCC Activities Were Simultaneously Adsorbed on Plastic Immobilized Monolayers of Antigen-Antibody Complexes[a]

Effector cell adsorptions[b]	*Number of LU/10^7 effector cells*	
	NC	*ADCC*
Control, not adsorbed	*190*	*250*
Adsorbed on:		
- plastic only	*185*	*240*
- immobilized immune complexes	*14*	*21*
- immobilized complexes coated with SpA[c]	*177*	*220*
- plastic only, coated with SpA	*202*	*264*

[a]*For details, see Kay* et al. *(1977)*

[b]*Suspensions of effector cells were incubated for 45 min on plastic surfaces which had been coated as indicated, and the nonadherent cells recovered from the surfaces were tested at multiple E/T ratios for NC and ADCC activity*

[c]*Staphylococcal protein A (SpA) was incubated at a concentration of 35μg/ml on the immobilized immune complexes*

soluble immune complexes were included in the cytotoxicity reactions; 2) effector cells were exposed to various enzymes; 3) SpA was included in the assays; or 4) FcR were modulated from the effector cell surfaces by overnight incubation with either soluble or insoluble complexes. Such "one-sided" effects may be relevant to *in vivo* functions, as will be discussed later.

1. Exposure of NK and K cells to soluble complexes. It was quite probable that, in the experiments described above, simultaneous inhibition of both NK and K cell functions by the macroscopic bEA or cEA complexes was due to stearic hindrance. Once the effector cells had bound EA to their FcR, they were unable to physically contact the surface membrane of the target cells. To avoid this problem, and to determine if NC, like ADCC, required free FcR for cytotoxicity, effector cells were preincubated for 40 min at 37°C with small, soluble TNP-antiTNP complexes (see legend, Figure 1), washed three times, and then tested for NC and ADCC. As shown in Figure 1, ADCC

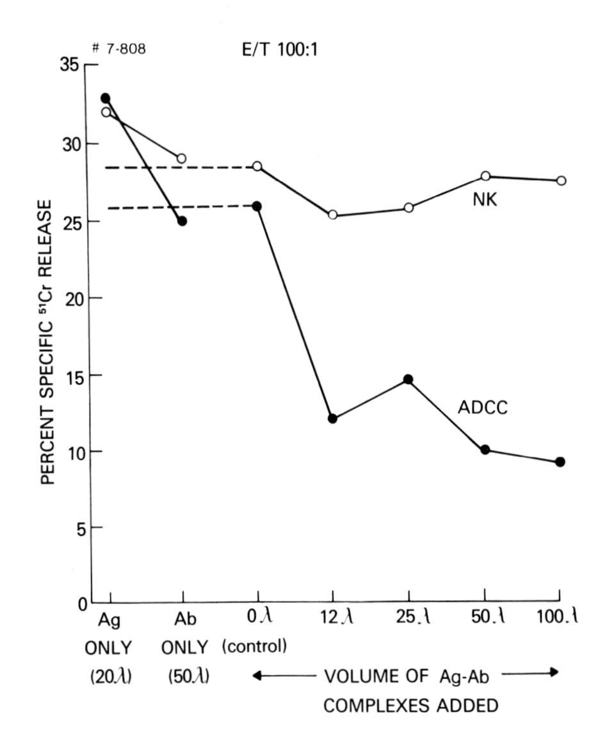

FIGURE 1. Lymphocytes were pretreated with increasing concentrations of TNP-rabbit antiTNP complexes for 40 min, 37°C; then washed 3X in medium before the CRA. NC (O-O), ADCC (●-●). Complexes were prepared as follows: 100 µl rabbit antiTNP, 1 mg/ml affinity purified; mixed with 40 µl TNP-BSA antigen, 0.6 mg/ml; and 60 µl PBS. After incubation at 37°C for 30 min, complexes were centrifuged before use to remove any gross aggregates.

activity, but not NC, was inhibited by pretreatment with soluble complexes. That the complexes had bound to the cells was confirmed by indirect immunofluorescence, and by failure of treated cells (but not of untreated controls) to form rosettes with bEA cells, as described in detail elsewhere (Kay *et al.*, 1979b). When soluble complexes were included in the assay, results were similar: ADCC was always significantly inhibited, while NC was only slightly, or not at all, depressed. Although this data confirms the requirement for free FcR by K cells, and does serve to distinguish an ADCC from an NC reaction, it does not completely address the role of FcR in NC, since any "arming antibodies", bound to the FcR *in vivo*, would not be blocked by this procedure.

2. Exposure to enzymes, and the concept of "arming" antibodies. While it is clear that FcR for IgG are quite resistant to the proteolytic effects of trypsin, evidence also suggests that the cytolytic mechanisms of NC and ADCC can be distinguished by exposure to this, and other, proteolytic enzymes (Kiuchi and Takasugi, 1976; Kay *et al.*, 1977; Nelson *et al.*, 1977; Perussia *et al.*, 1979). As shown in Table II, exposure of effector lymphocytes to mild proteolysis had little or no effect on ADCC (and, at times, even enhanced it), while, at the same time, such treatment completely and reproducibly abrogated NK cell activity. While the slight increase in ADCC following exposure to dilute proteases may reflect either a "clean up" of blocked FcR, or, perhaps, the uncovering of new FcR in the membrane, the abrogation of NC by all of the proteases is consistent with either of three quite different possibilities: either 1) the proteases are sufficiently damaging to the cells that they are turning off the metabolic activity (and thereby the cytolytic activity) of the effector cells (or, perhaps, even killing the cells); 2) NC is mediated by a unique trypsin-sensitive receptor, distinct from FcR, which expresses a considerable amount of target cell speci-

TABLE II. Effect of Various Enzymatic Digestions on NC and ADCC Activity By Effector Lymphocytes From Normal Human Blood

Enzyme	*Concentration*	*Percent ^{51}Cr release[a] in:*	
		NC	*ADCC*
None (control)	*medium only*	55	61
Trypsin	*>0.01 mg/ml*	*<15*	*>65*
α-chymotrypsin	*>0.01 mg/ml*	*<15*	*>70*
Pronase	*0.01 - 0.1 mg/ml*	*<28*	*>63*
"	*>1 mg/ml*	*<5*	*<25*
Subtilisin	*0.01 - 0.1 mg/ml*	*<39*	*>62*
"	*>1 mg/ml*	*<7*	*<19*

[a]*Effector lymphocyte suspensions were incubated with the various enzymes at the indicated concentrations for 30 min, at 37°C, washed 2X in RPMI 1640 + 30% FCS, and then tested at an E/T ratio of 50:1 (see Kay* et al., *1977)*

ficity; or else 3) NC may be mediated via trypsin-sensitive "cytophilic" or "arming" antibodies which are bound *in vivo* to the FcR of the NK cell (and thereby confer on the NK cell its *in vitro* specificities, thus making it a modified form of ADCC). With regard to the first point, K cells, active in ADCC and exposed to the same enzyme concentrations, are not at all inhibited (and are sometimes enhanced) by exposure to the proteases, so a generalized metabolic inhibition (or killing) by the enzymes is highly unlikely. Some investigators might argue that the loss of NC after exposure to proteases is evidence that NK cells are selectively lysed by the proteases, and are therefore separate from the K cell subset which remains intact. The fact that normal levels of NC are regenerated in protease-treated cultures after incubation at 37°C for from 24-72 hr (Kay *et al.*, 1977, 1979a; Nelson *et al.*, 1977; Perussia *et al.*, 1979) suggests that NK cells have not been selectively depleted by the proteases, but, rather, have only been temporarily modified by the enzymatic treatment.

Unfortunately, the second concept (that of a unique, trypsin-sensitive NK receptor, distinct from FcR), while being entirely consistent with this, and other, data, is also the most difficult to analyze. Data to be presented later will serve to strengthen this concept.

In support of the third potential interpretation of the enzyme data, Takasugi and colleagues reported that NC function, abrogated by exposure to trypsin, was frequently restored by incubation in either normal human sera, or in immune sera containing antibodies specific for the HLA antigens on the target cells (Takasugi *et al.*, 1977; Akira and Takasugi, 1977). Arguing against the concept that NK cells are armed *in vivo*, however, are recent data from our laboratory (Kay *et al.*, 1979a,b), as well as from Perlmann's (Troye *et al.*, 1977; Pape *et al.*, 1979), demonstrating that antibodies directed against human IgG (assuming that the "arming" antibodies are of the IgG type) did not inhibit NC when preincubated with the NK cells and washed out before the CRA. Further, preincubation of K562 target cells with any of a large group of sera from normal donors, all of whom had high levels of NC, failed to elevate NC compared to controls, and thereby failed to demonstrate the presence in these sera of enough arming antibodies with binding specificities for the target cells to generate an ADCC reaction (Kay *et al.*, 1979a).

On the other hand, Pape *et al.* (1979a) have reported that Fab and $F(ab')_2$ fragments of antihuman IgG antibodies, when incubated in the CRA with effectors and targets, partially inhibited NK cell activity, probably by binding to anti-target cell antibodies secreted during the incubation period of the assay. Since this partial inhibition was observed against only certain target cells, it was concluded that NC might be of two types: one being IgG-dependent, and the other being an IgG-independent mechanism (Pape *et al.*, 1979a). A major argument against this latter concept, however, still derives from the experiments with trypsin, i.e., if trypsin has little or no effect on FcR, and does not significantly alter a cell's metabolic machinery, why should NC -- being theoretically dependent on secretion of antibody -- be so easily abrogated by exposure to dilute proteases?

Were anti-target cell antibodies to be secreted during NC reactions, it should be possible to detect, or at least to block, such antibodies by appropriate procedures. In one such procedure, we included Staphylococcal protein A in the CRA.

3. Treatment of effector cells with Staphylococcal protein A (SpA). If antibodies with target specificity were either carried into the assay as arming antibodies on freshly isolated cells, or secreted during the incubation period of the CRA, two circumstances might be predicted. First, it might be expected that recovery of NC in culture by trypsinized lymphocytes could be prevented, or at least reduced, by exclusion of all antibody-producing SIg+ or C3R+ cells from the cell suspensions being cultured. In no experiment was such an inhibitory effect observed. NC recovered at about the same rate, whether or not B cells were present in the cultured effector cell suspensions (Ortaldo *et al.*, 1979).

Second, unless secreted antibody is attached directly to the appropriate target cell surface during intimate cell-cell contact, or is exclusively of an IgG3 subclass [shown by Troye *et al.* (1977) not to be the case], inclusion of SpA in the culture media would be expected to inhibit, not enhance, NC reactions which were dependent on such IgG. When included in the 4-hr CRA, SpA inhibited, in a dose-dependent manner, ADCC against the long-term, tissue-culture maintained Chang cell line sensitized with either rabbit or human antibodies (Kay *et al.*, 1979a), but it did not inhibit, and sometimes even enhanced, NC reactions which were simultaneously tested in parallel assays. This is in agreement with the studies of Pape *et al.* (1979a) who also reported that SpA was unable, at any concentration used, to inhibit NC against any of a variety of target cells.

Such data, taken together, would seem to argue against secretion of target-antigen-specific IgG antibody as a generalized mechanism for NC, particularly in view of what is known about the extremely small number of cells in any given lymphocyte suspension which can be expected to spontaneously secrete antibodies with specificity for a randomly chosen antigen (such as the NC target cell antigen). Furthermore, arguments that the presence of SpA in the culture medium actually induced IgG antibody secretion, thereby setting up an ADCC mechanism via an IgG-FcR bridge witn an effector cell, must take into account recent reports from one laboratory which indicate that soluble SpA, as a polyclonal B cell activator, induced synthesis of only IgM antibodies, not IgG, and that such induction was only seen with spleen cells, and not peripheral blood lymphocytes (Moller and Landwall, 1977; Ringden *et al.*, 1977).

After all is said and done, it remains remotely possible that human IgG, secreted by some cell in the effector cell suspension, and by chance having an anti-target cell specificity, is aggregated by the Spa in the culture medium. In its aggregated form, it can now efficiently bind to the FcR of the effector cells, thereby "arming" it with at least a few anti-target cell antibodies. By such a mechanism, SpA could conceivably promote, rather than hinder, NC reactions. While Sulica *et al.* (1976) have reported that, in an animal model system, high titered rabbit IgG was aggregated with SpA and used to arm nonimmune murine spleen cells with target-specific antibodies, we have as yet been unable to confirm this in an "all human" system. It is therefore possible that Pape's demonstration of partial inhibition of NC with Fab or $F(ab')_2$ fragments of anti-human IgG reflected not so much an interaction with secreted antibodies, as an interaction with a unique NK receptor, as mentioned earlier, distinct from FcR, and having something in its trypsin-sensitive structure which partially resembles a human immunoglobulin molecule.

4. Effect of various antilymphocyte antisera on NC and ADCC. Consistent with our concept that there might be a unique NK receptor on the surface of the NK cell are the results of a series of experiments in which effector cell suspensions were pretreated with various dilutions of antibodies with anti-lymphocyte specificities. In agreement with our earlier experiments using dilute proteolytic enzymes, or various concentrations of SpA, we observed that ADCC, but not NC, was strongly inhibited by exposure to these antisera (Table III). Particularly useful in these studies has been a human serum with potent anti-HLA activity derived from a patient (Io) who had been frequently transfused during treatments for Waldenstrom's macroglobulinemia (Kay *et al.*, 1979a). At serum dilutions ranging from 10^{-1} to 10^{-5}, ADCC, but not NC, was inhibited in direct proportion to the concentration of serum used to treat the effector cells (Figure 2; also, Kay *et al.*, 1979a). Similar in its effects was the rabbit anti-Chang cell antiserum. Inhibition of ADCC implied that these antibodies were binding to, or near, the FcR, on the effector cells. If sensitization, or cross-linking of lymphocytes into aggregates were the cause of the observed inhibition of ADCC (in a manner similar to cold-target inhibition), it is difficult to understand why NC

Table III. Relative Effect on NC and ADCC of Pretreatment[a] of Effector Cells With Various Antisera

Source	*Antiserum*	*Dilution*	*Number of LU/10[7] effector cells*	
			NC	*ADCC*
Control	*FCS control*	*1:10*	*120*	*160*
Rabbit	*Anti-Chang cells*	*1:50,000*	*130*	*<10*
Human	*Anti-HLA-(Io)*	*1:100*	*135*	*<10*
Human	*Anti-HLA-(Rp)*	*1:100*	*125*	*<10*
Horse	*Anti-lymphocyte*	*1:100*	*120*	*<10*

[a]*Effector cells were incubated 45 min at 37°C with indicated serum, washed 3X in medium, and tested in simultaneous assays for NC and ADCC at multiple E/T ratios.*

was not also efficiently inhibited, as when macroscopic complexes of EA were added to the CRA. Rather, it seemed that either 1) free FcR on the effector cells were being "masked" or physically perturbed by these antibodies, such that effective killer function was impaired, or 2) these antisera were not directly affecting FcR at all, but rather were combining with labile membrane antigens, causing membrane shedding of soluble antigen-antibody complexes which, in turn, were bound by FcR of neighboring cells, causing complete abrogation of ADCC function.

To confirm that these antisera caused blockage of FcR, and not their modulation from the cells, lymphocytes were coated with various dilutions of Io-anti-HLA serum, and then either tested for cytotoxic capacity directly, or tested after first being adsorbed onto plastic immobilized immune complexes (as described in Table I). We reasoned that, should FcR be blocked or modified by the antiserum (or complexes), the cells would not be able to adhere to the plate of immobilized complexes via their FcR. Natural killer activity (unaffected by the Io serum) should be detected in the recovered, nonadsorbed cells, in direct proportion to the concentration of serum used to treat the cells. This was confirmed, as shown in Figure 3. Of course, ADCC activity, blocked by the Io serum treatment, could not be detected in the recovered cell suspension. When Io serum-treated cells were subsequently exposed to trypsin, NK activity was, as expected, completely abrogated, but ADCC activity was partially restored, being consistent with the con-

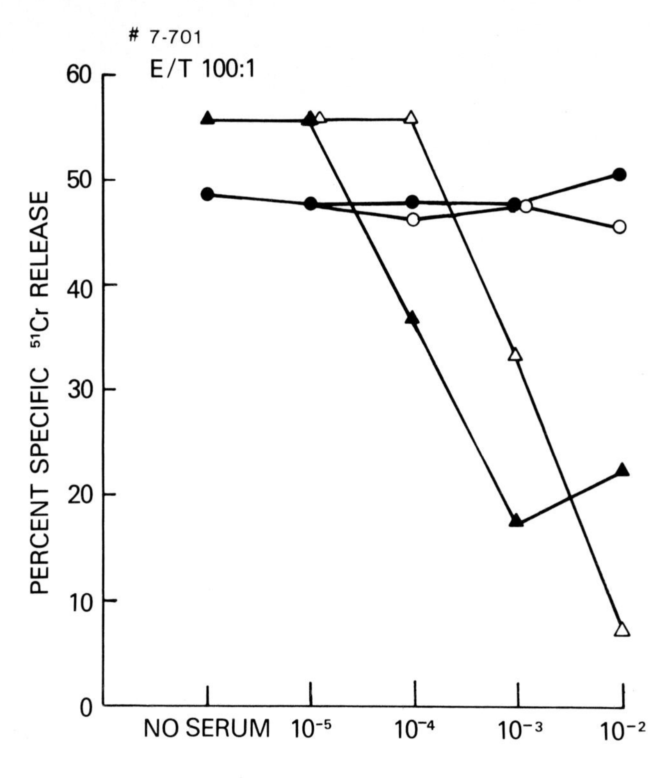

Figure 2. Cytolytic activity of effector cells after pretreatment with various dilutions of rabbit anti-Chang cell serum (NC,●—●; ADCC, ▲) or human anti-HLA-(Io) serum (NC,○—○; ADCC, △). E/T ratio was 100:1.

cept that trypsin had cleared some of the blocking antibodies or complexes from the FcR, making them available again for ADCC. Whatever the mechanism of action of these antisera, it remained clear that NC was not inhibited by blockade, or perturbation, of FcR. Since the question of FcR modulation had been raised by these experiments, we proceeded to investigate such a phenomenon directly.

5. *Modulation of Fc receptors.* In several recent reports it had been demonstrated that FcR could be modulated (induced to "shed") from effector cells by overnight incubation of cell suspensions with antigen-antibody complexes (Ziegler and Henney, 1977; Cordier *et al.*, 1977; Moretta *et al., 1978;* Bolhuis *et al.*, 1978). Modulation of FcR was confirmed by simultaneously monitoring treated cells for 1) ADCC function, and

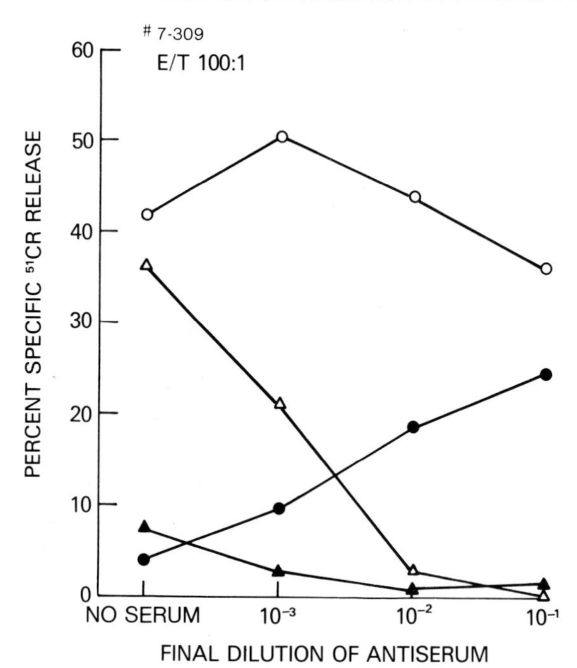

Figure 3. ADCC (○—○), but not NC (△—△), was inhibited by pretreatment of effector cells with increasing concentrations of human anti-HLA-(Io) serum. After exposure to the serum, cells were incubated on TNP-antiTNP monolayers (Kay et al., *1977) and recovered nonadherent cells were tested for cytotoxic activity. As shown, binding of NK cells (●—●) to antigen-antibody monolayers was inhibited by increasing the concentration of anti-HLA serum used to pretreat the cells.*

for 2)EA rosette formation. As shown in Figure 4 for a representative experiment, modulation of FcR completely abrogated ADCC activity, but, at the same time, only partially inhibited NC reactivity (approximate 40-70% reduction in activity, as determined by lytic units). That the reduction in ADCC was not due merely to blocking of the FcR by residual immune complexes was determined by exposing modulated cells to trypsin for 30 min at 37°C. Such treatment did not restore, or even partially raise, ADCC activity of modulated cells, but did restore rosette-forming capacity to non-modulated lymphocytes which had been previously reacted with immune complexes (Kay *et al.*, 1979b). Interestingly, the partial loss of NC which occurred after the modulation procedure could not be further reduced by adding additional immune complexes to the NC assay, nor could it be further depleted by adsorbing the modulated cells on plastic-immobilized complexes (Kay *et al.*, 1979b).

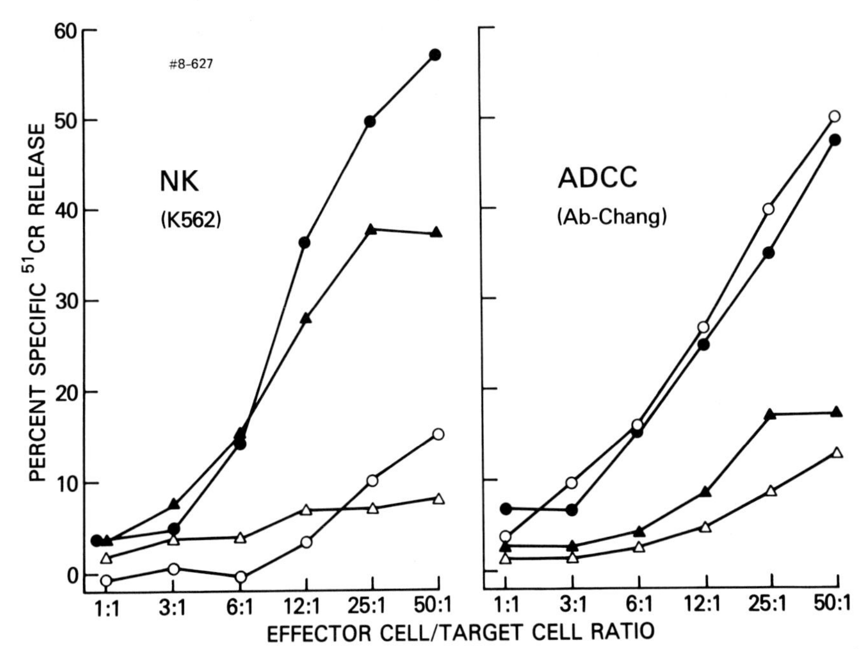

Figure 4. The effect on NC and ADCC cytolytic reactivities of incubating effector cells (2 x 10^6/ml) for 18 hr prior to the CRA with culture medium (●—●) or 7S-cEA immune complexes (▲). There were 10 erythrocytes per lymphocyte during the modulation procedure. Exposure to trypsin (0.125%) before (○—○), or after (△) modulation abrogated NC, and failed to restore ADCC activity to modulated cells.

As noted in Figure 4, exposure of modulated cells to trypsin (0.125%) failed to restore ADCC activity, thus demonstrating that the FcR had indeed been shed, and were not merely plugged with complexes. The strong natural cytotoxic reactivity which remained in the effector cell suspensions following modulation was, therefore, clearly independent of FcR, and therefore, also of IgG antibody. These results have been confirmed by the recent report of Pape *et al.* (1979b), who also reported that modulation of FcR from suspensions of effector T cells resulted in complete loss of ADCC function, but only partial loss of NC activity against K562.

IV. CONCLUSIONS

While both NC and ADCC functions reside in the same subpopulation of peripheral blood lymphocytes which bear FcR, it is not yet clear whether these functions represent distinct cellular subsets, or are the dual expression of a single cell type. It seems certain from the data discussed above that NC, as a cytotoxic phenomenon, is functionally distinct from ADCC, in that it does not require free FcR for its *in vitro* expression, and can, in fact, be expressed by cells which have shed all detectable FcR. Thus, our data are entirely consistent with the hypothesis that NC is mediated through a unique, and as yet undefined, "NK-receptor", which may have a trypsin-sensitive structure somewhat related to an IgG molecule.

It is interesting to speculate as to an *in vivo* function for this *in vitro* phenomenon. The presence of NK cell activity which can't be abrogated by FcR modulation, and which is independent of potential inhibition with soluble immune complexes, may help to provide a basis for an *in vivo* mechanism of immune surveillance against tumor growth in man that is not easily inhibited by circulating tumor-antigen-antibody complexes. While such a hypothesis remains speculative at this point, the data discussed above provide a basis for understanding the nature of the receptors involved in the cytolytic mechanisms of the NK and K cell(s).

ACKNOWLEDGMENTS

I want to express my sincere appreciation to Dr. Ronald Herberman for the opportunity to pursue, in his laboratory, the studies reported here.

REFERENCES

Akira, D., and Takasugi, M., *Int. J. Cancer 19:* 747 (1977).

Andersson, L.C., Nilsson, K., and Gahmberg, C.G., *Int. J. Cancer 23:* 143 (1979a).

Andersson, L.C., Jokinen, M., and Gahmberg., C.G., *Nature 278:*364 (1979b).

Arnaud-Battandier, F., Bundy, B.M., and Nelson, D.L., *Eur. J. Immunol. 8:* 400 (1978).

Barada, F.A., and Horwitz, D.A., *Arthritis Rheum. 21:* 543 (1978).

Bolhuis, R.L.H., Schuit, H.R.E., Nooyen, A.M., and Ronteltap, C.P.M., *Eur. J. Immunol. 8:*731 (1978).

Cordier, G., Samarut, C., and Revillard, J.-P., *J. Immunol. 119:* 1943 (1977).

deLandazuri, M.O., Silva, A., Alvarez, J., and Herberman, R.B., *J. Immunol. 123:*252 (1979).

Herberman, R.B., Nunn, M.E., Holden, H.T., and Lavrin, D.H., *Int. J. Cancer 16:* 230 (1975).

Herberman, R.B., Bartram, S., Haskill, J.S., Nunn, M.E., Holden, H.T., and West, W.H., *J. Immunol. 119:*322 (1977).

Herberman, R.B. and Holden, H.T., *Adv. Cancer Res. 27:* 305 (1978).

Hersey, P., Edwards, A., Edwards, J., Adams, E., Milton, G.W., and Nelson, D.S., *Int. J. Cancer 16:* 173 (1975).

Hersey, P., *Aust. N.Z.J. Med. 9:* 464 (1979).

Horwitz, D.A., Kight, N., Temple, A., and Allison, A.C., *Immunology 36:* 221 (1979).

Jondal, M., and Pross, H.F., *Int. J. Cancer 15:* 596 (1975).

Kay, H.D., Thota, H., and Sinkovics, J.G., *Clin. Immunol. Immunopathol. 5:* 218 (1976).

Kay, H.D., Bonnard, G.D., West, W.H., and Herberman, R.B., *J. Immunol. 118:* 2058 (1977).

Kay, H.D., Bonnard, G.D., and Herberman, R.B., *J. Immunol. 122:* 675 (1979a).

Kay, H.D., Fagnani, and Bonnard, G.D., *Int. J. Cancer 24:* 141 (1979b).

Kiessling, R., Klein, E., Pross, H., and Wigzell, H., *Eur. J. Immunol. 5:* 117 (1975).

Kiessling, R., and Haller, O., *in* "Contemporary Topics in Immunology" (N.L. Warner, ed.) Academic Press, New York, 8: 171 (1978).

Kiuchi, M., and Takasugi, M., *J. Natl. Cancer Inst., 56:* 575 (1976).

Lozzio, C.B., and Lozzio, B.B., *Blood 45:* 321 (1975).

MacLennan, I.C.M., *Transplant. Rev. 13:* 67 (1972).

Moller, G., and Landwall, P., *Scand. J. Immunol. 6:*357 (1977).

Moretta, L., Mingari, M.C., and Romanzi, C.A., *Nature (Lond.) 272:* 618 (1978).

Nelson, D.L., Bundy, B.M., and Strober, W., *J. Immunol. 119:* 1401 (1977).

Oehler, J.R., Lindsay, L.R., Nunn, M.E., and Herberman, R.B., *Int. J. Cancer 21:* 204 (1978).

Ojo, E., and Wigzell, H., *Scand. J. Immunol. 7:* 297 (1978).

Ortaldo, J.R., Bonnard, G.D., Kind, P.D., and Herberman, R.B., *J. Immunol. 122:*1489 (1979).

Ortaldo, J.R., MacDermott, R.P., Bonnard, G.D., Kind, P.D., and Herberman, R.B., *Cell. Immunol,* in press.

Pape, G.R., Troye, M., Axelsson, B., and Perlmann, P., *J. Immunol. 122:* 2251 (1979a).

Pape, G.R., Moretta, L., Troye, M., and Perlmann, P., *Scand. J. Immunol. 9:* 291 (1979b).

Parrillo, J.E., and Fauci, A.S., *Scand. J. Immunol. 8:* 99 (1978).

Perlmann, P., Perlmann, H., and Wigzell, H., *Transplant. Rev. 13:* 91 (1972).

Perussia, B., Trinchieri, G., and Cerottini, J.-C., *J. Immunol. 123:* 681 (1979).

Peter, H.H., Pavie-Fischer, J., Fridman, W.H., Aubert, C., Cesarini, J.-P., Roubin, R., and Kourilsky, F.M., *J. Immunol. 115:* 539 (1975).

Pross, H.F., and Baines, M.G., *Cancer Immunol. Immunother. 3:* 75 (1977).

Ringdén, O., Rynnel-Dagöö, B., Waterfield, E.M., Möller, E., and Möller, G., *Scand J. Immunol. 6:* 1159 (1977).

Roberts, M.M., and Greaves, M.F., *Brit. J. Haematol. 38:* 439 (1978).

Shaw, G.M., Levy, P.C., and LoBuglio, A.F., *J. Immunol. 121:* 573 (1978).

Shore, S.L., Melewicz, F.M., and Gordon, D.S., *J. Immunol. 118:* 558 (1977).

Sulica, A., Laky, M., Gherman, M., Ghettie, V., and Sjoquist, J., *Scand. J. Immunol. 5:* 1191 (1976).

Takasugi, J., Koide, Y., and Takasugi, M., *Eur. J. Immunol. 7:* 887 (1977).

Troye, M., Perlmann, P., Pape, G.R., Spiegelberg, H.L., Näslund, I., and Gidlov, A., *J. Immunol. 119:* 1061 (1977).

West, W.H., Cannon, G.B., Kay, H.D., Bonnard, G.D., and Herberman, R.B., *J. Immunol. 118:* 355 (1977).

Ziegler, H.K., and Henney, C.S., *J. Immunol. 119:* 1010 (1977).

NATURAL KILLING AND ANTIBODY-DEPENDENT CELLULAR CYTOTOXICITY: INDEPENDENT MECHANISMS MEDIATED BY OVERLAPPING CELL POPULATIONS

Hillel S. Koren
Pamela J. Jensen

Department of Microbiology and Immunology
Division of Immunology
Duke University Medical Center
Durham, North Carolina

CONTENTS

ABBREVIATIONS USED IN THIS PAPER:

NK = natural killing/killer
ADCC = antibody dependent cellular cytotoxicity
F_cR = F_c receptor
PBL = peripheral blood lymphocytes
XAγ = x-linked agammaglobulinemia
TNP = trinitrophenol
E:T = effector to target cell ratio

This work was supported by grants from the National Cancer Institute numbers CA-23354, T32-CA-09058. H.S.K. is a recepient of a Research Career Development Award CA-00581.

ISBN 0-12-341350-8

I. INTRODUCTION

The relationship between natural killing (NK) and antibody-dependent cellular cytotoxicity (ADCC) against tumor target cells is a controversial area (1-11). Physical separation of cells into subpopulations that can mediate exclusively either NK or ADCC has so far failed. Inability to separate the effector cells has prompted speculation that NK is actually a form of ADCC in which naturally occurring antibodies confer NK specificities by arming the effector cells *in vivo* via their F_c receptors (F_cR) (3,12-16).

However, there is indirect evidence that these activities are separate. Experiments involving treatment of effector cell populations with various enzymes (1) and pharmacologic reagents (10) demonstrate a differential sensitivity of NK and ADCC.

In this report we will summarize the data obtained from several *in vitro* systems currently employed in our laboratory.

Our results suggest that NK activity is antibody independent and that NK and ADCC are mediated by a single cell (K/NK).

The possibility remains however that, in at least some circumstances, a K cell which mediates only ADCC may also be present.

II. EVIDENCE AGAINST A ROLE FOR ANTIBODY IN NK

The effector cells responsible for NK and ADCC bear a close resemblance in that the cell type with the highest activity for NK and ADCC, on a per cell basis, is a non-T, non-B, non-adherent to plastic, F_cR+ cell (4,17,18). This has prompted speculation that NK is actually a form of ADCC in which naturally occurring antibodies confer NK specificities by "arming" K cells in vivo via F_cR (12-16). The purpose of this section is to examine the postulated role of antibody in conventional short-term NK assays *in vitro*.

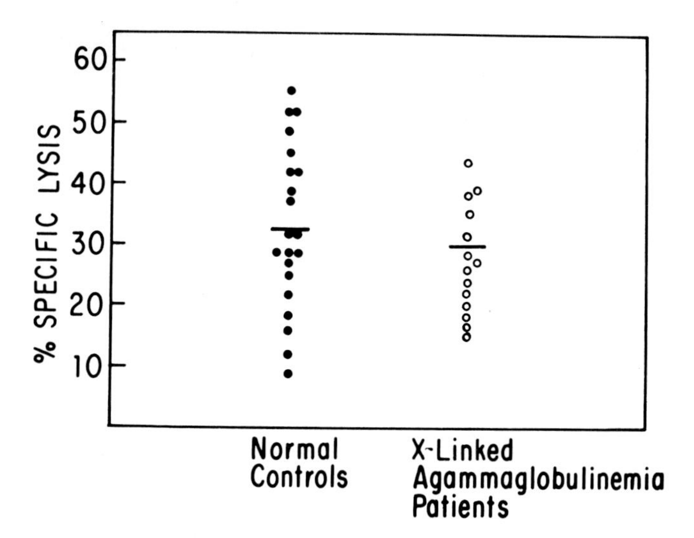

FIGURE 1. Distribution of NK activity against K562 by PBL of 14 normal donors and 21 X-linked agammaglobulinemia patients tested at an E:T of 20:1. The geometric means of the two groups are not significantly different based on respective log means and standard errors with an appropriate number of degrees of freedom.

A. NK of PBL From X-linked Agammaglobulinemia (XAγ) Patients

Patients with x-linked agammaglobulinemia (XAγ) have a total lack of B cells and circulating antibodies (19). PBL from fourteen of these patients have been tested, with lymphocytes from normal donors as controls, for NK activity over a period of two years (5). Figure 1 is a summary of this study, clearly showing that no significant difference in NK activity against K562 between these two groups exists. These data support the notion that NK is antibody independent. A similar study has been done by Pross et al. (20) who arrived at the same conclusions.

B. The Effect of Anti-Human Fab on NK

The possibility that lymphocytes "armed" by cytophilic antibodies *in vivo* may play a role in NK has also been addressed using a second experimental design. Fab fragments of rabbit anti-human Fab

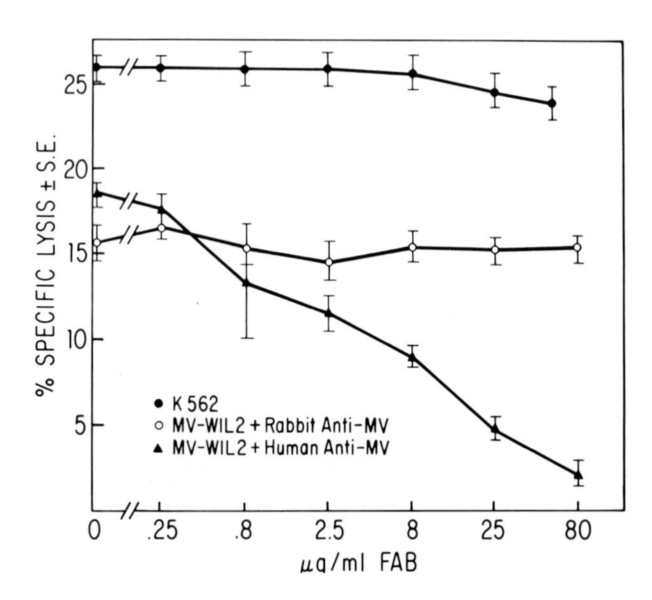

Figure 2. Effect of FAB on NK and ADCC. F_{ab} fragments of rabbit anti-human F_{ab} antibodies (FAB) were used in several concentrations by preincubating them with effector cells only for NK against K562 or with effector cells and antibodies in ADCC. For the ADCC assays a human lymphoblastoid cell line MV-WIL2, persistently infected with measles virus and relatively insensitive to human NK was employed. A rabbit anti-measles virus serum and a human serum with a high titer anti-measles virus activity obtained from a patient with a subacute sclerosing panencephalitis (SSPE) were used at the highest dilution still optimal in ADCC.
Weston et al., 1980

antibodies (FAB) were tested for their ability to block cytotoxicity against K562 (21). As control, FAB was tested simultaneously for its ability to block ADCC, using as the target a human lymphoid line persistently infected with measles virus (MV-WIL2) sensitized with either human or rabbit anti-measles virus sera (Figure 2). Cytotoxicity to K562 was not inhibited by FAB. In contrast, ADCC mediated by the human antiserum was strongly inhibited by FAB; however, ADCC mediated by the rabbit antiserum was unaffected by even the highest concentrations of FAB. Thus, NK against K562 was not affected by concentrations of F_{ab} fragments of anti-human F_{ab} which completely abrogated ADCC, indicating that antibodies from the lymphocyte donor were probably not required for NK.

These experiments are in agreement with those of Kay et al. (22), who used $F_{(ab')2}$ fragments of anti-IgG or anti-F_{ab} reagents in a similar study. These results are however in disagreement with those of Pape et al. (15,16) who did observe partial inhibition of NK against K562 by the addition of F_{ab} fragments of rabbit or goat anti-human IgG to their incubation mixtures. The reasons for this discrepancy are presently unclear but may be due to the differences in the reagents or test systems employed.

C. The Effect of Pronase and Autologous Serum on NK

To examine the possible role of natural antibodies in observed NK activities, we attempted to restore NK activities to lymphocytes which had been treated with pronase (23).

It was first necessary to establish the feasibility of an *in vitro* "arming" process using a reproducible model system. SB-TNP targets, which are relatively insensitive to NK, were found to be most suitable for this purpose. Thus, although SB-TNP targets are lysed to only a small extent by control lymphocytes, these same targets show dramatically increased lysis when the effectors are pretreated ("armed") with autologous serum with or without prior treatment with promase (Table I). Washing the "armed" effector cells three or four times at room temperature abolishes the enhanced activity due to treatment with serum. It should be noted that this "arming" activity was detected in the serum of every donor tested and that it was not observed when SB instead of SB-TNP targets were used; however, the exact nature of the arming factor has not yet been established.

When "armed" effectors as described above were tested against K562 targets (Table I) the initial loss of NK activity as a result of the pronase treatment was never completely regained in experiments with five out of six donors tested in this manner. Cells from one donor occasionally showed "arming-like" activity against K562. Therefore, this series of experiments also suggests that a

TABLE I. Cytotoxicity of Human PBL after Incubation in Autologous Serum against a TNP-Modified Target

Donor	Pronase Treatment[a]	Incubation with Serum[b]	Target (% specific lysis ±SE)	
			SB-TNP[c] 20:1	K562[c] 20:1
M.Q.	-	-	5.4±1.5	43.7±1.0
	-	FCS	1.6±1.6	37.7±3.1
	-	Autologous	13.4±2.4	36.5±2.4
M.Q.	+	-	4.4±3.4	7.7±0.6
	+	FCS	1.5±1.7	7.3±0.3
	+	Autologous	15.5±2.3	11.4±0.4
A.K.	-	-	2.6±0.6	34.4±0.8
	-	FCS	3.9±1.2	40.5±0.6
	-	Autologous	38.3±1.5	34.6±0.6
A.K.	+	-	1.8±0.9	8.7±0.4
	+	FCS	2.5±0.5	7.2±0.4
	+	Autologous	43.4±1.9	13.3±0.4

[a]Pronase-treated PBL were incubated for 30 min at 37°C with 0.1 mg/ml pronase. Untreated PBL were incubated in BSS+5% FCS for 30 min at 37°C.
[b]Both untreated and pronase-treated PBL were incubated in MEM+10% FCS, undiluted FCS or undiluted autologous serum for 3 hr at 37°C.
[c]^{51}Cr-labeled SB (modified with TNP) or K562 cells (1x10^4/well) were used as targets in a 3 hr ^{51}Cr release assay. % specific lysis was calculated as follows: $\frac{\text{Experimental CPM - Control CPM}}{\text{Maximum CPM - Control CPM}} \times 100$

Kall and Koren, 1979

major role of antibody in the conventionally described NK assay is unlikely.

Similar results were obtained in a miniature swine NK system (7). Using PBL as effectors and K562 as targets, initial NK activity was abolished by pronase treatment and was not restored upon incubation of those cells with autologous serum (24).

Our results are not in accord with those of Akira and Takasugi (12,13) and Koide et al. (14) but are in agreement with a similar series of experiments conducted by Kay et al. (22).

In spite of the conclusions derived from *in vitro* studies, it is still a reasonable possibility that the process of "arming" of F_cR+ NK cells can occur *in vivo* under some conditions and can therefore not be ruled out as an immunological phenomenon.

III. NK AND ADCC ARE MEDIATED BY DISTINCT MECHANISMS AND BY OVERLAPPING POPULATIONS OF EFFECTOR CELLS

One of the most intriguing and controversial questions in the NK area is whether NK and ADCC are mediated by the same or different effector cells. In this section we will describe several experimental approaches which address this central issue.

A. Attempts to Physically Separate NK and ADCC

In this line of experiments a combination of nylon column and rosetting separation techniques were used. Mononulcear cells obtained from PBL by Ficoll gradients were first depleted of plastic-adherent cells and then passed through nylon columns. Both the column non-adherent and adherent cells were then fractionated by conventional E-rosetting technique into T and non T cells. On occasions each of these fractions was further separated on the basis of their F_cR using antibody-coated erythrocytes (EA).

The data of a typical experiment are shown in Table II. The highest cytotoxic activities for both

TABLE II. ADCC and NK Activities of Human PBL Fractions

Effectors[b]	% Specific Lysis ±SE[a]					
	ADCC SB-TNP			NK K562		
	16:1	8:1	4:1	16:1	8:1	4:1
Macrophage depleted	9.2±0.9	6.0±0.8	2.2±0.7	16.2±1.5	8.6±1.0	3.3±1.4
Column passed	6.9±1.1	4.7±0.7	2.1±0.6	13.9±1.0	7.5±1.1	2.5±1.0
Column passed T	8.3±0.6	5.4±1.5	2.2±0.6	24.0±1.7	12.9±2.3	7.1±1.0
Column passed non-T	NT	25.4±0.9	15.6±0.6	NT	73.2±4.4	48.2±1.0
Column adherent	9.8±0.9	8.5±1.6	NT	22.9±2.8	8.7±0.9	4.7±1.2
Column adherent T	12.0±1.0	6.7±0.7	1.0±0.6	33.2±1.6	17.9±1.4	10.9±1.2
Column adherent non-T	NT	2.7±1.3	3.4±0.6	NT	6.1±1.3	2.0±1.0

[a]Effector cells were tested in a 4 hr ^{51}Cr release assay against two targets, SB-TNP and K562, calculations for % specific lysis were performed as described in Table I.
[b]Effector cells from a normal donor were macrophage depleted and incubated on nylon wool columns. The column passed cells (Cp) were incubated with SRC to obtain Cp-T and Cp non-T cells. Nylon adherent cells obtained by physical agitation of the column were also separated into T and non-T subsets. Red cells were removed by hypotonic lysis; the lymphocytes were tested after 18 hr incubation.

Kall and Koren, 1978

NK and ADCC on a per cell basis were obtained in the column passed non T cell fraction, though substantial activities were also obtained in the T cell fractions. Interestingly, the column adherent T cells had higher activity than the column passed T cells for both activities. Since the column adherent non-T fraction was not very active in either assay it is unlikely that the activities in the column adherent T cell fraction were due to contamination by the non-T cell fraction. Further fractionation experiments have shown that both the non-T and T effector cells in NK and ADCC were F_cR+ for the F_c portion of IgG (4), in agreement with the findings of other investigators (25,26). The data indicatethat the cellsmediating NK and ADCC comprise a heterogeneous subpopulation and that it is not possible, using conventional techniques, to isolate cells responsible for one or the other activity.

B. Disassociation of NK and ADCC

If NK cells do indeed recognize their targets in an antibody-independent manner, it should be possible to devise procedures based on the differences in recognition mechanisms to disassociate NK and ADCC activities. Cold cell competitive inhibition assays and a cellular immunoadsorbent technique were thus employed.

1. Cold Cell Competitive Inhibition of ADCC. Using the cold cell competitive inhibition assay, which is based on the assumption that cells with similar target structures will compete for the same receptor on the effector cell, we were able to demonstrate (Figure 3) that ^{51}Cr labeled ADCC targets (SB-TNP) can not be appreciably inhibited by several NK sensitive tumor cells (HSB and MOLT4) known to effectively inhibit NK (6). In contrast, ADCC was dramatically inhibited by two types of antibody complexed NK-sensitive target cells (SB-TNP) and TNP-modified chicken erythrocytes (CRC-TNP). The same targets when not complexed with antibody were not inhibitory. These results suggest that the recognition mechanisms of NK and ADCC are distinct. The fact that K562 cells did inhibit ADCC may be due to the presence of an F_cR on K562 cells

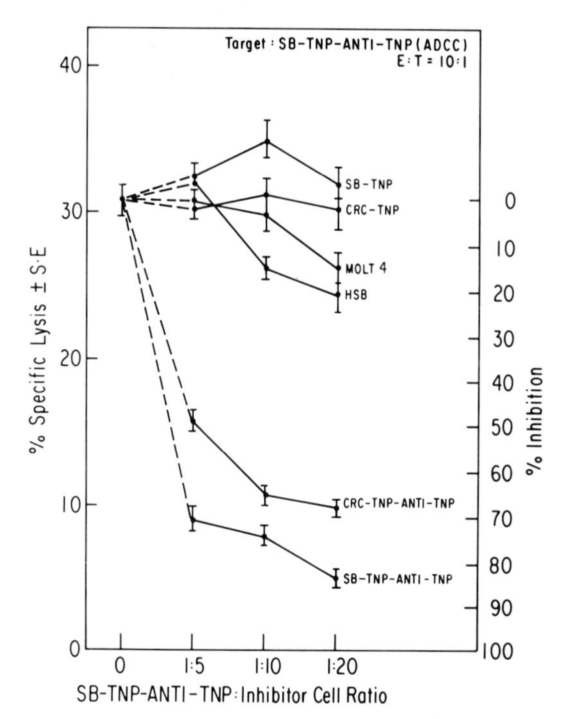

FIGURE 3. Competitive cell inhibition of ^{51}Cr labeled SB-TNP, anti-TNP coated (ADCC) by NK-sensitive tumor cells and antibody-coated competitors {SB-TNP and chicken red cells-TNP (CRC-TNP)}. The cytotoxic activity in a 2 hr assay at an E:T of 10:1 in the absence of inhibitor cells was 32.2% (=0% inhibition). % specific lysis was calculated as shown in Table I.

which can compete with the F_cR+ effector cells for the F_c portion of the added antibody. Alternative explanations (i.e. differences in the proportion of NK cells which recognize various targets and/or differences in affinities between the different NK targets and the effector cells) may also contribute to the observation. The use of an F_cR-negative K562 variant equally susceptible to NK might be helpful in distinguishing among the possibilities.

2. The Effect of Cellular Immunoadsorbents on NK and ADCC. The cellular immunoadsorption technique previously utilized to study the specificity of cytotoxic T lymphocytes (27,28) was employed to examine the relationship between NK and

ADCC. We have previously shown that this procedure can be used to selectively deplete PBL populations of NK effector cells (29). When NK and ADCC activities of control PBL and PBL non-adherent to a K562 monolayer were compared, results as shown in figure 4 were obtained. Both NK and ADCC activities were decreased in the non-adherent fraction, suggesting that the K562 monolayer was able to partially deplete the population not only of NK cells, but of K cells as well. Table III summarizes quantitatively the results obtained in experiments done as shown in figure 3 with several different donors. With four donors (represented by HK and DF in Table III), the K562 monolayers were consistently able to deplete NK activity against K562 to a significantly greater extent than ADCC. However, with two donors (represented by MQ in Table III), the extent of depletion of ADCC was not significantly different from that of NK in two out of three testings; in the third testing, however, NK was depleted significantly more than ADCC.

When analogous experiments were done with HSB monolayers, the extent of depletion of NK was greater than that of ADCC in every case.

The cellular immunoadsorbent studies have shown that with most individuals both K562 and HSB monolayers deplete NK against the homologous target to a greater extent than ADCC. However, in some cases the extent of depletion of NK and ADCC on K562 monolayers was equivalent. These observations are consistent with the hypothesis that NK and ADCC are mediated by the same cell, designated as K/NK. This cell bears an F_cR as well as one or more NK recognition sites; all K/NK cells can mediate ADCC but not all K/NK cells are capable of killing every NK-sensitive target. The type or types of NK recognition structures born by a given K/NK cell determine its NK target selectivity. In the cases where K562 monolayers depleted NK and ADCC equivalently, it would appear that a great majority, if not all, K/NK cells recognized K562, which is exceeding sensitive to NK and hence may bear a variety of NK determinants.

The possible existence in some populations of a K cell, i.e., a cell which mediates only ADCC and not NK, can not be refuted by the monolayer experiments. In fact, evidence suggesting that in some situations K cells in the absence of NK activity

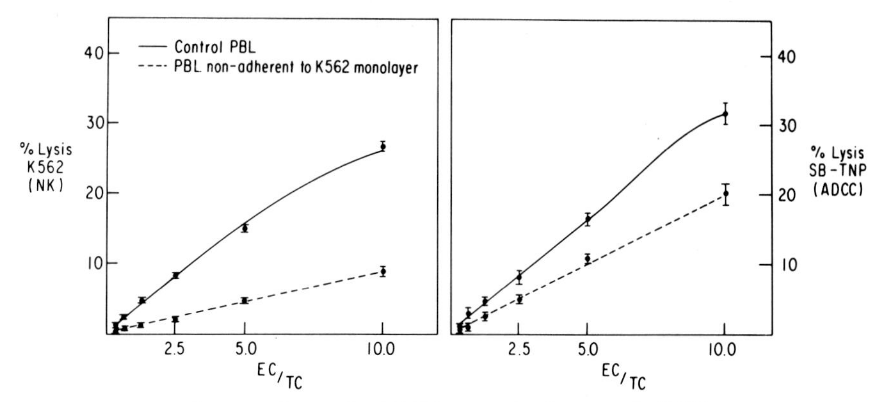

FIGURE 4. NK and ADCC activity of PBL non-adherent to a K562 monolayer. Control PBL (——) or PBL non-adherent to a K562 monolayer (----) were assayed for NK and ADCC activities at the indicated E:T ratios. The ^{51}Cr-release assay was carried out for 75 min. Spontaneous ^{51}Cr-release was 2.6% for K562 and 7.7% for SB-TNP. In the absence of antibody, the lysis of ^{51}Cr-SB-TNP at 5:1 E:T ratio was 0.4% ± 0.4. Jensen and Koren, 1980

TABLE III. Relative Depletion of NK and ADCC

Donor	Experiment	K562 Monolayer[b] Targets NK(K562) %Depletion[a]	ADCC(SB-TNP)	Significance
HK	1	74	45	p < .01
	2	86	58	p < .001
	3	83	56	p < .01
DF	1	66	37	p < .01
	2	67	40	p < .001
	3	82	34	p < .001
MQ	1	80	76	NS
	2	80	65	NS
	3	72	35	p < .01

[a]Control PBL and PBL non-adherent to K562 monolayers were tested for NK activity against K562 and for ADCC activity against SB-TNP in a 2 hr ^{51}Cr release assay. In each case specific lysis was determined for 5 or 6 E:T ratios and a slope calculated. %depletion was then calculated as follows:

$$1 - \frac{\text{slope of non-adherent PBL cutotoxic activity}}{\text{slope of control PBL cytotoxic activity}}$$

[b]For technical details describing the monolayer method, see the chapter by Jensen and Koren.

NS, not significant

Jensen and Koren, 1979

TABLE IV. NK and ADCC Activities in Peripheral Blood Mononuclear Cells of Colostrum-Deprived Piglets Obtained by Hysterectomy

Effector cells[a]			% Specific Lysis[b] ±SE			
		Hours in culture	ADCC (SB-TNP)		NK (K562)	
Exp.	Donor	prior to assay	100:1	50:1	100:1	50:1
1	Mother 3070-1	0	23.9±2.9	13.1±0.7	1.8±0.3	3.0±0.6
	Piglet 3070-1 Po-1	0	32.7±1.0	NT	0.4±0.3	NT
2	Mother 3070-1	18	31.0±3.0	11.2±0.5	7.0±0.6	5.2±0.5
	Piglet 3070-1 Po-1	18	46.9±0.5	NT	0.1±0.4	NT
3	Mother 3062-5	18	18.0±0.0	2.0±4.5	15.8±1.6	11.6±0.1
	Piglet 3062-5 Po-1	18	NT	NT	0.0±0.6	NT
	Piglet 3062-5 Po-3	18	19.0±2.4	NT	0.0±0.4	NT
4	Mother 3056-4	18	33.0±0.6	27.4±3.2	15.3±2.0	7.9±0.6
	Piglet 3056-4 Po-2	18	24.7±2.9	21.2±2.0	3.3±0.2	3.2±0.1
5	Mother 3037-5	18	52.5±2.5	36.3±7.6	36.0±1.2	21.3±1.0
	Piglet 3037-5 Po-1	18	28.5±0.3	NT	0.5±0.4	NT

NT, not tested
[a]PBL obtained from the piglets on the day of hysterectomy were tested in NK and ADCC immediately (as in exp. 1, 0hr) or incubated overnight first.
[b]NK and ADCC assays were 2½ hr long. % specific activity was calculated as shown in Table I. Incubation of pig effector cells with SB-TNP in the absence of anti-TNP serum did not result in a marked increase of cytolysis compared to medium control.
Koren et al., 1978

may also exist is presented below.

C. The Autonomous Existence of K Cells in the Minnesota Miniature Piglet

As mentioned earlier (Section II) PBL of adult Minnesota miniature pigs can mediate NK and ADCC against K562 and SB-TNP respectively (7). However, newborn piglets obtained by aseptic hysterectomy 3 days prior to full term and shown not to have any Ig were capable of mediating ADCC but totally lacked NK against K562 even when tested at an E:T ratio of 100:1 (Table IV). In some experiments feeding the piglets with colostrum for 2 days {which was sufficient to achieve maternal levels of Ig in the piglet (31)} still did not produce detectable NK activity (32). These data indicate that effector K cells mediating ADCC develop earlier in ontogeny than NK cells, and therefore suggest that at least in some stage of life a K cell with no NK activity may exist.

D. Single Expression of NK or ADCC in Disease States

We have observed that in certain pathological conditions NK and ADCC may sometimes be disassociated. Several explanations may exist to explain

TABLE V. Disassociation of NK and ADCC in Some Ovarian Cancer Patients

Expt.	Source of effector cells[a]	Targets % Specific Lysis ±SE NK(K562) 20:1	ADCC(SB-TNP) 20:1
1	PBL-control	25.5±2.3	43.0±2.3
	PBL-patient	1.7±0.2	15.3±1.9
	Ascites-patient	1.6±0.4	26.4±1.7
2	PBL-control	18.9±1.0	27.5±2.0
	PBL-patient	1.8±0.1	16.4±0.8
3	PBL-control	39.9±2.1	25.4±1.2
	PBL-patient	36.8±2.0	20.0±1.1
	Ascites-patient	13.3±1.5	1.3±0.2

[a]PBL of normal controls and PBL or lymphocytes isolated from the ascites of ovarian cancer patients obtained prior to surgery or treatment were used as effector cells in a 4 hr ^{51}Cr release assay against K562 and SB-TNP. % specific lysis was calculated as shown in Table I.

the partial deficiency in each case; however, the fact that either NK or ADCC can be mediated by lymphocytes of a given individual while the other activity is impaired further strengthens the notion that these activities are distinct and probably independent.

1. Ovarian Cancer Patients. During a study conducted to assess and compare NK and ADCC levels in ovarian cancer patients it was observed (Table V) that in 3 cases only one of the assayed activities was observed. The control donors' PBL were positive for both activities in every case. It should be noted that in most cases studied (Haskill and Koren, unpublished observation) both NK and ADCC were detectable in the PBL of these patients.

2. X-linked- agammaglobulinemia Patients. As mentioned above (Section IIA) PBL of patients with this immunodeficiency have normal levels of NK against K562 (Figure 1). However, we have previously reported that these patients have impaired ADCC (5). Further studies have shown that cells from these patients are capable of mediating ADCC if certain anti sera are employed. The results obtained with one XAγ patient and a control donor

TABLE VI. ADCC By X-linked Agamaglobulinemia (XAγ) Patients

Donor	Source and final dilution of anti-TNP serum		Targets % Specific Lysis[c] ±SE ADCC (SB-TNP) 20:1	10:1	5:1	NK(K562) 20:1
Control HK	-		3.0±1.0	2.0±0.5	0.9±0.2	58.7±1.9
"	Rabbit[a]	1:1000	41.2±1.3	35.9±1.0	25.7±0.8	
"	Balb/c[b]	1:40	31.5±0.6	20.2±1.1	13.1±0.8	
"	"	1:400	34.0±0.5	26.0±0.8	16.5±1.3	
"	"	1:800	34.2±0.5	24.2±1.1	16.1±1.1	
"	"	1:1600	32.2±0.9	27.5±3.6	14.7±0.7	
"	"	1:3200	23.2±0.6	15.1±1.1	10.8±0.7	
Patient SS(XAγ)	-		5.6±1.0	2.3±0.9	0.9±0.5	62.8±2.3
"	Rabbit[a]	1:1000	19.5±2.4	17.8±1.2	13.4±0.8	
"	Balb/c[b]	1:40	<1	<1	<1	
"	"	1:400	2.3±1.4	<1	<1	
"	"	1:800	1.7±1.7	<1	<1	
"	"	1:1600	3.0±1.7	<1	<1	
"	"	1:3200	2.7±1.7	<1	<1	

[a]Hyperimmune rabbit anti-TNP-KLH serum which was still active at a dilution of 10^{-5} with donor HK lost considerable ADCC activity with patient SS at that dilution.
[b]Hyperimmune serum from Balb/c mice immunized with TNP-modified M.tuberculosis organisms (strain H37Ra).
[c]PBL of control and XAγ patient were assayed for NK and ADCC activities in a 2 hr assay. % specific lysis was calculated as shown in Table I.

are presented in Table VI. Whereas the control donor exhibited ADCC activity with both the rabbit and mouse anti-TNP sera used, PBL of the XAγ patient had demonstrable ADCC activity with the rabbit anti-TNP serum, but not with a mouse (Balb/c) anti-TNP at any of the concentrations tested. Impaired ADCC activity by this group of patients was also observed when normal lymphocytes coated with a human anti-HLA serum were used as targets {data not shown and (33)} . The fact that under certain experimental conditions (Table VI) the ADCC activity of XAγ patients is impaired while their NK activity is intact (Figure 1 and Table VI) provides further evidence for the independence of NK and ADCC mechanisms.

IV. CONCLUDING REMARKS

The data presented in this paper clearly suggest that conventional *in vitro* NK assays do not involve the participation of antibodies. Evidence to substantiate this statment is derived from the following experimental models: 1. x-linked agammaglobulinemia patients (lacking B cells and circulating antibodies) exhibit NK activity, 2. anti-human F_{ab} does not affect NK against K562 but obliterates ADCC, and 3. autologous serum in all but one preparation studied does not "rearm" pronase treated effector cells against K562.

That NK and ADCC are distinct is further shown by the relative inefficiency of most NK-sensitive targets to block ADCC and the single expression of either NK or ADCC in some disease states. With regard to the nature of the effector cells, the monolayer adsorption experiments indicate that NK and ADCC are mediated by the same cell (K/NK). This cell bears an F_cR as well as one or more types of NK recognition structures and is therefore bifunctional. The finding that newborn piglets have only ADCC activity suggests the existence of a cell which mediates only ADCC and not NK in at least some stage of porcine life.

ACKNOWLEDGMENTS

The authors thank Dr. D. Bernard Amos for his interest and his support in providing the environment in which to carry out this work. Appreciation is expressed to Steven J. Anderson for his dedication and skillful help and to Linda Nash for typing and preparing this manuscript.

REFERENCES

1. Kay, H.D., Bonnard, G.D., West, W.H., and Herberman, R.B., J. Immunol. 118, 2058 (1977).
2. Nelson, D.L., Bundy, B.M., and Strober, W., J. Immunol. 119, 1401 (1977).
3. Koide, Y., and Takasugi, M., J. Natl. Cancer Inst. 59, 1099 (1977).
4. Kall, M.A.T., and Koren, H.S., Cell. Immunol. 40, 58 (1978).

5. Koren, H.S., Amos, D.B., and Buckley, R.H., J. Immunol. 120, 796 (1978).
6. Koren, H.S., and Williams, M.S., J. Immunol. 121, 1956 (1978).
7. Koren, H.S., Amos, D.B., and Kim. Y.B., Proc. Natl. Acad. Sci. U.S.A. 75, 5127 (1978).
8. Gupta, S., Fernandes, G., Nair, M., and Good, R.A., Proc. Natl. Acad. Sci. U.S.A. 75, 5137 (1978).
9. Ojo, E., and Wigzell, Scand. J. Immunol. 7, 297 (1978).
10. Parrillo, J.E., and Fauci, A.S., Clin. Exp. Immunol. 31, 116 (1978).
11. Santoni, A., Herberman, R.B., and Holden, H.T., J. Natl. Cancer Inst. 62, 109 (1979).
12. Akira, D., and Takasugi, M., Int. J. Cancer 19, 747 (1977).
13. Takasugi, J., Koide, Y., and Takasugi, M., Eur. J. Immunol. 7, 887 (1977).
14. Koide, Y., Kwok, R., and Takasugi, M., Int. J. Cancer 22, 546 (1978).
15. Pape, G.R., Troye, M., and Perlmann, P., J. Immunol. 118, 1925 (1977).
16. Pape, G., Troye, M., Axelsson, B., and Perlmann, P., J. Immunol. 122, 2251 (1979).
17. Jondal, M., and Pross, H., Int. J. Cancer 16, 173 (1975).
18. Bakacs, T., Gergely, P., and Klein, E., Cell. Immunol. 32, 317 (1977).
19. Schiff, R.I., Buckley, R.H., Gilbertsen, R.B., and Metzgar, R.S., J. Immunol. 112, 376 (1974).
20. Pross, H.F., Gupta, S., Good, R.A., and Baines, M.B., Cell. Immunol. 43, 160 (1979).
21. Weston, P.A., Levy, N., and Koren, H.S., submitted for publication.
22. Kay. D., Bonnard, G.D., and Herberman, R.B., J. Immunol. 122, 675 (1979).
23. Kall, M.A., and Koren, H.S., Cell. Immunol. 47, 57 (1979).
24. Huh, N.D., Kim, Y.B., Koren, H.S., and Amos, D.B., submitted for publication.
25. Gupta, S., Fernandes, G., Nair, M., and Good, R.A., Proc. Natl. Acad. Sci. U.S.A. 75, 5137 (1978).
26. Pichler, W.J., Gendelman, F.W., and Nelson, D.L., Cell. Immunol. 42, 410 (1979).

27. Stulting, R.D., and Berke, G., J. Exp. Med. 137, 932 (1973).
28. Stulting, R.D., Todd, III, R.F., and Amos, D.B., Cell. Immunol. 20, 54 (1975).
29. Jensen, P.J., Amos, D.B., and Koren, H.S., J. Immunol. 123, 1127 (1979).
30. Roder, J.C., Ahrlund-Richter, L., and Jondal, M., J. Exp. Med. 150, 471 (1979).
31. Kim, Y.B., and Watson, D.W., Ann. N.Y. Acad. Sci. 133, 727 (1966).
32. Kim, Y.B., Huh, N.D., Koren, H.S., and Amos, D.B., submitted for publication.
33. Sanal, S.O., and Buckley, R.H., J. Clin. Invest. 61, 1 (1978).

ARE SPONTANEOUS AND ANTIBODY-DEPENDENT LYSIS TWO DIFFERENT MECHANISMS OF CYTOTOXICITY MEDIATED BY THE SAME CELL?*

Bice Perussia
Daniela Santoli
Giorgio Trinchieri

The Wistar Institute of Anatomy and Biology
Philadelphia, Pennsylvania

Spontaneous and antibody-dependent cell-mediated cytotoxicity in lymphocytes obtained from different donors.

Lymphocytes obtained from the peripheral blood of normal donors, in absence of disease or any known or deliberate sensitization, are cytotoxic *in vitro* against unsensitized or IgG-antibody sensitized target cells. These two types of cytotoxic activity are referred to as spontaneous and antibody-dependent cell-mediated cytotoxicity (SpCMC and AbCMC) (Jondal and Pross, 1975). The effector lymphocytes are functionally distinct and defined as Natural Killer (NK) and Killer (K) cells, respectively (Jondal and Pross, 1975; West *et al*., 1977a). Cytotoxicity is commonly measured by ^{51}Cr-release assays, and it can be quantitated by calculating the absolute number of lytic units present in each lymphocyte preparation. One lytic unit is defined as the number of effector cells that kills 50% of the target cells during the test time (Cerottini and Brunner, 1976).

When peripheral blood lymphocytes from different donors are tested for their ability to mediate SpCMC and AbCMC, high variability is observed within the donors in the same experiment. Moreover, if the lymphocytes from one donor are tested several times, they will display slightly different degrees of cytotoxicity depending on the lymphocyte or the target cell preparations. The activity of lymphocytes from different donors in SpCMC and AbCMC can be compared only when they are tested under exactly the same experimental

The experimental work described in this paper was supported by NIH grants CA-20833, CA-10815, CA-43882 and NS-11036 and by the National Multiple Sclerosis Society.

ISBN 0-12-341350-8

conditions. A significant positive correlation was observed between SpCMC and AbCMC in repeated experiments with a large number of donors (Table I). These data suggest that either the same subpopulations of lymphocytes mediate both cytotoxic activities, or that common regulatory mechanisms affect the activity of two discrete populations of effector cells.

Various lymphocyte subsets were obtained by using different cell fractionation procedures, including adherence to nylon wool columns (Julius *et al.*, 1973), velocity sedimentation gradients, anti-Ig columns for immunoglobulin-bearing lymphocytes (Trinchieri *et al.*, 1978b), C3-Sepharose columns for C3b receptor-positive cells (Casali and Perussia, 1977; Perussia *et al.*, 1979a), monolayers of IgG-antibody-sensitized erythrocytes prepared on poly-L-lysine treated plastics for IgG-Fc receptor-positive cells (Kedar *et al.*, 1976; Perussia *et al.*, 1979b), or binding to sheep erythrocytes. It was not possible, with these techniques, to separate K cell activity from NK cell activity. Both activities are mediated by cells that are surface immunoglobulin-negative, C3b receptor-negative, IgG-Fc receptor-positive, medium-sized lymphocytes (Perussia *et al.*, 1979a; Santoli *et al.*, 1978; Trinchieri *et al.*, 1978c; West *et al.*, 1977a). The effector cells mediating both activities show a similar sensitivity to gamma ray irradiation (Perussia *et al.*, 1979a). About 50% of both activities, with some variability among different donors, is found in each of the lymphocyte fractions obtained by separating cells rosetting and non-rosetting with neuraminidase- or AET (2-aminoethyl isothiouronium bromide hybrobromide) treated sheep erythrocytes (Santoli *et al.*, 1978b; Trinchieri *et al.*, 1978b).

Effect on cytotoxicity of the interaction of IgG-Fc receptors with immune complexes.

K cell function requires the presence of intact IgG-Fc receptors on the effector cells for the interaction with antibody-sensitized target cells (Revillard *et al.*, 1975). The possible role of the receptors in NK cell activity remains unclear. AbCMC is inhibited by immune complexes, by aggregated IgG and by cell-bound IgG antibodies (Ziegler and Henney, 1975, 1977a; Ziegler *et al.*, 1977b). It has been shown in humans that also NK cell activity can be

TABLE 1. *Correlation Between K and NK Cell Activity in Lymphocyte Preparations from Different Donors*

Expt. Number	No. of Donors*	Correlation Coefficient† (r)	Level of Significance (P)
1	19	0.3308	0.1
2	13	0.7873	0.001
3	20	0.5493	0.01
4	20	0.8133	0.001
5	19	0.7248	0.001
6	19	0.6561	0.001
7	20	0.7241	0.001
8	18	0.4963	0.05
9	9	0.9384	0.001
10	27	0.6905	0.001
11	41	0.5774	0.001

*The numbers of donors tested for each single experiment are listed. NK cell activity was tested in an 18-hr ^{51}Cr-release assay using LN-SV cells (human fibroblasts, SV40-transformed) as target cells. K activity was tested in a 4-hr ^{51}Cr-release assay against human EB-P8 (EBV-transformed B cell line) target cells sensitized with human IgG anti-HLA antibodies (0.1 mg/ml) (Santoli et al., 1976).

†The correlation coefficient for each experiment was calculated by the number of lytic units/10^7 cells observed in each lymphocyte preparation. One lytic unit is defined by the number of effector cells that kill 50% of the target cells during the test time.

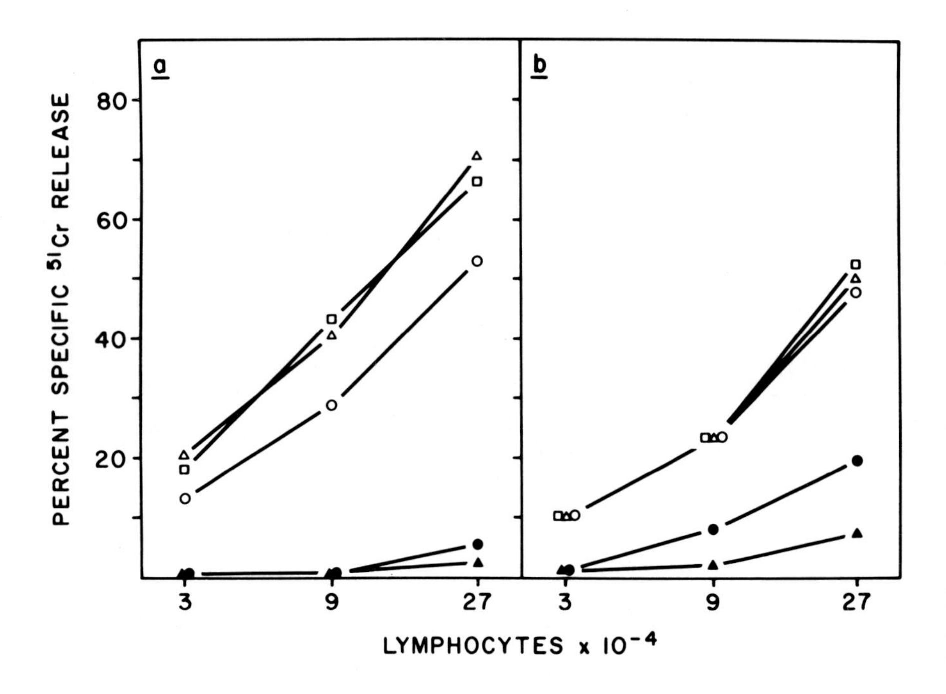

FIGURE 1. Effect of the interaction between IgG-Fc receptors and immune complexes on (a) antibody-dependent and (b) spontaneous cell-mediated cytotoxicity. Lymphocytes from one single donor were used as effector cells at different effector-to-target cell ratios, using 10^4 target cells/well in a 4-hr ^{51}Cr-release test performed in microtiter plates (Perussia et al., 1979b). (a) AbCMC was tested against L1210 mouse cell line sensitized with a rabbit anti-mouse antiserum (1:5000 final dilution); (b) SpCMC against K562 human erythroid cell line. Before testing, lymphocytes were incubated in normal medium, with particulate immune complexes, or with immobilized immune complexes. Particulate immune complexes were ox erythrocytes sensitized with a sub-agglutinating dilution of rabbit IgG anti-ox erythrocytes (EoxA7S). Unsensitized ox erythrocytes were used as controls. Lymphocytes and erythrocytes were mixed at a ratio of 1:40, centrifuged, and incubated 1 hr at 37°C. Erythrocytes were

inhibited by aggregated IgG (Bolhuis et al., 1978). In order to investigate the role of IgG-Fc receptors in SpCMC, we have chosen experimental conditions in which their expression at the cell surface is altered. When lymphocytes from normal donors were tested for their cytotoxic activity in the presence of particulate or immobilized immune complexes, AbCMC was completely abolished (Fig. 1a) and SpCMC was reduced, (Fig. 1b). Insoluble immune complexes (i.e., mouse Ig-rabbit anti-mouse Ig) also inhibited both the cytotoxic activities: the highest inhibition was obtained with immune complexes prepared in antibody excess (unpublished results). The inhibition of AbCMC is not simply due to a competitive blocking of the Fc receptors by immune complexes, but is associated with an irreversible functional disappearance (modulation) of the receptors (Revillard et al., 1975; Moretta et al., 1978; Perussia et al., 1979b). Capping or shedding of IgG-Fc receptors might occur after reaction with the immune complexes, so that receptors able to bind new immune complexes are not expressed on the cell surface. In this case, which is analogous to what has been described for other surface receptors, culturing of the cells should permit the re-expression of the receptor at cell surface. However, after reaction with immune complexes, lymphocytes are no longer able to mediate AbCMC (and SpCMC) and to form EA7S rosettes even when washed and incubated in vitro up to 4 days in tissue culture conditions (Perussia et al., 1979; Revillard et al., 1975). The ability to form EA7S rosettes and to mediate cytotoxicity is also not restored if the lymphocytes are treated with trypsin, an enzyme able

---

lysed by treatment with hypotonic medium, and the lymphocytes were washed once before testing. Immobolized immune complexes were rabbit IgG sensitized sheep erythrocytes (EA7S) monolayers prepared according to Kedar et al. (1974) on poly-L-lysine treated flat-bottom 96-well plates. Unsensitized Es monolayers were used as controls. □—□ control untreated lymphocytes; △—△ Eox-treated lymphocytes; ▲—▲ EoxA7S-treated lymphocytes; ○—○ lymphocytes on Es monolayers; ●—● lymphocytes on EsA7S monolayers.

to remove IgG bound to the receptors from the cell surface (Moretta _et al_., 1978). After reaction with immune complexes, cells were also treated with pronase in an attempt to digest completely the IgG-Fc receptors on the cell surface, and were then incubated at 37°C to allow resynthesis of the receptors. Cells treated in this way recovered neither functional IgG-Fc receptors nor cytotoxic activities, whereas an almost complete resynthesis was observed with pronase-treated lymphocytes which had not reacted with immune complexes (Perussia _et al_., 1979b). Modulation of IgG-Fc receptors was partially prevented when the cells were incubated with immune complexes in a Ca^{++}-free medium (Perussia _et al_., 1979b) or at low temperature (Cordier _et al_., 1977).

These experiments suggest that the modulation of IgG-Fc receptors takes place shortly after the reaction with immune complexes and involves more than mere "exhaustion" of the available receptors. It may require metabolic changes induced by interaction between the immune complexes and the IgG-Fc receptor and which may result in a modification of the functional state of the effector cells. The inhibition of SpCMC after reaction of lymphocytes with immune complexes might be due to a modification of the functional state of the effector cells that could not only induce modulation and block resynthesis of the IgG-Fc receptor, but could also affect other cellular mechanisms involved in SpCMC. The difference observed in the kinetics of AbCMC and SpCMC could help clarify the role of the IgG-Fc receptors. The rate of lysis of sensitized target cells by K cells increases up to 3 to 4 hr of incubation. After this period, no additional killing occurs even if fresh sensitized targets are added (Ziegler and Henney, 1975). Thus, the inactivation of K cell-dependent cytotoxic activity may be interpreted as the expression of the modulation of the IgG-Fc receptors, induced by the interaction between the effector cells and the sensitized target cells. On the contrary, the killing of unsensitized target cells increased linearly with time (Trinchieri _et al_., 1977), a result that is difficult to explain if one assumes that the IgG-Fc receptors play a direct role in SpCMC. Further, the modulation of the IgG-Fc receptors and inactivation of the cytotoxic lymphocytes would be expected to occur during effector-target cell interaction in SpCMC and, therefore, the kinetics of cytotoxicity should be the same as in AbCMC. The possibility that two distinct mechanisms, mediated by the same IgG-Fc receptor-bearing cells, are responsible for the antibody-dependent and for the spontaneous cell-mediated cytotoxicity must be considered.

Evidence against a role of IgG antibodies in the cytotoxicity mediated by NK cells.

The hypothesis that, at least in some experimental conditions, a single cytotoxic mechanism operates in both AbCMC and SpCMC, and that NK cell activity depends on the presence of cytophilic natural antibodies bound *in vivo* to the IgG-Fc receptors and directed against target cell surface antigens has been proposed by Koide and Takasugi (1977). Their proposal was based on the following experimental evidence: the treatment of effector cells with trypsin completely abolishes SpCMC, while leaving the expression of IgG-Fc receptors and the activity of the effector cells in AbCMC unaffected. The difference in the sensitivity of AbCMC and SpCMC to trypsin treatment has been interpreted as a result of the digestion of cytophilic antibodies absorbed to the NK cells. Experimental data showing the possibility of rendering the trypsin-treated lymphocytes cytotoxic by treatment with autologous serum have been presented (Akira and Takasugi, 1977). Recovery of cytotoxic activity, however, could not be reproduced by several researchers in various experimental conditions (Nelson *et al.*, 1977; Kay *et al.*, 1979). Both in a 4-hr and in an 18-hr ^{51}Cr-release assay against two different target cells, we were unable to reconstitute NK activity of trypsin-treated cells by incubation with autologous serum (Perussia *et al.*, 1979b). We were also unable to induce lymphocyte cytotoxicity against target cells, which are not lysed in SpCMC (e.g., P815Y mouse mastocytoma cells or L1210 mouse leukemia cells), by preincubating effector lymphocytes or trypsin-treated lymphocytes with hyperimmune antiserum at concentrations even higher than those able to induce very efficient AbCMC when used for target cell sensitization (unpublished results).

We have shown previously that rabbit-IgG or $F(ab')_2$ fragments of anti-human IgG efficiently inhibit AbCMC induced by human antibodies (Trinchieri et al., 1975). Troye et al. (1977) have also found that SpCMC against some tumor-derived target cells was partially inhibited by anti-human IgG reagents. Härfast et al. (1977), however, reported the inability of these reagents to inhibit SpCMC against mumps-infected target cells. This has been confirmed for a variety of target cells (Trinchieri et al., 1978c; Santoli et al., 1978; Kay et al., 1979). Troye et al. (1977), however, used the Fab' fragment of rabbit anti-human IgG antibodies instead of the $F(ab')_2$ used by the other researchers. It is difficult to explain why the divalent fragment, which effectively blocks all the cytotoxic assays of AbCMC, would not be able to inhibit SpCMC if NK cells do indeed recognize target cells through human natural antibodies bound to the IgG-Fc receptors.

The loss of the ability of trypsin-treated lymphocytes to mediate SpCMC is reversible when lymphocytes are incubated in tissue culture conditions for 18 hr (Perussia et al., 1979b). Although we were not able to restore the cytotoxic activity with a short treatment with autologous serum or hyperimmune anti-target serum, it was still possible that the recovery of SpCMC activity of trypsin-treated lymphocytes depended on antibodies synthesized in the cultures by B cells. However, an almost complete depletion of B cells from the lymphocyte population by two subsequent filtrations through nylon wool columns did not prevent the recovery of cytotoxicity (Fig. 2). The possibility that a few remaining B cells in the culture were able to secrete antibodies in sufficient amounts to arm NK cells was tested by adding anti-human $F(ab')_2$ reagents during the culture and the cytotoxic test. If the recovery of SpCMC activity was due to absorption of antibodies to the cells, it should have been possible to inhibit SpCMC with the rabbit $F(ab')_2$ anti-human $F(ab')_2$ reagent, which was used at concentrations 20 times higher than those sufficient to completely suppress AbCMC in a variety of target cells. As shown in Fig. 2, the anti-human $F(ab')_2$ reagent did not affect the recovery of the cytotoxic activity of trypsin-treated cells. These results suggest that NK cell activity requires some recognition structure(s) that act either independently of or in cooperation with the IgG-Fc receptors. Such structures are not IgG antibodies, are very sensitive to proteolytic enzymes and can be resynthesized in culture.

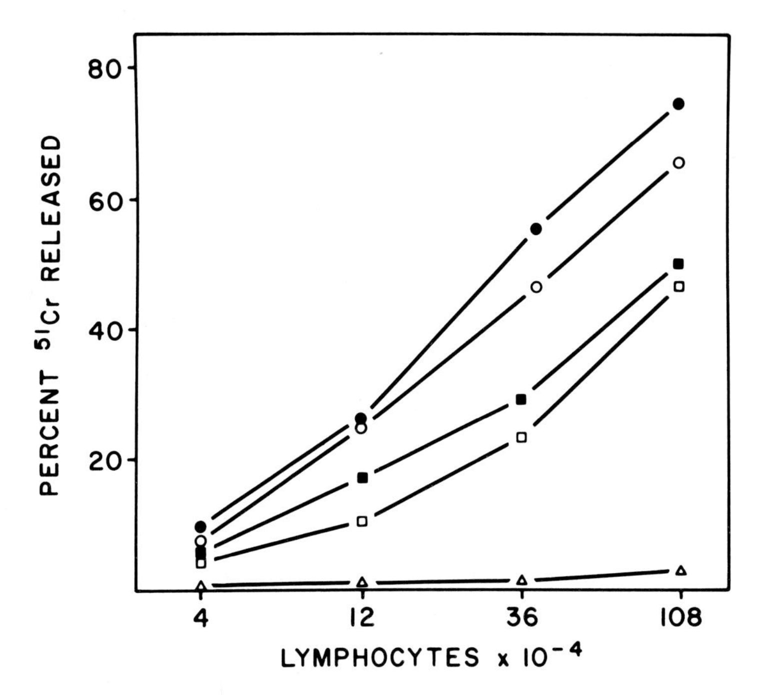

FIGURE 2. Inability of anti-human F(ab')$_2$ antibodies to prevent the recovery of SpCMC of trypsin-treated lymphocytes upon in vitro culture. Lymphocytes were filtered twice on nylon wool columns, according to Julius et al. (1973) in order to minimize the contamination with monocytes and B cells. They were treated with trypsin (Sigma, Bovine Trypsin type XI, 1 mg/ml/10^7 cells) for 20 min at 37°C, washed three times and tested for SpCMC against ^{51}Cr-labeled K562 target cells in a 4-hr assay. The assay was performed immediately after the enzymatic treatment, or after incubation of the cells at 37°C for 18 hr in media with or without rabbit F(ab')$_2$ IgG fragments anti-human IgG F(ab')$_2$ (Cappel, 100 µg/ml/2 x 10^6 cells). The cytotoxic test with the lymphocytes incubated with the anti-human F(ab')$_2$ reagent was performed in the presence of the same concentration of antiserum. ●—● control lymphocytes after 18 hr incubation in normal medium. ○—○ control lymphocytes incubated in medium containing anti-human F(ab')$_2$ anti-antibodies. △—△ trypsin treated lymphocytes. ■—■ trypsin treated lymphocytes incubated in medium containing anti-human F(ab')$_2$ antibodies.

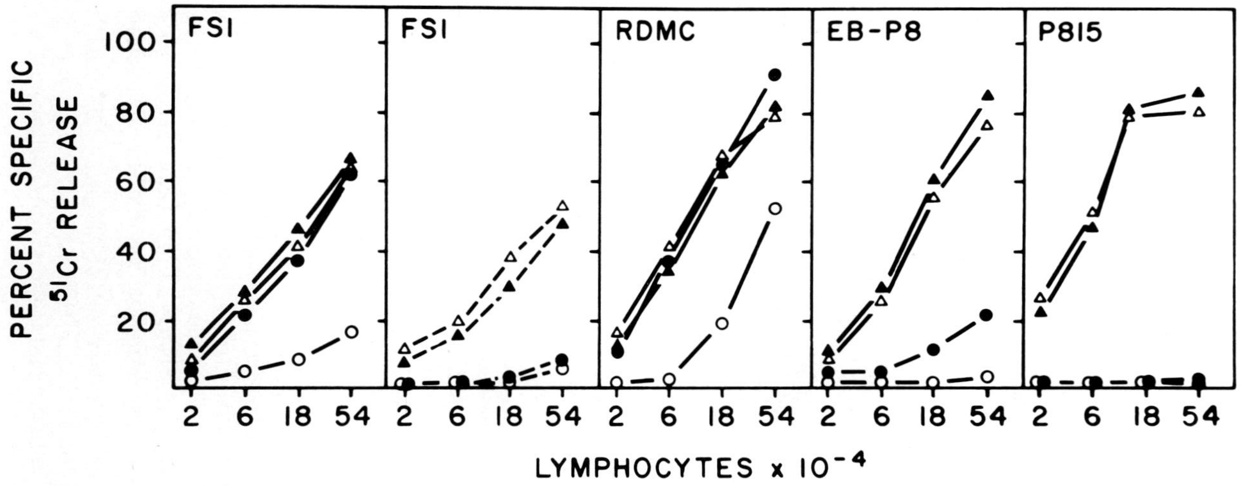

FSI

FSI

RDMC

EB-P8

P815

PERCENT SPECIFIC ^{51}Cr RELEASE

100 80 60 40 20

2 6 18 54 2 6 18 54 2 6 18 54 2 6 18 54 2 6 18 54

LYMPHOCYTES x 10^{-4}

FIGURE 3

Differential effect of interferon on K and NK cell activity.

We have shown that IF have a complex modulatory effect on the spontaneous cytotoxicity and that they affect both the activity of effector NK cells and the susceptibility to lysis of their target cells (Trinchieri et al., 1978a). The effect on the two partners of the cytotoxic reaction are paradoxically opposite: NK cell activity is several-fold enhanced, whereas certain target cells are protected by lysis.

All three known types of human IF (fibroblast and leukocyte type I, and type II) increase the human NK cell activity against different target cells up to 10-20 times. They also induce a proportional target cell resistance to lysis. In the same experimental conditions, the activity of K cells is either not enhanced or increased only 2 or 3 times

---

FIGURE 3. Differential effect of IF on spontaneous and antibody-dependent cell-mediated cytotoxicity. Lymphocytes obtained from one donor were incubated at 37°C for 18 hr in normal medium, or in medium containing partially purified fibroblast IF (1000 U/ml/5 x 10^6 cells; kindly provided by Dr. A. Billiau, Leuven, Belgium). After incubation, the lymphocytes were washed twice and tested for spontaneous and antibody-dependent cytotoxicity in a 4-hr ^{51}Cr-release assay against different target cells that were unsensitized or sensitized with specific antibodies. FS1 (human fetal skin fibroblast) and RDMC (rhabdomyosarcoma-derived human line) cells were used as target cells in monolayer (Santoli et al., 1978b). For sensitization, the monolayers were incubated with a 1:100 dilution of rabbit antiserum to human cells and washed before the test. EB-P8 (human EBV-transformed B cell line) and P815Y (murine BALB/c mastocytoma cell line) were tested as target cells in suspension and sensitized with 0.1 mg/ml human IgG anti-HLA antigens or with a 1:5000 dilution of rabbit anti-mouse cell antiserum, respectively. Immediately before the test, the lymphocytes used as effectors against FS1 target cells were also treated with trypsin under the same conditions described in the legend to Figure 2. ○—○, lymphocytes incubated in normal medium, tested against unsensitized target cells; ●—● , IF-treated lymphocytes, tested against unsensitized target cells; △—△ , lymphocytes incubated in normal medium, tested against IgG antibody-sensitized target cells; ▲—▲ IF-treated lymphocytes, tested against IgG antibody-sensitized target cells. Broken lines (----) refer to trypsin-treated lymphocytes.

(Herberman _et al_., 1979). The target cells used for testing K cell activity are also somewhat susceptible to NK activity. Treatment of lymphocytes with IF activates NK cells and may determine an increase in the background spontaneous cytotoxicity against unsensitized target cells: as a consequence, an apparent increase in the cytotoxicity against antibody-coated target cells is often observed. When target cells that are very susceptible to NK activity are used (e.g., FS1 and RDMC in Fig. 3), the increase in spontaneous cytotoxicity may mask the antibody-dependent cytotoxicity and, therefore, similar proportions of unsensitized and antibody-sensitized target cells are killed. When the lysis due to NK cells is abrogated by treatment of the effector cells with trypsin, no increase of the antibody-dependent cytotoxicity is observed over the control values (Fig. 3). When target cells not sensitive to NK cell-lysis are used (e.g., EB-P8 or P815Y in Fig. 3), no increase is observed. Identical results have been obtained using leukocyte type I and type II IF and IF-inducers such as influenza and Newcastle disease virus, instead of semipurified fibroblast-IF. Herberman _et al_. (1980), using more purified IF preparations, were able to show an increase in K cell activity, but this increase was always lower than that observed using K562 target cells, in which the NK cell enhancing effect of IF is usually limited.

In view of the possibility that both SpCMC and AbCMC are mediated by the same cell, we could interpret these data to suggest that IF is acting on NK cells at the recognition level, facilitating the contact between effector and target cells. In the presence of IgG antibodies on the target cells, the binding would be almost optimal due to the high affinity of the IgG-Fc receptors present on the effector cells. The enhancing effect of IF would then be only minimal. Interferons also mediate protection of target cells by acting at the recognition level, as demonstrated in competition experiments. In this case, there is a blocking effect (Trinchieri _et al_., 1978). Alternatively, IF could act by increasing the rate of killing, allowing each effector cell to lyse a higher number of target cells in the same time interval. In AbCMC the inactivation of the effector cells, due to a modification of the IgG-Fc receptors (Ziegler and Henney, 1975), probably occurs after the first round of lysis. An effect of IF on the rate of cytotoxicity would then be difficult to detect. The limited increase in AbCMC observed by Herberman et al. (1980) could be due to an additional effect on the recruitment of previously inactive cytotoxic cells.

The observation that IF has a protective effect on target cells for NK cytotoxicity, described in detail elsewhere in this volume, supports the hypothesis that the mechanisms of target cell recognition by K and NK cells are different. IF-treated fibroblasts become completely resistant to the cytotoxic effect of NK cells, but are lysed by K cells when sensitized with IgG antibodies. If one eliminates the unlikely possibility that IF specifically suppress the expression of the antigen(s) recognized by "natural cytophilic" antibodies, then these data argue against the possibility that recognition and lysis of target cells by NK cells is mediated by antibodies.

REFERENCES

Akira, D., and Takasugi, M. *Int. J. Cancer 19*,747-755 (1977).
Bolhuis, R.L.H., Shuit, H.R.E., Nooyen, A.M., and Routeltap, C.P.M., *Eur. J. Immunol. 8*,731-740 (1978).
Casali, P., and Perussia, B. *Clin. Exp. Immunol. 27*, 38-42, (1977).
Cerottini, J.-C., and Brunner, K.T., *Adv. Immunol. 18*,67-132, (1974).
Cordier, G., Samurut, C., and Revillard, J.P., *J. Immunol. 119*,1943-1968 (1977).
Harfast, B., Torbjörn, A., Stejskal, V., and Perlmann, P., *J. Immunol., 118*, 1132-1137 (1977).
Herberman, R.B., Ortaldo, J.R., and Bonnard, G.D. *Nature, 277*, 221-223 (1979).
Herberman, R.B., Ortaldo, J.R., Djeu, J.Y., Holden, H.T., and Jett, J. *NY Acad. Sci., in press* (1980).
Jondal, M., and Pross, H. *Int. J. Cancer, 15*,596-605 (1975).
Julius, M.H., Simpson, E., and Herzenberg, L.A., *Eur. J. Immunol. 3*,645-649 (1973).
Kay, H.D., Bonnard, G.D., West, W.W., and Herberman, R.B. *J. Immunol. 122*,675-685 (1979).
Kedar, E., DeLandazuri, M., and Bonavida, B.,*J. Immunol. 112*, 1231-1243 (1974).

Koide, Y., and Takasugi, M. *J. Natl. Cancer Inst. 59,* 1099-1105 (1977).
Moretta, L., Mingari, M.C., and Romanzi, C.A., *Nature 272,* 618-619 (1978).
Nelson, D.L., Bundy, B.M., and Strober, W., *J. Immunol. 119,* 1401-1405 (1977).
Perussia, B., Trinchieri, G., and Cerottini, J.-C., *Transplant. Proc. 11,* 793-795 (1979a).
Perussia, B., Trinchieri, G., and Cerottini, J.-C., *J. Immunol. 123,*681-687 (1979b).
Perussia, B., Santoli, D., and Trinchieri, G., *NY Acad. Sci. in press* (1980).
Revillard, J.P., Samarut, C., Cordier, G., and Brochier, J. in: "Membrane Receptors of Lymphocytes" (M. Seligman, J.L. Preud'Homme and F.M. Kourilsky, eds.), pp. 171-184. North Holland, Amsterdam.
Santoli, D., Trinchieri, G., Zmijewski, C.M., and Koprowski, H., *J. Immunol. 117,* 765-770 (1976).
Santoli, D., Trinchieri, G., and Koprowski, H., *J. Immunol. 121,* 532-538 (1978a).
Santoli, D., Trinchieri, G., Moretta, L., Zmijewski, C.M., and Koprowski, H., *Clin. Exp. Immunol. 33,* 309-318 (1978b).
Trinchieri, G., Bauman, P., DeMarchi, M., and Tökés, Z., *J. Immunol. 115,* 243-255 (1975).
Trinchieri, G., Santoli, D., Zmijewski, C.M., and Koprowski, H., *Transplant. Proc. 9,*881-884 (1977).
Trinchieri, G., Santoli, D., Dee, R.R., and Knowles, B.B. *J. Exp. Med. 147,* 1299-1313 (1978a).
Trinchieri, G., and Santoli, D., *J. Exp. Med. 147,* 1314-1333 (1978b).
Trinchieri, G., Santoli, D., and Koprowski, H., *J. Immunol. 120,* 1843-1855 (1978c).
Troye, M., Perlmann, P., Pape, G.R., Smegelberg, H.L., Näslund, J., and Gidlöf, A., *J. Immunol. 119,* 1061-1067 (1977).
West, W.H., Cannon, G.B., Kay, H.D., Bonnard, G.D., and Herberman, R.B., *J. Immunol. 118,* 355-361 (1977a).
West, W.H., Payne, S.M., Weese, J.L., and Herberman, R.B. *J. Immunol. 119,* 548-554 (1977b).
West, W.H., Boozen, R.B., and Herberman, R.B., *J. Immunol. 120,* 90-95 (1978).
Ziegler, H.K., and Henney, C.S., *J. Immunol. 115,* 1500-1504 (1975).
Ziegler, H.K., and Henney, C.S., *J. Immunol. 119,* 1010-1017 (1977a).
Ziegler, H.K., Geyer, C., and Henney, C.S., *J. Immunol. 119,* 1821-1829 (1977b).

A COMPARATIVE ANALYSIS OF THE NK CYTOLYTIC MECHANISM AND REGULATORY GENES [1]

John C. Roder
and
T. Haliotis

Department of Microbiology and Immunology
Queen's University
Kingston, Ontario
Canada K7L 3N6

I. THE LYTIC CYCLE

NK mediated cytolysis can be divided into 4 discrete stages: (i) recognition and binding to the target, (ii) triggering and activation of the lytic mechanism, (iii) lethal hit, and (iv) target cell death. ^{51}Cr release assays measure the end results of the entire cycle and an assay was required to dissect the earlier stages of target-effector interaction. Therefore we devised a target-binding-cell assay (TBC) to visualise target-effector contact (1, 2), based on earlier studies in the CTL system (3-5).

Investigations into the nature of the nylon non-adherent lymphocyte binding to target cells (TBC) revealed that the frequency of TBC and the level of lysis in a population were closely correlated in kinetics experiments and under varying biological conditions of age, organ site, genotype and target selectivity. The genes controlling the frequency of TBC were inherited in a dominant fashion and were linked to the H-2 complex as shown in backcross experiments. In addition, cell populations enriched or depleted in TBC by velocity sedimentation showed a corresponding increase or decrease in the ability to lyse YAC targets and the majority of single TBC isolated in droplets or monodispersed in agar killed the target to which they were attached. This suggests that (i) the majority of TBC detected are indeed NK cells, and (ii) the lytic event is independent of helper cells although the

[1] *Supported by the M.R.C. and N.C.I. of Canada*

ISBN 0-12-341350-8

involvement of soluble factors and helper or suppressor cells in the formation of TBC cannot be excluded. It is not yet known if NK cells can recycle to lyse several targets as in the CTL system (4). Binding to the target was found to be a necessary pre-requisite for lysis to occur. If cell contact was inhibited by EDTA, lysis was not observed and in kinetics experiments target cell binding was detectable 5-10 min prior to measurable cell damage. In addition, when both target cell binding and lysis were abolished by trypsinisation of the effector (or by papain and pronase) both functions regenerated in a parallel time course in the absence of cycloheximide which is compatible with the suggestion that binding occurs prior to lysis and is mediated by "protein like" cell surface "recognition" structures. Prolonged (3 hr) treatment with puromycin and cycloheximide alone also prevented TBC formation possibly by blocking the synthesis of the recognition receptor. One can speculate that H-2 linked genes controlling the TBC frequency might code for the putative NK recognition receptor.

Target-lymphocyte contact alone, irrespective of the effector cell properties, was not a sufficient condition for lysis since nylon retained spleen cells did not lyse the targets to which they attached. These results are reminiscent of findings in the CTL system but TBC in the NK system are unique. Whereas CTL are totally prevented from binding to target cells at low temperatures or in the presence of metabolic inhibitors (6, 7) NK cells do form stable contacts with the target in similar drug concentrations and binding is also evident at $0^{O}C$ (although less avid than at higher temperatures). This suggests that energy is required for binding by CTL but not NK cells.

Membrane and cytoskeleton integrity may also be important in the NK-target binding step. The aprotic dipolar solvent, dimethylsufoxide (DMSO), inhibited NK mediated binding (8). Although the mechanism of drug action is not entirely clear, this agent would be expected to destabilise the plasma membrane and lead to a disorganisation of integral membrane proteins, including recognition receptors (9). Secondary inhibition of the lytic phase could also occur if free radicals are involved since DMSO is also a free radical scavenger. In the CTL system DMSO inhibits the CTL-target contact phase (9) but its effects on the lytic step are controversial (9, 10). Cytochalasin B also inhibited TBC and lysis in the NK system but it was not possible to assess if the lytic stage was inhibited independently or by virtue of inhibition of the earlier TBC stage. In the CTL system, target binding but not the lytic step, is inhibited (reviewed in 11) and the available evidence favours the view that the relevant drug action involves disruption of microtubules (12) rather than secondary effects such as inhibition of glucose transport (13). Since tightly opposed interdigitating microvilli are observed in the area of NK-target contact (2), it is conceivable that such tertiary strengthening of the adhesion is dependent on cell motility and therefore requires intact microtubules. These results raise the possibility that membrane and cytoskeleton organisation may be important for NK-target binding. However, the free movement of integral membrane proteins may not be necessary since the protein cross-linking agent, glutaraldehyde, completely abolished lysis with only partial inhibition of the target binding phase (8).

The target cell requirements for step 1 in this target-effector interaction in the NK system are less well studied. However, biochemical isolation procedures have established that the NK-target "antigen" on the surface of target cells consists of up to three glycoprotein molecules of M.W. 120K-240K (14,15) as discussed above in the "Specificity" section. The expression of these target antigens may be blocked by interferon (16) and may be controlled by differentiation genes as suggested by studies of somatic cell hybrids between NK sensitive and insensitive targets (15). These structures are also cleaved by trypsin and pronase and turn over at a low rate (>3 hr), (Roder and Argov, unpublished observation). Energy metabolism does not appear to be important and in other systems it has been shown that neither protein synthesis, RNA or DNA synthesis is required and indeed, enucleated targets are lysed equally well by NK cells (140).

The triggering of NK cells (step 2), subsequent to making contact with the target cell, appears to involve two pathways which may or may not be linked, namely energy metabolism and the cyclic nucleotide system. The lytic phase of NK cytolysis was blocked by DNP, NaN_3 or low temperature (2) as observed for CTL mediated cytolysis (6, 10). CTL cytolysis was more temperature dependent than NK cytolysis (8) although as previously shown, CTL responding to a secondary challenge are less temperature dependent than primary CTL (11). Inhibitors of glycolysis such as iodoacetate and NaF also block the NK lytic phase which suggests that the energy necessary for NK lysis may be derived from both glycolysis and oxidative phosphorylation as in the CTL system (8). Dibutyryl cAMP (dB-cAMP) and the cAMP elevating agents, prostaglandin E_1, theophylline and histamine markedly suppressed NK cytolytic function with no effect on TBC formation (18). Conversely, dB-cGMP and carbamylcholine accelerated the rate of lysis to a small but significant degree and could compete with inhibitory doses of dB-cAMP to reduce the level of suppression thereby suggesting that the cAMP/cGMP ratio might be important in NK mediated lysis.

The mechanism by which cyclic nucleotides modulate NK cytolysis is unclear but perhaps the most attractive hypothesis is a "stimulus-secretion" model. Under this model, target-effector contact, via specific recognition structures, leads to an alteration in intracellular cyclic nucleotide levels which in turn triggers a lytic event in the effector cell. The observation that cAMP or cGMP active agents alter NK cytolysis with no effect on the target cell contact phase favours this sequence of events.

The nature of the lytic events (step 3) is entirely unclear but within the "stimulus-secretion" model of NK cytolysis we postulate that lysosomal enzymes may be the actual lytic moiety since (i) chloroquine a selective lysosomal inhibitor, inhibited NK cytolysis as well as lysosomal enzymes (8), (ii) the mutation on chromosome 13 of the mouse, beige, results in both defective lysosomal enzyme function and a profound impairment in the NK lytic mechanism, whereas the level of TBC are normal (19, 20) and (iii) the same concentrations and variety of agents which inhibit the lytic phase of NK cytolysis (cAMP, PGE_1, theophylline, histamine, high dose epiniphrine) (18) also inhibit lysosome secretion in cells (21) and conversely agents which increase lysosomal discharge (cGMP, carbamylcholine) significantly augment NK lysis; (iv) inhibitors of serine esterases, phenylmethylsulfonylfloride and diisopropylflorophosphate, inhibited NK cytolysis but not TBC formation (2) and (v) interferon enhances NK cytolysis (22) and is also known to augment IgE mediated histamine release from basophils (23) and therefore might also cause the release of lysosomal enzyme containing granules. If lysosomes are involved in target destruction, then a special localised mode of delivery is implicated since "innocent bystanders" were not killed in NK cytolytic experiments (8). These observations suggest that the lysosome dependent, "stimulus-secretion" model is worthy of further investigation in the NK system.

Although we favour a serine protease as the actual lytic moiety, others have argued that lymphotoxin (24-26) or complement (27) may be involved in cell-mediated cytolysis. Lymphotoxin has previously been an unlikely candidate at least in the T cell system since cytolysis can be completely inhibited under conditions which do not inhibit the production of lymphotoxin (28). Recently however more sensitive techniques have revealed that upon activation alloimmune T cells release large molecular weight aggregates of lymphotoxin which appear to be associated with specific T cell receptors (24). However, even if lymphotoxin is the lytic moiety, in the CTL system there is no reason to believe the same mechanism is involved in NK cytolysis, a priori. Some of the arguments which indirectly support the complement hypothesis are as follows: (i) Inhibitors of serine proteases block NK killing (2) and key enzymatic steps in the complement cascade, (ii) in retrospect there is a correlation between the ability of some cell lines to activate complement (29) and its susceptibility to NK mediated lysis, (iii) complement bridges have recently been demonstrated between cells (3), (iv) the kinetics of NK mediated killing and mode of cell death strongly resemble complement mediated lysis, (v) some unpublished observations suggest that anti-complement antibody to the terminal components may block killing by cytotoxic T lymphocytes, (vi) some forms of cytolysis such as ADCC are enhanced by complement (31). It is clear that more direct experiments are required to elucidate the lethal hit stage of NK cytolysis and to allow a choice between these competing hypothesis.

The effect of hormones on NK activity has also been investigated. Insulin had no effect in vitro on NK cells whereas CTL mediated cytolysis was boosted (18). Insulin is thought to act through the cGMP system (32) and we have shown that cGMP causes a small but significant enhancement of NK cell activity (18). Therefore, NK cells, which are small "resting" lymphocytes, may lack the insulin receptors found on activated CTL (33). Adrenalin had both augmenting and suppressive effects depending on the concentration (Roder and Klein, unpublished observation) whereas B-estradiol administered in vivo was suppressive (34).

A number of genes are almost certainly involved in the lytic cycle although their precise location in the scheme of events is unknown. H-2 linked genes on chromosome 17 determine the size of the NK pool and possibly code for the recognition receptor on NK cells although this remains speculative (1). Genes on chromosome 2, 5 and 21 in the human code for interferon production as well as elements involved in interferon action. In addition a gene, bg, on chromosome 13 in the mouse is involved in some post recognition event in the lytic cycle (see below), possibly related to lysosome function. Since interferon does not fully restore the bg defect then the interferon sensitive event probably occurs earlier in the lytic cycle.

II. THE BEIGE MUTATION IN THE MOUSE

Germ line mutations affecting defined cell populations are often valuable tools in elucidating the function of these cells in complex biological systems such as cytolysis. We have recently found that a mutant gene in the mouse called beige (bg^J), leads to a partial and selective impairment of naturally occurring killer lymphocytes (2), whereas other forms of cytolysis mediated by T cells, macrophages and promonocytes are apparently normal (35). This defect in NK cytolysis was predetermined at the level of progenitor cells in the bone marrow as revealed in radiation chimaeras (19). This impairment in NK function shown in ref. 19 could not be accounted for by an altered organ distribution, target selectivity or ontogenesis. Interferon could improve but not fully restore the response which suggests that the defect does not result from a lack of endogenous interferon stimulation in beige mice. The frequency of target binding cells was normal in all lymphoid organs (19) which suggests that the defect is intrinsic to the NK cell and does not involve an altered population size or an inability to recognise and interact with the target. Rather, the defect may lie within the lytic pathway subsequent to target cell contact. The bg gene provides the first defined genetic marker for sequencing the events involved in the cytolytic pathway and shows that the cytolytic mechanisms in different effector cell types are distinct.

The bg mutant also provided an opportunity to re-examine the relationship between NK and ADCC effector cells. ADCC against chicken erythrocytes was found normal in bg/bg mice (19). This form of cytolysis is mediated by a variety of different effectors including FcR^+, adherent cells in the mouse (36, 37) and monocytes or granulocytes in the human system (38). Therefore it is likely that the cytolytic function of these cell populations in the beige mouse is normal. Some of the ADCC against tumour cells is mediated by different lymphocytic effectors, called K cells (39), and this population is defective in beige mice. However ADCC against tumour cells mediated by promonocytes from beige mice was normal (35) which indicates that the NK/ADCC defect in beige lymphocytes is not simply due to a generalised failure in the ADCC mechanism against tumour cells. Since ADCC against P815 tumour cells was deficient in beige mice these observations strongly suggest that NK and K cells are identical. This view is supported by recent work showing

NK and K cells have similar properties (40). In addition antibody-coated, NK insensitive P815 cells compete with NK cytolysis of ^{51}Cr labelled YAC cells in a cold target inhibition assay (36). It would seem, therefore, that NK cells in the mouse are capable of lysing tumour cells by two independent recognition mechanisms; one antibody dependent and the other antibody independent.

III. THE HUMAN ANALOGUE OF THE BEIGE MUTATION

The beige mouse has been used for over 10 years as a model for the Chediak-Higashi syndrome in man (41). Both species exhibit abnormal leukocyte granulation and pigmentation, whereas their immune responsiveness is intact. If the defective NK gene in the beige mouse was closely linked or identical to the gene controlling leukocyte granulation then it was predicted that Chediak-Higashi patients should also have abnormal NK function.

Two patients carrying the rare, autosomal recessive CH gene were examined and found to have a profound defect (over 100 fold) in their ability to spontaneously lyse various tumor cells by antibody dependent or independent mechanisms (42). Other forms of killing mediated by monocytes, neutrophils and T cells was relatively normal. As found in the beige mouse, the ability of CH lymphocytes to bind to target cells was not impaired and therefore the defect in the human may also effect a post recognition event.

These two genes, bg and CH, may not only be important as defined genetic markers for sequencing the NK cytolytic pathway but they provide an opportunity to unequivocally assess the importance of the NK cell in surveillance against neoplasia. Preliminary studies show that the beige mouse is more susceptible to the growth and dissemination of transplantable tumors (43, 44) and CH patients surviving childhood infections almost invariably develop a lymphoproliferative disorder which may be malignant (45). It is becoming increasingly likely therefore that NK cells are involved in surveillance against at least some tumors.

IV. CONCLUSIONS

A picture of the NK cytolytic mechanism is emerging (Table 1) in which various genes control and regulate

TABLE I. Model of NK cytolysis

Steps	Relevant molecules structures or processes	Genes	Supporting system	Stimulators	Inhibitors
1. CONTACT	-surface protein recognition moiety (cation requirement)	chrom.17 H-2 linked (mouse)	protein synth. (E. metabolism not required)		-trypsin/pronase/papain -puromycin/cycloheximide -EDTA/DMSO
BINDING	-microvilli "engulfment"	?	cyto-skeleton		-cytochalasin B - colchicine
2. TRIGGER	-cAMP/cGMP	?	adenylate cyclase	cGMP carbamyl-choline	-cAMP/PGE1/theophylline -histamine/epinephrine
	-ATP?	?	-glycolysis -oxidative phosphorylation		-DNP -NaN_3NaF/iodoacetate
REGULATOR (interferon sensitive)	IF-production IF-receptor IF-target	chrom.5 (2) and chrom.21 (human)	-protein synthesis -ganglioside synthesis	-interferon -poly I:C -NDV -tilorone	anti-IF antibody
3. LETHAL HIT	-lysosomal enzymes	chrom.13 ch/bg gene	-golgi and secretory vesicles	-cGMP -carbamyl choline	- chloroquine - PMSF/DIFP - glutaraldehyde
4. TARGET DEATH	- colloid osmotic lysis				

This table combines data obtained in both human and mouse experimental systems. References are given in text.

PMSF, phenylmethylsufonylfluoride, and DIFP, diisopropylflorophosphate are inhibitors of serine proteases.

discrete steps in the lytic cycle. H-2 linked genes on chromosome 17 control the initial stage of target-effector recognition either through their regulation of population size and/or the putative recognition receptor itself. Surface glycoproteins, which are important for recognition, have been isolated from the target cell membrane. Target recognition is postulated to trigger the cyclic nucleotide system which turns on those energy pathways important in the activation of the actual lytic moiety (lysosomal enzymes?). These intervening steps are susceptible to the action of genes regulating the production of, or response to, interferon. Finally the terminal stages of the cycle, close to the lethal hit are regulated by the bg gene in the mouse and the CH gene in the human. This model is amenable to further investigation, and shows that the mechanism of NK cytolysis is distinct from that in T cells, promonocytes, macrophages/monocytes or neutrophils.

REFERENCES

1. Roder, J.C., and Kiessling,R.,*Scand. J. Immunol.8,135* (1978).
2. Roder, J. C., Kiessling, R., Biberfeld, P., and Andersson, B., *J. Immunol. 121*, 2509 (1978).
3. Ryser, J. E., Sordat, B., Cerottini, J.C., and Brunner, K.T. *Eur. J. Immunol. 7*, 110 (1977).
4. Zagury, D., Bernard, N., Thierness, N., Feldman, M., and Berke, G., *Eur. J. Immunol.* 5, 818 (1975).
5. Grimm, E.A. and Bonavida, B., *J. Immunol.119*, 1041(1977).
6. Berke, G., and Gabison, D., *Eur. J. Immunol.* 5, 671 (1975).
7. Martz, E. Cont. Top.Immunobiol. (ed.O. Stutman) Plenum Press, N.Y. vol. 7, 301 (1977).
8. Roder, J. C., Argov, S., Klein, M., Petersson, C., Kiessling, R., Andersson, K., and Hansson, M., *Immunol* (in press).
9. Walberg, G., Hiemstra, K., Burge, J., and Singler, R., *J. Immunol. 111*, 1435 (1973).
10. Goldstein, P., and Smith, E.T., Cont. Top. Immunobiol. (O. Stutman, ed.) Plenum Press, N.Y. 7,273 (1977).
11. Cerottini, J.C. and Brunner, K.T. In "B and T cells in immune recognition" (F. Loor and G. E. Roelants, edgs.) Wyley and Sons, Chichester Chpt. 14, 319 (1977).
12. Kalina, M., and Hollander, N., *Immunol. 29*,709 (1975).
13. Bubbers, J.E., and Henney, C.S., *J. Immunol. 115*, 145 (1975).
14. Roder, J.C., Rosen, A., Fenyo, E.M., and Troy, F.A. *Proc. Natl. Acad. Sci. 76*, 1405 (1979).
15. Roder, J.C., Ahrlund-Richter, L., and Jondal, M., *J. Exp. Med. 150*, 471 (1979).
16. Santoli, D., Trinchieri, G., and Koprowski, H., *J. Immunol. 121*, 532 (1978).
17. Siliciano, R., and Henney, C.S., *J. Immunol. 121*,186 (1978).
18. Roder, J.C., and Klein, M., *J. Immunol. 123*, 2785 (1979).
19. Roder, J.C., *J. Immunol. 123*, 2168 (1979).
20. Roder, J.C., and Duwe, A.K., Nature 278, 451 (1979).
21. Wismann, G., Goldstein .I., Hoffstein, S., and Tsung, P.K., *Ann. N.Y. Acad. Sci. 253*, 750 (1975).
22. Gidlund, M., Orn. A., Wigzell, H., Senik, A., and Gresser, I., Nature 273, 759 (1978).
23. Ida, S., Hooks, J.J., Siraganian, R.P., and Notkins,A.L., *J. Exp. Med. 145*, 892 (1977).
24. Hiserodt, J.C., Tiango, G., and Granger, G., *J. Immunol. 123*, 332 (1979).

25. Tsoukas, C.D., Rosenau, W., and Baxter, J.D. *J. Immunol.* *116*, 184 (1976).
26. Bonnard, G.D. In "Perspectives in Immunology" (Riethmuller G., Wernet, P., and Cudkowicz, G., eds.) Academic Press, N.Y. in press.
27. Mayer, M.M., *J. Immunol.* *119*, 1195 (1977).
28. Henney, C.S., Gaffney, J., and Bloom, B.R., *J. Exp. Med.* *140*, 837 (1974).
29. Yefenof, E., Klein, G., and Kvarnung, K. *Cell. Immunol.* *31*, 225 (1977).
30. Dierich, M., and Landen, B., *J. Exp. Med.* *146*, 1484 (1977).
31. Rouse, B.T., Grewal, A.S., and Babiuk, L.A., Nature 266, 456 (1977).
32. Strom, T.B., Bear, R., and Carpenter, C., Science 187, 1206 (1975).
33. Hildeman, J.H., and Strom, T.B., Nature 274, 62 (1978).
34. Seaman, W.E., Blackman, M.A., Ginghart, T.,Roubinian,J.R. Loeb, J.M., and Talal, N., *J. Immunol.* *121*, 2193 (1979).
35. Roder, J.C., Lohmann-Matthes, M.L., Domzig, W., and Wigzell, H., *J. Immunol.* *123*, 2174 (1979).
36. Ojo, E., and Wigzell, H., *Scand. J. Immunol.* *7*,297 (1978).
37. Kiessling, R., Petranyi, G., Karre, K., Jondal, M., Tracey, D., and Wigzell, H., *J. Exp. Med.* *143*, 112 (1976).
38. Nelson, D.L., Bundy, B.M., Pitchon, H.E., and Blease, R.M., *J. Immunol.* *117*, 1472 (1976).
39. Perlmann, P., and Cerottini, J.C., In "The Antigens" vol. 5 (Academic Press, N.Y.) in press.
40. Santoni, A., Herberman, R.B., and Holden, H.T., *J. Natl. Cancer Inst.* *62*, 109 (1979).
41. Windhorst, D.B. and Padgett, G., *J. Invest. Derm.* *60*, 529 (1973).
42. Roder, J.C., Haliotis, T., Klein, M., Korec, S., Jett, J., Ortaldo, J., Herberman, R.B., Katz, P., and Fauci, A.S., submitted.
43. Talmadge, J.E., Meyers, K., Prieur, D., and Starkey, J.R., submitted.
44. Karre, K., Klein, G.O., Kiessling, R., and Roder, J., submitted.
45. Dent, P.B., Fish, L.A., White, J.F., and Good, R.A., *Lab. Invest.* *15*, 1634 (1966).

SUMMARY: MECHANISM OF CYTOTOXICITY BY NK CELLS AND THEIR RELATIONSHIP TO K CELLS

One of the intriguing observations that has been made in the past two or three years with NK cells is their close relationship to K cells mediating antibody-dependent, cell-mediated cytotoxicity (ADCC). With the findings of many similarities in the characteristics of NK and K cells, and the suggestions that they may even be the same cells, there has been intensive investigation into the possibility that NK activity may represent a form of ADCC, mediated by K cells interacting via their Fc receptors for IgG ($Fc_{\gamma}R$) with natural antibodies to NK-susceptible target cells. The chapters in this section provide a detailed and up-to-date summary of much of the available information about this issue.

I. NK AND K CELLS IN SIMILAR OR IDENTICAL SUBPOPULATIONS

As reported previously (Kay *et al.*, 1977; Santoni, *et al.*, 1979a,b; Ojo and Wigzell, 1978; Landazuri *et al.*, 1979) and in several chapters in this and other sections of the book, an impressive body of evidence has accumulated, indicating many similarities between NK cells and K cells (summarized in Table I). In addition to the parallel expression of these activities under a variety of circumstances and much similarity in cell surface markers, recent data point directly towards the probability that the same effector cells can mediate NK and ADCC. This was first demonstrated by cold target inhibition studies, in which some unlabeled NK target cells could appreciably inhibit ADCC (Ojo and Wigzell, 1978; Landazuri *et al.*, 1979; chapter by Koren and Jensen). In addition, and even more convincingly, it has been possible to deplete much or almost all K cell activity by adsorption to monolayers of some NK-sensitive target cells. Thus, it appears appropriate to refer to most of the responsible effector cells as NK/K cells. The human NK/K cells appear to have the morphology of large granular lymphocytes (see chapters by Saksela and Timonen and by Herberman *et al.*, in Section IA).

ISBN 0-12-341350-8

TABLE I. Summary of Similarities between NK and K Cells

Effect of age	*In mice, activities absent at birth, peak at 5-9 weeks, then low; in humans, activities relatively stable.*
Expression among individuals	*Activities high in some mouse strains (e.g., CBA and nudes) and low in others (SJL, beige); some human donors high in both activities and others low.*
Organ distribution	*Activity in blood, spleen, peritoneal cavity, bone marrow; low in human tonsil and lymph nodes; absent in thymus.*
Cell surface markers	*In mice, low density of Thy 1 on portion of NK and K; NK1, Ly5 and FcγR on most; in humans, low affinity receptors for sheep erythrocytes on portion and virtually all susceptible to anti-T cell sera + C; all NK vs. K562 have detectable FcγR.*
Size and morphology	*In mice, both activities cofractionate on gradients; in humans, both are in population of large granular lymphocytes.*
In vitro *culture*	*Parallel lability in mice; in humans, parallel generation from FcγR-cells in cultures with fetal bovine serum or allogeneic cells.*
Regulating factors	*Most studies indicate boosting of both activities by interferon or interferon-inducers; both activities inhibited by prostaglandins E_1 or E_2.*
Cold target inhibition	*Some unlabeled NK target cells inhibit ADCC.*
Monolayer adsorption	*Depletion of most K cells as well as NK cells on some monolayers of NK targets.*
Effect of X-ray	*Similar degrees of sensitivity.*

Although most of both activities appear to be mediated by the same cells, there are indications that some effector cells may have one function without the other. Koren and Jensen report here that cells of newborn miniature pigs have ADCC but not NK activity and that some cancer patients have depressed NK activity but normal levels of ADCC. Similarly, Pandolfi *et al.* (1980) have found that the leukemic cells of a patient with T cell chronic lymphocytic leukemia had strong ADCC activity but no detectable NK activity, even after treatment with interferon. There have also been some patients with normal levels of NK activity but low ADCC (e.g. some of the agammaglobulinemic patients of Koren and Jensen), and NK effector cells in certain organs (see Eremin) or against some targets (see Bolhuis and Herberman *et al.*, in Section IA) that lack $Fc_{\gamma}R$. The nature of the effector cells with only one of these cytotoxic functions, and their relationship to NK/K cells, remains unclear. Some studies clearly indicate (as discussed below) that modulation of $Fc_{\gamma}R$ on NK/K cells causes loss of ADCC activity with at least partial retention of NK activity. It seems possible, as suggested by Koren and Jensen, that most or all of the apparent discrepancies between NK and K cells may be due to failure to express either NK receptors or functional $Fc_{\gamma}R$ at certain points in differentiation of NK/K cells. Alternatively, there may be small subpopulations of effector cells that are programmed to express only $Fc_{\gamma}R$ or NK receptors, but not both.

II. ROLE OF $Fc_{\gamma}R$ IN NK ACTIVITY

Two major hypotheses have been developed to directly link the association between NK and ADCC activities:

1) Armed K cell hypothesis: This hypothesis, initially formulated by Koide and Takasugi (1977) and summarized here by Kamiyama and Takasugi, may be stated as follows: NK activity is mediated by K cells that are armed *in vivo* by natural antibodies attached to their $Fc_{\gamma}R$. Most of the support for this hypothesis has come from experiments indicating that mild proteolytic treatment of human peripheral blood mononuclear cells causes decreased NK activity but normal or increased ADCC, and that incubation of the treated cells with autologous serum partially or completely restores cytotoxicity against NK-susceptible target cells.

2) Hypothesis of ADCC with natural antibodies secreted during cytotoxicity assay: This hypothesis has been put forward by Troye *et al.* (1977) and may be summarized as follows: The observed NK activity is due to secretion

during the cytotoxicity assay of IgG antibodies by B cells or plasma cells, with consequent sensitization of the target cells and ADCC by K cells. To date, such natural antibodies have not been isolated from culture supernatants and the experimental evidence in support of this hypothesis has been indirect: Fab or $F(ab')_2$ fragments of antibodies to human IgG, when added to cytotoxicity assays have been found to partially inhibit the lysis of some NK-susceptible target cells.

Since these hypotheses have been put forward, several groups have taken a variety of approaches to determine the role of natural antibodies and $Fc_{\gamma}R$ in NK activity. These hypotheses have considerable intellectual appeal, since they would provide simple explanations for the close associations between NK and K cells and would allow a coming together of the well-established area of natural humoral immunity with the recent indications of natural cell-mediated immunity. However, many inconsistencies with, or contradictions to, these unifying hypotheses have emerged. Despite all of the similarities between NK and K cells, a number of differences between NK and ADCC activities has been seen (summarized in Table II). The most central challenge to these hypotheses has been the evidence against the requirement for functional $Fc_{\gamma}R$ for full expression of NK activity. As described here

TABLE II. General Evidence against Mediation of NK Activity by ADCC with Natural IgG Antibodies

1. *Retention of at least some NK activity after modulation or shedding of $Fc\gamma R$.*

2. *Substantial levels of NK activity in some patients with sex-linked agammaglobulinemia.*

3. *High levels of NK activity in mice with hypogammaglobulinemia induced by anti-IgM.*

4. *No detectable requirement for B cells in in vitro generation of NK activity.*

5. *Blocking of ADCC but not NK activity by various anti-lymphocyte antibodies.*

6. *Treatment of some targets with interferon decreased their susceptibility to NK activity but did not affect susceptibility to ADCC.*

by Bolhuis, Kay, and Perussia *et al.*, and as also reported by Pape *et al.* (1979), modulation and apparent loss of $Fc_{\gamma}R$ by incubation with immune complexes results in complete loss of ADCC activity. In contrast, some or all of the NK activity remains. This has indicated that at least an appreciable portion of NK activity is independent of functional $Fc_{\gamma}R$ and appears to be mediated by other types of recognition structures on the effector cells. Furthermore, several situations have been found in which substantial or even high levels of NK activity occur in the absence of detectable B cells. The NK activity of congenitally agammaglobulinemic patients (see Koren and Jensen; Pross) and of anti-IgM induced hypogammaglobulinemia in mice (see Gidlund *et al.*) is difficult to reconcile with a central role for natural antibodies. In addition, Kay and Perussia *et al.* have observed that trypsinized human lymphocytes regain their NK activity upon culture, even after depletion of cells bearing surface immunoglobulins and C3 receptors and in the presence of $F(ab')_2$ fragments of anti-IgG antibodies. Parallel evidence for regeneration of NK activity of enzyme-treated mouse and rat cells, in the absence of detectable B cells, has also been reported (Shellam, 1977; Santoni *et al.*, 1979b). Similarly, Ortaldo and Herberman (see chapter in Section IC2) have observed the *in vitro* generation of NK activity from $Fc_{\gamma}R$ negative precursors, even after depletion of all detectable B cells. It should be noted, however, that the evidence related to lack of B cells *in vivo* or *in vitro* is not conclusive. The agammaglobulinemic patients and mice have not been documented to be totally deficient in IgG antibodies. Persistence of low levels of natural antibodies might be sufficient to account for the observed NK activity. Also, the procedures used to deplete B cells *in vitro* may not have been adequate to remove all IgG producing cells, since mature plasma cells may lack surface membrane immunoglobulins.

In regard to the two particular hypotheses involving a role of natural antibodies in NK activity, further problems or contradictions need to be dealt with. Evidence against the armed K cell hypothesis is summarized in Table III. A primary difficulty has been the inability of most investigators (see Kay; Koren and Jensen; Perussia *et al.*) to reproduce the arming of trypsinized effector cells that has been reported by Takasugi's group. As suggested by Kamiyama and Takasugi, these differences may be technical, possibly related to some damage of the effector cells by extensive trypsinization. However, Koren and Jensen failed to observe arming with most normal sera for NK activity under the same conditions that gave good arming for ADCC against TNP-treated target cells. Another approach to the question of

TABLE III. Evidence against Role of Armed K Cells in NK Activity

---

1. *Failure to block NK activity by pre-treatment of effector cells with anti-immunoglobulin, including anti-Fab, reagents.*
2. *Elution of cytophilic IgG did not decrease NK activity.*
3. *Inability to consistently rearm trypsinized effector cells.*
4. *Failure to demonstrate natural antibodies in sera that are able to sensitize NK-sensitive target cells for ADCC.*

---

armed K cells has been to treat the effector cells in ways expected to elute off the cytophilic IgG or to block its activity. Incubation of cells at 37°, under conditions shown to elute off most or all detectable IgG has failed to eliminate or even reduce NK activity (Kay *et al.*, 1979; A. Sulica and R. B. Herberman, unpublished observations). It would be necessary to argue that the arming by natural antibodies for NK is more resistant to such elution than most cytophilic IgG and that the residual small amounts of attached IgG are sufficient for full expression of cytotoxic activity. The failure to sensitize NK-susceptible target cells for ADCC with normal sera would require other special attributes for the arming antibodies, since for most antibodies active in ADCC, sensitization of target cells has given stronger or more consistent results than arming of effector cells. A further important point to consider is that even if arming of trypsinized cells by natural antibodies can be conclusively documented, it would be difficult to determine whether this is the mechanism responsible for NK activity. Although such data are consistent with the hypothesis, an alternative argument can be raised: Both natural antibodies and natural cell-mediated immunity may exist against similar or even identical specificities on tumors and other target cells. The receptors for NK activity may be independent of IgG and susceptible to inactivation by trypsin and other proteolytic enzymes. Treatment of trypsinized cells with sera containing natural IgG antibodies could arm for ADCC, but this would be a phenomenon separate from, but parallel to, the original NK activity.

As summarized in Table IV, there have also been a number of specific objections raised against the hypothesis of NK

TABLE IV. Evidence against Role in NK Activity of Antibodies Produced during Assay

---

1. *Inability to inhibit mouse NK activity by aggregated immunoglobulins or immune complexes or to inhibit human NK activity by small soluble immune complexes.*

2. *Loss of NK but not ADCC activity by trypsinization of effector cells.*

3. *Inability of protein A to inhibit human or mouse NK activity.*

4. *Inability to consistently demonstrate inhibition of human or mouse NK activity by addition to assay of Fab or $F(ab')_2$ fragments of anti-IgG or anti-Fab.*

---

activity being dependent on production of antibodies during the assay. Even the initiators of this hypothesis have recently reported that a portion of NK activity against K562 target cells appears independent of antibodies (Pape *et al.*, 1979). In addition, other investigators (see Bolhuis, Kay, Koren and Jensen, Perussia, *et al.*) have been unable to reproduce the partial inhibition of NK activity by adding of fragments of anti-immunoglobulin antibodies to the cytotoxicity assays. These differences might be attributable to the characteristics of the particular reagents and their degree of purity. One would expect that protein A should give consistent inhibition of activity dependent on secreted antibodies, since it can quite efficiently block ADCC. However, Sulica *et al.* (1976) has reported that under some conditions, addition of protein A can form complexes and facilitate arming with cytophilic IgG. Perhaps the strongest specific argument against a role of secreted antibodies is that trypsinization of effector cells causes a temporary loss of NK activity without interfering with $Fc_{\gamma}R$ or the function of K cells. While this would be compatible with the armed K cell hypothesis, it does not seem to easily fit the secreted antibody hypothesis. One would have to postulate that the function of cells responsible for antibody production are inhibited in some way by trypsinization. A further line of evidence against this hypothesis is related to the lack of inhibition of either human or mouse NK activity by small soluble immune complexes (see chapter by Kay). Aggregated immunoglobulins and larger soluble complexes have given partial but not complete inhibition (Bolhuis, Kay, Kamiyama and Takasugi, Perussia *et al.*). Only cellular immune complexes strongly inhibited NK activity. The observed inhibition by large complexes can probably be attributed to steric hindrance rather than a specific block of NK receptors, since complexes of all sizes completely inhibited ADCC activity.

Although there may be a role for $Fc_{\gamma}R$ and antibodies in NK activity, the general consensus appears to be that much or perhaps all of NK activity is mediated by effector cell structures separate from $Fc_{\gamma}R$. Thus, the $Fc_{\gamma}R$ would appear to be a good marker for most NK cells, when studied under usual conditions, but would not be required for NK activity.

III. SIMILARITIES IN MECHANISM OF LYSIS BY NK CELLS AND K CELLS

Even if NK and ADCC activities are dependent on separate receptors on the cell surface, one might anticipate that the NK/K cell would produce lysis by a common mechanism. Roder and Haliotis offer a model for cytolysis by NK cells and suggest that lysosomal enzymes and in particular, serine esterases, are involved in the lytic event. It will be important to further evaluate the various steps in their model and also determine if parallel information can be accumulated for ADCC. From their data, the main analogy between the mechanisms of NK and ADCC has come from studies of beige mice and patients with Chediak-Higashi syndrome. K cell activity was depressed to about the same extent as NK activity, consistent with a common defect in the mechanism of lysis. In addition, several other lines of evidence point to similarities in the mechanisms of NK and ADCC (summarized in Table V). Kamiyama and Takasugi have listed several similarities between these mechanisms. Optimal lysis was seen at 37°, reduced levels at room temperature, and no lysis at 4° despite binding of effector cells to targets. The requirement for energy for NK and ADCC was supported by inhibition with azide. They, and also Ortaldo *et al.* (see chapter in Section IC3), observed strong inhibition of both activities by puromycin. Kamiyama and Takasugi also noted parallel inhibition of NK and ADCC at high concentrations of mitomycin C and actinomycin D. Since Ortaldo *et al.* failed to observe inhibition with these agents under conditions sufficient to block DNA and RNA synthesis, respectively, the effects observed by Kamiyama and Takasugi were probably due to some toxicity. Kamiyama and Takasugi also found similar effects on NK and

TABLE V. Evidence for Similarities in Mechanism of Lysis by NK and K Cells

1. *Parallel effects of temperature on altering rate of cytotoxic activity.*
2. *Parallel effects by metabolic inhibitors.*
3. *Similar requirements for divalent cations.*
4. *Augmentation of activity by interferon.*
5. *Inhibition of activity by prostaglandins E_1 and E_2 and by NIF.*
6. *Kinetic analysis indicates NK and ADCC activities of each donor have same or similar K_M.*
7. *Decreased K cell as well as K activity in beige mice and patients with Chediak-Higashi syndrome.*

ADCC by EDTA and Ca and Mg. The only differences seen appeared to be due to some role of monocytes, in addition to K cells, in ADCC.

The observations by most authors (with the exception of Perussia *et al.*) that treatment of human or mouse effector cells with interferon resulted in augmentation of K cell activity, as well as NK activity, provide another indication for similar mechanisms of cytolysis. The parallel effects on regulation of activity are further supported by findings that prostaglandins E_1 and E_2 could inhibit NK activity (Brunda *et al.*; Roder and Haliotis), as well as ADCC (Droller *et al.*, 1978).

The application by Callewaert of enzyme kinetics to analysis of NK and ADCC activities provides another interesting approach to this question. He found that the K_M for cytotoxicity of each donor varied, but that for each donor the K_M for NK and ADCC were the same or at least not significantly different. This finding is consistent with a common lytic mechanism for NK and ADCC. However, it should be noted that the interpretation of the results is very much dependent on the assumptions made regarding the rate-limiting step and the possible model for lysis.

One difference between NK and ADCC that is not readily explained is the effect of pretreatment with corticosteroids.

In mice (Santoni *et al.*, 1979b) and in humans, corticosteroids caused depression of NK activity but had little or no effect on ADCC. Since the depression of NK activity appeared to be a reversible defect (Santoni *et al.*, 1979b) rather than a lytic effect, this does not contradict the other evidence for the similarity or identity of NK and K cells but rather suggests some point of difference in the two activities. This may provide a useful probe to better understand the relationship between the mechanisms of these two related forms of cytotoxicity.

REFERENCES

Droller, M. J., Schneider, M. V., and Perlmann, P. (1978). *Cell. Immunol. 39*. 165.

Kay, H. D., Bonnard, G. D., West, W. H., and Herberman, R. B. (1977). *J. Immunol. 118*. 2058.

Kay, H. D., Bonnard, G. D., and Herberman, R. B. (1979). *J. Immunol. 122* :675-685.

Koide, Y. and Takasugi, M. (1977). *J. Natl. Cancer Inst. 59:* 1009-1106.

Landazuri, M. O., Silva, A., Alvarez, J., and Herberman, R. B. (1979). *J. Immunol. 123:* 252-258, 402.

Ojo, E., and Wigzell, H. (1978). *Scand. J. Immunol. 7:* 297-306.

Pandolfi, F., Strong, D. M., Slease, R. B., Smith, M. L., Ortaldo, J. R., and Herberman, R. B. (1980). Submitted for publication.

Pape, G. R., Troye, M., Axelson, B., and Perlmann, P. (1979). *J. Immunol. 122:* 2251.

Santoni, A., Herberman, R. B., and Holden, H. T. (1979a). *J. Natl. Cancer Inst. 62:* 109-116, 356.

Santoni, A., Herberman, R. B., and Holden, H. T. (1979b). *J. Natl. Cancer Inst. 63:* 95-1003, 412.

Shellam, G. R. (1977). *Int. J. Cancer. 19:* 225-235.

Sulicia, A., Lakey, M., Gherman, M., Ghetie, V., and Sjoquist, J. (1976). *Scand. J. Immunol. 5:* 1191-1197.

Troye, M., Perlmann, P., Pape, G. R., Spiegelberg, H. L., Näslund, I., and Gidlöf, A. (1977). *J. Immunol. 119:* 1061-1069.

IMMUNOGENETICS OF NATURAL IMMUNITY [1]

Phyllis B. Blair

Department of Microbiology and Immunology and
the Cancer Research Laboratory
University of California
Berkeley, California

I. INTRODUCTION

A target often used for the assessment of natural killer activity in the mouse is the YAC-1 cell line, derived from an MuLV-induced lymphoma. Inbred strains of mice differ considerably in their ability to display natural killer activity against this target. Genetic analyses have revealed that this activity is under polygenic control with a major gene linked to the H-2 (reviewed in Kiessling and Wigzell, 1979).

In tests of reactivity *in vitro* against YAC-1 target cells the hybrids of crosses between high-responder and low-responder strains resemble the high responder parental strain (Kiessling *et al.*, 1975a; Kiessling *et al.*, 1975b; Petranyi *et al.*, 1975; Roder and Kiessling, 1978; Kiessling and Wigzell, 1979), and in backcross mice from a mating of responder (A x C57BL) hybrid females with males of the low responder A parental strain, a significant association of reactivity with the H-2 gene derived from the C57BL was found (Petranyi *et al.*, 1976). An H-2 associated responsiveness has also been observed in the backcross to the C57BL of hybrids from the C57BL x DBA mating, and, using congenic and recombinant lines, it has been possible to localize the gene to the D-end of the H-2 complex (Klein *et al.*, 1978).

[1] *This work was supported by research grants IM-69 from the American Cancer Society, Inc., and CA-05388 from the National Cancer Institute and by research funds of the University of California.*

ISBN 0-12-341350-8

In vivo observations on relative resistance to inoculations of YAC cells correlate well with the levels of natural killer activity detected *in vitro* in both hybrid (Kiessling *et al.*, 1975b; Klein *et al.*, 1978; Riccardi *et al.*, 1979; Petranyi *et al.*, 1976) and backcross mice; backcrosses to the A strain of hybrids from the A x C57BL mating (Kiessling *et al.*, 1975b; Petranyi *et al.*, 1976), and from the A x CBA mating (Petranyi *et al.*, 1976) have demonstrated a linkage to the H-2.

II. EXPERIMENTAL DESIGN

In the experiments reported here, natural killer activity against YAC-1 target cells of spleen cells from mice of 13 inbred strains and 5 hybrids was tested. All mice were derived from the colony of the Cancer Research Laboratory. Only female mice were used, and they were 9-10 weeks old at the time their spleens were harvested for assay. Mice from 3 standard inbred strains (C57BL, BALB/c, and I), from their hybrids, and from 10 recombinant inbred strains derived from them were available for analysis. Each recombinant inbred strain was derived from a cross between two of the parent strains by brother-sister matings of the F_1 and all subsequent generations. The recombinant inbred strains were used in these experiments after 20-30 generations of inbreeding. Five of the recombinant inbred strains carry the H-2 of the C57BL strain (4 derived from matings of C57BL females and I males, and one derived from the mating of a C57BL female with a BALB/c male), two carry the H-2 of the I strain, (one strain derived from mating a C57BL female with an I male, and the other by mating a BALB/c female with an I male), and two carry the H-2 of the BALB/c strain (one strain derived by mating a C57BL female with a BALB/c male, and the other by mating a BALB/c female with an I male). The characteristics of the 10 recombinant inbred strains (original parent strains, H-2, and coat color genes) are presented in Table I.

Natural killer activity of spleen cells was measured using the standard ^{51}Cr-release assay (Kiessling *et al.*, 1975a, 1975b; Petranyi *et al.*, 1975). The YAC-1 cell line obtained from the Sidney Farber Cancer Center, Boston, was used as the source of target cells. The cells ($1.0 - 3.0 \times 10^7$) were washed once, resuspended in 1.0 ml RPMI 1640 and labeled with 300-500 μCi ^{51}Cr for one hour at 37°C. The labeled cells were then washed twice and resuspended to a concentration of 1.0×10^6 cells/ml in complete medium (RPMI 1640 supplemented with 10% heat-inactivated fetal calf serum and 100 units/ml of penicillin/streptomycin). Spleen cells from each female were tested separately. The spleen cell suspensions were prepared in Hanks balanced salt solution and adjusted to a final contration of 2.5 x 10^7 cell/ml in complete medium. Spleen effector cells were added to the ^{51}Cr-labeled target cells in Nunclon-Delta Microtiter plates to give effector:target cell ratios of 25:1, 50:1 and 100:1. The final volume in each well was 200λ. The plates were centrifuged at 1200 rpm for 8 minutes and then incubated at 37°C for 4 hours. At the end of the incubation period the plates were centrifuged again, and 100λ of supernatant was removed from each well for counting. Total release was determined by incubating target cells alone in the presence of 1% SDS. Spontaneous release averaged 7.5%

TABLE I. Characteristics of Ten Recombinant Inbred Strains Derived from Matings of C57BL, I, or BALB/c mice.

Strain	*Original parental strain mating*	*H-2 Derived from*[a]	*Recessive coat color genes*
ABS-BI	*C57BL × I*	*C57BL*	*aabbss*
ADP-BI	*C57BL × I*	*C57BL*	*aaddpp*
AD-BI	*C57BL × I*	*C57BL*	*aadd*
AS-BI	*C57BL × I*	*C57BL*	*aass*
ADS-BI	*C57BL × I*	*C57BL*	*aaddss*
ABDS-BI	*C57BL × I*	*I*	*aabbddss*
B-BC	*C57BL × BALB/c*	*C57BL*	*bb*
AB-BC	*C57BL × BALB/c*	*BALB/c*	*aabb*
ABP-CI	*BALB/c × I*	*BALB/c*	*aabbpp*
BPS-CI	*BALB/c × I*	*I*	*bbppss*

[a]*The H-2 of each recombinant inbred strain was determined with mouse antisera using a facilitated hemagglutination technique (Danilovs, 1978).*

of the total release. Results of 6 replicate wells were averaged and are presented as "percent cytotoxicity" calculated as:

$$\frac{\textit{Experimental release - spontaneous release}}{\textit{Total release - spontaneous release}} \times 100$$

As expected, cytotoxicity levels were in general higher at the effector:target cell ratio of 100:1 than at the 50:1 ratio; responses at the 25:1 ratio (data not shown) were even lower. Data on natural killer activity for a few of these strains are also presented in another chapter in this book (see chapter by Blair *et al.*).

III. NATURAL KILLER ACTIVITY IN RECOMBINANT INBRED STRAINS

The three parental strains from which the recombinant inbred strains were derived differ greatly in their natural killer activity (Table II). Spleen cells from females of our subline of C57BL, which was obtained from Jackson Laboratories in 1936 and which is neither C57BL/6 nor C57BL/10 (Danilovs, 1978), show considerable reactivity on YAC-1 target cells whereas spleen cells from females of our BALB/c strain are intermediate in response and those from I females are only marginally active.

Reactivity of spleen cells from females of each recombinant inbred strain resembles that of the parental strain with which they share the H-2 allele (Table II). Thus, both of the recombinant strains which have retained the H-2 complex contributed to the original hybrids by the I strain show very little natural killer activity, as does the I. Those recombinants which carry the H-2 complex contributed to the original hybrids by the BALB/c strain resemble that strain in intermediate activity. The only high responders among the recombinant inbred strains are those which have retained the H-2 complex of the high responder C57BL strain.

These data also indicate the importance of modifier genes in determining the level of natural killer activity; there are considerable differences in the level of activity among the reactive strains carrying the C57BL H-2 complex (Table II). Two of them (both derived from crosses with the I strain) are more reactive than the parent C57BL strain; the others are less so.

TABLE II. Natural Killer Activity Against YAC-1 Target Cells of Spleen Cells from Normal Females of Three Original and Ten Recombinant Inbred Strains

Strain of Spleen Donor[a]	H-2 Derived from	Percent Cytotoxicity			
		50:1[b]		100:1[b]	
		Average	Range	Average	Range
C57BL	C57BL	13.9	8.7-18.3	21.1	11.1-27.9
ABS-BI	"	7.1	2.0-11.2	9.5	1.9-17.6
ADP-BI	"	9.6	5.8-15.1	13.2	6.0-20.2
B-BC	"	12.3	7.1-22.0	15.5	9.7-26.0
AD-BI	"	15.7	8.3-27.6	17.8	7.4-34.7
AS-BI	"	21.8	8.2-35.1	24.5	9.8-36.8
ADS-BI	"	20.1	10.2-28.5	25.2	14.7-33.0
BALB/c	BALB/c	7.3	5.2-10.2	6.2	5.2-7.0
ABP-CI	"	6.1	5.0-7.8	7.8	6.3-10.3
AB-BC	"	11.2	3.3-16.5	12.2	3.3-19.6
I	I	2.2	1.1-5.5	2.8	0.8-5.1
BPS-CI	"	1.8	0 - 3.8	2.6	1.1-4.8
ABDS-BI	"	4.6	0 - 7.6	7.2	2.8-10.5

[a]For each strain, 4-8 females 9-10 weeks old were tested.

[b]Effector:target cell ratio

IV. INCREASED NATURAL KILLER ACTIVITY IN HYBRID MICE

Natural killer activity of spleen cells from hybrid mice was also tested. All of the 5 types of hybrids tested were more reactive than either parental strain at one or both of the effector:target cell ratios (Table III).

Since the C57BL parental strain is a high responder, the increased activity in the three types of hybrid which have a C57BL parent is not dramatic. It is, however, statistically significant; comparing all three types of hybrids with the parental C57BL strain in a ranking of individual responses at

TABLE III. Natural Killer Activity of Spleen Cells from Normal Females of Three Inbred Strains and Their F_1 Hybrids

Spleen cell donor[a]	Percent Cytotoxicity			
	50:1[b]		100:1[b]	
	Average	Range	Average	Range
C57BL	13.9	8.7-18.3	21.1	11.1-27.9
BALB/c	7.3	5.2-10.2	6.2	5.2-7.0
I	2.2	1.1-5.5	2.8	0.8-5.1
I × C57BL	24.7	23.0-27.2	30.0	26.9-31.7
C57BL × I	14.3	10.8-18.4	20.4	14.6-24.3
C57BL × BALB/c	22.9	19.8-26.7	27.5	22.2-33.8
BALB/c × I	15.4	12.4-18.9	19.6	16.9-24.7
I × BALB/c	11.6	8.7-17.6	13.3	9.2-19.3

[a] *For each strain or hybrid, 3-6 females 9-10 weeks old were tested.*

[b] *Effector:target cell ratio*

the 50:1 effector:target cell ratio, a p value of <0.05 is obtained in the Mann Whitney U test.

The increased hybrid natural killer activity is clearly evident in the two reciprocal crosses involving the BALB/c and the I strains. There is no overlap between the level of natural killer activity in any of the hybrid females with that of any of the individuals from the two parental strains (Table IV); this difference is highly significant statistically by the Mann-Whitney U test.

V. IMPORTANCE OF H-2-LINKED AND OTHER GENES IN DETERMINING LEVELS OF NATURAL KILLER ACTIVITY

The data presented here on the reactivity against YAC-1 target cells of spleen cells from the C57BL, BALB/c and I strains, their hybrids, and 10 recombinant inbred strains derived from them, provide additional evidence for the role of H-2 linked factors in determining levels of natural killer

---

TABLE IV. Increased Natural Killer Activity in Hybrid Mice Compared with that of Individuals from Either Parental Strain

Level of Activity[a]	Number of females showing percent cytotoxicity at each level			
	BALB/c × I	I × BALB/c	BALB/c	I
24-	1			
20-23.9	1			
16-19.9	2	1		
12-15.9	1	1		
8-11.9		2		
4-7.9			4	2
0-3.9				4

[a] *Percent cytotoxicity produced by spleen cells at 100:1 effector:target cell ratio*

activity, for the role of modifier genes in controlling the level of this activity in the reactive strains, and for the increased activity, which can be more than additive, of hybrids compared to individuals of the inbred strains from which they were derived.

Mice from our strain of C57BL are high responders, those from our BALB/c strain are relatively low responders, and those from our I strain are very poor responders. Mice of each of the recombinant inbred lines demonstrated reactivity similar to that of the parental strain whose H-2 complex was carried by that recombinant inbred line. In addition, more than one non-H-2-linked modifier gene appeared to play an important role. This was especially evident in those recombinant inbred strains carrying the H-2 derived from the C57BL; of the 5 recombinant inbred strains derived from crosses with the I strain, two were considerably less reactive than the C57BL (ABS-BI and ADP-BI) and two were more reactive (AS-BI and ADS-BI).

A striking result was the increased natural killer activity in hybrids as compared with the parental strains. This was detectable in the hybrids which have a C57BL parent, as has been reported by others (Klein *et al.*, 1978; Kiessling *et al.*, 1975a; Roder and Kiessling, 1978). The increase in activity was much more dramatic, however, in the hybrids of two other strains, the BALB/c and the I. The levels of reactivity observed in these hybrids were much more than additive.

There is more than one possible explanation for this increased activity in the hybrids. As yet, we do not know if the H-2-associated natural killer activity is determined by single or multiple genes; thus the additive or synergistic reactivities observed in hybrids could be either a heterosis effect of alleles of a single H-2-linked gene or a complementation of alleles from more than one H-2-linked genes (Klein *et al.*, 1978; Kiessling and Wigzell, 1979). In addition, modifier genes on other chromosomes may be important; the I strain, for example, may contribute to its hybrids modifier gene alleles which are effective in increasing reactivity determined by the C57BL or BALB/c H-2-linked responder gene (or genes) even though the effect of these same alleles is not detectable in the I strain which carries a low-response H-2-linked gene.

ACKNOWLEDGMENTS

I am grateful to Martha Staskawicz, Judith Sam, and Mary Roderick for their participation in these studies and to Clara Else for preparation of the manuscript.

REFERENCES

Danilovs, J.A. 1978 The genetics of resistance to mammary tumor virus infection and tumorigenesis in C57BL/Crgl mice. Ph.D. dissertation, University of California, Berkeley.

Kiessling, R. & Wigzell, H. 1979 An analysis of the murine NK cell as to structure, function and biological relevance. *Immunological Rev. 44:* 165-208.

Kiessling, R., Klein, E. & Wigzell, H. 1975a Natural killer cells in the mouse. I. Cytotoxic cells with specificity for mouse Moloney leukemia cells. Specificity and distribution according to genotype. *Eur.J.Immunol.5:*112-117.

Kiessling, R., Petranyi, G., Klein, G. & Wigzell, H. 1975b Genetic variation of *in vitro* cytolytic activity and *in vivo* rejection potential of non-immunized semi-syngeneic mice against a mouse lymphoma line. *Int. J. Cancer 15:* 933-940.

Klein, G.O., Klein, G., Kiessling, R. & Kärre, K. 1978 H-2-associated control of natural cytotoxocity and hybrid resistance against RBL-5. *Immunogenetics 6:* 561-569.

Petranyi, G.G., Kiessling, R. & Klein, G. 1975 Genetic control of "natural" killer lymphocytes in the mouse. *Immunogenetics 2:* 53-61.

Petranyi, G.G., Kiessling, R., Povey, S., Klein, G., Herzenberg, L. & Wigzell, H. 1976 The genetic control of natural killer cell activity and its association with *in vivo* resistance against a Moloney lymphoma isograft. *Immunogenetics 3:* 15-28.

Riccardi, C., Puccetti, P., Santoni, A. & Herberman, R.B. 1979 Rapid *in vivo* assay of mouse natural killer cell activity. *J. Natl. Cancer Inst. 63:* 1041-1045.

Roder, J.C. & Kiessling, R. 1978 Target-effector interaction in the natural killer cell system. *Scand. J. Immunol. 8:* 135-144.

AUGMENTATION OF NATURAL KILLER CELL ACTIVITY OF BEIGE MICE BY INTERFERON AND INTERFERON INDUCERS

Michael J. Brunda[1]
Howard T. Holden
Ronald B. Herberman

Laboratory of Immunodiagnosis
National Cancer Institute
Bethesda, Maryland 20205

It has recently been reported that C57BL/6 (B6) mice, homozygous for the beige mutation have a complete defect in natural killer (NK) cell activity, in contrast to substantial NK reactivity in B6 or heterozygous mice (Roder and Duwe, 1979). Beige mice were previously studied because of their abnormal granulocytes which are deficient in neutral protease activity (Lutzner *et. al.*, 1967; Gallin *et. al.*, 1974, Vassalli *et. al.*, 1978, Johnson *et. al.*, 1979). Further studies, however, have demonstrated that T cells and macrophages of these mice have normal levels of cytolytic activity (Roder *et. al.*, 1979). The NK defect did not appear to be due to alterations in tissue distribution of NK cells, in age-related maturation of the response or in target cell specificity (Roder, 1979). Furthermore, no evidence for suppressor cells which inhibit NK activity in these mice has been found (Roder, 1979). Spleen cells from beige mice formed normal numbers of conjugates with NK-sensitive target cells, suggesting that the low NK activity in these mice might reflect a defect in lytic capacity as opposed to a failure to recognize target cells (Roder and Duwe, 1979; Roder, 1979).

Mice that have an absolute, but selective, defect in NK activity would be of great value in the study of the *in vivo* relevance of NK cells. We examined these mice for both their spontaneous and interferon (IF) augmented NK activity. As previously reported, these animals were found to have decreased

[1]*On temporary assignment from the National Jewish Hospital and Research Center, Denver, Colorado 80206*

ISBN 0-12-341350-8

NK activity compared to the B6 strain. However, in contrast to the prior studies (Roder and Duwe, 1979, Roder, 1979), the spontaneous NK activity of beige mice was usually significant and could be augmented, to a degree comparable to that found in other low NK strains, by IF and other agents that presumably induced IF.

The NK activity of spleen cells was assessed *in vitro* using YAC-1 target cells in a 4 hr ^{51}Cr release assay (Herberman *et al.*, 1975). The conditions used for the *in vivo* and *in vitro* augmentation of NK reactivity have been previously described (Herberman *et. al.*, 1977; Djeu *et. al.*, 1979b; Brunda *et. al.*, 1979).

The spontaneous and lymphocytic choriomeningitis virus (LCMV)-augmented NK activities of spleen cells from several strains of mice were initially evaluated. Spleen cells from B6 mice had considerable spontaneous reactivity against YAC-1 target cells (Table I). Although NK activity from beige mice was low, it was always significantly above the baseline control and similar to the activity found in other low NK strains. Following injection of LCMV, spleen cells from B6 mice had an augmented response. The reactivity of spleen cells from beige mice was appreciably increased after LCMV injection although not to the same levels as those of

TABLE I.--Spontaneous and LCMV-boosted NK Activity of Beige and Other Mouse Strains

	% Cytotoxicity[a]	
Strain	*Spontaneous*	*LCMV Augmented*[b]
C57BL/6	*35*	*45*
Beige	*10*	*25*
SJL/J	*14*	*28*
A/J	*7*	*31*

[a] *NK activity at 200/1 spleen cell/YAC-1 ratio.*
Mice injected IP three days before testing.

boosted B6. As with spontaneous activity, the levels of activity in beige mice after boosting were similar to those observed with other low NK strains. The ability to augment NK activity in beige mice was not limited to LCMV since *in vivo* administration of other IF-inducers, including polyinosinic-polycytidylic acid (poly I:C) and Newcastle disease virus (NDV) and IF itself, resulted in an increased NK activity (Table II).

NK activity of spleen cells from beige mice could also be boosted by *in vitro* incubation overnight with IF or poly I:C. As expected, the reactivity of B6 spleen cells incubated overnight in medium was higher than that of spleen cells from beige or SJL/J mice (Table III). Likewise, incubation of B6 spleen cells with either IF or poly I:C substantially augmented NK activity. When beige or SJL/J spleen cells were cultured with IF or poly I:C, small but significant increases in NK activity were observed. Consistent increases in reactivity were found in five other experiments (data not shown).

Our results have confirmed the finding that beige mice have substantially lower NK activity than the congenic B6 strain. The defect does not appear to be absolute since

TABLE II. In Vivo Augmentation of NK Cell Activity in Beige Mice by IF and IF Inducers.

Treatment[a]	*% Cytotoxicity*[b]
None	*16*
LCMV	*26*[c]
Poly I:C	*21*[c]
NDV	*30*[c]
IF	*23*[c]

[A] *Mice injected IP three days, 18 hr or 3 hr before testing with LCMV or NDV, Poly I:C or IF respectively.*

[b] *NK activity at 200/1 spleen cell/YAC-1 ratio.*

$P < 0.01$.

significant levels of spontaneous reactivity were found which were comparable to the levels observed in other low NK strains. When mice were injected with a number of agents that induce IF or with IF itself, substantial increases in NK activity were observed. Following incubation *in vitro* with IF or poly I:C, a modest but consistent increase in NK activity was found with spleen cells from beige or SJL/J mice, although this was a lower absolute increase than that seen with B6 spleen cells. Differences in the incubation requirements or in the optimal concentrations of stimulants might account for the smaller increases in NK activity of beige and SJL/J compared to B6 spleen cells observed *in vitro*. Augmentation of NK reactivity *in vivo* may have less stringent requirements resulting in more substantial increases in reactivity.

Since low levels of spontaneous NK activity are present in beige mice and can be augmented by IF and IF-inducers, these results indicate that beige mice have at least a partially functional lytic mechanism which can destroy NK-sensitive target cells. Therefore, the beige mouse should provide a useful tool for the study of NK cells but the fact that this defect is not absolute should be carefully considered in experiments utilizing these animals.

TABLE III. In Vitro Augmentation of NK Cell Activity by IF and Poly I:C.

	Treatment with:[a]		
Strain	*Medium*	*IF*	*Poly I:C*
C57BL/6	*30*[b]	*41*	*51*
Beige	*11*	*17*	*16*
SJL/J	*12*	*19*	*15*

[a] *Overnight incubation of spleen cells with medium containing 1,000 U/ml IF or 100 μg/ml of poly I:C.*

[b] *% cytotoxicity at 200/1 spleen cell/YAC-1 ratio.*

REFERENCES

Brunda, M. J., Herberman, R. B. and Holden, H. T. (1979). In preparation.

Djeu, J. Y., Heinbaugh, J. A., Holden, H. T. and Herberman, R. B. (1979a). *J. Immunol. 122,* 175.

Djeu, J. Y., Heinbaugh, J. A., Holden, H. T. and Herberman, R. B. (1979b). *J. Immunol. 22,* 182.

Gallin, J. I., Bujak, J. S., Patten, E. and Wolff, S. M. (1974). *Blood 43,* 201.

Herberman, R. B., Nunn, M. E. and Lavrin, D. H. (1975). *Int. J. Cancer 16,* 216.

Herberman, R. B., Nunn, M. E., Holden, H. T., Staal, S. and Djeu, J. Y. (1977). *Int. J. Cancer 19,* 555.

Herberman, R. B., Djeu, J. Y., Kay, H. D., Ortaldo, J. R., Riccardi, C., Bonnard, G. D., Holden, H. T., Fagnani, R., Santoni, A. and Puccetti, P. (1979). *Immunol. Rev. 44,* 43.

Johnson, K. J., Varani, J., Oliver, J., and Ward, P. A. (1979). *J. Immunol. 122,* 1807.

Lutzner, M. A., Lowrie, C. T. and Jordan, H. W. (1967). *J. Heredity 58,* 299.

Roder, J. C. (1979). *J. Immunol. 123,* 2168.

Roder, J. C. and Duwe, A. (1979). *Nature. 278,* 451.

Roder, J. C., Lohmann-Matthes, M.-L., Domzig, W. and Wigzell, H. (1979). *J. Immunol. 123,* 2174.

Vassalli, V. J., Granelli, A. P., Griscelli, C. and Reich, E. (1978). *J. Exp. Med. 147,* 1285.

MUTATIONS THAT INFLUENCE NATURAL CELL-MEDIATED CYTOTOXICITY IN RODENTS[1]

Edward A. Clark
Nancy T. Windsor
Jerrilyn C. Sturge
Thomas H. Stanton*

Department of Genetics,
Regional Primate Research Center,
and Department of Microbiology & Immunology*
University of Washington
Seattle, Washington

I. INTRODUCTION

The development and activation of natural cell-mediated cytotoxicity (NCMC) in mice is under complex polygenic control (Clark and Harmon, 1979). Early studies reported that inbred strains differ markedly in the level of natural killer (NK) cell activity they display against lymphoid targets (Kiessling _et al._, 1975; Herberman _et al._, 1975). Segregation analysis and linkage tests revealed that NCMC is controlled by at least two genes and specifically by a locus linked to the _H-2_ major immunogene complex on chromosome 17 (Petranyi _et al._, 1975, 1976). Mapping studies using _H-2_ congenic and intra-_H-2_ recombinant strains demonstrated that a locus within or very near the _H-2D_ region affects NK cell activity against EL-4 lymphoma targets (Harmon _et al._, 1977). This finding subsequently has been confirmed using more sensitive target cells such as YAC-1 (Klein _et al._, 1978; Kumar _et al._, 1979). The effect of the _H-2D_-associated locus is most pronounced when an additional non-_H-2_ gene(s) in the C57BL background is present. This suggests that complementing _H-2_ and non-_H-2_ genes may interact to augment NK cell activity (Klein _et al._, 1978; Clark _et al._, 1979).

[1]This work was supported by American Cancer Society grants CD-29 and IM-228, and by NIH grant RR 00166 to the Regional Primate Research Center.

ISBN 0-12-341350-8

With the possible exception of this H-2D-associated locus, segregation and linkage studies and application of inbred, congenic, and recombinant strains have not led to clear identification of NCMC regulatory loci. This in part reflects the variability of the NK cell phenotype, which is strongly influenced by environmental factors (Herberman et al., 1977; Clark et al., 1979). Examination of mutations known to affect the immune system, where homozygous and heterozygous littermates can be compared, has been a more fruitful approach. The nude mutation (nu, chromosome 11), for example, leads to augmentation of NK cell activity (Herberman et al., 1975; Kiessling et al., 1975) and has found wide application in NCMC studies. Recently Roder and Duwe (1979) reported that another mutation, beige (bg, chromosome 13) dramatically impairs the ability of NK cells to lyse tumor targets. NK cells in beige mice can be activated under certain conditions as discussed elsewhere in this volume.

Because mutations such as nu and bg are powerful tools for examining the regulation of complex phenotypes such as NCMC, we have attempted to identify other mutations affecting NK cell activity. We describe here two new loci, obese (ob) and lymphoproliferation (lpr), which influence NK cell levels. Two mutations leading to anemia, Steel Dickie (Sl^d) and viable dominant spotting (W^v), in the heterozygous state did not obviously alter the NCMC phenotype.

II. MATERIALS AND METHODS

A. Animals

Control C57BL/6J and the following mutant mouse stocks were obtained from the Jackson Laboratory, Bar Harbor, Maine: C57BL/6J-Sl^d/+ (Steel-Dickie anemia; Russell, 1970), C57BL/6J-W^v/+ (viable dominant spotting anemia; Russell, 1970), and C57BL/6-ob/ob (obese; Herberg and Coleman, 1977; Bray and York, 1979). Lean littermate controls (ob/+ or +/+) were obtained and tested concurently with obese homozygotes. Breeder pairs of MRL/MP, mutant MRL/MP-lpr/lpr (lymphoproliferation; Murphy and Roths, 1978), and BXSB mice were kindly provided by Dr. Edwin Murphy (The Jackson Laboratory), and bred in our breeding colony (T.H.S.). C3H/HeJ-bg^{2J}/+ and bg^{2J}/bg^{2J} breeder pairs were the generous gift of Dr. Eva Eicher (The Jackson Laboratory) and were bred in our colony. Obese Zucker rats with the fatty mutation (fa/fa) and lean littermate controls (fa/+ or +/+; Bray and York, 1979) were kindly provided by Dr. Stephen Woods (Department of Psychology, University of Washington). Breeder pairs of BALB/Kh and BALB/Kh-$H\text{-}2^{dm2}$ mutants were kindly provided by Dr. Roger

Melvold (Northwestern University). In all experiments age-, sex-, and environment-matched animals were used.

B. Activation of NCMC

Mice were inoculated with 1-2 x 10^8 viable Bacillus Calmette-Guerin (BCG, Pasteur strain, Trudeau Institute, Saranac Lake, N.Y.) by the intraperitoneal route (i.p.) following the method of Tracey *et al.* (1977). Four days later peritoneal exudate cells (PEC) or spleen cells were harvested and tested for NK activity.

C. Effector Cells

PEC were harvested by lavage of the peritoneal cavity following injection of 10 ml of cold Hanks balanced salt solution (HBSS) and aspiration of the exudate with a 25 ga needle. Spleens and lymph node cells were excised, gently teased into cold HBSS with 5% fetal bovine serum (FBS), and washed. Subsequently, erythrocytes in the cell pellet were lysed with distilled water (1 ml, 15 sec). After two additional washes, cell suspensions were passed through fine nylon gauze and resuspended in RPMI 1640 medium containing 15% decomplemented FBS, and viable cells were counted by trypan blue dye exclusion. Cell suspensions were invariably 85% viable and generally 95% viable with this method.

D. Cytolytic Assay

The NK cell cytolytic assay has been described previously (Clark *et al.*, 1979). In brief, graded doses of effector cells and 1 x 10^4 ^{51}Cr-labeled YAC-1 target cells were incubated in a total volume of 200 µl at 37°C (humidified incubator, 5% CO_2, 95% air) in round-bottomed microtiter plates (Linbro Microtest II, Flow Laboratories, Hamden, Conn.). After 4-5 hours, the plates were centrifuged (1 min, 300 g) and 100 µl supernatant aliquots were removed with a micropipette (Titertek, Flow Laboratories) for counting in a γ scintillation counter. Percent specific cytotoxicity was calculated using the formula 100 x (T-S)/(D-S) where T = test cpm; S = spontaneous release (media control) cpm; and D = cpm in detergent control wells. Assays were performed in triplicate and standard errors of the mean were $\leq$5%.

III. RESULTS

A. Variation of NK cell phenotype

Genetic analysis of the regulation of NCMC has been hampered by marked variability of the NK phenotype even in individuals of the same inbred strain (e.g., Petranyi *et al.*, 1976). Recently, we have found that specific pathogen-free (SPF) mice of a number of inbred strains have little or no natural killer activity (Clark *et al.*, 1979). After placement in a pathogenic environment, NK activity develops rapidly within 2-3 days, peaks, and then wanes within 2 weeks. This suggests that most, if not all, NK activity is induced by exogenous agents, most likely infectious agents or their antigenic products. Genetic analysis of NK activity in SPF animals recently exposed to pathogens paralleled previous findings.

These results emphasize the importance of environment-induced variations in genetic studies of NCMC. Comparisons of cagemates and homozygous and heterozygous littermates where possible may be the optimal approach for examining NCMC regulation. Alternatively, artificial activation of NK activity may reduce variation and facilitate typing individual animals for NK cell phenotypes. Selection of the appropriate target cell may also be an important variable. Variations in killing activity by an inbred strain against one target cell may be much less than against a readily lysed, perhaps hypersensitive target.

B. H-2 Gene Control of NCMC

Our previous studies with intra-*H-2* recombinants have shown that an *H-2D*-associated locus affects NK activity; other *H-2*-linked genes may be operative as well (Clark and Harmon, 1979). We have speculated that *H-2* genes may control NK cell activity in a manner analogous to the control of T cell activation by interacting with inducing agents and thereby somehow affecting their immunogenicity. Precise identification of the *H-2* gene(s) influencing NCMC is required in order to test this hypothesis. In a preliminary study we have compared the effect of two *H-2* mutations on NCMC levels. The results are suggestive but still inconclusive since littermate controls were not tested. In three experiments C57BL/6By mice displayed a mean of 48% NCMC (100:1 effector: target (E:T) ratio; range 32-71) against YAC-1 targets compared with 31% NK-mediated lysis in *H-2K* mutant C57BL/6-*H-2*^{bm1} spleen cell donors (range 26-38). Comparison of NCMC in BALB/Kh mice (mean NCMC 28% at 100:1 E:T ratio) and *H-2L* mutant mice BALB/Kh-*H-2*^{dm2} (mean NCMC 34%) revealed a slight but consistent difference. Further detailed studies of other *H-2* mutations are in progress.

TABLE I. NCMC in Anemic and Obese Mice

Donor Strain	E:T Ratio	% Cytotoxicity[a] in Experiment: 1	2	3	4	5	Mean ± S.D.
C57BL/6J	100:1	35	22	-	45	22	31 ± 11
normal	50:1	22	15	13	22	11	17 ± 5
Steel-Dickie	100:1	27	25	21	51	NT	31 ± 14
anemia (Sl^d/+)	50:1	17	17	12	34		20 ± 10
W^v/+ anemia	100:1	33	19	9	33	14	22 ± 11
	50:1	21	7	0	19	7	11 ± 9
Obese	100:1	11	13	-1	9	9	9 ± 6
ob/ob	50:1	7	6	2	10	1	5 ± 4
Lean littermate	100:1	22	19	14	29	20	21 ± 5
controls	50:1	15	10	11	23	16	15 ± 5

[a]Spleen effector cells from untreated environment- and age-matched female donors, YAC-1 target cells, 4 hr assay.

Spontaneous release = 6%, 9%, 12%, 16%, and 22% in experiments 1-5 respectively.

C. NCMC in Anemic and Obese Animals

Natural killer cells originate in the bone marrow, and NK activity is dictated by the strain of origin of bone marrow cells (Haller *et al.*, 1977). Therefore, we decided to assess the effect on NCMC of two mutations known to affect hematopoiesis. Steel-Dickie (Sl^d) is a semidominant mutation which in the heterozygous state produces a mild macrocytic anemia (Russell, 1970). The viable dominant spotting mutation (W^v) is an allele of the *W* locus which in the heterozygous state also leads to a mild macrocytic anemia (Russell, 1970) and, in addition, clearly decreases hemopoietic progenitor cells (Bennett *et al.*, 1968). The Sl^d mutation had no effect on NCMC in Sl^d/+ normal (Table I) or BCG-activated hosts (Table II) compared with that in matched wildtype controls. Mice bearing the W^v mutation had somewhat lower NK levels than normal C57BL/6, but the differences were not dramatic. The BCG-induced activity of PEC is at least as great in $W^v/+$ mice as in normal controls. Thus, neither of these two mutations in the heterozygous state strongly influence NK activity. Examination of homozygotes with severe anemia is in progress.

Obese mice (ob/ob) display reduced antibody responses to sheep erythrocytes (Shultz, 1978) and have an impaired ability to reject allografts (Sheena and Meade, 1978) or generate cytotoxic cells in vivo (Meade et al., 1979). In a series of experiments obese mice also had lower NK activity than lean littermate controls (Table I). Even after activation of NCMC by BCG, obese mice had reduced NK levels in PEC (Table II) or the spleen (data not shown).

To determine if the impairment of NK activity was a specific pleiotropic effect of the ob locus or a secondary effect subsequent to obesity, we compared NK levels in ob mice and obese Zucker rats; these rats are homozygous for the recessive fatty mutation (fa) which produces obesity but, unlike ob, does not produce hyperglycemia (Bray and York, 1979).

TABLE II. Activation of NCMC in Anemic and Obese Mice

Donor Strain	% Activated NCMC[a] in Experiment: 3		4		5		Mean
	-[b]	+[b]	-	+	-	+	+
C57/BL6J	2	35	0	34	0	41	37
Steel-anemia	10	35	2	40	NT		38
W^v-amemia	5	53	3	50	-4	36	46
obese	2	21	-2	23	0	18	21
ob?/+controls	4	52	4	39	NT		46

[a]NCMC assay with PEC cells, YAC-1 target cells; 4 hour assay; spontaneous release 7%, 14%, and 22% in experiments 3-5 respectively; Effector:Target ratios 40:1 (Exper 3-4) and 20:1 (Exper 5).

[b]- = untreated; + = inoculated i.p. 4 days previously with 1 x 10^8 (Exper 3) or 2 x 10^8 (Exper 4-5) live BCG.

TABLE III. NK Activity in obese and lean rats and mice

Spleen cell Donor		body weight	Cytotoxicity[1] against: YAC-1	L5178cl27v
Obese rat (fa/fa)	#1	459g	14.1	5.0
	#2	433g	26.0	9.2
Lean rat (fa?/+)	#1	199g	54.7	29.8
	#2	229g	37.0	17.1
Obese mouse (ob/ob)		—	16.0	3.0
Lean mouse (ob?/+)		—	43.6	11.4
normal C57BL/6		—	48.5	13.5

Results shown at 200:1 effector cell: target cell ratio. Spontaneous release in 4 hr assay YAC-1, 6.0%; L5178 Cl 27v, 6.6%.

As shown in Table III, obese rats, like obese mice, have impaired NK activity. As with NK cell-deficient beige mice (Roder and Duwe, 1979), obese mice have normal levels of target binding cells (Roder *et al.*, 1978) but have impaired NK lytic activity (E.A.C. and S. Pollack, in preparation).

D. Elevation of NCMC in a Lymphoproliferative Disorder

Recently, Murphy and Roths (1978) described a mutation in the MRL strain of mice called lymphoproliferation (*lpr*) which produces a striking lymphoproliferative disease in 2- to 3-month-old animals. Theofilopoulos *et al.* (1979a) have reported that the majority of the proliferating cells are T cells, yet significantly a subpopulation of $Lyt123^-$ $Thy1^+$ cells also increases with age in *lpr/lpr* mice. We thought that these cells might be a subpopulation of $Thy\text{-}1^+$ NK cells (Mattes *et al.*, 1979), and thus compared the NCMC in MRL/MP and MRL/MP-*lpr* mice (Table IV). NCMC levels were low in both normal and mutant young mice, and in general the MRL strain displayed very low NK activity compared with reactive strains such as CBA and C57BL/6 (data not shown). At about eight weeks of age, concurrent with the onset of lymphoproliferation, splenic and lymph node cell NK activity increased in MRL-*lpr* mutant mice compared

TABLE IV. Natural Cell-Mediated Cytotoxicity in MRL/n and MRL/1 Mice

Experiment	Age (Sex)	E:T Ratio	% Cytotoxicity[a]								
			MRL - +/+		MRL - 1pr/1pr		BXSB	bg/+		bg/bg	
			-[b]	+[b]	-	+	-	-	+	-	+
1	7 wks (male)	200:1	9	NT	5	NT	5	NT		NT	
		100:1	4		2		3				
2	8 wks (male)	200:1	15	NT	41	NT	NT	NT		NT	
		100:1	9		25						
3	9 wks (male)	200:1	9	21	26	29	NT	NT		NT	
		100:1	8	17	28	21					
4	10 wks (female)	200:1	11	20	30	26	NT	27	48	3	8
		100:1	8	13	19	20		20	42	1	4
5	11 wks (male)	200:1	6	NT	9	NT	0	NT		NT	
		100:1	4		7		1				

[a] Spleen cells from age-, sex-, and environment-matched mice; 1 x 10^4 YAC-1 target cells; 4 hour assay; spontaneous release = 24%, 14%, 9%, 6% and 6% in experiments 1-5 respectively.

[b] - = untreated; + = animals inoculated i.p. 4 days previously with 2 x 10^8 live BCG.

with wildtype controls. Although NCMC could be activated readily in MRL wildtype recipients, NK levels in the spleen were not dramatically altered in BCG-inoculated MRL-lpr hosts (Table IV). NCMC could be activated with the same protocol in C3H/HeJ-bg/+ heterozygotes but to a lesser extent in mutant beige recipients.

IV. DISCUSSION

In this study we have identified three new genes that affect natural cell-mediated cytotoxicity levels in rodents: obese (ob) and lymphoproliferation (lpr) in mice and fatty (fa) in rats. These findings illustrate that the natural killer cell phenotype as presently measured is under complex genetic control. Already, five mutations in mice have been shown to clearly influence NK levels (Table V) and additional unmapped loci have been implicated (Clark and Harmon, 1979). The polygenic control of NCMC may reflect distinct sites of gene action or, alternatively, underscore the complexity of the "natural killer" phenotype. Initial characterization of surface markers on NK cells suggests there may be more than one NK cell subpopulation. For example, Chun and coworkers (1979) found that two peaks of NK cell activity are generated in cultures containing tumor necrosis serum. The first peak of NCMC, like NK cells recently activated in vivo (Clark et al., 1979), is mediated by $Thy-1^-$ NK cells bearing the Qa-5 antigen. The later peak of activity is mediated principally by $Qa-5^-$ $Thy-1^+$ cells. The genetic control and ontogenetic relationship of these NK subsets remain to be elucidated.

The site of ob gene action on NCMC has not been identified. Because the frequency of target binding "NK" cells is not obviously reduced in obese mice (Clark and Pollack, in preparation), the obese mutation most likely affects the efficiency or lytic potential of NK cells rather than NK cell frequency or binding ability. Genetically obese Zucker rats also have impaired NK activity (Table IV). Like obese mice, these rats are obese, hyperinsulinemic, and hyperlipemic; unlike ob/ob animals, they are not hyperglycemic (Bray and York, 1979), indicating that hyperglycemia is not required for NCMC to be reduced. Obese mice reject allografts slower than lean controls and display reduced contact sensitivity responses and cytotoxic cell responses to allogeneic target cells (Sheena and Meade, 1978); however, graft-versus-host proliferative reactions are normal. Plasma corticosteroid levels are raised in obese mice (Herberg and Kley, 1975) and to a lesser extent in heterozygotes, which presumably could account for T cell and NK-cell immunodeficiency; corticosteroids are known to reduce NK activity both in vivo and in vitro (Hochman and Cudkowicz, 1977; Parillo and Fauci,

TABLE V. Mutant Genes in Rodents Affecting NCMC

Gene (Chromosome)	Gene Name	Effect on NCMC	References
bg (13)	beige	impaired lytic activity; some NCMC inducible	Roder and Duwe, 1979
ob (6)	obese	quantitative reduction in NCMC	this report
mi (6)	microphthalmia	decreased NCMC: Replacement of NK cell precursors by osteoproliferation	Seaman *et al.*, 1979
fa (?)	Fatty Zucker Rat	NCMC reduced	this report
nu (11)	nude	elevated NCMC accentuation of underlying phenotype	Herberman *et al.*, 1975; Kiessling *et. al.*, 1975
lpr (?)	lymphoproliferation	elevated NCMC	this report
H-2 (17)	major immunogene complex	*H-2* linked control; no marked effect in mutants tested to date	this report and see Clark and Harmon, 1979
W^v (5)	dominant spotting anemia	no marked effect in $W^v/+$	this report
Dh (1)	dominant hemimelia	no obvious effect	Herberman and Holden, 1978
Lps (14)	Lps response	no obvious effect	Roder *et al.*, 1979
Sl^d (10)	Steel-Dickie anemia	no obvious effect in $Sl^d/+$	this report
Xid (x)	X-linked immunodeficiency	no obvious effect	Herberman and Holden, 1978

1978). Zucker fa/fa rats have been reported to have normal levels of adrenal steroids in one study (Yukimura et al., 1978) and high levels of serum corticosterone in another (Martin et al., 1978). Another possibility is that the increased or abnormal lipogenesis in obese animals may impede critical membrane surface changes necessary for cytolysis following binding of NK cells to targets.

The augmentation of NCMC in MRL mice with lymphoproliferative disease could be due to clonal expansion of NK cells in MRL-lpr mice. It is tempting to speculate that the subpopulation of $Lyt123^{-}$ $Thy\text{-}1^{+}$ cells that increases markedly with age in lpr/lpr homozygotes (Theofilopoulos et al., 1979a) may be identical or related to NK cells. Alternatively, MRL-lpr mice may be more susceptible to infections or other exogenous agents which augment NCMC levels. This possibility is supported by our finding that NK levels were not dramatically augmented in MRL-lpr recipients by BCG inoculation, and presumably are already activated. Furthermore, NK activity in older MRL-lpr mice is not dramatically increased. Additional studies of the ontogeny of natural killer activity and TBC frequencies in normal and diseased mice should distinguish these alternatives. MRL/MP-lpr/lpr mice display normal cell-mediated lymphocytic (CML) activity against allogeneic targets, but spleen cells from animals with advanced disease are poor stimulators of CML reactions (Theofilopoulos et al., 1979b).

In summary, certain obese states impair NK cell activity. Mild macrocytic anemia has little or no effect on NK cell levels. The homozygous recessive mutation lpr, which produces pronounced lymphoproliferation, also augments NK activity.

ACKNOWLEDGMENTS

We thank Drs. E. Eicher, R. Melvold and E. Murphy for mice, Dr. Len Shultz for helpful discussion, and Dr. S. Woods for supplying Zucker rats.

REFERENCES

Bennett, M., Cudkowicz, G., Foster, R. S. Jr. and Metcalf, D. (1968). J. Cell. Physiol. 71, 211.

Bray, G. A., and York, D. A. (1979). Physiol. Rev. 59, 719.

Chun, M., Pasanen, V., Hammerling, U., Hammerling, G. F., and Hoffmann, M. K. (1979). J. Exp. Med. 150, 426.

Clark, E. A., and Harmon, R. C. (1980). Adv. Cancer Res. 31, in press.

Clark, E. A., Russell, P. H., Egghart, M., and Horton, M. A. (1979). Int. J. Cancer 24, 688.

Haller, O., Kiessling, R., Orn, A., and Wigzell, H. (1977). J. Exp. Med. 145, 1411.

Harmon, R. C., Clark, E. A., O'Toole, C., and Wicker, L. S. (1977). Immunogenetics 4, 601.

Herberg, L., and Coleman, D. L. (1977). Metabolism 26, 59.

Herberg, L., and Kley, H. K. (1975). Horm. Metab. Res. 7, 410.

Herberman, R. B., and Holden, H. T. (1978). Adv. Cancer Res. 27, 305.

Herberman, R. B., Nunn, M. E., Holden, H. T., Staal, S., and Djen, J. Y. (1977). Int. J. Cancer 19, 555.

Herberman, R. B., Nunn, M. E., and Lavrin, D. H. (1975). Int. J. Cancer 16, 216.

Hochman, P. S., and Cudkowicz, G. (1977). J. Immunol. 119, 2013.

Kiessling, R., Klein, E., and Wigzell, H. (1975). Eur. J. Immunol. 5, 112.

Klein, G. O., Klein, G., Kiessling, R., and Karre, K. (1978). Immunogenetics 6, 561.

Kumar, V., Luevano, E., and Bennett, M. (1979). J. Exp. Med. 150, 531.

Martin, R. J., Wangsness, P. J., and Gahagan, J. H. (1978). Horm. Metab. Res. 10, 187.

Mattes, M. J., Sharrow, S. O., Herberman, R. B., and Holden, H. T. (1979). J. Immunol. 123, 2851.

Meade, C. J., Sheena, J., and Martin, J. (1979). Int. Arch. Allerg. Appl. Immunol. 58, 121.

Murphy, E. D., and Roths, J. B. (1978). In "Genetic Control of Autoimmune Disease" (N. R. Rose, P. E. Bigazzi, and N. L. Warner, eds.), p. 207. Elsevier North Holland, New York.

Parillo, J. E., and Fauci, A. S. (1978). Scand. J. Immunol. 8, 99.

Petranyi, G. G., Kiessling, R., and Klein, G. (1975). Immunogenetics 2, 53.

Petranyi, G. G., Kiessling, R., Povey, S., Klein, G., Herzenberg, L., and Wigzell, H. (1976). Immunogenetics 3, 15.

Roder, J. C., and Duwe, A. (1979). Nature 278, 451.

Roder, J., Kiessling, R., Biberfeld, P., and Andersson, B. (1978). J. Immunol. 121, 2509.

Roder, J. C., Lohmann-Mattes, M. L., Domzig, W., Kiessling, R., and Haller, O. (1979). Eur. J. Immunol. 9, 283.

Russell, E. S. (1970). In "Regulation of Hematopoiesis. I. Red Cell Production" (A. S. Gordon, ed.), p. 649. Appleton-Century-Crofts, New York.

Seaman, W. E., Gindhart, T. D., Greenspan, J. S., Blackman, M. A., and Talal, N. (1979). J. Immunol. 122, 2541.

Sheena, J., and Meade, C. J. (1978). Int. Arch. Allerg. Appl. Immunol. 57, 263.

Shultz, L. D. (1979). In "Inbred and Genetically Defined Strains of Laboratory Animals. III." (P. L. Altman and D. D. Katz, eds.), p. 68. Federation of American Societies for Experimental Biology, Bethesda.

Theofilopoulos, A. N., Eisenberg, R. A., Bourdon, M., Crowell, J. S. Jr., and Dixon, F. J. (1979a). J. Exp. Med. 149, 516.

Theofilopoulos, A. N., Shawler, D. L., Katz, D. H., and Dixon, F. J. (1979b). J. Immunol. 122, 2319.

Tracey, D. E., Wolfe, S. A., Durdik, J. M., and Henney, C. S. (1977). J. Immunol. 119, 1145.

Yukimura, T., Bray, G. A., and Wolfsen, A. R. (1978). Endocrinology 103, 1924.

GENETIC INFLUENCES AFFECTING NATURAL CYTOTOXIC (NC) CELLS IN MICE[1]

Osias Stutman
Michael J. Cuttito

Cellular Immunobiology Section
Memorial Sloan-Kettering Cancer Center
New York, New York

I. INTRODUCTION

Like all our entries in this volume, this paper will describe comparisons between NK and NC cells for strain distribution of activity and possible genetic influences that affect reactivity against a determined tumor target. Based on strain distribution of activity it will become apparent that NC and NK have quite different patterns. In addition, genes within, or close to the Tla-Qa region in chromosome 17, which affects NC reactivity levels, have no apparent effects on NK activity (see Section III.B).

II. GENETIC INFLUENCES ON NATURAL CYTOTOXICITY IN MICE

The idea for a possible genetic control of natural cell-mediated cytotoxicity (CMC) against tumor targets, was derived from the variation in levels of in vitro CMC between different mouse strains, when tested against the same targets (1-39). It was also observed that F1 hybrids of "high" and

[1] *This work was supported by grants CA-08748, CA-15988, and CA-17818 of the National Institutes of Health and Grant IM-188 from the American Cancer Society.*

ISBN 0-12-341350-8

"low" strains consistently showed high levels of CMC, both for the NK (3-5, 8, 25, 37, 38) and NC systems (18). In some experiments the F1 hybrids showed higher NK levels than both parents (7, 24, 29), implying some form of genetic complementation. In addition, radiation chimeras of high and low responders had NK levels similar to the marrow donor (38, 39), suggesting that one of the possible sites for genetic control may be the NK-precursor compartment in marrow.

When a more formal genetic analysis was done with anti-YAC NK cells, the results in F1 hybrids backcrossed to high or low responder parents indicated polygenic control, which included linkage with an $H2^b$ factor (3, 4, 8). A similar complexity was observed with other lymphoma targets (17, 24), showing again, polygenic control with either some linkage to $H2^d$ (24) or to the D end of H2 and Hhl (17). From these studies, it was also concluded that in vivo resistance to low numbers of lymphoma cells, did correlate with the NK levels in F1 hybrids or H2-recombinant mice (3, 4, 8, 17, 24, 25, 38). Additional in vivo studies, using a larger number of lymphomas and solid tumors showed a very complex picture (25). Resistance was under a highly polymorphic genetic control, probably pseudoallelic, and showing in some cases (especially with lymphomas) some degree of H2 linkage (25). In summary, no simple genetic pattern can define NK activity levels.

As we indicated in our Chapter on "Characterization," spleen levels of NK (or NC) activity at a particular moment in time may be influenced by so many factors, that it is impossible at present writing to decide at what levels the genetic influences are acting. For example, although NK activity appears to be regulated by interferon (29, 37, 38), there is no clear correlation between If.1 and If.2, two genes that affect interferon levels (29, 41) and NK activity. For example, although low anti-YAC NK strains like A/J belong to the If.1-low group (40), CBA mice, which are the prototype high anti-YAC NK reactors (38), also belong to the If.1-low group (40). In addition, sublines from these same strains may fall either in the high or low If.1 categories (40-42), making the problem even more complex.

The beige mutation on chromosome 13 strongly influences NK levels of activity in spleen (30, 36), although NK activity can be detected in beige mice using longer CMC assays (G. Cudkowicz, personnal communication).

NK levels of activity also appear to be influenced by factors associated with the black coat color (3)* and with albino

**Erroneously termed "B (black) locus" in ref. 3, since the black coat color is determined by the "aa" phenotype at the agouti locus (43).*

(c) coat color (8), while no linkage was observed for 5 isozyme loci, the Igl locus, C5 serum activity (8) and anti-M-MuLV antibody responses (11). Variations in strain distribution and other functional properties between anti-YAC and anti-EL4 NK cells have been described (29). In addition, our own studies on NC levels of reactivity, show a very different strain distribution from NK cells (18 and also Section III). These differences in strain distribution and genetic control also support our thesis of an heterogeneous, although closely related, population of effector cells in natural CMC responses (see our Chapter on "Characterization").

Several studies have shown groupings of mouse strains into high, intermediate or low reactors, based on their in vitro natural CMC against different tumor targets (1-38). However, it is accepted that a high degree of individual variation between members of the same mouse strains is a common feature (2, 3, 7, 10, 12, 18, 37, 38) and that many of the strain differences in reactivity tend to disappear after augmentation of NK activity by different agents (10, 15, 16, 20, 22, 23, 29, 31, 32, 35, 37, 38). For example, the CMC by spleen cells from A/Sn mice, which are the prototype low reactor against YAC-1 targets, can vary from 8 to 25% (3) or even show "intermediate" values (30, 35). The same can be said about A.CA and other congenic lines in the A background (3, 9). However, it is generally accepted that when appropriate numbers of animals are tested, some general patterns of reactivity can be defined (38). On the other hand, comparisons of strain distribution of NK reactivity against different targets has shown quite variable patterns of activity, depending on the target cells used. For example, compare the data obtained with YAC-1 cells (2-4, 7-9, 11, 19, 22, 23, 30, 35, 36, 38) with that obtained with EL4 (17, 29, 31, 32), RBL-5 or RL♂1 (5, 7, 10, 12, 13, 33, 34), other lymphoma targets and P815 (1, 6-8, 10, 12, 14-16, 20, 31, 32, 37) or with solid tumors (12, 21). A few examples may be informative. With YAC-1 targets it is accepted that CBA/J mice are the prototype high, while A/Sn, A/J and congenic animals in the A background are the prototype low reactors, with C57Bl/6 and other strains in the "intermediate" range (38). On the other hand, CBA and C57Bl/6 are low reactors (lower than A/J) against EL4 targets (29, 32). BALB/c have been reported as "intermediate" against YAC-1 (2) and RBL-5 as well as other targets (7, 10, 12), while they are non-reactors against RL♂1 targets (5, 13, 33). Although in a review it was indicated that the strain patterns of reactivity against YAC-1 targets were also observed against other tumor targets (38), from the above remarks it is apparent that such generalization is questionable. Even the actual data for the above statement (38) does not support it, and suggests

TABLE I. Strain Distribution of NC Reactivity Against Different Tumor Targets

Tumor	CMC Reactivity of Different Strains[a]		
	High	Intermediate	Low
Meth A[b]	All strains		
Meth 113[b]	A/J, NZB	C3H/HeJ, I/St	BALB/c*, CBA/H*, DBA/2 , C57Bl/6, B10.D2, B10.A, C3H/Bi
Meth E4[b]	A/J, I/St	BALB/c*, CBA/H*, C3H/Bi, C3H/HeJ, B10.D2, B10.A.	DBA/2, C57Bl/6, C57Bl/10
Meth X[b]	C57Bl/5, DBA/2, C57Bl/10, CBA nude, BALB nude	A/J, NZB, B10.D2, B10.A, CBA/H, C3H/Bi, C3H/HeJ, I/St	BALB/c
Ta3Ha[c]	A/J, DBA/2	BALB/c, C3H/Bi, C3H/HeJ	C57Bl/6
EL4	I/St	BALB/c*, DBA/2, A/J, CBA/H*, C57Bl/6, C57Bl/10, B10.D2	C3H/HeJ, C3H/Bi
P815	C3H/Bi & He	BALB/c*, CBA/H*	A/J, DBA/2, C57Bl/6, C57Bl/10, B10.D2, B10.A, I/St
YAC-1[d]	CBA/J, C3H/St, C3H/J	C57Bl/6, C57Bl/10, DBA/2, C3H/HeJ	A/Sn, A/J, A.BY, A.CA, A.SW, AKR, 129
EL4[e]	NZB	B10.D2, B10.A	A/J, CBA/J, C57Bl/6, DBA/2

that some intrinsic properties of the targets or other factors may also be important, For example, A/Sn mice were low or negative against YCAB-1 and P815 (2), however, CBA (the prototype high NK strain) was also negative against those same targets (2, 9, 22, 26). As a matter of fact, P815 is generally accepted as an NK-resistant target by most (7, 15, 22, 26, 31, 32, 37) and has been reported as lacking the surface glycoproteins that may represent the putative target structures for NK target-binding cells (43). However, some selected mouse strains can show high activity against P815 targets (1, 32) and activity can be increased in all strains after BCG (15) or virus infections (31), but not by C. parvum administration (22). When the high NK CBA mice were tested against 7 other lymphoma targets, the high activity was observed only against YAC-1, with lower or negative values against the others (2). Similarly, CBA mice tested against a total of 19 tumors (9, 26) showed intermediate values against 8, with negative or low responses against the rest (9, 26). Thus, the generalization for a particular mouse strain as being a "universal" high or low responder against all targets is questionable, and cannot be explained, when the results do not fit the preconceived idea , by the intrinsic variation of the system (38). In addition, to some special properties of the targets, the strain dependency or genetic influence of NK activity, may be the result of influences acting at many still undefined levels, and the overall CMC may be the final result of these complex interactions.

III. STUDIES WITH NC CELLS

A. Strain Distribution of NC Activity

In Table I we show a summary of our studies on strain distribution of NC reactivity in spleen against 5 adherent tar-

---

Footnotes for Table I.

[a]*Strain classification based on values determined at 100:1 E:T ratios, using spleen cells from 2-3 month old mice, in 24 hr assay using 3H-proline pre-labelled targets, as described in 18. EL4 and P815 tested in artificial monolayers prepared as in ref. 44. Strains were classified as high if they showed CMC of 30% or higher, intermediate from 15 to 30% and low if lower than 15%. (*) indicated that nude mice in that background were also tested.*

[b]*Ref 18;* [c]*Ref. 25;* [d]*NK data for YAC as in ref. 38;* [e]*NK data for EL4 as in ref. 29.*

gets derived from solid tumors (Meth A, Meth 113, Meth E4, Meth X and Ta3Ha) and 2 artificial monolayers of tumors usually grown in suspension (EL4 and P815). For details on the "Meth" tumors see ref. 18. Ta2Ha is a mammary tumor of A/Sn origin obtained from Dr. George Klein (Karolinska Institute, Stockholm, Sweden). Ref. 18 also contains details on the origin of the mouse strains tested. The last two lines in Table I also present NK strain distribution for YAC (38) and EL4 (29) targets in suspension, based on the published literature.

From Table I it can be concluded that the patterns of high, intermediate and low NC reactivity for different mouse strains against different tumor targets, is quite heterogeneous. For example, A/J show high or intermediate NC activity against all adherent targets except P815. CBA/H mice show low NC activity against Meth 113 and intermediate activity against the other adherent targets. C57Bl/6 are low NC reactors against Meth 113, Meth E4, Ta3Ha and P815, intermediate reactors against EL4-adherent and high against Meth A and Meth X. The three examples selected are low, high and intermediate reactive strains respectively for NK activity against YAC targets in suspension (38).

Table I also shows that in most instances, the reactivity of nude and normal mice in BALB/c or CBA/H background is comparable (18). However, against Meth X, the nudes in both backgrounds gave consistently higher NC activity than the normal controls, as was observed with NK reactivity (2, 7, 21, 31, 32, 37).

Comparing the data for EL4-adherent versus EL4-suspension in Table I, it appears that the patterns are not identical, and that the physical presentation of the target may be important (for further discussion of suspension versus adherent, see our Chapter on "Characterization").

Using Moloney sarcoma virus-induced adherent tumor targets and a 3H-proline assay comparable to ours (38), strain variation was also observed. Of 4 targets studied, 2 were resistant to effector cells from BALB and C57Bl/6 origin, one was susceptible to cells from both strains and the fourth was resistant to BALB/c and susceptible to cells from C57Bl/6 and other strains (28), again pointing at a complex pattern of susceptibility-resistance.

B. *A More Detailed Study of NC Activity Against Meth 113 Targets*

With Meth 113 fibrosarcoma targets of BALB/c origin, only some strains showed high levels of NC activity and the F1 hybrids of high and low reactive strains showed dominance of the high NC reactivity (18). A more detailed strain distribution study is presented in Table II. Besides the fact that

Table II. Strain Distribution of NC Reactivity Against Meth 113 BALB/c targets: Correlation with Tla and Qa Type

Strain	*H2*	*Tla*	*Qa1*	*Qa2*	*Qa3*	*NC Activity*[b]
C57Bl/6 (J, Boy)	b	b	b	a	a	L (Low)
B6.Tla^a (Boy)	b	a	a	a	a	H (High)
B6.H2^k (Boy)	k	b	b	b	b	H
B6.Kl (Boy)	b	b	a?	b	b	H
C57Bl/10	b	b	b	a	a	L
Bl0.A	a	a	a	a	a	L
AKR (Boy)	k	b	b	b	b	H
C58	k	a	a	b	b	H
C3H/Bi	k	b	a	b	b	H
BALB/cJ	d	c	b	a	a	L
BALB/cByJ	d	c	b	b	b	H
NZB	d	a	a	a	b	H
DBA/2	d	c	a	a	a	L
A (J, Sn,Boy)	a	a	a	a	a	H
A.Tla^b (Boy)	a	b	b	a	a	H
A.CA	f	d	a	b	b	H
A.TH	t1	a	a	a	a	H
A.TL	t2	c	b	a	a	H
A.BY	b	c	b	a	a	H
A.SW	s	b	b	a	a	L

[a]*All the strains indicated by (Boy) were obtained from Dr. E.A. Boyse (Sloan-Kettering Institute), and all the other mice used were obtained from Jackson Laboratories (Bar Harbor, ME).*

[b]*Activity was tested with spleen cells from 2-3 month old animals of the different strains against 3H-proline prelabeled Meth 113 target cells in a 24 hr assay (18). Animals were considered "high" reactors when showing CMC levels of 35% or more at 100:1 effector:target ratios; "low" reactors were defined as animals showing 15% or less CMC at 100:1 E:T ratios. The C3H/BiUmc mice consistently showed intermediate values of approximately 30% CMC. These patterns of reactivity were defined using at least 3 to 6 experiments and testing 3-5 individual animals per test.*

A strain mice and sublines (with the exception of A.SW) are all high NC reactors, in contrast with the anti-YAC NK studies (38). Table II also showed some interesting correlations when congenic strains at either H2 and especially at the Tla-Qa region (45-58) were studied. For example, C57Bl/6 mice (B6) are low NC reactors, while congenic animals that have either the "a" allele at Tla (derived from A strain mice) or the "b" alleles at Qa2-Qa3 are high reactors*. Similarly, BALB/cJ and BALB/cByJ which differ only at the Qa2-Qa3 regions (47) show different NC reactivity, and the mice carrying the "b" alleles at Qa2-3 are high reactors. The same trend was observed with other $H2^d$ strains like NZB (which carries the "a" allele at Tla and the "b" allele at Qa3) and DBA/2. Thus, one may postulate that genes on or in the vicinity of Tla and Qa2-3 can affect by themselves the expression of levels of NC activity in spleen against Meth 113 targets. In addition, a correlation with some alleles of such genes, i.e. a, c and d at Tla, which are the "positive" alleles, and the negative ("b") alleles at Qa 2 and 3 appears to favor high NC levels. Such genes do not appear to influence NK activity against YAC or EL4 (our unpublished observations).

A strain mice are consistently high NC reactors against the Meth 113 target (18). Table II shows studies with some congenic strains derived directly or indirectly from the A background (42, 48). From these studies we can postulate that an additional undefined gene (or genes) from the A background affects NC levels, based especially on the results from B10.A (Table II, line 6) and A. Tla^b (Table II, line 15). The B10.A, which derived its H2 region from strain A, although having the "a" allele at Tla, are low responders, suggesting that the gene or genes from the A background are located either outside the H2-Tla region or on other chromosomes. Conversely, the A.Tla^b (whose Tla region was derived from B6 mice, 45), although having the "b" allele at Tla, are high reactors. Again suggesting that genes outside the region or on other chromosomes can affect NC levels. The case for A.CA and A.TH, fit the suggested role of Tla and Qa2-3, since the "d" allele of Tla is very similar to the "a" (48). On the other hand, the "c" allele at Tla plus the "A background" gene, results in

**The Tla region phenotypes can express different antigenic specificities, thus the "a" allele expresses Tl. 1, 2, 3 & 5; the "c" allele only Tl.2 and the "d" allele Tl. 1, 2 and 3. The "b" is the negative allele (45-47). Similarly, the Qa 1, 2 and 3 genes have two alleles, the "a" allele which expresses the Qa 1, 2 and 3 antigens respectively and the "b" allele which is the negative one (47).*

good NC activity (the "c" allele at Tla by itself, does not favor high NC levels as is exemplified by BALB/cJ and DBA/2 mice). Finally, the A.SW strain, although derived from A and having a Tla-Qa composition comparable to A.Tla^b is a low responder, which may represent the exception to the above genetic associations. In summary, although the formal genetic analysis of these observations using the appropriate crosses and backcrosses is just beginning in our laboratories, one may postulate at least three "genes" that may affect NC levels against Meth 113 targets: 1) the gene/s related to Tla and associated with the "positive" alleles; 2) the gene/s related to Qa2 and Qa3 and associated with the "negative" allele and 3) the gene/s related to the A background. Since Tla and Qa2-Qa3 are relatively closely linked genes located distally at the D end of H2 in chromosome 17 (45-58), it may well be that a still undefined gene or genes on that region may be the ones affecting NC levels of activity. Especially, due to the fact that under normal conditions Tla is an exclusive marker for intrathymic lymphocytes (45-47), it is difficult to imagine how such a gene by itself can affect peripheral levels of NC cells. On the other hand the Qa antigens are expressed on peripheral T cells (45-47). One possibility, presently under study, is that the effect of Qa2-3 on NC activity may be due to Qa2-3 "positive" T cells which may act as regulators or suppressors of NC activity.

The present strain distribution studies and their possible genetic patterns appear quite different from anti-YAC NK activity (2-4, 8, 38) as well as from the ^{89}Sr-resistant anti-EL4 NK activity (29) or any other studies with EL4 (2, 7, 9, 16, 17, 26, 31, 32, which also show differences with 29 as well as between studies) or any other NK targets (1-38). Again, pointing to heterogenous systems with different patterns of strain reactivity and possibly also, genetic control. In addition, the strain distribution of NC activity against Meth 113, does not fit with either the strain distribution of the capacity to develop BCG-induced tumoricidal macrophages (49) nor with the "high or "low" alleles at If-1 and If-2, which are some of the genes controlling interferon levels (40-42).

As was indicated above, more formal genetic analysis is required before assigning definite gene/s to the control of NC activity. However, the marked differences in NC activity between congenic strains differing only at relatively small chromosomal segments, appears as a first step to define such genetic controls.

ACKNOWLEDGMENTS

We would like to thank Drs. E.A. Boyse and F.W. Shen for discussions over these results as well as for providing the B6.Tla^a, B6.H2^k, B6.Kl, A.Tla^b, A and B6 mice. We would also like to thank Dr. Lorraine Flaherty for the long phone conversations over some of these results and Linda Stevenson for the preparation of the manuscript.

REFERENCES

1. Greenberg, A.H. and Playfair, J.H.L., Clin. Exp. Immunol. 16, 99 (1974).
2. Kiessling, R., Klein, E. and Wigzell, H., Eur. J. Immunol.
3. Petranyi, G.G., Kiessling, R. and Klein, G., Immunogenetics 2, 53 (1975).
4. Kiessling, R., Petranyi, G., Klein, G. and Wigzell, H. Int. J. Cancer 15, 933 (1975).
5. Sendo, F., Aoki, T., Boyse, E.A. and Buafo, C.F., J. Natl. Cancer Inst. 55, 603 (1975).
6. Zarling, J.M., Nowinski, R.C. and Bach, F.H., Proc. Natl. Acad. Sci. U.S.A. 72, 2780 (1975).
7. Herberman, R.B., Nunn, M.E. and Lavrin, D.H., Int. J. Cancer 16, 216 (1975).
8. Petranyi, G.G., Kiessling, R., Povey, S., Klein, G., Herzengerg, L. and Wigzell, H. Immunogenetics 3, 15 (1976).
9. Becker, S., Fenyo, E.M. and Klein, E., Eur. J. Immunol. 6, 882 (1976).
10. Herberman, R.B., Nunn, M.E., Holden, H.T., Staal, S. and Djeu, J.Y., Int. J. Cancer 19, 555 (1977).
11. Asjo, B., Kiessling, R., Klein, G. and Povey, S., Eur. J. Immunol. 6, 554 (1977).
12. Nunn, M.E., Herberman, R.B. and Holden, H.T., Int. J. Cancer 20, 381 (1977).
13. Glichmer, L., Shen, F.W. and Cantor, H., J. Exp. Med. 145, 1 (1977).
14. Lee, J.C. and Ihle, J.N., J. Immunol. 118, 928 (1977).
15. Tracey, D.E., Wolfe, S.A., Durdik, J.M. and Henney, C.S., J. Immunol. 119, 1145 (1977).
16. Welsh, Jr., R., and Zinkernagel, R.M., Nature 268, 646 (1977).
17. Harmon, R.C., Clark, E.A., O'Toole, C.O. and Wicker, L.S., Immunogenetics 4, 601 (1977).
18. Stutman, O., Paige, C.J. and Feo Figarella, E., J. Immunol 121, 1819 (1978).

19. Seaman, W.E., Blackman, M.A., Gindhart, T.D., Roubinian, J.R., Loeb, J.M. and Talal, N., J. Immunol. 121, 2193 (1978).
20. Welsh, Jr., R.M., J. Exp. Med. 148, 163 (1978).
21. Burton, R.C., Grail, D. and Warner, N.L., Brit. J. Cancer 37, 806 (1978).
22. Ojo, E., Haller, O., Kimura, A. and Wigzell, H., Int. J. Cancer 21, 444 (1978).
23. Gidlund, M., Orn, A., Wigzell, H., Senik, A. and Gresser, I. Nature 273, 759 (1978).
24. Klein, G.O., Klien, G., Kiessling, R. and Karre, K., Immunogenetics 6, 561 (1978).
25. Klein, G., Klein, G.O., Karre, K. and Kiessling, R., Immunogenetics 7, 391 (1978).
26. Hansson, M., Karre, K., Bakacs, T., Kiessling, R. and Klein, G., J. Immunol. 121, 6 (1978).
27. Roder, J.C. and Kiessling, R., Scand. J. Immunol. 8, 135 (1978).
28. Henin, Y., Gomard, E., Gisselbrecht, S. and Levy, J.P., Br. J. Cancer 39, 51 (1979).
29. Kumar, V., Luevano, E. and Bennett, M., J. Exp. Med. 150, 531 (1979).
30. Roder, J. and Duwe, A., Nature 278, 451 (1979).
31. Welsh, Jr., R.M., Zinkernagel, R.M. and Hallenbeck, L.A. J. Immunol. 122, 475 (1979).
32. Croker, B.P., Zinkernagel, R.M. and Dixon, F.J., Clin. Immunol. Immunopathol. 12, 410 (1979).
33. Cantor, H., Kassai, M., Shen, F.W., Leclerc, J.C. and Climcher, L., Immunol. Rev. 44, 3 (1979).
34. Santoni, A., Herberman, R.B. and Holden, H.T., J. Natl. Cancer Inst. 62, 109 (1979).
35. Lohmann-Mathes, M.L., Domzig, W. and Roder, J., J. Immunol. 123, 1883 (1979).
36. Roder, J.C., Lohmann-Mathes, M.L., Domzig, W. and Wig-Zell, H., J. Immunol. 123, 2174 (1979).
37. Herberman, R.D. and Holden, H.T., Adv. Cancer Res. 27, 305 (1978).
38. Kiessling, R. and Wigzell, H., Immunol. Rev. 44, 165 (197 (1979).
39. Haller, O., Kiessling, R., Orne, A. and Wigzell, H., J. Exp. Med. 145, 1411 (1977).
40. DeMaeyer, E., Jullien, P., DeMaeyer-Guignard, J. and Demant, P., Immunogenetics 2, 151 (1975).
41. DeMaeyer, E., DeMaeyer-Guignard, J., Hall, W.T. and Bailey, D.W., J. Gen. Virol. 23, 209 (1974).
42. Altman, P.L. and D. Dittmer Katz (ed.). Inbred and Genetically Defined Strains of Laboratory Animals. 1.Mouse and Rat. Federation of American Societies for Experi-

mental Biology, Bethesda, MD (1979).
43. Green, M., in "Biology of the Laboratory Mouse" (E.L. Green, ed.) p. 87. McGraw-Hill, New York (1966).
44. Stulting, R.D. and Berke, G., J. Exp. Med. 137, 932 (1973).
45. Stanton, T.H. and Boyse, E.A., Immunogenetics 3, 525 (1976).
46. Flaherty, L., Immunogenetics 3, 533 (1976).
47. Flaherty, L., in Origins of Inbred Mice" (E.C. Morse III, ed.) p. 409. Academic Press, New York (1978).
48. Klein, J., Flaherty, L., VandeBerg, J.L. and Shreffler, D.V., Immunogenetics 6, 489 (1978).
49. Meltzer, M.S., Ruco, L.P., Boraschi, D. and Nagy, C.A., J. Reticuloendothel. Soc. 26, 403 (1979).

Addendum

A recent paper by Clark et al. (Int. J. Cancer 24, 688, 1979) which was not available to us at the time of completion of the present manuscript, contains an extensive study of strain distribution of NK activity against YAC-1 targets. Although, in general, this study shows a strain distribution comparable to that described in ref. 38, some discrepancies are again apparent, i.e. DBA/2 are "low" in Clark et al. and "intermediate" in 38 and similar studies. From the comparisons of B10.A and other B10 congenics, and from Clark et al., the case for a regulatory gene on D-end of H2 appears to be quite strong.

SUMMARY: IMMUNOGENETIC REGULATION OF NK ACTIVITY

Immunogenetic factors have been shown to play an important role in determining the levels of NK activity. Most of the evidence has been obtained in studies of mice. In contrast, only fragmentary information is available on the immungenetics of rat and human NK activity. Therefore, the summary below is mainly restricted to mouse genetic factors but some comments are also included regarding the limited human data.

I. IMMUNOGENETIC FACTORS IN MICE

A. *Genes Affecting Levels of NK Activity*

NK activity varies substantially among the inbred strains of mice and several investigators have performed detailed studies on the genes linked to expression of this effector function and on the effects of various genetic mutations. It is clear that NK activity is under polygenic control and analysis is quite complex. There are also indications of different genetic factors affecting various subsets of natural effector cells. A good example of this is the findings of Stutman and Cuttito that the genetic factors affecting levels of NC activity are distinct from those affecting NK activity. Even among NK or NC cells, the target cells used appear to have a major influence on the genetic patterns. Such heterogeneity is compatible with the possibility of multiple clones or subsets of NK cells (see section ID), each under somewhat separate genetic control. A further difficulty in the genetic studies is that even among mice of the same age and inbred strain, there is often a rather wide range in NK activity. This necessitates testing large numbers of mice and even then, minor genetic influences may be difficult to discern because of overlapping values between groups.

ISBN 0-12-341350-8

As discussed in detail by Clark et al and by Blair, one major gene affecting the levels of NK activity is closely linked to the D region of the H2 locus. The non-H2 background also has been found to be important, with the H2-linked differences being most apparent on the C57BL background. It is of interest to note that although different genes appear to be associated with expression of NC activity, at least one is also on the same chromosome as the H2 locus, distal to the D end. Thus the same genetic region appears to be involved in both NK and NC activities.

In F_1 hybrids between most strains, high activity seems to be dominant. In fact, as pointed out by Clark et al and by Blair, some complementation often occurs, with NK activity being higher in the hybrids than in either parental strain. In some recent immunogenetic studies, M. Brunda and H. Holden (unpublished observations) have found one interesting exception to this pattern. F_1 hybrids between SJL and A/J, both low NK strains, also had low NK activity. These data suggest that some of the genes responsible for low activity in these two strains are the same.

Screening of mice with various genetic mutations had led to a number of interesting findings. As discussed in section IA, homozygous nude mice have substantially higher NK activity than euthymic mice with the same genetic background. Cudkowicz and Kaminsky observed that the low reactivity of SJL mice was largely overcome by introduction of nude genes. Similarly, E.Clark (personal communication) has found that mice homozygous for both nude and beige genes had appreciable levels of activity, in the same range as normal mice with the same genetic background. Stutman and Cuttito also found that nude mice with BALB/c or CBA/H backgrounds had higher NC activity against one target cell than the normal controls. It has been suggested that this increased natural reactivity of nude mice might be related to their greater difficulty in handling environmental pathogens, with consequent augmentation of cytotoxic activity by increased levels of interferon. However, high levels of NK activity have also been found in pathogen-free nude mice (e.g. Clark et al). Also, Stutman and Cuttito did not observe increased NC activity against other target cells.

The findings by Roder and his colleagues, that beige mice have selective deficits in NK activity, are quite important since this allows detailed studies on the in vivo role of NK cells in groups of mice differing at only one genetic locus. Although the influence of the beige gene was initially studied in mice with C67Bl/6 background, it also causes low NK activity in mice with other backgrounds (Cudkowicz and Kaminsky). Although the original studies suggested that beige mice had an absolute defect in NK activity, with no cytotoxicity even after treatment with interferon or interferon-inducers, several groups have subsequently found some NK activity, especially after boosting (Brunda et al, Durdik et al, Cudkowicz and Kaminsky). The deficit in reactivity of beige mice also was found to be considerably less marked in the long term cytotoxicity assay (Cudkowicz and Kaminsky). However, the levels of spontaneous activity in a 13 hr assay varied among different groups of beige mice (Cudkowicz and Kaminsky) and Burton failed to detect spontaneous NK activity against YAC-1 in a 16 hr. assay. The beige mutation only appears to affect NK activity, with natural reactivity against solid tumor target cells being in the normal range (Burton; Stutman and Cuttito). Since those targets require longer term assays, it may be argued that the time-dependent deficit described by Cudkowicz and Kaminsky is overcome. However, Burton found a major difference between YAC-1 and WEHI-165 target cells in susceptibility to lysis by beige NK cells, in assays of the same length.

Several other genetic mutations have been found to affect NK activity. In support of their suggestion of the NK depression associated with estradiol being due to sclerosis of the bone marrow, Seaman and Talal have found that mice bearing the mi gene, associated with osteopetrosis, have low NK activity. Clark et al have found an association between the obese gene and low NK activity. Clark et al also report some interesting findings in mice with the lpr mutation, that is associated with lymphoproliferative disease. At 8 weeks of age, at the onset of disease, NK activity was found to be increased and this was paralleled with an increased proportion of Thy 1 positive cells. Clark et al raise the intriguing possibility that the disease may represent an abnormal proliferation of NK cells. More studies on these mice, to explore this suggestion, are awaited.

B. *Possible Mechanisms for Genetic Control of NK Activity*

Genetic factors could affect NK activity in several different ways. They could: a) determine the number of NK cells or their precursors; b) determine factors affecting the rate of differentiation of NK cells or the efficiency of their lytic machinery; c) influence the responsiveness of NK cells to interferon (IF) or other regulatory signals; and d) determine the ability to produce IF in response to various stimuli.

The studies of Haller et al, showing that levels of NK activity in radiation chimeras are dependent on the reactivity of the strain donating the bone marrow, indicate that the main genetic control of NK activity is at the level of the NK cells or their precursors, rather then related to other factors in the host. From this, one would predict that genes affecting the ability to produce IF would only control NK activity if NK cells themselves or other hematopoietic cells in the donor bone marrow were responsible for the IF production. The finding that regulation of IF production by two genetic loci, If 1 and If 2, did not correlate with NK activity is consistent with this prediction, since nonlymphoid cells are probably the main producers of IF in response to the stimuli used.

The findings of Cudkowicz and Kaminsky indicate that in addition to intrisic low reactivity of NK cells of SJL mice, the host environment has an appreciable influence. In contrast to the results of Haller et al in other strains of mice, Cudkowicz and Kaminsky found that transfers of bone marrow from strains with high or intermediate NK activity into SJL irradiated recipients resulted in very low NK activity. Conversely, when SJL bone marrow cells were transferred into recipients with high or intermiate NK activity, intermediate reactivity was seen. It will be of interest to detemine whether the low reactivity associated with the SJL environment is due to some deficit in factors needed for inducing or maintaining NK activity, e.g. deficient IF production in response to some stimuli, or to some form of active inhibition or suppression of NK activity.

There have been suggestions that responsiveness of NK cells to IF may vary among inbred strains, with the activity of cells from mice of high NK strains being augmented more than that of cells from low strains (e.g. see Brunda et al; Cudkowicz and Kaminsky). Thus, this may be one important mechanism for genetic control of activity. However, this could be a secondary phenomenon, due either to differences in numbers of pre-NK cells able to respond to IF or in the lytic efficacy of IF-boosted cells. To distinguish between these latter two possibilities, enumeration of NK cells independent of lytic activity would be very helpful. Two approaches have been considered for this measurement: a) antibodies to NK cell associated cell surface antigens and b) formation of conjugates with NK-sensitive target cells. As discussed in section IA, both of these methods have potential limitations. Correlations between numbers of antigen-positive cells and genes affecting NK activity would only be expected to be helpful if the antibody reacted only with NK cells and their precursors. Likewise, if counts of conjugate-forming cells included appreciable numbers of cells unrelated to NK, misleading information could be obtained. Despite these possible problems, it is of interest that beige mice have been found to have normal numbers of conjugate-forming cells (Roder and Haliotis) and of NK1.1 positive cells (Tam *et al*). These data suggest that the deficit in beige mice is related to the suboptimal ability of their NK cells to produce lysis of target cells. In contrast to the findings in beige gene, Roder and Haliotis have reported low percentages of conjugate-forming cells in most strains of mice with low NK activity. These data have not yet been confirmed by studies with antisera to NK associated antigens.

II. IMMUNOGENETIC FACTORS IN MAN

All studies have shown considerable variation in levels of NK activity among normal donors. However, there have been almost no genetic analyses to determine the possible basis for such variations. Some reports have described associations of high or low activity with some HLA types (e.g. Santoli *et al*, 1976). However, these associations have not been extended to family studies, to determine if there is genetic linkage of NK expression with the HLA locus. There has also been a reported influence of sex on NK activity. Forbes *et al* did find males to have a trend toward higher activity, but although large numbers of donors were tested, this was not significant.

It is of much interest that one human genetic mutation has been associated with low NK activity. Two patients with Chediak-Higashi syndrome, which seems to be analogous with the abnormalities in beige mice, were found to have a profound and selective deficiency in NK and K cell activities (Roder and Haliotis). An important clue to the mechanism responsible for these deficits came from the observation that treatment of the patients' cells with cyclic guanosine monophosphate led to almost normal levels of NK activity (Katz *et al*, 1980).

REFERENCES

Katz, P., Roder, J., Herberman, R.B., and Fauci, A.S., *Clin. Research*, in press.

Santoli, D., Trinchieri, G., Zmijewski, C.M., and Koprowski, H., *J. Immunol.* 117, 765 (1976).

DEVELOPMENT OF NK ACTIVITY DURING *IN VITRO* CULTURE

Reinder Bolhuis

Rotterdam Radio-Therapy Institute,
Rotterdam;
and
Radiobiological Institute TNO,
P.O. Box 5815
2280 HV Rijswijk
The Netherlands

C. REGULATION OF ACTIVITY

2. Ontogeny and development in culture.

a. GENERAL

Many in vitro grown tumor cells and virus-infected cells are susceptible targets for lysis by natural killer (NK). The possible role of these NK-cells as an alternative immunosurveillance mechanism has drawn considerable attention. Transformed cells may express antigens not present on their normal counterparts but these antigens may be cross reactive with allo-antigens on normal cells of other individuals (1-5), e.g. foreign haplotypes against which specific cytotoxic T-lymphocytes (CTL) can be generated in a mixed lymphocyte culture (MLC) (6-8).

In vitro generation of CTL by MLC with a pool of allogeneic mononuclear cells obtained from 20 allogeneic individuals containing all CD determinants results in CTL that lyse lymphocyte target cells from individuals that differ with the CD antigens from the responding individual (9). Zarling and

The work presented here was supported by grant X-67 of the Dutch Cancer League, the "Koningin Wilhelmina Fonds".

Bach (5) showed that CTL obtained from MLC with only a pool of allogeneic normal cells as stimulator cells gave rise to effector cells cytotoxic to autologous lymphoblastoid cell lines (LCL) but not to autologous normal lymphocytes nor phytohaemagglutinin (PHA) induced blasts.

If MHC molecules, known to be responsible for transplantation immunity, would have evolved as recognition sites for immunosurveillance T lymphocytes that eliminate aberrant cells, one would expect at least a proportion of MLC generated cells, being cytotoxic to tumor cells and operationally defined as MLC generated NK (MLC-NK) cells, to be identical with CTL.

The characteristics of the different types of cytotoxic cells generated after MLC (CTL and MLC-NK cells) will be compared and related to those of "fresh" NK cells and K-cells (ADCC). Furthermore, data from the relationship of target cell structures for MLC-NK on tumor cells and lymphoid cells will be presented.

METHODS

The experiments described here compare the cytotoxic activities of human lymphocytes either cultured alone (A) or stimulated with a) autologous lymphocytes (A.A*); b) autologous plus allogeneic lymphocytes of one individual [A.(A+B)*]; c) allogeneic lymphocytes (A.B*); and d) a pool of lymphocytes of 20 allogeneic individuals (A.C.* pool 20). The CTL generated after MLC were tested on the following target cells: a. PHA transformed autologous lymphoblasts; b. PHA transformed allogeneic (stimulator) lymphoblasts; c. PHA transformed pooled allogeneic lymphoblasts; d. K-562 erythroleukemic cell line without detectable HL-A and Ia antigens, growing in suspension (10); e. T24 bladder carcinoma cells and HT-29 colon carcinoma cells, both being anchorage dependent (monolayer target cells); f. P-815 mouse mastocytoma and GRSL mouse mammary tumor cells, being not susceptible to NK cell lysis in a 4 h ^{51}Cr-release assay (IgG-P-815 cells are used in K cell (ADCC) assays) (Section I.A; this issue).
K-562 cells are highly susceptible to lysis by fresh NK cells in a 4 h ^{51}Cr-release assay and the monolayer target cells are susceptible to lysis by fresh NK cells in a 16-20 h ^{51}Cr-release assay.

Lymphocyte purification and fractionation techniques and methodology of the analysis of cell surface markers have been summarized before (Section I.A.; this issue).

MLC-procedure: The MLC procedure was performed as described elsewhere (11, 12): In brief, .2 times 10^6 per ml responder cells and .5 times 10^6 per ml ^{137}Cs-irradiated (2500 rad:*) stimulator cells in either 10 ml or 50 ml of RPMI-1640 + 20 % pooled heat-inactivated human AB serum obtained from young male donors (younger that 35 years). .6 mg/ml L-glutamine, 1 mg/ml $NaHCO_3$ and 100 E/ml penicilline and streptomycine were added to Greiner 25 cm^2 or Costar (3075), 75 cm^2 tissue culture flasks, respectively. The flasks were placed under an angle of 45° and incubated at 37° C in a humidified atmosphere of 95 % air and 5 % CO_2 for 6 days. After incubation, the cells were harvested, washed and used as effector cells.

Cytotoxicity assays for CML, (MLC-)NK-cell and K-cell (ADCC) reactivities: The cytotoxicity assays were carried out as described previously (12; Section I.A., this issue).

Target cell preparation for CML assay: Target cells were obtained from the same donors as used for the MLC procedure. The lymphocytes were cultured for 3 days in RPMI-1640 + 20 % human AB and on day 3, 50 ul of PHA-M (Difco Labs, Detroit, Michigan) was added to 10 x 10^6 lymphocytes in 10 ml medium to induce blast formation (6). On day 6-7, the target cells were collected and washed once, spinned at 150 g for 10 min and 1 x 10^6 target cells were incubated with 200 uCi of $Na_2{}^{51}CrO_4$ solution, specific activity 50-400 uCi per mg ^{51}Cr for 1 h at 37° C (Radiochemical Center, Amersham, England). ^{51}Cr-labelled target cells were washed 3 times and resuspended at .1 x 10^6 per ml.

Absorption of effector cells on a monolayer of target cells: For the depletion of immunologic specific CTL and of MLC induced NK-cells, the effector cells were absorbed out by monolayers of either lymphoid mononuclear cells of the target cell type or control lymphoid cells and on T24 or K562 tumor cell monolayers. The original technique has been described by De Silva and DeLandazuri (14) and used for adsorbing CTL and MLC-NK cells (11).

Cytotoxicity of peripheral blood lymphocytes after culturing and after MLC: When lymphocytes are cultured for 6 days in medium supplemented with human AB serum in the absence of irradiated (*) allogeneic stimulator cells, the NK-cell activity decreases although sometimes residual activity may be found (Tables I and II; 15, 16).

The responder lymphocytes of individual donors which are stimulated with a pool of 20 irradiated lymphocytes yield effector cells that exert a strong cytotoxicity against all cell lines tested. It is noteworthy that T24 tumor cells are lysed within 4 h by MLC-NK cells (Table I), whereas "fresh" NK cells lyse monolayer target cells only after a prolonged effector-target cell incubation time (16-18 h) (11, 12, 17).

Whereas it is known that the MLC-generated CTL are from the T-cell lineage (6-8), the nature of the MLC generated NK-cells killing the tumor cell lines is not determined and the question whether they relate to the NK-cells which are present in fresh human PBL is not firmly answered.

Relationship between MLC-generated CTL and NK-cells and between PHA lymphocyte blasts and tumor target cells: Zarling and Bach (5) demonstrated that sensitization of lymphocytes with a pool of normal mononuclear cells of 20 allogeneic donors gives rise to effector cells cytotoxic to autologous Epstein-Barr virus transformed lymphoblastoid cell lines (LCL), but not to autologous normal lymphocytes nor to PHA-induced blasts. Hence, the tumor target cell structures for MLC generated NK cells may be cross-reactive with allo-antigens (5). On the basis of this hypothesis one would expect that stimulation with a pool of normal allogeneic mononuclear cells would generate effector cell cytotoxic to a variety of tumor target cells and that the stimulation with cells derived from 1 individual donor would not regularly do so.

In order to investigate whether the high level of MLC-NK reactivity against all tumor cells tested was due to the presence of all CD determinants in the mixture of stimulator cells as is the case in a stimulator cell population of twenty randomly chosen donors ($C^*_{pool\ 20}$) (9), we also tested MLC-NK cells with stimulator cells obtained from 1 single donor (A.B*). Since the increased level of NK-cytotoxicity might (partly) be due to soluble factors produced by the, among themselves, allogeneic stimulator cells we also tested MLC-NK cells using a mixture of autologous and allogeneic mononuclear cells as stimulators [A.(A+B)*].

As can be seen from Table II, there is no consistent difference in the NK cell lytic capacity generated after an A.B*, A.(A+B)* or $A.C^*_{pool\ 20}$ type of MLC. On the average the lytic capacity of $A.C^*_{pool\ 20}$ being AB* $\geq$ A.(AB)* $\gg$ A.A* $\geq$ A cultured alone, i.e., the average per cent lysis ($\pm$ SD): 58 $\pm$ 14; 59 $\pm$ 10; 54 $\pm$ 18; 14 $\pm$ 18; 12 $\pm$ 11 (11). This result excludes that putative soluble factors produced by the allogeneic stimulator cells play a major role in lysis of the target cells.

Several conclusions can be drawn from these results: The A.B* MLC generated NK cell activity is more or less equal to that of $A.C^*_{pool\ 20}$ generated effector cells, thus the amount of different MHC antigens (HLA-D) expressed by the stimulator cell population seems to be of minor importance for the induction of MLC-NK cells. In general, A.B* generated CTL will specifically lyse mononuclear cells from donor B only and, for instance, not those of a donor C which is allogeneic to donor B. A.C*$_{pool\ 20}$ MLC generated CTL will kill lymphocytes of any individual, since the CTL are sensitized against all CD-determinants possible (4, 5, 12), i.e. more cytotoxic clones are proliferating and thus more CTL are produced. This and the observation that significantly more ^{14}C-thymidine is incorporated after pool than after A.B* (individual) stimulation (data not shown) without a similar increase in MLC-NK cell activity indicates that the rate of cell proliferation is not a crucial factor. Callewaert et al. (16) provided direct evidence for this conclusion. These authors recently reported that the NK-cell and K-cell activities are not abrogated by 5-bromodeoxyuridine (BUDR) and light treatment. This treatment results in destruction of dividing cells and hence results in elimination of CTL cells. These results suggest that MLC generated CTL are not identical with the MLC generated NK cells nor that there exists an antigenic relationship between the CD antigens on the mononuclear lymphoid target cells recognized by the CTL and the (antigenic) structures on the tumour cells recognized by the MLC generated NK cells. The chance that stimulator lymphoid cells from a randomly chosen donor would share determinants with all the tumor cells tested, including mouse tumor cells (see below) is neglectable. This lack of relationship is also suggested by the fact that T24 bladder cancer cells could not be tissue-typed (unpublished observations) and K-562 target cells lack detectable HLA and Ia antigens (10).

Analysis of the antigens involved in recognition by MLC generated CTL and NK cells: To further investigate the structural relationship of the MHC antigens and tumor associated antigens (TAA) we performed inhibition of CTL and MLC-NK reactivity using a cold target cell inhibition ^{51}Cr-release assay. As can be seen from Table III, the inhibition of ^{51}Cr-release by A.B*-CTL is most outspoken when the relevant stimulator (or C$_{pool\ 20}$, data not shown) competitor cells are added to the lytic assay but not by adding autologous competitor cells. Cells conpletely allogeneic to the labelled target cells do not inhibit either (data not shown). This demonstrates the well-known immunologic specificity of the CTL effector cells.

K-562 and T24 cells both inhibit the MLC-NK ^{51}Cr-release of both K-562 and T24 labelled target cells. K-562 cells is always the most efficient inhibitor in cross competition assays, i.e. in general as efficient as the relevant target

TABLE I

CELL MEDIATED LYMPHOLYSIS: EFFECT OF CULTURING AND OF AUTOLOGOUS AND "POOL" STIMULATION ON THE GENERATION OF NK CELLS

Effector cells	Target cells[a] K-562	T24		Mel-1	HT29	% E-RFC		% EA-RFC	
	4 h	4 h	20 h	20 h	20 h	before MLC	after MLC	before MLC	after MLC
A	9		14.2		-10.6	89		33	
AA*	0		16.9				23		
AF* pool 20	25	15.5	65.3	63.5	49.3		41		6
B	0		-3.3			90		30.2	
BB*	5		33.1				33		6
BF* pool 20	53	31.5	71.4	55.2	41.5		29		6
C	0		-7.2			82		38	
CC*	20		47.4				41		5
CF* pool 20	56	29.8	71.5	66.8	63.6		28		8
D			2.6	13.8		83		29	
DD*			35.0				42		7
DF* pool 20		25.9	70.7	84.4	73.4		32		5
D K-562		9.7	-2.5		-0.4				
E	11		15.2	27.8	-14.1	88		23	
EE*									
EF* pool 20	46	24.1	70.7	83.8	60.1		34		7
F[b]	64	8							
G[b]	49	7							

[a]Effector cell:target cell ratio 50:1; 4 h or 20 h ^{51}Cr-release assay at day in Cooke round bottom plates. Medium: RPMI-1640 supplemented with 20 mM Hepes; 1 g $NaHCO_3$/1; 4 mM glutamin, 1 % penicillin/streptomycin and 20 % pooled human AB serum.
[b]Frozen/stored lymphocytes of donors F and G tested on day 7.

TABLE II

CELL MEDIATED LYMPHOLYSIS: EFFECT OF DIFFERENT RESPONDER/STIMULATOR CELL COMBINATIONS ON THE INDUCTION OF CTL AND NK-CELL ACTIVITY

Effector cells	Targets[a] A-PHA	B-PHA	$C_{pool\ 20}$-PHA	K-562	T24 4 h	T24 20 h**
AA*[b]	- 5	- 3	-12	1	1	8
A(A,B)*	18f	15	18	60	49	100
AB*	17	14	19	66	54	95
AC*pool 20	18	18	19	67	64	107
	D-PHA	E-PHA	C_{pool5}-PHA			
DD*[b]	0	0	1	10	2	
D(D,E)*	9	38	29	65	50	
DE*	10	31	27	65	43	
DC*pool 5	2	7	17	46	18	

a ^{51}Cr-release assay in Cooke round bottom plates. Effector cell:target cell ratio 50:1.
b 2 x 10^6 responders + 5 x 10^6 stimulators of each donor;

cell. This is not the case in the reciprocal cross competition assays, i.e., the lysis of K-562 is inhibited by other tumor cells but to a lesser extent than by the K-562 cells themselves.

From Tables III A-C, it can be seen that heat inactivated mononuclear lymphoid cells do not inhibit the MLC generated NK-cell lysis of K-562 target cells. Both K-562 and T24 tumor cells do sometimes inhibit the specific lysis of A.B* and A.C* pool 20 CTL against B lymphoid target cells (Table III, A and B) and we have reported this finding (11, 12). We have data which suggest that this inhibition is due to the PHA induced susceptibility to lysis of lymphoblasts by MLC-NK cells (18). Our results differed from the experience of Seeley et

TABLE III

COLD TARGET CELL CROSS-INHIBITION ASSAYS

	Effector cell	Inhibitor cell	Inhibition target cell ratio	% ^{51}Cr-release target cells: A-PHA	B-PHA	K-562	T24	P815
A	A.C*pool 20			35	58	75	68	
		A-PHA	50 : 1		38	72	77	
			10 : 1		49	65	74	
		B-PHA	50 : 1		27	69	73	
			10 : 1		42	69	79	
		K-562	50 : 1		24	17	11	
			10 : 1		41	59	40	
		T24	50 : 1		27	41	9	
			10 : 1		38	62	20	
B	A.B*			14	47			34
		A-PHA	50 : 1		38			60
		B-PHA	50 : 1		15			57
		K-562	50 : 1		38			2
			25 : 1		37			3
			12 : 1		42			5
		P815	50 : 1		44			4
			25 : 1		45			6
			12 : 1		45			10
	B.A*			35	21			48
		A-PHA	50 : 1	10				64
		B-PHA	50 : 1	21				66
		K-562	50 : 1	10				1
			25 : 1	13				2
			12 : 1	15				5
		P815	50 : 1	22				5
			25 : 1	23				9
			12 : 1	25				16
C	A.B*			0	50	61		
		A-PHA	30 : 1		40	62		
			10 : 1		50	60		
		B-PHA	30 : 1		18	59		
			10 : 1		34	60		
		K-562	10 : 1		40	43		
	B.A*			54	0	35		
		A-PHA	30 : 1	21		34		
			10 : 1	42		34		
		B-PHA	30 : 1	54		32		
			10 : 1	56		32		
		K-562	30 : 1	49		2		
			10 : 1	53		8		

Effector:target cell ratio 50 : 1.
Spontaneous ^{51}Cr-release of PHA-lymphoblasts ranged from 9 - 19 per cent.
^{51}Cr-release of target cells in the presence of inhibition cells only was equal to medium control values.

al. (19). These investigators reported that K-562 cells did did not inhibit the lysis of lymphoblasts. Our experience, however, is that it may (Table III, A and B) or may not (Table III,C) occur, depending whether or not there is a high "anomalous" kill of autologous PHA lymphoblasts (11). In contrast to the findings of Zarling and Bach (5) we repeatedly, but not constantly, observed killing of autologous PHA blasts, especially after "pool" stimulation (Tables III,A and B). This anomalous killing has, however, been reported by others (20-22). The frequency of such anomalous kill depended on the PHA batch used to induce blast formation (unpublished observations). Control experiments taking irradiated A*.B* or A*.(A+B)* yielded no cytotoxic effector cells indicating that the lysis of autologous target cells was not caused by surviving irradiated (*) stimulator cells (data not shown). Addition of lymphoblasts or tumor inhibitor cells to labeled lymphoid target cells did not influence the per cent ^{51}Cr release from the target cells excluding non-immunologic factors such as physical crowding or changes in culture conditions to be the cause of inhibition.

If one, however, subtracts the percentages "anomalous" kill (A.B* on target A; B.A* on target B) from the percentages kill on the relevant target cell (A.B* on target B; B.A on target A), then it appears that these differences of percentage lysis equal the percentage lysis of the lymphoblasts in the presence of the K-562 and T24 inhibitor cells (Table III, A and B). When no anomalous kill of autologous target cells is encountered, no inhibition of immune specific lysis by K 562 and T24 inhibitor cells is observed (Table III,C). Hence, the per cent lysis of target cells by the relevant effector cells as measured in the CML (for instance, A.B* on B-PHA) may represent the sum of the immune specific lysis (by CTL) and the anomalous kill (h, MLC-NK). This only occurs when PHA transformation of the lymphoid target cells renders these cells susceptible to MLC-NK cell lysis. In that case, both PHA lymphoblast syngeneic to the CTL effector and MLC-NK tumor target cells can inhibit.

Table III also demonstrates that MLC-NK cells can lyse P-815 mouse mastocytoma cells in a 4 h ^{51}Cr-release assay. One has to bear in mind that these P-815 mouse tumor cells (like GRSL mouse leukemia tumor cells, see below) are not lysed by "fresh" human NK cells.

Occasionally, we found unlabeled lymphoblasts to significant enhance the lysis of ^{51}Cr-labeled P-815 target cells (Table III,B), although the unlabeled lymphoblasts did not influence the ^{51}Cr-release of labeled target cells as compared to medium controls. Recently, Callewaert et al. have reported enhancement of "fresh" NK cell lysis after addition of SB lymphoblast cells and "fresh" NK insensitive RPMI-7666 cells in similar inhibition studies (23). This may explain why PHA blasts, which (occasionally) might be susceptible to MLC-NK lysis, do inhibit labeled K-562 on T24 target cells. The net zero effect of addition of unlabeled PHA-lymphoblasts may be the result of the enhancement of lysis which is compensated by its inhibition of lysis. We have no explanation for this enhancement phenomenon. The inhibitor lymphoblasts by themselves had no effect on the per cent ^{51}Cr-release.

The nature of the data obtained in cross cold target cell inhibition assays of cell-mediated lysis are complex and need careful analysis to avoid erronous conclusions. The experimental results do, however, clearly show that the target cell structures for lysis on tumor by MLC-NK cells are different from the CD determinant for CTL on lymphocytes.

Absorption of MLC-induced CTL- and NK-cells on lymphocyte and tumor cell monolayers: To further substantiate this important conclusion we have chosen a different approach to analyse the CTL and MLC-NK effector cell-target cells interactions and specificities. For this purpose, we used the monolayer technique originally developed to study CTL. Cells with a specificity for a particular target cell will only adhere on a monolayer of that particular target cell or of cells with cross-reacting structures on their surface. We have studied the adherence properties of CTL and MLC-NK cells on monolayers of lymphoid cells, K-562 and T24 tumor target cells. This technique permits the investigation of the relationship between the recognition structures on lymphoid cells for CTL and on tumor target cells for MLC-NK on the one hand and the selectivity of MLC-NK cells for K-562 and T24 target cells on the other. Unseparated effector cells and effector cells incubated on control monolayers were tested simultaneously. Recoveries of effector cells from the monolayer varied from 60 to 90 per cent. A representative example of the depletion experiments is presented in Fig. 1.

As for the CTL, it can be seen in Fig. 1 that A.B* induced CTL can only be absorbed out on a donor B-lymphocyte monolayer and not on monolayers of control A lymphocytes, K-562 or T24 tumour cells. Similarly, in the reciprocal stimulation B.A*, effective depletion of effector cells is only seen when donor A-lymphocyte monolayers are used to absorb the effector cells (data not shown). The MLC-induced NK-cytolytic activity against both K-562 and T24 can effectively be absorbed out on either K-562 or T24 monolayers but not on lymphocyte monolayers. The NK-activity against K-562 is more effectively reduced by absorption on K-562 monolayers as compared to T24 monolayers but both K-562 as well as T24 monolayers are equally efficient in absorbing out the NK-cells reactive against T24 (Fig. 1). These results confirm our cold target cell inhibi-

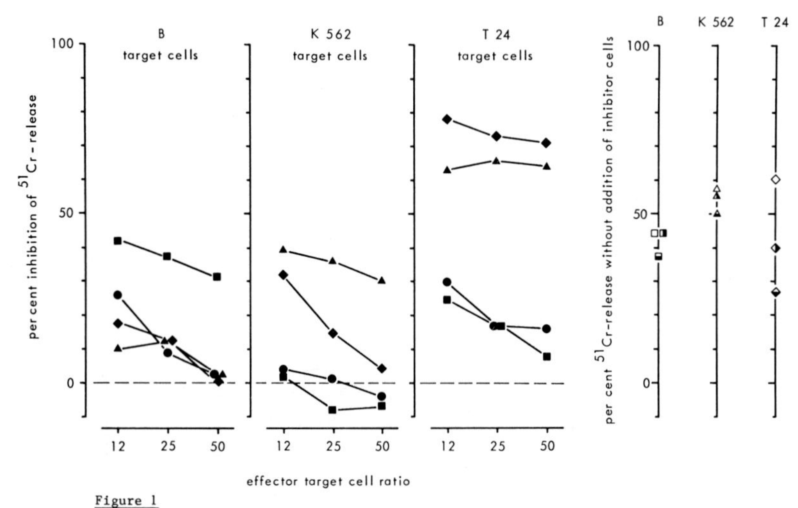

Figure 1

Monolayer of donor : A●; B■; K-562▲; T24◆.
The non-adherent fraction was tested on various eff.: t.c. ratios.
On the axis □◧⬓; △◭▲; ◇◈◆ represent the per cent ^{51}Cr-release before absorption of the effector cells A and B on targets A, B, K-562 and T24, respectively.

tion studies described above where it was demonstrated that K-562 cells can inhibit the lysis of T24 targets as efficiently as T24 whereas T24 is a less effective inhibitor of the lysis of K-562 target cells than K-562 cells themselves. The efficacy of the absorption on monolayers becomes more clear at higher effector to target cell ratios and this indicates the specificity of the absorption procedure. The tumor cell monolayer absorption experiments also revealed a slight reduction of cytotoxicity against PHA blasts, i.e. depletion on the tumor cell monolayers of non-specific effector cells (NK cells) against PHA blasts. The specific CTL cells are recovered.

A number of investigators recently reported on the enhancement of lysis by PBL of tumor target cells and autologous lymphoblastoid cell lines in K (ADCC) and NK cell assays, not only after stimulation of T cells with mitogens and FCS but also after MLC (24-27). The cytotoxic effects of the generated effector cells against autologous lymphoblastoid cell lines and autologous PHA transformed mononuclear cells was denoted as non-specific or anomalous killing (20-22).

Involvement of the IgG-FcR in the MLC-induced CTL and NK-cell lysis: We have shown that the percentage of EA-RFC present in MLC-stimulated lymphocytes is lower than that present in freshly isolated human peripheral blood lymphocytes confirming the data of Poros et al. (26, Table I). We and others have previously demonstrated that the IgG-FcR, although exexpressed on all NK-cells that are cytotoxic to K-562 cells (13, 28-30) and on a proportion of the NK cells reactive against anchorage dependent cells (13, 28) is not necessarily involved in the lytic process (13, 28, 29; Section 1.B, this issue). Our results demonstrate that a small proportion of MLC-generated NK-cells may bear IgG-FcR on their membrane but the IgG-FcR negative cells show significant lysis of K-562 independently confirming the independent findings of Poros et al. (30). Thus, depletion of residual IgG-FcR positive cells on immunocomplex monolayers does not or only slightly reduce the per cent lysis of target cells indicating that the CTL and MLC-NK cells do not express IgG-FcR (Fig. 2). This does not necessarily mean that the IgG-FcR negative cells are essentially different from the positive cells since we demonstrated that the IgG-FcR positive cells can be modulated leading to shedding of the IgG-FcR with loss of K-cell activity, whereas the NK-cell activity is retained (13, 28). Thus, the FcR-negative cells may represent the same NK cells, but in a physiological state where they have shed their IgG-FcR.

As shown the MLC-NK cells lyse human T24 and mouse P-815 and GRSL tumor cells a 4 h ^{51}Cr-release assay, whereas "fresh" NK cells lack this capacity. This strongly indicates that MLC-NK cells represent *de novo* generation of previously inactive progenitor cells which are present in human peripheral blood.

To illustrate this conclusion we have depleted Ficoll separated mononuclear cells of fresh NK cells by depleting the IgG-FcR positive cells. This NK-depleted cell fraction was used as responder cells in MLC. The MLC-generated effector cells were tested for CTL and MLC-NK reactivity. A representative experiment is shown in Fig. 3. This figure shows that depletion of IgG-FcR positive cells (and hence of the NK cells): a) does not influence the generation of immune specific CTL; b) MLC-NK cells can still be generated.

The fact that the MLC induced level of NK cell cytotoxicity of the EA-RFC depleted cell fraction may be lower as compared to that of the unseparated fraction may be due to the removal of an IgG-FcR positive accessory cell, necessary for optimal activation of NK cells after MLC or alternatively that at least two types of NK precursor cells are generated whereby the generation of at least one NK precursor is dependent on the presence of IgG-FcR positive accessory cells or, alternatively, possessing that receptor itself. It is noteworthy that human and (cross-species) mouse P-815 and GRSL

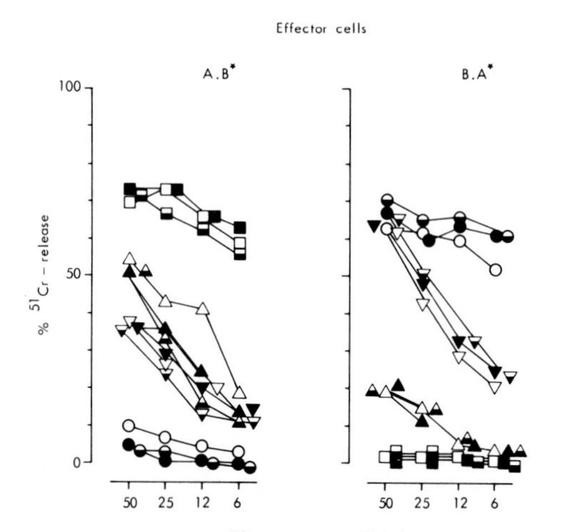

Figure 2:
The effect of EA-RFC depletion after MLC on the reactivity of CTL and NK cells. Unseparated effector cells: open symbols; EA-RFC depleted cells: closed symbols; cells separated on control monolayers: half open/closed symbols.
Target cells: ○, A-PHA; □, B-PHA; △, K-562; ▽, T24.

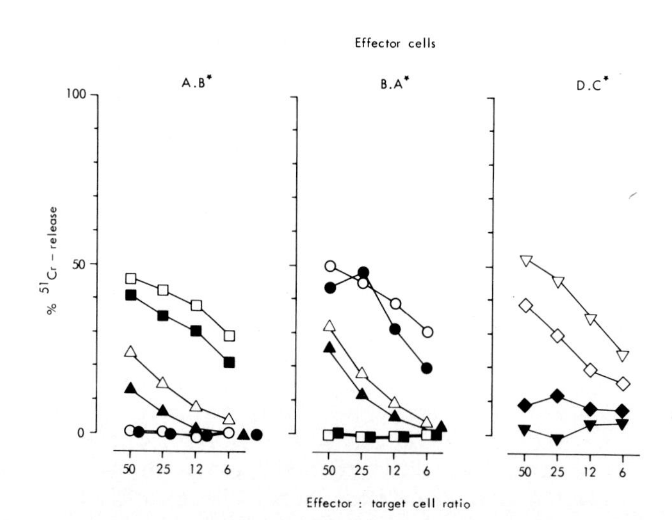

Figure 3:
The MLC induced generation of CTL and NK cells in unseparated (open symbols) and NK cell depleted, prior to MLC (closed symbols), cell populations.
Target cells: ○, A; □, B; △, K-562; ▽, P-815; ◇, GRSL.

tumor cell lines are readily lysed by MLC-NK cells but not by fresh NK cells. MLC-NK cells, generated in a population depleted of EA-IgG-FcR positive cells prior to MLC, only lyse the human target cells and not the (cross-species) mouse tumor target cells. This again suggests that the MLC-NK cells indeed represent a heterogeneous population. However, our small series of experiments do not allow a definite statement.

It can be concluded that:

a) the MLC generated NK cell killing of K-562 target cells is increased;
b) T24 target cells are lysed in a 4 h ^{51}Cr-release assay by MLC-NK but not by fresh NK cells;
c) P-815 and GRSL mouse tumor cells are lysed in a 4 h ^{51}Cr-release assay by MLC-NK but not by fresh NK cells, i.e. the target cell spectrum of MLC-NK cells is broader than that of "fresh" NK cells.
d) T24 cells can inhibit the lysis in a 4 h ^{51}Cr-release assay of K-562 labelled target cells by fresh and MLC-NK cells and vice versa;
e) K-562 and T24 target cells may inhibit the MLC-NK cell lysis of either K-562 or T24 labelled target cells and occasionally the CTL lysis of labelled mononuclear PHA-lymphoblasts in cold target inhibition assays. This latter inhibition is only the case when anomalous lysis of the PHA-blasts is observed, i.e., when the per cent lysis of blasts in CML in the sum of MLC-NK and immune specific (CTL) lysis of the PHA blasts;
f) lymphoid cells do not inhibit the NK-cell lysis of K-562 and T24 labelled target cells;
g) depletion of CTL on monolayer of either lymphoid or tumor cells can only be obtained on a monolayer of the relevant lymphoid cells;
h) absorption of MLC-NK cells reactive against K-562 or T24 target cells is successful using K-562 as well as T24 cell monolayers but not lymphoid monolayers. Monolayers of K-562 are the most efficient absorbens of MLC-NK.

ACKNOWLEDGEMENTS

The author wishes to thank Mr. C.P.M. Ronteltap, Mrs.A.M. Nooyen, Mrs. R. de Rooy for superb technical assistance. Mrs. M. van der Sman for inventive secretarial help.

REFERENCES

1. Martinis, J. and Bach, F.H. Transplantation 25, 1978, 39.
2. Intervenizzi, G. and Parmiani, G., Nature (Lond.) 254, 1975, 713.
3. Parmiani, G. and Intervenizzi, G. Int.J. Cancer 16, 1975, 756.
4. Martin, W.J., Gipson, T.C., Martin, S.E. and Rice, J.M. Science 194, 1976, 532.
5. Zarling, J.M. and Bach, F.H. J. Expt. Med. 147, 1978, 1334.
6. Lightbody, J., Bernoco, D., Miggiano, V.C. and Ceppelini, R. G. Bacteriol. Virol. Immunol. 64, 1971, 243.
7. Trinchieri, G., Bernoco, D., Curtoni, S.E., Miggiano,V.C. and Ceppelini, R. In: Histocompatibility Testing (J.Dausset and J. Colombani, eds.), Munksgaard, Copenhagen 1973.
8. Eijsvoogel, V.P., Du Bois, M.J.G., Melief, C.J.M., De Groot-Kooy, M.L., König, C., Van Rood, J.J., v. Leeuwen, A., Du Tort, E. and Schellekens, P.Th.A. In: Histocompatibility Testing (J. Dausset and J. Colombani, eds.), Munksgaard, Copenhagen, 1973.
9. Bach, M.L., Bach, F.H. and Zarling, J.M., Lancet 1, 1978, 20.
10. Drew, S.I., Terasaki, P.I., Billing, R.J., Bergh, O.J., Minowada, J. and Klein, E., Blood 49, 1977, 715.
11. Bolhuis, R.L.H., Submitted for publication.
12. Bolhuis, R.L.H. and Ronteltap, C.P.M., Immunol. Letters, in the press.
13. Bolhuis, R.L.H., Schuit, H.R.E., Nooyen, A.M. and Ronteltap, C.P.M., Eur. J. Immunol. 8, 1978, 731.
14. Silva, A. and Delandazuri, M.O. J. Immunol. Methods 23, 1978, 303.
15. Ortaldo, J.R., Bonnard, G.D. and Herbermann, R.B. J. Immunol. 119, 1977, 1351.
16. Callewaert, D.M., Lightbody, J.J., Kaplan, J., Joroszewski, J., Peterson, W.D. and Rosenberg, J.C., J. Immunol. 121, 1978, 81.
17. Bolhuis, R.L.H., Cancer Immunol. Immunother.2, 1977, 245.
18. Bolhuis, R.L.H., manuscript in preparation.
19. Seeley, J.K. and Golub, S.K. Am. Assoc. Cancer Res. 18, 1977, 174.
20. Lundgren, G., Zukoski, Ch.F. and Möller, G. Clin. Exp. Immunol. 3, 1968, 817.
21. Svedmyr, E.A., Deinhardt, F. and Klein, G. Int. J. Cancer 13, 1974, 891.
22. Butterworth, A.E. and Franks, D., Cell.Immunol. 16, 1975, 74.
23. Callewaert, D.M., Kaplan, J., Johnson, D.F. and Peterson, W.D., Cell. Immunother. 42, 1979, 103.

24. Nelson, D.L., Bundy, B.M., Pitchon, H.E., Blase, R.M. and Strober, W. J. Immunol. 117, 1976, 1472.
25. Ortaldo, J.R. and Bonnard, G.D. Fed.Proc. 36, 1977, 1325.
26. Poros, A. and Klein, E. Cell. Immunol. 64, 1978, 240.
27. Jondal, M. and Targan, S., J. Exp. Med. 148, 1978, 1621.
28. Bolhuis, R.L.H., Thesis Eramus University, Rotterdam, 1977.
29. Eremin, O., Ashby, J. and Stephens, J.P. Int. J. Cancer 21, 1978, 35.
30. Poros, A., Seeley, J.K., Klein, E. and Masucci, G. (1979) in the press.

In Vitro Development of Human NK Cells: Characteristics of Precursors and Effector Cells and Possible Cell Lineage

John Ortaldo
Ronald B. Herberman

Laboratory of Immunodiagnosis
National Cancer Institute
Bethesda, Maryland

INTRODUCTION

The presence of human natural cell-mediated cytotoxicity in mononuclear peripheral blood leukocytes of normal healthy donors has been extensively studied (1-4). Spontaneous cytotoxicity that was at first considered an artifact, recently has been shown to be due to a distinct subpopulation of cells, termed natural killer (NK) cells. NK cells and K cells, mediating antibody-dependent cellular cytotoxicity (ADCC), in fresh peripheral blood are Fc receptor positive (FcR+), complement receptor negative, surface membrane immunoglobulin negative (SmIg-) cells. (5-9). The majority of these NK and K cells have low affinity receptors for sheep erythrocytes (E), forming rosettes only when optimal conditions are used (8). However, E-SmIg- cells have been shown (6,8) to also have high NK activity. Moreover, with the optimal conditions used for E rosetting, many of the NK effector cells appear truly to lack receptors for E. This small population of E- NK cells may be a clue to the development of NK cells. As discussed below, this population may represent either a developmental stage or a distinct sub-population of NK cells.

We have recently reported (7,10) that NK and K cell activities persist in lymphocyte cultures supplemented with fetal calf serum, without additional antigenic stimulation from cell lines or mitogens. In addition, if only FcR-

ISBN 0-12-341350-8

depleted (FcR- lymphocytes were put into culture), FcR+ cells were spontaneously regenerated which had NK-like and K cell activities and this generation of cytotoxic effector cells was shown to be proliferation dependent. The effector cells generated in culture appear very similar, if not identical, to NK or K cells. They are FcR+, SmIg- and the majority have low affinity receptors for weak sheep red blood cell (SRBC). In addition, the NK-like activity is directed against specificities very similar to those recognized by NK cells (10).

The present report summarizes the available information on the nature of the cells required for development of cytotoxic activity, with emphasis on the cell type which is the precursor of NK and K cells, and on the conditions required for this process.

As previously described in detail (6,7,10) and summarized in Table 1, PBL depleted of FcR+ cells and incubated *in vitro* result in generation of FcR+, active NK and K cells. This observation provided an *in vitro* model for examining the cellular requirements for development or differentiation of NK and K cells from FcR- precursors. When various subpopulations of PBL were cultured by themselves, little or no regeneration of NK and K cell activity was seen. In contrast the mixture of E+ and E- cells led to the concomitant appearance of NK and K cell activities. Since the E- population, is heterogenous, composed of B cells, null cells, C receptor bearing cells, and monocytes, further fractionation was then performed to determine more precisely the cells required for the interaction with E+ cells. When E+ cells were mixed with various subpopulations of E- cells, only the combination of null cells plus E+ cells resulted in regeneration of NK and K cell cytotoxic activities. It thus appeared that cooperation between E+ and null cells was required for *in vitro* development of NK. To further define the nature of the cellular interactions, proliferation of the whole FcR- populations or of the E+ or null cell subpopulations were selective by blocked by pretreatment with x-ray or mitomycin C. Pretreatment of the PBL or the null cells inhibited development of reactivity, whereas treatment of E+ cells had no effect, indicating that only the null fraction needed to proliferate, whereas the E+ could cooperate without expansion. These results are consistent with the hypothesis that E+ T cells provide help for the proliferation and differentation into NK and K cells from precursors in the null cell subpopulation.

Table 1

Cells Required for In Vitro Generation of NK and K Cells

Cell Population[1]	*Activity on Day 7*	
	NK	*K*
PBL	+[2]	+
PBL depleted of FcR	+	+
Purified populations of		
(1) E rosette forming only	-	-
(2) Non-E rosette forming only	-	-
(3) Surface membrane Ig positive only	-	-
(4) Null only	-	-
Mixtures of[3]		
(1) + (2)	+	+
(1) + (3)	-	-
(1) + (4)	+	+

[1] *Approximately 1x10^6 cells/ml were cultured in RPMI-1640 plus 10% fetal bovine serum at 37 for 6-7 days.*

[2] *"+" indicates high levels of activity, equal to or higher than the activity of Day 0 PBL activity. "-" indicates low or undetectable activity.*

[3] *Mixtures contained 80% of (1), with a total of 1x10^6 cells/ml as described above.*

Since previous evidence from studies in mice and humans has indicated that NK cells may in the T cell lineage, studies were performed to determine whether the null cells involved in generation of NK activity had T cell associated antigens (6, 7,10,). As shown in Table 2, when E- cells were treated with specific heterologous anti-T cell serum plus complement and then mixed with E+ cells, little or no NK activity developed after culture. These results indicated that although the null cells, required for regeneration and presumably the NK precursors, although not possessing the ability to form rosettes with the SRBC (a marker for mature T cells), did possess T antigenic markers on their cell surface.

Table 2

Lack of In Vitro Generation of NK and K Cells after Pretreatment of E- cells with anti-T cell serum plus complement

Cell Population[1]	*Day 7 Activity*	
	NK	*K*
E+ only	-[2]	-
E- only	-	-
E+ plus E- treated with anti-T serum plus C	-	-
E+ plus E- treated with normal rabbit serum plus C	+	+
E+ plus E- treated with C only	+	+

[1]*See Table 1, footnote 1. E-rosette forming cells,(E+); non-E-rosette forming cells, (E-); complement, (C).*

[2]*See Table 1, footnote 2.*

An essential point in the use of this in vitro culture system as a model for differentiation of NK cells is that the effector cells which develop are indeed NK cells. Cytotoxic reactivity against K-562 target cells is not definite proof that this is a regenerated NK cell. Therefore, we have carefully compared the cellular characteristics and the specificity patterns of the cultured effector cells with those of fresh NK cells (10). These results are summarized in Table 3. No major differences in surface characteristics were seen between fresh and cultured NK cells. Minor changes were observed in that cultured NK cells were more adherent to rayon wool (removing approximately 10-30% of the activity), formed less avid rosettes and they weakly expressed Ia-like antigens . A very important point, indicated in Table 2 for the precursors and Table 3 for the effectors, was that the NK cells and their precursors expressed T cell associated antigens. This demonstrated that most of the precursors and effectors of in vitro generated NK activity were T antigen positive.

In addition to the cell surface characteristics of the cultured cells, if was also important to determine, whether the specificity pattern after regeneration was the same or

Table 3

Characteristics of NK cells and of cultured effector cells

	Fresh NK Cells	*Cultured Effector Cells*
Part of activity recovered in E+	*yes*	*yes*
Part of activity recovered in E-	*yes*	*yes*
Presence of receptor for Fc-IgG	*yes*	*yes*
Requirement for SmIg+ cells	*no*	*no*
Activity removed by depletion of C receptor-bearing cells	*no*	*no*
Sensitive to trypsin	*yes*	*yes*
Adherence to rayon wool	*no*	*weak*
Boosted by interferon	*yes*	*yes*
Activity sensitive to anti-T cell sera + C	*yes*	*yes*
Activity sensitive to anti-Ia-like sera + C	*no*	*weak*
Specificity patterns reproducible[1]	*yes*	*yes*

[1]*Cells were tested for their specificity pattern by cold-target inhibition. The cells from individual donors at Day 7 demonstrated patterns of specificity similar or identical to those of Day 0 PBL.*

similar to that of the fresh PBL. Fresh PBL were tested against a panel of NK susceptible targets using the cold target inhibition method (11). When PBL from the same donors were depleted of FcR+ cells and allowed to regenerate, their cytotoxicity in vitro, the pattern of reactivity for each individual was the same or very similar to that of the fresh PBL. Although the patterns of reactivity varied among donors, the fresh and cultured PBL of each gave parallel results. Taken together, the data on the characteristics of the cultured effector cells support the contention that these are newly generated NK cells, arising from FcR- precursors that circulate in the peripheral blood. In addition, the development of the same specificity pattern as seen with fresh NK cells suggests that the information needed for target cell recognition is inherent in these cells and does not depend on in vivo influences.

The data discussed above have been related solely to spontaneous NK/K activity in PBL or to NK/K cells that spontaneously developed in in vitro cultures in the presence of fetal calf serum. However NK-like activity has been reported to be generated in human serum plus a variety of stimulating agents (Table 4). NK-like cells have been reported to be generated in cultures of human cells stimulated with lymphoid cell lines (14,16-19), alloantigens (14,20), or mitogens (22, 23). In addition, supernatants from PHA-stimulated lymphocytes (24), have been shown to be capable of inducing and maintaining continued growth of T cells (25). In preliminary studies (21), we have detected NK-like activity by these cultured T cells. Each of these agents and also fetal bovine serum induce cellular proliferation in cultures and this may be the critical factor for development of NK activity.

Most of the effector cells generated _in vitro_ by stimuli other than fetal bovine serum have not yet been extensively examined in regard to their cell surface characteristics. Inferences about their relation to NK cells have been based mainly on their reactivity against NK-susceptible targets. Thus, further evidence will be needed to more definitely show

Table 4

Generation of NK-like cells in cultured lymphocytes with various stimuli

Stimuli	*Expression of FcR*	*Reference*
None (fetal calf serum)	*FcR+*	*Ortaldo (6,7,10) et al* *Treves (13) et al* *Seeley (14) et al* *Golub (15) et al*
LCL	*FcR-/or weak FcR*	*Poros (16) et al* *Stejskal (17) et al* *Seeley (14) et al* *Golub(18) et al* *Jondal (19) et al*
Alloantigens	*FcR+ (weak)*	*Ortaldo (20) et al* *Seeley (14) et al*
T cell growth factors, inducing continuous growth of T cells	*FcR?*	*Ortaldo (21) et al*
Mitogens	*FcR?*	*Stejskal (22,23) et al*

that the cultured effector cells are indeed NK cells. However, all of these results are consistent with our hypothesis that some proliferative signal is the minimal requirement for NK precursors to develop *in vitro* from FcR negative precursors. One could predict that the *in vitro* generated effector cells, regardless of stimulus, would be FcR positive. To the extent examined, the data on this point are somewhat conflictory (6,10,13-19). This may be due to variable and generally lower avidity of the FcR in cultured PBL. Data based on the use of EA-rosetting techniques to remove FcR positive cells and reliance on the same technique for monitoring the efficiency of depletion may not be adequate. The experience in our laboratory has been that the efficiency of FcR+ cell depletion by some techniques may not be complete and it is essential to monitor this by a more sensitive procedure. We have found that complete elimination of ADCC activity is a more sensitive indicator of depletion than is EA-rosetting. Thus conclusions about the presence or absence of FcR on cultured effector cells should be deferred until this has been more carefully analyzed. In general, more detailed analysis of a variety of addditional surface markers, specificity of cytotoxicity, and response to various immunopharmacological manipulations will be needed to better define the nature of the various cultured effector cells and their relationship to NK cells.

The *in vitro* system described here offers a model to examine factors involved in the development and differentiation of NK effector cells. Using antiserum to T cells provided evidence that the precursors to NK cells and mature NK cells are in a T cell lineage. This anti-T serum (24, and chapter by Kaplan and Callewaert in this book) has been shown to specifically kill T cells and abrogate their function and not detectably affect the numbers or function of B cells and monocytes. In the present study, precursors to NK cells in the E- fraction, fresh NK cells and day 7 *in vitro* regeneraated NK cells all were eliminated or inactivated by pretreatment with this antiserum and complement. It should be noted, however, that although all studies with this anti-T serum have indicated activity restricted to T cells, it might also react against a differentiation antigen common to immature cells of more than the T lineage. Thus, it is important to note that in addition to evidence with the anti-T serum, two additional lines of evidence regarding the T lineage of human NK cells exists. 1) The majority of fresh NK cells in PBL have been shown to form E-rosettes under optimal conditions and thus appear to have a low affinity receptor for E. 2) After 7 day *in vitro* regeneration, a small but distinct population of E-rosette forming NK cells can be found. The percentage of cells

(1)

Bone Marrow Stem Cells → Early T Lineage Cells (E−,FcR− T Ag+) —(T cell help) or Thymus→

→ NK/K Cell E−,FcR+ --------> NK/K Cell E+,FcR+

→ Mature T Cell (E++,FcR−)

(2)

Bone Marrow Stem Cells → Early T T Ag+ E−,FcR− → T Ag+,E− FcR+ → T Ag+,E+ FcR+ → Mature T (E++, T Ag+, FcR−)

----NK/K ACTIVITY----

(3)

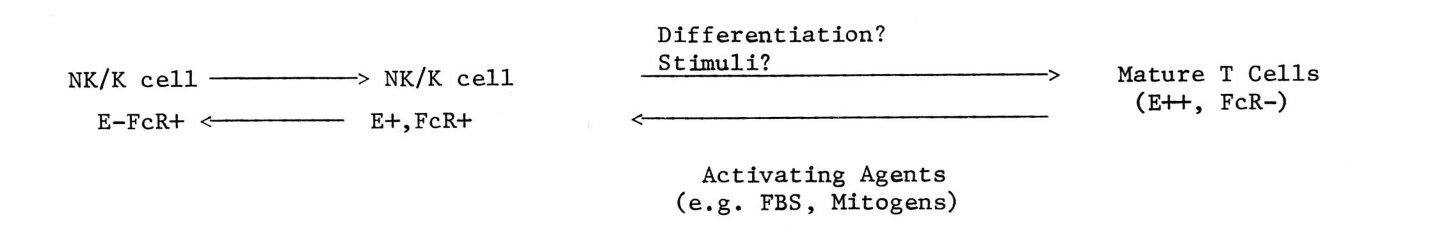

FIGURE 1.

MODELS FOR ONTOGENY OF NATURAL KILLER CELLS: Three proposed models for the development of NK cells. The following abbreviations are used: E+, sheep erythrocyte rosette-forming cells; E-, non-E-rosette forming; T Ag+, reactive with antisera to T cell associated antigens; FcR, receptor for the Fc portion of IgG. Dashed lines in model (1) indicate alternate pathways for development of E+ NK cells.

forming rosettes after this in vitro regeneration is usually less that 25%, considerably lower that that seen with fresh PBL(greater than 50%) and may be due to the lack of thymic influence. Although the ability to rosette is not universally accepted as a T cell marker, human lymphoid cells unrelated to T cells have not been shown to form rosettes even under optimal conditions.

A major question remains regarding the relationship between, 1) E- NK cells (those that have the general characteristics of L cells) (25); 2) E+,NK cells (those that are in the T-gamma population); and 3) mature T cells. It seems likely that E- cells could be become E+ and the heterogeneity in affinity of the receptors for E may reflect different points in the continuum of differentiation of NK cells. This would be consistent with the many similarities between L cells and T-gamma cells (6,7,10,26,27).

From the information available, some schemes for the differentiation of NK cells can be formulated (Figure 1). The initial precursors for NK cells appear to arise in the bone marrow, since it has been possible to reconstitute NK activity in irradiated or radioactive strontium-treated mice by transfer of bone marrow from normal donors (28,29). In regard to further differentiation, several possibilities would be consistent with our data on fresh and in vitro generated NK cells: 1) Although sharing common or related precursors, NK and mature T cells may differentiate along separate pathways, with no differentiation from one to the other (Figure 1, model 1). The two sub-populations of NK cells, E-,Fc+ and E+,Fc+ both appear to develop from precursors in the T lineage. Whether E-NK cells become E+ NK cells or are separate populations can not be answered at this time. According to this model, mature T cells would develop in a separate pathway and cytotoxic T cells would be developmentally quite distinct from NK cells. 2) NK cells may develop along the main pathway of differentiation to mature T cells (Figure 1, model 2). Expression of NK activity might then be a characteristic of cells during a certain period of T cell development, with this activity being lost as maturation of T cells continues and more specialized functions develop. According to this model, it would seem most likely that transition of E- NK cells to E+ NK cells is along this continuum of differentiation. Recent data (30) exists for in vitro shifts of T-gamma cell populations to T-mu and this would be consistent with Model 2. It is also possible that in response to certain stimuli or activating factors, mature T cells can develop into NK/K cells, as well as having differentiation in the opposite direction (Figure 1, model 3).

The data in our in vitro model are compatible with a transition from resting, mature T cells to activated NK/K cells if one considers the possibility that E+, FcR- mature T cells differentiate into NK cells with proliferating null cells playing the requisite accessory role. The recent report of Moretta (31), that in response to allogeneic cells in leukocyte cultures a high proportion of T-mu cells convert to E+ cells with Fc-gamma receptors, is quite consistent with this possibility.

At present, there is not sufficient information to cause us to clearly favor one or another of these alternative differentiation schemes. However, by further in vitro studies with selected subpopulations of NK cells and/or pre-NK cells, it should be possible to gather evidence regarding some of these questions. This approach seems quite promising for obtaining better insight into the ontogeny of NK and K cells and their relationship to mature T cells.

REFERENCES

1. Herberman, R.B., Djeu, J.Y., Kay, H.D., Ortaldo,J.R., Riccardi, C., Bonnard, G.D., Holden H.T., Fagani, R., Santoni, A. and Puccetti, P., Immunol. Rev. 44:43 (1979).
2. Saksela, E., Timonen, T., Ranki, A. and Hayry, P., Immunol. Rev. 44, 71 (1979).
3. Kiessling, R. and Wigzell, H., Immunol. Rev. 44, 165 (1979).
4. Santoli, D. and Kaprowski, H., Immunol. Rev. 44, 125 (1979).
5. West, W.H., Cannon, G.D., Kay, H.D., Bonnard, G.D., and Herberman, R.B., J. Immunol. 118, 355 (1977).
6. Ortaldo, J.R., MacDermott, R.D., Kind, P.D., Bonnard, G.D., and Herberman, R.B., Cell. Immunol. 48, 356 (1979).
7. Ortaldo, J.R., Bonnard, G.D., and Herberman, R.B. J. Immunol. 119, 1351 (1977).
8. West, W.H., in "Immunodiagnosis of Cancer" (R.B. Herberman and K.R. McIntire, eds.), p. 704. Marcel Dekker, Inc, New York, (1979).
9. Takasugi, M. and Mickey, M.R., J. Natl. Cancer Inst. 57, 255 (1976).
10. Ortaldo, J.R., Bonnard, G.D., Kind, P.D., and Herberman, R.B., J. Immunol. 122, 1489 (1979).
11. Ortaldo, J.R., Oldham, R.K., Cannon, G.D., and Herberman, R.B., J. Natl. Cancer Inst. 59, 77 (1977).
12. Kay, H.D., Fagnani, R., and Bonnard, G.D., Int. J. Cancer, in press.

13. Treves, A.J., Feldman, M., and Kaplan, H.S., J. Immunol. 119, 955 (1977).
14. Seeley, J.K. and Golub, S.H., J. Immunol., 120, 1415 (1978).
15. Golub, S.H., Golightly, M.G., and Zielski, J.V., Int. J. Cancer 24, 273 (1979).
16. Poros, A. and Klein E., Cell. Immunol. 41, 240 (1978).
17. Stejskal, V. and Perlmann, P., Eur. J. Immunol. 6, 347 (1976).
18. Golub, S.H., Hewetson, J.F., Svedmyr, E.A., and Singh S., Int. J. Cancer 10, 150 (1972).
19. Jondal, M. and Targan, S., J. Exp. Med. 148, 1621 (1978).
20. Ortaldo, J.R. and Bonnard, G.D., Fed. Proc. 36, 1325 (1977).
21. Ortaldo, J.R., Timonen, T., and Herberman, R.B., unpublished observation.
22. Stejskal, V.S., Holm, G., and Perlmann, P., Cell. Immunol. 8, 71 (1973).
23. Stejskal, V.S., Lindberg, S., Holm, G., and Perlmann, P., Cell. Immunol. 8, 82 (1973).
24. Kaplan, J. and Callewaert, D., J. Natl. Cancer Inst. 60, 961 (1978).
25. Horwitz, D.A. and Lobo, P.I., J. Clin. Invest. 56, 1464 (1975).
26. Horwitz, D.A., Cooper, M., and Carvalho, E., Clin. Immunol. Immunopathol. 14, 159 (1979).
27. Ferranini, M. and Grossi, C., Proceedings of the Serono Symposium on Thymus, Thymic Hormones and T Lymphocytes. Academic Press, in press.
28. Bennett, M., Baker, E.E., Eastcott, J.W., Kumar, V., and Yonkosky, J., J. Reticuloendth. Soc. 20, 71 (1976).
29. Haller, O., Kiessling, R., Orn, A., and Wigzell, H., J. Exp. Med. 145, 1411 (1977).
30. Pichler, W.J., Broder, S., Gendelmann, F.W., and Nelson, D., J. Immunol. 119, 955 (1978).
31. Moretta, L., Proceedings of the Symposium on Thymus, Thymic Hormones and T Lymphocytes. Academic Press, in press.

MLC-INDUCED CYTOTOXICITY AGAINST NK-SENSITIVE TARGETS

J. K. Seeley
K. Karre

Department of Tumor Biology
Karolinka Institute
Stockholm, Sweden

I. INTRODUCTION

A principal effector in natural cell mediated cytotoxicity against tumor targets has been identified as a particular subpopulation of lymphocytes termed natural killer (NK) cells (Herberman and Holden, 1978). Recently, there has been considerable interest in factors influencing the levels of NK activity. It has been found that inoculation with active tumor cells, (Herberman *et al.*, 1977) bacterial adjuvants (Wolfe *et al.*, 1976), or interferon inducers (Gidlund *et al.*, 1978) causes a rapid increase in cytotoxicity against NK sensitive targets. The effectors involved are not activated by a specific NK antigen, but apparently by the interferon induced by those agents (Herberman *et al.*, 1980). Furthermore, the effectors do not proliferate in response to the activating stimulus, nor do they produce memory cells, and thus are different from the classical antigen-activated cytotoxic T-lymphocytes (CTL) (Engers and MacDonald, 1976).

This work was supported by grants from the Swedish Cancer Society.

J. K. Seeley is a recipient of fellowships from the International Agency for Research on Cancer, Lyon, and the National Cancer Institute (No. F32 CA 06445-01) Public Health Service, U.S.A.

ISBN 0-12-341350-8

Several investigators have also observed that enhanced activity against NK sensitive targets accompanies specific immune responses to a variety of viruses (Welsh, 1978). For example, spleen cells from mice immunized with lymphocytic chorio meningitis (LCM) or ectromelia virus have enhanced NK-like activity which peaks on the third day several days before the appearance of the virus-specific CTL.

In some instances, positive identification of cytotoxic activity as NK has proven difficult because of a lack of known surface antigens or metabolic requirements expressed exclusively by NK effectors. Thus, investigators have relied on the characteristic pattern of NK target selectivity and a composite of functional and surface markers.

For example, the activity of endogenous mouse NK cells has the following properties (see Table IV): it can be detected in short-term cytotoxicity assays, does not require addition of immunoglobulin (Ig) or complement and is usually labile in culture at 37°C. The NK effectors express low levels of Thy 1 antigen, are surface Ig negative, express low affinity or undetectable receptors for the Fc portion of Ig (FcR) and are nonadherent, nonphagocytic, small to medium-sized lymphocytes (Kiessling and Wigzell, 1979).

The effector cells responsible for enhanced cytolytic activity during virus infections were found to have characteristics very similar to endogenous NK cells although they express more readily detectable Thy 1 antigen (Herberman *et al.*, 1978) and Fc receptors and are more adherent to nylon wool (Kiessling *et al.*, 1980). These effectors have been termed activated NK cells (Welsh, 1978).

As mentioned above, NK cells generally lose all or part of their activity after one day *in vitro* at 37°C. After a longer period, however, depending on the culture conditions, a cytolytic reactivity with NK-like target selectivity often reappears. We, and several other investigators, have reported this phenomenon in lymphocyte cultures containing allogeneic lymphocytes (MLC) (Seeley and Golub, 1977 and 1978 and Ortaldo and Bonnard, 1977), autologous or allogeneic cell lines (Jondal and Targan, 1978), or fetal calf serum (FCS) (Zielske and Golub, 1976 and Ortaldo and Bonnard, 1977).

The main focus of our work in the MLC system has been (1) to characterize the NK-like effectors (termed anomalous killers, or AK), (2) to distinguish between the AK cells and the allospecific CTL's and (3) to investigate the origin of the AK cells: are they boosted, endogenous NK cells, or are they activated from a precursor stage or from another lymphocyte subpopulation? The possibility that NK cells are boosted, or that NK precursors are activated early in an immune response would lend support to the theory that NK is a primary event in the complex immune response to antigens.

We present below a summary of our MLC results obtained thus far. For a detailed discussion of NK reactivity induced in other culture systems, we direct the reader to the chapters by Ortaldo and Herberman and by Burton.

II. CYTOTOXIC REACTIVITY INDUCED IN HUMAN MLC

A. General Features

During studies on the cytotoxic response induced in standard human MLC (with 20% human serum and mitomycin C (MMC)-treated stimulating cells) we found that the specificity detected was dependent on the type of target cell. With ^{51}Cr labelled Con A-induced lymphoblasts, allogeneic but not autologous targets were lysed. However, both autologous and allogeneic EBV-transformed lymphoblastoid cell lines (LCL) were sensitive to the same MLC generated effector cell population (Seeley and Golub, 1977). Since the auto-LCL targets shared no known antigens with the stimulating allogeneic lymphocytes we termed this reactivity anomalous killing (AK) (Seeley and Golub, 1978).

We have shown that AK occurs transiently, reaches a peak early and then declines as the allospecific effect peaks (Fig. 1). AK correlates with proliferation, as measured by ^{3}H-TdR incorporation (Seeley 78).

B. Target Cells Sensitive to Human AK

In addition to the autologous and allogeneic LCL targets just described, many other cultured cell lines could also be killed during this early phase of reactivity. This was apparently independent of histocompatibility relationships, or to antigens associated with T or B lymphocytes or with FCS (Seeley and Golub, 1979). The spectrum of susceptible targets and their relative sensitivities to the anomalous effectors resembled that described for endogenous NK cells (Table I). The most sensitive targets were K562 and T-lymphoblastoid cell lines.

C. AK and Allospecific Killers Have Different Patterns of Reactivity

Although the kinetic studies previously described indicate that at least two cytotoxic effects were activated in MLC, it was not clear if they were mediated by the same or

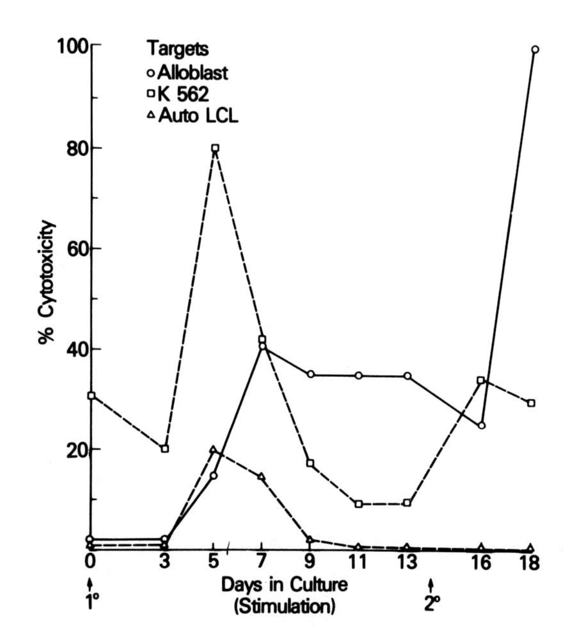

FIGURE 1. Time course of generation of allospecific cytotoxicity and AK in primary and secondary MLC. PBL from donor X and MMC-treated PBL from X or Y were cultured for 3 to 13 days. Some of the day 11 and 13 responders were restimulated with MMC-treated X (control) or Y PBL, for 2 or 4 days. The cultures were tested for cytotoxicity at 50:1 effector:target ratio against the alloblast (y) o—o, auto (x) LCL △—△, and K562 □—□.

distinct effector populations. This issue was investigated by cold target inhibition studies, as illustrated in a representative experiment in Figure 2. Cold K562 cells efficiently inhibited ^{51}Cr release from labelled K562 while allogeneic and autologous lymphocytes had no effect. Conversely, the allospecific (anti-y) cytotoxicity against the allo (y) Con A-induced blasts was inhibited by cold allo (y) lymphocytes but not by autologous (x) cells, nor by K562.

In similar experiments, allo and auto LCL were also used as cold competitors. A summary of all the inhibition experiments is presented in Table II. The specific CTL was inhibited when cells carrying the relevant HLA target antigens were added, whereas AK was inhibited by any of the cells that could serve as AK targets (summarized in Table 1). The efficiencies of the inhibitions varied and probably reflected the degree of sensitivity of the cells to the allo and AK effects.

TABLE I. Relative Sensitivity of Various Targets To Human Lymphocyte Effectors[a]

Effectors	Allogeneic		Autologous		Third party						
	Blasts[b]	LCL[c]	Blasts	LCL	Blasts	LCL	K562[d]	MOLT-4	HSB-II	SB[c]	Chang
Fresh	-[e]	-	-	-	-	-	++++	++++	++++	+	++
Control culture	-	-	-	-	-	-	++	++	++	-	-
MLC	+++	++++	+	+++	+	+++	+++++	+++++	+++++	++++	++++

[a]Purified lymphocytes were assayed fresh, or cultured in 10% human AB serum with MMC-treated autologous (control) or allogeneic (MLC lymphocytes) and tested in a 4 hr ^{51}Cr-release assay.

[b]Blasts - Con A stimulated lymphocytes from the MLC stimulator (allogeneic), responder (autologous), or an unrelated third party donor were cultured for 3 days in 10% AB serum with 1 µg/ml Con A. Before labelling, the blasts were washed with 0.1 M a-methyl mannoside.

[c]LCL - Epstein Barr Virus-transformed lymphoblastoid cell lines from normal B cells, maintained in 10% FCS and transferred to 10% AB serum for three weeks prior to testing as targets. SB is an LCL autologous to HBS-II (see d).

[d]Tumor cell lines K562 (myeloid leukemia), MOLT-4 (T-cell leukemia), HSB-II (T-cell leukemia) and Chang (Hepatoma) were cultured as in c.

[e]Level of cytotoxicity: - (0-5%), + (6-10%), ++ (11-20%), +++ (21-40%), ++++ (41-60%), +++++ (> 60%).

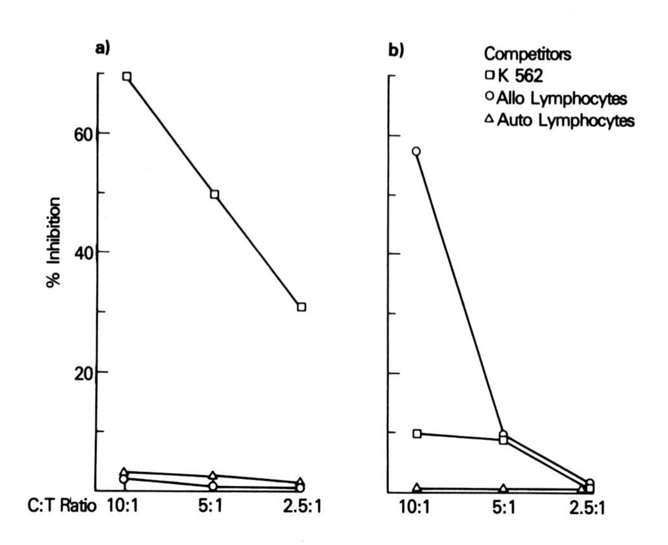

FIGURE 2. Cold target inhibition of 5-day MLC effectors (X vs Ym) in the AK and allospecific killing system. Various numbers of cold inhibitor cells were added to a mixture of 5-day MLC effectors and ^{51}Cr-labelled K562 (left panel) or allo (y) blasts (right panel) at a 40:1 effector:target ratio. Cytotoxicity in absence of inhibitors was 58% (allo) and 90% (K562).

Considered together, these results demonstrate that AK and the CTL effectors have distinct patterns of specificity. This is compatible with the hypothesis that the majority of the effectors responsible for specific killing and AK belong to two different populations: one directed against the sensitizing histocompatibility antigens, and the other directed against one or more target structures distinct from the alloantigens and present only on cultured cell lines. However, the possibility that the same cell population could show both AK and CTL activity is not ruled out.

From the cross-competition between the auto LCL and K562 and competition with the allo LCL, it appeared that the AK effectors may in part be directed against common target structures on these targets.

Existence of distinct patterns of specificity were also implied by the results from secondary cultures. MLC cells maintained in culture 14 days were resensitized with lymphocytes from the original allogeneic donor (Fig. 1). As expected for a secondary response, cytotoxic activity against

TABLE II. Cold Target Inhibition Pattern of AK and Allo-specific Killing

Inhibitors	*Cytotoxic activity, targets*			
	Allospecific		*AK*	
	allo blast	*allo LCL*	*K562*	*auto LCL*
Allolymphocytes	+	+	-	-
Allo LCL	+	+	+	+
K562	-	+	+	+
Auto LCL	-	+	+	+
Auto lymphocytes	-	-	-	-

+ Inhibition of 20% or more of the cytotoxicity produced in absence of inhibitors is considered positive.

the allo targets rapidly increased to 3-6 times that reached in the primary response. However, in this same culture, there was no activity against the auto LCL and little against K562 (Seeley, 1975). Thus, little AK activity accompanies a secondary allospecific CTL response.

These data led to our conclusion that AK cells are distinct from CTL. However, they offered no information about the origin of the AK effector cells.

D. Precursors of AK Cells

The majority of endogenous NK cells in human peripheral blood have a receptor for the Fc portion of IgG (FcγR). Thus, NK cells can be depleted or enriched by rosetting with IgG-coated erythrocytes (EA) (Bakacs, 1977), or by absorption and elution from immunocomplex-coated (IC) plates (Targan and Jondal, 1978). MLC's initiated with NK-enriched responders showed no evidence for induction of AK: the day 5 anti-K562 activity was lower than the original input activity (Fig. 3d). In contrast, AK could be generated from FcγR negative responders, originally depleted of endogenous NK reactivity (Fig. 3b and c).

Furthermore, AK could be induced from E rosette enriched, NK depleted responders (Fig. 3c, Seeley *et al.*, 1979 and Masucci *et al.*, 1980). Thus, it appears that at least part of the MLC-induced AK reactivity is derived from a population of FcγR negative, NK-inactive T cells.

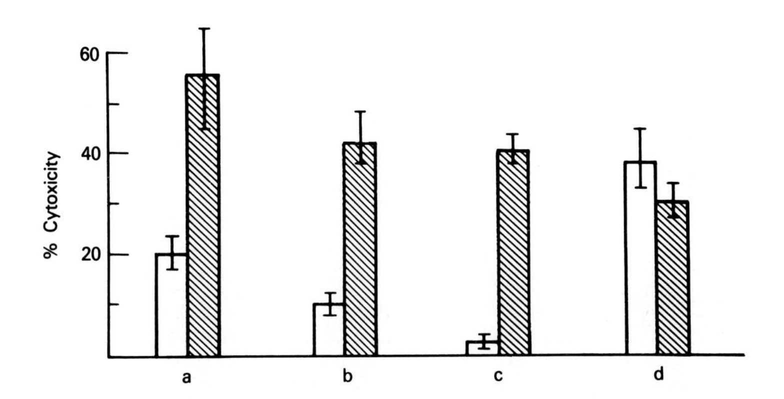

FIGURE 3. Anti-K562 activity of unfractionated (a), E rosette enriched (b), E rosette enriched, FcR depleted (c), or E rosette depleted, FcR enriched (d) lymphocytes. Open bars: fresh lymphocytes immediately after fractionation. Shaded bars: same lymphocyte subsets after 5-day sensitization in MLC. Effector:target ratio 30:1.

E. Characteristics of AK Effector Cell

In an unfractionated population of human PBL, about 20-30% of the cells bear FcγR. As mentioned above, most endogenous NK cells are FcγR positive. However, NK cells represent only a subfraction of these FcγR cells. In culture, the percentage of FcγR+ cells decreases, reaching 1-3% of the total cells in day 5 control culture and 2-8% of the MLC cells. In the control culture, the remaining anti-K562 activity can be depleted by absorption to IC plates, suggesting that FcγR+ residual NK cells are responsible. In contrast, the anti-K562 effect in MLC, that is, AK, is resistant to this treatment (Seeley *et al.*, 1979). Similarly, the ADCC levels in the IC-nonadherent MLC population were not significantly reduced, while the same technique abolished ADCC reactivity of fresh lymphocytes. This suggests that the FcγR on the MLC-induced K cells (ADCC effectors) were of low affinity, compared to that on the fresh K cells (Poros, *et al.*, 1980). Considered together, these data indicate that AK effectors activated in MLC were negative for the FcγR, or that they also had relatively low affinity receptors compared to endogenous NK cells.

F. Cytolytic Reactivity Induced in Other Culture Systems

It is interesting to compare this information on MLC-induced AK with the NK-like effects observed in several other culture systems. As in MLC, mixed cultures of lymphocytes and autologous LCL stimulators (AS) can give rise to cytotoxic reactivity against K562 and other NK sensitive targets. Again, as in MLC, this AK-like activity cannot be depleted by absorption to IC plates (Jondal and Targan, 1978). In contrast, lymphocytes stimulated with 10% fetal calf serum (FCS) (Ortaldo, 1979) or with irradiated K562 (cultures termed MKC)(Poros and Klein, 1978), produce an NK-like activity which can be depleted or partially depleted by such treatment and is therefore mediated by FcγR+ cells.

Golightly and Golub (1980) have found that the majority of MLC-induced AK effectors express Fc receptors for IgM (FcμR), while the FCS-activated effectors are negative. It may be, as suggested by those authors, that Fc receptors are not markers for a distinct NK subset, but should be considered markers for certain stages in the cell cycle or steps in a cell's maturation pathway.

G. Induction Requirements in Other Systems

Some clues regarding AK activation can be obtained by comparing the induction requirements in other culture systems. As mentioned above, MLC-induced AK can be generated from purified T cell responders, initially depleted of NK reactivity. This is also true of the autologous LCL stimulation (AS) system (Jondal and Targan, 1978). In contrast, no anti-K562 effect is induced in purified T cells stimulated with FCS (Ortaldo *et al.*, 1979) or with K562 (Masucci *et al.*, 1980). However, cytolytic activity can be induced in these systems if an Fc negative, T negative (Null) cell population is added to the T cells in the FCS cultures or if a supernatant from MLC is added to the T cells cocultured with K562 (MKC). Evidently, the T cells require certain factors and/or cell-cell cooperation which was provided in the MLC and AS systems, but was missing from the MKC and FCS cultures.

One possible explanation for these differences could be a requirement for T responders to interact with Ia-like B cell antigens, which are not provided by the HLA-negative K562. This interaction might by itself or through soluble mediators cause *de novo* or reexpression of NK activity in a subset of the T lymphocytes. Ortaldo proposed another explanation for the FCS system: the null cells may contain the NK precursors and may be activated upon cooperation with the T cells.

The precursor for interferon-induced human NK cells has recently been identified in a subpopulation of T cells which have morphologic characteristics of large granular lymphocytes (LGL) (Saksela *et al.*, 1979). It may be that the various different culture conditions described above provide interferon or similar inducing signals to this precursor. Indeed, supernatants from lymphocyte-LCL cocultures have been reported to enhance NK activity in normal lymphocytes (Koide and Takasugi, 1978). So far, we and other investigators have been unable to demonstrate such activity in MLC supernatants but this may be due to technical problems and requires further study.

It may be that NK like reactivity can be induced in several different lymphocyte subpopulations, requiring various different conditions for activation. Experiments using NK enriched and depleted responder populations are currently in progress to help resolve these possibilities.

III. MURINE MLC-INDUCED NK CELLS

All of the experiments discussed above were performed with human lymphocytes. Since the dynamics of cellular immunity have been studied more extensively in murine systems, it was of considerable interest to use mouse MLC to characterize the details of AK activity.

A. *General Features*

The results discussed here include experiments with (CBA x A), (C3H x A) or (DBA x A) F_1 hybrid spleen cells responding against irradiated C57BL spleen cells in ordinary MLC's (RPMI, 10% FCS). The resulting effectors were tested against C57BL derived tumor cells (e.g. RBL-5) as a measure of allospecific cytotoxicity. NK-sensitive targets semisyngeneic to, or sharing H-2 haplotype with the F_1 responder cells were used to detect AK.

A typical experiment illustrating the kinetics of the cytotoxic responses is shown in Figure 4. The NK activity of fresh NK cells against YAC-1 and MPC-11 declined rapidly during the first 24 hours of culture. Thereafter, cytotoxicity against both targets increased with a sharp peak on day 3, clearly preceding the peak of the allogeneic anti-RBL-5 response (4b) on day 4-5. The semisyngeneic NK-insensitive target P815 (4d) was not sensitive to the transient cytotoxicity. Instead, a later response, resembling the kinetics of the allospecific reactivity, was observed against P815 cells. Thus, in murine MLC, as in the human MLC, there is a transient

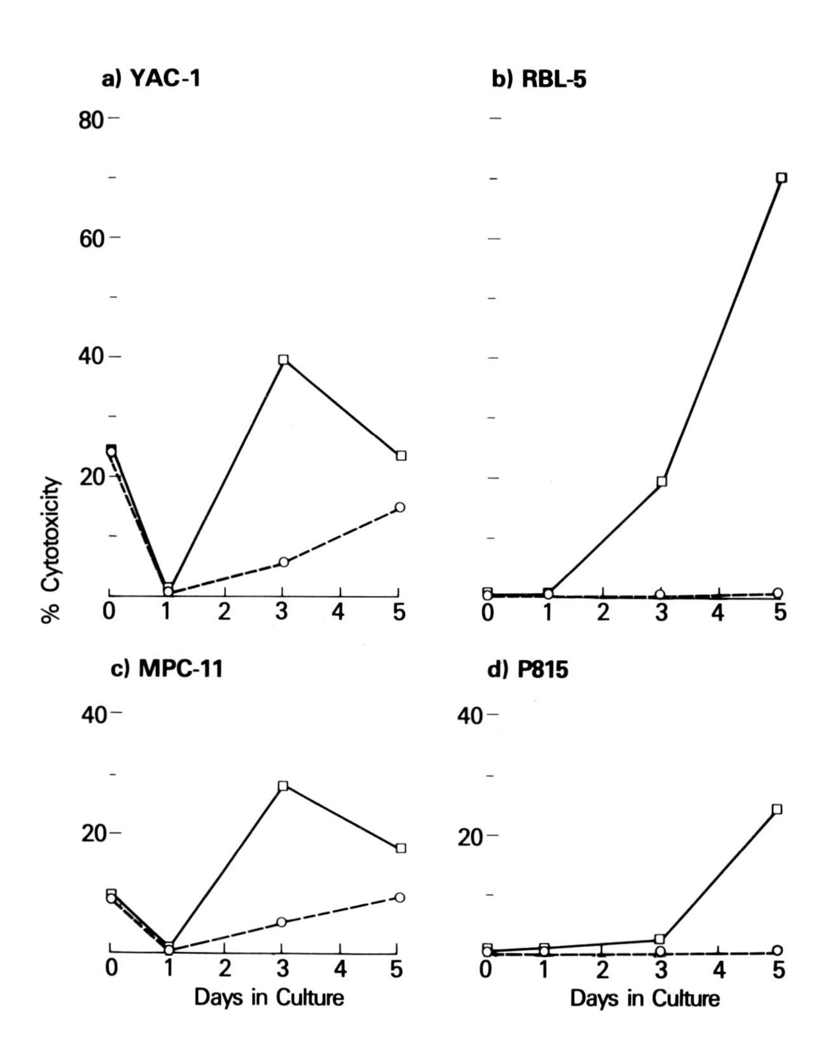

FIGURE 4. Kinetics of cytotoxic responses in MLC and control cultures of mouse spleen cells supplemented with 10% FCS. Effector cells from (DBA x A ↝ BLm) (H-2^{dxa} ↝ H-2^{b}) (solid lines) or (control) (dashed lines) cultures were assayed in a ^{51}Cr release assay against YAC (H-2^{a}), RBL-5 (H-2^{b}), MPC-11 (H-2^{d}), and P815 (H-2^{d}). E:T ratio was 50:1 and incubation time was 4 hrs.

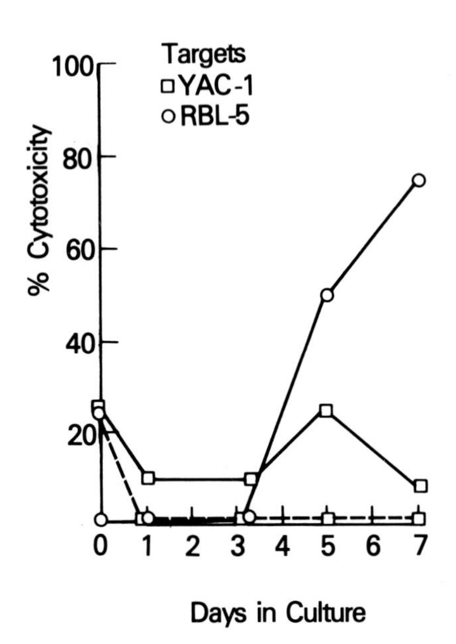

FIGURE 5. Kinetics of cytotoxic reactivity in MLC and control cultures of mouse spleen cells supplemented with 0.5% mouse serum. Assay and symbols as in Figure 4.

wave of cytotoxic reactivity against NK sensitive targets, which declines as the allospecific response increases.

Anti-YAC activity also reappeared in control cultures. It appeared more slowly and was always lower than that of the MLC's at day 3 (Karre and Seeley, 1979). By day 5, this reactivity was sometimes higher than that in the sensitized cultures. It is important to remember that control cultures contained FCS, which may possess several stimuli (antigenic or mitogenic). Indeed, the picture was different when cultures were supplemented with 0.5% autologous mouse serum as the only source of protein (Fig. 5). Here, cytotoxicity against NK sensitive targets reappeared only in the MLC with a peak around day 5, shortly before the peak of allospecific activity. Thus, AK as well as allo killing could be induced during MLC, in the absence of stimulatory serum. Although the two cytotoxic components were "delayed" relative to those in FCS supplemented cultures, the characteristic sequence was maintained: AK always precedes the allospecific response.

TABLE III. Effector Characteristics of NK and AK, CTL

	Fresh spleen	*MLC*	
Treatment	*Endogenous NK*	*AK*	*CTL*
Nylon wool	*enhanced*	*no effect*	*no effect*
1G Sedimentation (size)	*small-medium*	*large*	*large*
Density gradient (d)	*dense*	*light*	*light*
X Thy 1.2 + C' (serum dilution)	*5% reduction (1/25)*	*80% reduction (1/250)*	*100% reduction (1/2500)*

B. Characteristics of Effectors Generated in Murine MLC

In the following investigations designed to characterize the anomalous killers, we focused on the effectors derived from day 3-4 MLC's, since they have a strong cytotoxic activity against YAC-1 as well as classic CTL, activated against a known antigen ($H-2^b$). Table III summarizes the results comparing AK to the CTL and to endogenous NK effectors.

None of the cytotoxic activities can be depleted by techniques removing adherent or phagocytic cells. A small difference was observed in that fresh NK activity constantly showed enrichment after nylon wool treatment, whereas activity by cultured effectors (anomalous as well as allospecific) remained unaffected. Since 50-80% of the input cells are removed after passage over nylon wool, it may be tht the lack of enrichment reflects partial loss of anomalous and allospecific effectors.

NK and AK effectors also differ with respect to physical properties such as size and density. Fresh NK cells show some size heterogeneity, with cytotoxic activity recovered in all fractions after sedimentation at unit gravity. However, the majority of lytic units (80-90%) are in the fractions of small to medium sized lymphocytes. In contrast, anti-YAC activity in day 3 MLC's is recovered in the fast sedimenting fractions, also containing the large CTL-blasts (Karre and Seeley, 1979). Similarly, both AK and allospecific effectors are enriched in the light density layers of a BSA-gradient, whereas the activity of fresh NK cells distributes primarily in layers corresponding to high buoyant density. Taken together, these results indicate that AK effectors are large buoyant cells, in contrast to the small, dense endogenous NK effectors.

Finally, AK cells differed from NK in terms of detectable surface Thy 1.2 antigen. Reduction of AK activity by treatment with monoclonal anti-Thy serum and C' was 80%, i.e. intermediate between that of fresh NK and that of allospecific killer T cells.

Further reduction of AK could not be obtained with higher antiserum concentrations. Thus, the majority of AK cells expressed Thy 1 antigen. On the basis of fluorescent cell sorter experiments using a monoclonal anti-Thy 1.2, Mattes *et al.*, (1979) reported that there may be at least two subpopulations of NK cells: those which express Thy 1.2 and others which do not. This may also be true of AK cells.

As indicated above, a small proportion (less than 10%) of endogenous NK activity is mediated by larger, faster sedimenting cells. We considered the possibility that AK simply represents selective survival of these cells. However, this seemed unlikely, since they were as labile during the first 24 hours of culture as the total NK population and they were no more sensitive to anti-Thy 1.2 treatment (unpublished results).

C. Specificity of AK Cells Generated in Mouse MLC

Since the AK effectors bear some resemblance to the CTL, we used cold target inhibition experiments to investigate the possibility that AK might represent nonspecific background of the allogeneic response. As can be seen in Figure 6a (representing cells taken from day 4 in the experiment shown in Figure 4) RBL-5, although highly sensitive to the allospecific effect, did not cause any inhibition of anomalous killing against YAC. Conversely, YAC-1 and MPC-11, both sensitive to NK and AK, could inhibit the anti-YAC but not the anti-RBL-5 reactivity, mediated by the same MLC effectors (Fig. 5b). The NK-insensitive P815 was a poor competitor in both cases although it is semisyngeneic with the responders as are YAC and MPC-11. On the other hand, P815 self competed efficiently (data not shown), indicating that the anti-P815 activity represented a third component of cytolytic activity, distinct from allospecific and anomalous anti-YAC-1 activities.

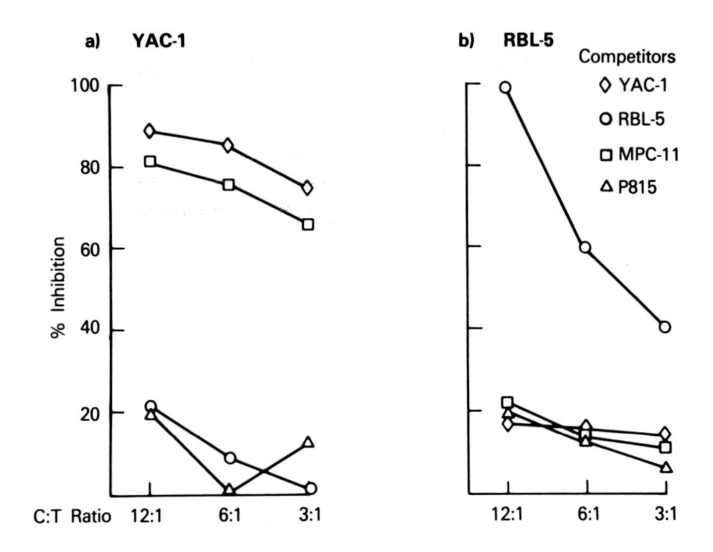

FIGURE 6. Cold target inhibition tests with day 4 MLC-derived effector cells from experiment depicted in Figure 4. E:T ratio = 20:1.

The lack of cross reactivity between AK and allospecific killing was confirmed also for effectors derived from MLC's in mouse serum, as shown in Figure 7. These competition patterns indicate that the antigens recognized by anomalous and allo specific effectors are quite distinct, as found previously in human MLC's.

The comparison between NK and anomalous killing was extended by testing against a panel of tumor cells of varying NK sensitivity (Karre and Seeley, 1979). The anomalous effectors from day 3 MLC's were thus found to lyse several targets in the same preferential order as NK cells, including ascites-derived mouse lymphoma cells and *in vitro* cultivated human tumors such as K562 and MOLT-4. Both of these are sensitive to the human NK and AK as pointed out in the previous section, further stressing the parallels between the murine and human systems.

Taken together, the crossreacting cold target inhibition pattern and the close correlation between AK and NK target selectivities strongly support the idea that these two reactivities are directed against the same surface components on the targets.

On the basis of target selectivity, AK effectors can be distinguished from the murine FCS-activated cytolytic effectors discussed earlier. The selectivity of those FCS-acti-

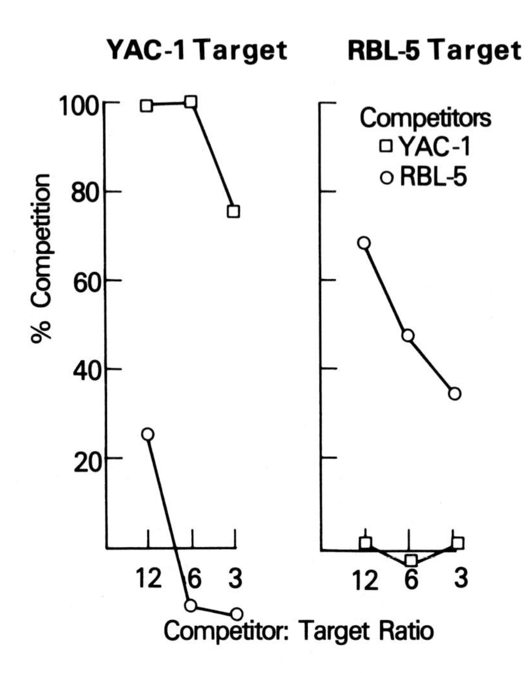

FIGURE 7. Cold target inhibition tests with day 4 MLC-derived effectors from experiment shown in Figure 5. E:T ratio = 20:1.

vated cells is controversial. When Peck *et al.*, (1977) investigated the specificity of day 6 FCS-stimulated spleen cells, they concluded that the effectors were restricted to altered, autologous H-2 determinants. This alteration did not seem to be related to FCS. Burton et al., (1977) also found that day 6 FCS cultured spleen cells could kill autologous tumor targets. However, in contrast to Peck's results, a wide range of unrelated cultured tumor targets were capable of inhibiting lysis. Similarly, Fogel *et al.*, (1978) reported sensitization to target-bound FCS determinants, resulting in unexpected cross reactivities between unrelated tumor targets.

Thus, a number of different cytotoxic activities may be induced in spleen cells cultured with FCS. Some of these may also be activated in the FCS-supplemented MLC system. However, the above-mentioned FCS-induced cytotoxic effect peaks much later than AK and seems to express different target selectivities. Therefore, as in the human systems, it appears that several different anti-tumor effects can develop in culture. However, anomalous killing appears to be the most closely related to natural killer activity.

VII. CONCLUSIONS

It is clear that very similar anomalous killer activities are generated in human and mouse MLC: in both there is an early, transient phase of cytotoxicity which displays NK target selectivity and does not cross-react with allo specific targets. In both systems, there is evidence that AK cells belong to the T cell lineage and that the phenotypic characteristics of AK effectors differ from those of endogenous NK cells (Table IV).

In considering the origin and activation mechanisms of the AK cells, three main possibilities seem most likely:

1) AK cells belong to the "NK lineage," arising from endogenous NK or non-lytic NK precursors. These cells might undergo the observed phenotypic changes (e.g. Thy 1.2 and FcγR expression) during *in vitro* culture, perhaps as a response to mitogenic factors or differentiation signals. Interferon has been shown to be involved in other *in vivo* and *in vitro* NK activation systems and may be involved in MLC-induced AK also. Experiments are currently in progress to compare the characteristics of MLC and interferon induced effectors, and to try inhibiting the expression of AK with anti-interferon sera, known to inhibit interferon induction of NK.

2) AK arise from cells normally not associated with NK cells. As discussed previously, there is considerable evidence that AK cells are large (or blastoid?) T cells. It is well known that a major proportion of the T cells during MLC become activated and proliferate (Engers and MacDonald, 1976). It is clear that the allospecific CTL effectors constitute only a small proportion of these cells. Many of the other activated cells bear markers (LyI) which are expressed on T helper cells (Cantor and Boyse, 1975), but the actual role, if any, for so many activated T cells in the MLC is not known. AK cells may be a subpopulation of those activated T cells which normally, or upon activation, express an NK receptor.

3) Although this seems the least likely alternative, AK may even be mediated by the allo-activated CTL early in the antigen-induced maturation process. If so, it is puzzling that the allo and AK targets do not cross inhibit. This might imply that there is reciprocal or mutually exclusive expression of the AK and allo receptors on the effectors at any one time.

Recent evidence from studies (Timonen *et al.*, 1979) of NK cells imply that the effectors express receptors by which they can bind to NK sensitive targets. It may be that this NK receptor structure is on many cells, but has only been detect on cells with cytotoxic potential, since this is the charac-

TABLE IV. Properties of NK, AK and CTL Cells[a]

Property	Effectors		
	NK[b]	AK	CTL
Activity in culture	Labile	Peak day 3-4	Peak day 5-7
Ag-induced memory	–[c]	–	+
Target selectivity	Broad range against tumor targets		Sensitizing target
Inhibition by cold targets	Cross inhibition with NK sensitive targets		Sensitizing target only
Phenotype			
T-cell antigen	+	++	++++
FcγR mouse	±	?	±
human	+	–	±
Surface Ig	–	–	–

TABLE IV. (Continued)

Property	*Effectors*		
	NK[b]	*AK*	*CTL*
Phagocytic	-	-	-
Adherent	-	$\underline{+}$	$\underline{+}$
Morphology			
mouse	*Small-medium lymphocyte*	*Large lymphocyte*	
human	*Medium-large lymphocyte*	*Large lymphocyte*	

[a] *Summary of cytotoxic reactivity and other properties as discussed in text.*
[b] *NK - Fresh lymphocyte effectors (mouse or human) against NK-sensitive targets (YAC-1 or K562, respectively).*
[c] *- characteristic not detectable.*
$\underline{+}$ *characteristic detected at low levels or is controversial.*
$+$ *characteristic regularly and clearly detectable.*

teristic measured in NK assays. The effectors responsible for AK may have this lytic capacity for only a short phase of their development and would therefore be elusive to characterization.

REFERENCES

Bakacs, T., Gergely, P., and Klein, E. (1977). *Cell Immunol. 32,* 317.

Burton, R. T., Chism, S. E., and Warner, N. L. (1977). *J. Immunol. 119,* 1329.

Cantor, H., and Boyse, E. A. (1975). *J. Exp. Med. 141,* 1390.

Engers, H. D., and MacDonald, H. R. (1976). *Contemp. Top. Immunobiol. 5,* 145.

Fogel, M., Segal, S., Gorelik, E., and Feldman, M. (1978). *Int. J. Cancer 22,* 329.

Gidlund, M., Orn, A., Wigzell, H., Senik A., and Gresser, I. (1978). *Nature 273,* 759.

Golightly, M., and Golub, S. H. (1980). Submitted for publication.

Herberman, R. B., Nunn, M. E., Holden, H. T., Staal, S., and Djeu, J. Y. (1977). *Int. J. Cancer 19,* 555.

Herberman, R. B., and Holden, H. T. (1978). Natural cell-mediated immunity. *In* "Advances in Cancer Research" (G. Klein and S. Weinhouse, eds.), Vol. 27, 305-377. Academic Press, New York, N.Y.

Herberman, R. B., Nunn, M. E., and Holden, H. J. (1978). *J. Immunol. 121,* 304.

Herberman, R. B., Ortaldo, J. R., Djeu, J. Y., Holden, H. T., Jett, J., Lang, N. P., and Pestka, F. (1980). *Ann. N.Y. Acad. Sci.,* in press.

Jondal, M., and Targan, S. (1978). *J. Exp. Med. 148,* 1621.

Karre, K., and Seeley, J. K. (1979). *J. Immunol. 123,* 1511.

Kiessling, R., and Wigzell, H. (1979). *Immunol. Rev. 44,* 165.

Kiessling, R., Eriksson, E., Hallenbeck, L., and Welsh, R. (1980). Submitted for publication.

Masucci, G., Poros, A., Seeley, J. K., Klein, E. (1980). *Cell. Immunol.,* in press.

Mattes, M. J., Sharrow, S. O., Herberman, R. B., and Holden, H. T. (1979). *J. Immunol. 123,* 2851.

Ortaldo, J. R., and Bonnard, G. D. (1977). *Fed. Proc. 35,* 1325.

Ortaldo, J. R., MacDermott, R. P., Bonnard, G. D., Kind, P. D., and Herberman, R. B. (1979). *Cell. Immunol. 48,* 356.

Peck, A. B., Anderson, L. C., and Wigzell, H. (1977). *J. Exp. Med. 145,* 802.

Poros, A., and Klein, E. (1978). *Cell. Immunol., 41,* 240.

Poros, A., Seeley, J. K., Masucci, G., and Klein, E. (1980). Submitted for publication.

Saksela, E., Timonen, T., and Cantell, K. (1979). *Scand. J. Immunol. 10,* 257.

Seeley, J. K., and Golub, S. H. (1977). *Am. Assoc. Cancer Res. 18,* 174.

Seeley, J. K., and Golub, S. H. (1978). *J. Immunol. 120,* 1415.

Seeley, J. K., Masucci, G., Poros, A., Klein, E., and Golub S. H. (1979). *J. Immunol. 123,* 1303.

Targan, S., and Jondal, M. (1978). *J. Immunol. Methods 22,* 123.

Timonen, T., Saksela, E., Ranki, A., and Hayry, P. (1979). *Cell. Immunol. 48,* 133.

Welsh, R. M. (1978). *Nature (London) 121,* 1631.

Wolfe, S. A., Tracey, D. E., and Henney, C. S. (1976). *Nature* (Lond.) *262,* 584.

Zielske, J. V., and Golub, S. H. (1976). *Int. J. Cancer 15,* 342.

SUMMARY: DEVELOPMENT OF NK ACTIVITY DURING IN VITRO CULTURE

There is as yet only rudimentary information on the steps involved in the development of active NK cells from their precursors. By their *in vivo* studies in mice, Haller *et al* have obtained evidence that NK cells develop from precursors in the bone marrow, but they did not define the stages betweeen the bone marrow stem cells and functional NK cells. Some additional insight has come from studies of augmentation of NK activity with interferon (IF), by the demonstration of phenotypic differences between spontaneous NK cells and the pre-NK cells responding to IF. However, as discussed in section IC3, the IF-responsive pre-NK cells are very similar to active NK cells and appear to already have receptors for recognizing their target cells. Such pre-NK cells are presumably just before active NK cells in the differentiation scheme and it is of interest to determine what earlier stages of maturation might exist. Virtually all of the data on this point has come from *in vitro* studies, in which there are indications that development of NK cells from phenotypically distinct precursors can occur. This fragmentary information is summarized below.

I. DEVELOPMENT OF MOUSE NK CELLS DURING CULTURE

Although spontaneous NK cell activity usually declines to very low levels upon *in vitro* culture at 37C, several investigators have observed that more prolonged culture can lead to reappearance of substantial cytotoxic activity, which has a specificity pattern very similar to that of NK cells. Such apparent development of NK cells *in vitro* has been observed in cultures of spleen cells alone in medium containing fetal bovine serum (FBS) or in mixed leukocyte cultures (MLC). Since some differences have been observed in these culture systems, they will be discussed separately below.

ISBN 0-12-341350-8

A. *Cultures in FBS*

Mouse spleen cells, cultured alone in medium containing FBS, have been found to develop cytotoxic activity against NK-sensitive target cells, with peak activity seen after 5-6 days (Burton; Seeley and Kärre). Comparable cultures of cells in medium with normal mouse serum did not develop any cytotoxic activity (Seeley and Kärre), suggesting that some factor in FBS stimulates the development of NK cells. As discussed by Koo and Hatzfeld, Chun et al (1979) found that Thy 1+ cells from euthymic mice were required at the beginning of culture in order for NK activity to develop. It is not clear from this study whether the Thy 1+ cells are the precursors for NK activity or are required as accessory cells. These data and the two alternative possibilities for a role of T cells are quite analogous to the human data (see below and Ortaldo and Herberman). The cells required for generation of effectors appear to be quite distinct from NK cells, being negative for Qa5 (Chun et al, 1979) and NK (Burton) antigens. Burton has also noted a difference between the cells required to develop NK cells reactive against lymphoma targets and those reactive against solid tumor targets. In the latter case, the precursor cells, as well as the effector cells, were resistant to treatment with anti-H2 plus complement.

The effector cells that developed in culture appeared to be similar to in vivo generated NK cells in their specificity and in showing some reactivity with antibodies to Thy 1. However, in contrast to fresh NK cells, the NK cells from cultures were resistant to treatment with anti-NK plus complement (Burton) or anti-Qa5 plus complement (Chun et al, 1979). It is difficult to determine the explanation for this. The natural effector cells reactive against solid tumor targets, both fresh and from cultures, are resistant to anti-NK and NK antigen negative effector cells may be a separate subset of cells. Alternatively, as suggested by environmentally-induced shifts in expression of other antigens on NK cells, expression of the NK or Qa5 antigens may vary with the state of activation or differentiation of the same cells. In this context, it is important to re-emphasize that the degree of expression of Thy 1 does not appear to be a reliable criterion for distinguishing between CTL and NK cells.

B. *Mixed Leukocyte Cultures*

Seeley and Kärre have performed detailed studies on the nature of cytotoxic effector cells that develop during mixed leukocyte cultures. In addition to the peak appearance of specifically immune CTL on day 5, transient reactivity on day 3 was seen against NK-sensitive target cells. The specificity of these early effector cells was different from that of CTL and was consistent with that of NK cells. With the stimulus of alloantigens, the presence of FBS in the medium did not appear to be required for development of these NK cells. The nature of the precursor cells and other possible cells that are needed for generation of NK cells in mouse MLC has not yet been defined. However, some information is available on the phenotype of the effectors. These cells appear to vary somewhat from the NK cells that develop in FBS-containing medium, being more sensitive to elimination by anti-Thy 1 plus complement. The cultured NK cells were also found to be larger and less dense than fresh NK cells.

II. DEVELOPMENT OF HUMAN NK CELLS DURING CULTURE

In *in vitro* studies with human cells, NK activity has also been generated in cultures in medium containing FBS or in MLC. As in the mouse, some differences between these culture systems have been noted in the cellular requirements for development of activity and in the effector cells. In addition, the characteristics of the involved human cells have been defined more extensively than in the mouse, thereby providing further evidence for development of NK cells from precursors with a disparate phenotype.

A. *Cultures in FBS*

Generation of NK cells by cultures of mononuclear cells by themselves in medium containing FBS has been studied extensively by Ortaldo and Herberman. Evidence for the development of new effector cells was provided by the observation that culture of cells lacking Fc_γ receptors, and thus concomitantly lacking detectable NK or ADCC activities, developed high levels of both activities after 4-5 days, with peak levels at days 6-7. Some factor(s) in FBS appeared to be required for this generation of effector cells. In regard to cellular requirements, some interaction between cells with E receptors and E receptor negative cells, bearing T cell associated antigens, was required. It was not possible to clearly determine which of these cell types was the precursor for the NK cells. Since proliferation of the E receptor negative cells, but not of the E receptor prositive, appeared to be required, it was postulated that the former subset contained the precursors and that the latter were accessory cells.

The effector cells that developed had the general characteristics of NK cells. Their specificity was quite similar and they shared some major cell surface characteristics. All of the cultured NK cells appeared to express Fc_{γ} receptors, since activity was efficiently depleted on monolayers of immune complexes. Some of the effector cells had detectable E receptors, but this portion seemed lower than with fresh NK cells. There were some other changes from fresh NK cells, with a small portion of the cultured effector cells being adherent to rayon and having detectable Ia antigens. The expression of Fc_{γ} receptors on the cultured NK cells provided a very useful marker for distinguishing these cells from <u>in vitro</u> generated CTL, since the latter had no detectable Fc_{γ} receptors.

B. Mixed Leukocyte and Other Mixed Cell Cultures

Seeley and Kärre, and Bolhuis reported detailed information on the cells involved in generation of NK cells in mixed cultures. Although they choose to refer to the effectors as anomolous killer (AK), they appear to have the expected specificity of NK cells. In contrast to the cultures in FBS, peak levels of NK activity were observed at day 3, several days before the peak of alloimmune CTL. This time of appearance corresponded to the peak of ^{3}H-thymidine incorporation into the cells, but no evidence was provided for a requirement for proliferation in the generation of the NK cells.

As with the cultures in FBS, NK cells could develop from Fc_{γ} receptor negative input cells. However, in contrast with the cultures in FBS, E receptor positive responder cells in MLC appeared sufficient for generation of NK cells. Mixed cultures with K562 stimulator cells gave results more similar to those in FBS cultures, since E receptor positive cells alone were not sufficient for development of NK cells (Seeley and Kärre). Despite this, the precursors for the effector cells appeared to be in the E receptor positive population, since addition of soluble factors from MLC provided the needed stimulus for development to proceed. These data suggest that the differences in cellular requirements in the various culture systems may be related to the need for accessory factors that can be produced in MLC, and possibly by proliferating E receptor negative cells in the cultures in FBS but not by K562.

The NK cells generated in MLC appear to differ from fresh NK cells and NK cells from cultures in FBS in regard to their expression of Fc_{γ} receptors. Neither Bolhuis nor Seeley and Kärre were able to deplete effector cells on immune complex monolayers. It is not clear whether these NK cells have low affinity Fc_γ receptors or lack them completely. It would be helpful to measure ADCC activity before and after adsorption on the monolayers, since this would be a sensitive method to determine the adequacy of depletion. Some cultured cells do appear to have low affinity Fc_γ receptors, with retention of ADCC activity after adsorption on immune complex monolayers (J. Ortaldo, unpublished observations). In any event, it appears that separation on immune complex monolayers of effector cells generated in MLC would not be a satisfactory procedure for clear discrimination between CTL and NK cells. Other procedures, particularly those based on the differences in specificity, would seem to be more reliable.

III. POSSIBLE RELATIONSHIP BETWEEN DIFFERENTIATION PATHWAYS OF NK CELLS AND T CELLS

Given the expression on NK cells of several markers associated with T cells (see section IA), it is of interest to consider where NK cells might be placed within the T cell lineage. From data on high expression of NK activity in nude or neonatally thymectomized mice, it has been thought that NK cells might be early or pre-T cells. It is an attractive concept to have early T lineage cells with NK activity and upon further maturation to have the development of more exquisitely specific cytotoxic T lymphocytes. The suggestion of Kaplan and Callewaert regarding the nature of the recognition structures on NK cells would fit with this hypothesis. However, as pointed out by Koo and Hatzfeld, mouse NK cells don't fit into the category of prothymocytes, since those are Thy 1-, Ly10+, and have receptors for peanut agglutinin (PNA), whereas a portion of NK cells are Thy 1+ and none have been found to have Ly10 antigen or PNA receptors. Also, if NK cells were typical early or pre-T cells, one might expect exposure to thymic hormones to induce further differentiation, with either loss of their cytotoxic activity or the expression of markers of more mature T cells on the effector cells. However, *in vitro* treatment with these hormones has yielded modest and rather inconsistent results (Gidlund *et al*, Herberman *et al*). The report by Koo and Hatzfeld of expression of Ly1 on some mouse NK cells suggests that they can express markers of more mature T cells; however, it is not known whether Ly1 might be detected on some lymphocytes of nude mice, if the same sensitive procedure with high titered monoclonal antibody were used. The data from the human studies also don't provide a clear picture as to where NK cells and their precursors might fit into the pathway of differentiation of T cells. The data of Ortaldo and Herberman are consistent with a differentiation of NK cells from T cell antigen +, E receptor negative cells to some NK cells with E receptors. However, as discussed above, to be reconciled with the data of Seeley and Kärre, one must postulate the precursors for NK cells to have a more mature phenotype, E receptor +, Fc_{γ} receptor -.

These difficulties in assigning a place for NK cells in the main pathway of differentiation of T cells may be due in part to our fragmentary knowledge of the steps in this pathway. Alternatively, and perhaps more likely, NK cells may be related to T cells but have their own discrete pathway of differentiation and never differentiate further into mature T cells with the typical features of those cells. A third possibility, supported by the data of Chun et al (1979) and of Seeley and Kärre, is that mature T cells may be activated by some stimuli to develop into NK cells (see chapters by Bloom et al and by Ortaldo and Herberman for more discussion regarding these alternative differentiation pathways). The recent ability to propagate selected populations of human and mouse NK cells in vitro, with the aid of T cell growth factor, should be very helpful in obtaining more detailed data on this important issue.

REFERENCES

Chun, M., Pasanen, V., Hämmerling, U., Hämmerling, G.F. and Hoffmann, M.K., J. Exp. Med. 150, 426 (1979).

INTERFERON AND NK CELLS IN RESISTANCE TO PERSISTENTLY VIRUS-INFECTED CELLS AND TUMORS

Barry Bloom[1]
Nagahiro Minato
Andrew Neighbour
Lola Reid[2]
Donald Marcus

Department of Microbiology and Immunology
Department of Cell Biology
Department of Pharmacology
Department of Medicine
Albert Einstein College of Medicine
Bronx, New York

The Problem

Most virus infections in man and experimental animals appear to follow an acute brief course that is restricted by an appropriate immune response. The principal immunological mechanisms known to be responsible for restriction of acute virus infection are antibodies, which act to prevent infection by neutralizing virus or restricting the spread of infection, and T-cell mediated cytotoxicity, which serves to lyse infected cells, hopefully aborting the infection. Nevertheless, it is quite clear that there are a number of diseases the etiology of which appears to be dependent on persistent virus infection. Subacute sclerosing panencephalitis, a chronic demyelinting disease caused by a measles-related virus, multiple sclerosis and lupus erythema-

[1]This research was supported by US Public Health Service grants AI 09807, AI 10702 from the National Institutes of Health, and RG 1006 from the National Multiple Sclerosis Society.
[2]This research was supported by US Public Health Service grant P30-CA1330.

ISBN 0-12-341350-8

tosus, both of unknown etiology, have epidemiological and serological attributes of persistent virus infections. Obviously, many types of cancer appear to be related to persistence of oncogenic viruses. The questions which these situations present are: (1) how such viruses manage to survive and persist in a host which has generated appropriate immune response to protect itself from the acute phase of virus infection; and (2) whether there exists an additional immunological mechanism, beyond the conventional immune responses, which can provide resistance to persistent virus infections. Rather extensive studies have been carried out on the mechanisms by which viruses establish a persistent state in host cells, exploring the role of DI particles (1), ts mutants (2) and interferon (3). On the other hand, very little is currently known about the nature of the host defense mechanisms against the persistent viral infections.

In this review, we present an experimental model in which the host response against virus infected tumor cells largely independent of the conventional immune responses can be studied. In this model, it will be shown that the "natural killer -interferon (NK-IF)" system is one of the critical factors in host defense against persistent viral infections and tumorigenesis. The detailed cellular events involved in the NK-IF system and their relationship to the immune system will be considered.

The Experimental Model.

We have chosen to examine the resistance of athymic nude mice to tumor cells persistently infected with a variety of viruses, since this provides a system in which mechanisms of natural resistance to persistent virus infection largely independent of antibody and T-cell functions can be explored. The model was appealing at a second level, because while nude mice have been extensively used in studies on tumorigenicity of human and animal tumors, it has become clear that nude mice are not totally immunodeficient, and a number of tumors fail to grow in the nude mouse host (4). This system thus provides a simple model for pursuing the mechanisms of natural resistance in nude mice to neoplastic cells.

In previous studies, we have reported that as few as 10-100 HeLa or BHK cells produce tumors in 100% of Balb/c nu/nu mice within 3 weeks. However, when these tumor cells were rendered persistently infected with a variety of RNA viruses, including vesicular stomatitis virus, measles, mumps, influenza, no evidence of tumor growth was observed when as many as 10^4 virus persistently infected (PI) cells were inoculated subcutaneously (5). When 10^4-10^7 virus PI cells were in-

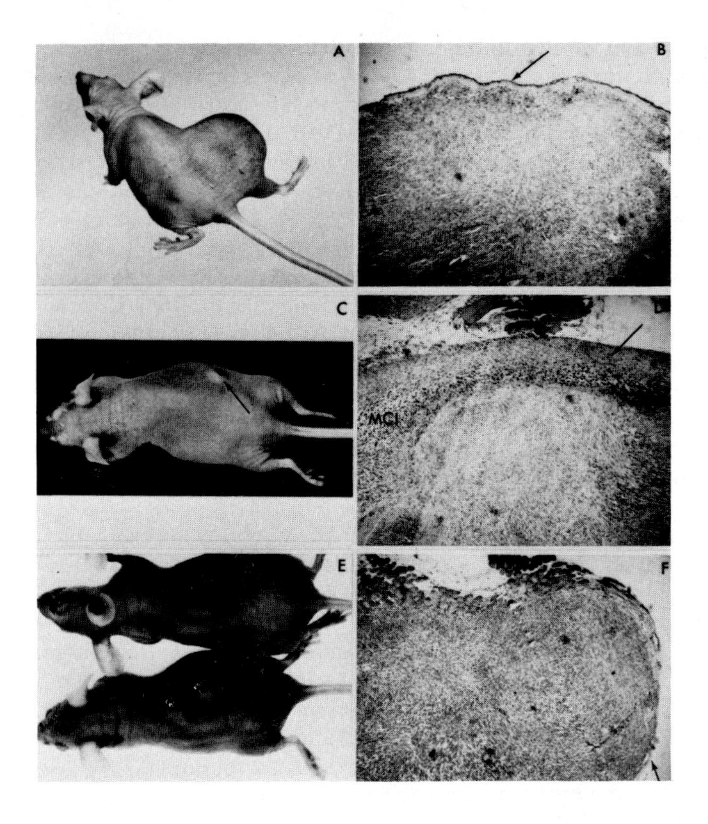

Figure 1. Neoplasms in BALB/c nude mice injected with BHK21 or BHK-VSV cells. A. The mouse was inoculated with 10^6 BHK21 cells subcutaneously. The tumor was initially palpable by 10 d, and the animal was moribund with the tumor by 6 wk. B. A section of a tumor produced in a nude mouse injected with 10^6 BHK21 cells. Note the thin but distinct fibrous capsule (arrow) infiltrated with a small population of mononuclear cells. The 8-µm paraffin section was stained with haematoxylin and eosin. Magnification: X 130. C. The mouse was inoculated with 10^6 BHK-VSV cells subcutaneously. The small neoplasm noted on the right side of the mouse(arrow) developed by the 4th wk after inoculation and persisted in this benign form for >6 mo. D.Section from a nodule produced in a nude mouse injected with 10^6 BHK-NWS flu cells. Similar results were obtained from tumors from injections with other virus P.I. cell lines. Note the thick fibrous capsyle(arrow) and the mononuclear infiltrate(MCI) surrounding the BHK-flu cells.

Reprinted from *J. Exp. Med. 149,* 1117, (1979).

jected, small nodules appeared which failed to develop into tumors and were maintained over a six month period. An illustration of these findings is shown in Fig. 1. Histological examination of the nodules revealed a marked round cell infiltration of nodules produced by virus PI tumor cells, with only very slight infiltration of the virus uninfected parental tumor cell sites (Fig. 1). The *in vivo* growth rates of the uninfected and virus persistently infected cells *in vitro* could not be distinguished, suggesting that the failure of the virus PI cells to form tumors in nude mice was not an intrinsic property of these cells, but rather a consequence of a host response to them. This was confirmed when it was shown that irradiation of nude mice with 550 r rendered them all susceptible to tumor growth.

The Effector Cell - The NK Cell.

The mechanism of resistance to virus PI tumor cells by nude mice was investigated by examining cytotoxic activity of spleen cells derived from normal nude mice *in vitro* against uninfected or virus PI infected tumor cell lines. The results of over 50 experiments unambiguously demonstrated: i) that uninfected BHK or HeLa cells are not subject to spontaneous cytotoxicity *in vitro*, whereas the same cells persistently infected with the above mentioned viruses are lysed to various degrees *in vitro*; ii) virus PI tumor cells stimulate interferon production *in vitro*, whereas uninfected parental cells do not (Table I).

TABLE I. Preferential Responsiveness of Normal Nude Mouse Spleen Cells In Vitro Against Virus P.I. Tumor Cells--Spontaneous Cytotoxicity and Interferon Production[a]

Tumor cells	*Cytotoxicity*	*IF Production*
	%	*units*
HeLa	*3.7*	*< 2*
HeLa-measles	*26.2*	*64*
HeLa-mumps	*26.3*	*16*
HeLa-VSV	*28.2*	*16*

[a]*The cytotoxicity of spleen cells against tumor cells was assayed by* ^{51}*Cr-release assay at 8 hr. The antiviral activity of the supernates of 24 hr mixed lymphocyte-tumor cell culture (MLTC) was assayed using the cytopathic inhibition test in L cells by VSV challenge. The L/T ratio was 100:1.*

Classical techniques used to enrich and deplete lymphocyte subpopulations from spleen cells were employed to characterize the cytotoxic effector cell, and the results indicated that the effector cell lacked the conventional characteristics of T-cells, B-cells or macrophages (6). For example, under conditions in which conventional anti-Thy 1.2 anti-serum + C eliminated over 90% of the mitogenic response to Con A, spontaneous cytotoxicity of nude mouse spleen cells for HeLa-measles targets was only partially affected. Passage of these spleens over nylon wool or treatment with anti-Ig + C were without effect. On this basis, it was reasonable to presume that the effector cell in nude mouse spleens capable of selectively lysing virus PI tumor cells had the characteristics generally associated with natural killer (NK) cells.

Using more refined reagents, however, it was possible to characterize the NK effector cells in this system as being positive for four surface markers (Table II). Using monoclonal anti-Thy 1.2 serum + C, the spontaneous cytotoxic activity for the virus PI target cells was consistently reduced by 30-35%, consistent with recent reports of Herberman (7)using a leukemia target cell system in which a portion of the effector

TABLE II. Summary of the Phenotypes of the NK Effector Cells as Determined by Complement-Mediated Cytolysis[a]

Antibody (species)	*Diminution of NK activity*	*NK Phenotype*
	%	
α-Thy 1.2 (hybridoma)	*30-40*	*+ and -*
α-Lyt 2.2 (mouse)	*0*	*-*
α-Lyt 3.2 (mouse)	*0*	*-*
α-Lyb 2.2 (mouse)	*0-10*	*-*
α-Ly 5.1 (mouse)	*70-100*	*+*
α-Qa 5 (hybridoma)	*100*	*+*
α-AsGm1 (rabbit)	*60-80*	*+*
α-Ig (goat)	*0*	*-*

[a]*The effect of antisera was determined using the mice as follows: Balb/C nude and +/+ for anti-Thy 1.2, anti-Lyb 2.2, anti-AsGm1, anti-Ly 5.1, and anti-Ig; CBA/J for anti-Thy 1.2, anti-AsGm1, anti-Ly 5.1, and anti-Ig; C57Bl/6 for anti-Thy 1.2, anti-Lyt 2.2 and Lyt 3.2 and anti-Qa 5. The results of several independent experiments are summarized.*

cells were found to be Thy 1+. Antisera which define two other differentiation antigens on lymphocytes, Ly 5, and Qa 5, in the presence of complement essentially totally abolished NK activity. While Ly 5 determinants appear to be present on a variety of cells of the lymphoid system, this serum appears to be lytic in the presence of complement only for T-cells and NK cells (8). In contrast, anti-Qa 5 serum is present on a small number of lymphoid cells, and essentially all cells with surface antigen appear to be susceptible to lysis in the presence of complement (9). This antigen appears to be found exclusively on T-cells and NK cells. In man, some NK cell activity appears to be present in a subpopulation of cells which possess receptors for sheep erythrocytes, a classical marker for T-cells (10). Consequently, while the effector cell in this system appears not to be a conventional T-cell, B-cell or macrophage, it is clearly not without interest that it shares several surface markers with cells of the T-lymphocyte series in mice and man.

Regulation of NK Activity.

In order to examine the specificity of the effector cell in this system, spontaneous cytotoxicity of spleen cells from animals challenged with uninfected or virus PI infected tumor cells was tested. For example, BHK cells, BHK-mumps and BHK-VSV cell lines were injected subcutaneously into nude mice, and the cytotoxic activity of spleen cells was assayed both on the homologous tumor cell and on a totally irrelevant target cell, HeLa-measles. Results summarized in Table III demonstrated that inoculation of nude mice with any virus PI cell line augmented cytotoxicity not only for that specific cell line, but for essentially any of the other virus PI cell lines. The augmentation of cytotoxic activity was found as early as two days and persisted at high levels for at least 35 days, differing in this respect from augmentation seen in conventional mice which waned after approximately 7 days(6). Of interest, no augmented cytotoxic activity was observed with spleen cells from nude mice which had been inoculated with uninfected tumor cells; if anything, there was a reproducible depression in NK activity in tumor bearing mice as compared with normal controls. These results clearly demonstrated the challenge of nude mice with virus PI cell lines non specifically enhanced NK activity for both specific and irrelevant virus PI targets.

We have previously reported (6), that in addition to the non-specific augmentation in NK activity, there may indeed exist a degree of specificity, or at least a high level of selectivity for specific virus infected target cells. The

Table III. Nonspecific Augmentation of NK Activity by Virus P.I. Tumor Cells But Not by Parental Tumor Cells[a]

Nude mice injected with,	*% Relative cytotoxicity against*	
	HeLa-measles	*HeLa-mumps*
	%	%
PBS	*100*	*100*
HeLa-measles (10^6)	*148*	*185*
BHK-mumps (10^6)	*142*	*n.t.*
BHK-VSV (10^6)	*164*	*n.t.*
BHK (10^6)	*30*	*n.t.*

[a]*Normal Balb/c nude mice were injected with 10^6 tumor cells or PBS subcutaneously. 15 days later, the cytotoxicity of their spleen cells was assayed against HeLa-measles or HeLa-mumps cells using ^{51}Cr-release assay at 8 hr at L/T ratio 50:1. The results were normalized relative to the cytotoxicity of the PBS-injected mice (=100%).*

possible specificity in effector cell activity was examined using cold competition experiments, in which the effectiveness of unlabeled target cells to compete with labeled target cells was examined. As summarized in Table IV, unlabeled HeLa-measles cells in ratios of 4:1-8:1 were able to block lysis of labeled HeLa-measles targets by 70%. At similar ratios, none of the uninfected or other virus PI target cell lines was able to block as efficiently as HeLa-measles. Similar results using HeLa-VSV targets were obtained. In any of the virus PI systems studied, the standard NK cell targets commonly used, YAC or K562, totally failed to inhibit killing of HeLa-measles targets. These experiments do not prove that the effector cells in this system have immunologic specificity, but they do demonstrate, at a minimum, that they are not totally non-specific.

The finding that any of the virus PI cell lines was capable of augmenting the cytotoxicity of spleen cells of nude mice even for irrelevant virus PI target cell lines, taken with the findings that interferon inducers or interferon have known regulatory activity for NK cells (11,12), strongly implicated interferon as the mediator of NK cell regulation. This was tested directly and unambiguously by treating spleen cells from normal nude mouse with mouse interferon purified to homogeneity ($4x10^9$ U/ml) by Dr. Peter Lengyel, Yale Uni-

Table IV. Cold Target Inhibition Tests of NK Activity of Normal Nude Mouse Spleen Cells against Various Target Cells[a]

Exp. No.	Labeled target cells	% Inhibition of the cytotoxicity by unlabeled				
		HeLa-Ms	HeLa-Mps	HeLa-VSV	BHK-Mps	BHK-VSV
I	HeLa-Ms	68	-	-	-	1
II	HeLa-Ms	21	-	2	0	9
III	HeLa-Ms	42	28	-	-	-
	HeLa-Mps	0	47	0	-	-
	YAC	0	-	-	-	-
	K562	0	-	-	-	-

[a] $2x10^4$ to $4x10^4$ of various unlabeled target cells were added to the $1x10^4$ of ^{51}Cr-labeled target cells, and then 10^6 of normal spleen cells were admixed for 8 hr. The results were expressed as % inhibition of the specific ^{51}Cr-release compared with that without any unlabeled target cells.

Table V. Effect of Chemically Purified Mouse Interferon In Vitro on NK Activity against Uninfected or Virus P.I. Tumor Cells[a]

Pretreatment of spleen cells	Cytotoxicity		
	HeLa	HeLa-VSV	HeLa-measles
	%	%	%
medium (30 min.)	-3.2	29.7	15.5
1,500 U IF (30 min.)	-5.9	48.0	36.1

[a] Normal nude mouse spleen cells were pretreated in vitro with medium or 1,500 units of chemically purified IF for 30 min., washed, and the cytotoxic activity was assayed on various target cells at 8 hr using ^{51}Cr-release assay. The interferon purified as described in ref. , had a specific activity of $2x10^9$ U/mg and was generously provided by Dr. Peter Lengyel, Yale University.

versity (13), in examining its effect on NK activity. The results shown in Table V indicate that purified mouse interferon, at a level of 1500 U/ml, significantly enhanced NK activity. Additional experiments indicated a parallel between the ability of virus PI cell lines to augment NK activity *in vitro* and their ability to induce detectable levels of interferon and the ability of antibodies against purified mouse interferon to abrogate the enhancement by interferon or interferon containing supernatants.

The critical test of whether interferon provides a major immunoregulatory role for the restriction of virus PI tumor cells *in vivo*, operating either through NK cells or other means, is currently being provided by experiments *in vivo* using antibodies to interferon generously provided by Drs. Kurt Paucker and Ion Gresser. Preliminary results of these experiments are summarized in Table VI, and indicate that treatment of nude mice with antibodies to mouse interferon permits BHK-mumps cells, which ordinarily fail to grow in these animals, to grow into tumors with high frequency. Obviously these experiments need to be expanded and extended to other tumors as well. Nevertheless, they indicate that interferon, possibly acting through NK cells, is critically involved in the resistance of athymic nude mice to the growth of virus PI tumor cell lines.

Table VI. Effect of Anti-Mouse IF Serum on the Growth of Virus P.I. Tumor Cells In Vivo in Nude Mice[a]

Tumors	*Treatment of mice*	*Mean tumor weight*
		g
BHK-mumps	*PBS 0.1 ml i.v.*	*0.22 ± 0.10*
	αIF (1:3) 0.1 ml i.v.	*1.21 ± 0.46*

[a]*Balb/c nude mice were injected with PBS or αIF at the same time with* 10^6 *BHK-mumps cells s.c. (each group, 6 mice), and 11 days later all mice were killed and the tumor weight was measured.*

Mode of Interferon Action.

It is well established that interferon and interferon inducers augment NK cell function (11,12). Yet, the current technical limitations on obtaining homogeneous populations of NK cells pose serious limitations to analysis of the mechanism by which interferon exerts its effects. The conventional view has been that interferon "activates" existing NK cells in much the same way that lymphokines can activate macrophages. An alternative view would be that interferon acts on a precursor of NK cells leading to the generation of increased numbers of NK cells. The ability to discriminate between these hypotheses at present depends on the usefulness of surface markers to distinguish NK cells. As indicated in Table II, there are two differentiation antigens associated with NK cells - Ly 5 and Qa 5. While Ly 5 is an antigen widely distributed among mononuclear cells, it appears that only T-cells and NK cells are lysed in the presence of complement with anti-Ly 5 antisera. In contrast, Qa 5 is found on a more restricted population of cells, and essentially all of these cells exhibiting this phenotype are lysed in the presence of complement. To elucidate the nature of the cell upon which interferon acts, we have treated the spleen cells from normal nude mice with anti-Ly 5 + C and anti-Qa 5 + C, as summarized in Table VII,

Table VII. Effect of Anti-Ly 5.1 and Anti-Qa 5 + C' Treatments on Endogenous NK Activity and Interferon-Mediated Induction of NK Activity[a]

Mouse strains	*Pretreatment of spleen cells*	*NK activity after the incubation*	
		medium	*interferon*
			%
Balb/c, nude	*C'*	*19*	*34*
	anti-Ly 5.1+C'	*3*	*24*
C57bl/c	*C'*	*15*	*31*
	anti-Qa 5+C'	*2*	*2*

[a]*Normal mouse spleen cells were pretreated with C' alone or with antiserum+C; washed, and then preincubated in vitro with medium or with interferon for 6 hr. The cytotoxicity on HeLa-measles cells were assayed using 8 hr* ^{51}*Cr-release assay.*

and then determined whether interferon has any ability to augment NK activity in these depleted populations. Both anti-Ly 5 and anti-Qa 5 in the presence of complement essentially totally eliminate NK activity. Treatment in the absence of complement, followed by washing, is without effect on the NK function of these cells. As shown in Table VII addition of purified mouse interferon ($2x10^9$ U/ml) generously provided by Dr. Peter Lengyel to anti-Qa 5 + C treated cells fails to result in any increase in NK activity. In contrast, addition of chemically purified interferon to NK cell depleted spleens treated with anti-Ly 5 + C results, within 1-3 hours,in a remarkable increase in NK activity. We believe that these experiments formally demonstrate that interferon can act on a non-functional precursor to NK cells and convert them to lytic effector cells. Our interpretation would be that both the precursor and NK cells share the Qa 5 antigen, and treatment with anti-Qa 5 + C eliminates both cell populations. Secondly, we would argue that NK cells are Ly 5+ whereas their precursors are Ly 5-. Consequently, removal of Ly 5 cells depletes the NK population, while the precursor population is unaffected, and can be induced by interferon treatment to differentiate into functional NK cells. That this is the case has been confirmed by the demonstration that anti-Ly 5 + C depleted cells, stimulated by interferon which leads to reappearance of functional NK cells, also results in a parallel increase in Ly 5+ cells. Retreatment of the anti-Ly 5 depleted cells exposed to interferon with anti-Ly 5 + C again removes all NK activity, indicating that interferon induces the expression not only of NK activity but the reappearance of the Ly 5 surface antigen in these experiments. In other experiments described elsewhere (14,15), we have provided evidence that it is the Ly 5^+ cell which produces interferon, and not the precursor, at least when stimulated by virus PI tumor cells.

Cell fractionation experiments on BSA density gradients also support the idea that NK effector cells and IF sensitive cells are different subpopulations or at different stages of differentiation. As shown in Fig. 2, endogenous NK activity of CBA spleen cells was found to have peak activity in fraction C, whereas the greatest augmentation of NK activity produced by IF pretreatment was found in fraction D.

Reality Testing.

1. *Role of interferon and NK cells in rejection of virus PI tumors in animals.* The experimental evidence which has accrued to date suggests a strong parallel between susceptibility to NK cell killing *in vitro* and failure of the virus

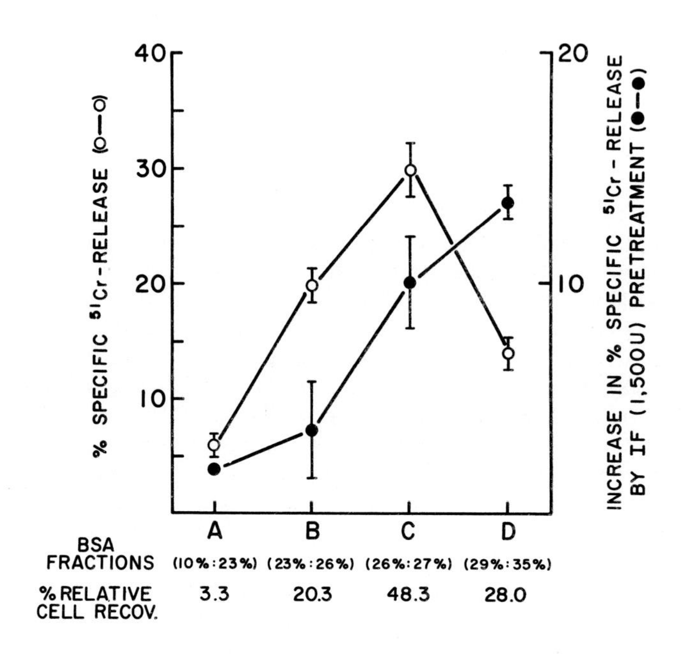

Figure 2. Endogenous NK activity and the induction of NK activity by interferon in vitro in different spleen cell fractions separated by BSA density gradient centrifugation. Normal CBA/J spleen cells were fractionated on discontinuous BSA gradients into four fractions: 10%/23% (A); 23%/26% (B); 26%/29% (C); and 29%/35% (D). A Portion of the spleen cells of each fraction were directly assayed for NK activity on Hela-Ms cells at an L/T ration of 100:1 for endogenous NK activity. Another was incubated in vitro with medium or 1,500 U interferon for 3hr prior to assay for NK activity. Induced NK activity was calculated as % specific ^{51}Cr-release after incubation with interferon minus % specific ^{51}Cr- release after incubation with medium , for each fraction.

PI tumor cell to produce tumors *in vivo*. It is also clear that interferon is a critical factor in the differentiation of NK cells, and, in data published elsewhere (14), all of the virus PI tumor cells examined are capable of inducing type I interferon upon coculture with spleen cells from nude mice. One of the critical tests of our conclusion that NK cells and interferon are responsible for the rejection of virus PI tumor cells *in vivo* is a model in which the ability of the virus PI tumor cell to elicit significant levels of interferon *in vivo* is impaired. We believe that we have preliminary evidence in at least one tumor system, namely BHK cells persistently infected with mumps, which supports the general conclusion. Nude mice were inoculated with either BHK cells or BHK-mumps cells. In the control animals, BHK cells grew in 9/9 nude mice to form tumors at 14 days, whereas BHK-mumps cells grew in 2/11. When comparable animals were treated with antibodies to mouse interferon, generously provided by Drs.Ion Gresser and Kurt Paucker, the virus PI tumor cells which were ordinarily unable to grow in nude mice, were found to grow in 12/12 animals. This formally demonstrates that interferon is critical to the rejection of some virus PI tumor cells *in vivo*, and since mouse interferon is unlikely to have direct growth inhibitory effects on hamster tumor cells, it is strongly suggested that the interferon is effective through the mediation of NK cells. While it must be acknowledged that there are a variety of immunologic mechanisms capable of restricting the growth of tumor cells, these experiments with virus PI tumor cells in the nude mouse suggest that the interferon-NK cell mechanism may well be of significance *in vivo*.

2. *Interferon production and NK cells in persistent virus infections in man.* If the interferon NK cell system is a significant immunological mechanism for restricting persistent virus infection and/or tumor cells, why, indeed, do viruses persist in man? While clearly a multiplicity of factors are involved in determining the outcome of infection or neoplasia, one correlate of our general view would be that a deficiency in interferon production or NK activity could be a predisposing factor for persistent virus infections in man. Both multiple sclerosis and systemic lupus erythematosus are human diseases generally viewed as having a persistent virus etiology, although the etiologic agent in neither disease has been identified with certainty; juvenile onset diabetes may be associated with virus infection but there is no evidence for viral persistence. We have examined the production of viral-induced interferon and NK activity of peripheral blood lymphocytes obtained from patients with these diseases, in order to ascertain whether any deficiency with respect to these two

functions existed in some of the patients (14,16). The results presented in Table VIII indicate that at least in some patients with these diseases, there is a depression in production of virus induced type I leukocyte interferon. Concommitantly, a significant proportion of donors in the MS and SLE patient group fail to exhibit spontaneous cytotoxicity on K562 acute myeloblastic leukemia cells. In addition, many patients in these groups are unresponsive to in vitro addition of NDV at least in regards to augmentation of NK activity. Clearly, these data should be expanded both within the disease categories already studied, and extended to other diseases, particularly neoplastic diseases. It will be important to analyze whether, in some patients or diseases, there is a primary defect in interferon production, or more particularly type I leukocyte interferon production, or a defect in NK function.

DISCUSSION

Interferon and the Differentiation of NK Cells.

Two hypotheses have been considered which could explain the immunoregulatory function of interferon on NK cell activity. First, interferon acts on NK cells and activates them to exert their cytolytic function, in a manner analogous to the activation of macrophages by products of activated lymphocytes. Alternatively, interferon may act on a biologically inactive precursor and facilitate its differentiation into functional NK cells. The data provided here unambiguously demonstrate that interferon can act on a non-functional precursor and, within a period 1-3 hours, initiate its differentiation into a functional NK cell. They do not, however, exclude the possibility that interferon may also act directly on NK cells to enhance their function. Functional NK cells are characterized as having surface Qa 5 and Ly 5 antigens, with a subpopulation exhibiting, in addition, the Thy 1.2 antigen. When NK activity was eliminated with treatment with anti-Ly 5 + C and the remaining cells treated with chemically purified interferon, NK activity reappeared in the nude spleen cell population, and all of the interferon induced NK cells expressed the Ly 5 surface alloantigen. In contrast, the precursor cell was found to be Ly 5- but Qa 5+. Treatment with anti-Qa 5 monoclonal antibodies + C eliminated both NK cells and the precursor, and no NK activity could be generated by addition of interferon.

In experiments to be presented elsewhere (15), we have observed a high degree of correlation between functional NK

Table VIII. Interferon Production and Natural Killer Activity in Normal and Various Patient Donor Groups

	DONOR GROUP			
	Normal	Systemic lupus erythematosus	Multiple sclerosis	Juvenile diabetes
a) NDV-induced[1] interferon				
Mean titer, units/ml	1,778	16	350	75
No. of donors	43	29	34	8
b) Natural killer activity				
Spontaneous cytotoxicity[2] No. positive/ no. tested	15/18	13/26	9/17	4/5
Augmented cytotoxicity[3] No. positive/ no. tested	12/14	1/17	9/16	not done

[1]Interferon harvested 48 hr after incubating $2x10^6$ PBL with a standard inoculum of inactivated NDV.

[2]Cytotoxicity of K562 cells by untreated PBL in a 5 hr ^{51}Cr-release assay: positive donors exhibited >1 lytic unit 30% per 10^6 PBL.

[3]Cytotoxicity of WI-L2 cells by PBL pretreated for 12 hr with a standard inoculum of inactivated NDV and tested in a 5 hr ^{51}Cr-release assay: positive donors scoured as above (untreated PBL from all donors failed to lyse WI-L2 under these assay conditions).

activity and production of interferon in mixed cultures between virus persistently infected tumor cells and mouse lymphocytes. In this system, the interferon producing cell possessed the Ly 5 surface antigen, and its precursor failed to produce interferon upon contact with virus PI cell lines. Thus the functional Qa 5+, Ly 5+ NK population also has the capability of producing interferon, which can act on Qa 5+, Ly 5-

precursors serving to recruit them into NK activity. Of particular interest in this regard are the recent observations of Saksala (17) that the human cell acted upon by IF appears to be a different subpopulation than that which exerts NK activity. Formally this process can be viewed as a positive feedback loop. Of interest will be the elucidation of the negative controls which regulate the process of differentiation of precursors into functional NK cells in the presence of interferon.

Two fundamental questions on the nature and fate of NK cells remain. The first concerns the mode of recognition of target structures or antigen. It is generally believed that NK cells lack immunologic specificity, yet a growing body of data including some involving cold competition inhibition of cytotoxicity assays suggest that there is at least a high degree of selectivity for appropriate targets, if not immunologic specificity (6,18). In order to explain this selectivity, one has to argue either: 1) that a variety of cells, neoplastically transformed or persistently infected with different viruses, acquire a common alteration of their cell surface which permits them to be recognized by NK cells. In this model, they would be seen as non-specific in the immunological sense but selective for a common surface structure; or, 2) NK cells have antigen specificity in a true immunologic sense. The difficulty in this model is its apparent inability to explain the non-specific reactivity of NK cells against such a wide variety of target cells. Since it is clear that interferon serves non-specifically to augment NK activity, its action may be viewed analogous to a polyclonal mitogen. Thus, interaction of a small subpopulation of virus specific NK cells with the appropriate virus could release interferon which would then serve to force the differentiation of a variety of clones capable of recognizing a variety of target antigens. In either case, the nature of the specific receptors on NK cells is of great importance, and currently under investigation in several laboratories (18).

The second fundamental question in the differentiation of NK cells is whether they represent an independent lymphocyte lineage or alternatively, intermediates in the differentiation of either T-cells, B-cells or macrophages. The present data reveal that NK cells share four surface alloantigens in the mouse in common with T-cells, namely Qa 5, Ly 5, AsGm1 (19) and, to a lesser extent, Thy 1. It is tempting to speculate that the NK cell is in fact a precursor to the cytotoxic T lymphocyte. One could argue, if it could be shown definitively that NK cells have antigen specific recognition, that the NK cell represents a T-cell precursor which possesses an antigen receptor but has not been histocompatibility restricted because it has not yet been processed by the thymus. The augmented NK activity present in nude mice could be explained by accumulation of NK cells, which might be viewed as T-cell precursors that are not processed by the thymus in a steady state fashion, as might be the case in conventional mice. One of several problems with this interpretation is the failure to detect any Lyt surface alloantigens on NK cells - they remain consistently negative for Ly 1 and Ly 2,3. It is tempting to speculate that NK cells, rather than representing the exclusive precursor of cytotoxic T-cells, might represent an "alternative pathway" to cytotoxic T lymphocyte activity. The alternative pathway would concern the differentiation of precursor cells into functional cytotoxic cells in the periphery, rather than in the thymus, and which would explain the presence of Thy 1 antigen on approximately 35% of NK cells in the nude mouse.

NK Cells, Interferon and Resistance to Persistent Virus Infections

As mentioned earlier, in the natural course of resistance to acute virus infections, antibodies would serve to neutralize virus and block spread of infection in cytotoxic cells and would function to lyse infected cells prior to maturation of virus, thereby aborting the infection. Were these systems ideally functional, persistent virus infection would be a rarity. It is quite unclear how common persistent virus infections which do not lead to disease really are, but they may be more common than generally thought.

Following infection with most lytic viruses, and probably some oncogenic viruses as well, interferon could be produced by a wide variety of host cells, including somatic cells, macrophages, B-cells, T-cells and NK cells. Our preliminary data and those of others (20) indicate that any of the species of interferon is capable of initiating the differentiation of NK functional activity. The preliminary studies presented here, together with studies on the effects of interferon inducers *in vivo* strongly suggest that amplification of NK activity is of considerable importance in resistance to virus infection and some tumors. The experiments of Schellekens *et al* (21) have demonstrated elegantly in a system in which interferon is ineffective at protecting cells against vaccinia infection *in vitro* that at least some of the protection *in vivo* must be provided by the host, presumably NK cells. In the case of the virus PI tumor cells presented here, it is worthy of note that BHK cells are hamster derived and unlikely to be affected by mouse interferon, due to the relatively high degree of species specific restriction of interferon. For these reasons, it may be inferred that a major part of the effectiveness of interferon *in vivo* depends upon its ability to amplify NK cells.

These findings raise a general question concerning the preexistence of functional NK cells. As is well known, there is a spontaneous cytotoxicity on NK susceptible targets of lymphocytes from a variety of tissues in both mice and humans. The question remains, however, whether these represent a normal circulation of preexistent functional NK cells, or whether all NK activity is dependent on the production of low levels of interferon stimulated by viruses or other environmental factors. Our preliminary data suggest that anti-interferon treatment of normal nude mice results in a marked diminution in spontaneous cytotoxicity, although it is at the moment unclear as to whether all NK activity can be eliminated by this treatment. These considerations, however, do raise a significant point in evaluating NK activity *in vitro* and relating it to the immunological status of patients. In experiments on virus PI tumor cell lines, spontaneous cytotoxicity *in vitro* was unaffected by the presence of anti-interferon antibodies for a period up to nine hours, and results under these conditions may be taken to indicate the level of preexistent NK activity in lymphocyte source. Using assays longer than nine hours, there was a marked inhibition of further development of NK activity, concomitant with the ability to detect interferon in the culture media. These observations suggest that in each system there will be a critical time in which preexistent NK activity can be determined, following which there is *in vitro* induction of additional NK activity by interferon produced *in vitro*. If the goal of the study is to assess the NK activity preexisting in patients, then it is important to be certain that *in vitro* induction and amplification are distinguished from preexisting NK activity.

Finally, if the interferon-NK system is of importance in restricting the persistence of viruses *in vivo*, it might be expected that patients suffering diseases believed to be of persistent viral etiology might have some deficiency in their ability either to generate interferon or functional NK cells. As summarized here, significant diminution in the ability of peripheral lymphocytes to produce interferon upon exposure to killed measles or Newcastle disease viruses was found in lymphocytes obtained from patients with multiple sclerosis and systemic lupus erythematosus, and possibly from patients with juvenile onset diabetes. Preliminary observations suggest a comparable decrease in NK activity, although the precise correlation between interferon production *in vitro* and NK activity remains to be established. A deficiency of NK activity in patients can obviously be attributed to a number of causes - particularly failure to produce interferon or failure to develop precursors or a failure of precursors to respond to interferon to become functional NK cells. Preliminary characterization of lymphocytes *in vitro* from patients with MS and SLE has indicated that all three possibilities appear to exist. Our preliminary data indicate that in the MS and SLE patient groups leukocytes from some patients fail to respond to interferon or interferon inducers. It is our view that it is of considerable importance to analyze the deficit in each patient, particularly if the use of interferon therapy is contemplated. If one of the objectives of interferon therapy for cancer or diseases of persistent virus etiology is to augment NK cell activity then at least some indication as to whether the NK cells or their precursors are responsive to exogenous interferon should be obtained before applying a long and very expensive course of interferon therapy. And obviously, in appropriate patients, it would seem also to be important to monitor both levels of interferon and levels of NK activity during treatment, in order to attempt to correlate clinical improvement with immunoregulatory effects of the interferon.

REFERENCES

1. Holland, J.J., and Villarreal, L.P. *Proc. Natl. Acad. Sci. 71,* 2956 (1974).
2. Preble, O.T., and Younger, J.S. *J. Infect. Dis. 131,* 467 (1975).
3. Rodriguez, J.E., and Henle, W. *J. Exp. Med. 119,* 895 (1964).
4. Reid. L., and Shin, S., *in* "The Nude Mouse in Experimental and Clinical Research" (J. Fogh and B. Giovanella, eds.), p. 313.
5. Reid, L, Jones, C., and Holland, J. *J. Gen. Virol. 42,* 609 (1979).
6. Minato, N., Bloom, B.R., Jones, C., Holland, J., and Reid, L.M. *J. Exp. Med. 149,* 1118 (1979).
7. Herberman, R.B., Nunn, M.E., and Holden, H.T. *J. Immunol. 121,* 304 (1978).
8. Cantor, H., Kasai, M., Shen, H.W., LeClerc, J.C., and Glincher, L. *Immunol. Revs. 44,* 1 (1979).
9. Hammerling, G., Hammerling, U, and Flaherty, L. *J. Exp. Med. 150,* 108 (1979).
10. Herberman, R.B., Djeu, J.Y., Kay, D. Ortaldo, J.R., Riccardi, C., Bonnard, G.D., Holden, H.T., Fagnani, R., Santoni, A., and Puccetti, P. *Immunological Rev. 44,* 43 (1979).

11. Gidlund, M., Orn, A., Wigzell, H., Senik, A., and Gresser, I. *Nature 237,* 759 (1978).
12. Trinchieri, G., Santoli, D., Dec, R.R., and Knowles, B.B. *J. Exp. Med. 147,* 1299 (1978).
13. Cabrer, B., Taira, H., Braeze, R.J., Kempe, T.D., Williams, K., Stattery, E., Konigsberg, W.H., and Langyel, P. *J. Biol. Chem. 254,* 3681 (1979).
14. Minato, N., Reid, L., Neighbour, A, and Bloom, B.R. *Annals of the N.Y. Acad. of Sci. In press.* (1980).
15. Minato, N., Reid, L., Bloom, B.R. *Submitted for publication.*
16. Neighbour, P.A., Grayzel, A., and Bloom, B.R. *Manuscript in preparation.*
17. Timonen, T., Ranki, A., Saksela, E., and Hayry, P. *Cell. Immunol. 48,* 121 (1979).
18. Roder, J.C., Ahrlund-Richiter, L., and Jondal, M. *J. Exp. Med. 150,* 471 (1979).
19. Stein, K.E., Schwarting, G.A., Naiki, M., and Marcus, D. M. *J. Exp. Med. 143,* 822 (1976).
20. Falcoff, E. *Annals of the N.Y. Acad. of Sci. In press.* (1980).
21. Schellekens, H., Weimar, W., Cantell, K., and Stitz, L. *Nature 278,* 742 (1979).

INTERFERON-INDEPENDENT ACTIVATION OF MURINE NATURAL KILLER CELL ACTIVITY

Michael J. Brunda[1]
Ronald B. Herberman
Howard T. Holden

Laboratory of Immunodiagnosis
National Cancer Institute
Bethesda, Maryland

Interferon (IF) and IF-inducers have been shown to cause a rapid augmentation of the cytotoxic activity of murine natural killer (NK) cells both in vivo and in vitro (Djeu et al, 1979; Gidlund et al, 1978; Herberman et al, 1977). Although this suggests a major role for IF, the possibility that NK reactivity can be activated by other mechanisms has not been excluded. In this communication we have summarized our studies on the rapid activation of NK activity by Helix pomatia (HP) lectin or by alloantibodies with specificity for NK cells. Activation by these stimuli appeared to be independent of IF production, suggesting the existence of alternative pathways for NK activation.

The results from several experiments are presented in Table I. Spleen cells from C57BL/6 (B6) nude mice have relatively low levels of spontaneous NK activity against human K562 target cells in a 4 hr ^{51}Cr release assay. When BALB/c anti-B6 antiserum (Ab) was added to the assay or when spleen cells were pretreated with Ab, a marked increase in cytotoxicity was found. Similar results have been previously reported using spleen cells from conventional euthymic mice (Saxena and Adler, 1979). Likewise, addition of HP lectin to the assay also resulted in enhanced cytotoxicity. Of particular inter-

[1]*On temporary assignment from the National Jewish Hospital and Research Center, Denver, Colorado.*

ISBN 0-12-341350-8

TABLE I. Augmentation of NK Activity by Ab or HP[a]

Effector cells	% Cytotoxicity			
	K562			YAC-1
	Alone	+Ab	+HP	Alone
Expt. 1				
B6 nu/nu	5	35	N.T.[b]	55
B6, >12 wk	1	6	N.T.	11
Expt. 2				
B6 nu/nu	18	N.T.	37	52
B6, >12 wk	1	N.T.	4	7

[a]*Splenic effector cells assayed against YAC-1 or K562 target cells at 100/1 effector/target cell ratio with BALB/c anti-B6 antiserum (1/20 dilution) or HP (50μg) added to assay.*

[b]*Not tested.*

est, binding sites for HP have been previously demonstrated on NK cells (Haller et al, 1978; Mattes and Holden, 1980). The Ab-and HP-mediated augmentation was 1) dependent on the concentration of Ab or lectin added, 2) independent of the presence of mature T cells, B cells or macrophages, and 3) demonstrable against both Fc receptor positive and negative xenogeneic human tumor cells and some allogeneic target cells (data not shown). The ability of Ab or HP to increase cytotoxicity against K562 target cells was directly related to the level of spontaneous NK activity against YAC-1 target cells. Thus, when spleen cells from older, euthymic mice were tested, little increase in cytotoxicity was observed following addition of Ab or HP. In contrast, IF readily augmented NK activity of spleen cells from older mice (Djeu et al, 1979; Herberman et al, 1977). These results suggested that the augmentation observed in this system was not mediated by IF.

Experiments were performed to examine in greater detail whether augmentation of NK activity by Ab and HP was independent of IF. First, supernatants from 4 hr cultures of B6 nude spleen cells with Ab or HP, in the presence of absence of K562 target cells, were tested for anti-viral activity. All supernatants lacked anti-viral activity, indicating the absence of detectable levels of IF. Second, spleen cells from nude mice were pretreated with emetine, an irreversible protein synthesis inhibitor, or actinomycin D, an irreversible inhibitor of RNA synthesis, and activation of cytotoxicity by Ab or HP

TABLE II. Effect of Inhibition of Protein or RNA Synthesis on Augmentation of NK Activity[a]

Treatment	*% Cytotoxicity*		
	Alone	*+Ab*	*+HP*
Medium	*8*	*37*	*30*
Emetine	*10*	*33*	*29*
Actinomycin D	*8*	*35*	*29*

[a]*B6 nu/nu spleen cells assayed against K562 target cells at 100/1 effector/target cell ratio with BALB/c anti-B6 anti-serum (1/60 dilution) or HP (50μg) added to assay. Spleen cells were pretreated for 1 hr prior to testing with medium, 10^5M emetine or 10 μg/ml actinomycin D.*

was measured. It has been previously reported that similar treatment of spleen cells with these drugs inhibited augmentation of NK activity by IF but had no effect on spontaneous NK activity (Holden et al, 1980; Djeu et al, 1980). As seen in Table II, no inhibition of Ab- or HP-mediated activation was found, suggesting that the mechanism of activation was different from that of IF boosting. Finally, in preliminary experiments the addition of rabbit anti-mouse IF (type I) serum to the assay did not decrease the augmentation of cytotoxicity by Ab or HP (data not shown). Anti-IF has been previously demonstrated to inhibit augmentation of NK activity by IF or IF-inducers (Djeu et al, 1979).

Our results clearly indicate that alloantibodies with specificities directed toward splenic effector cells or HP lectin, which binds to NK cells (Haller et al, 1978; Mattes and Holden, 1980), can readily augment NK-like activity. Although the mechanism of this activation is not understood, our results strongly suggest that this activation is not mediated through IF. An interesting speculation is that Ab or HP works directly on NK cells by modulating effector cell surfaces and thereby exposing receptors for target cells or by providing a signal which triggers increased NK cell activity. Future studies using this model system may help to clarify the role that substances other than IF, or processes independent of IF production, have on the activation of NK activity.

REFERENCES

1. Djeu, J.Y., Heinbaugh, J.A., Holden, H.T. and Herberman, R.B., J. Immunol. 122, 175 (1979).
2. Djeu, J.Y., Varesio, L., Holden, H.T., and Herberman, R.B., submitted (1980).
3. Gidlund, M.A., Orn, A., Wigzell, H., Senik, A., and Gresser, I., Nature 273, 759 (1978).
4. Haller, O., Gidlund, M., Hellstrom, U., Hammerstrom, S., and Wigzell, H., Eur. J. Immunol. 8, 765 (1978).
5. Herberman, R.B., Nunn, M.E., Holden, H.T., Staal, S., and Djeu, J.Y., Int. J. Cancer 19, 555 (1977).
6. Holden, H.T., Brunda, M.J., Herberman, R.B., and Djeu, J.Y., in "Proceedings of the Second International Lymphokine Workshop" in press.
7. Mattes, M.J. and Holden, H.T., submitted (1980).
8. Saxena, R.K. and Adler, W.H., J. Immunol. 123, 846 (1979).

ENHANCEMENT OF HUMAN NK ACTIVITY BY INTERFERON. *IN VIVO* AND *IN VITRO* STUDIES

Stefan Einhorn[1]

Radiumhemmet
Karolinska Hospital
Stockholm, Sweden

INTRODUCTION

During the last 15 years several animal studies have revealed that interferon (IF) can have antitumor effects against chemically or virally induced tumors as well as transplanted and spontaneously occurring tumors (Gresser, 1977). Due to these findings and the development of techniques for the production of large amounts of human IF from peripheral blood leukocytes (Strander and Cantell, 1966; Mogensen and Cantell, 1977) clinical trials with human IF have been initiated. These studies were started in Stockholm in 1969 and to date more than 200 tumor patients have been treated with human leukocyte IF at the Karolinska Hospital and other hospitals in Sweden (Strander, 1977). In several of the diseases studied, such as myeloma (Ideström et al., 1979; Mellstedt et al., 1979), Hodgkin's lymphoma (Blomgren et al., 1976) and juvenile laryngeal papilloma (Haglund et al., 1980) antitumor effects have been observed. Also at other clinics throughout the world beneficial effects due to IF therapy have been reported, for instance in non-Hodgkin's lymphoma (Merigan et al., 1978) and acute leukemia (Hill et al., 1979).

Although it is clear that IF preparations have antitumor effects in animals and, at least in some tumors, also in man, the mechanism(s) behind these effects are not understood. The

[1]*This work was supported by grants from the Swedish Cancer Society*

ISBN 0-12-341350-8

antitumor effects could be due to direct inhibition of tumor cell multiplication by IF (Paucker et al., 1962) and/or to indirect effects via, for instance, the immune system. Some support for a possible role of IF influence on host defense systems comes from a study by Gresser et al. (1972) in which tumor cells, resistant to IF *in vitro*, after transplantation to mice were found to be inhibited in their growth by IF preparations *in vivo*.

IF excerts a variety of effects on the immune system (Epstein, 1977) and to further investigate the possible role of IF as a regulator of immunological functions, studies have been initiated to evaluate the effect of *in vivo* administration of human leukocyte IF on different functions of the immune system in man. These studies are performed on tumor patients treated with human leukocyte IF at different hospitals in Stockholm. In this article I will present data on *in vitro* and *in vivo* effects of IF on the natural killer (NK) activity of peripheral lymphocytes.

IF INDUCED ENHANCEMENT OF NK ACTIVITY *IN VITRO*

In agreement with the findings by other workers (Trinchieri and Santoli, 1978), treatment of peripheral lymphocytes with partially purified human leukocyte IF (PIF, kindly provided by Dr K Cantell) *in vitro* significantly enhances their NK activity (Einhorn et al., 1978a). This is seen using a ^{51}Cr-release assay, a microcytotoxicity assay and an assay measuring inhibition of ^{3}H-thymidine uptake into cells. When fibroblast IF purified to homogeneity with regard to molecular weight (kindly provided by Dr E Knight, Jr) is used, an increase in NK activity is also observed (Einhorn, 1980), indicating that the enhancement of NK is due to IF and not to contaminating substances in the IF preparations.

When Chang cells are treated with IF a slight decrease in their sensitivity to NK killing is observed (Einhorn et al., 1979); a finding in agreement with a study by Trinchieri and Santoli (1978) in which they used a variety of tumor cells and fibroblasts. A decrease in sensitivity to killing is also observed with K562 cells pretreated with PIF or homogeneous fibroblast IF, indicating that this effect is also due to IF and not to contaminating substances in the preparations (unpublished observation).

IF INDUCED ENHANCEMENT OF NK ACTIVITY *IN VIVO*

A. First IF Injection

In a preliminary study NK activity was measured in five patients before and at different times after an intramuscular injection of 3 million units of PIF (Einhorn et al., 1978b). This study has now been extended and to date 40 patients with a variety of diseases, mainly myeloma, osteosarcoma and malignant melanoma, have been tested for NK cell activity before and after an injection of IF (Einhorn et al., 1980). Six h after the injection a slight decrease in NK activity is observed (figure 1). NK activity thereafter increases and reaches a peak at around 24 h, after which the activity decreases, although still above preinjection level at 48 h (figure 1). The time kinetics for IF induced increase in NK activity in man show similarities to that observed in mice (Senik et al., 1979).

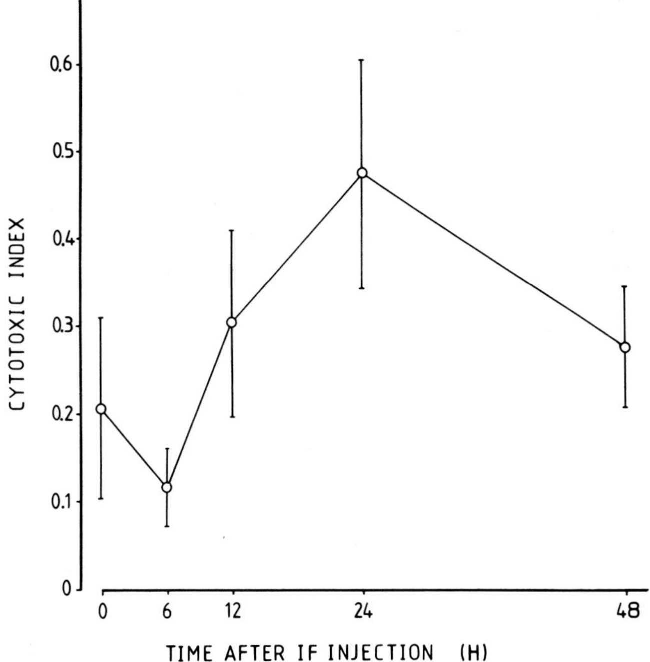

FIGURE 1. Change in NK activity after the first injection of PIF. Mean ± S.E. of five osteosarcoma patients. The data presented in this figure as well as in figures 2- 4 are based on a ^{51}Cr-release assay using Ficoll-Isopaque separated lymphocytes and Chang cells at a lymphocyte:target cell ratio of 50:1.

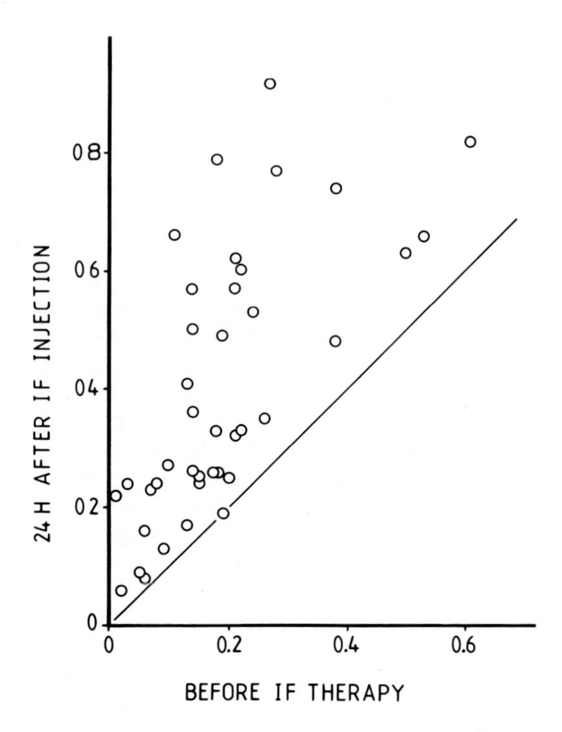

FIGURE 2. NK activity before and 24 h after the first PIF injection. Symbols denote individual patients.

In all 40 patients NK activity was measured before and 24 h after the first PIF injection. With few exceptions the NK activity increased (figure 2). The enhancement of NK activity *in vivo* is not significantly correlated to age, sex, previous therapy, disease or preinjection level of cytotoxicity. The observation that NK activity is increased after an intramuscular injection of PIF has recently been confirmed in patients with non-Hodgkin's lymphoma (Huddlestone et al., 1979).

B. Prolonged IF Therapy

When a second PIF injection is given 24 h after the first, the NK activity remains at an increased level. This is also seen after a third injection of IF and during prolonged IF therapy (3 million units/daily) the NK activity remains elevated for at least 6 months (figure 3). This is not attributable to a general recovery of NK activity due to a decrease in the patients' tumor load, since some of the patients did not respond clinically to IF therapy. The fact that the NK activity of once stimulated lymphocytes can be boosted again

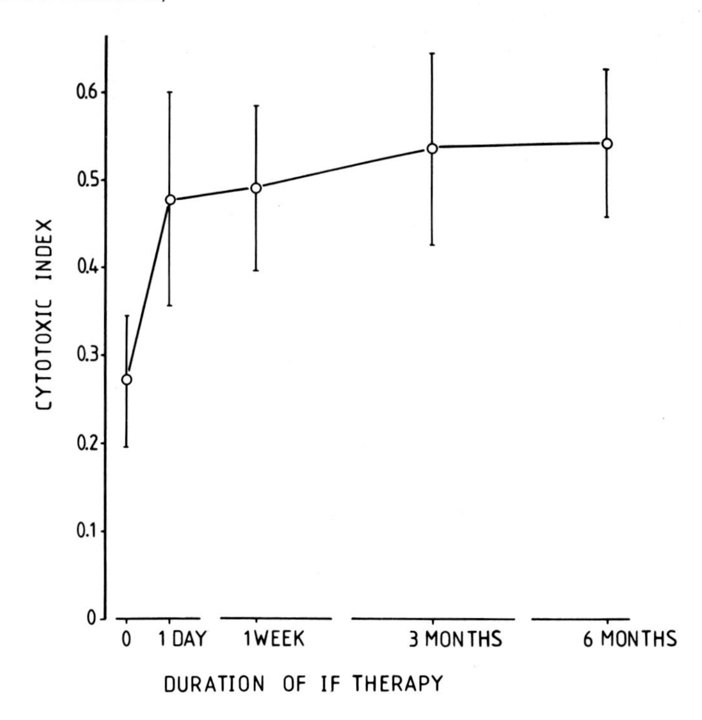

FIGURE 3. Change in NK activity during prolonged IF therapy. Mean ± S.E. of five patients (four myeloma, one malignant melanoma).

by IF has also been observed *in vitro* (unpublished observation) and in mice using tilorone as inducer (A. Örn, personal communication).

The NK cell activity of 15 patients was measured before and after 3 months of IF therapy. With few exceptions the NK activity was elevated during the IF therapy (figure 4).

C. Enhancement of NK Activity In Vitro During IF Therapy

When IF (30 units/ml) is added to the assay *in vitro* an increase in NK activity is observed in lymphocytes drawn prior to IF injection. This increase is correlated ($p < 0.05$) to the extent by which an IF injection enhances NK activity. Six to 48 h after an IF injection the ability of IF to enhance NK activity *in vitro* is decreased and with few exceptions the ability of IF to enhance NK activity *in vitro* remains low during prolonged IF therapy.

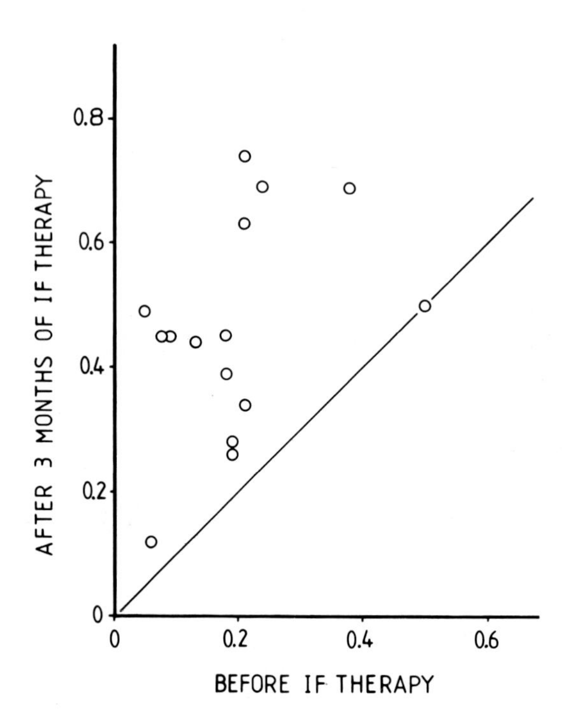

FIGURE 4. NK activity before and three months after initiation of IF therapy. Symbols denote individual patients.

CONCLUSIONS

Exposure of peripheral blood lymphocytes to IF *in vitro* increases their NK activity. The NK activity is also increased after an injection of IF and with daily IF injections this activity can be maintained at an increased level for at least six months. The susceptibility of target cells to NK killing is diminished by preincubation with IF. Although this effect is more pronounced in "normal" fibroblasts as compared to tumor cells (Trinchieri and Santoli, 1978), this finding may imply that the NK sensitivity of tumor cells can be diminished also *in vivo*. This observation may bear special relevance when high doses of exogeneous IF are administered *in vivo*.

Animal studies have suggested that the NK system may play a role in the host's defence against tumors (see chapter on *in vivo* role of NK cells). In man no conclusive proof has yet been presented for a role of the NK system in tumor immunity.

One way of possibly evaluating if the IF induced increase in NK activity is of benefit for the tumor patients is to study if the degree of IF induced enhancement of NK activity is correlated with the response of the tumor to IF therapy.

REFERENCES

1. Blomgren, H., Cantell, K., Johansson, B. Lagergren, C., Ringborg, U., and Strander, H., *Acta Med. Scand. 199*, 527 (1976).
2. Einhorn, S., *J. Clin. Lab. Immunol.* In press (1980).
3. Einhorn, S., Blomgren, H., and Strander, H., *Int. J. Cancer 22*, 405 (1978a).
4. Einhorn, S., Blomgren, H., and Strander, H., *Acta Med. Scand. 204*, 477 (1978b).
5. Einhorn, S., Blomgren, H., and Strander, H., *Cancer Letters 7*, 1 (1979).
6. Einhorn, S., Blomgren, H., and Strander, H., Manuscript in preparation.
7. Epstein, L., *in* "Interferons and their actions" (ed. W.E. Stewart), p. 91. CRC Press, Cleveland, (1977).
8. Gresser, I., *in* "Cancer - a comprehensive treatise" (F. Becker, ed.), *5*, p. 521. Plenum Press, New York, (1977).
9 Gresser, I., Maury, C., and Brouty-Boyé, D., *Nature 239*, 167 (1972).
10. Haglund, S., Lundquist, P-G., Cantell, K., and Strander, H., Manuscript in preparation.
11. Hill, N.O., Loeb, E., Pardue, A.S., Dorn, G.L., Khan, A., and Hill, J.M., *J. Clin. Hemat. Oncol. 9*, 137 (1979).
12. Huddlestone, J.R., Merigan, T.C., and Oldstone, M.B.A., *Nature 282*, 417 (1979).
13. Ideström, K., Cantell, K., Killander, D., Nilsson, K., Strander, H., and Willems, J., *Acta Med. Scand. 205*, 149 (1979).
14. Knight, E., Jr., *Proc. Nat. Acad. Sci. 73*, 520 (1976).
15. Mellstedt, H., Ahre, A., Björkholm, M., Holm, G., Johansson, B., and Strander, H., *Lancet 3*, 245 (1979).
16. Merigan, T.C., Sikora, K., Breeden, J.H., Levy, R., and Rosenberg, S.A., *N. Engl. J. Med. 299*, 1449 (1978).
17. Mogensen, E., and Cantell, K., *J. Pharmac. Ther. C. 1*, 369 (1977).
18. Paucker, K., Cantell, K., and Henle, W., *Virology 17*, 324 (1962).
19. Senik, A., Gresser, I., Maury, C., Gidlund, M., Örn, A., and Wiqzell, H., *Cell. Immunol. 44*, 186 (1979).

20. Strander, H., *Blut 35*, 277 (1977).
21. Strander, H., and Cantell, K., *Ann. Med. Exp. Fenn. 44*, 265 (1966).
22. Trinchieri, G., and Santoli, D., *J. Exp. Med. 147*, 1314 (1978).

REGULATORY FACTORS IN HUMAN NATURAL AND ANTIBODY-DEPENDENT CELL-MEDIATED CYTOTOXICITY[1]

Yukio Koide
Mitsuo Takasugi

Department of Surgery
UCLA School of Medicine
Los Angeles, California

I. HISTORICAL BACKGROUND

When lymphocytes from most individuals are tested against cultured target cells, a strong reactivity is observed which is now known as natural cell-mediated cytotoxicity (NCMC) (1-3). It has been suggested that NCMC has a surveillance or policing role against the development of tumors in the intact host. Support for this proposal is derived from studies of congenital athymic (nude) mice which lack T-cell immunity but nevertheless show high NCMC activity (4). Despite the deficiency, no increase in the incidence of spontaneous cancers is observed in these mice. They are also no more susceptible to the induction of tumors by chemical carcinogens than normal litter mates (5,6). More direct evidence for a protective role for NCMC was reported by Haller *et al.* who observed a correlation between resistance to tumor growth and NCMC (7). Thus, from the perspective of preventing the development of cancer, NCMC is of special interest to tumor immunologists.

Many investigators have characterized the effector cells responsible for human NCMC. The cell which is primarily responsible for NCMC is now known as the NK cell. In earlier studies, we described these cells as "N cells" and observed

[1]*This work was supported in part by contracts N01-CB 74133 from the Tumor Immunology Section and N01-CP43211 from the Biological Carcinogenesis Branch, Division of Cancer Cause and Prevention, National Cancer Institute.*

ISBN 0-12-341350-8

that they did not bear the conventional T-cell markers shown by high affinity rosetting with sheep red blood cells nor the B-cell markers of membrane-associated immunoglobulin and C'_3 receptors. They did possess receptors for the Fc portion of IgG immunoglobulins (8-10). It is still unclear if NK cells are derived from lymphoid, monocyte or other cell precursors. Other than their derivation from bone marrow progenitor cells, clarification of the developmental lineage is needed. For example, defects at the stem cell level, as in severe combined immunodeficiency, are accompanied by a loss of NCMC activity. On the other hand, patients with X-linked agammaglobulinemia, common variable immunodeficiency, and thymic aplasia have substantial levels of NCMC activity (11).

Although the nature of the effector cells is still clouded, understanding of the regulation of NCMC is advancing rapidly. Trinchieri *et al.* (12) first described the augmentation of NCMC by interferon (IF). This observation was supported by evidence in mice and rats that IF and IF inducers such as viruses, poly I:C, tilorone, and statolon markedly enhanced murine NCMC (13). We have also described an N-cell activating factor (NAF) which is produced by lymphocytes in response to stimulation by lymphoblastoid cell lines (14).

Suppression of NCMC has also been described employing spleen cells from young or experimentally-treated mice exhibiting low NCMC activity (15). In humans, we have observed a factor produced by lymphocytes cultured alone which suppresses NCMC (N-cell inhibitory factor or NIF). The supernatants containing NAF appear to include NIF as well. The levels of NAF and NIF seem to be especially important in the precise regulation of NCMC activity.

Most early studies in the culturing of lymphocytes were designed to achieve *in vitro* sensitization of lymphocytes to tumor-associated or histocompatibility antigens. In many of these studies, the criterion for successful sensitization was an increase in cytotoxic activity with little regard for the specificity. When NCMC was finally identified, it became clearer that most of this increased cytotoxicity was related to the NCMC phenomenon. In our early studies of the effector cell for NCMC, we observed that lymphocyte suspensions incubated at 37° C for one week maintained NCMC activity, whereas cells incubated at ambient temperature for a week lost most of their cytotoxic activity (8). We also observed that lymphocytes harvested from mixed lymphocyte culture (MLC) after the generation of specifically cytotoxic lymphocytes exhibited increased antibody-dependent cell-mediated cytotoxicity (ADCC) and NCMC-like reactions against target cells other than the stimulating cells (16). Zielske and Golub (17) and Ortaldo *et al.* (18) attributed the increased activity to the presence of fetal calf serum (FCS) in the culture medium. Moreover, Ortaldo *et al.* reported that effector cells depleted of Fc receptor-positive cells can also give rise to NCMC-like activity with reappearance of Fc receptors during culture. In our studies, enhanced NCMC during coculture was related more to allogeneic stimulation than to FCS since the effect was observed in media with human sera.

We also attempted to induce cytotoxic T lymphocytes against lymphoblastoid cell lines (LCL) through one-way MLC (19). In the induction of specifically cytotoxic lymphocytes against LCL through MLC, the specificity was difficult to demonstrate because of the presence of enhanced NCMC by the effector cells. Strong NCMC detected in the tests presented a high background with little selectivity. Therefore, application of the interaction and regression analyses to the results, together with competition studies, were necessary to detect specificity. Furthermore, the lymphocytes incubated with LCL showed a greater enhancement of cytotoxicity than when cultured alone, in agreement with more recent observations by Saksela *et al.* (19). We realized that a closer examination of the MLC system might provide some information about augmentation and suppression in the regulation of NCMC.

II. REGULATORY FACTORS IN SUPERNATANTS OF LYMPHOCYTE CULTURE

A. N-Cell Activating Factor (NAF)

1. Production and Testing of NAF. The level of human NCMC is augmented by a soluble mediator, NAF, produced by coculturing lymphocytes with mitomycin C treated Raji cells (14). NAF was assessed by incubating fresh lymphocytes in the cell-free supernatant containing the factor 37°C for 2 hours. The cells were washed and then tested for NCMC. The kinetics of NAF production were investigated by maintaining a lymphocyte-Raji coculture for 7 days with daily exchange of medium. The supernatants harvested daily were frozen immediately and tested simultaneously after the last harvest. We observed that NAF was detectable by the second day of culture, reaching peak activity on day 5. However, more recent results indicate that NAF is produced early in culture. This apparent discrepancy can be explained by the release of N-cell inhibitory factor (see Section IIIB) which is also produced during early culture.

The influence of HLA-A and -B loci antigens on NAF production was examined by testing four different LCL as stimulators and target cells. As shown in Table I, there is no significant influence of HLA-A and -B loci antigens since HSB-2 and SB, a

T- and a B-cell line derived from the same individual and carrying the same A and B loci antigens, produced supernatants with low and high NAF activity respectively. Daudi, with no A and B loci antigens, also stimulated the production of NAF. Moreover, NAF is unrelated to target specificities, i.e., NAF

TABLE I. HLA Relationships in Enhancement of NCMC by NAF

Effector cells	NAF producer	NAF stimulator		Percent cytotoxicity HSB-2	SB	CEM[a]
1. Aw24, Aw33, B5 B12	A11, A28, B12, Bw22	A1, A2, B12, B17	(HSB-2)	30	22	45
		A1, A2, B12, B17	(SB)	46	43	59
2. A1, Aw24 Bw37[c]	A2, Aw26, B18, B27[d]	A1, A2,	(HSB-2)			16
		A1, A2, B12, B17	(SB)			24
		A3, A10, B18, B17	(Raji)			29
		-------- --------	(Daudi)			21

Responder	Stimulator	Stimulation index[b]
1. Aw24, A233, B5, B12	$HSB\text{-}2_m$	0.6
	SB_m	13.6
	$Raji_m$	3.8

[a]CEM carries the HLA antigens A1, Aw30, B8, Bw40

[b]$\text{Stimulation index} = \frac{\text{cpm MLC}}{\text{cpm responder + cpm stimulator}}$

[c]172193

[d]172247

induced by Raji enhances NCMC equally against Raji and other target cells. Table I also shows that there was no restriction for the sharing of HLA-A and -B loci antigens between NAF producers and effector cells. NAF producer 172193 and effector 172247 shared no A and B loci antigens, yet enhancement of cytotoxicity by NAF was clearly seen.

B-cell lines are generally better inducers of NAF than are T-cell lines or K562. Among B-cell lines, Raji was the strongest inducer of NAF as observed also by Saksela *et al.* (20). Several studies have shown that B but not T lymphocytes stimulate MLC reactions (21), implying that NAF production may be dependent upon the MLC response and antigens controlled by the HLA-D locus. Although B-cell lines (Raji and SB) were usually better stimulators in MLC (Table I), NAF production did not always correlate with MLC reactivity. Raji, the strongest inducer of NAF, was still relatively weak in stimulating MLC. That human LCL in the coculture did not produce NAF was concluded from the absence of activity in supernatants from the culture of LCL. Also, several reagents are known to stimulate NAF and interferon production by lymphocytes. Moreover, treatment of lymphocytes with inhibitors of protein synthesis decreased NAF and interferon production while treatment of the LCL had little effect.

Agreement has not been reached on the population of cells producing NAF or interferon. In our studies, several cell separation techniques were employed to investigate the subset of lymphocytes responsible for synthesis and release of NAF. Passage of isolated lymphocytes through nylon wool or degalan bead columns coated with IgG anti-IgG complexes did not remove the major subset of lymphocytes that produced most of the factor. This was supported by indications that E- but not EAC-rosette forming cells produced the NAF. Thus it appears that T-cells are required, but further studies are needed to clarify whether a single, several or all subsets are involved in NAF production.

Because FCS has been reported to enhance cytotoxic activity during culture, we examined NAF activity in the supernatant from MLC between lymphocytes and LCL in medium supplemented with FCS or human serum. NAF activity was detected in media with human serum indicating the basic importance of allogeneic stimulation.

2. The Effect of NAF on ADCC. The similarity between NCMC and ADCC has been described by several investigators (22-25). Recent studies have suggested that several classes of cells are involved in both reactions. Still, it appears that the major effector subclass mediating NCMC and ADCC is either the same cell or very similar for most properties. Therefore, it was natural to study whether NAF enhances ADCC. As seen in Table II, effector cells treated with NAF showed enhanced ADCC as well as NCMC, further supporting the strong similarity between NK and K cells.

3. Chemical and Physical Properties. In order to determine the chemical nature of NAF, the supernatant containing the factor was treated with different enzymes (Table III). NAF activity was unaffected by DNase, RNase, and neuraminidase but was destroyed by trypsin. Several investigators, however, have reported that trypsin treatment of the effector cells decreased NCMC activity (9,24,26). To avoid the direct effect of trypsin on effector cells, the reactivity of trypsin on NAF was blocked with soybean trypsin inhibitor. Trypsin treatment of NAF resulted in a loss of enhancing activity. NAF was also tested for heat sensitivity. Aliquots of the NAF were heated at 40°, 60°, and 80° C for 1 hour and tested for their ability

TABLE II. The Effect of NAF and NIF in NCMC and ADCC

A. NAF

			Target system		
Effector cell	*NAF producer*	*NAF stimulator*	*CEM*	*NC37*	*ALS-treated lymphocytes*
163558	------	-----	*41*	*48*	*23*
	162420	*Raji*$_m$	*60*	*70*	*41*
163784	------	-----	*53*	*63*	*16*
	161373	*Raji*$_m$	*73*	*82*	*31*

B. NIF

Effector cell	*Factor*	*CEM*	*8402*	*ALS-treated lymphocytes*
196736	----------	*82*	*70*	*67*
	Pooled NIF	*45*	*58*	*25*

to augment NCMC against CEM target cells (Table IV). Noticeable losses of enhancing activity were observed at 60°C and a complete loss at 80°C. The supernatant containing NAF was then dialyzed against phosphate buffered saline (PBS) for 48 hours at 4°C and tested for its effect in NCMC. No loss of enhancing activity was observed (Table IV). Thus, NAF is a heat-sensitive, nondialyzable protein with a molecular weight greater than 12,000.

The supernatant containing NAF was concentrated to 1/5 its original volume by Amicon model 52 ultrafiltration cell using a PM-10 Diaflomembrane and applied to a Sephadex G-100 column. Eluates collected from the column were mixed immediately with

TABLE III. Effect of Enzyme Treatment

Effector cell no.	*Factor from*	*Enzyme treatment*	*Percent cytotoxicity*	
			CEM	*NC37*
165691	*Fresh medium*	*-----*	*17*	*ND*[g]
	164094, Raji$_m$	*-----*	*35*	*ND*
		DNase (0.1 mg/ml)[a]	*35*	*ND*
		RNase (0.1 mg/ml)[b]	*39*	*ND*
166322	*Fresh medium*	*-------------*	*48*	*46*
	164094, Raji$_m$	*-------------*	*67*	*68*
		Neuraminidase (20 u/ml)[c]	*65*	*63*
		Neuraminidase (40 u/ml)[d]	*67*	*66*
167825	*Fresh medium*	*-----*	*32*	*42*
	165917, Raji$_m$	*-----*	*57*	*74*
	Fresh medium	*Trypsin (250 ug/ml)*[e]	*32*	*45*
	165917, Raji$_m$	*Trypsin (250 ug/ml)*[f]	*33*	*52*

[a,b]*Factors were treated with DNase or RNase at 37°C for 1h*
[c,d]*Factors were treated with neuraminidase at 37°C for 1h*
[e,f]*Factors were treated with trypsin at 37°C for 2h and the trypsin reaction was stopped by adding 500 ug/ml soybean trypsin inhibitor.*
[g]*Not done*

TABLE IV. Differential Effects on Regulatory Factors

A. Temperature sensitivity

Temperature treatment of factor	*Percent cytotoxicity*	
	NAF activity against CEM	*NIF activity against CEM*
37° C	35	17
60° C	25	0
80° C	11	34
Original effector cell	17	61

B. Effect of Dialysis

Treatment of factor	*Percent cytotoxicity*	
	NAF activity against NC37	*NIF activity against NC37*
Factor (untreated)	52	4
Factor (dialyzed)	51	22
Original effector cell	25	22

an equal volume of fresh medium to prevent denaturation of the factor. Effector cells were incubated in each fraction and tested against target CEM for their effect on NCMC. NAF activity was observed in a single symmetrical peak eluted immediately following bovine serum albumin (BSA). Thus NAF has a molecular weight of less than 67,000 daltons.

4. Relation of NAF to Interferon (IF). The production of IF in response to tumor monolayer cell lines and its ability to augment NCMC were described by Trinchieri *et al.* (27). Support for such a role by IF in the regulation of NCMC was soon forthcoming. Injection of IF inducers, as well as IF itself, was found to increase NCMC activity in mice (28). This enhancement of NCMC activity by IF inducers could be inhibited by anti-IF antibody (13). Because of the similarity in the effect on NCMC by IF and NAF, we tested supernatants containing NAF for the presence of IF. Interferon was assessed as follows: G11 cells in the wells of the microtest plate (Falcon 3034, Oxnard, Calif.) were incubated with the supernatant for 1 day and then challenged with 5 ul vesicular stomatitis virus (VSV) at 1×10^7 PFU/ml. After an additional day of incubation, the test was terminated and remaining cells were counted by Quantimet image analysis (Imanco, Cambridge, England). The NAF preparation possessed IF activity and protected G11 cells from destruction by VSV. Heating of the supernatant for 1 hour at 60° C destroyed IF as well as NAF activity. When the same supernatants were tested for NAF and IF, a good correlation was observed, indicating that IF plays a major part in the enhancement of NCMC by NAF. Trinchieri *et al.* had reported that the molecular weight of IF was approximately 25,000 daltons (12). This is within our approximations for NAF. However, they failed to detect the boosting of ADCC by IF, whereas our NAF and the IF reported by Herberman *et al.* (29) enhance ADCC activity. This discrepancy is probably explained by the different ADCC systems used.

B. N-Cell Inhibitory Factor (NIF)

1. Production of NIF. Supernatants from MLC contain a number of lymphokines as well as NAF. Most of these lymphokines do not affect NCMC and ADCC activity and are distinguishable from NAF by various procedures. Recently, we observed another factor, N-cell inhibitory factor (NIF), which suppresses NCMC and ADCC and interferes with the detection of NAF activity. Conversely, the presence of NAF often obscures the detection of NIF. NIF is most readily detected in supernatants of lymphocytes cultured by themselves since interference by the induction of NAF is then reduced.

Table V shows the kinetics of NIF production. NIF appeared

TABLE V. Production of NIF

	Percent cytotoxicity against CEM by effector cells treated with supernatant collected on day:				
Original effector cell	*2*	*3*	*4*	*5*	*6*
75	*5*	*29*	*18*	*36*	*51*

early and by day 2 was present at near maximum levels. When the culture was continued longer than 4 days, activity declined because of decay of NIF or the accumulation of other factors which increased NCMC activity. NIF activity was again detectable after the supernatants were heated. Instability of the factor seems less likely to explain the decline in activity during culture since NIF appears to be resistant to heating. Incubating NIF at 60° C for 1 hour, a process which destroys NAF, did not impair NIF activity and even increased its effect, suggesting the presence of NAF in the supernatant (Table IV). At higher temperatures, NIF activity was partially destroyed.

NIF preparations were also dialyzed for 48 hours against 100 ml PBS (Table IV) and tested for inhibition of NCMC. In contrast to NAF, NIF was lost during dialysis. The presence of two factors with opposing effects introduces some problems in the study since the two effects need to be differentiated, but it provides a sensitive regulatory mechanism for the control of NCMC.

2. Effect of NIF on ADCC. NIF suppresses ADCC (Table II) as well as NCMC, further supporting the concept of identical effector cells for both reactions. Several preparations of NIF were pooled and heated at 60° C to exclude NAF activity. Inhibition of ADCC was observed in two target systems, anti-lymphocyte serum (ALS) treated lymphocytes and ALS-treated CEM. The ALS-treated lymphocyte target exhibited more exclusively ADCC since NCMC is rarely detected against lymphocyte target cells.

In conclusion, regulatory factors have been demonstrated in a variety of immunological phenomena, including antibody production and cellular immunity. NCMC and ADCC were also shown to be regulated by such controls. NAF and NIF produced by lymphocytes in culture possessed the opposing effects of enhancing and inhibiting NCMC and ADCC. IF, which increases NCMC and ADCC, is the basic component in the effect by NAF.

Both regulatory factors influence the activity of the effector cells rather than the specificity of NCMC (they are nonselective). Neither the augmenting capacity of NAF nor the inhibitory ability of NIF were related to the sensitivity of target cells. Although NAF is obtained from the supernatants of MLC, the mechanism of enhancement by NAF needs further investigation to examine whether it differs significantly from augmentation by merely incubating effector cells with allogeneic cells (16,19). Such treatments also induce or increase NCMC-like activity in effector suspensions even when NK cells are depleted initially. Thus, it appears that N(NK) cells undergo a developmental process from precursors.

Suppressor cells in murine NCMC have also been described recently (15,16). Spleen cells from young mice or mice treated with irradiation or hydrocortisone are capable of inhibiting NCMC. It is still unclear whether our NIF is a product of such suppressor cells or a product of other cells. Nevertheless, NCMC is not only specific but also strictly regulated by at least two factors with opposing effects which provide sensitive control over the reactions.

REFERENCES

1. Oldham, R. K., Djeu, J. Y., Cannon, G. B., Siwarski, D., and Herberman, R. B., *J. Natl. Cancer Inst. 55,* 1305 (1975).
2. Takasugi, M., Mickey, M. R., and Terasaki, P. I., *Cancer Res. 33,* 2898 (1973).
3. Takasugi, M., Mickey, M. R., and Terasaki, P. I., *J. Natl. Cancer Inst. 53,* 1527 (1974).
4. Herberman, R. B., Nunn, M. E., and Lavrin, D. H., *Int. J. Cancer 16,* 216 (1975).
5. Stutman, O., *Science 183,* 534 (1974).
6. Rygaard, J., and Poulsen, C. O., *Transpl. Rev. 28,* 43 (1976).
7. Haller, O., Hanson, M., Kiessling, R., and Wigzell, H., *Nature 270,* 609 (1977).
8. Kiuchi, M., and Takasugi, M., *J. Natl. Cancer Inst. 56,* 575 (1976).
9. Peter, H. H., Pavie-Fischer, J., Fridman, W. H., Aubert, C., Cesarini, J. P., Roubin, R., and Kourilski, F., *J. Immunol. 115,* 539 (1975).
10. Jondal, M., and Pross, H., *Int. J. Cancer 15,* 596 (1975).
11. Koren, H. S., Amos, D. B., and Buckley, R. H., *J. Immunol. 120,* 796 (1978).
12. Trinchieri, G., and Santoli, D., *J. Exp. Med. 147,* 1314 (1978).
13. Gidlund, M., Orn, A., Wigzell, H., Senik, A., and Gresser, I., *Nature 273,* 759 (1978).
14. Koide, Y., and Takasugi, M., *J. Immunol. 121,* 872 (1978).
15. Hochman, P. S., and Cudkowicz, G., *J. Immunol. 123,* 968 (1979).
16. Takasugi, M., Akira, D., and Mickey, M. R., in "Histocompatibility Testing" (F. Kissmeyer-Nielsen, ed.) p. 827. Munksgaard, Copenhagen, (1975).
17. Zielski, J. V., and Golub, S. H., *Cancer Res. 36,* 3842 (1976).

18. Ortaldo, J. R., Bonnard, G. D., and Herberman, R. B., *J. Immunol. 119,* 1351 (1977).
19. Koide, Y., and Takasugi, M., *J. Immunol. 117,* 1197 (1976).
20. Saksela, E., Timonen, T., Ranki, A., and Hayry, P., *Immunol. Rev. 44,* 71 (1979).
21. Opelz, G., Kiuchi, M., and Takasugi, M., *J. Immunogenetics 2,* 1 (1975).
22. Takasugi, M., Kiuchi, M., and Opelz, G., *Transpl. Proc. 9,* 789 (1977).
23. Koide, Y., and Takasugi, M., *J. Natl. Cancer Inst. 59,* 1099 (1977).
24. Kay, H. D., Bonnard, G. D., West, W. H., and Herberman, R. B., *J. Immunol. 118,* 2058 (1977).
25. Ortiz de Landazuri, M., Silva, A., Alvarez, J., and Herberman, R. B., *J. Immunol. 123,* 252 (1979).
26. Koide, Y., and Takasugi, M., *J. Natl. Cancer Inst. 59,* 1099 (1977).
27. Trinchieri, G., Santoli, D., and Koprowski, H., *J. Immunol. 120,* 1849 (1978).
28. Djeu, J., Heinbaugh, J., Holden, H. T., and Herberman, R. B., *J. Immunol. 122,* 175 (1979).
29. Herberman, R. B., Ortaldo, J. R., and Bonnard, G. D., *Nature 277,* 221 (1979).
30. Savory, C. A., and Lotsova, E., *J. Immunol. 120,* 239 (1978).

SPONTANEOUS CELL-MEDIATED CYTOTOXICITY (SCMC) AND SHORT-TERM MIXED LEUKOCYTE CULTURE (MLC):ROLE OF SOLUBLE FACTORS AND OF CELLULAR INTERACTIONS[1]

Wolfgang Leibold

Institute of Pathology, Veterinary School
Hannover, West-Germany

Rudolf Eife

Department of Pediatrics, University of München
München, West-Germany

Rainer Zawatzky
Holger Kirchner

Institute of Virus Research, German Cancer Research Center
Heidelberg, West-Germany

Hans H. Peter

Department of Clinical Immunological, Medical School
Hannover, West-Germany

I. INTRODUCTION

The spontaneous cell-mediated cytotoxicity (SCMC) has turned out to represent an autonomous part of the immune system with possible major implications in the control of differentiating and aberrant cells (for review see Herberman et al., 1979a;

[1] *Supported by the Deutsche Forschungsgemeinschaft: SFB 54 - C5, F2; SFB 37 - B7; Ki 165/3; Pe 151/6*

ISBN 0-12-341350-8

Kiessling and Haller, 1978; Kiessling and Wigzell, 1979; Leibold and Peter, 1978; Pross and Baines, 1977). In vivo it sensitively reacts to various influences, particularly to exogenous administration of virus, bacteria or cells (Svet-Moldavsky et al., 1973; Herberman et al., 1977), resulting in considerable alteration of the measurable SCMC capacity. Also in vitro different treatments of the effector cells might intensely change their cytotoxic behaviour. The isolation procedure might result in an enrichment of SCMC-effector cells (de Vries et al., 1975; Mukherji et al., 1975; Peter et al., 1976 b) or in a dissociation of effector from suppressor cells (Parkman and Rosen, 1976). In either case Saksela et al. (1977) considered a general activation of effector cells during the handling procedure, possibly by direct triggering of the lymphoid effector cells but more likely by activation of macrophages to produce SCMC augmenting factors. Indeed, various factors generated either by T-cells during spontaneous rosetting with sheep red blood cells (Mackler et al., 1977) or by rosette formation with C3-receptor bearing cells (O'Neill et al., 1975) or by culturing lymphnode cells (Brooks et al., 1976) were shown to considerably influence the outcome of SCMC reactions. Similar factors, produced by cocultivation of lymphoid cells with tumor cells or lymphoblastoid cell lines (LCL), have been characterized as lymphotoxin-like factor(s) (Peter et al., 1976 a) or as interferon (Trinchieri et al., 1977, 1978 a). Particularly interferon has meanwhile been reported to alter SCMC in vitro (Djeu et al., 1979a; Droller et al., 1979; Einhorn et al., 1978; Gidlund et al., 1978; Herberman et al., 1979b; Heron et al., 1979; Trinchieri et al., 1978b; Zarling et al., 1979). Production of such factors might be one reason for the discordant results concerning the loss, maintenance or increase of SCMC-activity during cultivation of effector cell populations (Kiuchi and Takasugi,1976; Leibold et al., 1978; Shellam, 1977).

In view of these influences on the variability of the SCMC-system and in order to properly evaluate SCMC-effects, the monitoring assay plus the factors and mechanisms involved become of essential importance. As the above factors are produced within 24 hours (h) (Trinchieri and Santoli, 1978) and we recently observed that considerable changes of SCMC pattern occur by cultivating effector cells for 5 and 6 days or treating them as responder population in 5 and 6 day mixed leukocyte culture (MLC) reactions (Leibold et al., 1978, 1979) we were prompted to study the effect on SCMC of supernates and of cells generated in 1 day-MLC reactions. Here we would like to present data obtained in human autologous and allogeneic short-term MLC combinations with particular emphasis on the role of interferon (IF) and lymphotoxin (LT) produced in these reactions.

II. MATERIALS AND METHODS

A. *Cell Lines, Media and Culture Conditions*

A panel of permanent human suspension cell lines was employed as stimulator or target cells. The panel comprised the T-cell lines CEM (Foley et al., 1965) and JM (Schneider et al., 1977), the erythroid leukemia cell line K 562 (Lozzio and Lozzio, 1975; Andersson et al., 1979) and the B-cell lines Kaplan (Schaadt et al., 1979), PDe-B-1 (Leibold et al., 1980) and AL, BL, CL, DL, GL, which were established in our laboratory from lymphocytes of the healthy donors A, B, C,D and G with the aid of transforming Epstein-Barr virus according to Menezes et al. (1975). The cell lines were propagated in vitro RPMI-1640 medium, supplemented with 18 mM sodium bicarbonate, 15 mM Hepes-buffer, 2 mM L-glutamine and 10 % heated (1h 56°C) fetal bovine serum. All stimulation and cytotoxic tests as well as preparations of supernates were exclusively performed in medium designated R-10H, which corresponded to the above medium but contained 10 % heated (1h 56°C) human AB^{+}-serum instead of fetal bovine serum and was further supplemented with 100 IU penicillin plus 100 µg streptomycin per ml. RD_{M}-10H. methionine-deficient R-10H medium, was exclusively used for labelling target cells with ^{75}Se (cf.II.G.). Washing procedures and dilutions were carried out in either R-10H or R-0 (R-10H without any serum content). All media were obtained from Seromed, München, West-Germany. Cultivation was consistently performed in 7 % CO_2 in air at 37° C.

B. *Preparation of Lymphoid Cells*

Lymphoid cells were separated from the peripheral blood of healthy human male donors (21 - 38 years of age) as recently described (Kalden et al., 1977). Briefly, fresh blood containing 10 U/ml of preservative free heparin was diluted with an equal volume of R-0 and separated on a discontinuous Ficoll-Isopaque gradient of 1.075 g/ml density for 20 min at 750 g at ambient temperature. The interphase cells were subsequently washed three times, at 500, 250 and 60 g, and designated "F"-preparation (F stands for Ficoll) of peripheral blood lymphoid cells (PBL). If not otherwise stated, this preparation was used throughout the experiments presented in this article. A further treatment at 37° C for 45 min with carbonyl iron (ferrum) and magnetism plus additional 60 min of incubation in Falcon tissue culture flasks removed most of the readily phagozytising and adhering cells. The resulting "FFF"-preparation (stands for Ficoll, Ferrum and Falcon) of PBL usually contained less than 2 % latex-phagozytising cells.

C. *Mixed Leukocyte Cultures (MLC)*

The procedure of Svedmyr et al. (1975) was used. As stimulator cells, served either F-preparations of PBL (S) or cell lines (L) after 30 min treatment at 37° C with 25 μg (S_m) or 100 μg (L_m) mitomycin C per ml R-0, respectively. Afterwards care was taken to remove the excess of mitomycin C by washing the cells 3 times in R-0, with an additional incubation for 10 min at 37° C after the second wash in order to avoid mitomycin C-effects in subsequent tests of the supernate, particularly in the lymphotoxin assay (cf. II.F.). As a standard procedure usually F-preparations of PBL as responder cells (R) were mixed with S_m or L_m in ratios of 1:1 or 5:1, respectively, and cultured for 22 - 38 h (1 d MLC) or 140 - 148 h (6 d MLC). Proliferation assays were carried out in round-bottom microtiter plates with quadruplicates of $5 \cdot 10^4$ R and $5 \cdot 10^4$ S_m or $1 \cdot 10^4$ L_m in a total volume of 175 μl/well. Each well was pulsed with 0.5 μCi of tritated thymidin (^{3}H-TdR) in 25 μl R-0 for the last 18 h of the assay time in order to measure DNA-synthesis as one parameter of cell proliferation.

D. *In Vitro Generation of Effector Cells and Supernates*

F-preparations of PBL were cultured either alone ($1 \cdot 10^6$/ml) or in autologous and allogeneic MLC-combinations ($5 \cdot 10^5$ R plus $5 \cdot 10^5$ S_m or $1 \cdot 10^5$ L_m/ml) in R-10H for 1 day at 37° C. Subsequently the cells were separated from the supernate by centrifugation (10 min at 200 g). While the cells were washed twice in R-10H and adjusted to serve as cytotoxic effector cells (cf.II.G.) the supernate was either passed through a sterile 0.45 μm filter or was respun at 1000 g to be free of any residual cells. Cell free supernates were stored at 4°C for immediate use in SCMC-assays or were frozen in sterile aliquots below -70°C until determination of their IF or LT content could be carried out.

E. *Interferon (IF) Assay*

Supernates were tested for their IF content by means of their ability to interfer with the replication of vesiculostomatitis virus (VSV, strain Indiana) in the monolayer cell line (Rita) of monkey kidney cells as described by Kirchner et al. (1979) and Peter et al. (1980). The results of this virus yield reduction assay are expressed either as the number of residual virus plaques or as units (U) of interferon.

F. Lymphotoxin (LT) Assay

LT-production was measured according to the methods published previously (Eife et al., 1974; 1979). The LT-activity was calculated as the percentage inhibition of target cell (HeLa)-DNA-synthesis by cell-free culture medium from stimulated, as compared to that from unstimulated lymphocytes:

$$\left(1 - \frac{\text{cpm (targets + experimental medium)}}{\text{cpm (targets + control medium)}}\right) \times 100$$

To determine the actual LT-content (in units/ml) for each sample, the percentage inhibition was compared with the corresponding value of a two-fold serially diluted standard LT-preparation. As standard LT served pooled crude supernates from mitogen activated cultures of lymphocytes from 150 normal donors, containing 500 LT-units per ml. One unit of LT was defined as the inhibitory activity present in 1 ml of cell-free supernate reducing the DNA-synthesis in target cells by 50 % in an 48 h assay.

G. Spontaneous Cell-Mediated Cytotoxicity (SCMC) Assay

Throughout these studies we employed the recently developed ^{75}Se-assay (Leibold and Bridge, 1979). As targets served cell lines (cf.II.A.) which had been labelled with 4 μCi ^{75}Se-selenomethionine (^{75}Se) per ml of RD_M-10H (cf.II.A.) for 22 h resulting in an uptake of 2 - 20 cpm per cell and a spontaneous isotope release of 0.8 - 1.8 % of the input per hour of subsequent cultivation. F- and FFF-preparations of PBL or cells generated in 1 d MLC (MLC-effectors, cf.II.D.) were used as effector cells. All tests were performed for 20 - 22 h in quadruplicates of $1 \cdot 10^3$ target cells (T) and different amounts ($8 \cdot 10^3$ - $2 \cdot 10^5$) of effector cells (E) in a total volume of 160 μl per U-shaped well in microtiter plates. When cell free supernates (cf.II.D.) were tested for their effect on SCMC, 25 μl uf supernate was added to 25 μl of effector cell suspension, and incubated at 37° C in humid atmosphere for 3 h before the targets were added and the volume was topped up with R-10H to 160 μl giving a 1:6.4 dilution of the supernate which remained in the assay. The assay was stopped by careful resuspension and subsequent pelleting of the cells before an aliquot of the cell free supernate of each well was harvested for measurement of the ^{75}Se-release in a γ-counter.

In order to evaluate the cytotoxic effect we considered three parameters. The *input*: all calculations were based exclusively on the entire input of radioactivity provided by the intact targets. The *OR:* during the time after the last wash of the targets and the actual start of the SCMC assay by placing the microtiter plates into the incubator, usually some radioactivity was spontaneously released into the medium, designated as "zero release" (OR). It was determined by pelleting the residual target cell suspension and harvesting 4 - 6 aliquots of the cell free supernate at the time of the actual start of the cytotoxic test. The *BR:* the spontaneous isotope release of the $1 \cdot 10^3$ targets incubated in 160 µl R-10H alone or in 160 µl R-10H containing 25 µl of relevant supernate was defined as "baseline release" (BR). We calculated the BR which took place during the actual assay time (t) by correcting for the OR:

$$(1)\quad \%\ BR_t = \frac{\text{cpm BR} - \text{cpm OR}}{\text{cpm input} - \text{cpm OR}} \times 100;$$

the "standardized specific release" (SSR) which was achieved during the actual assay time (t):

$$(2)\quad \%\ SSR_t = \frac{\text{cpm test} - \text{cpm BR}}{\text{cpm input} - \text{cpm OR}} \times 100.$$

However, the % SSR_t was only calculated when the replicates of the test release values were significantly different from that of the BR values (2 p usually less than 0.01 in a bilateral Student's t-test). Although providing relatively low figures, this method of calculation permitted reliable evaluation of significant cytotoxic activities of effector cells and comparisons of different tests, irrespective of the BR. Compared to the control effector cells the *alteration* of cytotoxicity due to the presence of supernate or to MLC-effectors in the assay was calculated as

$$(3)\quad \%\ \text{alteration} = \left(\frac{\%\text{SSR (test + supernate)}}{\%\text{SSR (test - supernate)}} - 1 \right) \times 100$$

III. RESULTS

A. *Discordance between SCMC-Effects and IF-Production in Short Term MLC*

In order to evaluate the role of IF produced during the calculation of effector and target cells in a 1 day SCMC-assay, we compared the spontaneous cytotoxic effect of human PBL on ^{75}Se-labelled autologous or allogeneic target cell lines with the amount of IF released into the supernate of a 1 day MLC of the same cell combination, under identical culture conditions.

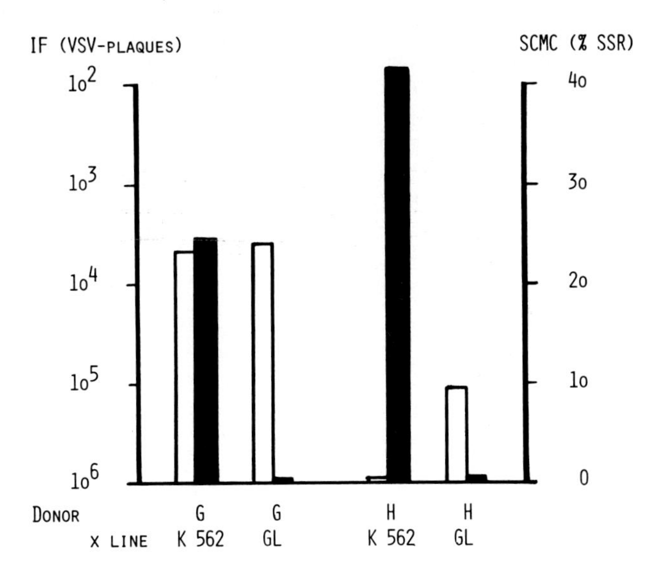

FIGURE 1. For legend cf. Figure 2.

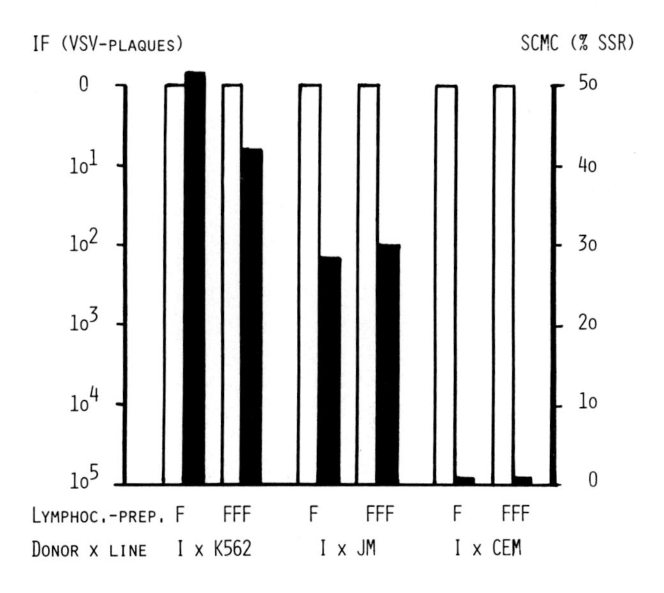

FIGURE 2. Interferon (IF)-production and SCMC in a 22 h assay. Open bars = IF, stimulator : responder = 5:1.Filled bars = SCMC, effector : target = 100:1. F and FFF (cf.II.B.) were different lymphocyte preparations from the same donor.

Although IF-production has been measured in supernates of 1 day MLC with up to 500 responder cells per 1 lymphoid line stimulator cell, the optimal IF-production in 1 day MLC and the best proliferative response in 6 d MLC was achieved with 2 - 10 responder cells per 1 lymphoid line stimulator cell (data not shown). To monitor both IF-production in MLC and SCMC at their optimal levels, we compared MLC with responder to stimulator ratios of 5:1, to SCMC with effector to target ratios between 8 and 200 : 1. In several experiments we found that for some E-T combinations there was no correlation between IF-production and SCMC-effect. Such a discordance is shown in Figure 1. In contrast to PBL from donor G which lysed K 562 in SCMC and produced detectable amounts of IF, the cocultivation of PBL from donor H with K 562 yielded much stronger SCMC but hardly any detectable IF. The opposite effect was seen with line GL which caused IF-production in PBL of the donors G and H but was not killed by any of them, although GL has been lysed under similar conditions by effector cells from other donors. Low IF-production (Fig. 1) was apparently not due to a lack of mature monocytes or macrophages, as the FFF-preparation of PBL, largely depleted of readily plastic-adhering and iron-phygozytosing cells, produced as much IF and displayed similar discordance with SCMC as the F-preparation (Fig. 2). Under comparable conditions the "discordant" target cell line CEM was frequently lysed by several human effectors (Leibold et al., 1980). Thus, apparently, neither was IF required for all E-T combinations in SCMC nor did high IF-production in the supernate always imply a positive SCMC-effect.

B. *Relationship of SCMC with IF- and LT-Production in Short Term MLC and with DNA-Synthesis in Long Term MLC*

In view of the discordance between SCMC and IF-production we compared them with the generation of lymphotoxin (LT) in short term MLC and with DNA-synthesis in 6 day MLC (Table I). In these experiments neither the stimulator lines nor the responder cells alone produced detectable amounts of IF or LT. Cocultivation for 22 h or 38 h of PBL with stimulator cells of the autologous or allogeneic leukocyte lines caused the production of slightly but not significantly differing amounts of IF and LT in the supernates. There was no convincing correlation between IF- and LT-production during 22 h or 38 h MLC and proliferative response after 6 day MLC. In contrast to DNA-synthesis the IF- and LT-production did not reveal any difference between autologous and allogeneic MLC. The comparison of Kaplan and K 562 as stimulator cells demonstrated best that high amounts of IF and LT can be generated in MLC within 1 day, unrelated to the degree of DNA-synthesis at day 6.

TABLE I. Relationships among DNA-Synthesis in 6 Day-MLC, Induction of Interferon and Lymphotoxin in 1 Day-MLC, and SCMC

Stimulator cells / Target cells	Day 1[c] IF (U/ml)	Day 1[c] LT (U/ml)	Day 6 Prolif. (dpm)	+ Responder cells	MLC[a] Day 1 IF (U/ml)	MLC[a] Day 1 LT (U/ml)	MLC[a] Day 6 Prolif. (dpm)	+ Effector cells	SCMC[b] Day 1 $2 \cdot 10^4$ (%SSR)	SCMC[b] Day 1 $2 \cdot 10^5$ (%SSR)
				A	o	o	55o			
				B	o	o	1,33o			
				C	o	o	28o			
AL	o	o	9o	A	5	22	16,14o	A	o	7.9
				B	15	79	1o2,o7o	B	o	o
BL	o	o	8o	A	1o	18	41,19o	A	o	o
				B	1o	14	8,89o	B	o	o
CL	o	o	7o	C	5	83	63,62o	C	o	o
DL	o	o	54o	C	15	179	112,94o	C	o	o
K562	o	o	56o	A	5o	79	2,9oo	A	27.4	57.2
				B	150	1o4	2,97o	B	15.o	47.1
				C	125	51o	3,98o	C	15.6	34.o
KP[d]	o	o	23o	A	5o	17o	98,83o	A	o	o
				B	25o	249	1o6,68o	B	o	o
				C	3o	347	128,59o	C	o	8.8

[a] Stimulator:responder = 1:5; [b] with $1 \cdot 10^3$ ^{75}Se-labelled targets
[c] Assay time; [d] Kaplan cell line.

Moreover, no correlation could be established between SCMC on one hand and short term IF- or LT-production and long term DNA-synthesis on the other one. This was shown in particular by the target lines AL, K 562, and Kaplan, which were recognized, at least by those effectors exerting a significant lysis on them. Neither the degree of lysis, nor the amount of IF or LT produced, nor the extent of DNA-synthesis fitted a uniform pattern.

C. *Alteration of SCMC by Short Term Culturing of Effector Cells*

In order to evaluate events occuring during cocultivation of effectors with target cells it was important to examine the influence of culturing the effector cells alone for 22 or 38 h. It resulted in hardly any generation of IF or LT but frequently in drastic alteration of their behaviour in subsequent SCMC. The results in Table II are representative of numerous experiments. They indicate that short term culturing of effector cells may increase their lytic capacity towards one target, decrease it towards another one and maintain it at a constant level for a third target. These alterations were apparently not due to measurable amounts of IF or LT. They could rather be explained by differential selection and/or modulation of various effector cell populations.

D. *Alteration of SCMC Effector Cells by Short Term MLC and by Supernates from it*

To further investigate effector cell alteration we cultured PBL from four donors (Tables III, IV) either alone and used them as control effector cells (A1, B1, C1, D1), or together with autologous or allogeneic stimulator cell lines for 38 h (A2-A5) or 22 h (C2-C5). Subsequently the corresponding cell-free supernates (SA1-SA5, SC1-SC5) were added to aliquots of control effectors 3 h prior to addition of the target cells. In parallel the MLC-cells (A2-A5, C2-C5) were washed, readjusted in fresh medium and tested as "MLC-effectors". Where significant lysis was provided by the control effector cells, the lytic activity of effectors incubated with supernates and that of MLC-effectors was expressed as percent alteration of cytotoxicity. Otherwise the cytotoxic effect was given as standardized specific isotope release (% SSR; cf.II.G.).
None of the supernates was toxic by itself to any of the targets tested (data not shown). Several aspects were indicated by results depicted in Tables III and IV:

1. There was a general trend towards enhanced cytotoxicity exerted by effector cells which where either pretreated with IF- and LT-rich supernates or cocultivated in MLC. In several E-T combinations (e.g. effectors AO and BO an the target Kaplan cf. Table II) no detectable SCMC occurred while IF and LT were efficiently produced in parallel MLC. If the corresponding effector cells (e.g. A1) where incubated with their own relevant supernate (e.g. SA5) significant induction (e.g. on the target Kaplan) or enhancement (e.g. on the targets BL and K 562) of the cytotoxic effect was found in the subsequent 22 h assay in comparison to the untreated control effector

TABLE II. Alteration of SCMC by Culturing the Effector Cells

Donor	A		B		C		D	
$2 \cdot 10^5$ Effectors	Ao	A1	Bo	B1	Co	C1	Do	D1
Preculturing (h)	o	38	o	38	o	22	o	22
Supernate content								
of IF (U/ml)	o	o	o	o	o	o	o	8
of LT (U/ml)	o	o	o	o	o	o	o	o
$1 \cdot 10^3$ Targets[a]								
AL	7.9[b]	8.4	o	8.7				
BL	o	5.1	o	8.o				
CL					o	o	13.9	o
DL					o	o	7.3	o
K 562	57.2	9.6	47.1	12.5	34.o	29.6	39.8	35.5
Kaplan	o	o	o	3.2	8.8	o	11.8	o

[a]Labelled with ^{75}Se; [b]%SSR obtained in a 22 h SCMC assay.

cells (e.g. A1). The enhancing effect of supernates was not restricted to autologous effectors; it also happened in allogeneic situations (e.g. SC2 enhanced the lytic capacity of the effector D1 against the target Kaplan, cf. Table IV).

2. The enhancement by IF- and LT-rich supernates was not uniform but varied with the E-T combination and the modulating treatment. A lack of recognition or "lytic susceptibility of targets" was reliably excluded in the tests shown, as cells from each donor killed each target at least once. In Table IV supernate SC2 exerted no influence on the effector cells C1 but induced significant cytotoxicity in D1 against the targets CL and Kaplan. However, D1 as well as C1 were able to lyse the targets CL, DL and Kaplan, provided the "right" supernate (e.g. SC4 or SC5) was added; this enhanced capacity of the effector cells varied with the target. While the effector population D1 was consistently more efficient in lysing the targets CL and Kaplan, the effector C; proved to be equally or even more cytotoxic against the targets DL and K 562 (Table IV).

3. Significant enhancement of cytotoxicity against K 562 was usually low or lacking if the untreated control effectors showed high (although still increasable) lytic capacity.If the control effectors were less cytotoxic against K 562 (e.g. in Table III), this was apparently not due to a lack of further lytic capacity as their activity could drastically be enhanced in MLC or by supernates.

4.Factor(s) other than IF and LT might be involved to explain the significant increase in cytotoxicity against BL by

TABLE III. Alteration of SCMC by 38 h MLC and by MLC-Supernates

38 h MLC[a] Responder	Stimulator	38 h Supernate Code	IF (U/ml)	LT (U/ml)		Effectors Code ($1 \cdot 10^5$)	Target Cells ($1 \cdot 10^3$) AL (%SSR)	BL (%SSR)	K 562 (%SSR)	Kaplan (%SSR)
A	-					A1	7.2	4.2	6.5	o
B	-					B1	6.1	6.6	1o.5	o
							Alteration	Alteration	Alteration	(%SSR)
A	-	SA1[b]	o	o	+	A1	o	98 %[c]	o	o
		SA1	"	"	+	B1	o	79 %	o	o
A	AL_m	-				A2	o	o	94 %	o
		SA2	5	22	+	A1	o	o	o	o
		SA2	"	"	+	B1	o	o	o	o
A	BL_m	-				A3	o	o	117 %	o
		SA3	1o	18	+	A1	o	o	1o6 %	o
		SA3	"	"	+	B1	o	o	93 %	o
A	K 562_m	-				A4	o	o	o	o
		SA4	5o	79	+	A1	1o4 %	15o %	3o8 %	3.3
		SA4	"	"	+	B1	148 %	85 %	165 %	4.8
A	$Kaplan_m$	-				A5	o	o	354 %	5.7
		SA5	5o	17o	+	A1	o	174 %	246 %	5.9
		SA5	"	"	+	B1	93 %	92 %	215 %	9.2

[a]Stimulator : responder = 1 : 5; [b]25 μl of supernate was added to 25 μl of effector cell suspension and incubated for 3 h prior to addition of the target cells; [c]significant alteration (2p less than o.o2 in a bilateral Student's t-test).

TABLE IV. Alteration of SCMC by 22 h MLC and by MLC-Supernates

22 h MLC[a] Responder	Stimulator	22 h Supernate Code	IF (U/ml)	LT (U/ml)		Effectors Code ($2 \cdot 10^5$)	Target Cells ($1 \cdot 10^3$) CL (%SSR)	DL (%SSR)	K 562 (%SSR)	Kaplan (%SSR)
C	-					C1	o	o	29.6	o
D	-					D1	o	o	35.5	o
							(%SSR)	(%SSR)	Alteration	(%SSR)
C	-	SC1[b]	o	o	+	C1	o	o	o	o
		SC1	"	"	+	D1	o	o	o	o
C	CL_m	-				C2	4.3	11.9	71 %[c]	o
		SC2	5	83	+	C1	o	o	o	o
		SC2	"	"	+	D1	7.5	o	o	9.3
C	DL_m	-				C3	9.6	15.4	62 %	1o.7
		SC3	15	179	+	C1	4.9	o	36 %	9.7
		SC3	"	"	+	D1	11.1	11.5	o	17.o
C	K 562_m	-				C4	1o.7	17.6	53 %	17.4
		SC4	125	51o	+	C1	13.5	13.6	37 %	17.o
		SC4	"	"	+	D1	23.7	14.5	o	22.o
C	$Kaplan_m$	-				C5	5.8	16.6	69 %	11.5
		SC5	3o	347	+	C1	5.4	15.4	64 %	14.7
		SC5	"	"	+	D1	2o.7	14.1	37 %	23.4

[a,b,c] cf. legend to Tab. III.

A1 and B1 after addition of the IF- and LT-negative supernate SA1. Similar enhancing effects have been observed in other E-T combinations.

5. Furthermore IF and LT might not be the predominant factors explaining the discordancy between the cytotoxic effect of distinct MLC-treated cells and of effector cells incubated with supernate of that same MLC. In Table III the MLC-effector A2 exerted significantly higher cytotoxicity than the control effector A1, while its IF- and LT-containing supernate SA2 was unable to augment the lytic capacity of A1 against K 562. In reverse, the MLC-effector A4 provided not more anti-K 562 cytotoxicity than the control A1, which, however, drastically increased its lytic effect in the presence of supernate SA4. Although not entirely excluded, residual K 562-stimulator cells acting as cold competitors in A4 were not the most likely explanation. A similar set up in Table IV resulted in significantly increased lysis of K 562 by the MLC-effector C4 in spite of the presence of cold K 562 stimulator cells. Further support for the discordant action of MLC-effectors and the related supernates was provided by the MLC-combinations C2 and C3 in Table IV and by results not shown. Thus, the MLC-effectors might have been activated or might act differently to the supernate augmented effector cells.

IV. DISCUSSION

Several investigators almost unanimously reported the decisive regulatory, usually enhancing influence of IF on SCMC (Djeu et al., 1979a,b; Droller et al., 1979; Einhorn et al., 1978; Gidlund et al.,1978; Herberman et al., 1979b; Heron et al., 1979; Lohmann-Matthes et al., 1979; Roder et al., 1978; Sato et al., 1979; Senik et al., 1979; Trinchieri et al.,1978a, b; Zarling et al., 1979). That tempted us to study the role of IF during the actual effector-target cell interaction in SCMC. Cocultivation of PBL with suspension line cells under comparable conditions for optimal IF-production in MLC, and for SCMC frequently resulted in both IF in the supernate and significant SCMC-effects. However, in several E-T combinations extreme discordancies between IF-production and SCMC were observed. In contrast to the hypothesis by Heberman et al.(1979a) claiming interferon to be required for the development of prekiller cells into active effector cells in SCMC, these results suggested IF not to be essential for the generation of active SCMC-effectors in all E-T combinations. This view was supported by cocultivations where significant SCMC occurred while low or no IF was detectable as well as by E-T combinations generating high amounts of IF in the absence of any SCMC effect, for which it was excluded that the lack of cytotoxicity was due to a lack of recognition of the targets by the effector cells. Thus, we extended the studies to the role of LT, reported to regulate cellular cytotoxicity (Lee and Lucas, 1976; Williams and Granger, 1973), particularly during interaction of PBL with tumor cells (Peter et al., 1976a). IF and LT, as defined by the monitoring assay used, showed no convincing differences in regard to their production in MLC and their functional influence in SCMC. Considering the cocultivation of effector and target cells in SCMC to be at the same time the starting period of the responder-stimulator interaction in MLC, we compared the SCMC-effect and the IF- and LT-production in short term cocultivation (22-38 h) with the proliferative response in 6 day MLC. The lack of correlation among SCMC, 6 day MLC response and production of IF and LT at day 1 confirmed and extended previous findings (Leibold et al., 1979). It suggested that various cell populations might be involved in the different processes studied. Furthermore they might be differently controlled, as in contrast to the proliferative response in 6 day MLC, no convincing difference was found between autologous and allogeneic combinations, neither in SCMC nor in IF- and LT-production.

As the IF- and LT-amounts produced during short term MLC (e.g. PBL of donor A with the allogeneic cell line BL, AxBL) did not necessarily correlate with the cytotoxic effect obtained in parallel SCMC (A against the target BL), it was of interest to compare whether the direct cocultivation of cells (AxBL) or the addition of their supernate (SAxBL) to the same effector (A) resulted in an altered SCMC-effect on the same target (BL) and against other ones. According to the previous experiences (Leibold et al., 1978) it was important to monitor alterations which may occur during cultivation of the effector cells alone. Remarkable changes in SCMC with cultured PBL were seen but they were never uniform for all targets or effectors. They varied considerably with the E-T combination and were not due to detectable amounts of IF or LT. None of the short term MLC supernates was toxic to any of the targets or to the effectors tested. In contrast to many E-T combinations which were not altered in their SCMC-effect, several others were significantly enhanced by the addition of supernates. The enhancement was usually stronger when the supernates contained higher amounts of IF or LT, but supernates with low or no IF or LT were also able to enhance the cytotoxic effect considerably. One might consider IF and LT to modulate SCMC, already in amounts below our levels of detection. Although not excluded, this would contradict Sato et al. (1979) who found 20 - 500 U/ml to be the enhancing range of IF-concentrations for human SCMC. Alternately, one might think of other biological functions of IF and LT which we were unable to assess by the present monitoring assays. Otherwise additional factors might be considered to be involved in the regulation of SCMC, which might be rapidly produced during E-T interaction, independently of IF and LT. Some of them might be the factors produced by T-cell enriched populations upon rosetting with sheep red blood cells (O'Neill et al., 1975) or after activation with Corynebacterium parvum (Peter et al., this volume).

If soluble factors, including IF and LT, are essential regulators for SCMC, one should assume that the cell populations producing such factors contain effector cells which act like their own supernate. E.g. the MLC-cells (AxBL) after washing should exert a comparable effect on a target CL as the effector A after addition of the cell free supernate (SA). As long as the MLC-effectors killed CL more strongly than A plus SA, one might consider the relevant enhancing factors to be insufficiently concentrated in the supernate. The reverse effect, showing augmenting activities in the supernate while the MLC-effector cells displayed no or non-enhanced cytotoxicity, argued against a decisive influence of stable soluble factors in the regulation of these MLC-effector cells. They might either be altered by the direct E-T cell contact or they might exert their cytotoxic activity via a different mechanism than the supernate activated effector cells. Whatever the various SCMC regulating factors and mechanisms might be, each alteration of the SCMC-capacity is essentially dependent on the inherent capacity of the effector cells from the individual donor to interact differently with various target cells.

V. SUMMARY

In order to study regulatory influence in the effector-target cell interaction in SCMC we investigated combinations of human PBL with autologous and allogeneic permanent suspension cell lines in 1 day SCMC and in 1 and 6 day MLC. The alteration of SCMC due to the influence of cellular interactions and of soluble factors, particularly of interferon (IF) and of lymphotoxin (LT), in supernates was monitored. In contrast to the proliferative response in 6 day MLC neither in SCMC nor in IF- and LT-production were reproducable differences between autologous and allogeneic effector-target (E-T) combinations observed. IF and LT, as defined by the monitoring assays employed, showed similar trends in respect to their production in MLC and their functional influence on SCMC.Neither of them, however, was essential for successfull SCMC in all E-T combinations. Our results indicate that SCMC-effects could be altered in three different ways: by cultivating the effector cells alone, by adding various soluble factors (including IF and LT) to them, or by direct cell to cell interaction. The alteration was not uniform, for all targets or in all effector cell populations. It depended essentially on the inherent capacity of the individual donor to respond to the modulating influences and to act differently with the various target cells.

ACKNOWLEDGMENTS

The expert technical assistance of Ms. A. Dietrich, S. Eulenberger, R. Yupanondh and Mr. S.P. Bridge is gratefully acknowledged. We thank Mr. S.P. Bridge for valuable editorial help and Ms. I. Jöhrens for dedicated typing of the manuscript.

REFERENCES

Andersson, L.C., Nilsson, K., and Gahmberg, C.G. (1979). *Int. J. Cancer 23,* 143.

Brooks, C.G., Rees, R.C., and Baldwin R.W. (1976). *Int. J. Cancer 18,* 778.

De Vries, J.E., Meyering, M., and van Dongen, A. (1975).*Int. J. Cancer 15,* 391.

Djeu, J.Y., Heinbaugh, J.A., Holden, H.T., and Herberman, R.B. (1979a). *J. Immunol. 122,* 175.

Djeu, J.Y., Heinbaugh, J.A., Holden, H.T., and Herberman, R.B. (1979b). *J. Immunol. 122,* 182.

Droller, M.J., Borg, H., and Perlmann, P. (1979). *Cell. Immunol. 47,* 248.

Eife, R.F., Eife, G.W., August, C.S., Kuhre, W., and Staehr-Johansen, K. (1974). *Cell. Immunol. 14,* 435.

Eife, G.W., Eife, R.F., and Brendel, W. (1979). *Cell. Immunol. 46,* 35.

Einhorn, S., Blomgren, H., and Strander, H. (1978). *Int. J. Cancer 22,* 405.

Foley, G.E., Lazarus, H., Farber, S., Uzman, B.G., Boon, B.A., and McCarthy, R.E. (1965). *Cancer 18,* 522.

Gidlund, M., Örn, A., Wigzell, H., Senik, A., and Gresser, I. (1978). *Nature 273,* 759.

Herberman, R.B., Nunn, M.E., Holden, H.T., Staal, S., and Djeu, J.Y. (1977). *Int. J. Cancer 19,* 555.

Herberman, R.B., Djeu, J.Y., Kay, D.H., Ortaldo, J.R., Riccardi, C., Bonnard, G.D., Holden, H.T., Fagnani, R., Santoni, A., and Puccetti, P., (1979a). *Immunological Rev. 44,* 43.

Herberman, R.B., Ortaldo, J.R., and Bonnard, G.D. (1979b). *Nature 277,* 221.

Heron, I., Hokland, M., Möller-Larsen, A., and Berg, K.(1979). *Cell. Immunol. 42,* 183.

Kalden, J.R., Peter, H.H., Roubin, R., and Cesarini,J.P.(1977). *Eur. J. Immunol. 8,* 537.

Kiessling, R.,and Haller,O.(1978).*Contemp.Top.Immunobiol.8,* 171.

Kiessling, R.,and Wigzell,H.(1979).*Immunol.Rev. 44,* 165.

Kirchner, H., Peter, H.H., Hirt, H.M., Zawatzky, R., Dallügge, H., and Bradstreet, P. (1979). *Immunobiol. 156,* 65.

Kiuchi,M.,and Takasugi,M.(1976).*J.Natl.Cancer Inst. 56,*575.

Lee, S., and Lucas, Z.J. (1976). *J. Immunol. 117,* 283.

Leibold, W., and Bridge, S. (1979). *Immunobiol. 155,* 287.

Leibold, W., and Peter,H.H. (1978). *Behring Inst.Mitt. 62,*144.

Leibold, W., Peter, H.H., and Gatti, R.A. (1978). *In:* "Manipulation of the immune response in cancer" (A. Mitchison, M. Landy, eds.), p. 185, Academic Press, New York.

Leibold, W., Gatti, R.A., Just, S., and Peter, H.H. (1979). *Transpl. Proc. 11,* 1393.

Leibold, W., Janotte, G., and Peter, H.H. *Scand. J. Immunol.* (in press)

Lohmann-Matthes, M.L., Domzig, W., and Roder, J. (1979). *J. Immunol. 123,* 1883.

Lozzio, C.B., and Lozzio, B.B. (1975). *Blood 45,* 321.

Mackler, B.F., O'Neill, P.A., and Meistrich, M. (1977). *Eur. J. Immunol. 7,* 55.

Menezes, J., Leibold, W., and Klein, G. (1975). *Exptl. Cell Res. 92,* 478.

Mukherji, B., Vassos, D., Flowers, A., Binder, S.C., and Nathenson, C. (1975). *Cancer Res. 35,* 3721.

O'Neill, P., Mackler, B.F., and Wyde, P. (1975). *Cell. Immunol. 20,* 33.

Parkman, R., and Rosen, F.S. (1976). *J. Exp. Med. 144,* 1520.

Peter,H.H.,Eife,R.F.,and Kalden,J.R.(1976a).*J.Immunol.116,*342.

Peter, H.H., Pavie-Fischer, J., Kalden, J.R., Roubin, R., Cesarini, J.P.,and Kourilsky,F.M.(1976b). *INSERM 57,*213.

Peter, H.H., Dallügge, H., Zawatzky, R., Euler, S., Leibold, W., and Kirchner, H. (submitted for publication).

Pross,H.F.,and Baines,M.G.(1977).*Cancer Immunol.Immunother.3,*75

Roder, J.C., Kiessling, R., Biberfeld, P., and Andersson, B. (1978). *J. Immunol. 121,* 2509.

Saksela,E.,Imir,T.,and Mäkelä,O.(1977).*Eur.J.Immunol. 7,*126.

Sato,T., Fuse,A., and Kuwata,T.(1979). *Cell.Immunol. 45,*458.

Schaadt, M., Kirchner, H., Fonatsch, C., and Diehl, V.(1979). *Int. J. Cancer 23,* 751.

Schneider, U., Schwenk, H.-U., and Bornkamm, G. (1977). *Int. J. Cancer 19,* 621.

Senik, A., Gresser, I., Maury, C., Gidlund, M., Örn, A., and Wigzell, H. (1979). *Cell. Immunol. 44,* 186.

Shellam, G.R. (1977). *Int. J. Cancer 19,* 225.

Svedmyr, E.A.J., Leibold, W., and Gatti, R.A. (1975). *Tissue Antigens 5,* 186.
Svet-Moldavsky, G.J., Nemirovskaya, B.M., Osipova,T.V., Slavina, E.G., Zinzar, S.N., Karmonova, N.V.,and Morozova, L.F. (1973). *Folia Biol. (Praha) 20,* 230.
Trinchieri,G., and Santoli, D. (1978). *J. Exp. Med. 147,* 1314.
Trinchieri,G., Santoli, D., and Knowles, B.B. (1977). *Nature 270,* 611.
Trinchieri,G., Santoli, D., Dee,R.R.,and Knowles, B.(1978a). *J. Exp. Med. 147,* 1299.
Trinchieri,G., Santoli, D., and Koprowski, H. (1978b). *J. Immunol. 120,* 1849.
Williams, T.W., and Granger,G.A. (1973). *Cell. Immunol. 6,*171.
Zarling, J.M., Eskra, L., Borden, E.C., Horoszewicz, J., and Carter, W.A. (1979). *J. Immunol. 123,* 63.

AUGMENTATION OF HUMAN NK AND ADCC BY INTERFERON

M. Moore
I. Kimber

Paterson Laboratories
Christie Hospital and Holt Radium Institute
Manchester M20 9BX
England

I. INTRODUCTION

There is currently much interest in the observation that the spontaneous cytotoxic activity of lymphoid cells in human peripheral blood against selected targets may be augmented by endogenous and exogenous interferon (IF) (refs 1 - 4). The relationship between natural killer (NK) activity and antibody dependent cellular cytotoxicity (ADCC) in this respect, has been controversial (1,2) not least because physical separation of the cells into subpopulations that can exclusively mediate either activity has so far proved elusive (5).

Approaches to this problem have employed targets which are susceptible to both spontaneous and antibody-dependent killing (2,6). In these circumstances, the question whether IF enhancement of ADCC actually reflects an effect on cells directly involved in this type of cytotoxicity, or enhancement of antibody-independent mechanisms is not invariably clear. In an attempt to circumvent this complication, we recently initiated studies in an ADCC system in which concomitant antibody-independent cytotoxicity was non-existent. The use of human erythrocytes as targets and antibodies directed against the blood group antigens A and Rh(D), fulfilled this criterion. Moreover, these targets had the additional advantage that more than one ADCC effector cell type could be studied, since the effector cell profile is determined by the nature of the antigen - antibody reaction at the cell surface. Accordingly, the effect of IF on lysis of anti-A treated human erythrocytes

ISBN 0-12-341350-8

(mediated exclusively by monocytes) and of anti-D treated erythrocytes (mediated by monocytes and lymphocytes) (7) were studied in parallel.

II. MATERIALS AND METHODS

Target Cells

Natural killer activity was assayed against several susceptible (K562, CCRF/CEM, Molt-4) and resistant (Raji, Bri 8) cell lines, which were routinely propagated as suspension cultures in RPMI medium containing 10% heat inactivated foetal calf serum (RPMI-FCS) and antibiotics.

ADCC was assayed against human red blood cells (HRBC) of phenotype A Rh(D)+ve, obtained from a single normal donor. HRBC were collected in a four-fold excess of citrate phosphate buffer, pH 6.9, and stored at 4°C for periods not exceeding 3 days.

Interferon

Human lymphoblastoid interferon (Type I), produced by Namalva cells was prepared and purified by Dr. K.H.Fantes (Wellcome Research Laboratories, Beckenham, Kent, England). The preparation (batch 479/602) used in this study was of specific activity 2.2×10^6 IU/mg protein. Units refer to British Standard Unit calibrated against Std B69/19 (Nat. Inst Biol. Stds. Controls, London, England). The interferon, which contained added human plasma protein as a stabilizer, was stored at -70°C. Freshly thawed material was diluted with RPMI FCS before use.

Effector Cell Preparation and Culture

Peripheral blood was drawn from normal donors into 5.27mM EDTA and mononuclear cells (PBMC) separated as described previously (8) using Ficoll-Paque (Pharmacia Fine Chemicals, Sweden) in the density centrifugation step. After washing, PBMC were suspended in HEPES-buffered Eagles MEM supplemented with 5% heat-inactivated foetal calf serum (MEM-FCS) (Flow Laboratories, Ltd. Scotland), their viability determined by trypsan blue exclusion and concentration adjusted to working levels (2 - 7×10^6 cells ml^{-1}).

PBMC were depleted of adherent cells by incubation on nylon fibre columns (8).

Differential counts were made on Jenner-Giemsa stained cytocentrifuge preparations. Quantitation of monocytes was facilitated by incubation of cell suspensions with 1.1μ polystyrene latex particles (Uniscience, Cambridge) for 45 minutes at 37°C before centrifugation. Non-specific esterase staining was carried out by the method of Yam et al (9). PBMC comprised 71 ± 9% lymphocytes and 27 ± 10% monocytes. Nylon passed cells ($PBMC^{\downarrow}$) consisted of 95 ± 4% lymphocytes and 3 ± 3% monocytes.

The conditions of culture for pretreatment of effector cells with IF were suspension of $3x10^6$ cells ml^{-1} in RPMI-FCS at 37°C in a humidified 5% CO_2atmosphere for 18 hours (unless otherwise stated). At the end of the incubation, cells were washed three times in Hank's balanced salt solution, pH 7.2, their viability re-assessed and resuspended in RPMI-FCS.

Antisera

Sera containing anti-A antibodies (of IgG class) were obtained from a single untransfused, nulliparous female donor of blood group O Rh(D)+ve.

Anti-D sera from group A donors were the gift of the Regional Blood Transfusion Service, Piccadilly, Manchester.

Sera were heat-inactivated for 60 minutes at 56°C and stored in small aliquots at -20°C until immediately before use. Optimal concentrations for cell-mediated haemolysis in the anti-A and anti-D systems were 1 - 2% and 10% (v/v) respectively.

Cytotoxicity Assay

Cultured target cells and trypsinized HRBC (ref. 10) were washed and labelled with 100 - 400μCi ^{51}Cr sodium chromate (Radiochemical Centre, Amersham, England) as previously described (8). Labelled targets (T) were then dispersed into tubes containing sensitizing antisera (where appropriate) and effector (E) cells at various E:T ratios. Interferon was also included where effectors had not been pretreated with the agent. Triplicate tubes were incubated for 6 or 18 hours at 37°C in a humidified atmosphere of 5% CO_2 in air. Assays were terminated by centrifugation and removal of supernatants which were counted separately from the residual supernatants and pellets, in a Searle model 1185 gamma counter. The percentage ^{51}Cr release was determined for each tube and percentage cytotoxicity calculated from the following formula:

$$\% \text{ cytotoxicity} = \frac{\%^{51}\text{Cr release in test} - \%^{51}\text{Cr release in control}}{\% \text{ maximum } ^{51}\text{Cr release} - \%^{51}\text{Cr release in control}} \times 100$$

Maximum isotope release was determined by addition of Triton X100 (1/100 dilution) and spontaneous release from control tubes containing target cells only (<10% for HRBC; 5-15% for cell lines). In assays of ADCC, controls routinely comprised target and effector cells without antiserum and targets and antiserum without effectors. In NK assays, controls were labelled targets alone.

III RESULTS

Augmentation of Natural Cytotoxicity by Interferon

In comparison with untreated PBMC, incubation of effectors and targets with IF (250 IU ml^{-1}) for 6 hours markedly augmented cytotoxicity against the susceptible targets K562,CCRF/CEM and Molt 4 (Table 1).

TABLE 1 Effect of Interferon on PBMC Cytotoxicity against Five Cell Lines

	Interferon Treatment								
	None			IF included in test **			Incubation with IF prior to test***		
Target Cells	20:1*	10:1	5:1	20:1	10:1	5:1	20:1	10:1	5:1
K562	33	24	14	46	40	33	64	56	50
CCRF/CEM	20	13	12	39	28	25	57	49	35
Molt 4	36	30	24	49	42	38	73	58	52
Raji	4	6	4	10	7	5	33	21	14
Bri 8	2	1	1	7	6	5	27	9	9

E:T ratio; **250 IU IF ml^{-1};*18 hours pretreatment with 250 IU IF ml^{-1}*

The B cell lines, Raji and Bri 8, resistant to untreated PBMC, revealed a measureable degree of susceptibility only after exposure of PBMC to IF.

To determine whether the action of IF was directly on effector cells, PBMC were preincubated for 18 hours with IF (250 IU ml^{-1}). Levels of cytotoxicity thereafter were even higher against all five cell lines (Table 1). This augmentation was IF dose dependent and could be detected at concentrations as low as 10 IU IF ml^{-1}, reaching a maximum between 100 and 500 IU IF ml^{-1} (Table 2).

TABLE 2 Interferon Dose-Dependence of PBMC Cytotoxicity against K562 Cells

Interferon Concentration (IU ml^{-1})	Percentage cytotoxicity at E:T ratios of:		
	20:1	10:1	5:1
0	45.9	28.5	15.2
10	48.4	31.4	17.0
50	57.1	37.9	22.1
100	56.6	39.4	22.9
250	66.1	35.9	25.5
500	66.8	41.1	24.9
1000	58.1	36.7	21.0

PBMC were incubated with IF for 18 hours prior to cytotoxicity testing

Significant enhancement of cytotoxicity was detectable after only one hours' preincubation with IF rising to a maximum at 6 hours (Table 3).

TABLE 3 PBMC Cytotoxicity against K562 Cells as a Function of Time of Pretreatment with Interferon (250 IU ml^{-1}).

Effector:target ratio	PBMC pretreatment period (hours)			
	0	1	6	18
20:1	18.4	40.9	62.1	60.7
10:1	17.5	29.6	46.9	41.5
5:1	NT	16.3	25.1	24.9

NT, not tested

Separation of lymphocyte subpopulations by sheep erythrocyte rosette formation and nylon column filtration demonstrated that the activities of IF treated and untreated cells were similarly distributed, suggesting that the major effect of IF is enhancement of the activity of pre-existing spontaneously cytotoxic cells (or their precursors) rather than the generation of new populations of effectors (4).

Augmentation of Antibody-Dependent Cellular Cytotoxicity by Interferon

In the anti-A system, HRBC revealed a pattern of lysis by PBMC which was dependent on the concentration of sensitizing antiserum (Table 4).

TABLE 4 Antibody-Dependent Cellular Cytotoxicity against Anti-A Sensitized HRBC Induced by PBMC in the Presence of Interferon

	Percentage cytotoxicity (±1SD) in presence of:		
Concentration of Anti-A serum (%)	0	200 IU IF	600 IU IF
0	0	0	0
0.25	1.9 ± 3.1	4.7	6.5 ± 3.2
0.5	6.8 ± 0.9	17.7 ± 1.9	14.1 ± 0.6
1.0	26.0 ± 3.8	32.8 ± 2.2	38.8 ± 1.3

E:T ratio 5:1

Addition of IF (200 and 600 IU) to the cytotoxicity assay increased the level of haemolysis at each antibody concentration. Under optimal conditions of HRBC sensitization (1% anti-A) the increase was from 26% to 39% (in the presence of 600 IU IF), representing a 50% enhancement of cytotoxicity. In the absence of sensitizing antibody, ^{51}Cr release from HRBC in the presence of effectors and interferon, was identical with (or less than) the spontaneous release from HRBC alone. Under the conditions of these experiments, therefore, no antibody-independent cytotoxicity against HRBC by untreated or IF-treated effectors could be demonstrated.

Essentially similar results were obtained in the anti-D system (Table 5). Under optimal conditions of HRBC sensitization (10% anti-D) the increase was from 36% to 57% (at 600 IU IF), corresponding to an enhancement of cytotoxicity of 55%. Again, effectors plus IF, but without antibody, induced no release of ^{51}Cr greater than that from HRBC alone. These data thus established that IF significantly enhanced cellular cytotoxic reactions which were dependent on antibodies with specificities for different antigens on the same target cell.

Further experiments were performed to determine whether the effect of IF in these systems, like that of natural cytotoxicity, involved a direct action on effector cells. For this purpose, PBMC were preincubated with interferon (200 IU ml^{-1}). The patterns of IF dose-dependence, and cytotoxicity as a function of IF pretreatment time were essentially similar to those for natural cytotoxicity (c.f. Tables 2 & 3).

TABLE 5 Antibody-Dependent Cellular Cytotoxicity against Anti-D Sensitized HRBC Induced by PBMC in the Presence of Interferon

Concentration of Anti-D serum (%)	Percentage cytotoxicity (±1SD) in presence of:		
	0	200 IU IF	600 IU IF
0	0	0	0
2.5	10.5 ± 5.0	36.4 ± 2.6	31.9 ± 2.4
5.0	28.7 ± 5.3	46.3 ± 2.0	44.9 ± 4.0
10.0	36.4 ± 4.2	55.6 ± 3.1	56.5 ± 1.6

E:T ratio 5:1

In both the anti-A and anti-D systems, the level of haemolysis induced by IF-pretreatment of effectors exceeded that by untreated effectors at most concentrations of sensitizing anti body (Table 6).

TABLE 6 Antibody-Dependent Cellular Cytotoxicity Induced by Untreated and IF-Pretreated PBMC

Antiserum/ Concentration (%)	Percentage cytotoxicity (±1SD) induced by:	
	Untreated PBMC	IF-pretreated PBMC
0	0	0
Anti-A/0.5	5.4 ± 0.1	6.3 ± 2.7
Anti-A/1.0	18.1 ± 1.1	25.3 ± 5.2
Anti-A/2.0	34.1 ± 4.9	47.1 ± 2.6
Anti-D/2.5	41.8 ± 3.9	69.2 ± 6.4
Anti-D/5.0	52.6 ± 3.6	84.1 ± 4.2
Anti-D/10.0	50.6 ± 10.5	83.3 ± 1.5

E:T ratio 7:1

Against HRBC optimally sensitized with anti-A, cytotoxicity was increased from 34% to 47%, representing an augmentation of 38%, and against HRBC sensitized with anti-D from 51% to 83%, an increase of 65%. These data thus showed that, in common with NK activity, augmentation of ADCC in these systems involves a direct action of IF on effector cells.

Since PBMC possess a potential for ADCC which is not restricted to one effector cell type, fractionation experiments were performed to determine the respective contribution of lymphocytes and monocytes to enhanced cytotoxicity by IF. The activity of unfractionated PBMC was potentiated against both anti-A and anti-D treated HRBC in accordance with previous experiments (Table 7).

TABLE 7 Comparison of ADCC against Sensitized HRBC and Spontaneous Killing of K562 Cells by Untreated and IF-Pretreated PBMC

Target Cells/ Antiserum	Percentage cytotoxicity induced by:			
	PBMC	$PBMC_{IF}$	$PBMC^{\downarrow}$	$PBMC^{\downarrow}_{IF}$
HBRC/anti-A	23.2 ± 3.1	46.1 ± 1.0	1.8 ± 0.6	1.3 ± 0.5
	22.9 ± 2.7	40.2 ± 5.8	0.6 ± 0.5	0.1 ± 0.1
HRBC/anti-D	53.8 ± 3.5	75.5 ± 1.1	38.8 ± 1.3	29.4 ± 2.7
	67.4 ± 1.1	90.0 ± 4.9	67.9 ± 7.5	80.0 ± 6.2
K562	13.4 ± 1.6	32.1 ± 4.2	23.0 ± 2.3	27.4 ± 0.4
	14.4 ± 3.2	36.4 ± 2.5	23.3 ± 4.0	30.2 ± 1.5

E:T ratio 5:1 The subscript $_{IF}$ denotes interferon pretreatment prior to fractionation and cytotoxicity testing. The superscript ↓ denotes depletion of adherent cells by passage over nylon wool.

In the anti-A system, passage of PBMC through nylon columns completely abolished ADCC, directly implicating the monocyte as the effector cell in this system. IF pretreatment of nylon passed effectors failed to restore this activity. In the anti-D system, nylon column passed effectors retained their ADCC capability, but this activity was not augmented by IF. These preliminary results therefore suggest that, whereas lymphocytes lyze HRBC sensitized with anti-D, significant enhancement of cytotoxicity by IF does not occur in the absence of monocytes. PBMC depleted of monocytes consistently lyzed K562 targets although the magnitude of the increase when pretreated with IF, was less than that for unfractionated PBMC.

IV DISCUSSION

Evidence has been presented which justify the conclusion that IF enhances the cytotoxic potential of effectors in PBMC for cultured cell lines and for antibody-sensitized HRBC. Concurrent studies utilizing Namalva IF preparations of different specific activity have shown that, at least as far as the NK activity against cell lines is concerned, the active principle is indeed interferon (4). The phenomena herein described, by deliberate experimental design, would appear to be the result of a direct action of IF on effector (or accessory) cells. This does not mean that IF cannot interact with target cells, since in experiments to be reported, it has been shown that they may actually be protected from lysis by IF-stimulated and unstimulated effectors. This finding probably accounts in part, for the fact that preincubation of effectors in IF resulted in enhancement of cytotoxicity against the cell lines invariably greater than when IF was included in the cytotoxicity assay.

Two cellular cytotoxicity systems were examined in this study. In the first, different cultured targets were lyzed to a variable extent, by effector cells possessing the characteristics of NK cells. These cells lack receptors for mature T or B lymphocytes, and are non phagocytic. Although they possess Fc receptors, they are generally believed to function in an antibody-independent manner (11).

In the second, the involvement of antibodies in the lytic process, is by definition, obligatory. These cells are also Fc receptor positive and immunological specificity is determined by interaction with the relevant target cell (12). Lymphoid cells, monocytes and neutrophils may function in this capacity (13),depending on the nature of the target cells and the antigen-antibody reaction at the cell surface. By a judicious choice of target cell (human erythrocyte) it was possible to develop systems for the study of IF augmentation of ADCC in which concomitant killing by NK cells was obviated. Pretreatment of PBMC with IF, or inclusion of the latter in the cytotoxicity tests, unequivocally increased the lysis of both anti-A and anti-D-sensitized HRBC.

Sensitization of A Rh(+ve) erythrocytes with non-immune anti-A serum mediates cytotoxicity which is induced exclusively by monocytes, via both extra and intra-cellular mechanisms (14). The relative contribution of these mechanisms to increased lysis by IF has not been elucidated, but enhancement of phagocytosis (15), leading to increased intra-cellular lysis is clearly one possibility.

Cytotoxicity by PBMC in the anti-D system, on the other hand, is induced by both monocytes and lymphocytes. Failure of IF to augment the cytotoxic activity of lymphocytes purified by passage through nylon wool suggests either that the presence of monocytes is required for optimal enhancement of ADCC mediated by K cells; or a direct action of IF on monocytes themselves. Our data also imply some degree of lymphocyte-monocyte interaction in natural cytotoxicity, on account of the fact that the enhancement by IF of the cytotoxicity of monocyte-depleted PBMC was less than that for the unfractionated effector population. The critical dependence of natural killing *in vitro* on accessory monocytes has been described (16).

In quantitative terms, the differences in responsiveness of purified lymphocytes to IF revealed by cytotoxicity against sensitized HRBC and K562 cells are presently too small to definitively attribute the two cytotoxicity phenomena to different effector subpopulations, or different functional attributes of the same population. The data do, however, establish that ADCC, as a cytotoxicity mechanism, is enhanced by interferon. The relative contribution of the different cell types involved must await the outcome of further experimentation.

ACKNOWLEDGMENTS

This study was supported by grants from the Medical Research Council and Cancer Research Campaign of Great Britain We are grateful to Ms. Wendy White for skilled technical assistance and also to Ms. Linda Corby for preparation of the manuscript.

REFERENCES

1. Trinchieri, G. and Santoli, D., J.Exp.Med. 147, 1314 (1978)
2. Herberman, R.B., Ortaldo, J.R. and Bonnard, G.D., Nature, 277, 221 (1979).
3. Zarling, J.M., Eskra, L., Borden, E.C., Horoszewicz, J. and Carter, W.A., J. Immunol., 123, 63, (1979).
4. Moore, M. and Potter, M.R. Brit. J. Cancer, 41, (in press) (1980).
5. Ozer, H., Strelkauskar, A.J., Callery, R.T. and Schlossman S.F., Europ. J. Immunol., 9, 112, (1979).
6. Droller, M.J., Borg, H. and Perlmann, P. Cell Immunol., 47, 248 (1979).
7. Kimber, I. and Moore, M. In preparation (1980).
8. Potter, M.R. and Moore, M. Immunology,37, 187 (1979).
9. Yam, L.T., Li, C.Y. and Crosby, W.H. Amer. J. Clin. Path. 55, 283 (1971).
10. Holm, G. Int. Arch. Allergy, 43, 671 (1972).
11. Herberman, R.B. and Holden, H.T. Adv. Cancer Res., 27, 305 (1978).
12. Perlmann, P., Perlmann, H., Larsson, A. and Wahlin, B., J. Reticuloendothelial Soc., 17, 241 (1978).
13. McDonald, H.R., Bonnard, G.D., Sordat, B. and Zawodnik, S.A., Scand. J. Immunol., 4, 487, (1975).

14. Hersey, P. Transplantation, 15, 282, (1973).
15. Huang, K., Donahoe, R.M., Gordon, F.B. and Dresser, H.R., Infect. Immun., 4, 581 (1971).
16. de Vries, J., Bont, W.S., Mendelsohn, J. and Rümke, P., Proc. Fourth European Immunology Meeting, Budapest, Hungary, p. 71 (abstract) (1978).

FACTORS CONTROLLING THE AUGMENTATION OF NATURAL KILLER CELLS

Anders Örn
Magnus Gidlund
Emmanuel Ojo[I]
Kjell-Olof Grönvik
Jan Andersson
Hans Wigzell

Department of Immunology,BMC
University of Uppsala
Uppsala,Sweden

Robert A.Murgita

Department of Microbiology and Immunology
Mc Gill University
Montreal,Canada

Anna Senik
Ion Gresser

Laboratories of Cellular Immunology and Viral Oncology
Institut de Recherches Scientifiques sur le Cancer
Villejuif,France

INTRODUCTION

Several parameters are known to in a significant manner regulate the levels of NK cell activity in the individual. Genetic differences between inbred strains of mice will result in the creation of "high" and "low" NK strains (I,2).The ageof

[I]*Present adress:University of Ife,Ife,Benin,Nigeria*

ISBN 0-12-341350-8

the mouse is critical in deciding the activity of NK cells with a sharp peak of activity residing approximately between 3 weeks and 3 months of age (I,2).In addition to this"normal" regulation of NK cells extraneous conditions involving viral or other infections (3-5) as well as injections with several adjuvants (6-8) can be shown to have drastic enhancing or sometimes inhibitory consequences for NK activities.When considering these regulatory effects it is now important to realize that the NK cell is in a quite direct manner linked to the bone marrow function (9,I0),and stem cells from the marrow seem quite decisive in determining NK levels.

In the present article we will discuss parameters involved in the augmentation of murine NK cells in vivo or in vitro. The presentation will be biased to contain our own results and views as parallel articles of other workers in the same area will be presented in this volume.

THE LEVEL OF AUGMENTATION IN RELATION TO NORMAL ACTIVITY

When discussing augmentation by various agents of NK cells in relation to normal NK levels in untreated mice it is of importance to establish the quantitative aspects in addition to qualitative questions.As mentioned several infections can cause a significant degree of NK enhancement in vivo.In table I are given exemples of the effect of NK activity by malarial infestation of mice.As seen Plasmodium chabaudi will in CBA mice (a relative resistant mouse strain) result in a rapid increase in NK levels.Total increase in lytic units in such malaria-infected spleens will frequently be in the order of 50-times the normal levels.Another point besides quantity in conditions of e.g. viral infections is time.It is thus now well known that viral infections may within a matter of hours lead to an increase in NK levels (3) indicating that the agents involved in the enhancement of NK activity must be produced within this time period.

Table I.Plasmodium chabaudi increases NK activity in mice.

Effector cells	*Specific target lysis(% lysis)*	
	Effector:target ratio	
	50:I	*25:I*
Normal spleen,CBA	*24%*	*I0%*
Normal peritoneal cells	*23%*	*not done*
Malarial spleen	*72%*	*49%*
Malarial peritoneal cells	*76%*	*not done*

Test 5 days after infection.YAC targets.4 hr chromium assay.

INTERFERON:THE MAJOR REGULATOR OF NK ACTIVITY

The rapid rate of NK induction and the variety of agents found able to enhance NK activity lead us in I977 to explore the possibility that interferon may be a common denominator for all these agents in the enhancement of NK activity.Our approach involved initially three steps:a)Testing several substances with known interferon inducing ability for their possible NK enhancing properties.b)Test interferon directly for NK activating properties.c)Use anti-interferon antisera to block possible positive effects achieved under a or b. Our efforts were quite successful and we could in a conclusive manner indicate interferon to be a major regulator of NK cells (II).Other groups did in parallel reach similar conclusions (I2-I4).Exemples of our own showing the relevance of interferon by these approaches are shown in table II.Note in this table that several agents (Newcastle Disease Virus,tilorone, statolon,poly-I:C and Corynebacterium parvum) with completely different molecular build up but with the common denominator of being good interferon inducers all functioned as efficient NK augmentors.Anti-interferon antibodies when tested on these agents did obliterate their NK enhancing abilities showing that indeed the interferon substance(s) was required for the process.Do also note that anti-interferon antibodies alone when present in the test had no decreasing effect on the normal NK activity.This we have also found in the human NK system using anti-human interferon antisera in clear contrast to other groups (I5,I6).Within the short time periods used active induction in vitro of interferon thereby regulating NK cells would not play any detectable role in our tests.

One may argue that the use of anti-interferon antisera in itself does not necessary prove that such antisera act via their content of anti-interferon antibodies.One may argue that such antisera in addition may contain antibodies specific for other components in the semi-pure interferon batches used for immunization.Anti-interferon hybridomas would here be required.

A series experiments using bone marrow chimeras and two different interferon inducers (NDV versus tilorone) in the strain combinations AKR and CBA make this possibility less likely .Here it could be shown that irradiated CBA or AKR mice repopulated with AKR marrow would fail to respond to tilorone either by interferon production or NK augmentation. In contrast,CBA or AKR mice repopulated with CBA marrow cells would respond to tilorone with both interferon (IF) and NK enhancement.All combinations produced IF and increased levels of NK cells using NDV,admittedly with AKR marrow reconstituted mice being lower (I,9).Results are shown in table III.

Table II. Effects in vivo or in vitro of interferon inducers, interferon and anti-interferon antisera on NK activity.

A. In vivo treated effector cells	Specific lysis (%lysis) Effector:target ratio		
	I00:I	50:I	25:I
CBA, normal, spleen	37	23	I3
CBA, NDV, spleen	73	62	52
CBA, normal spleen	53	40	26
CBA, tilorone, spleen	93	83	64
CBA, statolon, spleen	94	87	64
C57Bl, nude, normal spleen	45	30	I7
– " –, tilorone spleen	67	52	38
CBA, normal, spleen	32	20	I0
CBA, tilorone spleen	74	60	42
CBA, tilorone + anti-IF, spleen	44	28	I4
CBA, normal spleen	37	23	I3
CBA, IF-treatment, spleen	74	55	42
B. In vitro treated effector cells			
CBA, normal spleen	9	7	3
CBA, poly-I:C spleen	39	23	I2
CBA, normal spleen	I8	–	–
CBA, anti-IF, spleen	I7	–	–
CBA, IF + anti-IF, spleen	I7	–	–
CBA, IF, spleen	54%	–	–

Experiments carried out at peak levels of augmentation. For details of in vivo experiments (II, I7) and in vitro (I0, I8).

Table III. Linkage between inability to produce IF of AKR marrow cells when stimulated by tilorone and failure to show augmented NK ability. Spleen cells as effector cells.

Recipient	Marrow donors	Treatment	Specific lysis I00:I	IF
AKR	CBA	No	32,4	–
–"–	–"–	Tilorone	56,3	++
–"–	–"–	NDV	53,3	++
–"–	AKR	No	7,2	–
–"–	–"–	Tilorone	I2,I	–
CBA	AKR	No	9,2	–
–"–	–"–	Tilorone	8,4	–
–"–	–"–	NDV	I6,6	+
CBA, thx	AKR	No	I,3	–
CBA, thx	AKR	Tilorone	3,5	–
AKR, thx	CBA	No	29,2	–
AKR, thx	CBA	Tilorone	52,5	++

YAC target, 4 hr, chromium release assay. In vivo conditions as in table II (II, I7). thx=thymectomized. –=IF -titers below I0. +=average IF-titers 256. ++=average IF-titers 5I2.

INTERFERON:THE SOLE INDUCER OF NK ACTIVITY?

The preceeding results indicate that so far analyzed all agents capable of enhancing NK activities do seemingly act via interferon(s).One may speculate whether all NK activity is dependent upon interferon.Support for such a possibility come from two sorts of evidence.Mice reared under specific pathogen free conditions have been reported to be close to zero with regard to NK levels but would within days reach normal levels when put under normal,microbiological conditions (I9).Germfree mice have,however,by other workers been found to be relatively normal with regard to NK levels (Kiessling,R. and Herberman,R.B,personal information) so this issue is not quite settled.We have attempted to analyze this question in two ways:a) looking in the supernatants of IF-treated spleen cells for any secondary mediator(I8) without finding evidence for such molecules.b) Inoculating sheep-anti-mouse interferon antisera to normal mice and examining their NK activities several days later.Our results in this regard indicate a selective reduction in NK activity as will be shown in table IV.However,normal sheep serum will by itself as shown have some enhancing effect on NK cells which will make this reduction seem somewhat less efficient.Not included are data from mice tested only 2 days after antiserum inoculation where no reduction of NK activity was appearant indicating that the anti-interferon serum would require some critical time before exerting a measurable reduction.These two sets of data do indicate that interferon when tested as augmentor itself would not require a second,soluble mediator and that endogenous

Table IV.Anti-interferon antibodies:In vitro impact on "IF-induced supernatants" to enhance NK activity.In vivo impact on normal NK levels.

A.Anti-interferon will block "IF-supernatant" activity.

Effector cells	*Specific target lysis(in%)*
Normal spleen cells	*3,5%*
Spleen cells treated with IF +anti-IF	*3,5%*
Spleen cells treated with IF	*I8,6%*
Spleen cells,with "IF-sup"	*I2,0%*
Spleen cells, - " - +anti-IF	*3,0%*

B.Anti-interferon will reduce normal NK levels in vivo.

Effector cells	*Treatment*	*Specific target lysis*		
		I00:I	*50:I*	*25:I*
Spleen cells	*None*	*25,2*	*I9,I*	*I2,2*
- " -	*Normal sheep serum*	*28,0*	*I9,2*	*II,6*
- " -	*Anti-interferon-"-*	*2I,8*	*I4,3*	*8,0*

interferon may well be the final regulator of "normal" NK activities in vivo.Final proof for this would however require access to assays sensitive enough to allow the determination of endogenous interferon in normal sera.

The results in table IV may also require some technical information.The search for a secondary mediator (18) in the supernatants of IF-treated spleen cells was carried out using such supernatants obtained after 3 hours incubation in vitro. Such supernatants were then added to fresh spleen cells for another incubation period of 4 hours before testing for NK activity.Anti-interferon antisera were used in 10-fold excess to original IF added.The results do thus mean that only IF activity was detected in such supernatants assuming pure anti-IF action of the antiserum used.

INTERFERON WILL DIRECTLY INTERACT WITH NK OR NK-LIKE CELLS

Another way to approach the pathways of activation has been to explore if IF acts directly on NK (or pre-NK) cells to make them become more lytic.We will here only comment on our own studies.When analyzing the effect of IF in vitro it soon became clear that IF had a very rapid effect with regard to induction of a process leading to augmentation of NK activity (17).Here it could be shown that anti-IF serum which if added at time 0 with IF would completely block the augmentation of NK activity only had a partial effect if added minutes later.Later studies have in fact indicated 30 seconds contact with IF to be enough (18).This rapid effect would in itself indicate a direct hit with the eventual NK cell, in particular as the results in table IV would fail to indicate the induction of a second,soluble mediator.

That IF acts directly on cells with surface markers similar or identical to NK cells was proven by the use of normal spleen cells fractionated by various procedures before addition of IF in vitro.Removal of adherant cells using nylon wool columns,removal of T cells using anti-Thy-1 antibodies and complement or elimination of B cells and strong Fc-receptor positive cells by filtration through anti-Ig columns did all fail to have any impact on the ability to respond to augmentation by IF in vitro (18).As these fractionation procedures would leave a cell population largely devoid of most conventional cell types except NK cells these data are compatible with the view that IF has a direct effect on NK (or pre-NK cells with similar surface features as studied by these procedures) cells.

INTERFERON-INDUCED AUGMENTATION OF NK ACTIVITY REQUIRES PROTEIN AND RNA SYNTHESIS

The process of augmentation of NK activity can be shown to have metabolic requirements distinct from the lytic action of "normal" NK cells (18,20).Our own data in this regard are quite clearcut with regard to a distinction as to protein and RNA synthesis being required for augmentation but not for the lytic action of already existing NK cells.In contrast,DNA synthesis would not seem to be required for NK augmentation to occur which would fit with the increase taking place within matter of a few hours in vitro (17).Metabolic inhibitors used included cycloheximide for protein inhibition,actinomycin-D for RNA inhibition and Arabinoside-C for inhibition of DNA synthesis (18).From this and findings of others (20) we would conclude that IF augmentation is taking place using a metabolic machinery at least in part distinct from that of already existing NK cells.

MACROPHAGE ACTIVITY MAY HAVE SECONDARY IMPACTS ON NK LEVELS

T lymphocytes as well as macrophages have been implicated as possible suppressor cells for NK cells in vivo (20,21). This action may be exerted via several possible pathways as discussed elsewhere in this volume.The finding that IF is a major regulator of NK activities in vivo makes it possible that certain in vivo variations in NK activity may be due to a relative defiency of another cell type with regard to IF production.We have carried out some model experiments in this regard which we consider supporting such a possibility.PolyI:C is an interferon inducer considered to be dependent upon macrophages for its production (22 and own data).It is also known that newborn mice are very low in NK activity (23), and that they have "odd" macrophages (24).Alpha-fetoprotein is known to exert an immunosupressive action in T-dependent systems (25) but it is not known whether this protein (AFP) exerts its action directly on T lymphocytes or is functioning via action on another celltype,possibly macrophages.AFP can be studied in vitro on adult spleen cells in immune systems and will then inhibit and induce suppressor T cells of a kind which are normally found in the newborn mouse spleen (25).In the present system we have analyzed the effects of poly-I:C in relation to AFP and comparing the effects to those found when attempting to induce NK activity in newborn spleen cells.

Table V.AFP will make adult spleen cells to behave like newborn in their differential reaction patterns towards poly-I:C compared to IF as measured by NK activity.

A.AFP action on adult spleen cells

Poly-I:C	*IF*	*AFP*	*MSA*	*Specific lysis(I00:I)*
-	-	-	-	5,3%
25ug/ml	-	-	-	I8,2%
- " -	-	250ug/ml	-	6,0%
- " -	-	I25 -"-	-	8,4%
- " -	-	60 -"-	-	I5,5%
- " -	-	30 -"-	-	I7,6%
- " -	-	-	500 ug/ml	I7,9%
-	-	-	-	I0,9%
-	I00 IU/ml	-	-	23,4%
-	-"-	250ug/ml	-	I8,I%
-	-	-"-	-	7,I%

B.Differential action of IF and NDV versus poly-I:C on adult versus newborn spleen NK augmentation.

Effector cells (tested at I00:I)	*Activating agents*			
	None	*Poly-I:C 25ug/ml*	*NDV $I0^{5}$ IED*	*IF I00IU/ml*
Young adult spleen (I0 weeks)	*I5,3%*	*34,7%*	*33,2%*	*34,I%*
Newborn spleen (=2 days old)	*2,5%*	*2,7%*	*I0,7%*	*I2,9%*

Augmentation experiments carried out as described (I7). Target of lysis=YAC.=4hr chromium release assay

The results in table V do clearly show that AFP is a potent inhibitor of poly-I:C induced NK activation using adult spleen cells in vitro whereas the effect on IF induced augmentation was only marginal.Thus,AFP would seem to act at the level of IF induction by poly-I:C and preliminary results support such an interpretation.Trivial explanations such as direct binding of AFP to poly-I:C have been excluded.The relevance of this finding to that of newborn NK augmentation is a matter of speculation.It can be clearly shown in the newborn spleen augmentation data (26) that poly-I:C (and poly-A:U,data not shown) are completely without activity using newborn spleen targets.On the other hand other interferon inducers considered independent on macrophage activity such as NDV could be shown as efficient as IF itself.Thus,no doubt exist that newborn spleen cells have a deficiency,presumably at the level of the macrophage response to certain IF-inducers.Whether the fact that the same IF inducers are selectively afflicted by AFP would mean that the newborn macrophage deficiency is caused by endogenous AFP is a testable hypothesis.

The data would anyhow suggest that the reason why newborn

mice are so extremely low in NK activity may in part be due to a lack of a potentiating,IF-producing cell,presumably of macrophage origin.It would here be important to know whether the known impact of silica in vivo with regard to NK activity in adult mice (27) has a similar background.If the main source of endogenous interferon that we assume must exist in normal serum comes from macrophages the present findings may add to our understanding how NK cell levels may be under secondary control by other cell types.

PROLONGED AUGMENTATION OF NK ACTIVITY

Interferon action on NK cells may have beneficial effects in certain tumor or infectious diseases.It would here be of value to understand more about the possibilities to maintain high levels of NK activity in vivo by addition of various agents such as IF or IF-inducers.Likewise,availability of NK cells being maintained in vitro under augmenting conditions would be of both theoretical and possibly clinical interest. We have in the mouse been able to via repeated inoculations of an IF-inducer,tilorone,to in succession obtain repeated peaks of augmented NK activity.Thus,using this procedure we failed to exhaust the NK response machinery within the time span studied (two weeks).IF alone will do likewise and in the human patient systems it has been found that IF if added for several months will still maintain an increased level of NK activity in such human beings (28 and own data).

In vitro augmentation of NK cells has besides type I interferon and type I interferon-inducers also been reported to occur using mixed leukocyte cultures (29-30) or mitogens. Furthermore,use of supernatants from such cultures have been reported to allow propagation of NK cells both in the human (3I) and the mouse (32,33) system.We have just began an analysis of this in vitro system as to the parameters involved. Our attempts to repeat the initial findings,that is using supernatants from in this case mitogen-activated spleen cells to maintain murine NK cells have been quite successful as shown in table VI.Here it can be seen that TCGF (T cell blast growth maintaining factor) obtained from Con A induced supernatant of spleen cells can maintain NK cells (and also possibly also induce NK cells)for several days in a manner not found possible by us in vitro using type I interferon. TCGF was found equally efficient in nude spleen systems and was superior to ConA alone in effectuating the NK effect using normal spleen cell populations.Our attempts to define the active component in TCGF has so far failed to conclusively

Table VI. The effect of TCGF on the maintenance or appearance of cytolytic effector cells in nude and normal mouse spleen.

Effector cells	Augmenting agent	Day	Target lysis (in %)	
			P8I5	YAC
C57Bl/6 nude	Medium only	0	-I,3	I8,6
– " –	– " –	3	I,4	-0,8
– " –	Con A	3	-I,0	0,2
– " –	TCGF	3	0,8	I6,9
– " –	ConA +TCGF	3	I,3	I6,2
C57Bl/6 normal	Medium only	0	-0,5	8,5
– " –	– " –	3	-0,5	-0,3
– " –	Con A	3	I,5	2,8
– " –	TCGF	3	0,6	I2,7
– " –	Con A +TCGF	3	II,0	20,5

For details see 33. Using PHA as a glue supposedly detecting polyclonally activated cytotoxic T lymphocytes no lysis was observed against P8I5 using nude spleen effector cells whereas the last three groups using normal spleen cells yielded lysis at the levels of 9, II and 5I % respectively. Thus, in parallel to NK cell there was also an appearance of killer T cells.

prove that this component is immune interferon. In some tests immune interferon has been present in such culture fluids lacking NK augmenting properties. Still we consider immune or type II interferon a highly viable candidate participating in this prolonged augmentation system. Further experiments are here obviously necessary to define the conditions which seem to activate and maintain NK cells for prolonged periods of time (the table VI does only include day 3 values but NK lytic activities increase in subsequent days if further TCGF is provided). The results of Nabel and Cantor indicating the possibility of creating NK lines by the use of certain TCGF-containing media (personal communication) in the mouse would indicate the feasibility of obtaining well defined conditions for select subsets of immunocompetent cells.

In conclusion, augmentation of NK activities above the normal levels for prolonged periods of time would seem possible both in vivo and in vitro. Analysis of such systems should allow a more definite molecular and cellular understanding of NK cell regulation.

SUMMARY

The natural killer cells have certain features of a select but primitive killer cell. Its sole regulator may be interferon. In vivo regulation of NK activity under normal conditions may in part be under secondary regulation by another cell type making interferon.The NK system is able to sustain itself at a high level of activity for prolonged periods of time if properly supported.

ACKLOWLEDGMENTS

The present work was supported by grants from the Swedish Cancer Society,I.N.S.E.R.M (ATP 78-9I,44.77/79/I3/I6),by the NIH contract NOI-CB-64033 and by the MRC of Canada grant MA 6470.

REFERENCES

I)Kiessling,R.,Klein,E,.and Wigzell,H,.*Eur.J.Immunol.*,*5*,II2,(I975).
2)Herberman,R.B.,Nunn,M.E.,and Lavrin,D.H.,*Int.J.Cancer*,*I6*,2I6,(I975).
3)Welsh,R.M.,and Zinkernagel,R.M.,*Nature*,*268*,646,(I977).
4)Herberman,R.B.,Nunn,M.E.,Holden,H.T.,Staal,S.,and Djeu,J.Y.,*Int.J.Cancer*,*I9*,555,(I977)
5)Minato,N.,Bloom,B.R.,Jones,C.,Holland,J.,and Reid,L.M.,*J.Exp.Med.*,*I49*,III7,(I979).
6)Wolfe,S.E.,Tracey,D.E.,and Henney,C.S.,*Nature*,*262*,584,(I976)
7)Ojo,E.,Haller,O.,Kimura,A.,and Wigzell,H.,*Int.J.Cancer*,*2I*,444,(I978).
8)Herberman,R.B.,and Holden,H.T.,*Adv.Cancer Res.*,*27*,305,(I978)
9)Riesenfeld,I.,Örn,A.,Gidlund,M.,Axberg,I.,Alm,G.,and Wigzell H.,*Int.J.Cancer*,in press.
I0)Haller,O.,Kiessling,R.,Örn,A.,and Wigzell,H.,*J.Exp.Med.*,*I45* I4II,(I977).
II)Gidlund,M.,Örn,A.,Wigzell,H.,Senik,A.,and Gresser,I.,*Nature* *273*,759,(I978).
I2)Trinchieri,G.Santoli,D.,Dee,R.R.,and Knowles,B.B.,*J.Exp.Med* *I47*,I299,(I978).
I3)Djeu,J.Y.,Heinbaugh,J.A.,Holden,H.T.,and Herberman,R.B.,*J.Immunol.*,*I22*,I75,(I979).
I4)Welsh,R.M.,*J.Exp.Med.*,*I48*,I63,(I978).
I5)Herberman,R.B.,Ortaldo,J.R.,and Bonnard,G.D.,*Nature*,*277*,22I,(I979).
I6)Ohmori,K.,Kawata,M.,Okumura,K.,Kuwata,T.,and Tada,T.,*Immunology Letters*,*I*,57,(I979).

I7)Senik,A.,Gresser,I.,Maury,C.,Gidlund,M.,Örn,A.,and Wigzell H,,*Cell.Immunol.,44*,I86,(I979)
I8)Senik,A.,Kolb,J.P.,Örn,A.,and Gidlund,M.,*Scand.J.Immunol.,* in press.
I9)Clark,E.A.,Russell,P.H.,Egghart,M.,and Horton,M.,*Int.J. Cancer,*in press.
20)Herberman,R.B.,Djeu,J.Y.,Kay,H.D.,Ortaldo,J.R.,Riccardi,C. Bonnard,G.D.,Holden,H.T.,Fagnani,R.,Santoni,A.,and Puccetti,P *Immunol.Rev.,44,*43,I979.
2I)Hochman,P.S.,Cudkowicz,G.,and Dausset,J.,*J.Nat.Cancer Inst 6I,*265,(I978)
22)Djeu,J.Y.,Heinbaugh,J.A.,Holden,H.T.,and Herberman,R.B., *J.Immunol.,I22,*I82,(I979)
23)Kiessling,R.,and Wigzell,H.,*Immunol.Rev.,44,*I65,(I979)
24)Landahl,C.A.,*Eur.J.Immunol.,6,*I30,I976.
25)Murgita,R.A.,Goidl,E.A.,Kontiainen,S.,Beverly,P.C. and Wigzell,H.,*Proc.Nat.Acad.Sci.,USA,75,*2897,I978.
26)Örn,A.,to be published.
27)Kiessling,R.,Hochman,P.S.,Haller,O.,Wigzell,H.,Shearer,G., and Cudkowicz,G.,*Eur.J.Immunol.,7,*655,(I977).
28)Einhorn,S.,Blomgren,H.,and Strander,H.,*Acta Med.Scand.,20,* 477,(I978).
29)Ortaldo,J.R.,Bonnard,G.D.,Kind,P.D.,and Herberman,R.B. *J.Immunol.,I22,*I489,(I979).
30)Kärre,K.,and Seeley,J.K.,*J.Immunol.,I23,*I5II,(I979).
3I)Bonnard,G.D.,personal communication.
32)Nabel,G.,and Cantor,H.,personal communication.
33)Grönvik,K.O.,and Andersson,J.,*Immunol.Rev.,in press.*

CHARACTERISTICS OF AUGMENTATION BY INTERFERON OF CELL-MEDIATED CYTOTOXICITY

John R. Ortaldo
Ronald B. Herberman

Laboratory of Immunodiagnosis
National Cancer Institute
Bethesda, Maryland

Julie Y. Djeu

Bureau of Biologics
Bethesda, Maryland

INTRODUCTION

The recent discovery of human and rodent natural cell-mediated cytotoxicity has added yet another mechanism by which a host may resist invasion by tumor cells, foreign cell grafts or infectious agents (see reviews 1,2).

In the mouse the effector cells mediating this natural killer (NK) activity are distinct from mature T cells, B cells, or macrophages. NK activity becomes readily detectable in normal mice about 3 weeks of age. After peak levels of reactivity are reached at 5-8 weeks, there is a decline to low spontaneous levels by about 12 weeks of age. However, mouse NK activity is readily augmented with tumor cells (3,4), allogeneic normal cells (3,4), bacterial products or viruses (3, 4,5-9). With each type of inoculation, the peak level of NK activity is found to usually coincide with the time of appearance of serum interferon (IF). Regardless of the type of stimulus, the augmentation of mouse NK activity appears to be mediated through the induction of IF.

ISBN 0-12-341350-8

In the human system, spontaneous NK effector cells are present throughout life. These cells are characteristically Fc receptor positive, complement receptor negative, negative for surface membrane immunoglobulin, non-phagocytic, and non-adherent. Since human NK cells express T related antigens (10-12) and the majority rosette weakly with sheep red blood cells, they are thought to be in the T cell lineage. As in the case of mouse NK activity, human NK activity can be augmented significantly above the high levels that spontaneously exist in peripheral blood lymphocytes, by treatment with IF in vitro (13,14) or with poly I:C (15). The augmentation of human NK cells with IF results in effector cells with the characterisics of spontaneous NK cells (FcR+, nonphagocytic, surface membrane immunoglobulin negative and the majority havng receptors for sheep erythrocytes). In addition to its influence on other immune functions, (16) IF clearly is involved in the positive regulation of NK activitiy. It is therefore important to analyze the mechanism by which this regulation takes place and to better understand the role of NK *in vivo*. The present report summarizes a series of recent studies on the characteristics of interaction of IF with NK cells and subsequent metabolic requiremnets for the augmentation of mouse and human NK activity.

CHARACTERISTICS OF AUGMENTATION OF NK ACTIVITY BY IF

Detailed studies on the characteristics of the interaction of IF with human (17) and mouse (18) NK cells have been performed. Similar observations have been made with NK cells of both species and the major findings are summarized in Table 1. Pretreatment of lymphocytes with IF, and then washing prior to testing in a 4-hr ^{51}Cr release assay, results in agumentation. Significant levels of boosting have been seen consistently after exposure of either mouse or human lymphocytes to IF for only 5-10 minutes. Peak augmentation occurred after exposure to IF for 10-30 minutes, with levels of reactivity remaining on a plateau when longer periods were studied. The interaction with IF could take place at 4 C as well as at 37 C, with no appreciable differences seen in resultant levels of boosting. Thus, the initial interaction of IF with NK effector cells appeared to be a rapid and temperature independent pendent process and the subsequent events leading to the development of cytotoxicity did not require the continued presence of IF. Evidence that antisera to IF could abrogate the action of IF (subsequent boosting) provided positive evidence for the direct role of IF. These observations are con-

Table 1

Characteristics of Augmentation of NK activity by IF

Features	*Human*	*Mouse*
Pretreatment of cells with IF sufficient and presence during cytotoxicity assay not required	*yes*	*yes*
Necessary interaction with IF:		
occurs rapidly,within minutes	*yes*	*yes*
is temperature independent	*yes*	*yes*
IF action blocked by antiserum to IF	*yes*	*yes*
Augmented activity can be detected within 1-2 hours at 37 C	*yes*	*yes*
Augmentation persists for days	*yes*	*yes*
Boosted by human leukocyte, lymphoblastoid and fibroblast (type I) IF	*yes*	*no*
Boosted by mouse Type I & II IF	*no*	*yes*
Augmentation with purified IF occurs in apparent absence of accessory cells	*yes*	*yes*

sistent with an initial binding of IF to cellular receptors. However, since receptors for IF have not been formally demonstrated, it is possible that some other type of triggering is induced by IF. When IF-pretreated lymphocytes were tested for cytotoxicity, the kinetics were similar to those of spontaneous NK activity. Lysis of target cells was first detected after a lag of 1-2 hours, and at each time point thereafter in the 4 hour assay, the levels of cytotoxicity were higher that those produced by untreated lymphocytes. The augmentation, once begun, remained elevated for 24 to 36 hours in human cells in vitro and for a similar time period in vivo in mice. Pure human leukocyte IF augmented human NK activity to the same extent as partially purified fibroblast or leukocyte IF, thus eliminating the possibility that augmentation was due to some contaminating agent.

METABOLIC REQUIREMENTS FOR AUGMENTATION OF NK ACTIVITY

To determine the metabolic processes required for development of augmented NK activity after treatment with IF, the effects of a variety of metabolic inhibitors were evaluated with both mouse (18) and human (19) NK cells. These results are summarized in Table 2. To evaluate the requirement for DNA

Table 2

Effects of Metabolic Inhibitors on Augmentation of NK Activity by IF

Inhibition of:	*Treatment Time*	*Inhibition of Augmentation of NK Activity by Drug Treatment*	
		Human	*Mouse*
DNA synthesis	*before IF*	*no*	*no*
DNA synthesis	*after IF*	*no*	*no*
RNA synthesis	*before IF*	*yes*	*yes*
RNA synthesis	*after IF*[1]	*yes*	*yes*
Irreversible			
Protein synthesis	*before IF*	*yes*[2]	*yes*
Protein synthesis	*after IF*[3]	*yes*[2]	*yes*
Reversible			
Protein synthesis	*before IF*	*yes*[2]	*no*
Protein synthesis	*during IF*	*yes*[2]	*no*
Protein synthesis	*after IF*	*yes*[2]	*yes*

[1] *Only within 4 hours*

[2] *But interpretation complicated by inhibition also of spontaneous NK (see text)*

[3] *Only within 6 hours*

synthesis in the augmentation of NK activity, lymphoid cells were treated with DNA synthesis inhibitors (x-ray or mitomycin C) prior to IF treatment. Cells treated in such a manner showed little ^{3}H-thymidine incorporation even after stimulation with mitogens, but they still developed increased NK activity in response to IF. The requirement for RNA synthesis was examined by using actinomycin D, an irreversible inhibitor of RNA synthesis, either prior to or after IF treatment. When RNA synthesis was inhibited before IF treatment, no augmentation was seen. Inhibition of augmentation was also seen when

RNA synthesis was blocked within about 4 hours of IF treatment. Later treatment with actinomycin no longer affected the boosted activity. These data indicate that a period of RNA synthesis is required for development and maintenance of augmented NK activity but then the increased reactivity becomes independent of further RNA synthesis. The examination of the requirement for protein synthesis was a logical next step. In this one area, the data regarding the human and mouse effector cells differed substantially. Cytotoxicity by the human spontaneous effector cells was found to be strongly inhibited by reversible (puromycin) or irreversible (emetine) protein synthesis inhibitors. Similarly, after treatment with IF, inhibition of protein synthesis resulted in little or no detectable activity. Since the baseline NK activity was highly susceptible to these inhibitors, it was not possible to separately assess the requirement for protein synthesis in augmentation by IF. In contrast, a clearer picture could be obtained with mouse NK cells since the spontaneous NK activity was unaffected by protein synthesis inhibition. This enabled us to adequately examine the requirement for protein synthesis in IF boosting of mouse NK activity. If irreversible inhibitors (emetine or pactamycin) were used either before or immediately after IF exposure, no augmentation occurred. By using a reversible inhibitor (puromycin) , it was possible to determine the exact period in which protein synthesis was required. Treatment of cells with puromycin before or simultaneous with IF, followed by washing, did not interfere with boosting. In contrast, when puromycin was added within 8 hours after exposure to IF and was left in the medium during the assay, no augmentation was detected. Later addition of puromycin did not interfere with the increased activity. Thus, the ability of the mouse NK cells to interact with IF does not appear to require new production of protein. This would be consistent with the binding of IF to previously formed cellular receptors for IF. The subsequent steps involved in generation and maintenance of augmented activity are dependent on new protein synthesis, for a period somewhat longer than that required for RNA synthesis.

In the rodent system, NK activity can be rapidly augmented *in vivo* by agents that have the ability to induce high levels of serum IF. Viruses, tumor cells and poly I:C boosted NK activity above baseline levels at a time which coincided with the induction of peak levels of serum IF. When spleen cells were harvested at the time of peak of *in vivo* augmentation and treated with DNA, RNA or protein synthesis inhibitors, no interference with the boosted activity was seen (Table 3). These data indicate that *in vivo*-boosted mouse

Table 3

Effects of Metabolic Inhibitors on NK Activity of In Vivo Augmented Mouse Spleen Cells

Boosting Agent	*Time of peak Augmentation*	*Effect of in vitro incubation with synthesis inhibitors of:*		
		DNA	*RNA*	*Protein*
Virus (LCM,Influenza A or cytomegalo-)	*3 days*	*none*	*none*	*none*
NK-sensitive Tumor cells	*24 hours*	*none*	*none*	*none*
Poly I:C	*15 hrs*	*none*	*none*	*none*

effector cells (20), at the height of activity, have acquired all the necessary machinery for target cell lysis and the early events blocked by inhibitors of RNA or protein synthesis are no longer essential for maintaining the augmented state. Since the effector cells had probably been exposed to IF for at least several hours in vivo, these data seem compatible with those obtained in experiments with in vitro boosted cells.

POSSIBLE MODELS FOR MECHANISM OF AUGMENTATION OF NK ACTIVITY BY IF

The analysis of the metabolic requirements provided some insight into the mechansim of boosting of NK activity by IF. The data are compatible with the hypothesis that IF binds to receptors on NK or pre-NK cells and thereby triggers the cells to produce new messenger RNA and then in turn new protein(s) that are involved in the cytotoxic activity of NK cells. This requisite protein(s) may be relatively stable or long-lived, since by 6 hours after treatment with IF, the boosted state seemed to be stable and independent of new RNA or protein synthesis. The data also indicate that augmentation of NK activity does not require any cellular proliferation, but rather some change in the metabolic state of preexisting cells.

These observations and the proposed mechanism for the IF effect on NK activity are similar to those that are already well known for the induction of antiviral resistance by IF (16). Viral resistance in host cells can be induced after a brief contact with IF at $4^{o}C$ or $37^{o}C$ (21). In addition, the establishment of the antiviral state is readily blocked by actinomycin D and inhibitors of protein synthesis, suggesting that new messenger RNA synthesis is required for transcription and translation into antiviral protein(s) or enzyme(s) (16). In the last few years at least 3 enzymes have been discovered which contribute to the antiviral resistance of cells. The enzymes appear to act by inhibiting translation of viral messenger RNA into proteins. A protein kinase(s) has been identified which, in the presence of double-stranded RNA and ATP, phosphorylates an initiator factor to an inactive form, resulting in the decrease of methionine-tRNA binding to 40S ribosomes (22). Another enzyme is an oligoadenylate synthetase, also dependent on double-stranded RNA and ATP, for the synthesis of (2'-5')pppApApA that activates an endonuclease to degrade mRNA (23-25). A third enzyme, phosphodiesterase, does not depend on double-stranded RNA and degrades the cytosine-cytosine-adenosyl-terminus of tRNA, thereby producing tRNA-reversible inhibition of polypeptide chain elongation (26).

Recently, it has been shown that cells incubated with IF showed a 2-3 hr lag in the generation of protein kinase (27). This lag in protein synthesis is similar to that seen in the detection of augmentation of the lytic activity of NK cells. The appearance of several proteins, which are enhanced by IF and are susceptible to actinomycin D (28), displayed a characteristic affinity for double-stranded RNA like the enzymes described in antiviral resistance. The need for new RNA synthesis was time-dependent, since actinomycin D was no longer inhibitory after the cells had been pretreated with IF for 4 hrs. These findings suggest that the biochemical events involved in augmentation of NK activity may be similar to those involved in the induction of antiviral resistance by IF. IF may therefore act via a common pathway to alter a variety of cellular functions.

The evidence that IF induces augmentation of NK activity, not by induction of proliferation of NK cells but by stimulation of new RNA and protein sythesis in cells, leaves further questions as to the nature of the induced change. IF might induce the differentation of pre-NK cells into mature NK cells or might activate or enhance the lytic activity of pre-existing NK cells. The IF-induced proteins might be 1) receptors or recognition structures on NK effector cells, or 2) lytic components or enzymes that are required for, or involved in cytolysis. There are precedents for both possibilities. Treatment of mouse lymphocytes with IF has been shown to induce increased H-2K and H-2D antigens on the cell membrane (29). Production of lytic enzymes may also take place similar to the above mentioned induction of enzymes that inhibit translation of viral proteins in IF-treated cells.

Alternative models for IF-induced augmentation of NK activity are shown in Figure 1. The available data suggests that NK cells arise from precursor stem cells (11,12 and our chapter in IC2), initially coming from the bone marrow (30), and after some proliferation develop into intermediate 'pre-NK' cells. Further defferentiation, from pre-NK cells to active NK cells, might involve the sequential development of some essential components in the lytic machinery and of receptors for recognition of target cells. IF may facilitate or be required for production of either or both types of proteins (effects a and/or b). Alternatively, the maturation of pre-NK to NK cells may be IF-independent with IF acting to increase the lytic efficiency of these cells (effect c) rather than increase the number of NK cells. Again one could divide the possible effects into an increase in some components in the lytic machinery and an increase in the number or avidity of receptors. These various possible effects of IF are not mutually exclusive and IF may be involved both in the generation of more mature NK cells and in increasing the lytic activity of NK cells. At the present time, the evidence in support of each mechanism for IF action is inconclusive. Preliminary attempts to determine the possible effects of IF on induction of more receptors for target cells have given divergent results, with Roder (31) finding no increase in the number of mouse lympho cytes forming conjugates to NK-sensitivie target cells, but with Timonen and Saksela (32) observing an IF-induced augmentation of NK activity by non-conjugate-forming lymphocytes. Bloom et.al. (33) have demonstrated an IF-mediated induction of Ly 5.1 antigen on mouse NK cells. This appears to support the differentiative role of IF. However, since there is no evidence for the involvement of Ly 5.1 in the recognition or lytic processes of NK cells, such interesting results do not directly bear on the alternatives that we have formulated.

The proposed models appear to identify specific possible points for action of IF and further research can be directed towards validation of one or more of these mechanisms for

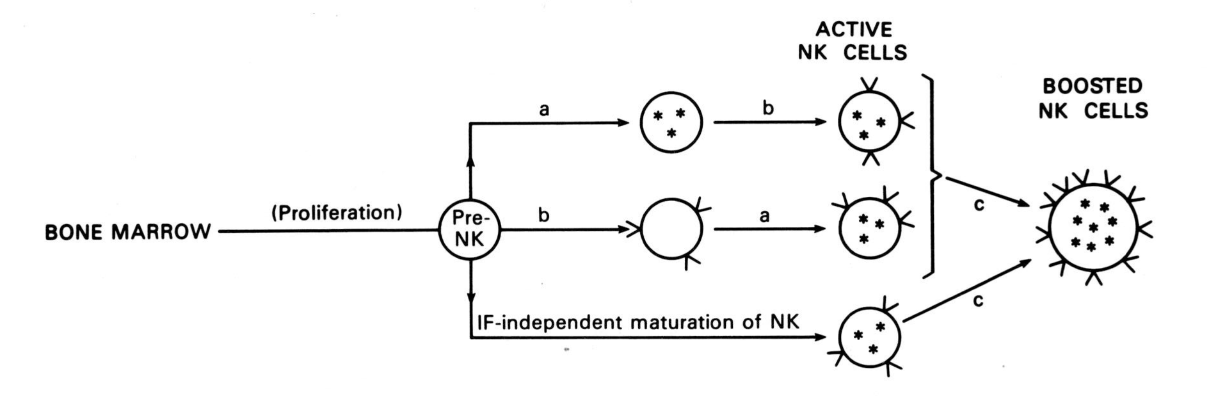

FIGURE I *Models for IF Augmentation of NK Cells.*

Functionally active NK cells may be induced by IF from inactive pre-NK cells via development of lytic machinery (*) and/or receptors for target cells (V) (effects a and/or b). Alternatively, mature NK cells may develop from pre-NK cells by IF-independent differentiation steps and IF may then induce increased activation of the effectors (effect c), by increasing the number of receptors and/or lytic machinery proteins. Also indicated is that these alternative are not mutually exclusive, i.e., effect c may occur in addition to effects a and/or b.

agumentation of NK activity. By preparation of highly enriched or pure populations of NK cells or pre-NK cells, it should be possible to experimentally approach these questions.

EFFECTS OF IF ON VARIOUS TYPES OF CYTOTOXIC EFFECTOR CELLS

One approach to obtain insight into the mechanism of IF augmentation of NK activity has been to examine the spectrum of activity of IF on various types of cytotoxic effector cells. If the main action of IF were to induce specific receptors for recognition and binding to target cells, one might expect IF to similarly affect the receptors for target cell recognition on other types of effector cells, but to have no effect on effector cells that do not require such receptors for their activity. Alternatively, if IF acts mainly on the lytic machinery, one would expect to see similar effects on effector cells having the same cytotoxic mechanism.

Since NK and K cells seem to be very similar, if not identical cells, but appear to function via different cell surface receptors, we have been particularly interested in determining the effects of IF on antibody-dependent cell-mediated cytotoxicity (ADCC). Partially purified human leukocyte and fibroblast IF and pure leukocyte IF, have been found to substantially augment ADCC activity against antibody-coated Chang cells (14,34). It was possible that the apparent boost of ADCC was actually due to augmentation of NK activity against the target cells, acting synergistically with antibodies to give high levels of cytotoxicity. To resolve this, we performed experiments with several target cells that were completely resistant to lysis by human NK cells, even after boosting with IF (mouse tumor lines and chicken erythrocytes) (35). With each target cell, IF treatment of the effector cells induced augmentation of ADCC. It was also possible to treat the lymphocytes with trypsin, which is known to inhibit NK activity but not affect the Fc receptors or ADCC activity. When such trypsinized cells were treated with IF, appreciable augmentation of ADCC was still seen (35). We had yet another opportunity to examine the effects of IF on human ADCC when we observed that leukemic cells from a patient with T cell chronic lymphocytic leukemia had strong ADCC activity in the absence of detectable NK activity (36). Treatment of these leukemic cells with IF substantially augmented ADCC but did not induce any detectable NK activity.

Studies on ADCC by mouse spleen cells, against tumor target cells resistant to NK activity (EL-4), have given comparable results. Pretreatment of the cells with purified IF and *in vivo* boosting of NK activity with virus caused a clear augmentation in ADCC activity compared to control groups (Djeu, unpublished observation). Taken together, our data strongly support the conclusion that IF can augment ADCC as well as NK activity. Since IF boosted ADCC activity of a subpopulation of FcR+ human cells as well as unfractionated mononuclear cells, these observations point toward some effect of IF on lytic machinery common to NK and ADCC, rather than, or in addition to, an effect on cell surface receptors.

Table 4 summarizes our results with other human effector cells. Pure leukocyte IF (34), as well as partially purified fibroblast IF (15), significantly augmented cytolytic activity by peripheral blood monocytes. However, in contrast to the need for only a brief preincubation of NK and K cells with IF, optimal boosting by IF of monocyte-mediated cytolysis required the presence of IF during the 48 hr cytotoxicity assay (15). IF also augmented lectin-induced cell-mediated cytotoxicity (LICC) (37). It was of particular interest that the most dramatic effect was on the subpopulation of E rosetting cells with gamma FcR, with IF inducing a shift from very low activity to high levels. Augmentation of NK activity by IF was also strongest with this subpopulation of cells. This latter observation makes it unlikely that IF is involved in the possible differentiation of non-E-rosetting to rosetting NK cells (see our chapter in IC2).

The rapid effects of IF on LICC, as well as on NK and ADCC in the same subpopulation, further supports the hypothesis of IF acting on a common lytic process. This is consistant with our results that, using Michaelis-Menton kinetics analysis on NK and K effectors, the maximum velocity (Vmax) is increased in the absence of any change in binding affinity (Km). The boosting by IF of monocyte-mediated cytolysis might be taken as an indication of a similar lytic mechanism, but the different time course requirements for the effects on monocytes leaves open the possibility of a different mechanism of action on those effector cells.

Treatment with IF had no effect on reactivity against the relevent PHA-blasts by specific cytotoxic T cells generated in mixed lymphocyte culture. This treatment did augment reactivity against K562 target cells, but this was presumably due to an effect on the NK cells generated during the cultures. IF also had no effect on the cytostatic activity of normal granulocytes, in a 24 hour assay of incorporation of ^{3}H-thymidine by mouse tumor cells (Korec, S. unpublished observation). The

Table 4

Effects of IF on Cytotoxic Reactivity of Various Human Effector Cells

Effector Cells[1]	*Effect*
NK cells	*Boost*
E+, FcR+	*Boost (relatively strong)*
E-, FcR+	*Boost (relatively weak)*
K cells versus variety of antibody-coated targets	*Boost*
Monocytes	*Boost*
Lectin-inducted cytotoxicity	*Boost*
E+, FcR+	*Boost (very strong)*
E+, FcR-	*Boost (relatively weak)*
After Mixed Lymphocyte Culture	
versus K562	*Boost*
versus PHA blasts	*No Effect*
Granulocyte-mediated Cytostasis	*No Effect*

[1] *E+, cells forming rosettes with sheep erythrocytes; E-, cells not forming rosettes with sheep erythrocytes; FcR+, cells with receptors for the Fc portion of IgG; FcR-, cells lacking this FcR; and CRBC, chicken erythrocytes.*

lack of effect of IF on the activity of cytotoxic T cells, which require specific receptors for interaction with target cells, and on granulocytes, which lack any apparent specificity, seems most compatible with these effector cells having cytotoxic mechanisms disparate from those of IF-augmentable effector cells.

CONCLUSIONS

Treatment of mouse or human lymphocytes with IF for a brief period of time leads to substantial augmentation of NK and K cell activities. The metabolic events involved in boosting of NK activity appear very similar to those previously found for induction of aniviral resistance by IF. Cellular proliferation was not required for complete augmentation of cytotoxicity, but for several hours after exposure of IF, active RNA and protein synthesis was needed. This strongly suggests that IF induces the formation of one or more new proteins that play an important role in the cytotoxic activity of NK cells. It is as yet unclear whether IF acts mainly to induce differentiation of pre-NK cells to active NK cells or to increase the lytic efficiency of pre-existing mature NK cells. The ability of IF to also augment ADCC and LICC suggests that it may have an effect on some components of the lytic machinery that are common to all three forms of cytotoxicity.

REFERENCES

1. Herberman, R.B., Djeu, J.Y., Kay, H.D., Ortaldo, J.R., Riccardi, C., Bonnard, G.D., Holden, H.T., Fagnani, R., Santoni, A. and Puccetti, P., Immunol. Rev. 44, 43 (1979).
2. Cudkowicz, G., and Hochman, P.S., Immunol. Rev. 44, 169 (1979).
3. Herberman, R.B., Nunn, M.E., Holden, H.T., Staal, S. and Djeu, J.Y., Int. J. Cancer 19, 555 (1977).
4. Djeu, J.Y., Huang, K.Y. and Herberman, R.B., J. Exp. Med. (in press).
5. Tracey, D.E., Wolfe, S.A., Durdic, J.M., and Henney, C.S., J. Immunol. 119, 1145 (1977).
6. Welsh, R.M. and Zinkernagel, R.M., Nature 268, 646 (1977).
7. Quinnan, G.V., and Manischewitz, J.E., J. Exp. Med. (in press).
8. Djeu, J.Y., Heinbaugh, J.A., Holden, H.T., and Herberman, R.B., J. Immunol. 122, 175 (1979).
9. Gidlund, M.A., Örn, A., Wigzell, H., Senik, A. and Gresser, I., Nature 273, 759 (1979).
10. Bonnard, G.D. and West, W.H., in "Immunodiagnosis of Cancer, Part 2" (R.B. Herberman and K.R. McIntire, eds.), p. 1032. Marcel Dekker Publishers, New York, (1979).

11. Ortaldo, J.R., MacDermott, R.P., Bonnard, G.D., Kind, P.D., and Herberman, R.B., Cell. Immunol. 48, 356 (1979).
12. Ortaldo, J.R., Bonnard, G.D., Kind, P.D., and Herberman, R.B., J. Immunol. 122, 1489 (1979).
13. Trinchieri, G., and Santoli, D., J. Exp. Med. 147, 1314, (1978).
14. Herberman, R.B., Ortaldo, J.R., and Bonnard, G.D., Nature 277, 221 (1979).
15. Jett, J.R., Montavoni, A., and Herberman, R.B., Cell. Immunol. (in press).
16. Stewart, W.E., in "Interferons and their Actions" CRC Press, Clevland (1977).
17. Ortaldo, J.R., Lang, N.P., and Herberman, R.B., (submitted for publication).
18. Djeu, J.Y., Varesio, L., Holden, H.T., and Herberman, R.B., (submitted for publication).
19. Ortaldo, J.R., Phillips, W.P., and Herberman, R.B., (submitted for publication).
20. Djeu, J.Y. and Herberman, R.B., (submitted for publication).
21. Dianzani, F., and Baron, S., Proc. Soc. Exp. Biol. Med. 155, 562 (1977).
22. Chernajovsky, Y., Kimchi, A., Schmidt, A., Ailberstein, A., and Revel, M., Eur. J. Biochem. 96, 35 (1979).
23. Kerr, I.M., and Brown, R.E., Proc. Nat. Acad. Sci. 75, 256 (1978).
24. Ratner, L., Wiegand, R.C., Farrell, P.J., Sen, G.C., Cabrer, B., and Lengyel, P., Biochem. Biophys. Res. Comm. 81, 947 (1978).
25. Baglioni, C., Minks, M.A., and Maroney, P.A., Nature 273, 684 (1978).
26. Schmidt, A., Chernajovsky, Y., Shulman, L., Federman, P., Berissi, H., and Revel, M., Proc. Nat. Acad. Sci. 76, 4788 (1979).
27. Revel, M., Shulman, L., Schmidt, A., Fradin, A. and Kimichi, A., Proc. Natl. Acad. Sci. (in press).
28. Gupta, S.L., Rubin, B.Y., and Holmes, S.L., Proc. Natl. Acad. Sci. 76, 4817 (1979).
29. Vignaux, F. and Gresser, I., J. Immunol. 118, 721 (1977).
30. Bennett, M., Baker, E.E., Eastcott, J.W., Kumar, V., and Yonkosky, J., J. Reticuloendth. Soc. 20, 71 (1976).
31. Roder, J.C., J. Immunol. 23, 2168 (1979).
32. Timonen T. and Sakesela, E., Proc. N.Y. Acad. Sci. (in press).
33. Bloom, B.R., Minato, N., Neighbour, P.A., and Reid, L., Proc. N.Y. Acad. Sci. (in press).
34. Herberman, R.B., Crtaldo, J.R., Jett, J.R., Rubenstein, M., and Pestka, S., (submitted for publication).

35. Ortaldo, J.R., Petska, S., Slease, R.B., Rubenstein, M., and Herberman, R.B., (submitted for publication).
36. Pandolfo, F., Strong, D.M., Slease, R.B., Smith, M.L., Ortaldo, J.R., and Herberman, R.B., (submitted for publication).
37. Lang, N.P., Ortaldo, J.R., and Herberman, R.B., (submitted for publication).

SPONTANEOUS CELL-MEDIATED CYTOTOXICITY (SCMC): ENHANCEMENT BY INTERFERONS AND CORYNEBACTERIUM PARVUM INDUCED T-CELL FACTOR(S) LACKING ANTIVIRAL ACTIVITY §

Hans H. Peter, Helga Dallügge,
Susanne Euler

Abteilung für klinische Immunologie
und Transfusionsmedizin
Dept. Innere Medizin, Med. Hochschule
D-3000 Hannover, GFR

Holger Kirchner, Rainer Zawatzsky

Institut für Virusforschung
Deutsches Krebsforschungsinstitut
D-6900 Heidelberg, GFR

Wolfgang Leibold

Tierärztliche Hochschule Hannover,
D-3000 Hannover, GFR

§) Supported by DFG grants Pe 151/6, Ki 165/3, SFB 54/C2, F2.

ISBN 0-12-341350-8

TABLE OF CONTENT

Footnotes to Page 1: Abbreviations used in the text.

CP: Corynebacterium parvum. E, EA, EAC: Reagents for rosette formation tests: Erythrocyte, antibody, complement. EDTA:
F: Lymphocytes isolated by Ficoll-Hypaque density gradient. FFF: 'F' lymphocytes depleted of iron phagocytosing and plastic adherent cells. FFF-Nylon: 'FFF' lymphocytes treated in addition by passage through nylon wool column. FFF-Nylon-anti-Ig: 'FFF-Nylon' lymphocytes passed in addition through Ig-anti-Ig column. FIF: interferon induced in fibroblasts. IF: interferon. LSR: lymphocyte separating reagent. MLTC: mixed lymphocyte tumor cell reaction. NK: natural killing. PFU: Plaque forming unit. RPMI-ABS, -FCS: Medium RPMI 1640 supplemented with either 10 % heated fetal calf serum or 10 % heated AB serum SCMC: spontaneous cell-mediated cytotoxicity. SIg: surface immunoglobulin. TIF: Tumor cell induced interferon. VSV: vesicular stomatitis virus.

I. INTRODUCTION

Following first reports by Svet-Moldavsky et al (1967) and Borecky et al (1971) on the generation of interferon (IF) during lymphocyte target cell interactions, Trinchieri et al (1978 a, b) established the important role of tumor cell induced IF (TIF) as a major enhancing factor for natural killer (NK) cell activity. It was suggested that the ability of different tumor cell lines to induce IF production in effector lymphocytes is directly related to the selectivity and the degree of cytotoxicity observed against various target cell lines (Trinchieri et al 1978). By now, several other groups (Gidlund et al 1978, Herbermann et al 1979, Djeu et al 1979, Heron et al 1979) have confirmed the role of IF in spontaneous cell-mediated cytotoxicity (SCMC). Highly purified human fibroblast IF (FIF) was recently shown to augment SCMC not only against tumor cell lines but also against fresh leukemic cells (Zarling et al 1979), and first clinical trials are under way to evaluate the anti-tumor effect of IF in vivo (Strander et al 1978).

In the present study we extended previous experiments on a "lymphotoxin-like mediator" generated in SCMC reactions against the IGR3 melanoma cell line (Peter et al 1976). As predicted by Trinchieri et al (1978a) our supernatants from mixed lymphocyte tumor cell cultures (MLTC) contained high levels of anti-viral activity, which has been identified as type 1 IF (Peter et al 1980). Conditions influencing 'endogeneous' IF production and activation of NK cells during SCMC reactions were examined. Furthermore, the enhancing effect of 'exogeneous' human IF on NK cells was confirmed and a new type of NK enhancing factor is described being produced by highly purified T cells upon stimulation with Corynebacterium parvum (CP). This factor is lacking anti-viral activity and seems to preferentially enhance certain selective effector-target combinations.

II. MATERIALS AND METHODS

A. <u>Cell Lines.</u> Standard cell culture conditions and Eagle's minimal essential medium (MEM) supplemented with 10 % heated fetal calf serum (MEM-FCS; all products from Seromed München and Flow Laboratories,

Bonn, GFR) were employed for maintaining the human erythroid leukemia line K562 (Lozzio and Lozzio 1975), the murine leukemia L1210 and the human melanoma IGR3 (Peter et al 1975). The monolayer line IGR3 was suspended prior to use by 3 minute treatment with 0.05 % trypsin and 0.02 % EDTA (Grand Island Biological Cat. No 530).

B. Lymphocyte Isolation and Characterisation. Blood lymphocytes were isolated from 10 healthy male and 4 female donors (20 to 47 years old) according to a previously described separation protocol (Kalden et al 1977, Peter et al 1980). Briefly, defibrinated blood was diluted with saline and LSR (carbonyl iron suspension, Technicon Co., Frankfurt, GFR) at ratios of 3:2:1, respectively. Following a 30 min rotation at room temperature and 45 min of incubation at 37°C in Falcon tissue culture flasks (No 3024) a monocyte depleted cell population was isolated in Ficoll-Hypaque gradients (Böyum 1968) and referred to as fraction FFF (stands for Ferrum, Falcon plastics and Ficoll). The cells were washed twice and resuspended in Medium RPMI 1640 (Seromed München, GFR) supplemented either with 10 % FCS (RPMI-FCS) or 10 % AB serum (RPMI-ABS). In several experiments additional separation steps were performed. A crude lymphocyte enriched population (fraction F) was obtained by separating defibrinated blood on Ficoll-Hypaque gradients. Furthermore, 100 - 150 x 10^6 FFF lymphocytes were incubated for 30 min at 37°C in 5 ml packed nylon wool columns (Greaves et al 1976). The nylon non-adherent cells (fraction-FFF-nylon) were separated either directly into E- and non-E rosetting cells or passed first through an Ig-anti-Ig column (fraction FFF-nylon-anti-Ig) and then separated into T enriched and Null enriched populations (Kalden et al 1977, Peter et al 1980).

In the various lymphocyte preparations E-, EA-, EAC-rosettes formation, surface membrane Ig (SIg) Latex phagocytosis and diffuse unspecific esterase staining were determined according to previously described techniques (Kalden et al 1977; Rajvanshi et al 1979; Peter et al 1980).

C. Reagents

Corynebacterium parvum (CP), strain CN 6134, a formalin-killed suspension (7 mg dry weight/ml) from Burroughs Wellcome, Beckenham Kent, U.K., was used at a final concentration of 140 ug/ml for IF production (Kirchner et al 1979). Human Fibroblast (Diploid) Interferon (FIF), Charge No 8, 2.1 x 10^6 IU/ml, was a gift of Dr. Rentschler GmbH, Laupheim GFR.

Tumor cell induced leukocyte Interferon (TIF). 50 x 10^6 normal FFF lymphocytes were mixed with 5 x 10^6 tumor cells (K562, IGR3 or L1210) and incubated in 50 ml of RPMI-ABS for 36 hrs at 37°C. Cell free culture supernatants were collected, filtered through 0.22 um Millipore filters and tested for anti-viral activity and SCMC enhancing capacity. Human Leukocyte Reference Interferon induced by Sendai virus was kindly provided by the NIH, Bethesda, Maryland (Ref. No.-G-023-901-257 NIAID).

D. Interferon (IF) Production Cultures. The various lymphocyte fractions were adjusted to 10^6 cell per ml in RPMI-FCS or RPMI-ABS. Aliquots of one ml were placed in Falcon tissue culture tubes (No. 2054) togehter with 0.1 ml of IF inducer suspension containing either 10^5 living tumor cells or 140 ug of CP. In a first series of experiments the kinetics of IF production were studied using cultures of lymphocyte subpopulations exposed for 6, 12, 24 and 36 hrs to tumor cells (K562, IGR3, L1210) or CP. Subsequently IF production cultures were run in parallel to SCMC assays using the same tumor cells as IF inducer and SCMC targets. In these experiments identical culture conditions and incubation periods of 6 or 12 hrs were chosen for both SCMC assays and IF production cultures. IF secreted during the SCMC assays was referred to as "endogenous TIF" as opposed to "exogeneous IF" which was added to SCMC assays to test for enhancement of cytotoxicity. Culture supernatants containing IF were tested for remnants of IF inducers by admixing aliquots of 0.1 ml to fresh lymphocyte suspensions and incubate for 24 hrs as described above for IF production cultures. The procedure was referred to as test for "interferonogenicity" of culture supernatants.

E. Interferon (IF) Assay and Characterization of TIF. Leukocyte culture supernatants were tested for their ability to interfere with the replication of

Vesicular Stomatitis Virus (VSV; strain Indiana) in a permanent line of monkey kidney cells Rita. A highly sensitive virus yield reduction assay was employed (Stewart 1979; Kirchner et al 1979; Peter et al 1980).

The anti-viral activities released into the supernatants of MLTCs were subjected to several treatments: a. Centrifugation at 100.000 x g for 2 hrs. b. Treatment with trypsin (0.2 mg/ml) for one hour at 37 ^{o}C followed by the addition of FCS to stop the reaction. c. Dialysis at pH 2.0 in a glycin/HCl buffer for 24 hrs and subsequent overnight neutralization by dialysis at pH 7.4 in Hank's balanced salt solution. d. Heating to 37 ^{o}C and 56 ^{o}C for one hour. e. Testing for antiviral activity on both monkey kidney cells (Rita) and mouse fibroblasts (L-929).

F. <u>Spontaneous cell-mediated cytotoxicity (SCMC).</u> Spontaneous or natural cytotoxicity of lymphocytes was measured in a previously described ^{51}Cr release assay against K562, IGR3 and L1210 targets (Peter et al 1975; Rajvanshi et al 1979). Six and 12 hours tests were performed as triplicates in round bottom microculture plates (Linbro Co.). 10^4 chromium labelled target cells were incubated with 10 to 25 x 10^4 effector lymphocytes in a total volume of 0.2 ml at 37 ^{o}C and 5 % CO_2. Endogeneous TIF was determined in parallel microplate or tube cultures set up under identical conditions with unlabeled tumor cells. Exogeneous IF or culture supernatants from MLTCs and CP stimulated lymphocyte cultures were added in a final dilution of 1:2 either at the beginning of the test or after 6 hrs. In other experiments effector or target cells were preincubated in IF for one hour, washed once and then added to the test. Prior to and following incubation at 37 ^{o}C the SCMC microplates were spun for 2 min at 200 x g. The Skatron disposible supernate collecting device (DSC, Titertek, Flow Laboratories, Bonn GFR) was used to harvest the tests. Results were expressed as per cent specific ^{51}Cr release calculated as follows: (cpm_{test} $-cpm_{spontaneous}$):(cpm_{total} $-cpm_{spontaneous}$) x 100. The effect of exogeneous IF on NK cell activity was expressed as per cent increase of specific cytotoxicity: (SCMC ⊕IF - SCMC ⊖IF) : (SCMC ⊖IF) x 100.

III. RESULTS

A. Studies on the Producer Cell and the Type of IF Generated in Human Leukocyte Cultures Exposed to Tumor Cells or CP. The appearance of anti-viral activity in MLTCs and leukocyte cultures stimulated with CP was first investigated in kinetic studies. The simultaneous use of different lymphocyte subpopulations allowed additional conclusions as to the producer cell of TIF and CP induced IF. Figure 1 illustrates the results of a typical experiment. There was a striking similarity in the lymphocyte subpopulation requirments for the production of IF induced by tumor cells and CP. The T cell enriched populations were invariably ineffective in response to these inducers, whereas fractions F, FFF-nylon, FFF-nylon-anti-Ig and the Null cell enriched populations were excellent IF producers. In the great majority of the experiments IF was detectable between 6 and 12 hrs and became maximal between 12 and 24 hrs. L1210 and to a lesser extent K562 were exceptional in that they induced very rapidly high concentrations of IF in unfractionated (F) and monocyte depleted populations (FFF-Nylon) followed by a decrease of anti-viral activity by 24 hrs. The possibility that part of the generated TIF may be produced by tumor cells instead of lymphocytes has previously been excluded for the three tumor lines employed in this study (Peter et al 1980). According to the biochemical properties summarized in Table 1, TIF corresponds to type 1 IF as has already been shown for CP induced IF (Kirchner et al 1979).

B. Conditions Influencing the Generation of IF and SCMC in MLTCs. Having demonstrated the requirment of Null lymphocyte containing subpopulations for the production of TIF (Figure 1), it was of interest to find out if in a given MLTC NK cell activity would run in parallel to endogeneous TIF. Typical results selected from 7 experiments are shown in Table 2. As can be seen T cells were equally poor SCMC effectors as TIF producers, whereas non-T cells exhibited good activities in both assays. However, depending on the serum supplementation and the target cells employed a boost of T cell mediated SCMC and TIF production was repeatedly noted (Table 2, Exp. A) Thus, T cells co-cultured with K562 in RPMI-FCS

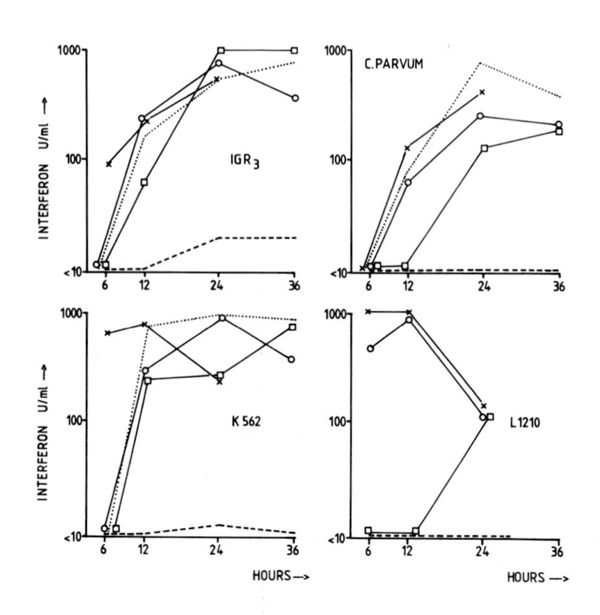

Figure 1:

Kinetics of tumor cell induced IF production by human lymphocyte subpopulations exposed to three tumor cell lines (two allogeneic - K562, IGR3 - and one xenogeneic - L1210) and CP. The following lymphocyte preparations were examined. a) Fraction F (x ——— x), a Ficoll-Hypaque isolated crude lymphocyte preparation. b) Fraction FFF-Nylon (o ——— o) was depleted of readily phagocytosing cells by iron treatment, plastic surface adherence and passage through a nylon fiber column. c) Fraction FFF-Nylon-anti-Ig (□ ——— □) was additionally passed through an Ig-anti-Ig column to remove B cells and Fc+ lymphocytes. d) T enriched (--------) was prepared from FFF-Nylon-anti-Ig by E-rosette formation and subsequent sedimentation in a Ficoll-Hypaque gradient. e) Null enriched fraction (........) corresponds to the non-E-rosetting cells of fraction FFF-Nylon-anti-Ig.

Table 1: CHARACTERIZATION OF INTERFERON PRODUCED IN MIXED CULTURES OF HUMAN LYMPHOCYTES AND ALLOGENEIC OR XENOGENEIC TUMOR CELLS[+)]

Tumor Lines	Treatment of Culture Supernates						
	None	Centrifugation (100.000xg/2hrs)	$56^{\circ}C/1hr$	Dialysis (pH2/24hrs)	Trypsin (0.2mg/ml)	$37^{\circ}C/1hr$	Dialysis (pH7.4/ 24hrs)
IGR3	900[§]	800	400	375	<5	900	450
K562	700	650	450	400	<5	800	520
L1210	750	700	350	450	<5	850	430
NIH Reference Interferon[++]	500	400	390	450	<5	500	450

+) 10^6 human leukocytes (fraction F) were co-cultured with 10^5 tumor cells in 1 ml RPMI-ABS for 24 hrs. The culture supernates were tested for IF (see also "Materials and Methods").

++) See "Materials and Methods".

§) Interferon activity expressed in IU/ml.

produced significantly higher TIF and NK cell activity than in RPMI-ABS, whereas the reverse was always true for MLTCs of T cells and IGR3 melanoma cells.

A dissociation of TIF production and SCMC was consistently found in the lymphocyte fraction that had been passed through nylon wool and Ig-anti-Ig columns (Fraction FFF-Nylon-anti-Ig). As can be seen in Table 2 (Exp. B) this cell fraction was depleted for B cells, monocytes and Fc-receptor bearing cells and enriched for T and Null cells. While being still capable of producing TIF the cells had almost completely lost their SCMC activity. A second passage through Ig-anti-Ig columns was necessary to remove also the TIF producing lymphocytes. Similarly, the Null fractions obtained after depletion of T cells, B cells monocytes and Fc-receptor positive cells were excellent TIF producers but exhibited only moderate SCMC. These findings suggest the requirement of Fc-receptor pos.Null or T cells for the full display of SCMC but not for the production of TIF.

Another interesting dissociation between endogenous TIF and SCMC was noted in two kinetic experiments shown in Table 3. In both experiments SCMC preceeded the maximal appearance of TIF. Moreover, the secretion of high levels of endogenous TIF seemed to impede NK activity. In the case of the L1210 target the very early generation of high TIF levels may be responsible for the comparatively low susceptibility to NK lysis of this target.

C. <u>Enhancement of SCMC by Exogenous IF.</u>

Table 4 summarizes results of SCMC assays against K562, IGR3 and L1210. Besides various concentrations of human FIF, three batches of human TIF (s. Materials and Methods) were also examined for SCMC enhancing activity. The IF preparations were either added directly into the test or used for preincubating effector and target cells. Up to 80 % of SCMC enhancement was measured. SCMC against IGR3 and L1210 was quite regularly enhanced by FIF and TIF whereas K562 was mostly resistant to NK enhancing factors. An exception of this rule was found when target cells were preincubated in IF and then exposed to effector lymphocytes. Under these conditions both allogeneic lines K562 and IGR3 were significantly increased in their susceptibility to NK lysis

Table 2: TUMOR CELL INDUCED INTERFERON AND SCMC: ROLE OF LYMPHOCYTE SUBPOPULATIONS AND SERUM SUPPLEMENTATION

Lymphocyte Fractions[+]	Cell Surface Markers[+]						12 Hours M L T C (L/T 10:1)[++]			
	E	EA	EAC	SIg	Latex ANAE	Serum Suppl.	K562 SCMC	K562 TIF	IGR3 SCMC	IGR3 TIF
A. FFF-Nylon	78[x]	12	7	5	1	10%FCS	57[&]	820[§]	24	820
						10%ABS	44	820	55	1000
T Enriched	88	6	2	1	0	10%FCS	25	162	8	10
						10%ABS	10	90	29	180
B. F	66	15	25	10	23	10%FCS	64	240	29	400
FFF-Nylon	70	8	7	4	1	"	62	1000	34	680
FFF-Nylon-1x-anti-Ig	85	2	1	0	0	"	6	240	9	1000
FFF-Nylon-2x-anti-Ig	94	0	0	0	0	"	n.t.	<5	n.t.	8
T Enriched	89[a]	1	1	0	0	"	0	40	1	45
Null Enriched	20[a]	1	n.t.	4	1	"	26	1000	7	480

+) For details see "Materials and Methods".
++) SCMC and endogenous TIF were determined in parallel microplate cultures.
x) Per cent of 200 evaluated cells. &) Per cent specific ^{51}Cr release. §) IU/ml of interferon.
a) Re-rosetting values after over night incubation at 37°C. Immediately after separation the Null enriched fraction contained 5% E-rosettes. n.t. not tested

Table 3: TUMOR CELL INDUCED INTERFERON AND SCMC: KINETIC ASPECTS

Exp. No.	Lymphocyte Donor Initials, Sex, Age	Targets	L/T Ratio	6 Hours		12 Hours	
				SCMC[+]	IF[++]	SCMC[+]	IF[++]
11	F.B.,m,29	K562	16:1	34	<5	42	540
		IGR3	16:1	12	<5	11	100
		L1210	16:1	10	1000	9	1000
12	K.C.,f,25[&]	K562	10:1	32	200	12	1000
		IGR3	20:1	11	20	17	1000

+) SCMC assays and IF production cultures were run in parallel under strictly identical conditions: Microplate cultures, 0.2 ml total volume, FFF effector lymphocytes, RPMI-FCS. For details see "Materials and Methods". SCMC is expressed as per cent specific ^{51}Cr release.

++) Interferon expressed in IU/ml.

&) Corresponds to donor No 6 of Table 6.

whereas the xenogeneic L1210 leukemia remained unaffected.

In Table 5 cell free culture supernatants were harvested from 6 and 12 hrs MLTCs of normal FFF lymphocytes stimulated with K562, IGR3 and L1210 cells. After determination of anti-viral activity the supernatants were added back to SCMC tests involving fresh lymphocytes from the same donor and ^{51}Cr labelled K562, IGR3 or L1210 targets. Addition of the supernatants at the beginning of the SCMC assay caused a significant increase of cytotoxicity against IGR3 and L1210 but not against K562. The increase of cytotoxicity could be roughly correlated to the TIF content of the added supernatants. SCMC enhancing activity was, however, no longer detectable when the supernatants were added 6 hrs after the beginning of the test. This observation suggests that NK cells once engaged into effector-target interactions become refractory to enhancing factors such as IF.

D. Corynebacterium Parvum (CP) Induced SCMC Enhancing Factor(s). CP has been found to be a potent inducer of type 1 IF in human leukocyte cultures (Kirchner et al 1979; Vilcek et al 1979) provided the culture medium was supplemented with ABS (Peter et al 1980). When cultures were run in RPMI-FCS considerable lower anti-viral activity was induced (Peter et al 1980) and lymphocytes (fraction FFF) from one out of 10 healthy donors failed even to produce any IF in RPMI-FCS after stimulation with CP (Table 6, donor No 6, K.C.,f,25). The same lymphocytes were, however, perfectly capable to produce TIF in FCS supplemented medium (Table 3). Surprisingly the CP induced and IF negative culture supernatant still enhanced SCMC in certain effector-target combinations (Table 6). The entire checkerboard presented in Table 6 shows results from an experiment involving 4 SCMC effectors (fraction FFF), two targets (IGR3, L1210) and 10 previously generated supernatants from CP stimulated lymphocytes cultures including those from the 4 SCMC effectors (donor No 6, 7, 8, 10). In the presence of CP induced supernatants effector lymphocytes from donors No 6 and 7 exhibited significantly enhanced SCMC against both targets whereas donors No 8 and 10 produced only enhancement against L1210 or IGR3, respectively. No obvious relationship could be

Table 4: ENHANCEMENT OF SCMC BY EXOGENOUS INTERFERON (IF)

IF Added to SCMC Assay		SCMC[+]								
Source	Activity (IU/ml)	K562 (L/T 10:1)			IGR3 (L/T 20:1)			L1210 (L/T 10:1)		
		A	B	C	A	B	C	A	B	C
Controls[§]	0	23[&]	25	25	20	20	20	13	22	25
Fibroblast IF	$2x10^3$	+30[a]			+80			+69		
"	$2x10^4$	+9	-8	+40	+45	-5	+20	+85	+23	0
"	$2x10^5$	-9			-5			+46		
MLTC, IGR3	$3x10^2$	-9	-20	+44	-15	+25	+85	+46	+14	-12
" , K562	$4x10^2$	-4	-28		+30	+50		+46	+18	
" , L1210	$4x10^2$	0	-16		+25	+25		+60	+18	

+) A, IF was added to the assay. B, preincubation of the effector cells in IF prior to SCMC assay. C, Preincubation of target cells in IF. For details see "Materials and Methods".

§) RPMI-FCS, supernates from cultures of tumor cells or lymphocytes alone.

&) Per cent specific ^{51}Cr release.

a) Per cent increase of specific cytotoxicity above controls.

Table 5: ENHANCEMENT OF SCMC BY EXOGENOUS TIF DERIVED FROM LYMPHOCYTES AUTOLOGOUS TO THE EFFECTORS

Supernatant[+]	Added to SCMC:	S C M C Assay (L/T 16:1)[+] At the beginning			After 6 Hours		
MLTC Cource[+]	Exogenous TIF (IU/ml)	IGR3[++]	K562[++]	L1210[++]	IGR3[++]	K562[++]	L1210[++]
IGR3, 6 hrs	2.000	31[&]	1	44	-7	7	-6
IGR3, 12 hrs	10.000	69	0	103	9	-4	-6
K562, 6 hrs	3.000	48	7	63	13	1	-18
K562, 12 hrs	10.000	31	-5	75	6	0	-12
L1210, 6 hrs	60	24	1	37	0	3	-18
L1210,12 hrs	10.000	44	-3	62	6	-8	-12
Controls[§]	5	29[a]	69	16	31	72	16
		2.000[b]	2.000	500	2.000	2.000	500

+) Lymphocytes (fraction FFF) from a healthy donor (P.H.,m,37) were mixed with the indicated tumor lines at a 16:1 L/T ratio and cultured for 6 and 12 hrs. The cell free supernates were collected and added in a final dilution of 1:2 to SCMC assays performed 2 days later with freshly prepared effector lymphocytes from the same donor.

++) Targets for SCMC assay. &) Per cent increase of specific cytotoxicity above controls.

§) RPMI-FCS, supernatants from tumor cells or lymphocytes cultured alone.

a) Per cent specific ^{51}Cr release. b) Endogenous TIF in IU/ml produced during SCMC assay.

established between IF content of the culture supernatants and their SCMC enhancing activity. The data were interpreted as being consonant with the existence of an IF independent SCMC enhancing factor in supernatants of human leukocyte cultures stimulated for 24 hrs with 140 ug of CP. To corroborate this finding cell separation experiments were performed designed to identify the producer cell of this factor. The essential results of these experiments are summarized in Figure 1 and Table 7. Whereas lymphocyte preparations containing Null cells (fractions F, FFF, FFF-Nylon, FFF-Nylon-anti-Ig and the Null enriched fraction) produced IF in response to CP, highly purified T cells secreted a supernatant factor(s) which lacked anti-viral activity but still enhanced SCMC against certain tumor targets (IGR3 and L1210, but not K562). For the sake of simplicity Table 7 shows only results with target IGR3. As can be seen CP induced T cell supernatants from both FCS and ABS supplemented cultures contained no anti-viral activity,did not induce IF in fresh FFF lymphocytes but significantly enhanced SCMC. Since this enhancement could not be explained by an increased endogenous TIF production during the SCMC reaction the generation of an NK enhancing factor distinct from IF had to be assumed in CP stimulated T cell cultures.

IV. DISCUSSION

The interest of immulogists in IF rose markedly since it became evident that leukocytes produce anti-viral activity as a result of immune specific or non-specific interactions with a wide range of IF inducers (Wheelock 1965; Stewart 1979; Falcoff 1972). Based on physico-chemical properties two classes of IF have been identified in human leukocyte cultures: The acid and heat-stabile type 1 IF corresponding to the classical virus induced fibroblast IF and the acid and heat labile type 2 IF, being exclusively produced after specific interaction of antigens or mitogens with the relevant immunocompetent cells (Stewart 1979). In previous studies our group has identified Null lymphocytes as producer cells of type 1 IF in human leukocyte cultures stimulated with Herpes simplex virus, CP or tumor cells (Kirchner et al 1979; Peter et al 198o). This finding was of a certain interest in

Table 6: CP INDUCED INTERFERON AND SCMC ENHANCING ACTIVITY IN HUMAN LYMPHOCYTE CULTURES

Supernatants+ Added to SCMC		12 Hours S C M C+ (L/T 20:1)							
Lymphocyte Donors	IF Content	No 6,K.C.f.25++		No 7,P.H.m.37		No 8,F.K.m.31		No 10,S.E.f.24	
Initials, Sex, Age	(IU/ml)	L1210§	IGR3	L1210	IGR3	L1210	IGR3	L1210	IGR3
No 1,L.S.,m.39	50	80&	93	56	46	31	11	-8	55
No 2,A.G.,m,42	50	65	79	68	61	29	0	-2	38
No 3,S.M.,f,20	155	32	62	45	47	47	-2	-9	26
No 4,H.B.,m,47	35	41	57	39	30	30	-7	-9	36
No 5,J.C.,m,36	200	48	72	69	42	50	-2	-2	25
No 6,K.C.,f,25	<5	39	53	41	17	23	-9	-11	17
No 7,P.H.,m,37	50	38	71	23	37	48	-2	1	21
No 8,F.K.,m,31	10	36	51	37	25	26	-9	-12	23
No 9,H.D.,f,25	55	45	53	36	43	23	-9	-10	25
No10,S.E.,f,24	40	48	85	56	41	35	-1	9	33

+) 10^6 lymphocytes (fraction FFF) from healthy donors were cultured with 140 ug of CP for 24 hrs in 1 ml of RPMI-FCS. The supernatants were stored at $-70^{\circ}C$ and added two days later to SCMC assays in a final dilution of 1:2.

++) Effector cells (fraction FFF)

§) ^{51}Cr labelled target cells.

&) Per cent increase of specific cytotoxicity.

Table 7: ENHANCEMENT OF SCMC BY CP INDUCED T CELL FACTOR(S) LACKING ANTI-VIRAL ACTIVITY

Original Culture	Supernatant[+] Added to SCMC: IF Content (IU/ml)	Supernatant[+] Added to SCMC: Interferonogenicity[&] (IU/ml)	"Endogenous TIF"[§] (IU/ml)	SCMC[++] (Target: IGR3) % Specific ^{51}Cr Release	(% Increase)
RPMI-FCS	0	0	1000	8	
Controls	<5	<5	160-185	9-10	
T cells[x] + CP	<5	<5	230	29	(190)
T cells + IGR3	<5	<5	370	16	(60)
RPMI-ABS	0	0	1000	15	
Controls	<5	<5	330-1000	18-20	
T cells + CP	<5	<5	820	42	(110)
T cells + IGR3	180	240	1000	37	(85)

+) Supernatants from 24 hrs IF production cultures supplemented with FCS or ABS. Controls comprised cultures of highly purified T cells, IGR3 or CP alone. The cell free supernatants were added to the SCMC reactions in a final dilution of 1:2.

x) For isolation procedure see "Materials and Methods", 90 % E; <1 % SIg; <1 % Latex

&) Capacity of supernatants (+) to induce SCMC effectors for IF production in the absence of targets.

++) Spontaneous cell-mediated cytotoxicity, 12 hrs assay, effector cells (fraction FFF) from donor No 6 (K.C.f,25), L/T ratio 25:1. For details see "Materials and Methods".

§) Tumor cell induced IF produced during SCMC assay.

view of the established role of Fc receptor positive Null cells as SCMC effectors and the recent finding that IF augments NK cell activity (Trinchieri et al 1978b; Droller et al 1979; Herberman et al 1979). Following our previous report on a "lymphotoxin-like mediator" produced in human MLTCs (Peter et al 1976) Trinchieri et al (1978a) discovered type 1 IF in the culture supernatants of human MLTCs. Table 1 confirms this finding and extends it to the three tumor lines used in this study. The possibility that in MLTCs the tumor cells by themselves may produce IF has been delt with in depth and can be excluded for the line K562, IGR3 and L1210 (Peter et al 1980). Obscure remains, however, the actual tumor cell structure that induces TIF. Besides tumor associated membrane antigens, the recently discovered NK target structures (Roder et al 1979) and artificial antigens introduced by unknown virus or mycoplasma infections (Sokhey et al 1977) have to be considered. Although regular mycoplasma controls did not reveal an overt contamination of our cultures the questionable reliability of such negative tests is well known. Evidence was provided that serum supplementation with FCS or ABS may depress or enhance SCMC against a given tumor target and cause a concommittant change of endogeneous TIF production. The use of lymphocyte subpopulations led to the disclosure of a dissociation between endogenous TIF production and SCMC. In accordance with Trinchieri et al (1978a) the major population responsible for TIF production in human MLTCs was a nylon-nonadherent, E-rosette negative, SIg negative lymphoid cell type which in our hands could not be removed by a single passage through Ig-anti-Ig columns (Table 2). The effluent cell population from these columns was greatly depleted of B cells, Latex phagocytosing monocytes and Fc-receptor positive cells; it showed a strong decrease of SCMC but exhibited almost an unreduced capacity to produce TIF. Separation into T and Null cell enriched populations clearly localized the IF producing cells in the Null cell fraction. A second passage through Ig-anti-Ig columns removed also the TIF producing cells suggesting that they may be distinguished from NK cells by the absence or the reduced expression and avidity of Fc-receptors. Taking into consideration the recent work of Lohmann-Matthes et al (1978, 1979; Domzig and

Lohmann-Matthes 1979) and the previous finding that human Null cells are highly enriched for hemopoietic precursors (Oehl et al 1977, 1978; Richman et al 1978) we would favor the hypothesis that TIF producers and NK cells in human MLTCs represent different stages of monocyte differentiation. Thereby IF production appears to lead the chain of events, followed by the expression of Fc receptors, the display of cytotoxicity and finally the maturation to phagocytosing monocytes. The capacity to produce IF doesn't necessarily have to be lost during this differentiation process since there is good evidence that promonocytes and mature mononuclear phagocytes may also produce IF in response to certain inducers (Roberts et al 1979; Borecky et al 1972; Neumann and Sorg 1977; Lohmann-Matthes et al 1979).

Trinchieri et al (1978b) have shown that TIF while enhancing SCMC may at the same time modulate the target cell susceptibility to lysis. Due to the species specificity of IF, in allogeneic lymphocyte tumor cell combinations the endogenously produced TIF may bind to both target and effector cells thus rendering their lytic interaction more efficient. In xenogeneic combinations TIF may bind only to the lymphocyte causing only moderate SCMC activity but allowing higher levels of IF to appear in the supernatant (Table 3). The results presented in Table 4 with target cell preincubation in IF would support this view. Preincubation of K562 and IGR3 in human FIF or TIF enhanced the subsequent action of NK cells, whereas no such enhancement was noted for L1210 cells preincubated in human IF. The argument that SCMC enhancement by preincubating the target cells in culture supernatant or IF preparations may be due to natural antibodies is not valid since virus infected fibroblasts do not produce antibodies and the supernatants from IGR3 stimulated lymphocyte cultures have already been shown to possess NK enhancing activity not related to IG (Peter et al 1976).

For unexplained reasons K562 was in many experiments resistant to the SCMC enhancing effect of exogenous TIF particulary when added into the test system or used to preincubate the effector cells. SCMC against K562 could, however, be enhanced by FIF as has also be shown by Zarling et al (1979). IGR3 and L1210 were both excellent targets to measure the NK enhancing effects of exogenous IF (Table 4 and 5). Interestingly no SCMC enhancement was noted when TIF from culture supernatants was added 6 hours after the SCMC reaction had been started (Table 5). At present this observation is difficult to interpret. It could mean that once SCMC effector cells are engaged in target cell lysis they become resistant to the enhancing effects of IF. On the other hand, the phenomenon brings into mind the well known hyporesponsiveness of various cell cultures to secondary IF induction discussed in detail by Stewart (1979).

A potentially important and new aspect of the NK reaction is the discovery of a CP induced T cell factor(s) which enhances SCMC but lacks anti-viral activity. If confirmed this factor would represent after natural antibody - a B cell product - (Troye et al 1977) and type 1 IF - a Null cell product - (Trinchieri et al 1978; Kirchner et al 1979; Peter et al 1980) the first T cell product that has been shown to augment NK cell activity. A peculiarity of this factor is its selective activity in certain effector-target combinations. It is feasible that similar T cell factors may also be induced by other stimulants perhaps also by tumor cells. A future task will be to dissect NK reactions for the contributions of different mediators. For the CP induced T cell factor the combination of FCS supplemented medium and highly purified T cells assured no overlap with IF production. Contamination with natural antibodies has not yet been excluded but appears unlikely considering the highly purified T cell preparations used to produce the factor and its selectivity for certain target-effector combinations. Currently several possibilities as to the biological meaning of this factor are discussed. a) It may still hide minute amounts of IF or IF related structures (e.g. IF precursor molecules) (Stewart 1979) not detectable with the highly sensitive virus yield-reduction assay. b) Various T cell factors have to be considered such as specific and unspecific macrophage cytotoxic factors (Evans et al 1972; Lohmann-Matthes et al 1973), unspecific T helper cell factor (Schimpel 1972; Watson et al 1979) or antigen specific T cell factors (Taussig et al 1975). Further immunological and biochemical characterization of T cell factors enhancing SCMC are currently in progress in our laboratory.

V. SUMMARY

Human blood lymphocytes exposed for 6 to 24 hours 'in vitro' to tumor cells (K562, IGR3, L1210) and Corynebacterium parvum (CP) produced high levels of anti-viral activity which was identified as type 1 interferon (IF). Lymphocyte fractionation procedures involving iron/plastic treatment, nylon wool columns, Ig-anti-Ig columns and E-rosette separation led to the identification of Null cells as highly efficient producers of type 1 IF. In mixed lymphocyte tumor cell cultures (MLTC) tumor cell induced IF (TIF) roughly parallel spontaneous cell-mediated cytotoxicity (SCMC) and both activities could be modulated together by altering serum supplementation and lymphocyte subpopulations. Evidence is, however, presented that TIF is at least partly produced by a Fc-receptor negative Null cell subset whereas SCMC requires Fc-receptor positive Null cells. Addition of 'exogenous' TIF or human fibroblast IF (FIF) to an MLTC enhanced SCMC to varying degres depending on the target cells used and the mode of addition chosen (direct admixture to the test at time zero or 6 hours later versus target or effector preincubation in IF). Highly purified T cells known to be inefficient SCMC effectors were also found to be poor IF producers in response to tumor cells and CP. However, upon stimulation with CP purified T cells produced an SCMC enhancing factor(s) which lacked anti-viral activity and preferentially enhanced killing in certain selective effector-target combinations. The significance of this first T cell factor involved in SCMC is discussed.

ACKNOWLEDGEMENTS

The autors appreciate the dedicated and competent technical assistance of Ms. A. Serbin, B. Lange and I. Roth (Hannover) and Ms. M. Keyssner, C.Kleinicke and H. Rogg (Heidelberg). Excellent secretarial assistance was provided by Ms. M. Nolte.

VI. REFERENCES

Böyum,A. (1968). Scand.J.Clin.Lab.Invest.(suppl.) 97, 1-8.

Borecky,L.,Fuchsberger,N.,Zemla,J., and Lackovic,V. (1971). Europ.J.Immunol. 2, 213-216.

Borecky,L.,Lackovic,V.,Fuchsberger,N.,and Hajnicka, V. (1974). In "Activation of Macrophages"(Eds. Wagner,W.H.,and Hahn,H.)Excerpta Medica, Amsterdam, pp. 111-122.

Djeu,J.Y.,Heinbaugh,J.A.,Holden,H.T.,and Herberman, R.B. (1979). J.Immunol. 122, 175.

Domzig,W.,and Lohmann-Matthes,M.L. (1979). Europ.J. Immunol. 9, 267.

Droller,M.J., Borg,H., and Perlmann,P. (1979). Cell. Immunol. 47, 248-260.

Evans.R.,Grant,C.K.,Cox,H.,Steele,K.,and Alexander, P. (1972). J.exp.Med. 136, 1318-1322.

Falcoff,R. (1972). J.gen.Virol. 16, 251-253.

Gidlund,M.,Orn,A.,Wigzell,H.,Senik,A.,and Gressner, I. (1978). Nature 273, 759.

Greaves,M.F.,Janossy,G.,and Curtis,P. (1976). In "In vitro Methods in cell-mediated and tumor immunity (Bloom,B.,and David,J.R.,eds) pp.217-230, Academic Press, New York.

Herberman,R.B.,Ortaldo,J.,and Bonnard,G.D. (1979). Nature 277, 221.

Heron,I.,Hokland,M.,Moller-Larsen,A.,and Berg,K. (1979). Cell.Immunol. 42, 183-187.

Kalden,J.R.,Peter,H.H.,Roubin,R.,and Cesarini,J.P. (1977). Europ.J.Immunol. 8, 537-543.

Kirchner,H.,Peter,H.H.,Hirt,H.M.,Zawatzky,R., Dallügge,H.,and Bradstreet,P. (1979). Immunobiol. 156, 65-75.

Lohmann-Matthes,M.L.,Ziegler,F.G.,and Fischer,H. (1973). Europ.J.Immunol. 3, 56-61.

Lohmann-Matthes,M.L.,and Domzig,W. (1979). Europ.J. Immunol. 9, 261-268.

Lohmann-Matthes,M.L.,Domzig,W.,andRoder,J. (1979). J.Immunol. 123, 1883-1886.

Lozzio,C.B.,and Lozzio,B.B. (1975). Blood 45,321-324

Neumann,C.,and Sorg,C.(1977).Europ.J.Immunol. 7,719.

Oehl,S.,Schäfer,U.W.,Boecker,W.R.,Kalden,J.R. and Peter,H.H. (1977). Z.Immun.Forsch. 152, 423-430.

Oehl,S.,Peter,H.H.,Kalden,J.R.,Boecker,W.R.,Schäfer, U.W.,Cesarini,J.P.,and Schmidt,C.G. (1978). In "Human lymphocyte differentiation: Its application to cancer" (Serrou,B.,and Rosenfeld,C., eds.), pp. 161-168. INSERM Symposium No.8, Elsevier,N.Holland.

Peter,H.H.,Pavie-Fischer,J.,Friedman,W.H.,Aubert,C., Cesarini,J.P.,Roubin,R.,and Kourilsky,F.M. (1975). J.Immunol. 115, 539-548.
Peter,H.H.,Eife,R.F.,and Kalden,J.R. (1976). J.Immunol. 116, 342-348.
Peter,H.H.,Dallügge,H.,Zawatzky,R.,Euler,S.,Leibold, W.,and Kirchner,H. (1980). Europ.J.Immunol.(In press)
Rajvanshi,V.,Peter,H.H.,and Avenarius,H.J. (1979). Z.Immun.Forsch. 155, 330-337.
Richman,L.M.,Chess,L.,and Yankee,R.A. (1978). Blood 51, 1-8.
Roberts,N.J.,Douglas,R.G.,Simons,R.M.,and Diamond, M.E. (1979). J.Immunol. 123, 365-369.
Roder,J.C.,Rosen,A.,Fenyo,E.M., and Troy,F.A.(1979). Proc.Natl.Acad.Sci. USA. 76, 1405-1409.
Schimpl,A.,and Wecker,E. (1972). Nature New Biol. 237, 15.
Sokhey,J.,Solovlev,A.I.,and Vasilieva,V.I. (1977). Acta Virol. 21, 485-490.
Stewart,W.E. (1979)."The interferon system", Springer Verlag, Wien, New York.
Strander,H.,Cantell,K.,Ingimarsson,S.,Jakobsson,P.A. Nilsonne,U.,and Soderberg,G. (1977). Forgarty Intern. Center Proc. 28, 377-380.
Svet-Modavsky,G.J.,Chernyakhovskaya,I.,and Yu,I. (1967). Nature 215, 1299-1300.
Taussig,M.J.,Munro,A.J.,Campbell,R.,David,C.S.,and Staines,N.A. (1975). J.exp.Med. 142, 694-704.
Trinchieri,G.,Santoli,D.,Dee,R.R.,and Knowles,B. (1978a). J.exp.Med. 147, 1299-1313.
Trinchieri,G.,and Santoli,D. (1978b). J.exp.Med. 147, 1314-1333.
Trinchieri,G.,Santoli,D.,and Koprowski,H. (1978c). J.Immunol. 120, 1849-1855.
Troye,M.,Perlmann,P.,Pape,G.R.,Spiegelberg,H.J., Näslund,I.,and Gidlöf,A. (1977). J.Immunol. 119, 1061-1067.
Vilcek,J.,Volvovitz,F.,and Havell,E.A. (1979). Abstract, 2nd Int.Lymphokine Workshop, New York.
Watson,J.,Aarden,L.A.,Shaw,J.,and Peatkau,V.(1979). J.Immunol. 122, 1633-1638.
Wheelock,E.F. (1965). Science 149, 310-311.
Zarling,J.M.,Eskra,L.,Borden,E.C.,Horoszewicz,J., and Carter,W.A. (1979). J.Immunol. 123, 63-70.

MODULATION OF NATURAL CYTOTOXICITY IN MAN BY BCG AND FIBROBLAST INTERFERON

Gert Riethmüller
*Gerd R. Pape**
Martin R. Hadam
Johannes G. Saal

Institut für Immunologie
and
* Medizinische Klinik II
Ludwig-Maximilians-Universität
München, F.R. Germany

I. INTRODUCTION

Among the various genetically controlled mechanisms of natural resistance spontaneous cytotoxic cells (natural killer (NK) cells)seem to play an important role as effector cells against infection and malignancy. As reviewed recently (Cudkowicz and Hochman 1979, Herberman et al 1979) experimental evidence exists that the activity of NK-cells is modulated by several types of regulator cells. As internal mediators of regulation prostaglandins and interferon have been considered. These mediators may be involved in various ways when NK - activity is influenced by bacterial adjuvants in vivo. From the in-vitro-work of Cudkowicz and Hochman (1979), one can deduce that a delicate balance exists between factors stimulating or suppressing NK-activity. As in other homeostatic systems of agonists and antagonists, overstimulation in one direction may result in paradoxical adverse reactions. A clinical study of BCG-treatment in patients with primary melanoma offered the possibility to study the time and dose kinetics of NK-activity under the influence of such a bacterial adjuvant. Analogously, the treatment of chronic hepatitis patients with fibroblast interferon allowed us to study longitudinally the influence of this mediator on NK-activity directly.

ISBN 0-12-341350-8

Earlier studies (Riethmüller et al, 1975) had shown that cell mediated cytotoxicity was increased in a group of patients which had been treated for several months with BCG. For the mouse it had been clearly shown that BCG and Corynebacterium parvum induce a rapid increase of NK-activity (Wolfe et al 1976) in spleen cells and peritoneal exsudate cells. When examining NK-activity immediately after BCG-application in patients we had seen distinct suppression of NK-activity as well as stimulation of activity (Saal et al, 1977).
At that time no easy explanation for this two discrepant patterns of cytotoxic response could be given. For further elucidation of these types of cytotoxic responses the dose of BCG applied was varied for the individual patient.

II. THE EXPERIMENTAL SYSTEM

Essentially two tests were applied to measure NK-activity of human peripheral blood lymphocytes: A short-term ^{51}chromium-release assay was used for the K-562 human leukemic cell line as target, provided kindly by Peter Perlmann, Stockholm. As sensitive longterm test the ^{3}H-proline release test was applied which had been shown to be rather versatile for all types of human tumor cells due to the high labelling index obtained with ^{3}H-proline and due to its low, spontaneous release. (Saal et al, 1976) For the ^{3}H-proline test mostly melanoma cell lines were used which were established from primary melanomas and adapted to growth in human AB sera under strict avoidance of all animal sera. Non-adherent lymphocytes (NAL) were isolated from heparinized blood by Ficoll-Urovison centrifugation. Adherent cells were removed by an incubation on plastic surfaces and by filtration through nylon wool columns.

III. THE PATIENTS

Only those melanoma patients free from clinically detectable tumor recurrencies were elected for monitoring dose- and time-dependent effects of BCG on NK-activity. As dosage of percutaneous BCG administration has remained a considerable problem for immune-stimulatory trials particular care was taken to apply the various dilutions of the fresh Pasteur vaccine (BCG Immuno F) in equal volumes to a defined sacrification wound, 32 cm long, induced with a 12 gauge cannula through a plexiglass mask.
Human fibroblast interferon (Fa. Rentschler, Laupheim) was injected intravenously or given as intravenous infusion to patients with chronic aggressive hepatitis.

The specific activity of interferon varied between 10^6 to 10^7 units/mg protein. The preparation was found to increase natural cytotoxicity of NAL in a dose-dependent fashion in vitro. NK-activity was monitored longitudinally in three patients.

IV. MONITORING OF NK-AKTIVITY UNDER BCG-TREATMENT

It was a prerequisite for any longitudinal monitoring of NK-activity to examine how stable the cytotoxic activity was expressed in patients during an uneventful phase of their disease. As demonstrated in Table I in four patients NK-activity remained rather stable during an observation period of 14 days, though the individual levels of activity were quite different from each other. When normal healthy donors were tested over a period of several months variation of NK-activity was greater; - however, for the individual donor the level of activity was rather characteristic.

TABLE I

NK-ACTIVITY IN UNSTIMULATED MELANOMA PATIENTS

Patient	*consecutive days*				
	0	*2*	*4*	*6*	*15*
1	*30**	*27*	*29*	*28*	*29*
2	*42*	*41*	*43*	*--*	*42*
3	*50*	*49*	*51*	*--*	*49*
4	*60*	*58*	*59*		

** NK-activity expressed as lytic units per 10^7 cells. Lytic units are arbitrarily defined as the number of effector cells required to obtain 25 % of target cells lysis. Always three effector/target cell ratios were tested in triplicates.*

Target cell susceptibility was not found to be drastically changing over longer periods, this holds true particularly when the 40h ^{3}H-proline test was applied. This finding was strenghthened by unchanged sensitivity of tumor cells to human antibodies detected in some patients sera with an ADCC test.

After scarification with 10^8 organisms of BCG a drastic change of NK-activity occurred. As demonstrated in Figure 1 for two melanoma patients, NK-activity against an autologous tumor cell was decreased to a strikingly similar degree as the cytotoxicity against an allogeneic melanoma cell. This parallel pattern of cytotoxic effects to allogeneic and autologous tumor cells points to NK cells as being the actual effector cells modulated by BCG.

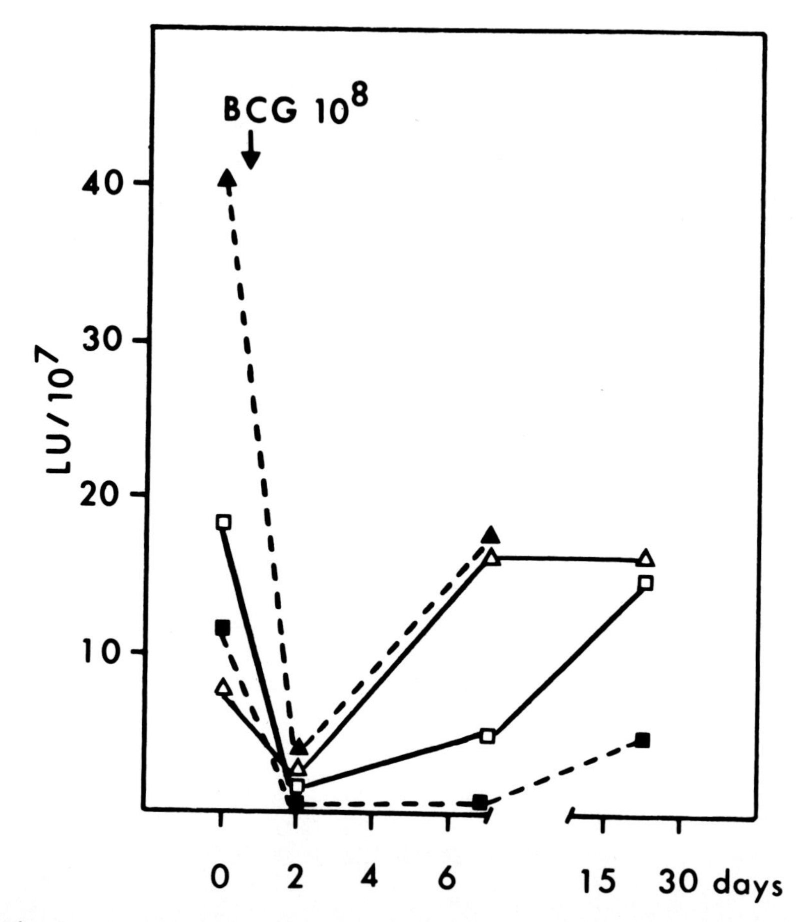

Figure 1. Influence of BCG administration on natural cytotoxicity directed against autologous (---) or homologous (——) melanoma cells tested in melanoma patients Ho (square symbols) and Ju (triangels).

Independently, it had been shown that increased or decreased cytotoxicity after BCG was abolished when the non-adherent lymphocytes were passed through an Ig-anti-Ig Degalan column.

It seemed possible that dose-dependent effects were responsible for the observed suppression or stimulation of NK-activity. To test this hypothesis three different doses - 10^6, 10^7 and 10^8 BCG organisms - were administered at weekly intervals to single melanoma patients.
A total of 7 patients were treated so far according to a regimen starting with either the high dose (10^8 organisms) or the low dose (10^6 organisms). One batch of BCG Pasteur was used for all simultaneously treated patients. Thus, the NK-activity at three different effector/target ratios was tested in each patient immediately prior to and at day 2 and 6 after BCG administration. From the results obtained a distinct dose-related pattern emerged in so far that after administration of 10^8 organisms a distinct suppression of NK-activity occurred (Fig. 3)

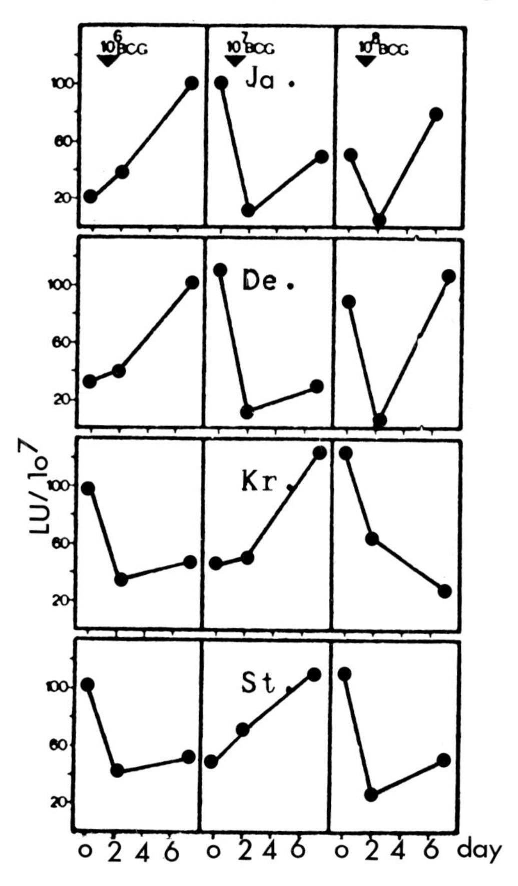

Figure 3. Effects of 10^6, 10^7, or 10^8 BCG organisms per week on NK-activity in patients Ja, De, Kr, and St. Cytotoxicity expressed in lytic units as described.

When more patients were monitored after administration of the standard dose of 10^8 BCG organisms essentially two characteristic patterns of cytotoxic responses were observed. Out of 18 tested patients 14 showed a dramatic decrease of NK-activity which reached its nadir at 48 to 72 hours after BCG administration. Only 4 out of 18 patients responded with a steep increase reaching a maximum after 48 to 72 hours. As can be seen from Fig. 2 (taken from J. Saal et al, 1979) the two patterns of responses appear rather symmetrical. The original pre-BCG level may be reached as early as on the sixth day after scarification.

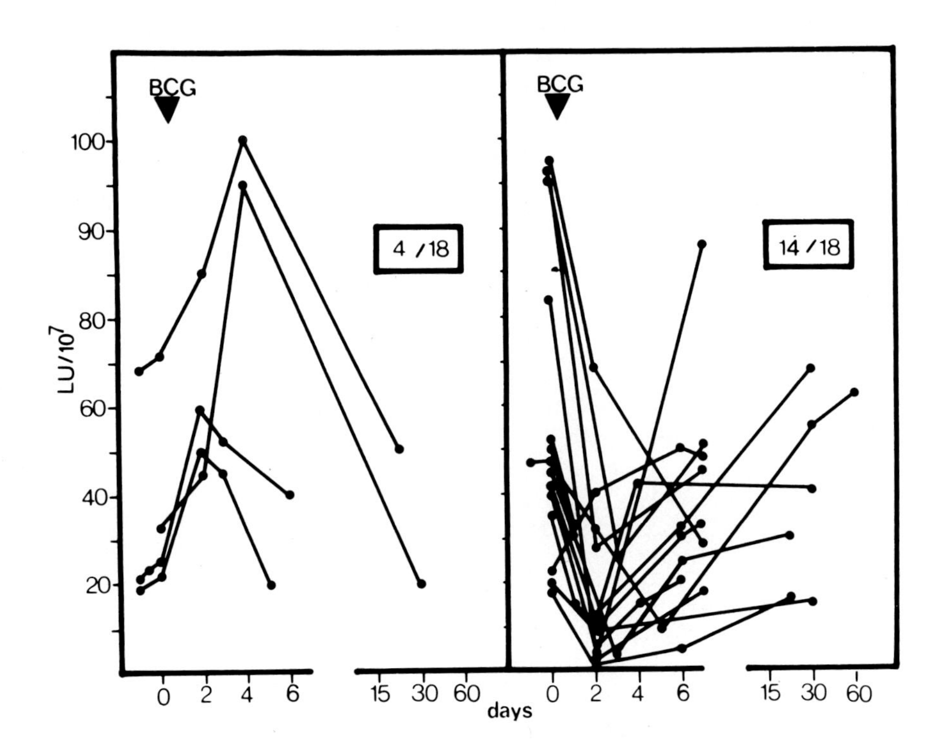

Figure 2. Short term effects of percutaneous BCG (10^8 organisms) on NK-activity in 18 patients with primary melanoma. Panel on the right side: 14/18 showing suppression of NK - activity. Left side: 4/18 exhibiting increase of NK-activity.

After lower doses of BCG, stimulation of NK-activity was observed. As demonstrated in Fig. 3 there seems to be a rather narrow dose range for some patients within which stimulation of NK-activity is obtained.

As demonstrated earlier (Saal et al 1979) the increased cytotoxicity was not found to be directed against all tested target cells. In some cases the increased cytotoxic response was found only on melanoma cell lines and not on target cells derived from various carcinomas. A general lower susceptibility could hardly account for this difference since these non melanoma cells were lysed equally well by lymphocytes of a larger panel of various donors (Saal et al 1979).

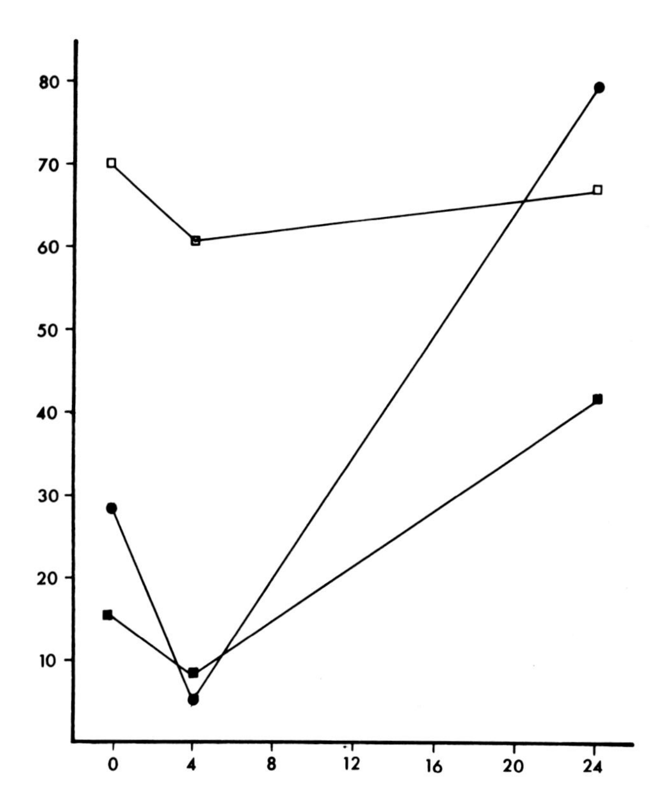

Figure 4. Short-term effects of intravenous injection of fibroblast interferon on NK activity of PBL. Patient Ki(■—■) and patient Ro(●—●) after first injection of 4x106 units. Patient Ki after fourth injection of $10x10^6$ units interferon (□—□). Abscissa: hours after interferon injection. Ordinate: percentage ^{51}Cr release from K562 target cells, corrected for release in medium controls (5%) at lymphocyte target ratio 50:1, time of incubation 4 hours.

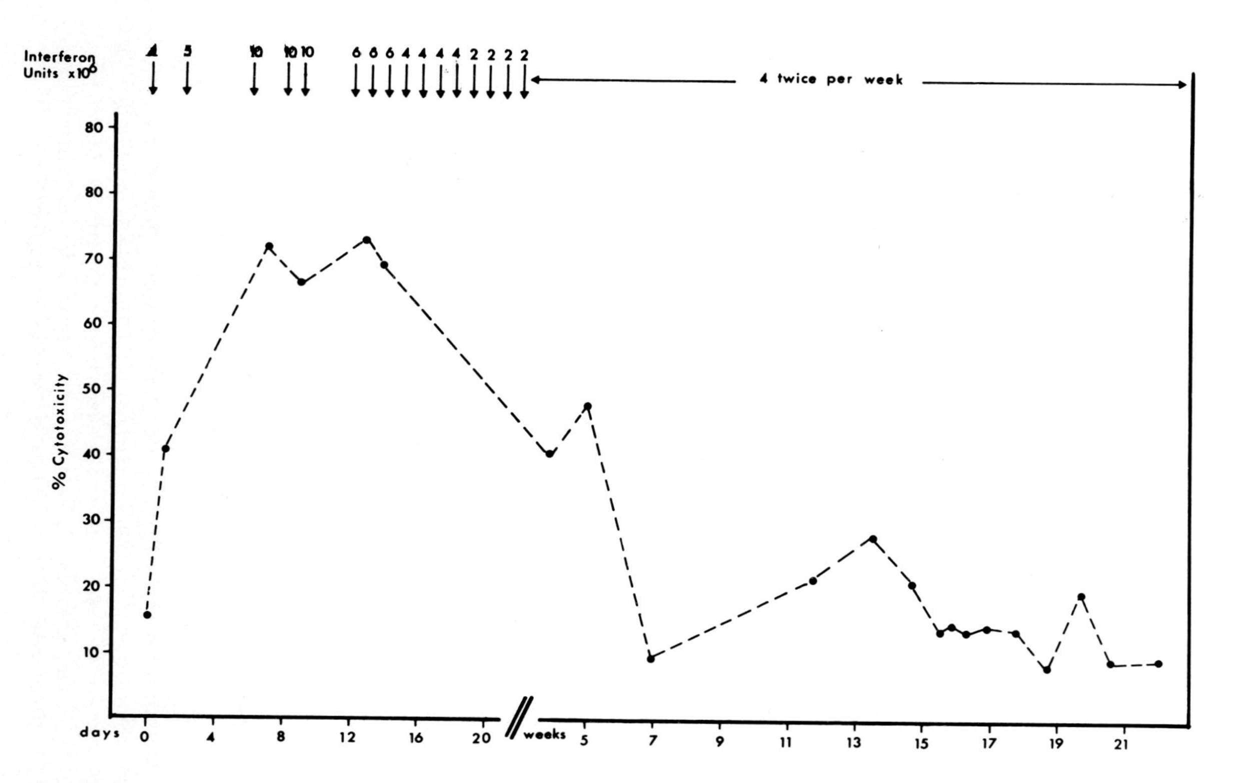

Figure 5. Natural cytotoxicity in a patient with chronic aggressive hepatitis treated with human fibroblast interferon at the indicated intervals. Target cell: K562. ^{51}Cr-release is given in percent for 50:1 effector/target cell ratio. For details see Fig.4.

V. SHORT AND LONG TERM EFFECTS ON NK-ACTIVITY UNDER INTERFERON TREATMENT

Besides its antiproliferative cellular activity on tumor cells, interferon has profound influences on the immune system. During the last years the stimulatory effect of interferon on cell-mediated cytotoxicity has gained particular interest. Thus, interferon induces readily natural cytotoxicity in vitro (Trinchieri and Santoli 1978; Herberman et al 1979). A clinical trial in which patients with chronic aggressive hepatitis (CAH) were treated with human fibroblast interferon offered the chance to study whether this type of interferon had any effects on NK-activity in vivo. Since interferon was administered over longer periods of time with different doses short term as well as long term influences on NK-activity could be monitored.

After a first single intravenous dose of interferon ($4x10^6$ units) NK-activity showed a distinct drop when tested at 4 hours after injection (Fig. 4). At 24 hours after interferon application, NK-activity was increased two to three fold compared with pretreatment levels. The short term decrease in NK-activity was also observed after a single dose at a later stage of interferon treatment when cytotoxicity had reached peak levels. As demonstrated in Figure 5, under repeated daily injections of interferon NK-activity was increased to peak acitvitites which so far had not been observed with human peripheral blood lymphocytes.

The plateau of maximal cytotoxicity was reached after doses ranging from 5 to $10x10^6$ units per application. When the daily dose was reduced from $6x10^6$ to $2x10^6$ units a decrease ensued. After prolonged treatment with even lower doses of interferon, $4x10^6$ units twice per week, NK activity returned to pretreatment level.

VI. CONCLUDING REMARKS

As far as time kinetics of BCG effects on NK-acitvity are concerned the findings in man resemble those obtained in mice. However, in view of the strong restriction of NK-activity by organ compartments one may not base too firm conclusions on a comparison of human circulating cytotoxic cells with murine NK cells derived from the peritoneal cavity or from the spleen. When doses of BCG in mice and men are compared the most striking finding is the extremely low dose of organisms at which systemic effects in men occur. As Ruitenberg et al have recently shown (personal communication) in mice a dose as high as $7.5x10^6$ culturable organisms of the BCG-RIV strain still stimulates peritoneal NK cells at the fourth day after i.p. injection.

As to the cause of the rapid and short-lasting suppression seen in many individuals after higher doses of BCG only speculations are possible at he present time. One is tempted to attribute thes antagonistic effects of the bacterial adjuvant not to direct influences on the effector cells but to effects on regulatory cells such as macrophages which have been shown to play a dualistic role either as stimulators or suppressors of hemopoiesis depending on the degree of activation (Moore and Kurland 1979). As suggested by Moore and Kurland prostaglandins of the E series and colony-stimulating factors elaborated both by macrophages may act as opposing regulatory mediators of hemopoetic cell proliferation. In the NK system where macrophages have been involved as regulatory cells interferon may be one of the enhancing factors opposing prostaglandins (Oehler and Herberman 1978). The positive and negative effects after BCG seen so far are comparable with a system which under perturbed circumstances may react according to the relative levels of its intrinsic inhibitors or promotors. It remains to be shown whether maturation of effector cells from precursors is the underlying mechanism or whether levels of activity in effector cells are affected. From the work of Trinchieri et al. (1978) and Herberman et al. (1979) the in vitro effect of interferon on NK-activity could be explained by an enhanced transit from precursors to mature effector cells. Since antibody to interferon could obviate the enhancement of NK-activity it was inferred that interferon itself was the responsible factor.

Recently, it had also been demonstrated in mice that interferon causes increments of NK-activity in vivo (Gidlund et al. 1978). Similarly, Einhorn et al. (1978) and Huddlestone et al. (1979) observed stimulation of NK activity in tumor patients treated with leucocyte interferon. Since interferon preparations derived from buffy coat leucocytes may contain besides immune interferon also other kinds of lymphokine-like material it was of interest to study the effects of virus induced fibroblast interferon on NK-activity in man.

As reported here, the intravenous injection of the fibroblast interferon resulted in a characteristic pattern of NK-activiy exhibiting a so far unexplained early drop, irrespective of whether the interferon was injected for the first time or whether a repeated single dose was monitored.

Under prolonged treatment conditions the plateau of maximal activity was rather impressive. However, this peak activity declined under reduced doses of interferon. It is quite noticeable that the same donor who responded with a several fold increase of cytotoxicity after the first dose showed only a slight enhancement when tested after 4 months of consecutive treatment. In both instances the same single dose of interferon had been administered.

At the present time it is premature to draw final conclusions on the correlation between therapeutic effects of interferon and the observed changes in natural cytotoxicity of circulating lymphocytes. Considering the wealth of experimental data assigning a decisive role to natural cytotoxicity in the defense against infection and malignancy the hope is justified that interferon as one of the possible internal regulators of this system may open up new avenues of therapy to these so far unsolved clinical problems.

ACKNOWLEDGEMENTS:

We thank Jutta Döhrmann and Friederike Frank for expert technical help. The cooperation of Professor J. Eisenburg is gratefully acknowledged.

This work was supported by the Deutsche Forschungsgemeinschaft Grant No. Pa 212/3 and Ri 174/9 and SFB 37.

REFERENCES

Cudkovicz, G., and Hochman, P. S., Immunol.Reviews 44, 13 (1979).

Einhorn, S., Blomgren, H., and Strander, H., Acta med. scand. 20, 477 (1978).

Herberman, R. B., Djeu, I. Y., Kay, H. D., Ortaldo, J. R., Riccardi, C., Bonnard, G. D., Holden, H. T., Fagnani, R., Santoni, A., and Pucetti, P., Immunol. Reviews 44, 43 (1979).

Herberman, R. B., Ortaldo, J. R., and Bonnard, G. D., Nature 277, 223 (1979).

Gidlund, M., Örn, A., Wigzell, H., Senik, A., and Gresser, I., Nature 273, 259 (1978).

Huddlestone, J. R., Merigan, T. C. jr., and Oldstone, M. B. A., Nature 282, 417 (1979).

Moore, M. A. S., and Kurland, J. I., in "Natural and induced cell-mediated cytotoxicity" (G. Riethmüller, P. Wernet, and G. Cudkovicz, eds.), p. 191. Academic Press, New York, (1979).

Oehler, J. R., and Herberman, R.B., Int. J. Cancer 21, 221 (1978).

Riethmüller, G., Saal, J.G., Rieber, E. P., Ehinger, H., Schnellen, B., and Riethmüller, D., Transplantation Proc. 7, 495 (1975).

Saal, J. G., Rieber, E. P., and Riethmüller, G., Scand. J. Immunol. 5, 455 (1976).

Saal, J. G., Riethmüller, G., Rieber, E. P., Hadam, M., Ehinger, H., and Schneider, W., Cancer Immunol. Immunother. 3, 27 (1977).

Saal, J. G., Riethmüller, G., Hadam, M. R., Rieber, E. P., and Fleiner, J. M., in "Natural and induced cell-mediated cytotoxicity" (G. Riethmüller, P. Wernet, and G. Cudkovicz, eds.), p. 89. Academic Press, New York, (1979).

Trinchieri, G., and Santoli, D., J. Exp. Med. 147, 1314 (1978).

Wolfe, S. A., Tracey, D. E., and Henney, C. S., Nature 262, 584 (1976).

REGULATION OF HUMAN NATURAL KILLER ACTIVITY BY INTERFERON

Eero Saksela[1]
Tuomo Timonen
Ismo Virtanen

Department of Pathology
University of Helsinki
Finland

Kari Cantell

Central Public Health Laboratory
Helsinki, Finland

I. INTRODUCTION

Interferon is released from human blood mononuclear cells as a result of contact with established, mainly tumor derived cell line cells (1,2) or with cells persistently infected with viruses (3). Interferon strongly augments the natural killer cell (NK) activity (4) and it appears to play a central role in the genesis of active cytotoxic NK cells from inactive "pre-NK" precursor cells (5). Therefore, the crucial step in the regulation of NK activity may be the release of interferon from its producer cell(s). Trinchieri et al. (4) have suggested that the producer cells are surface nonadherent lymphocytes with receptors for the Fc part of IgG molecule as also suggested by Peter et al. (6) in their earlier experiments on soluble mediators of NK ac-

[1]*Supported by grant No. 1 RO 1 CA 23809-1 from the National Cancer Institute, NIH, Bethesda, Md.*

ISBN 0-12-341350-8

tivity against human melanoma target cells. On the other hand, interferon induced by polyinosinic-polycytidylic acid appears to be derived from monocyte-macrophages (7), and virus-induced interferon synthesis may be dependent on B-lymphocytes (8). Interferon-mediated regulation of the NK activity may therefore occur in a variety of conditions, but of particular interest is the possibility that the tumor-cell induced interferon might be derived from NK cells themselves (9) and thus create an internal amplification system of positive feed-back type within the NK system itself as we have suggested in the human (9,10) and Bloom et al. in the mouse (11). In the present communication we review briefly the human data forming the basis of this contention.

II. AUGMENTATION OF FETAL FIBROBLAST ADSORBED ELUTED CELLS

Fetal fibroblasts are unable to induce interferon synthesis in human lymphocytes (1,12). When they are used as adsorbants and the eluted cells tested for cytotoxicity on susceptible target cells, an enrichment of NK activity can be seen as discussed elsewhere in this volume. The remaining cells are greatly depleted of natural killer activity but the activity can be augmented by exogenously added interferon as shown in Figure 1. We have interpreted these data to indicate that fetal fibroblast adsorption removes the initially cytotoxic NK cells ("mature" NK cells) but leaves behind a population rapidly augmentable by interferon to full cytotoxic activity. We have termed such cells "pre-NK" cells in analogy with the findings of Herberman et al. (5) in the mouse system. The step leading to activation of human "pre-NK" cells is independent of DNA synthesis but requires RNA and protein synthesis (13). Morphologically the "pre-NK" cells as well as "mature" NK cells are large granular lymphocytes as indicated by conjugate analyses (14).

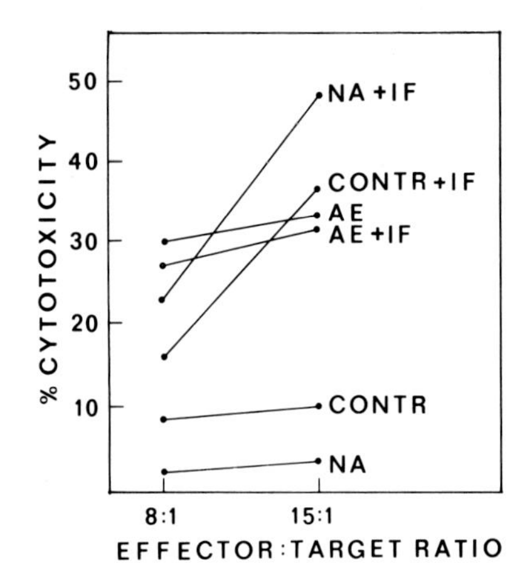

FIGURE 1. Effect of interferon on the cytotoxic activity of "mature" NK cell enriched (AE) and depleted (NA) populations. Contr. = input cells. Interferon (1000 IU/ml) added 18h prior to an 4h chromium release assay on K-562 cells.

III. TARGET CELL INDUCED INTERFERON SYNTHESIS OF FRACTIONATED CELLS

Exposure of the fibroblast adsorbed eluted effector cell fractions to interferon-inducing target cells, such as K-562, leads to augmentation of the activity of the "pre-NK" cells and this may be inhibited by anti-interferon antiserum (12). The crucial question is what is the cell type responsible for the interferon synthesis required for the activation. When the interferon titers are measured in the supernatants of the "mature" NK cell enriched and depleted fractions, the highest titers are always obtained in the "mature" NK cell fractions as shown in Table I. These fractions contain cells with LGL morphology in an enriched incidence, but they contain also other lymphoid cell types and occasional monocytes. We have shown that cells of the monocyte-macrophage series are unable to produce interferon at contact with inducing target cell types (9), but in order to differentiate between the various lymphocyte types as candidates for the interferon production other fractionation methods had to be devised.

TABLE I. The K-562 induced interferon production of effector cells enriched or depleted for "mature" NK cells by adsorption elution with fetal fibroblasts[1]

	Depleted	*Enriched*
Interferon titre[2]	*Not measurable*	*350*
Cytotoxicity (15:1)[3]	*12*	*48*
Differential[4]		
LGL	*15*	*43*
MSL+SL	*85*	*56*
Mon	*0*	*1*

[1] *Mean of three experiments*
[2] *International units per 10^6 cells as measured by VSV plaque reduction usage*
[3] *^{51}Cr release in percent from K-562 cells. 4 h assay with 15:1 effector:target ratio*
[4] *Percent of LGL = large granular lymphocytes; MSL = medium-sized lymphocytes; SL = small lymphocytes; Mon = monocytes*

Density gradient centrifugations using discontinuous Percoll gradients (15) resulted in an efficient separation of LGL and other lymphocyte types. The lower density fraction contained 80-90% pure LGL as compared to the higher density fractions containing practically 100% small and medium sized lymphocytes. When these fractions were exposed to interferon inducing target cells, such as K-562, interferon production could only be obtained from the LGL containing fractions (Fig. 2). As LGL are also the mediators of NK activity in human blood, these results suggested that NK cells themselves are the producers of interferon at tumor cell contact. Elimination of the NK activity and LGL by incubation in sodium butyrate, led also to the extinction of the interferon producing capacity (9) adding further weight to this contention.

To analyse directly the morphology of the cells producing interferon as a result of contact with K-562 cells we applied indirect immunofluorescence methods using a potent sheep anti human leukocyte interferon antiserum. Using techniques shown previously to be effective in detecting rapidly secreted

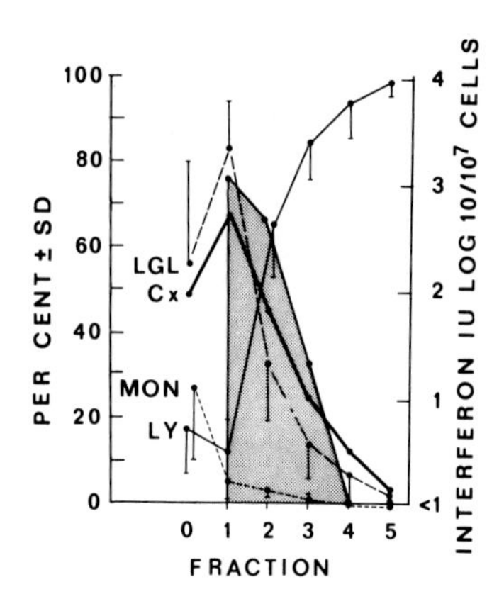

FIGURE 2. Interferon production (shaded area) of Percoll fractionated human lymphocytes during an 18h co-culture with K-562 cells. Relationship to NK-activity (Cx), percentage of large granular lymphocytes (LGL), other lymphocytes (Ly) and monocytes (Mon) in the same fractions are also shown.

proteins in cells, we were able to show intensive cytoplasmic fluorescence in Percoll purified LGL populations after 6 hrs contact with K-562 cells (9). The fluorescing cells had the morphology of LGL and their incidence was 30-50% at the peak of 6 hrs coinciding with the first demonstrable interferon in the supernatant. Only an occasional monocyte was fluorescent in the non-augmented population. The immunofluorescence was detected at low, 1:2000-4000 concentration of the antiserum and it was neutralized at close to the calculated equivalence by the most purified leukocyte interferon preparations that we had available. We believe, therefore that the results demonstrated directly that lymphocytes of LGL morphology, presumably NK cells, are able to produce interferon after stimulation with K-562 cells (Fig. 3).

CONCLUDING REMARKS

All the data are compatible with the conclusion that large granular lymphocytes (LGL) are responsible for the interferon synthesis in human blood

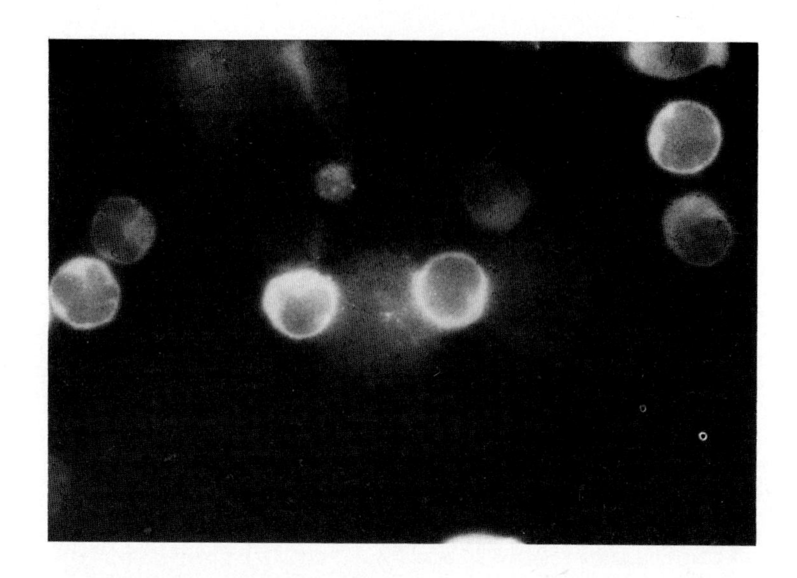

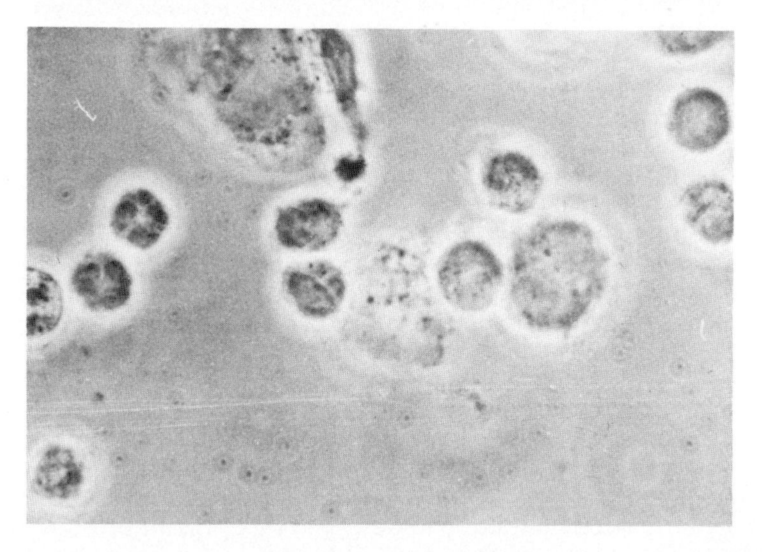

FIGURE 3. Cells from Percoll fraction No. 1 containing 86% LGL co-cultured with K-562 cells for 6h. 2.5% paraformaldehyde fixed, 0.05% triton treated cells reacted with sheep anti-interferon antiserum (450 000 neutralizing units per ml. 1:2000 dilution) and stained with fluorescein-coupled anti-sheep antiserum (upper panel). The same field is shown in phase contrast (lower panel). Note bright cytoplasmic fluorescence of LGL with characteristic granules visible in phase contrast.

lymphocyte populations co-cultured with certain, mostly tumor-derived target cells. LGL are also responsible for the natural killer activity in human blood. We have not been able to separate the interferon-producing ability and NK activity with any of the fractionation procedures suggesting that both activities may be mediated by the same cells. Enrichment of the "mature" NK cells with fetal fibroblast adsorption elution concentrated also the interferon producing cells in this fraction suggesting that among the LGL the "mature" NK cells might be those capable of interferon synthesis at contact with tumor cells. Interferon does not augment the cytotoxic activity of the "mature" NK cells but exerts its action by recruitment of initially non-cytotoxic "pre-NK" cells to full killer activity. The results thus suggest an internal amplification mechanism operating within the NK system itself as illustrated schematically in Fig. 4. Upon contact with tumor cells or persistently virus-infected cells "mature" NK cells release interferon, which in

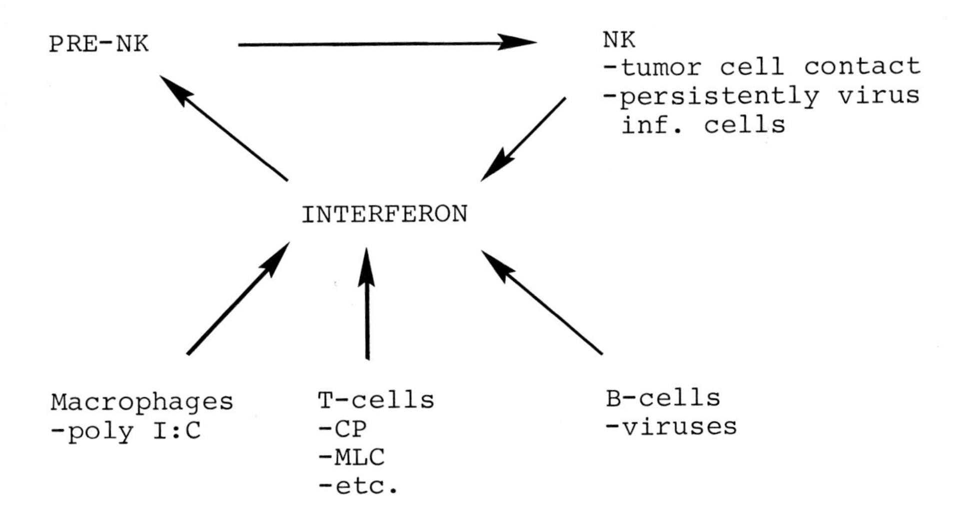

FIGURE 4. Schematic representation of various pathways operating in the regulation of human NK cell activity. Note the suggested "loop" of internal amplification within the NK-system itself.

turn recruits "pre-NK" cells to cytotoxic activity. Whether the activated "pre-NK" cells also acquire the capacity to produce interferon and further amplify the response is not known although there is some evidence pointing to that direction. In any case, such a positive feed back type of regulation mechanism operating with the NK cell system itself could provide an effective, rapidly recruitable primary resistance mechanism against tumor cells as well as virus infected cells.

ACKNOWLEDGEMENTS

The technical assistance of Ms. Maija-Liisa Mäntylä and Pirkko Kalliomäki is gratefully acknowledged.

REFERENCES

1. Trinchieri, G., Santoli, D., and Knowles, B. B. *Nature* 270, 611 (1977).
2. Trinchieri, G., Santoli, D., Dee, R. R., and Knowles, B. B., *J. Exp. Med.* 147, 1299 (1978).
3. Herberman, R. B., and Holden, H. T., *Adv. Cancer Res.* 27, 305 (1978).
4. Trinchieri, G., and Santoli, D., *J. Exp. Med.* 147, 1314 (1978).
5. Herberman, R. B., Nunn, M. E., Holden, H. T., Staal, S., and Djeu, J.Y., *Int. J. Cancer* 19, 555 (1977).
6. Peter, H. H., Pavie-Fischer, J., Fridman, W. H., Aubert, C., Cesarini, J., Roubin, R., and Kourilsky, F. M., *J. Immunol.* 115, 539 (1975).
7. Djeu, J. Y., Heinbaugh, J. A., Holden, H. T., and Herberman, R. B., *J. Immunol.* 122, 182 (1979).
8. Yamaguchi, T., Handa, K., Shimizu, Y., Abo, T., and Kumagai, K., *J. Immunol.* 118, 1931 (1977).
9. Timonen, T., Saksela, E., and Cantell, K., *Eur. J. Immunol.* (1979) (in press).
10. Saksela, E., Timonen, T., and Cantell, K., *Ann. N.Y. Acad. Sci* (1979) (in press).
11. Bloom, B. R., Minato, P. A., Neighbour, P. A., and Reid, L., *Ann. N.Y. Acad. Sci* (1979) (in press).

12. Saksela, E., Timonen, T., and Cantell, K., *Scand. J. Immunol.* 10, 257 (1979).
13. Carpén, O., and Saksela, E., (1979) (in preparation).
14. Timonen, T., Saksela, E., Ranki, A., Häyry, P., *Cell. Immunol.* 48, 133 (1979).
15. Timonen, T., and Saksela, E., *J. Immunol. Methods* (1979) (submitted).

SPONTANEOUS CELL-MEDIATED CYTOTOXICITY: MODULATION BY INTERFERON*

Giorgio Trinchieri
Bice Perussia
Daniela Santoli

The Wistar Institute of Anatomy and Biology
Philadelphia, Pennsylvania

Production of interferon in cultures of lymphocytes with cell lines and its role in enhancing natural killer cell activity.

Interferons (IF) are small glycoproteins produced by different cellular types upon virus infection or other stimuli. IF were originally described as inhibitors of virus replication in infected cells. In addition to antiviral activity, IF molecules also have an effect on cellular functions. The activity of several cell types involved in specific and non-specific immune reactions is either suppressed or enhanced by IF. We have shown that IF have a complex role in the spontaneous cytotoxicity mediated by effector lymphocytes which are usually referred to as natural killer or NK cells. NK cells are present in the peripheral blood or other lymphoid organs of normal donors in the absence of disease or of any known or deliberate sensitization (Trinchieri and Santoli, 1978; Trinchieri et al., 1978b; Santoli et al., 1976).

When lymphocytes are cultured with most tumor-derived or virus-infected cell lines, they rapidly release an antiviral substance with the characteristics of leukocyte type I (viral) IF (Trinchieri et al., 1977, 1978a). IF appears in the supernatant of these cultures at 3 to 4 hr of incubation, and maximum antiviral activity is reached at 18 to 24 hr. A more detailed description of this phenomenon and of the producer and the inducer cells is reported in another section of this book. Most of the target cells that

The experimental work described in this paper has been supported by NIH grants CA-20833, CA-10815, CA 43882 and NS-11036 and by the National Multiple Sclerosis Society.

ISBN 0-12-341350-8

TABLE I. *Human Cell Lines: Ability to Induce Interferon When Cultured with Lymphocytes and Susceptibility to the Interferon-Induced Resistance to Cytotoxic Lymphocytes and Inhibition of Viral Replication*

Cell line	Origin	Units of Interferon Induced* (mean ± Standard Error)	Inhibition of cytotoxicity†	Inhibition of viral replication**
			%	
FS1	Fetal skin fibroblasts	<1	92	4.0
Pa	Skin fibroblasts	<1	86	3.6
LR-1	Newborn brain	<1	82	3.3
WI38	Fetal lung fibroblasts	<1	62	3.0
MRC5	Fetal lung fibroblasts	<1	40	1.8
LN-SV	Skin, SV40-transformed	<1	77	3.0
W18.VA2	Lung, SV40-transformed	<1	75	2.1
S1054TR	Brain, SV40-transformed	193 ± 137	20	<0.3
SW690	Melanoma	850 ± 552	75	2.4
SW691	Melanoma	6,000 ± 3,000	13	<0.3
SW480	Colorectal carcinoma	125 ± 0	24	<0.3
D98 (HeLa)	Cervical carcinoma	312 ± 165	30	<0.3
HT1080	Fibrosarcoma	<1	15	0.6
RDMC	Rhabdomyosarcoma	3,494 ± 1,008	18	<0.3
K562	Myeloid leukemia	972 ± 0†	68	Not done

are commonly used for testing human NK cell activity are capable of inducing IF in lymphocytes (Table I). As discussed below IF exert a rapid enhancing effect on the cytotoxicity mediated by NK cells. In the culture of lymphocytes with IF-inducing cell lines, an increase in the rate of cytotoxicity appears concomitantly with antiviral activity in the supernatant (Fig. 1). The effect on cytotoxicity of the endogenous IF produced in the culture can be indirectly evaluated in two experimental systems. In one, the cytotoxicity on normal fibroblasts (non-IF-inducers) can be compared with that on virus-infected fibroblasts (IF-inducers) (as described elsewhere) (Santoli *et al.*, 1978). In the other, cytotoxicity of freshly separated lymphocytes (good IF-producers) is compared with that of lymphocytes preincubated at 37°C *in vitro* for 24 hr, which lose their IF-producing ability when cultured with inducer cell lines (Trinchieri *et al.*, 1978b). The results of the latter protocol are shown in Fig. 2. In an 18-hr test using target cell lines that are unable to induce IF, lymphocytes display the same level of cytotoxicity if tested as effector cells immediately after separation or following a preincubation of 24 hr at 37°C. No antiviral activity is detected in the medium of these cultures. When IF-inducing target cell lines are used, the level of antiviral activity is high after 18 hr of incubation of the cells with fresh lymphocytes. No

---

*Anti-viral units in the supernate (24 hr incubation of mixed cultures of monolayer of the cell line with human lymphocytes; four or more different lymphocyte preparations tested for each cell line).

†Average percent inhibition of cytotoxicity. After treatment with interferon (18 hr, 10^3 anti-viral U), cells from the various lines were tested as targets against two different preparations of effector lymphocytes (stimulated by 10^3 anti-viral U of NDV-induced lymphocyte interferon, 18 hr).

**Log_{10} of the reciprocal of the dilution of a lymphocyte interferon preparation (NDV-induced, 10^4 anti-viral reference U) inhibiting 50% of the cytopathic effect of VSV on monolayer of the cell line.

†IF induction was not observed with some sublines of K562.

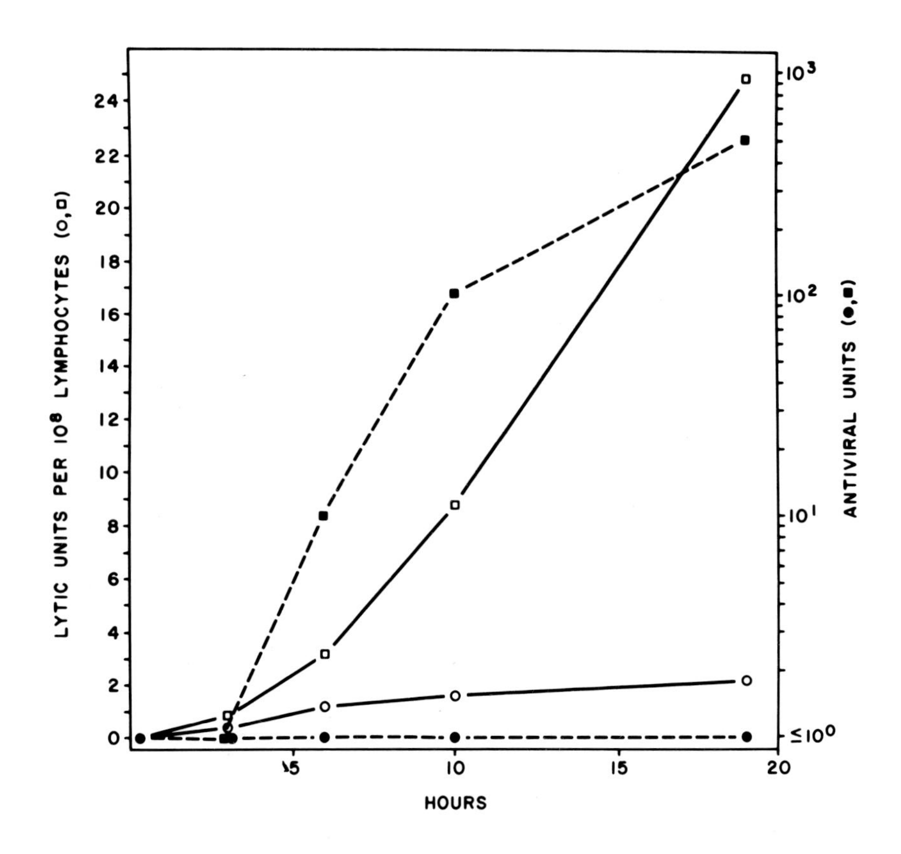

FIGURE 1. Kinetics of spontaneous cell-mediated cytotoxicity and induction of antiviral activity in the supernatants of effector lymphocyte-target cell cultures. One lytic unit represents the number of human peripheral blood lymphocytes required to induce 50% specific ^{51}Cr release, as determined by dose response curves obtained testing different numbers of effector cells. The antiviral activity was measured in the supernatants of the cultures containing the highest concentration of lymphocytes (5×10^6 lymphocytes/ml, 0.2 ml culture, ratio lymphocytes to target cells, 50:1). Antiviral titers of the supernatants were measured by inhibition of the cytopathic effect of vesicular stomatitis virus on a monolayer of human fetal skin fibroblasts. One antiviral unit is equivalent to approximately 1 reference unit of the NIH Human Reference Interferon A-023-901-527. □ cytotoxicity on RDMC target cells; Δ cytotoxicity on fetal skin fibroblasts (RS1); ■ antiviral activity in the supernatant of lymphocytes - RDMC mixed cultures; ● antiviral activity in supernatant of lymphocytes - FS1 mixed cultures.

IF, however, is produced when incubated lymphocytes are used as effector cells. The cytotoxicity of incubated lymphocytes on IF-inducing target cells (measured in 50% lytic units) is reduced to 10 to 20% of that mediated by fresh lymphocytes. These results suggest that when fresh lymphocytes are tested as effector cells against IF-inducing target cells, the enhancing effect of the IF released in the culture medium is responsible for up to 90% of the total cytotoxicity observed. Santoli _et al_. (1978) obtained similar results with virus-infected target cells. The effect of endogenous IF depends on the length of the incubation and is not observed in short-term assays (less than 4 hr). The different target cell lines displayed a different pattern of reactivity when cultured lymphocytes, instead of fresh lymphocytes, were used as effector cells. Susceptibility of the different target cell lines to lysis is, however, similar when incubated lymphocytes or lymphocytes activated by pretreatment with IF are used as effector cells (Trinchieri _et al_., 1978b). For example, IF-inducing RDMC cells are killed 6 times more efficiently than FS-2 fibroblasts by fresh lymphocytes, but only slightly more efficiently by lymphocytes cultured for 24 hr at 37°C (Fig. 2). Lymphocytes were much more efficient effector cells when preincubated with IF; however, different target cells were lysed by both types of effector cells in almost the same rank of susceptibility. There was also much less variability in the susceptibility to lysis of the target cells with IF-stimulated lymphocytes than with fresh or cultured ones. These results suggest that IF enhance the activity of NK cells without altering their apparent specificity, although the enhancing effect _in vitro_ is more apparent in target cell lines of intermediate susceptibility to lysis (e.g., normal fibroblasts) than in the highly susceptible ones (e.g., K562).

Pretreatment of lymphocytes with IF or IF-inducers.

The enhancing effect of IF on NK activity can be readily demonstrated and quantitated by preincubating lymphocytes in the presence of known IF preparations and then testing them in a cytotoxic assay not affected by the production of endogenous IF. This requires a short-term assay (less than 4 hr) and/or the use of target cell lines unable to induce IF. The IF produced in the mixed culture of lymphocytes and cell lines has the molecular and biological characteristics of virus-induced type I leukocyte IF (Trinchieri _et al_., 1978a). All three known types of human IF (fibroblast and leukocyte types I and II) increase human NK cell activity

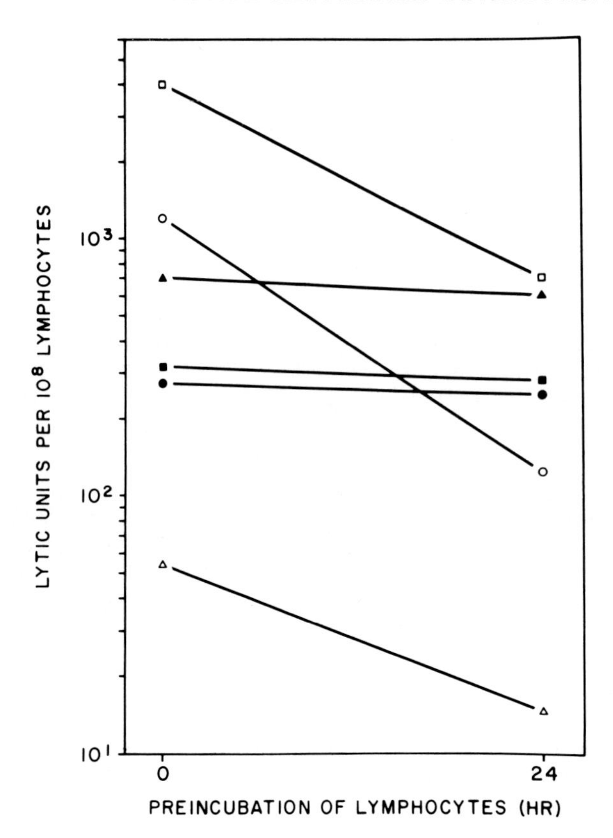

FIGURE 2. Effect of preincubation at 37°C on the ability of human lymphocytes to lyse various target cell lines. The lymphocytes were tested immediately after separation (time 0) or were incubated at 37°C for 24 hr and then tested as effector cells against the various cell lines in an 18 hr ^{51}Cr-release assay. The target cell lines indicated with open symbols are IF inducers when cocultured with lymphocytes. IF can be detected in the supernatant of the cytotoxic test only when fresh lymphocytes are used as effectors against these lines. No IF can be detected in the supernatant of the test with non-inducing target cell lines (closed symbols) or, with any cell lines, when lymphocytes preincubated for 24 hr at 37°C are used as effectors. [] *rhabdomyosarcoma-derived line (RDMC),* 0 *D98 (HeLa) cells,*▲ *human fetal skin fibroblasts (FS2),* ■ *human skin fibroblasts, SV40-transformed (LN-SV),* ● *human fibroblasts, SV40-transformed (W18VA2)* Δ *melanoma-derived cell line (SW690).*

to a similar extent as shown in Fig. 3 (Perussia et al., 1980). The use of electrophoretically homogenous leukocyte IF in defferent laboratories (Heron et al., 1979 and Herberman et al., 1980) has clearly shown that the same

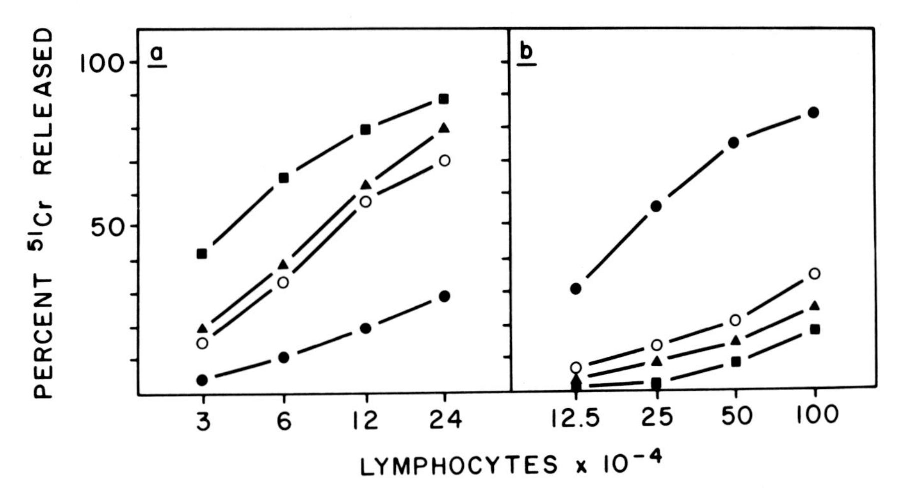

FIGURE 3. Effect of IF in enhancing NK cell cytotoxicity (a) and in protecting their target cells (b). (a) Peripheral blood lymphocytes (5 x 10^6 cell/ml in RPMI 1640 supplemented with 10% fetal bovine serum) were incubated 18 hr at 37°C in the presence of 1,000 antiviral units/ml of human fibroblast IF (partially purified, kindly provided by Dr. A. Billiau, Leuven, Belgium), 1,000 U/ml of leukocyte type I (from Newcastle disease virus-induced human lymphocytes) or 250 U/ml of leukocyte type II IF (supernatant from secondary human mixed lymphocyte cultures at the 2nd day after restimulation). NK cell-mediated cytotoxicity was tested at different effector-to-target cell ratios against human rhabdomyosarcoma-derived cells in 4-hr ^{51}Cr-release assay. ●----●, lymphocytes preincubated in medium; O----O, lymphocytes preincubated with leukocyte type I IF;Δ----Δ , fibroblast IF; □---□ , leukocyte type II IF. (b) Fetal skin fibroblasts, preincubated 18 hr at 37°C in medium or in the presence of the three different types of IF described above, were tested as target cells using human peripheral blood lymphocytes pretreated with 1,000 U/ml of human fibroblast IF as effector cells, in a 18-hr ^{51}Cr-release assay. ●----●, target cells preincubated in medium; O----O, target cells preincubated with leukocyte type I IF;Δ----Δ , fibroblast IF and □---□ leukocyte type II IF. Reproduced with permission from Perussia et al. (1980).

molecules in IF preparations are responsible for both the antiviral activity and the enhancing effect on cytotoxicity. When lymphocytes were pretreated for 18 hr with IF preparations, washed and tested as effector cells against several different target cell lines, they displayed a cytotoxic efficiency up to 20-fold higher than that of untreated lymphocytes. The increase in the non-specific cytotoxicity

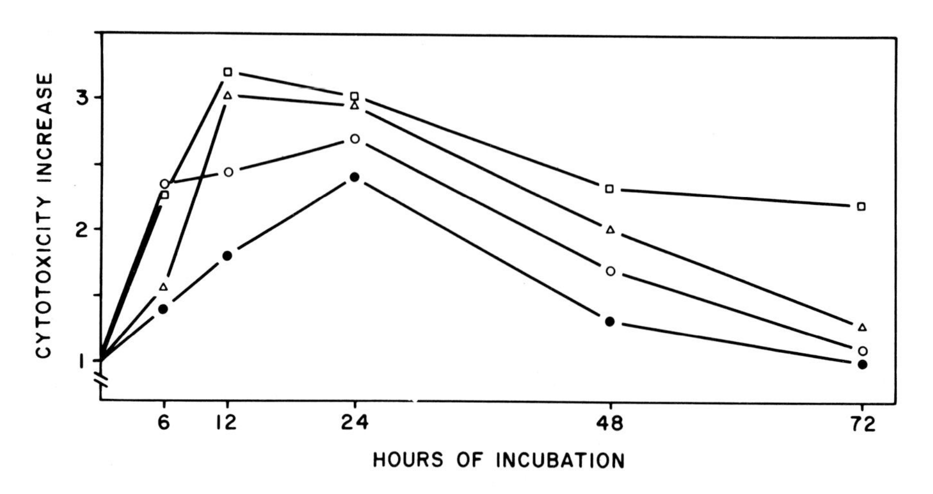

FIGURE 4. Time course of stimulation of cytotoxic lymphocytes by IF and IF-inducers. Human lymphocytes (5 x 10^6/ml, 2 ml/cultures) were incubated for the indicated times in the presence of medium with or without IF or IF-inducers and tested as effector cells against RDMC target cells in a 4-hr cytotoxic test. The cytotoxicity increase indicates the ratio between the lytic units observed with lymphocytes preincubated with IF or IF-inducers and the lytic units of lymphocytes incubated in normal medium. Lymphocytes were preincubated in presence of ● Newcastle disease virus-induced leukocyte IF (10^3 units); □ human B cell lines EB-P8 (lymphocytes to lymphoid cell ratio, 10:1); Δ [poly (rI) - poly (rC)] (50 μg/ml) and 0 Hong Kong strain of influenza A virus (85 HAU/ml).

of human lymphocytes cultured in the presence of IF was quantitatively comparable or higher than that observed upon stimulation of lymphocytes with optimal concentrations of phytohemagglutinin (PHA). The enhancement of cytotoxicity was dependent on the dose of IF added to the culture; a twofold increase was obtained with about 10 antiviral units of leukocyte type I interferon (Trinchieri and Santoli, 1978). IF-inducers were also very effective in enhancing cytotoxicity when preincubated with lymphocytes: this effect was observed with viruses (Santoli et al., 1978), inducing cell lines and a synthetic inducer [poly (rI) - poly (rC)] (Trinchieri et al., 1978b). Though cytotoxicity increased after only a few hours of incubation at 37°C either with IF or with IF-inducers, the maximum level was reached when lymphocytes had been preincubated for 24 to 48 hr as shown in Fig. 4 (Trinchieri et al., 1978b). IF binding to lymphocytes appears to be independent of temperature, and the presence of IF is required for only a few minutes. However, subsequent incubation at 37°C and the active synthesis of cellular protein and RNA are necessary in order to detect the enhancing effect (Herberman et al., 1980). These data show that IF act by inducing complex metabolic alterations in the effector cells. IF do not simply provide a bridge between effector and target cells, as suggested by Perlmann and Holm (1969) in the case of IgG induction of antibody-dependent cell-mediated cytotoxicity, and by Cerottini and Brunner (1974) in the case of mitogen induction of lysis of non-specific target cells during the efferent phase of T-cell-mediated cytotoxicity. IF can act either at the single effector cell level or by recruiting previously inactive cytotoxic cells. If are only able to enhance the cytotoxicity of the lymphocyte subpopulations that originally contain NK activity (Trinchieri and Santoli, 1978; Santoli et al., 1978). Those subpopulations that do not contain NK cells (B cells, Fc receptor-negative "null" cells and IgG-Fc receptor-negative T cells) do not acquire cytotoxic activity when exposed to IF (Trinchieri and Santoli, 1978). Saksela et al. (1979) have demonstrated, however, that once active NK cells have been removed by absorption on bead-attached fibroblasts, a cell population devoid of NK activity is obtained. However, "pre-NK" cells can be demonstrated in this population since cytotoxic activity returns following treatment with IF.

There is still the question of whether IF induce activation of NK cells by facilitating effector-target recognition or by increasing the activity of cellular factors involved in the cytolytic mechanism of cytotoxicity. Perussia et al. have described elsewhere in this volume their approach to this problem by comparing the effect of IF on the activity of NK cells and of the antibody-dependent effector cells. More direct information can be obtained by analyzing the effect of IF on the cytotoxicity of single lymphocytes. This involves studying the kinetics of cytotoxicity of lymphocytes which, after adherence to the target cells, are cultured in semisolid medium (Targan and Dorey, 1980 and our unpublished results). Lymphocytes and target cells (K562) are mixed at a ratio 1:1, incubated for a few minutes to allow cell-cell contact, plated in 1% agarose and stained with trypan blue to detect dead target cells. Percentage of conjugates in which target cells are killed is scored at various time intervals. The treatment of lymphocytes with IF does not significantly increase the number of lymphocytes binding to the target cells (about 9%); the number of target cells lysed in the effector-target cell conjugates increases 20% to 35% when IF-treated effector cells are used; and, more notably, the rate of cytotoxicity is much faster with IF-treated lymphocytes (the maximum number of target cells lysed is reached in less than 30 min) than with untreated lymphocytes (maximum reached at about 3 hr). These results suggest that, at least with very susceptible target cell lines like K562, IF act mainly by increasing the rate of killing, and allow each effector cells to lyse a higher number of target cells in the same time interval. These data, however, also suggest the possibility of recruitment of "pre-NK" cells, by conveying cytotoxic ability on cells that originally could only bind to the target cells, and do not exclude the possibility that cytotoxic cells are also generated from the cells originally unable to recognize and to bind to the target cells. The possibility that the effect of IF on NK cells was dependent on the increased expression of histocompatibility antigens induced by IF on lymphocytes was tested by using radiolabeled monoclonal antibodies to HLA antigens (Heron *et al*., 1978). In preliminary experiments, Perussia *et al*. (1980) have found no correlation between the increase of cytotoxicity and the enhancement of the expression of HLA antigens.

Inhibition of target cell susceptibility to lysis by pretreatment with interferon.

The effect of IF-pretreatment of target cells is paradoxically opposite to that obtained by pretreating effector cells. Target cells that had been preincubated in the presence of IF became resistant to the cytotoxic effect of NK cells (Trinchieri and Santoli, 1978). Incubation of fibroblasts with 10^3 antiviral units of IF had no toxic effect on the cells. The preincubation of fibroblast (FS1) target cells with IF induced up to 98% protection against the cytotoxicity mediated either by fresh or IF-stimulated human lymphocytes (Table I and Fig. 3b). This was true for all the three known types of human IF (Perussia *et al*., 1980). The inhibition of target cell susceptibility to lysis was dose dependent: 1 to 2 antiviral units of IF were required for 50% inhibition of cytotoxicity on FS1 target cells. The antiviral and the target protective titers correlated significantly in all IF preparations tested. A mock IF preparation and mouse IF were unable to induce resistance in human target cells. The protective activity in preparation of type I leukocyte IF was resistant to pH 2.0, destroyed by treatment with trypsin, and was eluted from a Sephadex G200 column in a peak with an approximate mol. wt. of 25,000, together with the antiviral activity (Trinchieri and Santoli, 1978). To reach the maximum level of inhibition, it was necessary to preincubate the target cells for several hours. The presence of IF was not required for the entire period.

Treatment of fibroblasts for 30 min with IF, and subsequent incubation for 24 hr without IF induced an 85% inhibition of cytotoxicity, whereas pretreatment for 30 min immediately before the test induced only 35% inhibition (Trinchieri and Santoli, 1978). The induction of resistance to lysis upon treatment with IF was prevented by concurrent treatment of FS1 cells with actinomycin D or cycloheximide, suggesting the requirement of both protein and RNA synthesis for the induction of resistance. Virus infection of the target cells with influenza A (Fig. 5) and vaccinia viruses also prevented the induction of most of the resistance in FS1 cells, possibly due to the inhibitory effect of virus replication on cellular protein synthesis. Fifteen different cell lines have been tested for IF-mediated induction of resistance to NK cell activity (Table I and Fig. 5) (Trinchieri and Santoli, 1978). Fibroblasts are susceptible to both the

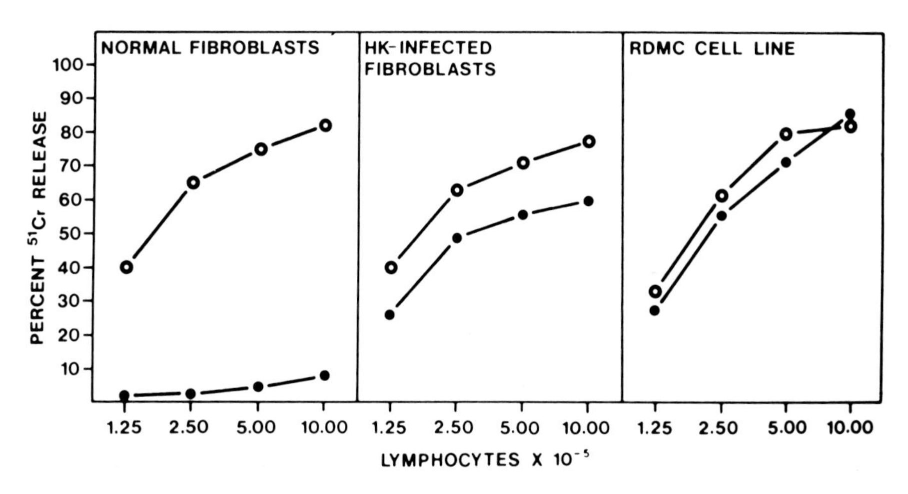

FIGURE 5. Ability of IF to protect different types of target cells from lysis mediated by NK cells. Human lymphocytes were incubated with 500 antiviral units of leukocyte IF for 18 hr at 37°C and washed. They were then used at different concentrations as effector cells in a ^{51}Cr-release assay against normal fetal skin fibroblasts, fibroblasts infected with Hong Kong strain of influenza A virus and a human rhabdomyosarcoma-derived cell line (RDMC). The target cells were untreated (O) or incubated before the test for 18 hr at 37°C in the presence of 500 antiviral units of human leukocyte IF (●). Reproduced with permission from Trinchieri et al. (1979).

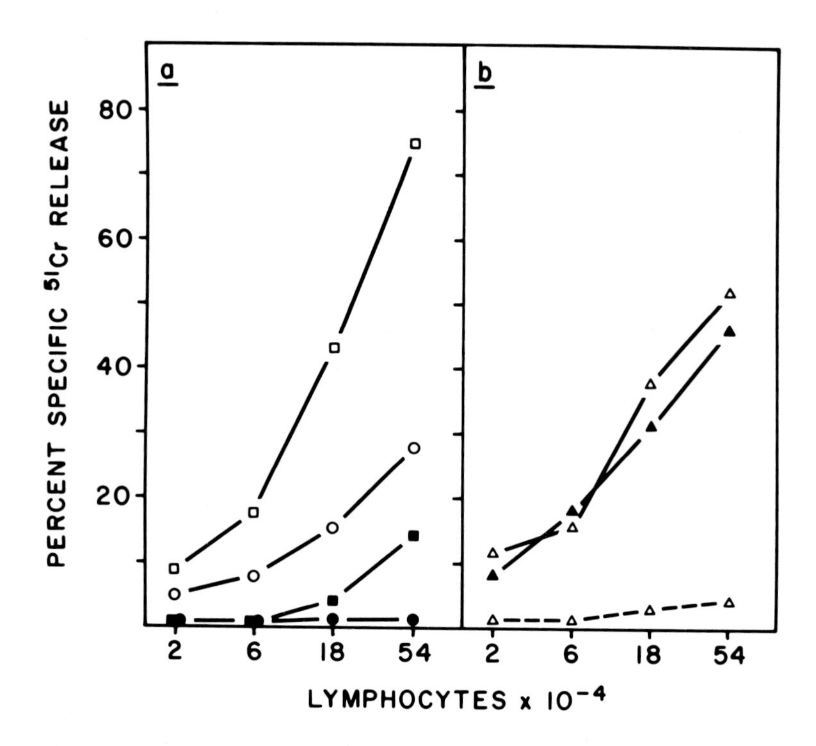

FIGURE 6. IF-treated target cells are protected against spontaneous cytotoxicity of human lymphocytes but not against antibody-dependent cell-mediated cytotoxicity. a) Lymphocytes were incubated for 18 hr at 37°C in medium or in the presence of 500 U of human fibroblast IF. They were then tested in an 18-hr assay against fibroblast (FS1) target cells preincubated in medium or in presence of 500 U of IF. O----O untreated lymphocytes, untreated target, □---□ IF-treated lymphocytes, untreated target, ●-----●, untreated lymphocytes, IF-treated target, ■---■ IF-treated lymphocytes, IF-treated target. b) Lymphocytes were treated with trypsin (1 mg/ml, 20 min, 37°C) and then tested for cytotoxicity against IF-treated or untreated fibroblast target sensitized with rabbit anti-human cell antiserum (4-hr test). Δ------Δ , untreated target cells, no antiserum, Δ----Δ untreated target cells sensitized with the rabbit antiserum, ▲----▲ IF-treated target cells sensitized with the rabbit antiserum.

antiviral and target-protecting activity of IF. When various SV40-transformed or tumor-derived cell lines were tested, a variable susceptibility to IF was observed in different lines. All the tumor-derived lines tested, however, were not susceptible to either the antiviral or the target protective activity of IF, with the exception of the melanoma-derived SW690 line. A significant positive correlation was observed between cell line susceptibility to the antiviral and to the target protecting activity of IF ($r = 0.954$, $p < 0.001$).

Interferon-treated target cells are inefficient inhibitors in competitive cold-target inhibition experiments, suggesting that the treatment leads to cell surface changes affecting recognition of NK cells (Trinchieri and Santoli, 1978). The protective effect appears specific for the cytotoxicity mediated by NK cells. The IF-treated IgG antibody-sensitized target cells are lysed by antibody-dependent effector cells as well as untreated cells (Fig. 6). In repeated experiments, IF-treated and untreated FS1 cells were equally susceptible to mouse anti-human cytotoxic T cells (Trinchieri and Santoli, 1978). The IF-treated target cells were only partially protected against PHA-induced cytotoxic human lymphocytes. PHA, however, probably stimulated both cytotoxic T cells and NK cells (Bonavida _et al_., 1977).

Does IF have a central role in the regulation of in vivo NK cell defensive activity?

The enhancing effect of IF and IF-inducers on NK activity has been demonstrated _in vivo_ in the mouse (Giglund _et al_., 1978), in the rat (Oehler _et al_., 1978) and in humans (Emodi G., personal communication). We have found (unpublished results) that during the growth of the transplantable mastocytoma P815Y in syngeneic DBA/2 mice, IF is present at a level of 50 to 1000 antiviral units (when the tumor load reaches 10^8 cells) in the ascitic fluid. The tumor cell obtained at that time does not permit the replication of vesicular stomatitis virus (VSV) nor is it lysed by the non-specific cytotoxic lymphocytes that are mixed with the tumor cells and which can be separated by velocity sedimentation (Biddison and Palmer, 1977). After 24 hr of incubation _in vitro_, the tumor cells regained both the ability to replicate VSV and the susceptibility to lysis.

The enhancing effect of IF on NK cells is non-specific and, with the limitations discussed above, IF-stimulated NK cells kill any target cells, including autologous cells. The protective effect of IF on target cells offers a possible explanation of the paradoxical existance in vivo of NK cells which can also efficiently lyse normal autologous cells in vitro, (Santoli et al., 1976). Normal fibroblasts are generally more susceptible to the antiviral and target cell protecting activities of IF than cultured tumor cells or virus-infected cells. IF, by stimulating very efficient non-specific cytotoxic cells and by simultaneously protecting normal cells from lysis, might render the NK system an inducible selective defense mechanism against tumor cells or virus-infected cells. However, some tumor cell lines e.g., SW690 in Table I and P815Y maintain their susceptibility to the IF target protecting activity. In this case, IF may furnish an efficient escape mechanism to the tumor by protecting the cells from lysis. Mouse spleen cells from apparently healthy animals and, occasionally, human peripheral blood lymphocytes, spontaneously secrete low levels of IF. This suggests the continual presence of physiologically active IF in small amounts which could possibly maintain the activity of the NK cells in vivo (Trinchieri and Santoli, 1978; Herberman et al. 1979). As schematically depicted in Fig. 7, the damage induced by these NK cells to normal

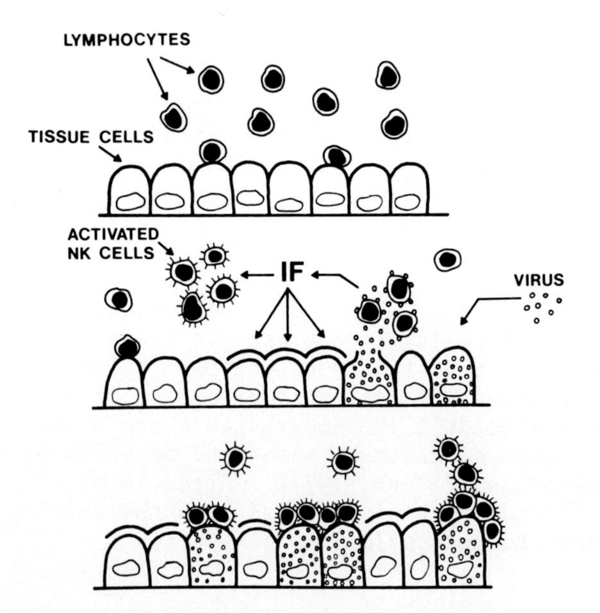

FIGURE 7. Model of the possible participation of NK cells in vivo in the defensive processes against virus infection. Reproduced with permission from Trinchieri et al. (1979).

tissue cells would be extremely reduced due to the limited susceptibility to lysis of normal tissue cells and to their ability to competitively inhibit NK cell activity. When an IF-inducing pathological alteration, such as a virus infection, occurs in a part of the organism (Fig. 7, center), cytotoxicity of NK cells would be greatly enhanced by IF and at the same time, normal tissue cells would be protected. The cytotoxicity of the NK cells on the virus-infected cells could be greatly enhanced not only due to the increased activity of the NK cells, but also because IF render "normal" tissue cells unable to compete for NK cells (Fig. 7, bottom). The two effects of IF on cytotoxicity, which *in vitro* are apparently antagonistic, could therefore act synergistically *in vivo* and concentrate NK cell activity on virus-infected cells (Fig. 7), or on other pathological cell types. Although this description of the defensive process is still mostly speculative, the information obtained from *in vitro* experimentation with human cells and the promising results from some *in vivo* experiments using animal models, make the original interpretation of spontaneous CMC as a technical artifact unlikely. These studies are beginning to elucidate the possible participation of the NK cells in the defensive system of the organism.

REFERENCES

Biddison, W.E., and Palmer, J.C., *Proc. Natl. Acad. Sci. USA 74*, 329-333 (1977).

Bonavida, B.A., Robins, A., and Saxons, A., *Transplantation 23*, 261-270 (1977).

Cerottini, J.-C., and Brunner, K.T., *Adv. Immunol. 18*, 67-132 (1974).

Giglund, M., Örn, A., Wigzell, H., Senik, A., and Gresser, I., *Nature 273*, 759-761 (1978).

Herberman, R.B., Ortaldo, J.R., and Bonnard, G.D., *Nature 277*, 221-223 (1979).

Herberman, R.B., Ortaldo, J.R., Djeu, J.Y., Holden, H.T., and Jett, J., *Ann. N.Y. Acad. Sci. in press* (1980).

Heron, I., Hokland, M., and Berg, K., *Proc. Natl. Acad. Sci. USA 75*, 6215-6219 (1978).

Heron, I., Hokland, A., Moller-Larsen, A., and Berg, K., *Cellular Immunol. 42*, 183-187 (1979).

Oehler, R.J., Lindsay, L.R., and Nunn, M.E., *Cancer 21*, 210-214 (1978).

Perlmann, P., and Holm, G., *Adv. Immunol. 11*, 117-131 (1969).

Perussia, B., Santoli, D., and Trinchieri, G., *Ann. N.Y. Acad. Sci. in press* (1980).

Santoli, D., Trinchieri, G., Zmijewski, C.M., and Koprowski, H., *J. Immunol. 117*, 765-770 (1976).

Santoli, D., Trinchieri, G., and Koprowski, H., *J. Immunol. 121*, 532-538 (1978).

Saksela, E., Timonen, T., and Cantell, K., *Scand. J. Immunol. 10*, 257-266 (1979).

Targan, S., and Dorey, F., *J. Immunol. in press* (1980).

Trinchieri, G., and Santoli, D., *J. Exp. Med. 147*, 1314-1333 (1978).

Trinchieri, G., Santoli, D., and Knowles, B.B., *Nature 270*, 611-612 (1977).

Trinchieri, G., Santoli, D., Dee, R.R., and Knowles, B., *J. Exp. Med. 147*, 1299-1313 (1978a).

Trinchieri, G., Santoli, D., and Koprowski, H., *J. Immunol. 120*, 1849-1855 (1978b).

Trinchieri, G., Perussia, B., Santoli, D., and Cerottini, J.-C., *Transplat. Proc. XI*, 807-810 (1979).

ACTIVATED NATURAL KILLER CELLS INDUCED DURING THE LYMPHOCYTIC CHORIOMENINGITIS VIRUS INFECTION IN MICE

Raymond M. Welsh, Jr.

Department of Immunopathology
Scripps Clinic and Research Foundation
La Jolla, California

Rolf W. Kiessling

Department of Tumor Biology
Karolinska Institute
Stockholm, Sweden

I. INTRODUCTION

The lymphocytic choriomeningitis virus (LCMV) infection of mice has uniquely contributed to theories on viral persistence (1), immunological tolerance (2), immune response disease (3), virus-induced immune complex disease (4,5), cytotoxic T-cell killing (6), and the role of H-2 in the immune response (7). It is only appropriate that this model was used for the initial studies on NK cell activation by virus infections (8-11), though NK cell activation was simultaneously discovered in other virus systems as well (12,13).

LCMV produces two distinctly different diseases in mice. Young or adult mice acutely infected with LCMV develop a high interferon response in lymphoid organs (14,15), a marked deficiency in hematopoiesis (15), macrophage activation (16), and a potent virus-specific H-2 restricted cytotoxic T-cell response (6,7). These mice either recover from the infection with lasting immunity or else develop fatal immunopathological lesions (6). In contrast, mice infected congenitally or within 24 hours of birth become life-long persistent virus carriers and usually succumb to a slow degenerative disease associated with virus-antibody-complement immune complex deposits and lymphoid infiltrations of many of the body's tis-

ISBN 0-12-341350-8

sues (4,5,17). LCMV carrier mice are reported to have no hematopoietic dysfunction, macrophage activation, LCMV-specific cytotoxic T cells, or elevated interferon levels (reviewed 18), though a recent report suggests that interferon may be made during the first week of the persistent carrier infection (19).

In this chapter we will examine (1) the factors contributing to the activation of the NK cell during the LCMV infection, (2) the altered properties of the activated cell when compared to the cytotoxic T cell and the unactivated "endogenous" NK cell, and (3) the possible role NK cells may play during the acute and persistent infections.

II. INDUCTION OF ACTIVATED NK CELLS DURING THE LCMV INFECTION

A. *Acute Infection in Adult Mice*

Infection of C3H/St mice intraperitoneally with 2×10^4 plaque forming units of LCMV, strain Armstrong, induces activated NK cells and virus specific cytotoxic T cells, which peak on the third and seventh day of infection, respectively (8,11). Depending on the dose, inoculation route, and strain of mouse, the relative peaks in these two activities may vary (11, Welsh and Zinkernagel, unpublished). Table I is a composite of several experiments showing the development of a "nonspecific" (NK cell) cytotoxicity against several types of target cells and a specific (T cell) cytotoxicity against LCMV-infected L-929 cells. Effector cells in the NK peak lysed target cells previously insensitive to lysis by endogenous NK cells and also caused augmented lysis against cells normally considered sensitive to endogenous effectors (YAC-1 cells). Similar enhancements in NK cell activity were found in every tested strain of mouse, including T cell-deficient nude mice (8,9), B cell-deficient CBA/N x DBA_2 mice (11), and C57BL6 mice carrying the beige mutation (20), a mutation reported to be associated with very low NK cell activity (21).

TABLE I. Induction of Cytotoxic Cells in Adult C3H/St Mice Infected with LCMV

Day post-infection	L-929	% Lysis caused by spleen cells L-929(LCMV)	F-9	SWR/J	Vero	YAC-1	Spleen IF[1]
0	2	0	6	-3	9	20	<4
1	8	5	11	16	26	-	128
2	23	20	34	42	38	49	512
3	33	30	59	32	36	65	400
4	20	21	43	35	31	-	80
5	20	32	38	24	45	-	12
6	14	43	41	-	-	56	-
7	15	81	34	-	-	-	40
8	8	83	20	-	-	-	<4
10	2	28	4	-	-	27	-
12	3	23	-	-	-	-	-
14	1	13	-	-	-	-	-

These data are a composite of a number of experiments using 4-6 week old male mice. Effector to target ratios are 100:1 except for YAC-1 targets, which are 25:1. SWR/J targets are primary peritoneal macrophages (see 21). F-9 cells lack H-2 expression (44). For details see 11,22.

[1] *Interferon units per spleen*

B. *Association of NK Activity with the Interferon Response*

The LCMV-induced activation of NK cells appears to be mediated by interferon (11), which has been shown by us and others (23) to activate mouse NK cells. Levels of interferon and NK activity in the spleen correlate well during the LCMV infection (11, Table I), and direct activation of NK cells <u>in vivo</u> by interferon was shown by injecting mice intraperitoneally with relatively low doses (500-2000 units) of interferon Type I preparations (11). In these experiments the activation of NK cells was locally confined to the peritoneal environment but not the spleen. Others have reported

NK cell induction by interferon in vivo, but these were systemic inductions requiring several orders of magnitude more interferon (23). Using the intraperitoneal injection method, we have also been able to activate NK cells with preparations of mouse serum containing interferon Type II, prepared by BCG hyperimmunization. These sera contained no detectable interferon Type I, and the inducing activity was totally eliminated by treatment of the serum with pH 2 (Welsh, Creasey, and Merigan, unpublished data). The significance of this is that during a virus infection NK cells may be activated by interferon produced by the virus-infected cell or produced by immune lymphoid cells responding to the viral infection.

C. *Interferon Production and NK Cell Activity In Vitro*

The peak in interferon activity in spleen homogenates is at 2 or 3 days postinfection, but if lymphoid cells are isolated from spleens and put in culture, considerably more interferon is produced by cells from spleens 6 days postinfection than from spleens 2 or 3 days postinfection (Table II). This suggests that a significant portion of the interferon produced in spleens early in the infection may be associated with cells other than lymphoid cells. The interferon-producing lymphoid cell two days

TABLE II. NK Activity in Cultured Leukocytes from LCMV-Infected C3H/St Mice

Day post-infection	Spleen cells % Lysis			IF[1]	Peritoneal cells % Lysis	IF
	F-9	L-929	L-929(LCMV)		F-9	
0	0	0	-2	-	3	-
2	-5	0	-3	8	7	-
3	0	1	1	-	-	5
4	0	0	1	-	-1	-
5	27	-	9	-	-	-
6	33	15	56	1024	37	128
8	12	11	60	-	13	-
10	6	4	28	-	3	-
14	0	5	8	-	0	-

[1]*Interferon units per ml produced after incubation of* 10^7 *spleen cells or* 5×10^6 *peritoneal cells per ml for 36 H.*

postinfection adheres to nylon and glass wool columns and is depleted from spleen leukocyte populations with iron filings and a magnet, suggesting that it may be a macrophage (24). In contrast, about half of the interferon producing cell activity in the day 6 leukocytes is not adherent to nylon wool. If cells are cultured at 37°C overnight before assay, the NK activity during the first 4 days postinfection is abolished. However, both spleen and peritoneal cells have a culture stable peak of NK activity on the sixth day postinfection (Table II). This correlates with the induction of the cytotoxic T cell response, and significant levels of interferon are produced in the culture at that time. Numerous experiments to be published (24) indicate that this culture stable "nonspecific" cell is an NK cell stabilized or continually activated in culture by interferon. We hypothesize that the expanding clones of T cells may secrete interferon which will in turn activate the NK cells in culture. Consistent with this hypothesis is the fact that athymic nude mice do not produce a culture-stable NK cell in this manner (24).

D. *NK Cell Activation in LCMV-Immune Mice*

Mice immunized with LCMV do not develop an activated NK cell response when challenged with a similar dose of virus (11). This fact is not surprising, since interferon production is usually low during secondary virus infections (25). The NK cells can still be activated, however, because injection of LCMV immune mice with Pichinde virus will induce NK cells. The reciprocal is true: Pichinde virus does not induce NK cells in Pichinde virus-immune mice but LCMV does. Whether very high doses of virus could induce NK cells in mice immune to that virus has not been tested.

E. *Age Distribution and NK Activity in LCMV Carrier Mice*

NK activity can be induced by LCMV to the highest degree in mice 5 to 10 weeks of age (11), correlating with earlier reports on age related peaks of endogenous NK activity (26,27). LCMV can, however, activate NK cells in mice infected within 24 hours of birth, though the activity is low (11). LCMV-persistently infected carrier mice do not have activated NK cells but do have normal levels of endogenous NK cell activity (28).

III. CHARACTERIZATION OF THE LCMV-INDUCED ACTIVATED NK CELL

A. *Comparison Between the Induced NK and the Cytotoxic T Cells*

Table III compares the properties of the LCMV-induced activated NK cell with the LCMV-specific cytotoxic T cell. Neither cell expresses surface immunoglobulin, adheres significantly to plastic, or is phagocytic (11). Both have surface theta antigen, but the cytotoxic T cell has considerably more, as judged by its sensitivity to lysis by antibody to theta antigen plus complement (22,29,30). Both can be passed through columns of nylon wool, but the activated NK cell is partially adherent and loses some activity after passage, in contrast to T cells, which gain activity (11). NK cells can be activated, though at reduced levels, in mice receiving 1000 R of X-irradiation, indicating that proliferation of NK cells is not required for activation (11). The isotope ^{89}Strontium, which, as an analog of calcium, deposits in the bone marrow and destroys developing cells in that microenvironment, significantly but not totally reduces the levels of NK cell activation (11). Others have shown that endogenous NK activity can be inhibited by this treatment (31). The LCMV-induced NK cell tends to be unstable in culture, losing over 80% activity within 5 hours of incubation at 37°C, while the T cell activity is stable in culture (8, Table I & II). The stability of NK cells *in vitro* is subject to considerable variation, however, at least partially reflecting the amount of interferon that is produced in the culture.

TABLE III. Comparison of the Properties of the LCMV-Induced NK and Cytotoxic T Cells

	NK	T
Plastic adherent	no	no
Phagocytic	no	no
Surface immunoglobulin	no	no
Surface theta	yes (low)	yes (high)
Nylon wool adherence	partially depleted	enriched
Induced in nude mice	yes	no
Induced in newborn mice	yes	no
Induced in X-ray (1000 R) mice	yes (reduced)	no
Induced in ^{89}Strontium mice	yes (very reduced)	yes (near normal)
Virus specific killing	no	yes
H-2 restricted killing	no	yes
Stability in culture	labile	stable

B. *Comparison Between the Endogenous and Activated NK Cells*

In contrast to some reports published by other laboratories (9,32,33), we have found significant differences in the properties of activated vs. endogenous NK cells (29). The most striking differences are those in adherence properties (Table IV). While endogenous NK cell activity is enriched on a cell-to-cell basis by passage through columns of nylon wool, the LCMV-induced NK activity is partially reduced (Table IVA). This difference in nylon wool adherence can easily be observed if both endogenous and activated cells are used in the same experiment. Without doing this, day-to-day fluctuations in nylon wool columns could lead to other interpretations. Activated NK cells are considerably more adherent to monolayers of antibody-coated erythrocytes, suggesting an increase in the number or avidity of Fc receptors expressed on the NK cell membrane (Table IVB). Confirmation that the EA adherence is due to Fc receptors was shown by blocking experiments with Staphylococcus A protein, which binds to the Fc region of IgG (34). This protein inhibited the

EA monolayer reduction of NK activity in the induced cells (Table IVC). EA monolayers did not significantly deplete NK activity in preparations of nylon wool-passed activated NK cells, indicating that the cells expressing EA adherence, i.e., Fc receptors, also bound to the nylon wool (Table IVD).

TABLE IV. Adherence Properties of LCMV-Induced Activated NK Cells from C3H/St Mouse Spleens

			% Lysis	
			Endogenous NK	Activated NK
Exp. A.	Untreated		11	42
	Nylon passed		23	19
Exp. B.	Untreated		27	60
	E depleted		39	54
	EA depleted		42	29
Exp. C.	Untreated		57	51
	E depleted		49	61
	EA depleted		45	30
	EA depleted + Staph A		52	51
Exp. D.	Unpassed:	untreated		83
		E depleted		81
		EA depleted		44
	Nylon passed:	untreated		59
		E depleted		68
		EA depleted		61

Numbers refer to microcytotoxicity assays using spleen cells depleted by the various treatments. E and EA depletions were done on monolayers of erythrocytes.

The phenomenon of increased nylon wool and EA adherence by activated NK cells may be due to either or both of two possibilities: 1. activation may cause NK cells to express more Fc receptors and become more nylon wool adherent; or 2. previously inactive cells which express these adherence properties become activated. While we have not conclusively resolved this question at this time, we favor the second hypothesis for several reasons. First, the experiments listed in Table IV can be reproduced using cells activated by a one hour exposure to interferon *in vitro* (29). It seems unlikely that an increase in Fc receptor expression could be induced in so short a period of time. Second, statistical analysis of cytotoxicity curves in our laboratories suggests that there is an increase in the number of cytotoxic effector cells after activation. Third, preliminary results suggest that the activity of nylon wool adherent cells is enhanced by interferon more so than that of the nonadherent cells, though the activity of the nonadherent cells is also augmented by this treatment. Roder *et al.*, (35) concluded that there was no increase in the number of NK cells binding to YAC-1 targets after *in vivo* activation with poly I:C, but these experiments used lymphocytes after passage through nylon wool, which would remove many of the induced cells, not known to be nylon wool adherent at that time.

TABLE IV. Properties of Endogenous vs. LCMV-Induced Activated NK Cells

	Endogenous	Activated
Nylon wool	Relatively nonadherent	Relatively adherent
EA monolayers	Relatively nonadherent	Relatively adherent
Theta antigen	Low levels	Higher levels: less than T cells
Size	Small to medium lymphocyte	Small to medium with some activity in larger cells
Target specificity	Restricted	Relatively unrestricted

LCMV-activated NK cells were reported by Herberman *et al.*, (30) to be more sensitive than endogenous NK cells to lysis by antibody to theta antigen plus complement, and we have confirmed this observation (29). The most plausible interpretation of these results is that the activated cell expressed more theta antigen, but this has not yet been confirmed by other techniques.

Using the Beckman centrifugal elutriation technique to separate cells on the basis of size, we have found differences between the endogenous and activated NK cell preparations (29). While most NK activity in both endogenous and activated preparations was associated with fractions containing small to medium size lymphocytes, NK activity on a cell-to-cell basis in the large cell fractions was proportionally much greater in activated NK cell populations than in controls. While some of this activity was associated with blast size cells, it is not known if NK cell blastogenesis is induced during the LCMV infection.

Table V summarizes the differences we have observed between populations of endogenous and LCMV-induced activated NK cells.

IV. ROLE OF NK CELLS DURING THE LCMV INFECTION

The role of NK cells in virus infections in vivo has thus far received little attention. The virus-specific cytotoxic cell most commonly studied in the mouse has been the T cell, and, in the LCMV system, transfer of immune T cells into infected animals was shown to mediate immunopathology (6) as well as virus clearance (36). LCMV induces high levels of NK cells in athymic nude mice, but these mice produce more infectious virus than heterozygous littermates and fail to clear the infection (11). Nevertheless, due to the profound augmentation of NK activity during the acute infection, experiments were designed to test any possible role of NK cells in the LCMV system.

A. *Failure to Demonstrate LCMV-Specific Killing*

LCMV acutely infected, persistently infected, or uninfected L-929 cells displayed comparable sensitivities to NK cells. In assays from 4 to 16 hours, endogenous NK cells failed to lyse any of these targets, and LCMV-induced NK cells lysed each target at identical levels (8,37, Table I). Since C3H/St mouse macrophages resist lysis by syngeneic activated NK cells, we examined whether LCMV-infection of those targets could confer any sensitivity to them, and it did not (22). In cold target competition experiments, LCMV-infected L-929 cells and uninfected L-929 cells competed equally well against radiolabeled L-929 cell targets, indicating no preferential binding of NK cells to the virus-infected target. Thus, there is no in vitro evidence that NK cells may selectively bind to or lyse LCMV-infected cells.

Attempts by us to demonstrate significant levels of LCMV-specific K cell killing, using guinea pig or mouse antibody to LCMV against L-929 cells have thus far been unsuccessful, even though anti-H-2^k antiserum mediates K cell killing against those same targets (37). We do not know the reason for this, since similarly LCMV-infected cells can be lysed by the same antibody source plus complement (38).

B. *Failure of the Beige Mutation to Influence LCMV Synthesis In Vivo*

The beige mutation in mice confers a comparatively very low NK cell reactivity to C57BL6 mice (21). The LCMV infection induces some NK activity in homozygous bg/bg mice, but this activity is considerably lower than that in heterozygous bg/+ controls (20). We hypothesized that the virus-induced interferon activation would cause NK cells in a localized area of infection to nonselectively lyse cells and thereby restrict the synthesis of virus in the early stages of infection. This seemed a feasible hypothesis, since activated NK cells can lyse isologous primary fibroblasts, and since the beige mutation has proven useful for in vivo studies on NK-mediated tumor resistance (39,40). However, during the first 3 days postinfection, spleen titers of LCMV in bg/bg mice did not differ significantly from bg/+ controls, despite marked differences of NK activity and similar levels of interferon (20). These experiments therefore failed to support the hypothesis that NK cells are important in controlling the early stages of the LCMV infection in mice. An ADCC mechanism of NK cells may be significant at later stages of infection when antibody is made, but as noted above (III.A.), ADCC has not yet been demonstrated in the murine LCMV system.

C. *NK Cells in LCMV-Carrier Mice*

NK cells are not activated in LCMV-carrier mice (at least in the spleen), and there is no evidence that they play a significant role in the immunopathology of the chronic disease. However, considerable amounts of anti-viral antibody are produced in these mice (41), and many of the organs are infiltrated with lymphocytes (17). If LCMV-specific K cell lysis occurred in vivo, then a considerable portion of the chronic injury may be due to NK-like cells having K cell capacities.

D. *The Effect of LCMV Infection on Tumor Growth*

It has been known for a number of years that acute LCMV infection of mice results in a markedly reduced incidence of spontaneously occurring leukemias in AKR mice and of tumors arising from transplanted lymphatic leukemia cells (42). In a limited number of cases some human cancer patients have been treated with LCMV infection with some success (43). Padnos and Molomut (42) gave evidence suggesting that LCMV-induced interferon was responsible for the anti-tumor effect. Whether the anti-tumor effect was due directly to interferon or indirectly through activation of cells such as NK cells or macrophages was not determined.

V. CONCLUSIONS

LCMV is a potent inducer of activated NK cells in mice. The activation appears to be mediated by the interferon induced in lymphoid organs during the infection. Several cell types may be involved in interferon production in vivo, and they vary with the time after infection. The LCMV-induced activated NK cells differ from endogenous NK cells in that they express increased adherence to nylon wool, higher levels of Fc receptors, higher levels of theta antigen, and, to a limited degree, some increase in size. The activated NK cells lyse a much greater range of target cells but show no selectivity in lysing LCMV-infected targets. LCMV-carrier mice do not have an elevated NK cell response, nor do LCMV immune mice after a secondary LCMV challenge. While the LCMV infection is a marked NK cell inducer and may be useful in anti-tumor studie the available evidence at this time fails to support the hypothe sis that NK cells play a major role in the pathogenesis of the

LCMV infection in vivo.

ACKNOWLEDGMENTS

This is publication number 1992 from the Department of Immunopathology, Scripps Clinic and Research Foundation, La Jolla, CA. We thank Ms. Linda Hallenbeck and Erene Eriksson for technical assistance, Ms. Laura Taxel for preparation of the manuscript, and Dr. M.B.A. Oldstone for support.

REFERENCES

1. Traub, E., *J. Exp. Med. 64,* 183 (1936).
2. Burnet, F.M., and Fenner, F., The Production of Antibodies. Monograph of the Walter and Eliza Hall Institute, p. 142, MacMillan Company of Australia Pty. LTD., Melbourne, (1949).
3. Rowe, W.P., *Res. Rep. Naval Med. Res. Inst. 12,* 167 (1954).
4. Oldstone, M.B.A., and Dixon, F.J., *Science 158,* 1193 (1967).
5. Oldstone, M.B.A., and Dixon, F.J., *J. Exp. Med. 129,* 483 (1969).
6. Cole, G.A., Nathanson, N., and Prendergast, R.A., *Nature 238,* 335 (1972).
7. Zinkernagel, R.M., and Doherty, P.C., *Nature 248,* 701 (1974).
8. Welsh, R.M., and Zinkernagel, R.M., *Nature 268,* 646 (1977).
9. Herberman, R.B., Nunn, M.E., Holden, H.T., Staal, S., and Djeu, J.V., *Int. J. Cancer 19,* 555 (1977).
10. Nunn, M.E., Herberman, R.B., and Holden, H.T., *Int. J. Cancer 20,* 381 (1977).
11. Welsh, R.M., *J. Exp. Med. 148,* 163 (1978).
12. MacFarland, R.I., Burns, W.H., and White, D.O., *J. Immunol. 119,* 1569 (1977).
13. Wong, C.Y., Woodruff, J.J., and Woodruff, J.F., *J. Immunol. 119,* 591 (1977).
14. Merigan, T.C., Oldstone, M.B.A., and Welsh, R.M., *Nature 268,* 67 (1977).
15. Bro-Jorgensen, K., and Knudtzon, S., *Blood 49,* 47 (1977).
16. Blanden, R.V., and Mims, C.A., *Aust. J. Exp. Biol. Med. Sci. 51,* 393 (1973).
17. Oldstone, M.B.A., and Dixon, F.J., *J. Immunol. 105,* 829 (1970).

18. Buchmeier, M.J., Welsh, R.M., Dutko, F.J., and M.B.A. Oldstone, *Adv. Immunol., in press,* (1980).
19. Riviere, Y., Gresser, I., Guillon, J.-C., and Tovey, M.G., *Proc. Soc. Natl. Acad. Sci. USA 74,* 2135 (1977).
20. Welsh, R.M., and Kiessling, R., *Scand. J. Immunol., in press,* (1979).
21. Roder, J., and Duwe, A.K., *Nature 278,* 451 (1979).
22. Welsh, R.M., Zinkernagel, R.M., and Hallenbeck, L.A., *J. Immunol. 122,* 475 (1979).
23. Gidlund, M., Orn, A., Wigzell, H., Senik, A., and Gresser, I., *Nature 273,* 759 (1978).
24. Welsh, R.M., and Doe, W.F., manuscript in preparation.
25. Baron, S., *J. Gen. Physiol. 56,* 193 (1970).
26. Kiessling, R., Klein, E., and Wigzell, H., *Eur. J. Immunol. 5,* 112 (1975).
27. Herberman, R.B., Nunn, M.F., and Lavrin, D.H., *Int. J. Cancer 16,* 230 (1975).
28. Hansson, M., Kiessling, R., and Welsh, R.M., manuscript submitted for publication.
29. Kiessling, R., Eriksson, E., Hallenbeck, L.A., and Welsh, R.M., manuscript submitted for publication.
30. Herberman, R.B., Nunn, M.E., and Holden, H.J., *J. Immunol. 121,* 304 (1978).
31. Haller, O., and Wigzell, H., *J. Immunol. 118,* 1503 (1977).
32. Senik, A., Gresser, I., Maury, C., Gidlund, M., Orn, A., and Wigzell, H., *Cellular Immunol. 44,* 186 (1979).
33. Wolfe, S.A., Tracey, D.E., and Henney, C.S., *J. Immunol. 119,* 1152 (1977).
34. Kay, H.D., Bonnard, G.D., West, W.H., and Herberman, R.B., *J. Immunol. 118,* 2058 (1977).
35. Roder, J.C., Kiessling, R., Biberfeld, P., and Andersson, B., *J. Immunol. 121,* 2509 (1978).
36. Zinkernagel, R.M., and Welsh, R.M., *J. Immunol. 117,* 1495 (1976).
37. Welsh, R.M., and Hallenbeck, L.A., *J. Immunol., in press,* (1980).
38. Welsh, R.M., and Oldstone, M.B.A., *J. Exp. Med. 145,* 1449 (1977).
39. Talmadge, J.E., Meyers, K.M., Prieur, D.J., and Starky, J.R., manuscript submitted for publication.
40. Karre, K., Klein, G., Kiessling, R., and Klein, G., *J. Exp. Med., in press* (1979).
41. Buchmeier, M.J., Elder, J.H., and Oldstone, M.B.A., *Virology 89,* 133 (1978).

42. Padnos, M., and Molomut, N., *in* "Lymphocytic Choriomeningitis Virus and Other Arenaviruses" (F. Lehmann-Grube, ed.), p. 151. Springer-Verlag, New York (1973).
43. Webb, H.E., Molomut, N., Padnos, M., and Wetherlyemin, G., *Clin. Oncol. 1*, 157 (1975).
44. Vitetta, E.S., Artzt, K., Bennett, D., and Jacob, F., *Proc. Natl. Acad. Sci. USA 72*, 3215 (1975).

AUGMENTATION OF HUMAN NATURAL KILLER CELL ACTIVITY BY PURIFIED INTERFERON AND POLYRIBONUCLEOTIDES[1]

Joyce M. Zarling[2]

Department of Human Oncology and the
Immunobiology Research Center
University of Wisconsin
Madison, Wisconsin

I. INTRODUCTION

Lymphocytes from normal mice (1-4), rats (5-7) and humans (8-12) spontaneously lyse a variety of tumor cell lines. This spontaneous cytotoxicity is mediated by lymphocytes referred to as natural killer (NK) cells which express receptors for the Fc portion of IgG (13,14). Since a correlation exists between the level of NK activity of lymphocytes from mice of different strains and resistance to in vivo leukemia cell challenges (15,16), it has been suggested that NK cells may play a central role in resistance to neoplastic development (16,12).

Recently there has been considerable interest in finding means to enhance NK cell activity; much of this is discussed in other chapters. Briefly, polyinosinic:polycytidylic acid ($rI_n \cdot rC_n$), Bacille Calmette-Guérin, statolon, many viruses and some tumor cells augment mouse NK activity (17-21). Since these agents all induce interferon (IF), it has been postulated that augmentation of NK cell activity

[1]This work was supported by USPHS research grants CA-20409, CA-14520, CA-14801, CA-15502 and GM-16066.

[2]J.M. Zarling is a Scholar of the Leukemia Society of America. Present address: Department of Laboratory Medicine and Pathology, Box 198 Mayo Memorial Building, University of Minnesota, Minneapolis, Minnesota 55455.

ISBN 0-12-341350-8

by these agents may be due to the IF which is induced. Evidence in favor of this hypothesis derives from findings that IF-containing preparations can augment mouse NK activity (17,19). Additionally, human IF preparations (22) and IF containing supernatants from human lymphocytes cultured with certain tumor cells augment human NK cell activity (23). However, whether the effect of the various human IF preparations on NK activity was due to IF itself was not clear since the IF preparations used were not highly purified; further, IF preparations of leukocyte origin often contain other lymphokines and, in the case of virus-induced IF, products of viral infection (24).

In this chapter, recent studies (25,26) done in collaboration with Drs. W. Carter, J. Horoszewicz, J. Greene and P. Ts'o will be reviewed concerning the ability of IF and polyribonucleotides to augment human NK cell activity. Results presented here indicate that highly purified human fibroblast IF (HFIF) augments NK cell activity against K562 leukemia cells and activates NK cells to lyse fresh leukemia cells from many patients without concommitant lysis of normal lymphocytes or bone marrow cells. Results of the studies with polyribonucleotides support the contention that they augment NK activity by inducing IF; further, a clinically promising non-toxic analogue of $rI_n \cdot rC_n$, namely $rI_n \cdot r(C_{12},U)_n$, increases human NK cell activity.

II. AUGMENTATION OF HUMAN NK CELL ACTIVITY BY PURIFIED HUMAN FIBROBLAST INTERFERON (HFIF)

In this section the effect of highly purified HFIF (2×10^7 Units/mg protein) induced by $rI_n \cdot rC_n$, on human NK cell activity (25) are reviewed. Specifically presented are the effects of varying concentrations of HFIF, the kinetics of augmentation of NK cell activity by HFIF and characteristics of the cells required for HFIF induced augmentation of cytotoxicity against the K562 leukemia cell line (27) which is highly sensitive to NK cell-mediated lysis (10,28).

A. Effect of Varying Concentrations of HFIF on Augmentation of NK Cell Activity

HFIF treatment of mononuclear cells from individuals differing in initial NK cell activity resulted in marked augmentation of cytotoxicity against K562 cells (Table I). The concentrations of HFIF causing maximal augmentation of cytotoxicity varied among individuals. For example, maximal enhancement of cytotoxic activity occurred when cells from individual B were pretreated with 150 U HFIF/ml. In contrast, with cells from individual A who initially had low NK cell activity, pretreatment with 250 U/ml resulted in a greater degree of augmentation than did pretreatment with 150 U/ml. Cells pretreated with 600 U/ml were not more cytotoxic, and often were less cytotoxic, than cells pretreated with 250 U HFIF/ml (data not shown).

The findings that human NK activity is augmented by highly purified HFIF strengthens the contention that the IF protein itself is responsible for increasing NK cell activity. The IF preparation used for these studies was induced from fibroblasts by $rI_n \cdot rC_n$ and lacks virus products and lymphokines that may be present in the leukocyte IF

TABLE I. Effect of Varying Concentrations of HFIF on Human NK Cell Activity[a]

E:T ratio	% Specific ^{51}Cr Release from K562 Cells				
	Mock HFIF[c] treated	HFIF[b] treated (U/ml)			
		0	40	150	250
A 40:1	5.8	6.4	9.7	17.7	35.1
B 40:1	32.1	31.0	36.0	50.0	49.9
D 100:1		33.2		63.7	
25:1		12.5		30.5	

[a]Mononuclear cells from individuals A, B and D were pretreated for 16 hr with mock HFIF (equivalent to 250 U/ml) or HFIF (0-250 U/ml) in RPMI 1640 medium containing 20% normal human serum. The effector cells were washed and tested against ^{51}Cr labeled K562 target cells in 6 hour ^{51}Cr release assays as previously described (25).

[b]HFIF, produced in human diploid foreskin fibroblasts by a superinduction procedure (29,30) using $rI_n \cdot rC_n$, was assayed as described (31) and its potency expressed in International Reference Units (U). The crude HFIF was purified by Concanavalin A agarose affinity chromatography (32) and phenyl sepharose chromatography to a specific activity of 2×10^7 U/mg protein (33) prior to lyophilization.

[c]The mock HFIF control, which lacks antiviral activity, was prepared and purified in a manner identical to HFIF, except that during the superinduction procedure no $rI_n \cdot rC_n$ was added. (Modified from Zarling et al. 1979 with permission from the Journal of Immunology).

preparations previously used (17,19,22,23); further, our IF preparation was more highly purified than any human IF previously used for such studies.

B. Kinetics of Augmentation of NK Cell Activity by HFIF

Results of an experiment in which cells were treated with HFIF for 0 to 120 minutes demonstrate that one hour of treatment is sufficient for markedly increasing cytotoxicity against K562 cells (Fig. 1). In this experiment there was a three fold increase in cytotoxicity of cells treated with HFIF for 60 or 120 minutes; 31% ^{51}Cr was released from K562 cells by HFIF pretreated cells at an effector:target ratio of 8:1 whereas a ratio of 25:1 was required for untreated cells to mediate the same amount of ^{51}Cr release. With several other individuals tested, 2.5 to 5 fold increases in cytotoxicity were observed after treatment of cells for one hour with HFIF. Other effects of interferon, such as the antiviral (34) and antiproliferative (35) effects, are also triggered by brief exposure

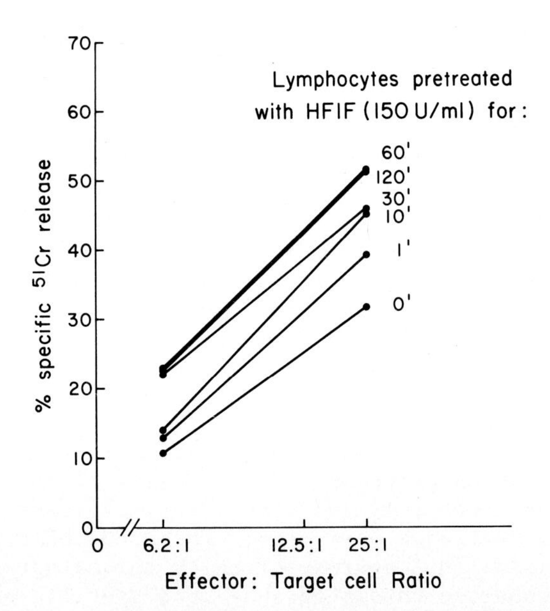

FIGURE 1. Effect of varying HFIF pretreatment time on cytotoxicity against K562 cells. Lymphocytes treated with HFIF for 0 to 120 minutes, were washed extensively and tested for cytotoxicity against ^{51}Cr labeled K562 cells in a 5 hour ^{51}Cr release assay. (From Zarling et al. 1979, with permission from the Journal of Immunology).

of cells to IF.

C. Cellular Requirements for Augmentation of Cytotoxicity by HFIF

It was previously reported that human NK cells express receptors for the Fc portion of IgG (referred to as FcR+ cells) (14). In order to determine whether augmentation of cytotoxicity by HFIF was also mediated by FcR+ cells, HFIF treated cells were depleted of FcR+ cells prior to testing for cytotoxicity against K562 cells. The results shown in Table II indicate that removal of FcR+ cells, from either untreated or HFIF treated cells, resulted in marked reduction of cytotoxicity against K562 cells. Since no monocytes were present in the nonadherent cells isolated from flasks that had been incubated with or without HFIF for 16 hours, lysis of K562 cells was clearly mediated by FcR+ lymphocytes, rather than by monocytes. In contrast to our findings that the HFIF increased cytotoxicity is mediated by FcR+ lymphocytes, we (25) and others (37) have found that cytotoxic T lymphocytes are FcR-. Thus, although IF has been shown to activate tumoricidal effects in macrophages (38) and increase the generation and cytotoxic activity of cytotoxic T lymphocytes (39-41), results shown here indicate that lymphocytes with characteristics of NK cells are those responsible for the enhanced lysis of K562 cells by HFIF treated cells.

TABLE II. Natural and HFIF Augmented Lysis of K562 Cells is Mediated by FcR+ Cells[a]

Effector cells pre-treated with HFIF	% Specific ^{51}Cr release from K562 cells ± S.D.	
U/ml	FcR+ cell depletion[b]	
	Before	After
0	39.1 ± 4.1	3.1 ± 1.1
200	75.3 ± 4.7	17.0 ± 2.1

[a]Mononuclear cells were cultured with or without HFIF for 16 hr. Untreated and treated effector cells were then washed and tested for cytotoxic activity before and after depletion of FcR+ cells on monolayers of sheep red blood cells (E) coated with anti-E IgG as detailed previously (36). Effector:target cell ratio = 30:1. (Modified from Zarling, et al. 1979 with permission from the Journal of Immunology).

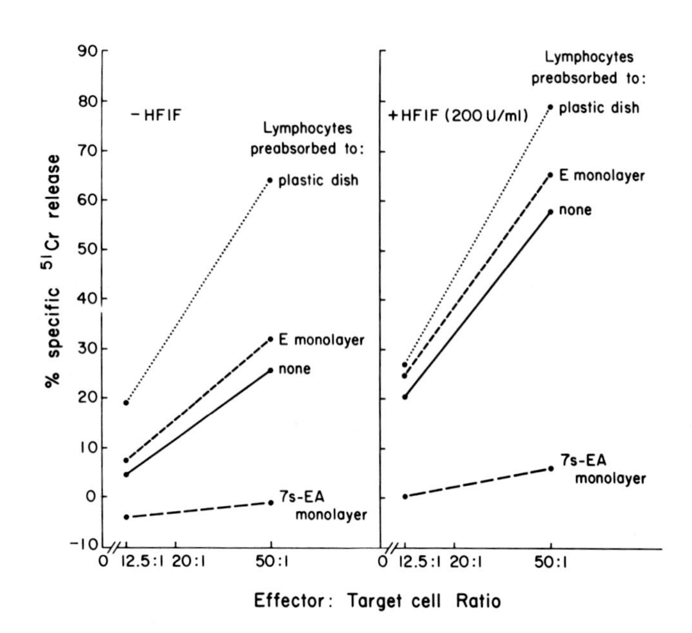

FIGURE 2. FcR+ lymphocytes are required for HFIF augmentation of cytotoxicity against K562 cells. Unfractionated mononuclear cells (●——●), non-adherent cells recovered from plastic dishes (●……●), from E monolayers (●---●) and from E monolayers coated with anti-E IgG (7S-EA) (●— —●) were incubated for 16 hr with or without HFIF. The effector cells were washed and tested for cytotoxicity against ^{51}Cr labeled K562 target cells in a 5 hr ^{51}Cr release assay. Non-adherent mononuclear cells recovered from plastic dishes and from E monolayers coated with anti-E 7S IgG, were devoid of monocytes. (Modified from Zarling et al. 1979 with permission from the Journal of Immunology).

In order to determine whether HFIF augments cytotoxicity of pre-existing FcR+ lymphocytes or causes the conversion of FcR- to FcR+ cytotoxic cells, mononuclear cells were depleted of FcR+ cells prior to treatment with HFIF. Removal of FcR+ cells prior to culturing the non-adherent cells in medium with or without HFIF, resulted in no detectable cytotoxicity against K562 cells (Fig. 2). Adsorption of mononuclear cells to non-antibody coated monolayers failed to decrease natural or HFIF augmented cytotoxicity. Although human mononuclear cells depleted of FcR+ cells prior to culture in fetal calf serum acquire cytotoxic activity against K562 cells (42), HFIF does not render FcR- cells cytotoxic. Monocytes were not required for augmentation of cytotoxicity by HFIF since removal of adherent cells, by adsorption to plastic dishes, did not prevent the augmentation of cytotoxicity by HFIF.

III. CYTOTOXIC EFFECTS OF HFIF ACTIVATED NK CELLS ON NORMAL CELLS AND HUMAN LEUKEMIA CELLS

NK cells have been suspected of playing a role in preventing tumor growth in vivo, based on several observations. First, athymic nude mice have high NK activity and are resistant to challenge with some tumor cell lines (12). Second, mice of strains with high NK activity are more resistant to in vivo challenge with NK sensitive leukemia cell lines than are mice of strains with low NK activity (15). Third, F_1 hybrid mice, irradiated and repopulated with bone marrow from donors with high NK activity, are more resistant to *in vivo* lymphoma cell challenge than are mice repopulated with bone marrow cells from donors with low NK activity (16). Since NK activity is predetermined at the level of the bone marrow donor (43), these results suggest that NK cells play a major role in the *in vivo* resistance to development of tumors by NK sensitive lines. Crucial for the hypothesis that NK cells may play a role in eliminating spontaneously arising malignant cells would be the demonstration that malignant cells, that have not been established as cell lines or adapted to tissue culture, can be killed by activated NK cells. In this section, results are presented showing that HFIF activated NK cells do not lyse normal lymphocytes or bone marrow cells but do lyse leukemic cells from many patients.

A. Failure of HFIF Activated NK Cells to Lyse Normal Cells

First, in order to determine whether HFIF would activate lymphocytes to non-specifically lyse any normal cells (like that which occurs in mitogen-dependent cytotoxicity using alloantigen-activated cells) HFIF treated lymphocytes were tested for their ability to lyse normal lymphocytes or Con A blasts, both of which are lysed by alloactivated T cells (44). Results shown in Table III confirm previous findings (9) that mononuclear cells are

TABLE III. Failure of HFIF Treated Cells to Lyse Normal Lymphocytes or Con A Blasts[a]

Effector cells	% Specific ^{51}Cr Release				
	C's lymphocytes	C's Con A blasts	F's lymphocytes	F's Con A blasts	K562
C-IF	-6.1	-6.4	-4.0	7.0	45.2
C+IF	-5.0	-12.2	-5.7	-5.4	59.8
F-IF	-3.2	-7.1	-2.4	3.2	46.4
F+IF	-3.4	-6.0	-3.4	0.1	68.9

[a]Mononuclear cells from individuals C and F were treated for 16 hr with 0 or 150 U/ml HFIF. Washed effector cells were tested for cytotoxicity against the target cells in 7 hour ^{51}Cr release assays. Effector:target cell ratio on lymphocytes and Con A blasts = 150:1 and on K562 cells = 37:1. Negative values indicate that the amount of ^{51}Cr released in the presence of effector cells was less than that spontaneously released in medium. (Modified from Zarling et al. 1979 with permission from the Journal of Immunology).

not spontaneously cytotoxic for normal lymphocytes or mitogen induced blasts and, in addition, indicate that HFIF treated cells do not lyse either autologous or allogeneic normal lymphocytes or Con A blasts even at ratios of 150 effector cells per target cell.

We have also observed that ^{51}Cr labeled normal human bone marrow cells are not lysed by HFIF activated NK cells. However, since bone marrow cells isolated from ficoll-hypaque gradients are very heterogeneous, the possibility was considered that activated NK cells might cause lysis of erythroid or myeloid colony forming cells which would not be detected by ^{51}Cr release assays due to the low percentage of these cells in the target cell population. Thus, experiments were performed to determine whether HFIF activated NK cells, when admixed with bone marrow cells, would reduce the number of erythroid colonies (CFU-E) or myeloid colonies (CFU-C) formed. As shown in Table IV, the number of colonies formed by bone marrow cells preincubated with HFIF treated mononuclear cells was not reduced from the number of colonies formed in the presence of untreated mononuclear cells; in some cases, the number of colonies was actually increased. The untreated and HFIF treated effector cells were γ-irradiated immediate-

TABLE IV. Failure of HFIF Activated NK Cells to Inhibit Erythroid or Myeloid Colony Formation by Autologous Bone Marrow Cells[a]

	Effector cells	No. colonies per plate erythroid (CFU-E)	myeloid (CFU-C)
Exp. A	A-IF	43	39
	A+IF	43	35.5
	B-IF	64.5	78.5
	B+IF	73.5	80
	C-IF	56	41.5
	C+IF	55	75.5
Exp. B	D-IF	30.5	23
	D+IF	48	24.5
	E-IF	43	33
	E+IF	39	42.5

[a]Mononuclear cells from individuals A through E cultured without HFIF (-IF) or with 200 U/ml HFIF (+IF) for 16 hr were exposed to 2000R γ-irradiation. The irradiated effector cells were then incubated with Ficoll-Hypaque isolated autologous bone marrow cells for 5 hr at 37°C at an effector:bone marrow cell ratio of 20:1 (Exp. A) or 40:1 (Exp. B). The mixed cells were plated for erythroid colony (CFU-E) and myeloid colony (CFU-C) formation as previously detailed (45,46). Irradiated lymphocytes, plated without bone marrow cells formed 0-2 colonies per plate. Values shown are the mean no. of colonies on duplicate plates.

ly prior to their admixture with the bone marrow cells to prevent colony formation by the colony forming cells present in the peripheral blood. The failure of irradiated activated NK cells to eradicate colony forming cells can not be attributed to a loss of NK activity following irradiation since lysis of K562 cells was not reduced following exposure of untreated or HFIF treated effector cells to 2000R.

B. Lysis of Fresh Human Leukemia Cells by HFIF Activated NK Cells

Untreated and HFIF treated lymphocytes were compared for their ability to lyse fresh human leukemia cells (Table V). Untreated lymphocytes from none of the individuals tested lysed leukemic cells from any of the 17

TABLE V. Ability of HFIF Treated Lymphocytes to Lyse Fresh Human Leukemia Cells

HFIF treated cells from individual	% Specific ^{51}Cr released from leukemic cells by HFIF treated lymphocytes[a] AML cells													CML cells				K562[b]
	1	2	3	4	5	6	7	8	9	10	11	12	13	14	15	16	17	
I	1	19	16	12	7													60 (13)
J	0	1	3	1	-1													72 (62)
K						21	3	16	15								15	81 (42)
L						2	-3	3	5								1	37 (30)
O	-1						1			3	3	8	8	-2	24	2		47 (31)
P	0						17			3	37	19	26	24	41	41		71 (62)

[a]Mononuclear cells from normal individuals I through P were cultured with or without HFIF (200 U/ml) and tested for their ability to lyse ^{51}Cr labeled AML (acute myelogenous leukemia) and CML (chronic myelogenous leukemia) cells from patients numbered 1 to 17, at an effector: target cell ratio of 150:1 in 7 hr ^{51}Cr release assays. The values shown represent the % ^{51}Cr released from leukemia cells by HFIF treated cells after subtracting the % ^{51}Cr released by untreated cells. The ^{51}Cr released from the fresh leukemia cells by untreated cells ranged from -3.2 to 3.4%.

[b]HFIF treated and untreated cells were tested for cytotoxicity against K562 cells at an effector:target cell ratio of 37:1. Values in parentheses are the % ^{51}Cr released from K562 cells by untreated cells. (Modified from Zarling, et al. 1979, with permission from the Journal of Immunology).

patients. These results agree with previous findings that very rarely are normal lymphocytes cytotoxic for fresh leukemia cells (28,47, Zarling, unpublished observations). In contrast, HFIF treated lymphocytes from several individuals tested caused at least 10%, and up to 40% specific ^{51}Cr release from many of the patients' leukemia cells. Acute myelogenous leukemia (AML) cells from 9 of 13 patients were lysed by HFIF treated cells from individual I, K or P and leukemia cells from all three patients in blast crisis with chronic myelogenous leukemia (CML) were lysed by HFIF treated lymphocytes from individual P. Chronic lymphocytic leukemia cells are also susceptible to lysis by HFIF activated NK cells (25).

Although the number of individuals used as donors of effector cells and the total number of patients' leukemia cells tested were relatively small (Table V), it appears that individuals may vary in the ability of their HFIF treated lymphocytes to lyse leukemia cells that have not been adapted to tissue culture. For example, although HFIF boosted anti-K562 NK activity in cells of individuals J and P, cells of P, after HFIF treatment, were cytotoxic for 7 of 9 patients' leukemia cells, whereas HFIF treated cells of J were not cytotoxic for any of the patients' leukemic cells tested.

The findings that HFIF augments anti-K562 cytotoxicity in all individuals tested but does not activate all individuals' lymphocytes to lyse fresh human leukemia cells may be explained as follows. Although FcR+ cells are required both for augmenting anti-K562 killing and for inducing cytotoxicity against fresh leukemia cells (25), the FcR+ cells may be functionally distinct populations that vary in number or in response to HFIF among different individuals. The HFIF activated NK cells that lyse K562 cells and those that lyse fresh leukemia cells may be directed against different target specificities; individuals may vary with regard to whether they possess IF inducible NK cells directed against targets on various leukemia cells.

Support for the contention that different subpopulations of NK cells exist which are directed against different targets expressed on tumor cells is derived from findings that NK lysis of a ^{51}Cr labeled cell line is generally blocked to a higher degree by the addition of unlabeled cells of that particular line as compared to other cell lines (28,48,49). Although the results in Table V show, for example, that HFIF treated cells from individual P lysed 7 of 9 different patients' leukemia cells, it has not been determined whether the activated NK cells are directed against a common target(s) on the various patients' cells or whether leukemic cells of each patient express a unique target. Results of cell-blocking experiments, where HFIF treated cells are tested for their ability to lyse ^{51}Cr labeled leukemia cells from one patient in the presence of unlabeled leukemia target cells from other patients, should help answer this question.

IV. AUGMENTATION OF HUMAN NK CELLS ACTIVITY BY POLYRIBONUCLEOTIDES

As discussed above, human IF augments the generation of cytotoxic T lymphocytes (39,40) and activates NK cells (22,23,25), both of which may retard tumor growth. Further, since purified IF is non-toxic (50,51) it might be an ideal immunotherapeutic agent. However widespread use of exogenous IF is limited by the supply of IF and its purification costs. Use of the inexpensively synthesized potent IF inducer, $rI_n \cdot rC_n$, would bypass these problems; however, $rI_n \cdot rC_n$ causes many toxic effects including fever, reduced hemopoesis and coagulation defects (52-55). Furthermore, $rI_n \cdot rC_n$ induces antibodies directed against ds RNAs and can activate latent autoimmune disease (for review see 56).

To overcome the adverse effects of $rI_n \cdot rC_n$, Ts'o, Carter and colleagues synthesized several non-toxic analogues of $rI_n \cdot rC_n$, and, in so doing, elucidated the structural requirements of polynucleotide complexes to induce IF. Briefly, the duplex must have a minimum molecular weight of both strands, a sufficient degree of resistance to nucleases to allow the IF triggering step, and a minimum cluster of base-pairs to give the required double-helical regions (57,58). $rI_n \cdot rC_n$ modified by complete substitution of the ribosyl residues with either the corresponding deoxy (dC or dI) or 2'-O-methyl (mC or mI) analogues do not induce IF (58). In contrast, $rI_n \cdot rC_n$ molecules with slight alterations that do not induce overall configurational changes and preserve small regions of ribosyl double-helicity, do induce IF. For example, when bases such as U or G are inserted at different intervals into the $r(C)_n$ strand, the resulting duplexes contain mismatched regions. Certain of these mismatched analogues, including $rI_n \cdot r(C_{12},U)_n$ and $rI_n \cdot r(C_{29},G)_n$ are fully capable of inducing IF yet do not cause the toxic effects ascribed to $rI_n \cdot rC_n$ (53-55,57,58). Their reduced toxicity is partly due to the fact that the mismatched analogues are more susceptible to endonucleases which allows initiation of IF induction but rapid degradation ensues before toxic effects are induced.

The focus of the study (26) reviewed in this section was to assess the effects of various polyribonucleotides on human NK cell activity. We first asked whether $rI_n \cdot rC_n$ which augments mouse NK cell activity (17) would augment human NK cell activity and, second, whether the structural requirements of dsRNAs for augmenting human NK cell activity corresponded with those required for inducing IF. Finally, we determined whether non-toxic mismatched analogues of $rI_n \cdot rC_n$ could augment NK cell activity. The polynucleotide complexes used in these studies were prepared as previously detailed (53,57,58).

A. Augmentation of Human NK Cell Activity by $rI_n \cdot rC_n$

Shown in Table VI are results indicating that treatment of human mononuclear cells for 24 hours with $rI_n \cdot rC_n$ results in marked augmentation of cytotoxicity against K562 leukemia cells. At an effector to target cell ratio of 10:1, untreated cells mediated 47.1% ^{51}Cr release whereas cells treated for 24 hours with $rI_n \cdot rC_n$ mediated 70.3% ^{51}Cr release. Augmentation of cytotoxicity was also observed following 4 hrs treatment with $rI_n \cdot rC_n$ whereas no augmentation occurred following treatment for 1 hour. In contrast, human NK cell activity is augmented following treatment of mononuclear cells for less than one hour with purified interferon (Fig. 1). The absence of augmentation of NK cell activity following 1 hour treatment with $rI_n \cdot rC_n$

TABLE VI. Kinetics of Augmentation of Human NK Cell Activity by $rI_n \cdot rC_n$ [a]

Treatment period	% Specific ^{51}Cr release from K562 cells ± S.D.	
	Untreated	$rI_n \cdot rC_n$ treated
1 hr	47.1 ± 4.8	45.3 ± 2.7
4 hr	46.1 ± 4.4	62.0 ± 4.8
24 hr	47.1 ± 4.8	70.3 ± 6.5

[a] Mononuclear cells were incubated with or without $rI_n \cdot rC_n$ (120 ug/ml) for 1 to 24 hours. The effector cells were washed, resuspended in fresh medium and tested for cytotoxicity against ^{51}Cr labeled K562 cells using an effector:target cell ratio of 10:1. (Modified from Zarling et al. 1980, with permission from the Journal of Immunology).

is consistant with the known time requirements for formation, processing and translation of new IF mRNA transcripts for IF production (59). Results shown in Table VII indicate that exposure of cells to $rI_n \cdot rC_n$ for thirty minutes, followed by prolonged incubation of pretreated cells, results in the same degree of augmentation of cytotoxicity as does exposure for 6 hours or longer. These findings agree with previous results that short exposure of cells to $rI_n \cdot rC_n$, followed by several hours incubation, results in IF induction (60) and support the hypothesis that $rI_n \cdot rC_n$ augments cytotoxic activity through IF induction.

As discussed above, FcR+ lymphocytes are required for HFIF augmentation of cytotoxicity against K562 cells and fresh human leukemia cells. $rI_n \cdot rC_n$ likewise augments cytotoxicity of FcR+ lymphocytes based on the following observations. First, no esterase-positive cells were detected in the non-adherent effector cells isolated from flasks after treatment with $rI_n \cdot rC_n$ indicating that the effector cells are not macrophages. Second, results shown in Figure 3 demonstrate that cells depleted of those expressing receptors for the Fc portion of IgG, but not IgM, do not become cytotoxic following treatment with $rI_n \cdot rC_n$.

B. Correlation Between the Ability of Polyribonucleotides to Augment NK Cell Activity with Their Ability to Induce IF

The availability of analogues of $rI_n \cdot rC_n$ that vary in their ability to induce IF enabled a determination of

TABLE VII. Time Required for Exposure to $rI_n \cdot rC_n$ for Subsequent Augmentation of NK Cell Activity

E:T ratio	% Specific ^{51}Cr release from K562 Cells ± S.D. Cells pretreated with $rI_n \cdot rC_n$ for 0 min	30 min	6 hr
30:1	47.9 ± 4.9	61.5 ± 5.7	64.9 ± 4.0
7.5:1	24.2 ± 3.2	35.1 ± 3.1	36.3 ± 2.7

[a]Mononuclear cells were cultured with rIn·rCn (100 μg/ml) for 0 min, 30 min or 6 hr. The cells were washed, resuspended in fresh medium and incubated overnight prior to testing for cytotoxicity against K562 cells. (Modified from Zarling et al. 1980, with permission from the Journal of Immunology).

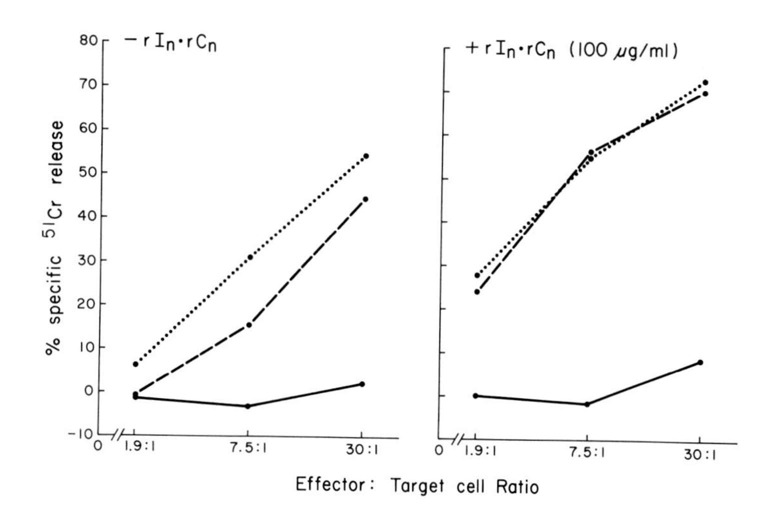

FIGURE 3. Requirement for cells expressing IgG Fc receptors for $rI_n \cdot rC_n$ augmented cytotoxicity. Unfractionated mononuclear cells (●– –●), and non-adherent cells recovered from E monolayers coated with anti-E IgG (●——●), or coated with anti-E IgM (●····●) were cultured overnight with or without $rI_n \cdot rC_n$. The cells were washed and tested for cytotoxicity against ^{51}Cr labeled K562 target cells. (From Zarling et al. 1980 with permission from the Journal of Immunology).

whether the structural requirements of dsRNA for augmenting NK activity are the same as those for inducing IF. Results of several experiments, summarized in Table VIII, in which mononuclear cells of different individuals were treated with $rI_n \cdot rC_n$ or $rI_n \cdot r(C_{12},U)_n$ demonstrate that both IF inducers augmented NK activity by approximately two-fold; further, another IF-inducing non-toxic analogue, $rI_n \cdot r(C_{29},G)_n$, was found equally effective in boosting NK activity (26). In contrast, the methylated analogue, $rI_n \cdot mC_n$, failed to boost NK activity and, in some cases, $rI_n \cdot mC_n$ treated cells were less cytotoxic than untreated cells (Table VIII). Thus, the ability of polyribonucleotides to augment human NK cell activity correlates with their known ability to induce IF. Combining the findings concerning the kinetics of augmentation of human NK cell activity by $rI_n \cdot rC_n$ and the absence in augmentation of NK cell activity by an $rI_n \cdot rC_n$ analogue ($rI_n \cdot mC_n$) which fails to induce IF, it is concluded that polyribonucleotides may augment NK cell activity exclusively through IF induction. With regard to clinical relevance, since both non-toxic analogues, $rI_n \cdot r(C_{12},U)_n$ as well as $rI_n \cdot r(C_{29},G)_n$, increase NK cell activity it can be concluded that the ability of polyribonucleotides to augment NK cell activity can be separated from their ability to manifest the toxic effects ascribed to $rI_n \cdot rC_n$.

TABLE VIII. Correlation Between the Ability of Polyribonucleotides to Induce IF and Increase NK Cell Activity[a]

Effector cell pretreatment (125 μg/ml)	NK activity after treatment		No. individuals >1.5 fold increase/ no. individuals tested
	mean	range	
$rI_n \cdot rC_n$ (inducer)	2.4	1.5-4.0	10/10
$rI_n \cdot r(C_{12},U)_n$ (inducer)	2.1	1.4-2.7	8/9
$rI_n \cdot mC_n$ (non-inducer)	0.9	0.6-1.0[b]	0/6

[a]Mononuclear cells, pretreated for 2 hr with or without polyribonucleotides were washed and incubated overnight in fresh medium prior to testing for cytotoxicity against K562 cells. Values shown represent the increase or decrease in NK activity following treatment, based on the ratio of the number of untreated to the number of treated effector cells required to cause an equal level of ^{51}Cr release from K562 cells.

[b]Values of 1.0 or <1.0 indicate that treated cells were equal to or less cytotoxic than untreated cells from the same individual. (Modified from Zarling et al. 1980, with permission from the Journal of Immunology).

V. CONCLUDING REMARKS

Following the discovery of NK cells and the demonstration that they play a role in resistance to in vivo tumor cell challenge, there has been much interest in elucidating means to augment NK cell activity. Results presented in other chapters indicate that IF and several IF inducers, previously shown to exert anti-tumor effects in vivo, enhance NK cell activity. Results presented in this chapter demonstrate that both highly purified human fibroblast IF and the polyribonucleotides which induce IF enhance human NK cell activity.

Regarding potential clinical usefullness of administering NK cell activating agents to cancer patients, the following criteria should be established. First, the agents considered for boosting NK activity should be relatively non-toxic in man. Second, cancer patients' lymphocytes must be responsive to the NK cell activator in vivo. Third, the patients' malignant cells, but not normal cells, should be susceptible to lysis by their activated NK cells. Concerning these points, we have shown that highly purified HFIF as well as $rI_n \cdot r(C_{12},U)_n$, both of which are non-toxic in vivo, augment human NK cell activity and that the activated NK cells are not cytotoxic for normal lymphocytes or bone marrow cells. Administration of IF to cancer patients has recently been reported to rapidly enhance NK cell activity (61,62) thus demonstrating that cancer patients' NK cells are responsive to IF activation in vivo. Further, our findings that many patients' leukemia cells, which have not been adapted to tissue culture, are lysed by activated NK cells reveal that susceptibility to lysis by activated human NK cells is not restricted to tumor cells established as lines. Accordingly, all of these observations, together with results of preliminary clinical trials showing that IF treatment can prevent relapse in osteosarcoma patients (63) and can induce regressions in lymphoma patients (64), point strongly to the possibility that activated NK cells may contribute to eradication of malignant cells in man.

It should be pointed out that the ability of HFIF to augment NK cell activity against highly NK sensitive K562 cells was not predictive of whether the activated NK cells would lyse fresh leukemia cells. Thus, in attempts to predict possible clinical benefit from augmenting NK cell activity in a given patient, it may prove worthwhile to ascertain whether the patient's in vitro activated NK cells are rendered cytotoxic for autochthonous malignant cells.

ACKNOWLEDGMENTS

The author is indebted to Drs. William Carter, Julius Horoszewicz, Susan Leong, Ernest Borden, James Greene and Paul Ts'o for their collaboration in these studies. The technical assistance of James Schlais, Linda Eskra and Jean Martin and expert preparation of this text by Cindy Smith are gratefully acknowledged.

REFERENCES

1. Zarling, J.M., Nowinski, R.C., and Bach, F.H., Proc. Natl. Acad. Sci. 72, 2780 (1975).
2. Herberman, R.B., Nunn, M.E., and Lavrin, D.H., Int. J. Cancer 16, 216 (1975).
3. Kiessling, R., Klein, E., and Wigzell, H., Eur. J. Immunol. 5, 112 (1975).
4. Sendo, F., Aoki, T., Boyse, E.A., and Buofo, C.K., J. Nat. Cancer Inst. 55, 603 (1975).
5. Nunn, M.E., Djeu, J.Y., Glaser, M., Lavrin, D.H., and Herberman, R.B., J. Nat. Cancer Inst. 56, 393 (1976).
6. Shellam, G.R., Int. J. Cancer 19, 225 (1977).
7. Oehler, J.R., Lindsay, L.R., Nunn, M.E., and Herberman, R.B., Int. J. Cancer 21, 204 (1978).
8. Takasugi, M., Mickey, M.R., and Terasaki, P.I., Cancer Res. 33, 2898 (1973).
9. McCoy, J.L., Herberman, R.B., Rosenberg, E.B., Donnelly, F.C., Levine, P.H., and Alford, C., Natl. Cancer Inst. Monogr. 37, 59 (1973).
10. Rosenberg, E.B., McCoy, J.L., Green, S.S., Donnelly, F.C., Siwarski, D.F., Levine, P.H., and Herberman, R.B., J. Natl. Cancer Inst. 52, 345 (1974).
11. Pross, H.F., and Jondal, M., Clin. Exp. Immunol. 21, 226 (1975).
12. Herberman, R.B., Djeu, J.Y., Kay, H.D., Ortaldo, J.R., Riccardi, C., Bonnard, G.D., Holden, H.T., Fagnani, R., Santoni A., and Puccetti, P., Immunol. Rev., 44, 43 (1978).
13. Herberman, R.B., Bartram, S., Haskill, J.S., Nunn, M., Holden H.T., and West, W.H., J. Immunol. 119, 322, (1977).
14. West, W.H., Cannon, G.B., Kay, H.D., Bonnard, G.D., and Herberman, R.B., J. of Immunol. 118, 355 (1977).
15. Kiessling, R., Petrányi, G.G., Klein, G., and Wigzell, H., Int. J. Cancer 15, 933, (1975).
16. Haller, O., Hansson, M., Kiessling, R., and Wigzell, H., Nature 270, 609 (1977).
17. Djeu, J.Y., Heinbaugh, J.A., Holden, H.T., and Herberman, R.B., J. Immunol. 122, 175 (1979).
18. Wolfe, S.A., Tracey, D.E., and Henney, C.S., Nature 262, 584, (1976).
19. Gidlund, M., Orn, A., Wigzell, H., Senik, A., and Gresser, I., Nature 273, 759 (1978).
20. Welsch, R.M., J. Exp. Med. 148, 163 (1978).

21. Herberman, R.B., Nunn, M.E., Holden, H.T., Staal, S., Djeu J.Y., Int. J. Cancer 19, 555 (1977).
22. Herberman, R.R., Ortaldo, J.R., and Bonnard, G.D., Nature 277, 221 (1979).
23. Trinchieri, G., Santoli, D., Dee, R.R., and Knowles, B.B., J. Exp. Med. 147, 1299 (1978).
24. Strander, H., Cantell, K., Carlström, G., and Jakobsson, P.A., J. Natl. Cancer Inst. 51, 733, (1973).
25. Zarling, J.M., Eskra, L., Borden, E.C., Horoszewicz, J., and Carter, W.A., J. Immunol. 123, 63 (1979).
26. Zarling, J.M., Schlais, J., Eskra, L., Greene, J., Ts'o, P.O.P., and Carter, W.A., J. Immunol., in press (1980).
27. Lozzio, B.B., Machado, E.A., Lozzio, C.B., and Lair, S., J. Exp. Med. 143, 225 (1976).
28. Ortaldo, J., Oldham, R.K., Cannon, G.L., and Herberman, R.B., J. Natl. Cancer Inst. 59, 77 (1977).
29. Havell, E.A., and Vilcek, J., Antimicrob. Agents Chemother. 2, 476 (1972).
30. Horoszewicz, J.S., Leong, S.S., Ito, M., Di Berardino, L.A., and Carter, W.A., Infect. Immun. 19, 720 (1978).
31. Borden, E.C., and Leonhardt, P.H., J. Lab. Clin. Med. 89, 1036 (1977).
32. Davey, M.W., Sulkowski, E., and Carter, W.A., Biochemistry 15, 704 (1976).
33. Horoszewicz, J.S., Karakousis, C., Leong, S., Holyoke, E., Ito, M., Buffest, R.F., and Carter, W.A., Cancer Treatment Rep. 62, 1897 (1978).
34. Pitha, P.M., and Carter, W.A., Nature New Biology 234, 105 (1978).
35. Pfeffer, L.M., Murphy, J.S., and Tamm, I., Exp. Cell Res., in press, (1979).
36. Kedar, E.M., Ortiz de Landazuri, M., and Bonavida, B., J. Immunol. 112, 1231 (1974).
37. Ortaldo, J.R., and Bonnard, G.D., Fed. Proc. 36, 1325 (1977).
38. Schultz, R.M., Papamatheakis, J.D., and Chirigos, M.A., Sci. 197, 674 (1977).
39. Heron, I., Berg, K., and Cantell, K., J. Immunol. 117, 1370 (1976).
40. Zarling, J.M., Sosman, J., Eskra, L., Borden, E.C., Horoszewicz, J.S., and Carter, W.A., J. Immunol. 121, 2002 (1978).
41. Lindahl, P., Leary, P., and Gresser, I., Proc. Natl. Acad. Sci. 69, 721 (1972).
42. Ortaldo, J.R., Bonnard, G.D., and Herberman, R.B., J. Immunol. 119, 1351 (1977).
43. Haller, O., Kiessling, R., Orn A., and Wigzell, H., J. Exp. Med. 145, 1411 (1977).

44. Sondel, P.M., and Bach, F.H., J. Exp. Med. 142, 1339 (1975).
45. Iscove, N.N., and Sieber, F., Exp. Hematol. 3, 32 (1975).
46. Metcalf, D., Recent Results in Cancer Res. 61, 12 (1977).
47. Rosenberg, E.B., Herberman, R.B., Levine, P.H., Halterman, R.H., McCoy, J.L., and Wunderlich, J.R., Int. J. Cancer 9, 648 (1972).
48. Kiessling, R., Klein, E., Pross, H., and Wigzell, H., Eur. J. Immunol. 5, 117 (1975).
49. Takasugi, M., Koide, Y., Akira, D., and Ramseyer, A., Int. J. Cancer 19, 291 (1977).
50. Carter, W.A., and Horoszewicz, J.S., Pharmacol. Therapeut., in press, (1979).
51. Carter, W.A., Dolen, J.G., Leong, S.S., Horoszewicz, J.S., Vladutin, A.D., Lebowitz, A.I., and Nolan, J.P., Cancer Letters 7, 249, (1979).
52. Freeman, A.I., Al-Bussam, N., O'Malley, J.A., Stutzman, L., Bjornsson, S., and Carter, W.A., J. Med. Virol. 1, 79, (1977).
53. Ts'o, P.O.P., Alderfer, J.L., Levy, J., Marshall, L.W., O'Malley, J., Horoszewicz, J.S., and Carter, W.A., Molec. Pharm. 12, 299, (1976).
54. Carter, W.A., O'Malley, J.A., Beeson, M., Cunnington, P., Kelvin, A., Vere-Hodge, A., Alderfer, J.L. and Ts'o, P.O.P., Molec. Pharm. 12, 440, (1976).
55. O'Malley, J.A., Leong, S.S., Horoszewicz, J.S., Carter, W.A., Alderfer, J.L., and Ts'o, P.O.P., Molec. Pharm. 15, 140, (1979).
56. Carter, W.A., and DeClercq, E., Science 186, 1172, (1974).
57. Carter, W.A., Pitha, P.M., Marshall, L.W., Tazawa, I., Tazawa, S., and Ts'o, P.O.P., J. Mol. Biol. 70, 567, (1972).
58. Greene, J.J., Alderfer, J.L., Tzazwa, I., Tazawa, S., Ts'o, P.O.P., O'Malley, J.A. and Carter, W.A., Biochem. 17, 4214, (1978).
59. Greene, J.J., Dreffenbach, C.W., and Ts'o, P.O.P., Nature 271, 81, (1978).
60. Pitha, P.M., Marshall, L.W., and Carter, W.A., J. Gen. Virol. 15, 89, (1972).
61. Einhorn, S., Blomgren, H., and Strander, H., Acta Med. Scand. 20, 477, (1978).
62. Huddlestone, J.R., Merigan, T.C., and Oldstone, M.B.A., Nature 282, 417, (1979).
63. Strander, H., Blut 35, 277, (1977).
64. Merigan, T.C., Sikora, K., Breeden, J.H., Levy, R., and Rosenberg, S.A., New Engl. J. Med. 299, 1449, (1978).

SUMMARY: AUGMENTATION OF NK ACTIVITY

In the past few years, it has become clear that NK activity can be substantially augmented above the spontaneous levels. In some cases, the augmentation has been quite striking, with rapid induction of high levels of cytotoxicity in individuals with low or undectable natural activity. Since the demonstration that interferon (IF) plays a central role in this augmentation of NK activity, there has been very rapid progress in our underatanding of the details of positive regulation of this effector function.

I. MEDIATORS OF BOOSTING OF NK ACTIVITY

A. *Role of Interferon*

A wide variety of agents has been shown to be able to rapidly augment mouse, rat and human NK activity and these are summarized in Table I. One feature in common to all these materials is their ability to induce IF. Furthermore, the time required to induce peak boosting of NK activity has been very similar to that needed for peak levels of IF. *In vivo* or *in vitro* treatment of NK cells with preparations of partially purified IF were also found to augment NK reactivity. These observations have led to the strong presumption that augmentation of NK activity is mediated by IF. However, despite the strong evidence pointing to a central role of IF, there was some underlying concern that some other mediator might actually be responsible. The IF-inducers and other boosting cells can have multiple effects on the immune system, and the content of IF in the partially purified IF preparations is actually 1% or less of the total protein. The possiblility of the NK boosting factor being a contaiminent of IF preparations now has been excluded, by evidence that small amounts of homogeneous human leukocyte (Herberman *et al*) and fibroblast (Einhorn) IF and mouse IF (Bloom *et al*) can strongly augment NK activity.

ISBN 0-12-341350-8

TABLE I. Agents Demonstrated to Augment NK Activity

Agent	Time for peak effect	Type of interferon induced
Variety of RNA and DNA viruses (main exception: most type C and B oncornaviruses)	3 days	type I
Double stranded RNA (e.g. poly I:C)	12-18 hrs.	type I
Other synthetic IF-inducers (e.g. tilorone, pyran copolymer)	2-3 days	type I
Bacteria		
C. parvum	*in vivo*, mouse: 3 days	type I
	in vitro, mouse: 1 day	type I
	human: ?1 day or 5-7 days	? type I
BCG	3-5 days	type I
Bacterial products		
Endotoxins	3-6 hrs.	type I
Staph. protein A	18 hrs.	?
Lentinan (β glucan)	1-3 days	?
Tumor cells and normal cells	*in vivo*, mouse: 1-3 days	probably type II
	in vitro, human: 12-24 hrs.	type I
Interferon	1-4 hrs	type I and type II

B. Possible Involvement of Other Mediators

Now that it appears certain that IF is a major mediator of augmentation of NK activity, an important remaining question is whether it is the sole positive regulator in this system or whether other factors may also exist. This issue is not entirely settled and it appears that other mediators or mechanisms of augmentation may exist. However, it will be necessary to examine each possible case and carefully rule out some involvement of IF. The NK activating factor (NAF) described by Koide and Takasugi, produced by culture of human lymphoid cells with B lymphoblastoid cell lines, appears now to be type I IF. However, Peter et al and Leibold et al suggest that some of the augmenting activity induced by culture of human cells with C. parvum or cell lines may be mediated by a factor(s) separate from IF. Although cultures of unseparated peripheral blood mononuclear cells or null cells with C. parvum in medium containing human serum resulted in parallel appearance of NK boosting activity and IF, stimulation of T cells or cultures in medium containing fetal bovine serum resulted in strong boosting activity but low or undetectable levels of IF. Leibold et al also found some supernates that augmented NK activity but had little or no detectable IF. Further studies on these situations seem warranted, since it is possible that the active augmenting factor is IF but that other constituents of such culture supernatants are interfering with detection of antiviral activity. It would be of much interest to determine whether the boosting activity of supernatants without detectable IF could be abrogated by addition of anti-IF antibodies.

The recent studies of Brunda et al appear to provide more definite indications for an IF-independent mechanism for augmentation of NK activity. Pretreatment of normal mouse spleen cells with certain alloantisera or other antisera, or with some lectins, has caused substantial augmentation in NK activity. In addition to the lack of association of this effect with production of detectable amounts of IF, antibodies to IF and inhibitors of protein synthesis, that can fully block boosting by IF or IF-inducers, have had no effect on boosting by such materials. It seems likely that binding of some antibodies or lectins to the surface of NK cells can directly activate or augment their activity. An alternative possibility is that these agents stimulate the production of another lymphokine that is in turn responsible for the augmentation of NK activity.

II. CHARACTERISTICS OF BOOSTING OF NK ACTIVITY BY IF

There appears to be agreement by most of the contributors regarding the main characteristics of boosting of NK activity by IF. Experiments with different concentrations of IF have usually demonstrated a dose response relationship. However, the levels of IF required for boosting have varied somewhat among recipients. In some cases, as little as 10 units of IF have produced significant augmentation. Along this line, Welsh and Kiessling have mentioned evidence for local effects of low doses of IF, with intraperitoneal inoculation boosting the activity of peritoneal but not spleen cells. Similar regional effects have been noted by Riccardi et al (section IC4) in their studies with pyran copolymer and adriamycin. It seems possible that an agent could induce substantial local augmentation in the absence of detectable circulating levels of IF.

IF appears to only have to be in contact with NK cells for a few minutes but the actual development of augmented cytotoxic activity does not become apparent for at least 1-2 hrs. The increase in reactivity is independent of cell proliferation but is dependent on new RNA and protein synthesis. The observations indicate that the following sequence takes place: rapid binding of IF to cellular receptors or some other initial triggering of the cells, followed by synthesis of one or more proteins that are required for cytotoxic activity.

There appear to be definite upper limits to the levels of NK activity that can be produced by IF. Thus, in mice, the magnitude of augmentation has been greater in recipients with low spontaneous levels of activity, whereas only modest boosting has been in mice at their peak of spontaneous activity. Similarly, Einhorn shows here that boosted NK cells from patients receiving IF are less responsive to in vitro treatment with IF. One possible explanation for these observations is that IF-treated cells become refractory to further treatments with IF. In rodent systems, there is little information on this point. There have been few efforts to maintain boosted levels of NK activity in mice or rats, but some experiments in my laboratory and by Orn et al have indicated that after repeated treatments with some agents, levels may remain augmented for 1-2 weeks. The human studies of Riethmuller et al and of Einhorn suggest that continued in vivo administration of IF can cause a rapid and sustained elevation in NK activity. The only concern with these promising data is that usually only one pretreatment level has been checked and, if not truly representative of the range of spontaneous activity in the patient, could lead to a false impression of a sustained rise thereafter. To better document this important point, it would be very helpful to have additional pretreatment tests on patients receiving IF and also to perform parallel serial monitoring of comparable patients not receiving IF.

There are a few suggestive indications that another form of refractoriness to boosting by IF may occur. Saksela et al observed that cells which adhered to and were then eluted from fetal fibroblasts were not boosted by IF, even though the fetal fibroblasts were unable to induce detectable production of IF. Similarly, Silva et al (1980) found that formation of conjugates with target cells immediately after brief pretreatment with IF prevented the development of augmented NK activity. These data suggest that binding of NK cells to targets induces a resistance to the boosting effects of IF. The data of Peter et al, indicating that addition of IF at hour 6 or later during a 12 hr cytotoxicity assay failed to induce augmentation of cytotoxicity, would also be consistent with this hypothesis. It will be of interest to further investigate this phenomenon, to determine its mechanism and how persistent it is.

Most investigators have concluded that IF acts directly on effector cells and no accessory cells are required (e.g. see Orn et al, Ortaldo et al, Zarling). However, Moore et al observed that removal of monocytes interfered with the boosting by IF of antibody-dependent cell-mediated cytotoxicity (ADCC) against anti-D coated human erythrocytes. They suggest that an accessory cell was required for appreciable boosting of the effector cells. However, their data could also be attributed to the involvement of both monocytes and NK/K cells as effectors in this system, with only the monocyte effectors being IF-responsive.

III. NATURE OF THE EFFECTOR CELLS THAT IF ACTS UPON

NK activity is clearly not the only effector function that can be augmented by IF. It was reported several years ago that the reactivity of alloimmune cytotoxic T cells in mice was boosted by IF, and since then evidence has been presented for augmentation by IF of monocyte-mediated cytotoxicity, ADCC, and lectin-induced cell-mediated cytotoxicity (for summary of much of these data see Herberman et al, 1980). A common feature to all human effector cells that have been found to be augmented strongly by IF is their possession of Fc_{γ} receptors.

Since NK cells and K cells mediating ADCC against tumor targets appear to be in the same subpopulation and are probably identical (see section IB), it is of particular interest to consider the effects of IF on the activity of K cells. This remains a controversial issue, with Trinchieri _et al_ and also Heron _et al_ (1979) observing strong augmentation of NK activity in the absence of appreciable effects on ADCC. In contrast, several groups have documented substantial augmentation of ADCC against a range of target cells, from the same and xenogeneic species (Koide and Takasugi, Moore _et al_, Ortaldo _et al_). The reasons for these discrepant reports are not clear. It seems possible that the differences may lie in the IF preparations used for boosting. Some might contain materials that selectively interfere with the augmentation of ADCC. Some direct comparative experiments between laboratories should help to resolve this important issue.

In regard to NK activity itself, it is important to determine whether the effects of IF are on already mature NK cells or on pre-NK cells. Although considerable evidence points toward the latter possibility, of IF-induced differentiation from pre-NK cells to NK cells, some data also indicate a possible effect on augmenting the cytotoxic levels of already active NK cells or of switching on activity in mature NK cells. Table II summarizes some of the evidence in support of each of these hypotheses. Studies on the effects of various immunopharmacologic agents first pointed to major differences in the phenotype of spontaneous NK cells and of the cells responsive to NK-boosting agents (Oehler _et al_, 1978; Djeu _et al_, 1979). Spontaneous NK activity was strongly inhibited by treatment with cyclophosphamide, hydrocortisone or x-ray, whereas these treatments failed to block augmentation of NK activity by poly I:C. In regard to morphology and cell surface receptors, there have been some similarities between NK cells and the cells responsive to IF. As with NK cells, human cells responding to IF have been shown to be Fc_{γ} receptor positive and within the population of large granular lymphocytes (Herberman _et al_ in section IA, Ortaldo _et al_, Zarling). However, as discussed below there are also a number of differences in the cell surface characteristics between spontaneous NK cells and augmented NK cells. The most clearcut change in markers on mouse NK cells after IF treatment has been the appearance of Ly5 antigen (Bloom _et al_). Spontaneous NK cells and IF-augmented NK cells have been shown to be Ly5 positive, whereas the cells responding to IF have no detectable expres-

TABLE II. Mechanism of Augmentation of NK Activity by IF

A. *Evidence for Differentiation from Pre-NK cells to NK Cells.*
   1. *Differences in phenotype of spontaneous NK cells and cells responding to IF.*
      a. *IF-responsive rat and mouse cells resistant to pharmocologic agents and NK cell sensitive.*
      b. *Change in cell surface markers (e.g. Ly5).*
   2. *Activation by IF of human cells not forming conjugates with fetal fibroblasts.*
   3. *In human single cell agarose assay, report of IF-induced increased proportion of lytic conjugate-forming cells.*

B. *Evidence for Increase in Activity of Mature NK Cells.*
   1. *No change in precentage of lymphoid cells forming conjugates with NK-susceptible target cells.*
   2. *In human single cell agarose assay, mainly increased rate of lysis of target cells.*
   3. *By enzyme kinetic analysis, no change in binding constant but increase in velocity of reaction.*

sion of this antigen. Although it seems clear from these studies that there are substantial differences in the characteristics of NK cells and the cells responding to IF or IF-inducers, it is uncertain how closely related these differences are to the characteristics required for cytotoxic activity. It is possible that an IF-induced change in state of functional NK cells, from low to high activity, could be accompanied by the observed changes in phenotype. As discussed in detail in the chapter by Ortaldo et al, the most relevant issues in regard to the mechanism of IF-induced augmentation of NK activity are whether IF induces the expression of target cell-recognition receptors or of the required lytic machinery on pre-NK cells or whether it activates cells with pre-existing recognition and lytic structures. Although the observations by Saksela et al, that human cells not forming conjugates with fetal fibroblasts developed cytotoxicity against K562 after IF treatment, suggested that IF induced differentiation of new NK cells, the interpretation is confounded by the use of different targets for conjugate-formations and for the cytotoxicity assay. In fact, some of the cells nonadherent to fetal fibroblasts formed conjugates with K562 even prior to treatment with IF. Furthermore, the studies directly examining the proportion of mouse or human cells forming conjugates with NK-susceptible target cells have shown no change after treatment with IF (Roder; Trinchieri et al; Silva et al, 1980; T. Timonen, J. Ortaldo and R.

Herberman, unpublished observations). Thus, it appears that the cells responding to IF have a pre-existing ability to recognize their targets.

It is more difficult to assess whether the cells responding to IF already have all of the requisite lytic machinery. There are clearly situations in which IF can induce high activity in cells with no detectable pre-existing activity. These include cells from newborn or older mice, and mouse cells after treatment with anti-Ly5 plus complement. Although this suggests the induction by IF of some factors essential for lysis or a switch-on of inactive cells, these data could also be explained by just quantitative changes. Before IF treatment, the NK cells could be functional but at such low levels that their activity is undetectable above the background isotope release or they could require a longer period to produce lysis of target cells. Several groups have recently tried to analyze this question with human NK cells, using the single cell agarose cytotoxicity assay. Although this technique is potentially powerful for evaluating this point, it is also technically demanding and somewhat subjective. The results obtained thus far have appeared to be contradictory. Silva _et al_ (1980) performed their assay for up to 3 hrs. and observed that a higher proportion of IF-treated conjugate-forming cells were lytic for their targets when compared to untreated NK cells. In contrast, Trinchieri _et al_ observed mainly an increase in the rate of lysis. Timonen, Ortaldo and Herberman (unpublished observations) have observed that about one-half to two-thirds of large granular lymphocytes forming conjugates with K562 caused lysis of the targets, with plateau levels occurring by 12-24 hrs., and pretreatment with IF caused somewhat more rapid lysis but also an increase in the proportion of lysed target cells in conjugates, to close to 100%. Analysis of spontaneous or IF-augmented human NK activity by enzyme kinetics indicated only a change in the velocity of the reaction, Vmax (Ortaldo _et al_).

From the data discussed above, it should be apparent that there are considerable disagreements and uncertainties regarding the mechanism of augmentation of NK activity by IF. Complete resolution of this issue may have to await the determination of the biochemical nature of the NK-relevant proteins induced by IF and of the factors involved in the lytic machinery of NK cells. Despite these remaining questions, some insight into the relationship of the IF-responsive cells to the active NK cell appears to be emerging. They have some differences in phenotype, yet are quite similar in a number of respects. If an IF-driven differentiation step is required for activation of NK cells, it clearly does not involve the complete steps in differentiation from precursors that are described in section IC2. The IF-responsive cell already appears to have the needed recognition structures for binding to its targets, is Fc$_\gamma$ receptor positive, in the human has the same morphology as NK cells, and the transition to NK cells does not require any expansion in cell numbers.

IV. POSSIBLE ROLE OF IF IN DEVELOPMENT OF SPONTANEOUS NK ACTIVITY

With the strong evidence for the major, if not exclusive role, of IF as the mediator of augmentation of NK activity, one needs to consider the question of whether it is also involved in the natural development of cytotoxic activity. Although it has been difficult to clearly determine whether there is an absolute requirement for IF in the ontogeny of NK cells, there is increasing evidence for its playing a substantial role in determining the levels of spontaneous activity.

A. *Evidence for Role of IF in NK Activity of Mice and Rats*

As discussed earlier, mice and rats that are raised under conventional conditions have a quite characteristic time course for development of NK activity, with transient expression for some period between 3 and 10 weeks of age. Although it was initially thought that the absence of reactivity in very young mice was due to insufficient maturation, the observations that newborns can develop NK activity after treatment with IF or some IF-inducers (e.g. see Orn et al, Welsh and Kiessling) indicated that the necessary NK or pre-NK cells were already present. Orn et al suggest an interesting alternative explanation for the unreactivity during the early postnatal period. Such mice still have appreciable levels of circulating alpha-fetoprotein, which appears to block IF production by macrophages. This would fit with other indications that macrophages play an important role in the development and maintenance of NK activity. Macrophages are required for induction of IF production by poly I:C in mice and rats (Djeu et al, 1979; Oehler et al, 1978). In addition, several groups have observed that treatment of mice or rats with macrophage toxic agents, silica or carrageenan, results in appreciable depression in spontaneous NK activity.

More direct evidence for the role of IF in development or maintenance of spontaneous NK activity in mice has come from experiments involving *in vivo* administration of antibodies to IF. While one inoculation has not affected activity, repeated doses over several days caused a modest decrease in NK activity of normal mice (Orn *et al*). Bloom *et al* report a more marked reduction of NK activity by such treatment in nude mice. The data from *in vitro* studies with anti-IF are compatible with these *in vivo* observations. Whereas the presence of the antibodies in a short term cytotoxicity assay has not interfered with NK activity, Bloom *et al* found some reduction in assays of more than 9 hrs with virus-infected target cells. It will be of interest to determine whether *in vivo* treatment with anti-IF, begun prior to 3 weeks of age, could completely prevent the development of spontaneous NK activity. The main limitation for performing such a study is the current paucity of potent antisera.

If IF is important in spontaneous NK activity, what is the stimulus for its production? Early studies indicated that NK activity was detectable in germfree mice and rats, suggesting the lack of a requirement of environmental pathogens for the development of NK activity. However, Clark's recent study of pathogen-free mice, with very low activity until shortly after exposure to a conventional environment, clearly raises the possibility that environmental factors are responsible for induction of IF and subsequent appearance of NK activity. Although my group has failed to observe depressed spontaneous NK activity in pathogen-free mice living in a virus-free environment, we have made observations in rats that are similar to those of Clark. The apparent discrepancies could be due to differences in diet or other environmental factors, since not only viable microbial agents but also their products, e.g. endotoxins, can stimulate IF production and NK activity.

A further question, for which virtually no information is available, is why NK activity in conventionally housed mice and rats usually declines to low levels after 10-12 weeks of age. Certainly, such animals continue to be exposed to a variety of IF-inducing agents in their environment. However, by that age, immunity has already developed to most common pathogens which in turn may limit their proliferation and the level of stimulus for production of IF. It would be very helpful to have more sensitive assays for circulating levels of IF, to directly determine the kinetics of its spontaneous appearance and persistence.

B. *Evidence for Role of IF in Human NK Activity*

One of the major characteristics that distinguishes human NK activity from that in rodents is the fairly stable levels of activity over long periods of time. This suggests that the regulatory controls are substantially different and it is of interest to reconsider this in the light of a possible central role for IF. One intriguing possibility is that in humans as well as in mice and rats, *in vivo* NK activity in adults is at low levels but is rapidly inducible *in vitro* upon incubation with target cells that stimulate IF production. As discussed in section IA (Herberman *et al*), the decline with age of NK activity in rats is not apparent when the effector cells are precultured overnight or when the assay period is prolonged. Thus the main distinction between regulation of rodent and human NK activity might be the rapidity of *in vitro* IF production and consequent stimulation of NK activity. This possibility is supported by the observations of Trinchieri *et al*, indicating that up to 90% of the NK reactivity against IF-inducing target cells appears due to *in vitro* production of IF. In addition, the inhibition of spontaneous human NK activity by high concentrations of anti-IF or by inhibitors of protein synthesis (Ortaldo *et al*) could be attributed to the ability of these treatments to interfere with *in vitro* stimulation by IF. However, NK activity has been detected, mainly in overnight assays, against target cells that do not appear to stimulate IF production (Leibold *et al*, Saksela *et al*, Trinchieri *et al*). It will be of interest to re-examine the age kinetics of human NK activity in short term assays with NK-susceptible but non-IF-inducing target cells, to determine what proportion of NK activity is indeed "spontaneous."

C. *Characteristics of IF-boosted NK Cells as Compared to Spontaneous NK Cells*

In the context of this discussion on the role of IF in the induction of spontaneous NK activity, it is worthwhile to consider the comparative characteristics of the spontaneous and IF-induced effector cells. If the mechanism for their generation were the same, one might predict that all characteristics would be identical. Although there are many similarities in their features, it has become clear that there are some differences which need to be accounted for. Several groups have observed that a higher proportion of augmented NK cells in mice are adherent to nylon or other columns (Herberman *et al*, Tai and Warner, Welsh and Kiessling). The avidity of the Fc_γ receptors and the proportion of cells expressing Thy 1 antigen also seem to be greater with boosted mouse NK cells.

Bloom _et al_ have also noted that some boosted mouse NK cells are larger than spontaneous NK cells. A further major difference, discussed in detail in section ID, is the reactivity of boosted cells against a broader range of target cells. It is not possible to completely reconcile these differences with the hypothesis that spontaneous NK activity is also IF-induced. However, the apparent discrepancies may be a reflection of the interval between stimulation by IF and testing. There are indications that treatment with IF can cause alterations in the phenotype of NK cells that are more transient than the augmented activity. For example, within the first few hours after treatment _in vitro_ with IF, cytotoxic activity can be appreciably reduced by inhibitors of RNA or protein synthesis (Ortaldo _et al_). Although this might appear to be a clear difference from the resistance of spontaneous NK activity to these agents, the same treatments at later times after _in vitro_ or _in vivo_ augmentation had not effect.

V. EFFECTS OF IF ON TARGET CELLS

A further dimension to the effects of IF on NK activity is the effects of this cytokine on NK-susceptible target cells. This has been analyzed most extensively by Trinchieri _et al_, who found that treatment of target cells rather than effector cells with IF frequently causes decreased levels of lysis. This effect has been seen with most normal target cells, some SV40-transformed cells, and two tumor lines (K562 and a melanoma line). Thus susceptibility to this protective effect of IF varies considerably among targets and does not seem to correlate well with the normal versus transformed phenotype. Einhorn has obtained similar protective effects with K562 and Chang target cells and Hansson _et al_ and Welsh and Kiessling have observed IF-induced protection of various mouse normal and tumor target cells. In contrast, Peter _et al_ have observed that pretreatment of K562 or a melanoma line with IF resulted in increased susceptibility to lysis. The reason for this apparent discrepancy is not clear but might be related to differences in the sublines of K562. The failure of Peter _et al_ to see increased lysis of K562 after pretreatment of effector cells is clearly divergent from the results of several other groups, and supports the possibility for some major differences in their line.

The mechanism responsible for alteration by IF in susceptibility of some target cells to lysis by NK cells is obscure. However, Trinchieri _et al_, Hansson _et al_, and Welsh and

Kiessling provide data from cold target inhibition experiments, suggesting a decrease in expression of NK-related antigens. The change in the targets also has been found to require RNA and protein synthesis, and appears to require a period of several hrs to reach maximal differences (Welsh and Kiessling).

Regardless of the mechanism, it seems clear that this is another effect to consider in regard to the action of IF on NK activity. For *in vitro* studies, it would seem desirable to avoid addition of IF to the assay itself, since the results would depend on the balance between possible opposing effects on the effector cells and target cells. The protective effects of IF on target cells also have important implications for *in vivo* studies with IF. Depending on whether the treatment first affects NK or tumor cells, and the susceptibility of the particular tumor to IF-induced protection, IF administration conceivably could interfere with, rather than augment, NK mediated resistance against tumor growth. It should be noted, however, that no information on the protective effects of IF on primary autochthonous tumors has yet been obtained.

REFERENCES

Djeu, J.Y., Heinbaugh, J., Vieira, W.D., Holden, H.T., and Herberman, R.B., *Immunopharmacolocy* 1, 231 (1979),

Herberman, R.B., Ortaldo, J.R., Djeu, J.Y.. Holden, H.T., Jett, J., Lang, N.P., and Pestka, S., *Ann. NY Acad. Sci.* in press.

Heron, I., Hokland, M., Möller-Larsen, A., and Berg, K., *Cell. Immunol.* 43, 183 (1979).

Oehler, J.R. and Herberman, R.B., *Int. J. Cancer* 21, 221 (1978).

Silva, A., Bonavida, B., and Targan, S., submitted for publication (1980).

PROSTAGLANDIN-MEDIATED INHIBITION OF MURINE NATURAL KILLER CELL ACTIVITY

Michael J. Brunda[1]
Howard T. Holden

Laboratory of Immunodiagnosis
National Cancer Institute
Bethesda, Maryland

It has been suggested that natural killer (NK) cells may be important as effector cells in immuno-surveillance against neoplastic cells (Herberman and Holden, 1978) and in natural resistance to allogeneic and semi-syngeneic parental transplants of hemopoietic cells (Cudkowicz and Hochman, 1979). In addition, a variety of normal cells are susceptible to NK activity *in vitro* (Nunn *et al.*, 1977; Welch and Zinkernagel, 1977) and, although the *in vivo* significance of this reactivity is not known, one possibility is that differentiation or control of various cell subpopulations could be influenced by NK cells. Because of these activities, it is important to have a thorough understanding of the manner in which NK activity is regulated and of the types of interactions that NK cells have with other lymphoid cells. Such knowledge could permit the modulation of NK activity *in vivo* resulting in a subsequent benefit to the host.

Multiple variables influence the level of murine NK activity. In most strains of mice, peak activity is present at 6 to 8 weeks while reactivity is low at birth and after 12 weeks of age (Herberman *et al.*, 1975; Kiessling *et al.*, 1975). High levels of spontaneous reactivity have been found in all strains of athymic nude mice while NK activity ranging from low to high has been found with various strains of euthymic mice (Herberman *et al.*, 1975; Kiessling *et al.*, 1975; Herberman and Holden, 1978). Interferon (IF) or IF-

[1] *On temporary assignment from the National Jewish Hospital and Research Center, Denver, Colorado.*

ISBN 0-12-341350-8

inducers can rapidly augment spontaneous levels of NK activity *in vivo* or *in vitro* (Herberman *et al.*, 1977; Oehler *et al.*, 1978; Djeu *et al.*, 1979a, 1979b; Gidlund *et al.*, 1978). The role of IF in the generation of spontaneous NK reactivity has not been fully established but it has been reported that environmental stimulation is necessary for the development of NK activity (Clark *et al.*, 1979). It is plausible that a variety of environmental stimuli can trigger IF production which then mediates the generation of spontaneous NK activity.

On the other hand, following a variety of experimental treatments, the level of murine NK reactivity has been found to be reduced. Tumor-bearing mice have been reported to have significantly lower splenic NK activity when compared to agematched normal mice (Herberman *et al.*, 1975; Becker and Klein, 1976). At certain times after injection of a number of immunomodulating agents, e.g., *Corynebacterium parvum* (Ojo *et al.*, 1978; Savary and Lotzova, 1978), glucan (Lotzova and Gutterman, 1979), silica (Djeu *et al.*, 1979), carrageenan (Cudkowicz and Hochman, 1979; Djeu *et al.*, 1979c) or cyclophosphamide (Djeu *et al.*, 1979c), a marked reduction in NK activity has been observed. Total body irradiation (Cudkowicz and Hochman, 1979) and chronic administration of β -estradiol (Seaman *et al.*, 1978, 1979) also have resulted in reduced reactivity. The mechanism(s) of suppression in these situations has not been established although several laboratories have reported that suppressor cells in mice treated by some of these protocols, such as mice injected with *C. parvum,* or hydrocortisone (Hochman and Cudkowicz, 1979; Cudkowicz and Hochman, 1979; Savary and Lotzova, 1978), could inhibit the cytolytic reactivities of NK cells *in vitro*. However, other laboratories (Ojo *et al.*, 1978; Seaman *et al.*, 1978) have failed to demonstrate suppressor cells in mice with reduced NK reactivity.

Our interest in the regulation of NK activity centers on the mechanism(s) which mediates the depression of NK reactivity *in vivo* in mice treated by some of these protocols. Interestingly, in association with depressed NK reactivity, mice injected with *C. parvum* (Grimm *et al.*, 1978) or mice bearing certain tumors (Humes *et al.*, 1974; Strausser and Humes, 1975; Pelus and Strausser, 1976; Lynch *et al.*, 1978) have been observed to produce increased amounts of prostaglandins (PGs). PGs have been previously shown to inhibit a variety of immunological reactivities including lymphocyte proliferation (Goodwin *et al.*, 1977; Webb and Nowowiejski, 1978), antibody formation (Plescia *et al.*, 1975), lymphokine production (Gordon *et al.*, 1976), and T cell (Henney *et al.*, 1972; Strom *et al.*, 1973) and macrophage-mediated (Schultz *et al.*, 1978) cytotoxicity. Recently, it was also reported that PGE can inhibit the spontaneous cytotoxicity of human peripheral blood lymphocytes against tumor target cells (Droller *et al.*, 1978a, 1978b) and that murine NK activity was inhibited by substances including PGE that increased intracellular concentrations of cyclic AMP (Roder and Klein, 1979). Since PGs can suppress certain immune reactivities and their production is increased in mice with depressed NK activity, we examined the *in vitro* and *in vivo* role of these substances as regulators of NK activity.

NK activity of murine spleen cells was assessed *in vitro* using a 4 hr ^{51}Cr release assay (Herberman *et al.*, 1975; Brunda *et al.*, 1979). The target cells used included YAC-1, RL♂1 and RBL-5, grown in stationary suspension culture as previously described (Brunda *et al.*, 1979).

The inhibition of splenic NK activity caused by the addition of exogenous PGs is presented in Table I. At a concentration of 10^{-6}M, PGE_1 and PGE_2 markedly depressed NK cell cytotoxicity. PGA_1 and PGA_2 also reduced cytotoxicity while PGB_1 and PGB_2 caused only a slight inhibition in these responses. In contrast, $PGF_{1\alpha}$ and $PGF_{2\alpha}$ caused no reduction in NK reactivity. The inhibition by PGE_1 and PGE_2 was dependent on the concentration of PG added to the culture and the suppression of NK activity by PGs could be obtained at all effector to target cell ratios (Brunda *et al.*, 1979). In addition, the PG-mediated inhibition was also observed when either spleen cells from athymic nude mice or nylon wool passed spleen cells were used as effector cells, indicating that a) neither T cells, B cells or macrophages were required

TABLE I. Effect of Prostaglandins on Murine NK Activity[a]

PG added to culture	*% Cytotoxicity*
None	*31*
PGE_1	*16*
PGE_2	*16*
PGA_1	*20*
PGA_2	*20*
PGB_1	*26*
PGB_2	*27*
$PGF_{1\alpha}$	*32*
$PGF_{2\alpha}$	*30*

[a]*NK activity of CBA/J spleen cells against RL♂1 targets at 100/1 ratio, with addition of 10^{-6}M PG to the assay.*

for PG mediated depression of NK activity and b) NK cells were directly affected by PG (Brunda *et al.*, 1979; unpublished observations).

The ability of PGs to inhibit the NK activity of one group of normal spleen cells against several target cells was tested to determine whether the inhibition of NK reactivity varied with the target cell used to measure cytotoxicity. As seen in Table II, NK activity against RL♂1 target cells, as previously demonstrated, was inhibited by addition of 10^{-6}M PGE_1 or PGE_2. A similar pattern of suppressed NK reactivity was found when more sensitive, YAC-1, or less sensitive, RBL-5, target cells were employed to measure cytotoxicity. With all 3 target cells, no inhibition was observed when $PGF_{1\alpha}$ or $PGF_{2\alpha}$ was added to the culture. These results indicate that PG-mediated inhibition of NK activity was independent of the target cell used.

Since in the preceding experiments PGs were added directly to the cytotoxicity assay, we next evaluated whether pretreatment of effector cells with PGs would result in inhibition of NK activity. Spleen cells were incubated with medium or PGs for 30 min., washed, and then tested for cytotoxicity against RL♂1 target cells (Table III). As in prior experiments, addition of PGE_1 or PGE_2 directly to the assay resulted in suppression of NK reactivity. However, following pretreatment of the effector cells, there was little or no inhibition of cytotoxicity. Addition of PGE_1 or PGE_2 to the assay with these pretreated spleen cells again resulted in reduced NK activity. These results indicate that PG-mediated suppression was reversible, with optimal effects obtained only when PG was present during the assay.

TABLE II. Prostaglandin-Mediated Inhibition of NK Activity against Different Target Cells[a]

PG added to culture	*% Cytotoxicity*		
	RL♂1	*YAC-1*	*RBL-5*
None	19	42	9
PGE_1	9	25	3
PGE_2	9	27	3
$PGF_{1\alpha}$	16	42	8
$PGF_{2\alpha}$	17	39	7

[a]*PGs (10^{-6}M) were added to the culture of CBA/J spleen cells and target cells at 100/1 effector/target cell ratio.*

TABLE III. Pretreatment of Effector Cells with PGs: Effect on NK Activity[a]

Pretreatment with	*Prostaglandin added to assay* (10^{-6}*M*)		
	None	*PGE*$_1$	*PGE*$_2$
Media	*31*	*15*	*16*
PGE$_1$	*25*	*11*	*N.T.*[b]
PGE$_2$	*28*	*N.T.*	*13*

[a]*NK activity of CBA/J spleen cells against RLô1 target cells at a 200/1 ratio.*
[b]*Not tested.*

As noted earlier, IF and IF inducers rapidly augmented NK activity both *in vitro* and *in vivo* (Herberman *et al.*, 1977; Oehler *et al.*, 1978; Djeu *et al.*, 1979a, 1979b; Gidlund *et al.*, 1978). It is possible that part of the explanation for this augmentation might be the ability of IF to modulate NK cells such that they do not respond to inhibitory signals which regulate their activity. Since PGs suppressed NK reactivity, we determined their effect on NK cells that had been stimulated by IF. As shown in Table IV, spleen cells from 6 week old mice had a high level of NK activity but this reactivity was reduced in 12 week old mice. Following treatment *in vitro* with IF for 1 hr, an enhanced cytotoxic response was found. When PGE_2 was added to the cultures, a comparable inhibition of cytotoxicity was observed. Similar results were obtained, regardless of whether the data were expressed as the percent cytotoxicity at a particular effector to target cell ratio or as the percent inhibition of response calculated on the basis of lytic units. To examine further the influence of PGs on augmented NK activity, 12 week old mice were injected with lymphocytic choriomeningitis virus (LCMV), a potent augmentor of NK activity (Herberman *et al.*, 1977) and an IF inducer (Riviere *et al.*, 1977; Merigann *et al.*, 1977), and the reactivity of their spleen cells was examined *in vitro* in the presence or absence of PGs (Table V). Addition of PGE_1 or PGE_2 markedly suppressed NK activity but the addition of $PGF_{1\alpha}$ or $PGF_{2\alpha}$ to the culture had no effect on the cytotoxicity expressed by these effector cells. Thus, *in vivo* or *in vitro* augmented NK cytotoxicity was inhibited by PGs to an extent similar to that of spontaneous NK cell activity.

TABLE IV. Prostaglandin-Mediated Inhibition of Effector Cells Augmented by Interferon In Vitro[a]

Age of mice	*IF treatment*	*PG added to assay*		*% Inhibition of response*[b]
		None	PGE_2	
6 wk	-	34	19	49
12 wk	-	14	N.T.[c]	N.T.
12 wk	+	26	16	44

[a]*NK cytotoxicity of CBA/J spleen cells against RLô1 target cells at 67/1 ratio with addition of* 10^{-6}*M PG.*
[b]*Based on lytic unit calculation.*
[c]*Not tested.*

TABLE V. Prostaglandin Mediated Inhibition of Effector Cells Augmented by LCMV In Vivo[a]

PG added to culture (10^{-6}*M*)	*% Cytotoxicity*
None	24
PGE_1	10
PGE_2	12
$PGF_{1\alpha}$	22
$PGF_{2\alpha}$	28

[a]*NK cytotoxicity of spleen cells from >12 wk old CBA/J mice, injected 3 days before with LCMV, against RLô1 target cells at 50/1 ratio.*

Although IF did not interfere with the response of NK cells to the inhibitory influence of PGs, it has been previously demonstrated that other lymphoid cells changed their sensitivity to PG-mediated inhibition upon *in vitro* incubation. For example, the cytotoxicity of alloimmune T cells generated *in vitro*, in contrast to *in vivo*-induced cytotoxic T cells, was not suppressed by PGE (Plaut, 1979). Likewise, peripheral blood lymphocytes lost their sensitivity to PGE-mediated inhibition of PHA-induced blastogenesis when they were first incubated overnight at 37°C (Goodwin *et al.*, 1977), a result that has correlated with the loss of receptors for PGE on these cells (Goodwin *et al.*, 1979). Therefore, it was of interest to determine whether NK cells might also lose their sensitivity to PG-mediated inhibition following *in vitro* incubation (Table VI). Murine NK cells have been previously reported to become inactivated when incubated at 37°C (Herberman *et al.*, 1975) but this inactivation can be minimized when the culture conditions were modified (Djeu *et al.*, 1979b). As in prior experiments, noncultured spleen cells exhibited good NK activity which could be inhibited by the addition of PGE_2. In contrast, when spleen cells were incubated overnight at 37°C, they retained much of their NK activity but addition of PGE_2 to the assay resulted in almost no inhibition of cytotoxicity. Spleen cells incubated overnight at 4°C retained both their NK activity and their susceptibility to PG-mediated suppression. These results indicate that there is a temperature dependent modulation of NK cells following overnight incubation such that these spleen cells become resistant to PG-mediated inhibition of NK activity.

As indicated earlier, there are several experimental situations which result in depressed NK activity. Although mice injected with tumor cells exhibited a transient increase in NK activity (Herberman *et al.*, 1977), there is a marked depression in this function at later time points (Herberman *et al.*, 1975; Becker and Klein, 1976). In addition, it has

TABLE VI. Effect of In Vitro *Culture of Effector Cells on Prostaglandin-Mediated Inhibition of NK Activity*[a]

Preculture	*PG added to assay*		*% Inhibition of Response*[b]
	None	*PGE_2 (10^{-6}M)*	
None	25	11	77
37°C	16	15	13
4°C	24	12	58

[a]*% cytotoxicity of CBA/J spleen cells, after culture overnight at 37°C or 4°C, against RLδ1 target cells at 22/1 ratio.*

[b]*Based on lytic unit calculation.*

also been reported that mice bearing certain tumors, such as those induced by murine sarcoma virus (MSV), produce increased amounts of PGs (Humes *et al.*, 1974; Strausser and Humes, 1975; Pelus and Strausser, 1976; Lynch *et al.*, 1978). Since NK reactivity of spleen cells could be markedly suppressed by PGs *in vivo*, we wondered whether the production of PG *in vivo* could also account for the depressed reactivity. To test this hypothesis, mice were injected with MSV and also treated with indomethacin, a potent inhibitor of PG synthesis, in their drinking water for 7 days before their spleen cells were assayed for NK activity. As shown in Table VII, mice bearing MSV-induced tumors had depressed NK activity compared to age-matched normal mice in agreement with earlier reports (Herberman *et al.*, 1975; Becker and Klein, 1976). When spleen cells from MSV tumor-bearing mice that had received indomethacin were tested, a partial or, in some experiments, a complete restoration of activity was observed in both euthymic or athymic mice.

To examine further the restoration of NK reactivity, a second inhibitor of PG synthesis, aspirin, was injected into MSV tumor-bearing mice 18 hr before testing of their spleen cells (Table VIII). Again, a marked restoration of activity was found in both euthymic and athymic, nude mice. Injection of aspirin or administration of indomethacin to normal mice resulted in little or no increase in NK activity. Although aspirin restored NK activity in MSV tumor-bearing mice in most experiments (12 of 18 experiments) some variability in the results was obtained. However, in general, it appears

TABLE VII. Effect of Indomethacin on NK Activity of Spleen Cells from Tumor-Bearing Mice[a]

Treatment	*% Cytotoxicity*	
	CBA/J	*Swiss nu/nu*
None	*19*	*34*
Indomethacin	*27*	*34*
MSV	*10*	*17*
MSV & Indomethacin	*25*	*26*

[a]*CBA/J or Swiss nu/nu mice were injected with MSV on day 0, started on indomethacin (20 μg/ml) in their drinking water on day 7 and tested for NK activity on day 14, against YAC-1 at 200/1 ratio.*

TABLE VIII. Effect of Aspirin on NK Cytotoxicity of Spleen Cells from Tumor-Bearing Mice[a]

Treatment	*% Cytotoxicity*	
	CBA/J	*Swiss nu/nu*
None	*41*	*55*
Aspirin	*36*	*47*
MSV	*17*	*32*
MSV & Aspirin	*33*	*52*

[a]*CBA/J or Swiss nu/nu mice were injected with MSV on day 0, injected with 10 μg aspirin intraperitoneally on day 13 and tested for NK activity on day 14 against YAC-1 at 200/1 ratio.*

that inhibition of PG synthesis resulted in restoration of NK activity in MSV tumor-bearing mice.

PG production has been implicated in growth of MSV tumors since administration of indomethacin to mice resulted in suppression of tumor development and growth (Humes *et al.*, 1974; Strausser and Humes, 1975). Since indomethacin can also restore NK activity, it is possible that at least a portion of the suppressed tumor growth previously observed was mediated by NK cells. To examine the effect of indomethacin on the growth of MSV-induced tumors, mice were injected with the virus and on the same day begun on indomethacin in their drinking water. When mice were injected with the regressor MSV strain, tumors developed and then spontaneously regressed. When mice were also treated with indomethacin, a much lower tumor incidence and smaller tumor size were found than in mice receiving no indomethacin (Table IX,A); these results are in agreement with prior studies (Humes *et al.*, 1974; Strausser and Humes, 1975). When mice were injected with a progressor strain of MSV (Takeichi *et al.*, 1978), over half of the mice developed progressively growing tumors. When treated with indomethacin, no mice developed progressive tumors and tumor growth, as measured by maximum tumor size, was inhibited. (Table IX,B).

TABLE IX. Effect of Indomethacin on MSV-Induced Tumor Growth[a]

A. Regressor Virus

Indomethacin	*Tumor incidence*	*Maximum tumor size*
-	*14/15*[b]	*4+*
+	*3/15*	*1/2+*

B. Progressor Virus

Indomethacin	*Tumor incidence*		*Maximum tumor size*
	Day 9	*Day 93*	
-	*9/9*	*5/9*	*4+*
+	*1/9*	*0/9*	*1/2+*

[a]*CBA/J (6 wk old) mice were injected with MSV intramuscularly.*

[b]*No. mice with tumors/no. mice injected.*

CONCLUDING REMARKS

Our data clearly indicate that PGs have a marked inhibitory effect on NK activity *in vitro* with PGs of the E series causing the largest decrease in activity. However, a complete inhibition of NK cytotoxicity by PGs was never achieved using nontoxic concentrations of PG (Brunda *et al.*, 1979). One explanation for this is that a subpopulation of NK cells lack PG receptors (Goodwin *et al.*, 1979) and are therefore resistant to PG-mediated inhibition. An NK cell subpopulation which lacks PG receptors might be an important set of effector cells, in particular, when dealing with a tumor that secretes or stimulates host cells to produce increased amounts of PGs.

Maximal inhibition of NK cytotoxicity occurred when PGs were present throughout the assay while pretreatment of effector cells resulted in little inhibition. Because of this finding, the effect of PG may have been on the target cells. However, this possibility was excluded by the studies using effector cells that had been cultured overnight. No decrease in NK activity was observed when PGE was added to effector cells that had been incubated for 18 hr at 37°C while the activity of effector cells cultured at 4°C was inhibited by PGE. Since the same target cells were used to test each group, it is clear that the effect of PG was on the effector cells.

It has been previously reported that *in vitro* incubation causes cells to become resistant to the inhibitory effect of PGE both with mitogen induced proliferation of human peripheral blood lymphocytes (Goodwin *et al.*, 1977) and with *in vivo*-generated cytotoxic murine T cells (Plaut, 1979). Our data indicated that murine NK cells can also be modulated in like manner upon *in vitro* culture. The reason for the resistance to PGE-mediated inhibition is not known, although human peripheral blood lymphocytes lose their receptors for PGE in culture (Goodwin *et al.*, 1979). The failure to inhibit may, therefore, be due to the inability of PGE to bind to the effector cells. However, in the cytotoxic murine T cell model, agents other than PGE which increase cyclic AMP levels also do not suppress cytotoxicity of *in vitro* generated effector T cells (Plaut, 1979). In contrast to the modulation induced by *in vivo* culture, IF, which augments NK activity, has no apparent effect on PG-mediated inhibition. The ability of environmental conditions to render NK cells unresponsive to PG could be an important factor in the regulation of NK activity *in vivo*.

To examine the possible *in vivo* regulation of NK activity by PGs, we chose a model system, mice bearing MSV-induced tumors, where depressed splenic NK activity had been demonstrated (Herberman *et al.*, 1975; Becker and Klein, 1976) and where tumor-bearing mice have been shown to produce elevated levels of PGE (Humes *et al.*, 1974; Strausser and Humes, 1975). Two inhibitors of PG synthesis, indomethacin and aspirin, were administered to MSV-tumor-bearing mice and their NK activity assessed. In most experiments, a complete or partial restoration of NK activity was observed with the spleen cells from tumor-bearing mice. The restoration of activity did not appear to be due to stimulation of NK activity, as seen with IF and IF-inducers, since indomethacin and aspirin had little effect on the NK activity of normal mice. The most direct explanation for these results is that the PG synthesis inhibitors suppress the increased production of PGs in MSV-tumor-bearing mice and that, therefore, the negative effect of PGs on splenic NK activity in these mice is reversed. Some variability in restoration of activity was observed and may reflect a failure to depress PG synthesis sufficiently to restore reactivity. PG synthesis might be influenced by factors such as tumor growth rate or environmental stimulation and might vary among animals. Another explanation for the experimental variation might be that other regulatory mechanisms, such as suppressor cells that function independently of PG production, may operate in tumor-bearing mice.

Suppressor cells for NK activity have been reported in mice treated with a number of agents including *C. parvum* and hydrocortisone (Cudkowicz and Hochman, 1979; Hochman and Cudkowicz, 1979; Savary and Lotzova, 1978). One possibility that should be examined is that suppressor cells induced by some of these protocols may produce PGs in culture, which then inhibit NK activity of spleen cells from normal mice. In contrast, suppressor cells induced by other treatments could work independently of PG production, thereby resulting in regulation of NK activity by several pathways.

The *in vivo* influence of PGs on NK activity might be of particular significance since NK cells are considered a possible candidate effector cell for immunosurveillance (Herberman and Holden, 1978; Kiessling and Haller, 1978). In our studies, indomethacin caused suppressed tumor growth and lowered tumor incidence in mice injected with regressor or progressor MSV. In other studies, indomethacin or aspirin were found to inhibit tumor growth or augment the antitumor effects of other immunostimulants such as *C. parvum* or BCG (Plescia *et al.*, 1975; Lynch *et al.*, 1978; Lynch and Salomon, 1979). These antitumor effects could have been mediated by NK cells whose activity had been restored by inhibiting PG synthesis.

In summary, our results indicate that PGs have a marked inhibitory effect on NK activity *in vitro* and suggest that PGs can regulate NK reactivity *in vivo* in MSV-tumor-bearing mice. Future studies may define this inhibition in more precise terms and give us a better understanding of the regulation of NK activity and the interaction of NK lymphocytes with other normal and malignant cells.

REFERENCES

Becker, S., and Klein, E. (1976). *Eur. J. Immunol. 6,* 892.

Brunda, M. J., Herberman, R. B., and Holden, H. T. (1980). *J. Immunol.* (In Press)

Cudkowicz, G., and Hochman, P. S. (1979). *Immunol. Rev. 44,* 13.

Djeu, J. Y., Heinbaugh, J. A., Holden, H. T., and Herberman, R. B. (1979a). *J. Immunol. 122,* 175.

Djeu, J. Y., Heinbaugh, J. A., Holden, H. T., and Herberman, R. B. (1979b). *J. Immunol. 122,* 182.

Djeu, J. Y., Heinbaugh, J. A., Viera, W. D., Holden, H. T., and Herberman, R. B. (1979c). *Immunopharmacology 1,* 231.

Droller, M. J., Perlmann, P., and Schneider, M. U. (1978a). *Cell. Immunol. 39,* 154.

Droller, M. J., Schneider, M. U., and Perlmann, P. (1978b). *Cell. Immunol. 39,* 165.

Gidlund, M. A., Orn, A., Wigzell, H., Senik, A., and Gresser, I. (1978). *Nature 273,* 759.

Goodwin, J. S., Bankhurst, A. D., and Messner, R. P. (1977). *J. Exp. Med. 146,* 1719.

Goodwin, J. S., Wiek, A., Lewis, M., Bankhurst, A. D., and Williams, R. C., Jr. (1979). *Cell. Immunol. 43,* 150.

Gordon, D., Bray, M. A., and Morley, J. (1976). *Nature 262,* 401.

Grimm, W., Seitz, M. Kirchner, H., and Gemsa, D. (1978). *Cell. Immunol. 40,* 419.

Henney, C. S., Bourne, H. R., and Lichtenstein, L. M. (1972). *J. Immunol. 108,* 1.26.

Herberman, R. B., and Holden, H. T. (1978). *Adv. Cancer Res. 27,* 305.

Herberman, R. B., Nunn, M. E., and Lavrin, D.H. (1975). *Int. J. Cancer 16,* 216.

Herberman, R. B., Nunn, M. E., Holden, H. T. Staal, S., and Djeu, J. Y. (1977). *Int. J. Cancer 19,* 555.

Hochman, P. S., and Cudkowicz, G. (1979). *J. Immunol. 123,* 968.

Holden, H. T., Oldham, R. K., Ortaldo, J. R., and Herberman, R. B. (1977). *J. Natl. Cancer Inst. 58,* 611.

Humes, J. L., Cupo, J. J., Jr., and Strausser, H. R. (1974). *Prostaglandins 6,* 463.

Kiessling, R., and Haller, O. (1978). *Contemp. Topics Immunobiol. 8,* 171.

Kiessling, R., Klein, E., and Wigzell, H. (1975). *Eur. J. Immunol. 5,* 112.

Lotzova, E., and Gutterman, J. U. (1979). *J. Immunol. 123,* 607.

Lynch, N. R., and Salomon, J. C. (1979). *J. Immunol. 123,* 607.

Lynch, N. R., Castes, M., Astoin, M., and Salomon, J. C. (1978). *Br. J. Cancer 38,* 503.

Merigan, T. C., Oldstone, M. B. A., and Welch, R. M. (1977). *Nature 268,* 67.

Nunn, M. E., Herberman, R. B., and Holden, H. T. (1977). *Int. J. Cancer 20,* 381.

Oehler, J. R., Lindsay, L. R., Nunn, M. E., Holden, H. T., and Herberman, R. B. (1978). *Int. J. Cancer 21,* 210.

Ojo, E., Haller, O., Kimura, A., and Wigzell, H. (1978). *Int. J. Cancer 21,* 444.

Pelus, L. M., and Strausser, H. R. (1976). *Int. J. Cancer 18,* 653.

Plaut, M. (1979). *J. Immunol. 123,* 692.

Plescia, O. J., Smith, A. H., and Grinwich, K. (1975). *Proc. Natl. Acad. Sci. 72,* 1848.

Riviere, Y., Gresser, I., Guillon, J. C., and Tovey, M. G. (1977). *Proc. Natl. Acad. Sci. 74,* 2135.

Roder, J. C., and Klein, M. (1979). *J. Immunol. 123,* 2785.

Savary, C. A., and Lotzova, E. (1978). *J. Immunol. 123,* 239.

Schultz, R. M., Pavlidis, N. A., Slylos, W. A., and Chirigos, M. A. (1978). *Science 202,* 320.

Seaman, W. E., Blackman, M. A., Gindhardt, T., Raubinian, J. R. Loeb, J. M., and Talal, N. (1978). *J. Immunol. 121,* 2193.

Seaman, W. E., Gindhardt, T. D., Greenspan, J. S., Blackman, M. A., and Talal, N. (1979). *J. Immunol. 122,* 2541.

Strausser, H. R., and Humes, J. L. (1975). *Int. J. Cancer 15,* 724.

Strom, T. B., Carpenter, C. B., Garovoy, M. R., Austen, K. F., Merrill, J. P., and Kaliner, M. (1973). *J. Exp. Med. 138,* 381.

Webb, D. R., and Nowowiejski, I. (1978). *Cell. Immunol. 41,* 72.

Welch, R. M., and Zinkernagel, R. M. (1977). *Nature 268,* 646.

C.PARVUM-MEDIATED SUPPRESSION OF THE PHENOMENON OF NATURAL KILLING AND ITS ANALYSIS

Eva Lotzová

Department of Developmental Therapeutics
The University of Texas System Cancer Center
M.D. Anderson Hospital and Tumor Institute
Houston, Texas

The association of natural killing levels with susceptibility to leukemias in murine system, together with the avid reactivity of natural killer (NK) cells to multifarious tumor targets led to the implication of these cells in immunosurveillance to malignancies and in resistance to already established tumors. The suggested anti-tumor potential of natural immunity motivated us to study the effect of various clinically pertinent immunomodulating and chemotherapeutic agents on the phenomenon of natural killing. One of the first agents, from the group of immunomodulators, we studied systematically was *Corynebacterium parvum (C.parvum)*. *C.parvum* attracted our interest firstly, for its extensive clinical application and secondly, for its frequently diverse effects on various limbs of immunity, resulting either in immune potentiation or immune depression (1-4). Moreover, the mechanism of *C.parvum* action and its target has been vaguely understood and it was reasonable to speculate that NK cells could be one of its targets.

I. TIME-DEPENDENT, *C.PARVUM*-MEDIATED AND SPLEEN-RESTRICTED DECLINE IN NATURAL KILIER CELL ACTIVITIES

In the first series of experiments we have studied the time-dependent effect of single intravenous injection of 0.5mg

This work was supported by Grant CA 21062 from NCI.

ISBN 0-12-341350-8

of formalin-killed *C.parvum* (Burroughs Wellcome, Co., Research Triangle Park, N.C.) on NK cell cytotoxicity of various murine lympho-hemopoietic tissues. Allogeneic T cell lymphoma, YAC-1 was used as a target tissue and $B6DF_1$ female mice as spleen donors. It can be clearly seen from Table I that no change in splenic natural killing was observed on day 3 post *C.parvum* inoculation; the percent of cytotoxicity was comparable to that of untreated, syngeneic mice. However, at later time intervals after *C.parvum* injection severe and relatively long-lasting decline in splenic NK cell cytotoxicity was detected. Splenic NK cell depression was in these particular series of experiments detected first on day 5 and lasted until day 21 post *C.parvum* inoculation. There was a time-dependent variability in the degree of NK cell depression; it was relatively weak on days 5 (56%),21 (37%) and stronger on day 7 through 17 (66-82%). On day 28,NK cell cytotoxicity of *C.parvum* treated mice returned to normal levels. It is certainly evident that NK cell depression required a certain time elapse before expression, the fact which suggests that induction of suppressor cells could have been necessary.

C.parvum-dependent depression of NK cell killing was not restricted to mice of $B6DF_1$ genotype since similar decrease in NK cell cytotoxicity was exerted by Balb/c and C57BL/6 (data are not shown) and $(B6xA)F_1$ mice (5-6). In fact, in the latter strain combination of mice suppression appeared to be even stronger and persisted longer. Moreover, before depression occurred, NK cell cytotoxicity was significantly increased (on day 3) in this strain combination, the observation compatible with that of Herberman et al., who first reported increase in NK cell activities after intraperitoneal injection of *C.parvum* (7-8). These observations indicate rather wide spread occurrence of *C.parvum* initiated suppression phenomenon between various mouse strains. Even though the decline in NK cell cytotoxicity was always induced by *C.parvum*, there was a slight variability between experiments with regard to its first appearance and its duration; the time range for appearance of depression ranged from 5-7 days and the range of its duration from 17-31 days. The strength and duration of *C.parvum*-caused NK cell depression appeared also to be mouse strain dependent.

Several possibilities could explain decline in NK cell cytoxicity in *C.parvum* inoculated mice; firstly,mobilization of NK cells to other lympho-hemopoietic tissues and consequently their depletion in the spleen. Secondly, NK cells could be diluted by the increase of other splenic cell populations that are known to be augmented by *C.parvum* (9). Indeed, the splenic cellularity is significantly increased after *C.parvum* injection. Thirdly, depressed NK cell activities could be caused by the presence of regulatory cell(s) controlling, in

TABLE I. Effect of C.Parvum on Natural Killing Expressed by Various Murine Lympho-Hemopoietic Tissues

Days Post C.Parvum[b]	Mean Percent of Natural Cytotoxicity ± S.E.[a,c]			
	Spleen	Thymus	Lymph Nodes	Bone Marrow
None	42.9±1.4(38)	0.4±0.5(35)	10.8±1.5(34)	20.0±1.2(35)
3	47.8±4.1(7)	2.0±1.5(5)	18.8±1.6(5)	47.2±5.0(5)
5	19.0±2.4(6)	4.0±1.8(6)	8.8±2.5(6)	10.5±1.5(6)
7	11.4±1.6(8)	4.2±2.5(6)	19.5±3.4(4)	12.5±3.0(6)
9	14.3±2.6(10)	4.3±3.3(6)	11.4±4.1(5)	18.3±2.3(6)
11	11.0±1.6(8)	6.0±1.7(6)	9.6±1.5(5)	18.8±1.6(6)
13	7.8±1.7(6)	4.3±2.5(6)	7.0±1.8(6)	18.5±1.9(6)
15	11.3±1.5(7)	7.9±2.0(6)	9.6±2.0(6)	24.0±2.6(6)
17	14.7±2.6(6)	6.3±3.0(6)	9.3±2.9(6)	26.5±4.1(6)
21	27.3±2.6(6)	13.0±3.7(6)	13.8±2.0(6)	32.4±4.6(6)
28	35.0±5.5(6)	8.5±1.8(6)	16.7±4.2(6)	35.0±4.8(6)

[a] 2×10^4 YAC-1 target cells were incubated with various tissues of $B6DF_1$ mice in 1:50 T:E ratio for 16 hrs; the number of animals in each group is indicated in parenthesis.

[b] Individual mice were injected with 0.5mg of C.parvum, i.v.

[c] Significant decrease in splenic NK cell cytotoxicity of C.parvum treated mice was observed on days 5-21 ($P<0.001$), increase in thymic NK cell killing was observed from day 3 through day 28 ($P<0.02$ to <0.05; bone marrow NK cell cytotoxicity increased significantly on days 3, 21 and 28 ($P<0.001$) and decreased on day 5 ($P<0.005$) and natural killing in lymph nodes increased significantly on days 3, 7 and 28 ($P<0.02$ to <0.05).

this particular system suppressing, NK cell activities, and finally, *C.parvum* could exert direct effect on NK cells, resulting in their destruction. To test the first possibility, we have studied NK cell activities in other lympho-hemopoietic tissues at several time intervals post *C.parvum* injection. These data are illustrated in Table I; there was an increase in thymic NK cell activity at all time intervals post *C.parvum* administration, including, however, also the time interval at which spleen NK cell cytotoxicity was not changed; thus, suggesting the lack of correlation between increase in thymic and decrease in splenic NK cells. In fact, at the peak of thymic NK cell activities (day 21) spleen was suppressed only marginally. There was an increase in lymph node cytotoxicity on day 3, 7 and 28, and again at two of these three time intervals splenic NK cytotoxicity was not changed, the fact excluding migration of NK cells to lymph nodes. Bone marrow natural killing was increased significantly on day 3, 21 and 28 (at the time where there was normal splenic NK cell cytotoxicity) and decreased on day 5,at which time also spleen was expressing low NK cell activities. Because of the compatible NK cell pattern between spleen and bone marrow,migration of splenic NK cells to bone marrow is excluded. It could be argued that low NK cell activities observed on day 10 may reflect the arrest of NK cell precursors (that are known to originate in bone marrow) and influence thus, the influx of NK cells to the spleen. As a consequence the splenic NK cell cytotoxicity would be low after day 10. However, this possibility is excluded experimentally as will be shown later. Migration of NK cells to other lympho-hemopoietic tissues was not obviously responsible for low splenic NK cell activities. We have not tested NK cell activities in peripheral blood after *C.parvum* administration,however, no change in this tissue after *C.parvum* treatment was reported by Ojo et al., (10) who confirmed our observations on splenic NK cell suppression after *C.parvum* treatment (5-6). To explore the posibility that dilution of NK cells,by increased numbers of other cell types stimulated by *C.parvum*,could be responsible for decline in NK cell activities, we made comparison between increase in splenic cellularity and NK cytotoxicity (data are not shown). We have found that degree of the decrease of natural killing was several times greater than the increase in splenic cellularity. Moreover, on day 3, spleen cellularity was already increased more than two times and there was no change in NK cell cytotoxicity, and furthermore, congenitally athymic mice, that do not express *C.parvum* dependent NK cells suppression (as will be shown later) also experience splenomegaly.

II. DEMONSTRATION OF SUPPRESSOR CELLS IN *C.PARVUM* INJECTED MICE

We further investigated whether the decline in NK cell cytotoxicity was not caused by suppressor cell activities that could have been induced by *C.parvum* treatment. One of the simple experimental approaches to determine the presence of suppressor cells in *C.parvum* treated mice, was to mix splenocytes of untreated mice with syngeneic splenocytes (to avoid any suppression due to histoincompatibility) of *C.parvum* injected mice. Experiments of this nature were performed and are illustrated in Table II. It is apparent from presented experimental data that splenocytes of mice that received *C.parvum* injection, and consequently expressed depression of NK cell killing, were also effective in suppressing significantly NK cell cytotoxicity of untreated syngeneic mice of the same genotype (see days 7 to 15). On the contrary, at the time when no decline in NK cell activity was detected (i.e. day 3 and 21), no suppression in mixtures was observed. On day 17, although there was still a significant decrease in NK cell cytotoxicity of *C.parvum* treated mice, their splenocytes did not exert any significant suppression in mixtures, an observation indicating that *in vivo* suppression appears to be stronger than suppression *in vitro*. This fact is also evident by the degree of suppression present in *C.parvum* treated splenocytes versus mixtures. For instance, suppression of NK cell cytotoxicity in *C.parvum* inoculated mice ranged from 71 to 96%, whereas an efficiency to suppress NK cell cytotoxicity in mixtures ranged from 42 to 64%. Data in Table II indicate also that suppression in mixtures was not caused by any nonspecific factors,such as suboptimal culture conditions since 1) it was expressed only at the time of *C.parvum* suppression and 2) control cell population, containing the same T:E ratio (1:100) as mixtures, did not exert any decrease in NK cell cytotoxicity. It is pertinent to mention here that even though there was not a linear relationship between the number of splenocytes and cytotoxicity at 1:50 and 1:100 T:E ratios there was never suppression at the latter ratio (see Table II). In fact, NK cell cytotoxicity reached a plateau at 1:50 T:E ratio. Despite the strong evidence against nonspecific suppression, we have provided in other series of studies, further control for mixing experiments, i.e. we added to the spleens of normal $B6DF_1$ mice various types of syngeneic splenocytes:a) *C.parvum* treated,b) normal heat-killed and c) NK cell-blank (adherent) populations obtained by double adherence on nylon wool columns, according to the slightly modified method described by Julius (11). The results of two different experiments of this nature are il-

TABLE II. *Time-Dependent and C.Parvum Mediated Suppression of Natural Killing*

Days Post C.Parvum	T:E Ratio	Mean Percent of Splenic NK Cell Cytotoxicity ± S.E.[a,b]		
		Untreated	C.Parvum Treated	Mixtures
3	1:50	47.5±5.0(5)	53.6±7.0(5)	
	1:100	45.6±7.0(5)	62.6±7.3(5)	55.0±5.9(5)
7	1:50	31.2±3.6(5)	4.4±0.8(5)	
	1:100	34.2±2.4(5)	3.2±1.8(5)	15.2±2.3(5)
9	1:50	25.0±0.4(4)	1.0±0.9(5)	
	1:100	28.5±2.5(4)	1.0±0.6(4)	10.2±2.1(4)
11	1:50	40.0±3.0(4)	9.5±3.2(4)	
	1:100	39.0±6.0(4)	6.7±2.7(4)	22.2±2.7(4)
13	1:50	28.3±1.8(3)	1.8±0.8(3)	
	1:100	29.0±4.4(3)	1.5±0.5(3)	11.3±3.4(3)
15	1:50	52.5±4.6(4)	10.0±2.7(4)	
	1:100	51.5±4.8(4)	10.0±5.7(4)	29.7±3.0(4)
17	1:50	41.6±3.1(4)	12.1±1.6(4)	
	1:100	39.8±2.9(4)	13.7±3.1(4)	31.7±2.1(4)
21	1:50	37.2±2.1(4)	39.1±4.6(4)	
	1:100	38.9±3.6(4)	31.7±2.0(4)	41.0±2.6(4)

[a] 4×10^4 YAC-1 target cells were incubated with untreated splenocytes, C.parvum injected splenocytes of $B6DF_1$ mice or with mixtures of both (1:1 ratio) for 16 hrs; the final T:E ratio in mixtures was 1:100.

[b] NK cytotoxicity of C.parvum splenocytes was suppressed on days 7–17 ($P<0.001$) and that of mixtures on days 7–15 ($P<0.005$).

lustrated in Fig. I. It is clearly indicated that neither heat-killed nor NK cell-blank population of splenocytes was effective in suppressing natural killing of normal splenocytes, even though there was a slight decrease in NK cell cytotoxicity when NK cell-blank splenocytes (in the first experiment) and heat-killed splenocytes (in the second experiment) were added to untreated cells in the highest ratio. In contrast, *C.parvum* treated splenocytes exerted strong suppression. The suppressive effect of *C.parvum* splenocytes was evident already at suppressor-to-effector (S:E) cell ratio of 0.12 (P values >0.05 to >0.02 for experiments 1 and 2, respectively) and degree of suppression increased with increased S:E ratio and was maximal in 1:1 S:E ratio (P values ranged from <0.005 to <0.01).

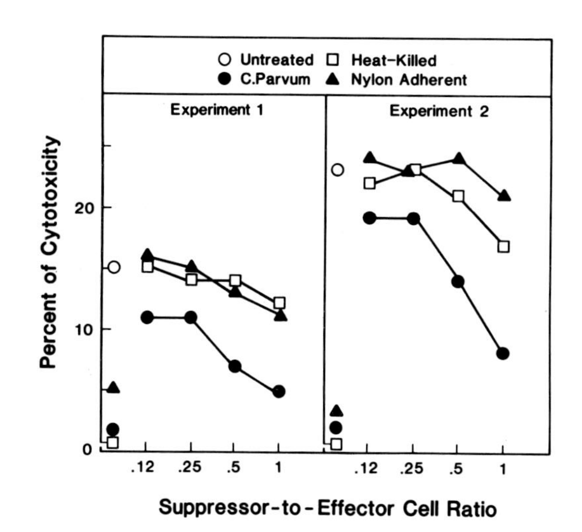

FIGURE I. Effect of Various Cell Populations on Natural Killing of Untreated B6DF$_1$ Mice. 4x10^4 YAC-1 target cells were incubated with C.parvum treated, normal heat-killed, NK cell-blank (adherent) splenocytes or mixtures of normal splenocytes and a various doses of above indicated splenocytes for 4 hrs; T:E ratio was 1:50. 0.5mg of C.parvum was injected i.v., 10 days before NK cell test.

To determine whether suppression of NK cell cytotoxicity in *C.parvum* injected mice was expressed solely to YAC-1 target cells, or also to other target tissues, we have tested *C.parvum* treated mice also against two xenogeneic targets, i.e. human lymphoblastoid cell line, CEM and human B cell line, BL. Table III illustrates clearly that NK cell activities of *C.parvum* injected mice were depressed also to xenogeneic target tissues, an indication that suppression is not restricted to a single NK cell clone.

Even though the suppressor cells were detected in *C.parvum* treated mice, it was still plausible that two concomitant and independent phenomenona, could occur in *C.parvum* injected mice, i.e. lack of NK cells (caused by the direct effect of *C.parvum*) and in addition to it the induction of suppressor cells, regulating various immune phenomena between others, suppressing also NK cells. The crucial experiment in this regard was to determine whether NK cells are present or not in *C.parvum* treated mice. To explore this question, we have approached a simple Ficoll-Hypaque gradient (specific gravity 1.08) separation since this technique has been shown previously to allow separation of suppressor cells from effector cells (12-13).

TABLE III. C.Parvum Suppresses Murine NK Cell Activity to Human Tissues

Source of NK Cells	Percent of Cytotoxicity at T:E ratio[a,b]			
	CEM		BL	
	1:50	1:100	1:50	1:100
Untreated	12.8±2.8	12.5±3.5	22.0±5.2	18.0±3.8
C.parvum[b]	1.2±0.2	1.0±0.0	1.2±0.5	0.2±0.2
Mixtures	--------	4.7±0.3	---------	7.0±1.0

[a] 4×10^4 target cells were incubated with untreated and C.parvum treated $B6DF_1$ splenocytes or mixtures of both for 4 hrs; 4-5 mice are represented in each group.

[b] C.parvum was injected i.v., in the dose of 0.5mg/mouse, 10 days before NK cell assay.

[c] P values between cytotoxicity of untreated splenocytes and C.parvum treated splenocytes were <0.001 and untreated splenocytes and mixtures were <0.02.

In Fig.II is shown pool of data of 2 representative experiments. It can be seen in the first part of the Fig. that unseparated, *C.parvum* treated splenocytes of $B6DF_1$ mice expressed only 17% of NKcell cytotoxicity of splenocytes from untreated mice, i.e. they showed 83% suppression of NK cell activity (both, 1:50 and 1:100 ratios are shown). Furthermore, the same

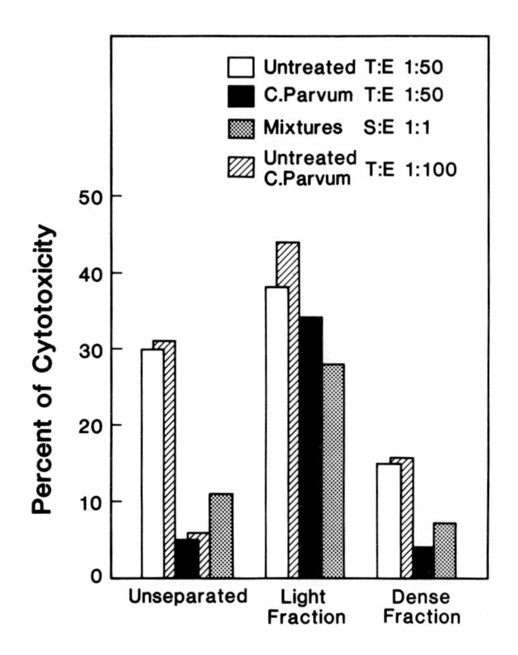

FIGURE II. Ficoll-Hypaque Gradient Separation of Untreated and C.Parvum Treated Splenocytes of $B6DF_1$ Mice.

$4x10^4$ YAC-1 target cells was incubated with untreated or C.parvum injected splenocytes or mixtures of both,for 4 hrs. In mixtures, the untreated splenocytes were always unseparated and final T:E ratio was 1:100. C.parvum was injected i.v., in the dose of 0.5mg, 10 days before NK cell test.

cell population was effective in suppressing NK cell killing of syngeneic splenocytes (63% suppression). The NK cell cytotoxicity of *C.parvum* injected mice however, changed drastically when light fraction obtained after Ficoll-Hypaque gradient separation was tested. Most of the suppression of *C.parvum* splenocytes was removed, since the degree of NK cell killing was close to normal splenocytes,subjected to the same Ficoll-Hypaque separation procedure (89% of normal in contrast to 11% of normal in unseparated,*C.parvum* treated mice). Actually, there was not statistically significant difference between NK cell cytotoxicity of these two groups. Similarly, in mixtures of unseparated normal splenocytes and light-fraction- *C.parvum* splenocytes,suppression was reduced from 63% to 7%. These data indicate that most of the suppressor cells were removed from the light fraction. The increase in NK cell activity of *C.parvum* treated mice could not have been caused by a simple NK cell enrichment by Ficoll-Hypaque procedure, since the enrichment of NK cell activity in untreated mice was only 1.3 fold, whereas that of *C.parvum* treated mice was 6.8 fold. When dense fraction obtained after Ficoll-Hypaque centrifugation was tested for NK cell cytotoxicity, only 50% of cytotoxicity was detected in untreated mice in comparison to unseparated splenocytes of the same mice. In contrast to light fraction,in heavy fraction the suppression of NK cell activity in *C.parvum* treated mice was still evident and their splenocytes possessed even higher ability to suppress in mixtures (suppression of *C.parvum* mice was 73% and that in mixtures 77%). These data provide evidence for the presence of NK cells in *C.parvum* injected mice and support the observation that NK cells are regulated by suppressor cells (which can be removed by Ficoll-Hypaque fractionation).

It is difficult at this point to speculate as to the nature of the suppressor cells removed by Ficoll-Hypaque gradient, however, it appears that T cells were depleted in light fraction,as determined by the response of light fraction-recovered cells to PHA mitogen. These data are in accordance with report of other investigators, describing removal of suppressor T cells from light fraction and their presence in dense fraction after Ficoll-Hypaque density fractionation (12).

III. CHARACTERIZATION OF SUPPRESSOR CELLS

Since the observation that NK cell cytotoxicity is regulated by suppressor cells,could be of utmost importance in cancer as well as in transplantation immunobiology, we proceeded further in their characterization. At first we tested the sensitivity of suppressor cells to various agents and treatments. These experiments are illustrated in Table IV. Suppressor cells were found not only to be resistant to, but to be enriched for by treatment with cortisone (2.5mg/mouse, i.p), cytoxan (350mg/kg, i.p.), irradiation, administered *in vivo* in the range of 1100-3000R and exposure to various types of carrageenans *in vitro* (10μg/0.1ml). Furthermore, they were not sensitive to silica, administered either *in vivo* (5mg/mouse, i.v.) or *in vitro*, (25μg/0.1ml), rabbit anti-mouse IgG serum and complement (14) or heat killing (56°C for 30 min.). They could not be removed by carbonyl iron technique or by adherence to glass or plastic. The fact that antimacrophage agents,

TABLE IV. Failure of Various Agents to Remove Suppression

Treatment of Suppressor Cells	*% Suppression of NK Cell Activity by C.Parvum Treated Splenocytes*[a,b]	
	Treated	*Untreated*
Cortisone	82[c]	59
Silica-in vivo	52	54
Silica-in vitro	48	52
Carrageenan-in vitro		
Seakem	69[c]	45
Lambda	80[c]	45
Iota	81[c]	45
Kappa	63[c]	45
Cytoxan	86[c]	54
Radiation-in vivo		
1100R	75[c]	57
3000R	79[c]	51
Rabbit anti-Mouse IgG & C'	60	57
Carbonyl Iron	46	49
Adherence	61	51
Heat-Killing	57	63

[a] *$4x10^4$ YAC-1 target cells were incubated with mixtures of normal and C.parvum treated or untreated splenocytes in 1:1 ratio, for 4 hrs. The final T:E ratio was 1:100; 5-6 mice are represented in each group.*

[b] *0.5mg of C.parvum was injected, i.v., 10-11 days before NK test. $B6DF_1$ mice were employed in these experiments.*

[c] *Cytotoxicity of treated mice showed statistically significant difference from that of untreated mice (P values range from <0.001 to <0.005).*

silica and carrageenan did not remove or at least decreased degree of suppression (in fact carrageenans even increased it), together with the observation that neither carbonyl iron nor adherent techniques removed suppression, eliminated involvement of mature macrophages in suppression phenomenon. The lack of anti-mouse IgG to prevent NK cell suppression,while preventing the response to B cell mitogens coupled with the evidence that B cells were indeed eliminated by anti IgG treatment (as established by immunofluorescence studies) indicates that B cells are not the suppressors. This statement is supported by the observation that Ficoll-Hypaque density separation did not appear to reduce the number of B cells present in the light fraction, whereas it removed suppression.

To test the involvement of T cells as the possible suppressor cell candidates, we have used advantage of congenitally athymic mice that lack mature T cell functions. If suppressor cells were mature T cells,or were at some level mature T cell dependent, it would be expected that athymic mice would not be sensitive to *C.parvum* induced suppression. Athymic Balb/c mice were injected with 0.5mg of *C.parvum*, i.v. and their NK cell cytotoxicity was tested at different time intervals afterwards. As indicated clearly in Table V, decrease in NK cell cytotoxicity was not detected at any time post bacteria injection. In addition, spleen cells of *C.parvum*-treated

TABLE V. C.Parvum Does Not Induce Suppression in Congenitally Athymic Mice

Days Post C.parvum	*Mean Percent of NK Cytotoxicity ± S.E.*[a]		
	Untreated	*C.Parvum*	*Mixtures*
1	22.7±4.6	33.2±4.1	ND
3	36.8±5.8	35.9±4.0	47.0±9.0
6	16.3±5.3	19.3±6.7	24.5±5.5
9	30.7±8.9	22.7±2.1	23.7±9.5
14	25.5±3.7	22.8±3.7	19.4±1.5
21	35.0±0.0	25.8±5.4	36.0±0.4

[a]$4x10^4$ YAC-1 target cells were incubated with splenocytes of untreated or C.parvum injected (0.5mg,i.v.) congenitally athymic Balb/c mice (1:50 T:E ratio) or mixtures of both (1:1 S:E ratio, final T:E ratio 1:100) for 16 hrs. 3-6 mice are represented in each group.

athymic mice did not exert any negative influence on NK cell cytotoxicity of untreated mice of the same genotype. It could be aruged that the lack of suppression induction could be due to the lack of sensitivity of Balb/c strain of mice to *C.parvum*. This argument is, however, excluded by our unpublished observations indicating that suppression could be induced in Balb/c mice lacking the nude gene. The failure of athymic mice to express NK cell suppression after *C.parvum* inoculation associates T cells with suppression. We have further tested T cell enriched population of *C.parvum* treated mice, obtained by nylon wool filtration for its effectiveness to suppress NK cell cytotoxicty of untreated spleen cells. Results of these experiments are illustrated in Table VI. The nylon wool nonadherent population contained >70% of T cells, as determined by immunoflourescence technique. It is evident from the presented data that T cell enriched fraction of *C.parvum* treated splenocytes suppressed NK cell cytotoxicity of untreated cells to the same or higher degree as did the population of unseparated splenocytes. This observation sustains the possibility of T cell involvement in NK cell suppression. However, apparently contradictory is the observation that the adherent population presumably deprived of T cells after nylon wool filtration possesses also, although to a lesser degree, suppressive capacity. This discrepancy is however, explained by our unpublished immunofluorescence studies, indicating the presence of sig-

TABLE VI. Effect of Nylon Wool Filtration on Suppressor Cell Activities

Type of C.Parvum Splenocytes in Mixtures[b]	*Suppression of NK Activity by C.Parvum Splenocytes (%)*[a]	
	Exp. 1	*Exp. 2*
Unseparated	*76*	*58*
Nylon Wool Nonadherent	*76*	*88*
Nylon Wool Adherent	*66*	*46*

[a] *$4x10^4$ YAC-1 target cells were incubated with mixtures of untreated and various types of C.parvum injected splenocytes in 1:1 ratio for 4 hrs; the final T:E ratio was 1:100. $B6DF_1$ mice were used in these experiments.*

[b] *0.5mg of C.parvum was injected i.v., 10 days before NK cell test.*

nificant numbers of T cells in nylon wool adherent fraction of *C.parvum* treated mice. This observation is not unfamiliar since the presence of T cells in nylon wool adherent fraction has been claimed by many, and reported by some investigators (15).

To further characterize the suppressor cells present in *C.parvum* injected mice, we have employed Sephadex G-10 filtration technique,according to Ly and Mishell (16). Using this method, we separated *C.parvum* splenocytes into adherent and nonadherent population, and then tested these two cell populations, as well as unseparated splenocytes for anti-NK cells suppressive capacity,in mixing experiments. Unseparated splenocytes of *C.parvum* injected mice (not mixed with untreated spleen cells) were also tested in these experiments, in order to evidence the presence of suppression in these mice. Representative experiment is illustrated in the left part of Fig. III. It is apparent that NK cell activity of untreated mice was sharply reduced when unseparated *C.parvum* splenocytes or their adherent fraction, obtained after Sephadex G-10 filtration,was employed (% of suppression was 67% and 73%, respectively). In fact, Sephadex G-10 adherent fraction expressed slightly higher suppression than unseparated *C.parvum* spleen cells, indicating that suppressor cells adhere to Sephadex G-10 columns.On the contrary, NK cell suppression decreased from 67% to only 20% ($P<0.001$) when nonadherent fraction after G-10 filtration was added to normal untreated spleen cells. Despite their adherence to G-10 columns,suppressor cells do not appear to be macrophages because of the lack of glass and plastic adherent properties and insensitivity to antimacrophage agents, silica and carrageenan. Furthermore, macrophages could be eliminated, as suppression mediators, on the basis of their normal numbers in light fraction after Ficoll-Hypaque density gradient, in which fraction most of suppression was removed, and on the basis of their minority in nylon wool nonadherent fraction, in which the suppression was strongly expressed. To obtain the information as to the type of *C.parvum* splenocytes present in adherent fraction after Sephadex G-10 filtration, we performed immunoflourescence evaluation. We have found that adherent fraction of *C.parvum* treated spleen cells contained besides macrophages and B cells,high numbers of T cells (twice as much as nonadherent). These data further suggest that T cell adherent to G-10,is involved in suppression. In the final set of our studies we have treated *C.parvum* splenocytes before addition to the mixtures with antisera (and complement) directed against T cell surface antigen, Thy-1.2 or with complement only (control) to determine whether suppressor cells were Thy-1.2 positive. It can be seen in the right part of Fig. III that there was a significant, but incomplete

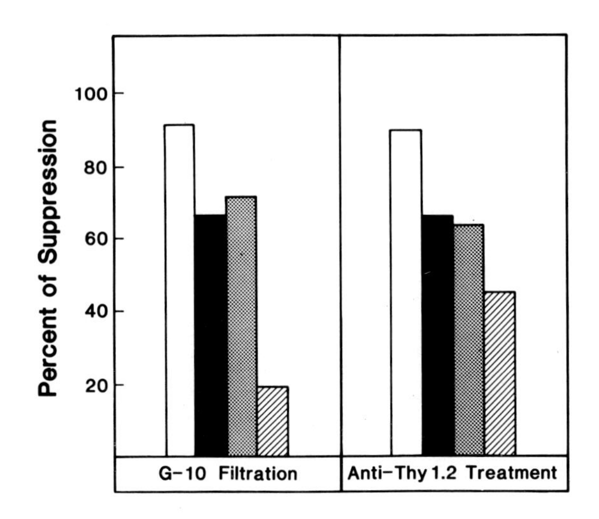

FIGURE III. Effect of Sephadex G-10 Filtration and Anti-Thy 1.2 Treatment on C.Parvum-Mediated Suppressive Activity. $4x10^4$ YAC-1 target cells were incubated with untreated C.parvum splenocytes ; or mixtures of normal splenocytes and untreated C.parvum splenocytes ■, G-10 adherent C.parvum splenocytes ▒, G-10 nonadherent C.parvum splenocytes ▨, complement-treated C.parvum splenocytes ▒, and anti-Thy 1.2 treated C.parvum splenocytes ▨; C.parvum was injected in the dose of 0.5 mg i.v., 11 days before NK test. $B6DF_1$ mice were employed in these experiments.

removal of suppressive capacity of *C.parvum* treated splenocytes after treatment with antisera directed against T cells. Suppression decreased from 66% (before treatment) to 45% (after treatment). This decrease was statistically significant (P value <0.01). In contrast, treatment of *C.parvum* injected splenocytes with complement did not exert any effect on the capacity to suppress; the degree of suppression was comparable to splenocytes of untreated *C.parvum* injected mice. Even though there was a decrease in the suppression after treatment with T cell antisera, greater reduction in suppression would be expected, if suppressor cells were T cells, expressing optimal amount of Thy-1.2 antigen. Several possibilities can explain the incomplete abrogation of suppressive effect by anti-T cell-directed antisera. Suppressor T cells may express low amount of Thy-1.2 antigen on their surface. The antisera may be relatively inefficient, i.e. they may destroy only certain percent of suppressor cells; in fact the efficiency of various preparations of antisera obtained from commercial sources fluctuates appreciably, with regard to the splenic T cell killing (as measured by microcytotoxicity test); the range is between 10-25%. We are currently testing the effect of monoclonal anti Thy-1.2 antibodies, that are more reliable in this regard. The difficulty in removing the suppressor cells with anti-Thy 1.2 antiserum could be also due to the involvement of another cell population, except of T cell, in suppression.

IV. CONCLUDING REMARKS

We have described *C.parvum*-induced (and/or augmented) suppressor cells, regulating NK cell activities, in murine spleen. Anti-NK cell directed suppressive activity was associated with the relatively dense, radioresistant and long-lived cells, nonadherent to glass or plastic, but adherent to Sephadex G-10 and present in both, adherent (in lower numbers) and nonadherent (in higher numbers) fraction obtained after nylon wool filtration. Suppressor cells were further insensitive to cortisone, cytoxan, antimacrophage agents, silica and carrageenan, treatment with anti-mouse immunoglobulin & complement and carbonyl iron. Suppressive effect was dependent on mature T cell function (since it was not expressed in congenitally athymic mice) and was partially sensitive to antisera directed against T cell antigen, Thy-1.2. Suppression was not dependent on viable suppressor cells, since heat-treatment (56°C, 30 min.) did not ablate suppressive action, however, it was time dependent; it was more powerful after longer incubation of suppressor cell with effector cells. Effectiveness of *C.parvum* splenocytes to suppress NK cell cytotoxicity of normal splenocytes was completely reversed by Ficoll-Hypaque gradient centrifugation and almost ablated by Sephadex G-10 filtration. Classical B cells and macrophages were eliminated as potential suppressor cell candidates because there was lack of correlation between their presence (absence) and expression of (lack of) suppression. On the contrary, removal of T cells correlated closely with removal of suppression and vice versa, their augmentation with increase in suppression. For instance, no suppression was expressed in athymic mice (lacking T cells) and was increased in nylon wool nonadherent population (composed of majority of T cells). Furthermore, suppressive activity of *C.parvum* treated mice was removed by adherence on Sephadex G-10 columns,in which fraction majority of T cells resided (as established by immunofluourescence). Also, in light fraction after Ficoll-Hypaque centrifugation, T cells appeared to be in a minority. The fact that anti-Thy-1.2 treatment was only partially effective does not invalidate T cell involvement in suppressor activity, since the T cell may express a low amount of Thy-1.2 surface antigen. Even though the T cells are strongly indicated in suppression, contribution of other cell population to the suppressive phenomenon, cannot be completely eliminated.

After our initial observation on *C.parvum*-induced suppression (5-6) Ojo et al., (10) reported likewise, decline in murine NK cell activities after i.v. injection of *C.parvum*. However, in contrast to our studies, these investigators were unable to detect suppression in mixing experiments. Several explanations can account for the failure to observe suppressive effect.As has been mentioned earlier, suppressive capacity *in vitro* is less sensitive than that *in vivo* and therefore, most optimal conditions are required for its expression. It is not only critical to attain optimal suppressor-to-effector cell ratio but also, to maintain optimal target-to-effector (and suppressor) cell ratio. Moreover, the dose of *C.parvum* and the strain of mice is also critical for suppression induction, duration and its strength. Both of these factors were different in our experiments and those of Ojo et al. In addition, these investigators employed in mixing experiments allogeneic (even though H-2 compatible) system, whereas our system was purely syngeneic. These are a few of several possibilities which could be responsible for the incompatibility in experimental data between these two laboratories.

REFERENCES

1. Adlam, C., and Scott, M.T., *J. Med. Microbiol. 6*, 261 (1973).
2. Pimm, M.V., and Baldwin, R.W., *Nature (Lond.) 254*, 77 (1975).
3. Scott, M.T., *Cell. Immunol. 5*, 459 (1972).
4. Kirchner, H., Glaser, M., and Herberman, R.B.,*Nature (Lond.) 257*, 396 (1975).
5. Lotzová, E., and Savary, C.A., *Biomedicine 27*, 341 (1977)

6. Savary, C.A., and Lotzová, E., *J. Immunol. 120*, 231 (1978).
7. Herberman, R.B., Nunn, M.E., Holden, H.T., Staal, S., and Djeu, J. Y., *Int. J. Cancer 19*, 555 (1977).
8. Oehler, J.R., Lindsay, L.R., Nunn, M.E., Holden, H.T., and Herberman, R.B., *Int. J. Cancer 21*, 210 (1978).
9. Castro, J.E., *Eur. J. Cancer, 10*, 115 (1974).
10. Ojo, E., Haller, O., Kimura, A., and Wigzell, H., *Int. J. Cancer 21*, 444 (1978).
11. Julius, S.A., Tracey, D.E., and Henney, C.S., *Nature 262*, 584 (1976).
12. Takei, F., Levy, J.G., and Kilburn, D. G., *J. Immunol. 118*, 412 (1977).
13. Pope, B.L., Whitney, R.B., and Levy, J.G., *J. Immunol. 120*, 2033 (1978).
14. Kilburn, D.G., Smith, J. B and Gorczynski, R.M., *Eur. J. Immunol. 4*, 784 (1974).
15. Cerny, J., and Stiller, R.A., *J. Immunol. 115*, 943 (1975).
16. Ly, L.A., and Mishell, R.I., *J. Immunol. Methods 5*, 239, (1974).

INHIBITION AS WELL AS AUGMENTATION OF MOUSE NK ACTIVITY BY PYRAN COPOLYMER AND ADRIAMYCIN

Angela Santoni[1]
Carlo Riccardi
T. Barlozzari

Institute of Pharmacology
University of Perugia, Perugia, Italy

Ronald B. Herberman

Laboratory of Immunodiagnosis
National Cancer Institute
Bethesda, Maryland

I. INTRODUCTION

Much evidence suggests that natural killer (NK) activity is a highly regulated system. Many agents have been found to affect the levels of NK activity, by acting either directly on NK cells or their precursors, or on the accessory or suppressor cell populations. Soluble mediators, as well as regulatory cells, have been found to be involved in the regulation of natural cytotoxicity. Interferon (IF) appears to play a major role in activating or augmenting NK activity (Djeu *et al.*, 1979a; Gidlund *et al.*, 1978) and prostaglandins can inhibit NK activity (Droller *et al.*, 1978; Brunda and Holden, this book). Macrophages appear to play an accessory role in maintaining the spontaneous levels of NK activity in mice and rats, since treatment with selective antimacrophage agents, silica and carrageenan, caused a decline in the levels of natural cytotoxicity (Djeu *et al.*, 1979c; Oehler and Herberman, 1978). Macrophages have only been shown to be required for the

[1]*This work was supported by Progetto Finalizzato "Controllo della crescita neoplastica, no. 79.00668.96, CNR, Italy*

ISBN 0-12-341350-8

augmentation of activity of mouse and rat NK activity by poly I:C (Djeu *et al.*, 1979b; Herberman *et al.*, section 1A, this book). Cells capable of inhibiting the lytic activity of mouse NK cells have also been generated in a variety of circumstances (treatment with carrageenan, hydrocortisone, X-rays, ^{89}Sr, *C. parvum)* (Hochman and Cudkowicz, 1978; Cudkowicz and Hochman, 1979; Hochman *et al.*, 1978; Savary and Lotzova, 1978). There has been some suggestion that macrophages may be involved in depression of NK activity, since inhibition of NK activity was associated with activation of macrophages, following treatment with pyran copolymer or adriamycin, and adherent cells from adriamycin-treated mice were found to suppress the NK activity of normal spleen cells (Puccetti *et al.*, 1980; Riccardi *et al.*, 1979; Santoni *et al.*, 1980). These inhibitory effects on NK activity have been of particular interest since the same agents have also been shown to be able to augment NK activity (Santoni et al, 1979; 1980). We have, therefore, studied in more detail the regulatory effects of these agents on NK cells and this chapter summarizes our results.

II. AUGMENTATION OF NK ACTIVITY BY PYRAN COPOLYMER AND BY ADRIAMYCIN

Pyran is a potent inducer of IF (Merigan *et al.*, 1967) and as with a variety of other IF-inducers, has been found to augment mouse NK activity (Santoni *et al.*, 1979). The conditions under which NK activity is boosted by pyran are summarized in Table I. Peak levels of cytotoxic activity have been detected at day 3, the time of peak circulating levels of IF. As with poly I:C, this augmentation may be mediated via production of IF by macrophages, since mice pretreated with silica were not boosted well by pyran (Puccetti *et al.*, 1980). It should be noted that augmentation of NK activity by pyran was not invariably seen. Boosting of the reactivity of spleen cells was seen only in mice at a time when their spontaneous NK activity was low. At 4-8 weeks of age, when peak spontaneous NK activity occurs, little or no boosting of splenic NK activity has been seen. In contrast, with peritoneal cells, that have low spontaneous activity at all ages, boosting of NK activity was observed in young as well as in older mice. However, boosting of peritoneal activity was not seen after IV inoculation of pyran, possibly due to failure of sufficient levels of the agent or of circulatory IF to enter the peritoneal cavity. Alternatively, few NK or pre-NK cells may reside in the peritoneal cavity and high NK activity may only develop at this site upon influx of NK cells after IP inoculation of a stimulating agent.

Intraperitoneal inoculation of adriamycin (ADM) was also found to result in boosting of NK activity (Santoni *et al.*,

TABLE I. Conditions for Boosting or Inhibition of NK Activity by Pyran Copolymer or Adriamycin

	Pyran copolymer		Adriamycin	
Kinetics	Boosting of NK maximal at day 3, decline by day 5	Depression first seen day 5, maximal day 7, persists about 2 weeks	No effect in spleen at day 1; Boosting in peritoneal cavity (low) at 1-6 days	Maximal depression in spleen (high) at day 3 and usually normal by day 6
Age and organ of recipients	Boost in spleen at <3-4 weeks and ≥ 12 weeks (low)[a] Boost in peritoneal cavity both at 4-8 weeks (low) and ≥ 12 weeks (low)	Depression in spleen at 4-8 weeks (high)	At day 3 after IV, marked depression in spleen (high) but increase in lymph node (intermediate) and bone marrow (low); depression can be induced in older as well as in young mice with high NK activity	
Strain of recipients	Higher boost at ≥ 12 weeks in high NK strains (low)	Depression observed in spleens of high NK strains but not in SJL, a low NK strain	Strong boost in peritoneal cavity (low) similar in high and low NK strains	Depression observed in spleens of SJL, a low NK strain, as well as in high NK strain
Route of administration	IP: boost in spleen and peritoneal cavity IV: boost in spleen but not peritoneal cavity		Boosting in peritoneal cavity after IP but not after IV	Depression in spleen more marked after IP than IV
Dose of agent	Boosting similar at all doses between 2.5 and 225 mg/kg	Depression only at ≥ 25 mg/kg		Depression at ≥ 10 mg/kg
Adherent suppressor cells for NK	Not detectable at day 3	Detectable at day 7	Not detectable at day 3	Detectable at day 7

[a]In parenthesis are indicated the levels of spontaneous NK activity at time of testing.

1980), within 1-3 days and peaking at around day 6 (Table I). The mechanism for this effect is unclear, since we have been unable to detect the induction of circulating levels of IF. It is possible, however, that ADM may induce the local release or production of IF in the peritoneal cavity, sufficient for activation of resident cells. Alternatively, ADM may in some other way activate NK cells or stimulate the migration of circulating NK cells into the peritoneal cavity, lymph nodes and bone marow. This last possibility might account for the failure of this drug to induce boosting of NK cells in the spleen, even after IV inoculation.

III. INHIBITION OF NK ACTIVITY BY PYRAN COPOLYMER AND BY ADM

In some situations, these agents have been found to cause appreciable depression of NK activity (Table I). With pyran, the conditions required for this inhibition are quite different from those associated with boosting. Depressed NK activity occurs later, being first detectable at day 5, becoming maximal at day 7, and then persisting for a long period. The depression has only been seen after inoculation of high doses of pyran and only in the spleens of mice with high spontaneous levels of NK activity. Pyran has not inhibited the splenic NK activity of SJL mice, which have low reactivity even at 4-8 weeks of age.

Depression of NK activity by ADM has also only been observed in the spleen, but unlike pyran, this effect appears to be independent of the spontaneous levels of splenic NK activity. Similar degrees of inhibition have been seen not only in young mice with high NK activity, but also in older mice or SJL mice, that have low levels of NK activity.

IV. POSSIBLE ASSOCIATION OF MACROPHAGE ACTIVATION WITH THE DEPRESSION OF NK ACTIVITY BY THESE AGENTS

At times and under conditions when depression of splenic NK activity has been observed after administration of pyran or ADM, increased cytostatic activity against tumor target cells by macrophages has been detected (Puccetti *et al.*, 1980; Santoni *et al.*, 1980). Some of the features of this macrophage activation are summarized in Table II. The doses of the agents that induced cytostatic activity corresponded to the doses associated with depressed NK activity. However, this association between depressed NK activity and augmented cytostatic activity of macrophages was not complete. Activated

TABLE II. *Conditions for Activation by Pyran or Adriamycin of Macrophage - Mediated Cytostasis of Tumor Cells*

	Pyran copolymer	Adriamycin
Kinetics	First detected at day 5 and maximal at day 7	Strong activity at days 3 and 6
Route of administration	Highest in peritoneal cavity after IP, but both IP and IV induce higher activity in peritoneal cavity than in spleen	Strong activity in peritoneal cavity after IP route, and in spleen after IV
Doses of agent	Only detected at $\geq$ 25 mg/kg	Activity detected after 10 or 18 mg/kg

macrophages were detected in the peritoneal cavity as well as in the spleen, and their activity after pyran inoculation returned to baseline levels long before the recovery of splenic NK activity. Data from an experiment with ADM that are representative of this association are shown in Table III. Nevertheless, the ability of both agents to affect macrophage activity as well as inhibit NK activity led us to investigate whether activated macrophages might be involved in regulating NK activity. In the experiment shown in Fig. 1, pyran caused an initial boost of NK activity at day 3, followed by depressed NK activity through day 39. In contrast, the high levels of macrophage-mediated cytostatic activity began to return to normal low levels after day 11 and were not significantly above normal at days 25-39.

V. SUPPRESSION OF NK ACTIVITY BY MACROPHAGES FROM PYRAN OR ADM-TREATED MICE

To directly examine whether macrophages in the spleens of mice treated with pyran or ADM might account for the depressed NK activity in that organ, mixture experiments were performed by essentially the same procedure as previously described by Cudkowicz and Hochman (1979). Table IV summarizes the data from a representative experiment with pyran-treated mice. As usual, the spleen cells of mice treated 7 days earlier with pyran had depressed NK activity when compared to that of age-matched untreated mice. Mixture of the spleen cells from the pyran-treated mice with those of normal mice resulted in a substantial inhibition of activity (from 21.2 to 12.8%). This inhibitory activity was associated with the adherent cells in the pyran-treated spleen. After treatment of the adherent spleen cells with carbonyl iron plus magnet, little

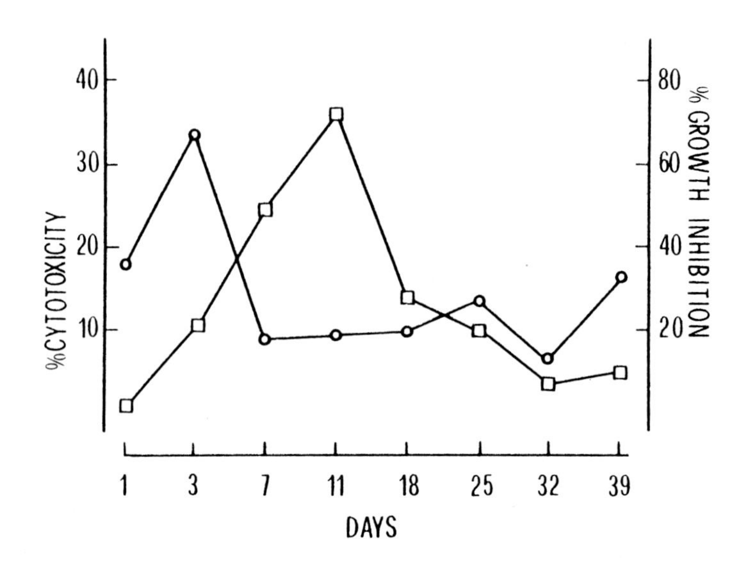

Figure 1. Kinetics of the effect of pyran copolymer (75 mg/kg IV) on NK activity (o—o) and macrophage-mediated cytostatic activity (□-□) of 12 wk old BD2F$_1$ mice. Spleen cells were tested for NK activity in a 4 hr ^{51}Cr release assay against YAC-1, E/T of 100:1; at this ratio the percent of cytotoxicity of untreated controls was 25.4. Cytostatic activity was measured by testing adherent spleen cells against K562 target cells at an E/T of 20:1; at this ratio the % growth inhibition of the untreated control was 8.7.

or no suppressor activity remained. The adherent and phagocytic properties of the suppressor cells indicated that they were macrophages. Furthermore, the suppressor activity was radioresistant, being essentially unaffected by treatment of the cells with 2000 R. The decreased activity of normal spleen cells in the presence of the cells from the pyran-treated mice could not be attributed to a simple crowding effect, since equal numbers of thymus cells or of adherent cells from normal mice caused substantially less inhibition. Similar results were obtained with spleen cells from ADM treated mice An example of such data is shown in Table V. The depressed NK activity of spleen cells from ADM-treated mice was accompanied by suppressor activity of the adherent spleen cells. Suppression was quite profound at a 4:1 suppressor:effector cell ratio and was still significant at a 1:1 ratio.

As was suggested by the decrease in macrophage-mediated cytostasis at more than day 11 after treatment with pyran (Fig. 1), adherent spleen cells from mice treated more than

TABLE III. Effect of ADM-treatment on NK and Macrophage-mediated Cytostatic Activities

Treatment	*% Cytotoxicity*[a]	*% Growth inhibition*[b]
None	*30.5*	*30.1*
ADM 18mg/kg IP, day-3	*18.2*	*65.2*

[a]*NK activity of 10 wk old $BD2F_1$ mouse spleen cells was tested in a 4 hr ^{51}Cr release assay against YAC-1 target cells at ratio of 100:1.*

[b]*Plastic adherent spleen cells were tested for macrophage-mediated cytostasis (^3H-thymidine uptake assay) against K562 tumor cells at ratio of 20:1.*

two weeks earlier with pyran had little or no suppressor activity. This suggests that additional mechanisms are involved in the maintenance of depressed NK activity. However, it is possible that the direct measurement of NK activity in the spleen is a more sensitive index of suppressor cell activity, or that after a period of suppression, it may take several days or weeks for NK cells to fully recover their activity.

VI. CONCLUDING REMARKS

The data obtained in our studies with pyran and ADM indicate that one can not simply categorize agents as being stimulatory or inhibitory for NK activity. Depending on the conditions of treatment, either effect may be seen with the same agent. These results are similar to those previously reported for *C. parvum* (Ojo *et al.*, 1978), with augmentation by that agent being seen after IP inoculation, but inhibition after IV inoculation. In addition to the treatment protocol affecting the direction of the effects on NK activity, our results further indicate that the status of the recipient can be an important variable. The ability of NK or pre-NK cells to be boosted by IF or other agents may vary with their physiological state. There already is evidence that after

TABLE IV. Suppression of NK Activity by Adherent Cells from pyran-treated, 8 week-old BD2F$_1$ Mice.

Effector cells	Cells tested for Suppressor activity[a]	% Cytotoxicity
Spleen, normal		21.2
Spleen, pyran day-7[b]		6.7
Thymus, normal		2.4
Adherent spleen, normal		4.4
Adherent spleen, pyran day-7		1.4
Spleen, normal	Thymus, normal	17.8
	Adherent spleen, normal	21.5
	Adherent spleen, pyran day-7	12.8
	Iron-treated adherent spleen, pyran day-7	19.0
	Irradiated[c] adherent spleen, pyran day-7	13.1

[a]Cells tested for ability to suppress NK activity of normal spleen cells (in 4 hr ^{51}Cr release assay against 5 x 10^3 YAC-1 at 50:1 effector:target cell ratio in round-bottom Limbro microtiter plates by mixture at suppressor:effector cell ratio of 4:1.

[b]Pyran treatment was 75 mg/kg, IV

[c]Adherent spleen cells were exposed to 2000 R, delivered by a ^{60}Co Irradiator (Hot Spot MKIV, Harwell, England).

augmentation to a given level of activity, further exposure of NK cells to IF leads to little or no additional increase

TABLE V. Suppression of NK activity by adherent cells from Adriamycin-treated 10 week-old BD2F$_1$ mice.

Effector cells	*Suppressor cells (ratio of suppressors: effectors)*	*% Cytotoxicity*[a]
Spleen, normal		*26.5*
Spleen, ADM day-3[b]		*12.5*
Thymus, normal		*1.0*
Adherent spleen, normal		*4.8*
Adherent spleen, ADM day-3		*1.0*
Spleen, normal	*Thymus, normal(4:1)*	*22.6*
	(1:1)	*22.6*
	Adherent spleen, normal (4:1)	*26.3*
	(1:1)	*28.9*
	Adherent spleen, ADM day-3 (4:1)	*7.5*
	(1:1)	*14.7*

[a]*As in Table IV.*

[b]*ADM (18 mg/kg, IP) was injected 3 days before assay.*

in activity. The frequent failure of pyran to induce a detectable boost in the splenic activity of young mice of a high detectable boost in the splenic activity of young mice of a high NK strain may be explained by their recent activation to a maximal state of activity, probably by endogenously or environmentally-induced IF. Similarly, the susceptibility of NK cells to suppression may vary with the functional status of the cells. As reported by Brunda and Holden in this section, overnight culture of NK cells renders them resistant to inhibition by prostaglandins. In addition, the failure of pyran to induce inhibition of NK activity in some mice may be due in part to differences in the susceptibility to induction of suppressor cells. With the use of the suppressor cell assay and the testing of various mice for suppressor activity and responsiveness of their NK cells to suppression, it should be possible to dissect out the factors involved in the range of results that we have observed.

The effects of ADM on NK activity are of interest from an additional standpoint. They indicate that one can no longer think of the effects of a chemotherapeutic agent on a component of the immune system only in terms of inhibition or lack of inhibition of their function. Clearly, under some circumstances, it appears that such agents may cause increased functional activity. Further, as has been seen with inhibitory effects of some agents on other immune functions, depression of NK activity may be attributable not only to direct toxic effects on the effector cells but also to effects on the function of regulatory cells. Although the mechanisms underlying the effects of ADM remain to be determined, these findings may serve as a model for examination of the effects of other drugs on NK activity.

It is also important to point out that the effects described here regarding *in vitro* NK activity have been found to be accompanied by parallel effects on the rapid *in vivo* clearance of IV inoculated radiolabeled tumor cells (see our chapter in section IF). At times when pyran was found to boost splenic NK activity, there was also increased clearance from the lungs and conversely, when splenic NK activity was depressed after pyran administration, the clearance of tumor cells from the lungs was reduced. Thus, the effects of these agents on regulation of NK activity appear to be directly relevant to shifts in *in vivo* natural resistance of the host to tumor growth.

REFERENCES

Cudkowicz, G., and Hochman, P. S. (1979). *Immunol. Rev. 44,* 13.

Djeu, J. Y., Heinbaugh, J. A., Holden, H. T. and Herberman, R. B. (1979a). *J. Immunol. 122,* 175.

Djeu, J. Y., Heinbaugh, J. A., Holden, H. T., and Herberman, R. B. (1979b) *J. Immunol., 122,* 182.

Djeu, J. Y., Heinbaugh, J. A., Vieira, W., Holden, H. T., and Herberman, R. B. *(1979c). Immunopharmacology. 1, 231.*

Droller, M. J., Schneider, M. V., and Perlmann, P. (1978). *Cell. Immunol.* 39, 165.

Gidlund, M., Orn, A., Wigzell, H., Senik, A., and Gresser, I. (1978) *Nature 273,* 759.

Herberman, R. B., Nunn, H. E., Holden, H. T., Staal, S., and Djeu, J. Y. (1977). *Int. J. Cancer 19,* 555.

Hochman, P. S., and Cudkowicz, G. (1978) *J. Immunol. 123,* 968.

Hochman, P. S., Cudkowicz, G., and Dausset, J. J. (1978). *J. Natl. Cancer Inst.* 265.

Mantovani, A., Luini, W., Peri, G., Vacchi, A., and Spreafico, F. (1978). *J. Natl. Cancer Inst. 61,* 1255.

Merigan, T. C. (1967). *Nature 214,* 416.

Oehler, J. R., and Herberman, R. B. (1978) *Int. J. Cancer* 21, 221.

Ojo, E, Haller, O., Kimura, A. and Wigzell, H. (1978). *Int. J. Cancer 21,* 444.

Puccetti, P., Santoni, A., Riccardi, E., Holden, H. T., and Herberman, R. B. (1980). *Int. J. Cancer.* In press.

Riccardi, C., Santoni, A., Barlozzari, T., Puccetti, P., Sorci, V., and Herbermann, R. B. (1979). *Proc. Soc. Am. Cancer Res. 20,* 250.

Santoni, A., Puccetti, P., Riccardi, C., Herberman, R. B., and Bonmassar, E. (1979). *Int. J. Cancer 24,* 656.

Santoni, A., Riccardi, C., Sorci, V., and Herberman, R. B. (1980). *J. Immunol. in press*

Savary, A. C., and Lotzova, E. (1978) *J. Immunol. 120,* 233.

THE EFFECT OF 17β-ESTRADIOL ON NATURAL KILLING IN THE MOUSE

William E. Seaman
Norman Talal

Immunology/Arthritis Section
Veterans Administration Medical Center
and the
University of California, San Francisco,
California

I. INTRODUCTION

Natural killing can be markedly reduced in mice by the sustained administration of 17β-estradiol at high levels (1,2). This phenomenon is not seen in response to physiologic levels of estrogen; we find no difference in levels of natural killing between male and female mice (1), and there is no loss of natural killing during pregnancy, when levels of estrogen are high (unpublished). Nonetheless, the reduction of natural killing by estrogen may prove useful as a probe for understanding the regulation of natural killing and for examining the effects of natural killer (NK) cell depletion *in vivo*.

II. METHODS

A. *Administration of Hormone*

To achieve sustained high levels of estrogen in mice, we utilize sealed Silastic tubes containing powdered estrogen. Small molecules such as estrogen diffuse through the tubing at a constant rate (3). When a tube is implanted subcutaneously, high levels of circulating hormone are

ISBN 0-12-341350-8

achieved within 24 hours and are sustained for at least several months, depending on the size of the implant. We use 2 cm of tubing with an inner diameter of 0.062 inches and an outer diameter of 0.125 inches (Dow-Corning, Midland, Mich, catalogue no. 602-285). The central 1.5 cm of the tube is filled with approximately 15 mg of anhydrous 17β-estradiol (Sigma, St. Louis, Mo, catalogue no. E-8875). The tubing is closed at one end by inserting a wooden applicator stick. The cone from a Pasteur pippete is used to deliver the powdered hormone into the other end of the tube which is then also closed with a wooden stick. The sticks are cut, leaving a small plug in either end of the tube, and both ends are sealed with Silastic adhesive (Dow, Corning, no. 891). The adhesive is allowed to dry at 20° C for 48 hours before the implant is used. Serum 17β-estradiol in mice bearing an implant of this size is approximately 180-200 ng/ml (kindly performed by Dr. William Crowley). Levels in normal mice vary with estrus, but the mean is less than 20 ng/ml.

To insert an implant, mice are anesthetized with Nembutal, given intraperitoneally. A 1 cm incision is made through the skin across the lower spine, about 1.5 cm above the tail. A blunt probe is inserted cephalad to lyse the subcutaneous tissue over the back, creating a pouch for the implant. After the implant is inserted, the incision is closed with suture or with metal clips. The instruments and the implants are clean but not sterile. Operative mortality is almost nonexistent. For our experiments, implants were placed at age 4 weeks. For control mice, an empty implant was inserted.

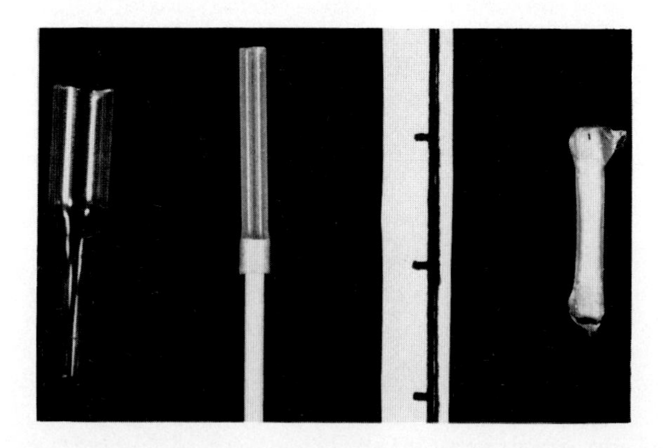

FIGURE 1. Equipment for making hormone implants. Left to right: cone from Pasteur pippete for loading hormone, tubing with one end closed by wooden stick, scale to measure length of tubing to be filled (here 1.5 cm), completed (sealed) tube containing hormone.

B. Natural Killing

Natural killing by spleen cells was assessed against YAC-1 in a 5-hour ^{51}Cr-release assay as previously described (1). Killing in the assay is enhanced by removal of immunoglobulin-bearing cells or adherent cells but is ablated by pretreatment of the effectors with antiserum to NK-1 (4). Monoclonal antibody to Thy-1 in high concentration will partially reduce killing

III. EFFECTS OF 17β-ESTRADIOL ON NATURAL KILLING

The effect of estradiol on natural killing requires several weeks, as demonstrated in Figure 2. There is little change in natural killing after 2 weeks of estrogen, but natural killing is substantially reduced after 4-6 weeks. Because 17β-estradiol does not affect natural killing for at least 2 weeks, it is unlikely that it is toxic to mature NK cells. This conclusion is supported by the observation that 17β-estradiol does not alter natural killing *in vitro* in concentrations up to 10 μg/ml (not shown).

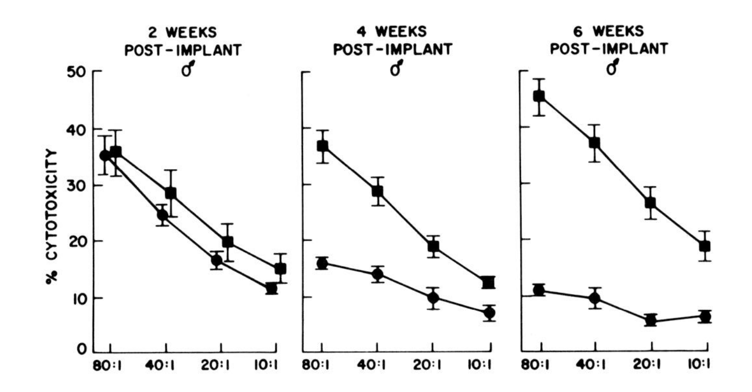

FIGURE 2. Time course of the effect of 17β-estradiol on natural killing by spleen cells from male NZB/NZW mice treated at four weeks. Circles, estrogen-treated mice; squares, sham-treated mice. (From Seaman, W.E., et al., J. Immunol., 121, 2193 (1978). By permission.)

The effect of 17β-estradiol on natural killing can be demonstrated in either sex and is unaffected by prior castration of male or female mice (which does not itself alter natural killing) (1). To date, all strains tested show a reduction in killing after 6 weeks of estrogen. Androgen (5α-methyltestosterone) has little or no effect (1).

If the estrogen implant is removed, natural killing recovers. Figure 3 demonstrates the recovery of natural killing in mice that have been treated for 6 weeks and then had the implant removed.

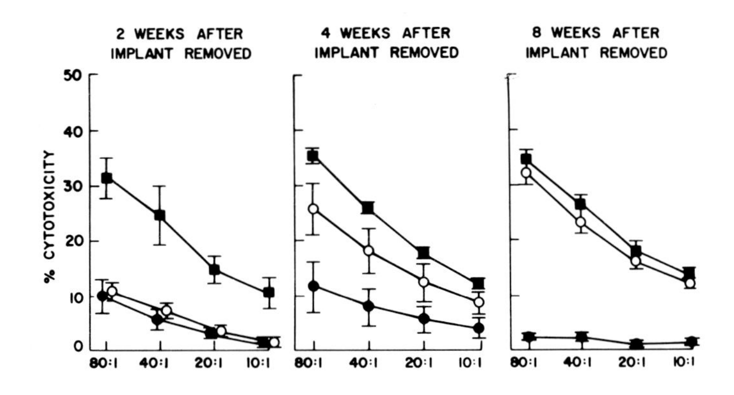

FIGURE 3. Recovery of natural killing following treatment with 17β-estradiol. NZB/NZW mice were given an estradiol implant for 6 weeks, after which the implant was removed (open circles) or left in place (closed circles). Sham mice received an empty implant that was removed after six weeks (squares). (From Seaman, W.E., et al., J. Immunol., 121, 2193 (1978). By permission.)

IV. INVESTIGATIONS INTO THE CAUSE OF REDUCED NATURAL KILLING IN MICE TREATED WITH 17β-ESTRADIOL

A. *Reduced Killing Is Not Due to Dilution of Effector Cells*

The loss of natural killing from the spleens of estrogen-treated mice is not due to the dilution of NK cells by other cells. As discussed later, the spleen in estrogen-treated mice does enlarge due to an increase in extramedullary hematopoiesis. However, the increase in size appears to be due entirely to an increase in red cells which, in our assay, are lysed prior to testing for natural killing. The splenic white cell counts for estrogen-treated mice were slightly, though not significantly, less than counts for controls. Moreover, natural killing by lymph node cells is reduced by estrogen, even though the lymph nodes are not enlarged.

B. *Estradiol Does Not Block Interferon Production*

The loss of natural killing in estrogen-treated mice is not due to an inability to generate interferon, which is known to stimulate natural killing (5-7). When BALB/c mice that had been treated with estrogen for 6 weeks were given 50 μg of polyinosine•polycytosine (Poly I•C) intravenously, interferon was stimulated to levels that equaled or exceeded those in sham-treated mice given Poly I•C (8). In the sham-treated mice, this increase was associated with a marked rise in natural killing, but killing in estrogen-treated mice was not significantly stimulated. Poly I•C stimulates interferon to detectable levels for less than 24 hours, so a single injection does not provide a sustained stimulus to natural killing. In recent experiments (unpublished), we have found that footpad injection of *Herpes simplex* virus leads to an increase in natural killing by spleen cells from estrogen-treated mice over the course of several days. Presumably this is because of sustained stimulation of interferon. The levels of natural killing achieved in estrogen-treated mice are, however, much less than levels in sham-treated mice infected with virus.

It has been suggested that (human) NK cells are themselves a source of interferon (9). Our results suggest that in the mouse either NK cells are not the major source of interferon in response to Poly I•C or estrogens can block cytotoxicity by NK cells without blocking their production of interferon.

C. Estradiol Does Not Induce Suppression of Natural Killing

We have been unable to demonstrate a humoral or a cellular suppressor of natural killing in estrogen-treated mice. Hochman and Cudkowicz have provided evidence for a cellular suppressor of natural killing in the spleens from mice treated with hydrocortisone, γ-irradiation, ^{89}strontium (^{89}Sr), or ι-carageenan, all of which lower natural killing (10,11). The demonstration of this suppressor cell requires an excess of spleen cells bearing the suppressor. When present in an excess of 4:1, spleen cells from estrogen-treated mice at times reduce killing by normal cells, but the effect is inconstant and never substantial (not shown). From these results, it would seem that estrogen-treated mice differ from most other models for reducing natural killing in that they lack a cellular suppressor of natural killing. It is possible, however, that the suppression of killing in other models actually represents cold-target inhibition by a "natural" target for natural killing. In accord with this possibility, Hansson, *et al.*, have demonstrated the presence of a "natural" target for natural killing in the thymus and, to a lesser extent, in the spleen (12). The target can block natural killing of tumor targets (13). Levels of the "natural" target vary inversely with natural killing, which would explain an increase in cold-target inhibition whenever natural killing is lowered. The target described by Hansson, *et al.*, appears to a lymphocyte, while the suppressor cell described by Hochman and Cudkowicz has features of a macrophage. These cells may therefore not be the same. If, however, cold-target inhibition does increase when natural killing is lowered, then estrogens must reduce levels of the "natural" target, since we found little or no cold-target inhibition by spleen cells from mice treated with estrogen.

D. Thymus not Required for the Effect of Estradiol

The effect of estrogen on natural killing is not completely selective. Another notable effect is involution of the thymus. It is difficult to find the thymic remnant in mice that have received an estradiol implant for 6 weeks. (The effects of estrogen on peripheral T cell function are discussed later.) The loss of natural killing in response to estradiol does not, however, require the thymus. Estradiol is active in suppressing natural killing in mice that have been thymectomized within 24 hours of birth (1).

E. Loss of Natural Killing in Relation to the Effects of Estradiol on Bone and the Bone Marrow

High doses of estrogen dramatically stimulate endosteal new bone formation in mice (14). In our studies, new bone formation was shown to be favored at sites adjacent to hematopoietic ("red") marrow as opposed to fatty ("yellow") marrow (2). Thus, estrogen appears to act on the marrow to induce new bone. As shown in Figure 4, the bone encroaches on the marrow and eventually replaces it. Hematopoiesis is

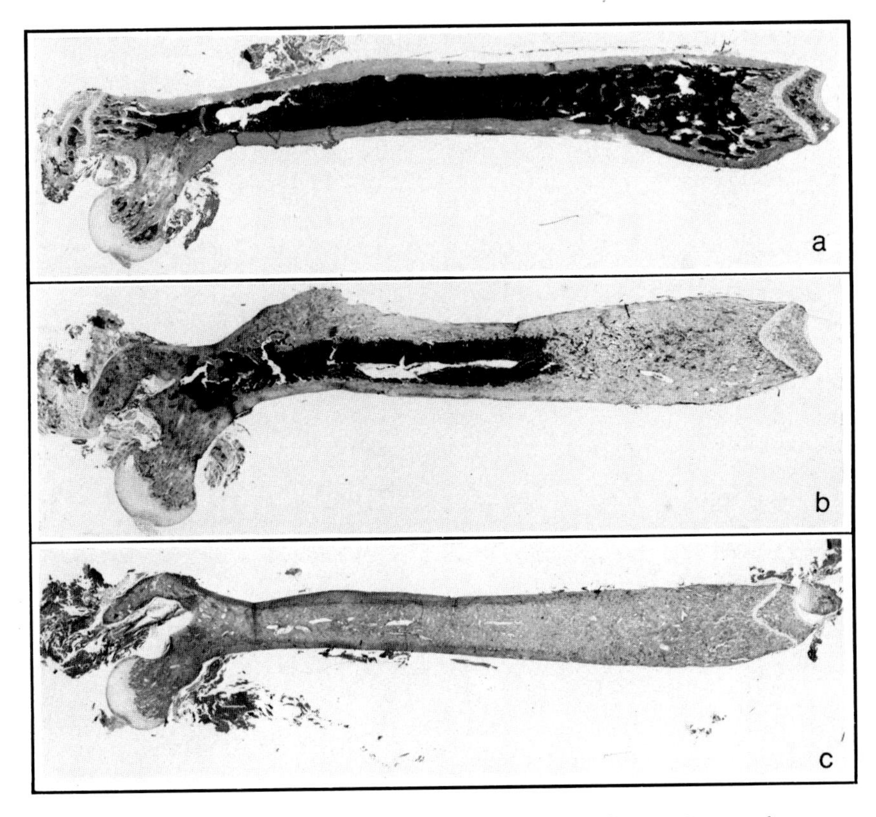

FIGURE 4. Effect of 17β-estradiol on bone formation in femurs from NZB/NZW mice treated at 4 weeks: (a) sham implant for 6 weeks (normal), (b) estradiol for 2 weeks showing endosteal new bone formation with encroachment on the marrow, (c) estradiol for 6 weeks, showing total replacement of the marrow by bone. Photos courtesy of Dr. T.D. Gindhart. (From Seaman, W.E., et al., J. Immunol., 122, 2541 (1979). By permission.)

assumed by the spleen, but myelopoiesis is only partially sustained. In mice given estrogen for 6 weeks, the peripheral red cell count is unchanged, but the white cell count falls by almost 50%, due largely to an 80% loss of polymorphonuclear cells (unpublished results).

NK cells are thought to depend on the bone marrow for their continued generation. This concept is based on the sensitivity of natural killing to the *in vivo* administration of ^{89}Sr, a bone-seeking radionuclide with high-energy β-emission (15,16). Treatment of mice with ^{89}Sr leads to marrow fibrosis, with relatively less effect on other reticuloendothelial organs. Hematopoiesis and, to a lesser extent, myelopoiesis are assumed by the spleen. T and B cell function as well as macrophage function remain relatively intact (15). Natural killing, however, is not sustained and has therefore been termed "marrow dependent". Estrogens might therefore reduce natural killing because they lead to a loss of marrow. In accord with this hypothesis, estradiol also reduces genetic resistance to bone marrow transplantation, another ^{89}Sr-sensitive function (2). However, we have found that estradiol reduces natural killing more rapidly than it reduces marrow volume, and natural killing recovers more rapidly than the marrow when estrogens are discontinued (2). Moreover, the concept of marrow dependence is as yet unproven. Kumar, *et al.*, have recently demonstrated that NK cells (or target binding cells, at least) are present in ^{89}Sr-treated mice but the cells are unable to lyse targets (18). This argues against a simple depletion of NK cells by ^{89}Sr.

In sum estradiol may reduce natural killing through a toxic effect on the marrow, but the evidence is circumstantial.

V. OTHER EFFECTS OF ESTRADIOL ON THE IMMUNE SYSTEM IN MICE

In order to assess the selectivity of 17β-estradiol for natural killing, we have begun to examine other aspects of immunity in estrogen-treated CBA/J and NZB/NZW mice.

Previous studies of the effects of estrogen on the immune system have produced varied results due, in part, to variation in species, strain, and/or protocol. In general, however, estrogens appear to increase humoral immunity and to decrease cellular immunity (19-21). In our experiments, mice were again given 17β-estradiol for 6 weeks beginning at 4 weeks. The results, although incomplete, also demonstrate an increase in humoral immunity and a reduction in some aspects of cellular immunity.

A. Response to Mitogens

Figure 5 demonstrates the response to mitogens of spleen cells from estrogen-treated female CBA mice. The response to the B cell mitogen, lipopolysaccharide (LPS) was slightly but significantly enhanced in estrogen-treated mice, while the response to the T cell mitogens phytohemagglutinin (PHA) and concanavalin A (Con A) was unaltered. Our colleague, Michael Dauphinée, has been examining the effects of estrogen on the response to mitogens by spleen cells from autoimmune NZB/NZW mice. In contrast to the findings with CBA mice, he finds a

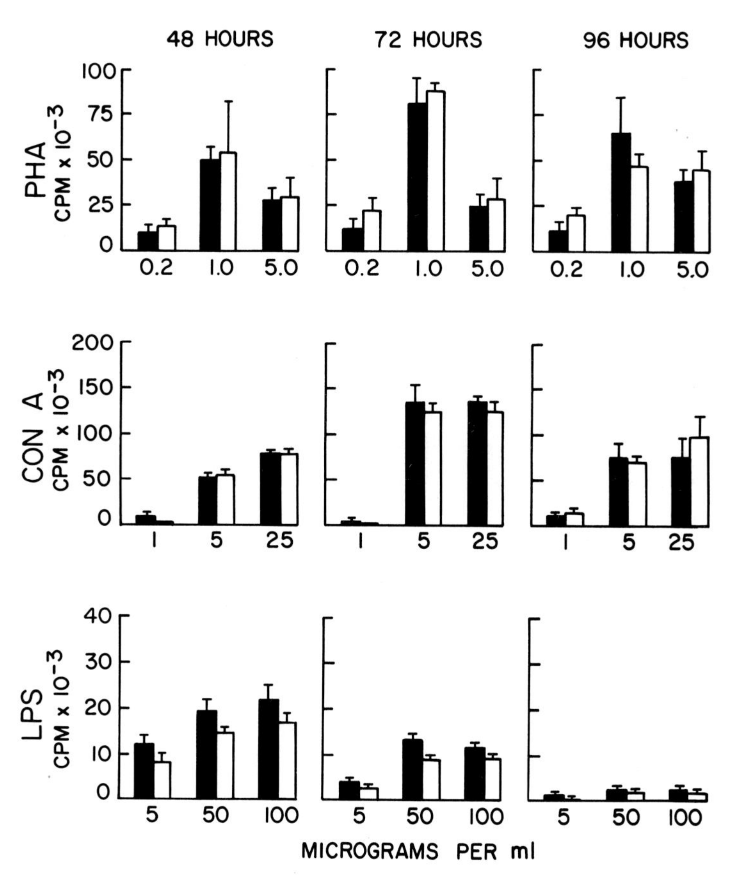

FIGURE 5. Response to mitogens by spleen cells from estradiol-treated CBA mice (dark bars) vs. sham-treated mice (open bars). 5 x 10^4 cells were incubated in 200 µl RPMI 1640 with 10% horse serum and pulsed with 10 µCi ^{3}H-thymidine 8 hours prior to harvesting.

reduced response to both PHA and Con A. It remains to be seen if this difference is related to the immune dysregulation in NZB/NZW mice or represents strain variation on another basis.

B. Plaque-forming Cell Response to Immunization

Mice treated with estradiol had a significant increase in the splenic plaque-forming cell (PFC) response to immunization with sheep red cells. Both direct and indirect plaques were increased about two-fold, whether expressed as PFC/10^6 cells or as PFC/spleen. The increase was seen in CBA, NZB/NZW, DBA/2, and C57BL/6 mice (results not shown).

C. Cytotoxicity by T Lymphocytes

Estrogens partially suppressed cytotoxicity mediated by T cells in CBA mice (Figure 6). The effect of estrogen on T cell cytotoxicity was not as great as its effect on natural killing.

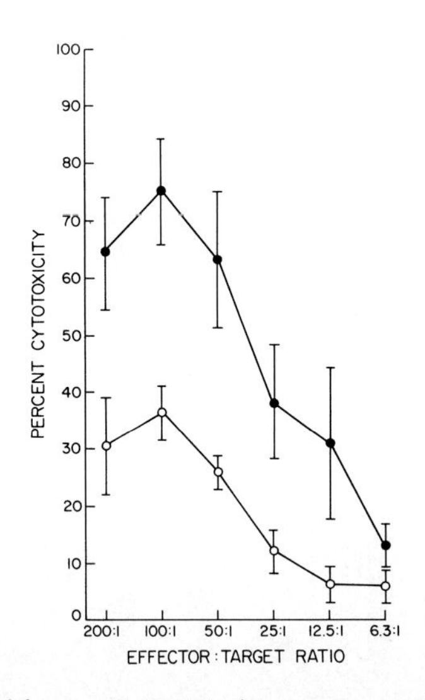

FIGURE 6. Killing of P815 (a mastocytoma from DBA/2 mice) by spleen cells from CBA/J mice that had been immunized with 6 x 10^7 irradiated tumor cells one week before. Killing by cells from estrogen-treated mice (open circles) was less than controls (closed circles) as assessed by ^{51}Cr-release over 18 hours. Killing was sensitive to anti-Thy-1 and required prior immunization.

D. Mixed Lymphocyte Reaction

We have examined the effects of estradiol on the mixed lymphocyte reaction only in NZB/NZW mice. When NZB/NZW spleen cells were tested against C57BL/6 cells, the mixed lymphocyte reaction was significantly reduced at days 4 and 5 (not shown).

E. Antibody-Dependent Cell-Mediated Cytotoxicity

Estradiol did not alter antibody-dependent cell-mediated cytotoxicity (ADCC) by either CBA or NZB/NZW spleen cells when tested with rabbit antiserum against chicken red cells (Figure 7). The cytotoxic cells in this assay are primarily macrophages rather than killer lymphocytes (K cells) (22). In light of evidence that K cells and NK cells may be the same (23), we would like to examine the effects of estradiol on ADCC against nucleated targets using mouse antiserum, an assay that is dependent on K cells. Unfortunately, we have has no success in establishing this assay.

F. Macrophage Function

Macrophages appear to function normally in mice treated with estrogen in that they are able to support a response to mitogens and to immunization and are effective killers in

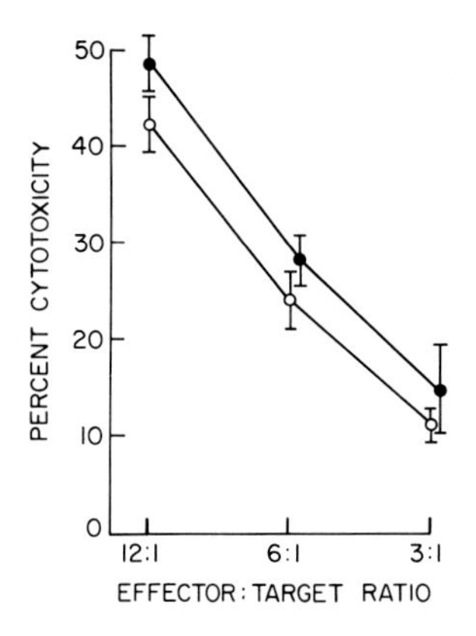

FIGURE 7. ADCC against chicken red cells by spleen cells from CBA mice treated with estradiol (open circles) or with a sham implant (closed circles) as assessed by release of ^{51}Cr over 6 hours. Rabbit antiserum to chicken red cells was used at 1:10,000.

ADCC. In addition, we found no reduction in the number of peritoneal macrophages induced by thioglycollate or by sodium periodate in estrogen-treated mice (unpublished results). The elicited cells were equal to controls in the biosynthesis and release of proteins, including neutral proteases (kindly performed by Dr. Zena Werb, UCSF).

G. *Summary of Effects of Estradiol on Immunity*

In summary, macrophage function and humoral immunity are apparently intact in mice treated with estradiol for 6 weeks. However, certain T cell functions are reduced, notably cytotoxicity and the mixed lymphocyte reaction. The production of interferon is normal.

VI. NATURAL KILLING AND AUTOIMMUNITY

Estrogens accelerate autoimmunity in NZB/NZW mice. Could the effect of estrogens on autoimmunity relate to their effect on natural killing? We examined the course of autoimmunity in NZB/NZW mice given ^{89}Sr to reduce natural killing. In this instance, a reduction in natural killing was associated with a decrease in autoimmunity as assessed by antibodies to DNA, by proteinuria, and by renal histology (24). Thus estrogen and ^{89}Sr have opposing effects on autoimmunity despite similar effects on natural killing. We suspect that estrogens exacerbate autoimmunity through their effect on T cells rather than their effect on NK cells.

ACKNOWLEDGMENTS

We wish to acknowledge the important collaborative efforts of Marcia A. Blackman, Thomas D. Gindhart, John S. Greenspan, Jirayr Roubinian, Thomas C. Merigan, and John M. Loeb.

REFERENCES

1. Seaman, W.E., Blackman, M.A., Gindhart, T.D., Roubinian, J.R., Loeb, J.M., and Talal, N., *J. Immunol. 121*, 2193 (1978).

2. Seaman, W.E., Gindhart, T.D., Greenspan, J.S., Blackman, M.A., and Talal, N., *J. Immunol. 122*, 2541 (1979).
3. Roubinian, J.R., Talal, N., Greenspan, J.S., Goodman, J.R., and Siiteri, P.K., *J. Exp. Med. 147*, 1568 (1978).
4. Glimcher, L., Shen, F.W., and Cantor, H., *J. Exp. Med. 145*, 1 (1977).
5. Chernyakhovskaya, I.Y., Slavina, E.G., and Svet-Moldavsky, G.J., *Nature 228*, 71 (1970).
6. Senik, A., Gresser, I., Maury, C., Gidlund, M., Orn, A., and Wigzell, H., *Cell. Immunol. 44*, 186 (1979).
7. Herberman, R.B., Djeu, J.Y., Ortaldo, J.R., Holden, H.T., West., W.H., and Bonnard, G.D., *Cancer Treat. Rep. 62*, 1893 (1978).
8. Seaman, W.E., Merigan, T.C., and Talal, N., *J. Immunol. 123*, 2903 (1979).
9. Santoli, D., and Kaprowski, H., *Immunological Rev. 44*, 125 (1979).
10. Cudkowicz, G., and Hochman, P.S., *Immunological Rev. 44*, 13 (1979).
11. Hochman, P.S., and Cudkowicz, G., *J. Immunol. 123*, 968 (1979).
12. Hansson, M., Kiessling, R., Andersson, B., Kärre, K., and Roder, J., *Nature 278*, 174 (1979).
13. Hansson, M., Kärre, K., Kiessling, R., Roder, J., Andersson, B., and Hayryr, P, *J. Immunol. 123*, 765 (1979).
14. Urist, M.R., Budy, A.M., and McLean, F.C., *J. Bone Joint Surg. (U.S.A.), 32-A*, 143 (1950).
15. Bennett, M., Baker, E., Eastcott, J.W., Kumar, V., and Yonkosky, D., *J. Reticuloendothel. Soc. 20*, 71 (1976).
16. Haller, O., and Wigzell, H., *J. Immunol. 118*, 1503 (1977).
17. Kumar, V., Bennett, M., and Eckner, R.J., *J. Exp. Med. 139*, 1093 (1974).
18. Kumar, V., Ben-Ezra, J., Bennett, M., and Sonnenfeld, G., *J. Immunol. 123*, 1832 (1979).
19. von Haam, E., and Rosenfeld, I., *J. Immunol. 43*, 109 (1942).
20. Kappas, A., and Palmer, R., *Pharmacol. Rev. 15*, 123 (1963).
21. Eidinger, D., and Garrett, T.J., *J. Exp. Med. 136*, 1098 (1972).
22. Pollack, S.B., Nelson, K., and Crausz, J.D., *J. Immunol. 116*, 944 (1976).
23. Ojo, E., and Wigzell, H., *Scand. J. Immunol. 7*, 297 (1978).
24. Seaman, W.E., Blackman, M.A., Greenspan, J.S., and Talal, N., *J. Immunol. 124*, in press (1980).

SUMMARY: SUPPRESSION OR INHIBITION OF NK ACTIVITY

There are increasing indications that NK activity is a well regulated system, subject to inhibitory controls as well as to activating or augmenting signals. In contrast to the situation with augmentation of NK activity, where the effects of most agents can be attributed to a single mediator, interferon (IF), inhibition of NK activity may result from a variety of mechanisms. It is worthwhile to first consider what mechanisms of inhibition might be involved and then to discuss the evidence related to the various inhibitory agents.

I. POSSIBLE MECHANISMS FOR INHIBITION OF NK ACTIVITY

Inhibitory effects on NK activity can be categorized according to at least five different mechanisms:

a. *Depletion of NK cells or their precursors.* A number of drugs and other treatments have been thought to act by direct toxic effects on NK cells or their stem cells. However, in most cases, the evidence has been indirect. Interpretation has usually been limited by the need to rely solely on changes in activity, without accompanying data on the cells themselves. One of the most direct pieces of evidence for depletion of NK cells has come from studies of the in vitro effects of butyrate on human NK cells (Saksela et al). Along with loss of NK activity, there was a substantial loss of viability of the treated cells and a disappearance of large granular lymphocytes (LGL). However, even these data are not conclusive. It is known that butyrate can induce differentiation of various hematopoietic cells and it seems possible that the observed effects on NK activity were due to a shift from LGL with NK activity to cells with differing morphology and perhaps function. The cells killed by butyrate may actually have been unrelated to NK cells. It will be of interest to repeat these studies with highly enriched populations of LGL. Likewise, studies of the effects of various other treatments on

ISBN 0-12-341350-8

enriched or purified populations of NK cells are most likely to provide convincing evidence for direct toxic effects, rather than the other possible mechanisms for inhibition.

b. Direct inhibition of function of NK cells. As discussed above, irreversible inactivation of NK cells would be quite difficult to distinguish from actual elimination of NK cells. However, it should be possible, particularly with enriched cell populations, to separately evaluate effects of treatments on the ability of NK cells to bind to targets and to cause lysis. Clearer evidence for this mechanism has already come from treatments that produce reversible inhibition of NK activity. The effects of prostaglandins seem to fall into this category, since they can cause potent inhibition of activity but only when left in the cytotoxicity assay. The NIF of Koide and Takasugi, which is found at 1-2 days after culture of human lymphocytes by themselves, may be similar and in fact, it seems likely that the observed effects may be due to prostaglandins produced by some of the cultured cells. Some of the effects of hydrocortisone (HC) on NK activity may be attributable to inhibition of NK function. The differential effects of corticosteroids on NK and K cell activities (Parillo and Fauci, 1978) and the reappearance of NK activity of HC-treated mice after overnight incubation of cells (Santoni et al, 1979) are more consistent with this possibility than with depletion of NK cells or induction of suppressor cells by HC.

c. Inhibition by suppressor cells. Several groups of investigators have obtained evidence for a role of suppressor cells in inhibition of NK activity (e.g. see Cudkowicz et al, Lotzova, Santoni et al). However, these have been difficult to detect and study in detail and therefore as yet little is known about their nature or mechanism of action. In regard to the cell type(s) of NK suppressor cells, insufficient information is available. The suppressor cells induced by various treatments (C. parvum, pyran copolymer, adriamycin) have been found to be adherent, but other suppressor cells (e.g. of newborn mice) were not. The suppressor cells induced by pyran copolymer appeared to be phagocytic as well as adherent and therefore were presumed to be macrophages. In contrast, Lotzova has suggested that T cells are involved in the suppression induced by C. parvum. Suppression was not seen in nude mice, there was a partial reduction in suppressor activity by treatment of the cells with anti-Thy 1 plus complement, and treatment with silica, carrageenan, or carbonyl iron had no effect. This postulated role of T cells in suppression of

NK activity is controversial, since Cudkowicz et al found suppressor activity in nude mice as well as in euthymic mice.

The mechanism for inhibition of NK activity by suppressor cells is also uncertain. Production of prostaglandins is one possibility which would be compatible with the data of Brunda and Holden. However, they did not demonstrate a role for suppressor cells in the inhibition associated with tumor-bearing mice. A link between these mechanisms seems likely, since Gerson has found evidence for suppressor cells in an analogous system. It will be of interest to determine whether inhibitors of prostaglandin synthesis will be able to reverse the depression of NK activity in the very situations where suppressor cells have been demonstrated. Other possible mechanisms for inhibition of NK activity by suppressor cells include: 1) nonfunctional NK cells, e.g. cells with receptors for binding to target cells but lacking an active lytic mechanism, and 2) cold target inhibition by a subpopulation of normal cells that express antigens recognized by NK cells. Some of the depression of NK activity in tumors or other sites in tumor-bearing individuals may similarly be due to cold target inhibition by neoplastic cells.

d. Depletion or inhibition of function of accessory cells. There is evidence that macrophages can act as accessory cells for activation of NK cells, due to their ability to produce IF in response to certain stimuli, e.g. poly I:C (Djeu et al, 1979a). The depression of spontaneous NK activity in mice and rats within 24 hrs after treatment with silica or carrageenan (Djeu et al, 1979b; Oehler and Herberman, 1978) also could be explained by this mechanism. Orn et al suggest that this may be the mechanism for the lack of NK activity in newborn mice, with the ability of macrophages to spontaneously produce IF inhibited by high circulating levels of alpha-fetoprotein.

e. Redistribution or sequestration of NK cells. This possibility has been raised mainly in regard to the depression of NK activity in tumor-bearing individuals. As discussed in section IE, this does not appear to be the major explanation for low activity in tumor bearers. However, it is conceivable that other treatments could cause a shift of NK cells from the spleen or blood and thereby produce the impression of depressed activity.

II. INHIBITORY EFFECTS OF VARIOUS TYPES OF TREATMENTS

A rather wide variety of *in vivo* treatments have been associated with depression in NK activity. Most of these treatments produce a range of effects on the immune system, only some of which may be related to inhibition of NK activity. However, some treatments producing inhibition of NK activity, e.g. estradiol, are more selective and therefore may be of considerable use in the evaluation of the role of NK cells in immune surveillance against tumors. Some of the treatments have also been shown to have selective effects on some aspects of natural cellular immunity. For example, x-irradiation and cyclophosphamide may inhibit spontaneous NK activity but have little or no effect on the ability to augment NK activity with IF-inducers (Oehler and Herberman, 1978; Djeu *et al*, 1979b). Also, Stutman *et al* have found that most agents that depressed NK activity had little or no inhibitory effects on NC cells. These differential effects may be due to divergent properties of subsets of natural effector cells, which may be related, at least in part, to the state of activation of the cells. Another complexity to be considered in regard to the inhibitory effects of some agents is that they may operate via more than one mechanism, depending on the conditions of treatment.

Cudkowicz *et al* have detected suppressor cells in newborn mice and in mice treated with radiation, hydrocortisone, carrageenan or some other agents. They and Lotzova also detected the presence of suppressor cells in mice with low NK activity after IV treatment with *C. parvum*. Since other mechanisms for depression of NK activity have been suggested for some of these treatments, it will be important to determine the *in vivo* role of the suppressor cells in these various situations. Determination of the effects of transfer of NK cells into mice with low NK activity should be quite helpful. Reconstitution of reactivity would favor a deficiency of NK cells in the recipients, whereas persistence of low NK activity despite infusion of large numbers of active effector cells would be more consistent with a dominant *in vivo* role of suppressor cells.

Inhibition of NK activity by pyran copolymer also has been associated with the presence of suppressor cells (Santoni *et al*). However, these do not seem to be the sole explanation for depressed activity after pyran treatment, since suppressors have been detected only during the early period of reduced NK activity. It remains to be determined whether the presence of suppressor cells for a period of time results in irreversible depression of NK activity or whether a separate mechanism is responsible for the later phase of depressed activity.

The findings of Seaman and Talal on the long-lasting and selective depression of NK activity by β-estradiol are of much interest, especially since this is accompanied by decreased *in vivo* clearance of tumor cells (Riccardi *et al*). In contrast to some other treatments, responsiveness to augmentation by IF as well as spontaneous NK activity was depressed by estradiol. They found no evidence for a role of suppressor cells or for direct inhibition of NK cells, and suggest that the low activity is due to toxic effects on bone marrow stem cells. However, it should be noted that this conclusion is based on circumstantial evidence. Recent *in vitro* studies in my laboratory have indicated another estrogenic compound, diethylstilbestrol, can directly inhibit spontaneous NK activity and boosting by IF (M. Hargrove and R.B. Herberman, unpublished observations).

III. OPPOSITE EFFECTS ON NK ACTIVITY BY SOME AGENTS AND POSSIBLE MECHANISMS

In considering the effects of some agents on NK activity, it is important to note that either augmentation or inhibition can be produced, depending on a variety of circumstances. Such opposite effects by the same agent have been seen with *C. parvum*, BCG, pyran copolymer, poly I:C, adriamycin, and glucan. The route of inoculation appears to be an important variable with some agents (e.g. *C. parvum*, glucan), with depression of NK activity mainly associated with IV inoculation. It is possible that, depending on the route, different cells come in contact with the agent and consequently different effects may be seen. This is not the entire explanation since treatment by the same route, with the same dose of an agent, can result in either augmentation or depression of activity. This may in part be related to differences in the kinetics of augmentating and depressive effects. Augmentation tends to occur early, within 1-4 days after treatment, whereas induction of depression tends to occur later. With the macrophage activating agents, this may be related to the more rapid induction of IF production than the activation of suppressor activity. Also, as seen with pyran copolymer and adriamycin (Santoni *et al*) in mice and with BCG, *C. parvum* and poly I:C in cancer patients (Riethmuller *et al*; R.B. Herberman, G. Cannon and J. Jett, unpublished observations), the status of the recipients may in some way determine the direction of the effect of the same treatment on NK activity. There are some indications that this may be related to the baseline levels of activity of NK cells and suppressor cells. At various sites and times, NK cells may vary both in their responsiveness to augmentation by IF (e.g., see Einhorn) and to depression (e.g. see Brunda and Holden regarding failure of prostaglandins to inhibit activity of NK cells after culture overnight). Similarly, macrophages or other suppressor cells may vary in their ability to be activated. Much more information seems required in this area, before one could predict with confidence the magnitude of response, or even the direction, of a particular *in vivo* treatment. Such efforts have important practical implications, since the clinical results of immunotherapy may depend, at least in part, on the effects on NK activity.

REFERENCES

Djeu, J.Y., Heinbaugh, J.A., Holden, H.T., and Herberman, R.B. *J. Immunol.* 122, 182 (1979a).

Djeu, J.Y., Heinbaugh, J., Vieira, W.D., Holden, H.T., and Herberman, R.B., *Immunopharmacology* 1, 231 (1979b).

Oehler, J.R. and Herberman, R.B., *Int. J. Cancer* 21, 221 (1978).

Parillo, J.E. and Fauci, A.S., *Clin. Exp. Immunol.* 31, 116 (1978).

Santoni, A., Herberman, R.B., and Holden, H.T., *J. Natl. Cancer Inst.* 63, 995 (1979).

COMPARISON OF NATURAL IMMUNITY TO MTV AND NATURAL KILLER REACTIVITY [1]

Phyllis B. Blair
Mary Ann Lane[2]
Candace Newby
Martha O. Staskawicz
Judith Sam
Virginia Joyce

Department of Microbiology and Immunology,
and the Cancer Research Laboratory
University of California
Berkeley, California

I. NATURAL CELLULAR CYTOTOXICITY DETECTED BY USE OF MTV-EXPRESSING TARGET CELLS

A. *Introduction*

The existence of natural killer activity in several species, including the mouse, is well recognized and has been amply documented and reviewed (Herberman and Holden, 1978; Herberman *et al.*, 1979; Beverly and Knight, 1979). The nature of this cytotoxic activity and its relationship to specific immunologic activities such as antibody-dependent cell-mediated (ADCM) cytotoxicity (Koide *et al.*, 1978; Takasugi and Akira, 1979; Santoni *et al.*, 1979; de Landazieri *et al.*, 1979; Pape *et al.*, 1979; Roder *et al.*, 1979) remain as matters of some controversy, however. A basic question is whether

[1] *This work was supported by research grants IM-69 from the American Cancer Society, Inc., and CA-05388 from the National Cancer Institute, and by research funds of the University of California.*

[2] *Present address: Division of Tumor Immunology, Sidney Farber Cancer Center, Boston, Massachussetts.*

ISBN 0-12-341350-8

natural killer activity, or at least some of what is identified as such, involves specific antigen recognition for any or all of the antigenicities expressed on the cell culture lines usually used as targets in natural killer assays.

One class of antigenicities often present on the mouse cell lines routinely used as natural killer targets are antigens associated with oncogenic viruses such as murine leukemia virus (MuLV) and murine mammary tumor virus (MTV). Mice are normally exposed to these oncogenic viruses, and therefore may possess specific immunologic reactivity, T-cell and/or antibody, to some of the viral antigens. The possibility exists, therefore, that in tests in which comprehensive controls are not included, specific T-cell cytotoxicity or ADCM cytotoxicity (the antibody either already bound to the effector cells or else secreted in culture) to viral antigens expressed on the target cells could be interpreted as natural killer activity. This possibility has already been explored for MuLV-related antigenicity; natural immunity has been clearly documented (Hirsch *et al.*, 1975; Callahan *et al.*, 1979; Kende *et al.*, 1979; Stockert *et al.*, 1979) but attempts to correlate this natural immunity with natural killer activity against targets expressing MuLV-associated antigenicities have produced conflicting results (Asjo *et al.*, 1977; Kelloff *et al.*, 1979; Becker *et al.*, 1978; Hatzfeld *et al.*, 1979; Herberman *et al.*, 1977).

In the experiments reported here, we have asked if there is any correlation between natural killer activity and induced specific immunity to MTV. Levels of natural killer activity against a commonly used target cell line, YAC-1, which expresses MTV antigenicity have been compared with the specific T-cell and non-T-cell ADCM immunologic reactivities to MTV-associated antigens on MTV-induced mammary tumor target cells which are detectable in the 2-day microcytotoxicity assay. Both normal and immunologically manipulated female mice of several strains were tested,and we found that their spleen cells had reactivities in the natural killer assay which did not correlate with the anti-MTV activity. Neonatal infection with MTV did not significantly affect natural killer activity. Specific immunization with MTV resulted in humoral immune responses to MTV detectable in immunodiffusion assay but did not significantly affect natural killer activity within the same time period. A non-specific immunologic manipulation, transient immunosuppression induced by injection of antithymocyte globulin (ATG), which we have shown to produce specific ADCM cytotoxic immunity to MTV, did not produce an increase in natural killer activity. Nevertheless, the presence of MTV-associated antigens on the YAC-1 target cells could be demonstrated; complement-mediated cell lysis occurred following treatment with goat antiserum to MTV gp52. Thus, even though YAC-1 cells express MTV antigenicity, specific natural T-cell or ADCM cytotoxic immunity to MTV appears to play little role in the cytotoxicity detectable under the conditions of a standard natural killer assay and levels of specific immunity are not directly related to levels of natural killer activity.

B. *Reactivity to MTV-Expressing Primary Mammary Tumor Target Cells Measured in Long-Term Microcytotoxicity Assay*

1. Previous Observations. In a series of publications we have described the immune reactivity of the BALB/cfC3H mouse, neonatally infected with MTV, to the MTV-associated antigens expressed on isologous mammary tumor cells. Response to these antigens occurs during the first month of life (Blair, 1976). The response, measured by spleen cell activity in microcytotoxicity assay, is relatively low-level, but in this sensitive assay it reaches statistically significant levels in most of the females tested (Blair *et al.*, 1974). The spleen cell cytotoxicity or cytostasis of these virgin females, which is dependent upon the presence of T cells (Lane *et al.*,1975), is not expressed until the second half of the 42 hour culture period (Blair and Lane, 1975a). Parity alters the immunologic picture; the level of T-cell cytotoxic activity increases as number of pregnancies increases (Blair, 1976). Spleen cells from multiparous BALB/cfC3H females exhibit, in addition, an ADCM cytotoxicity which is expressed within a few hours in the assay, and which is not dependent upon the presence of T cells (Blair and Lane, 1975a). Virgin BALB/cfC3H females also can develop a strong ADCM cytotoxic reactivity if they are experimentally manipulated; transient immunosuppression with antithymocyte globulin (ATG) effectively induces this ADCM cytotoxicity, which develops after the females recover from the immunosuppression and remains readily detectable for months (Blair and Lane, 1977; Blair, in press).

Specific immune reactivity to MTV antigens is not limited to those BALB/c mice neonatally infected with exogenous MTV; those exposed to MTV-infected mice are also specifically reactive, and the reactivity is ADCM cytotoxicity (Lane *et al.*, 1975). The usual modes of transmission of infectious exogenous MTV from one mouse to another are prenatal transfer (genomic and gametic), milk transfer, and transfer from male to female during copulation. In addition, MTV, at least as an antigenic moiety, can also be transmitted to BALB/c mice from infected mice during residence in the mouse colony. We first reported in 1974 (Blair and Lane, 1974) that specific immune reactivity to antigens of the mammary tumor virus (MTV) develops in uninfected adult BALB/c females which are raised in the same room with MTV-infected females, that BALB/c females raised from birth in isolation remained unreactive, and that such isolated females developed specific spleen cell cytotoxic reactivity shortly after the introduction of an MTV-infected female into their cage. Tagliabue and associates (1978) have also provided evidence of this horizontal exposure to MTV; they reported that BALB/c mice exposed to MTV-infected mice possessed immunologic reactivity to MTV antigens in MIF assay, whereas BALB/c mice maintained in isolation did not respond. In our BALB/c strain, the colony-raised females do not make responses detectable in the microcytotoxicity assay during the first three months of life, although by 14 weeks of age all of the females possess strong ADCM cytotoxic activity. We cannot yet explain this lack of cytotoxic response to MTV antigens in the young BALB/c female. It is sex-limited, as BALB/c males are reactive when younger (Blair, 1976), and in addition, it appears to be genetically controlled, since as we will report here, females of another strain are responsive at younger ages. Further, the unresponsiveness of the young BALB/c females can be altered; after immunization with MTV-producing isogeneic mammary tumor cells, they produce a strong cytotoxic spleen cell response (Yagi *et al.*, 1978). They also normally respond at younger ages in assays which measure lymphocyte stimulation rather than cytotoxicity (Lopez *et al.*, 1978).

The non-T-cell cytotoxic activity which develops in parous BALB/cfC3H females, in ATG-treated virgin BALB/cfC3H females, and in horizontally-exposed adult BALB/c females is of particular interest because, if we had not analyzed the specificity of the reaction and shown the participation of antibody secreted in culture, the activity might have been interpreted as an example of natural killer activity. We first demonstrated (Lane *et al.*, 1975) that neither T-cells nor B-cells were the effectors; samples of cells retained in nylon wool columns (consisting predominantly of B-cells) did not kill the target cells whereas the passaged cells, treated with antiserum and complement to remove T-cells, were active. We then hypothesized that although B-cells apparently had no direct cytotoxic activity in our system, the few B-cells which passed through the nylon wool columns might be supplying specific antibody *in vitro*, and that the cytotoxicity observed was thus antibody-mediated. In supernatant transfer experiments, we found that B-cells from these spleens did indeed release antibody specific for the target tumor cells in culture (Blair and Lane, 1975b). We also demonstrated that a very small number of B-cells (perhaps only one) from an immunologically reactive donor could be added to a population of inactive but recruitable spleen cells to provide the specificity. We did this by mixing a small number of B cells with an excess number of recruitable cells in a dilution series. Extrapolating from studies on the release of antibody in other systems (Perlmann and Holm, 1969), we anticipated that a single specific B-cell in a well of the assay plate could, during the culture period, release enough antibody for maximal activation of recruitable cells. The results of the cell-mixing experiments indicate that this expectation was correct. In experiments in which limiting dilutions of antibody secreting cells were used a few test wells showed maximal cytotoxic activity and the rest showed none (Blair and Lane, 1975b). We estimated from our data that about 1% of the B-cells in the spleen secrete antibody specific for MTV. Another source of immunologic specificity in the non-T-cell ADCM cytotoxicity may be spleen cells already armed with antibody; we have as yet no direct evidence for this.

The target antigen(s) detected in our microcytotoxicity assay are those of the MTV virion, since both T-cell and non-T-cell cytotoxic activities can be blocked by pretreatment of the spleen cells with MTV virions (Blair *et al.*, 1975). Such direct blocking of receptors can inhibit T-cells as well as antibody armed non-T-cells, and B-cell activity can be blocked by antigen-induced inhibition of antibody secretion (Schrader and Nossal, 1974). As controls, we used MuLV virions, MuLV-producing mammary tumor target cells and effector cells from MuLV-immunized donors. The MuLV virions could block the activity of spleen cells from MuLV-immunized donors against MuLV-expressing target cells but could not block the response in the MTV system, and vice versa. Lymphoid cells may be a target for infection (and thus possibly for inactivation) by both MTV and MuLV, but the blocking in these experiments was not random; each oncornavirus, MTV or MuLV, was effective in blocking spleen cell activity only against target cells expressing that virus and not the other.

2. *Experimental Design.* Cytotoxic activity against MTV-induced and MTV-expressing primary mammary tumor target cells was measured in the 42 hour microcytotoxicity assay which we have used extensively. The assay procedure has been described and its specificity for the detection of immune responses directed against MTV-associated antigens has been documented (Blair *et al.*, 1974, 1975). Target tumor cells were obtained from primary cultures of MTV-induced mammary tumors from

hybrid (C57BL x I) females which had been neonatally infected with MTV by foster-nursing on C3H females. Tumor cells in 20 μl medium (RPMI 1640, 20% fetal calf serum, 10 μg insulin, and antibiotics) were seeded in Falcon microtest 3034 plates and incubated at $37^{\circ}C$ in a humidified atmosphere. After 24 hours, adhering cells were counted, the medium was changed and spleen cells were added at a ratio of 100 spleen cells to one target tumor cell. At the end of the 42 hour culture period, each well of the plate was washed twice in saline, and the remaining cells were fixed, stained, and counted. For each spleen cell preparation, the average number of cells in six replicate wells was calculated. In comparisons of mice with each other and with controls, differences were considered statistically significant only if there was no overlap in the ranges of individual well cell counts ($p = <0.005$ by the Mann-Whitney U test). To allow combination of data from several experiments for presentation, data have been converted to "percent cytotoxicity" calculated as:

$$\frac{\text{Average number of cells in six control wells} - \text{Average number of cells in six experimental wells}}{\text{Average number of cells in six control wells}} \times 100$$

All calculations of statistical significance, however, have been carried out on the raw data. Control wells were those to which no spleen cells were added or which received spleen cells from donors not exposed to MTV or unresponsive to MTV antigens; the two types of controls result in similar target cell survival.

Spleen cells were obtained from female mice of the C57BL and the I strains, and from female hybrids of the C57BL x I cross; until use, all animals were maintained in cages without filter-tops to provide horizontal exposure to MTV antigenicity from MTV-infected mice also maintained in the colony, as previously described for BALB/c mice. Spleen cells from each female were tested separately. The spleen cells were washed twice, and the red blood cells lysed by the addition of 0.8% NH_4Cl. The remaining cells were incubated in medium on a slant for 2 hours at $37^{\circ}C$ to permit macrophages to adhere to the plastic substrate. Cells remaining in suspension were pelleted and resuspended in fresh medium, counted, diluted, and added to target tumor cells in the microtest plates. In all experiments, the mammary tumor target cells and effector cells were syngeneic or semi-syngeneic.

C. *Reactivity to YAC-1 Cells Measured in Short-Term ^{51}Cr-Release Assay*

1. *Experimental Design.* For both these experiments and the ones using the microcytotoxicity assay, all mice were derived from the colony of the Cancer Research Laboratory at the University of California, Berkeley. The BALB/c, C3H, C57BL, I and BALB/cfC3H are maintained as inbred strains in the colony. The BALB/cfDBA subline was created by foster-nursing BALB/c pups on DBA/2/Crgl lactating females. The recombinant inbred strains, ABP-CI, ABDS-BI, BPS-CI, and AB-BC, which are described in detail elsewhere in this book (see chapter by Blair), were developed by brother-sister matings of F_1 hybrids and subsequent generations from crosses of BALB/c, C57BL, or I mice, and were 20-30 generations old at the time these experiments were performed. Only female mice were used, and they were 9-10 weeks old at the time of testing for natural killer activity unless otherwise indicated.

Natural killer activity of spleen cells was measured using the standard ^{51}Cr-release assay (Becker *et al.*, 1978; Ojo *et al.*, 1978; Hochman and Cudkowicz, 1979). The YAC-1 cell line, obtained from the Sidney Farber Cancer Center, Boston, was used as the source of target cells. Spleen cells from each female were tested separately. The cells ($1.0 - 3.0 \times 10^7$) were washed once, resuspended in 1.0 ml RPMI 1640 and labeled with 300-500 μCi ^{51}Cr for one hour at 37°C. The labeled cells were then washed twice and resuspended to a concentration of 1.0×10^6 cells/ml in complete medium (RPMI 1640, 10% heat-inactivated fetal calf serum and antibiotics). The spleen cell suspensions were prepared in Hanks balanced salt solution and adjusted to a final concentration of 2.5×10^7 cells/ml in complete medium. Spleen effector cells were added to the ^{51}Cr-labeled target cells in Nunclon-Delta Microtiter plates to give effector:target cell ratios of 25:1, 50:1 and 100:1. The final volume in each well was 200λ. The plates were centrifuged at 1200 rpm for 8 minutes and then incubated at 37°C for 4 hours. At the end of the incubation period the plates were centrifuged again, and 100λ of supernatant was removed from each well for counting. Total release was determined by incubating target cells alone in the presence of 1% SDS. Spontaneous release averaged 7.5% of the total release. Results of 6 replicate wells were averaged and are presented as "percent cytotoxicity" calculated as:

$$\frac{\textit{Experimental release - spontaneous release}}{\textit{Total release - spontaneous release}} \times 100$$

The data on natural killer activity for a few of the groups are also presented in another article in this book (Blair).

2. *Demonstration of MTV Antigenicity on YAC-1 Cells.* The presence of MuLV antigenicity on YAC-1 cells has been documented by others (Becker *et al.*, 1978), as has the presence of MTV antigenicity (Lane *et al.*, unpublished observatons). We have further established that MTV gp52 antigenicity is expressed on the YAC-1 cells maintained in this laboratory (Table I). Negative controls for this experiment included an antiserum against Sendai virus. The YAC-1 target cells were tested for the presence of MTV antigenicity in a two step antibody and complement ^{51}Cr-release assay. The sera tested included goat anti-gp52, mouse anti-Sendai virus (both obtained from the Office of Program Logistics and Resources, NCI) and normal mouse serum (NMS). All sera were heat-inactivated for 30 minutes at 56°C prior to use. The target cells were labeled with ^{51}Cr as described above and seeded into Nunclon-Delta microtiter plates at a density of 2.5 x 10^{4} cells/well. Antisera were diluted in RPMI 1640 containing 10% heat-inactivated fetal calf serum and incubated with YAC-1 cells for one hour at 37°C. Following a wash to remove unbound antibody, the target cells were incubated with fresh guinea pig complement for 40 minutes at 37°C. At the end of the incubation period the plates were centrifuged

TABLE I. Detection of MTV Antigenicity on YAC-1 Cells Using Antibody to MTV gp52 plus Complement. Target cells were labeled with ^{51}Cr and percent lysis was calculated from the release of ^{51}Cr into the supernatant.

Serum Dilution	*Percent Lysis*		
	Anti-gp52 Antiserum	*Normal Mouse Serum*	*Anti-Sendai Antiserum*
1:2	*39.4*	*0.6*	*2.8*
1:4	*38.6*	*0.6*	*1.0*
1:8	*25.3*	*0.6*	*0.9*
1:16	*16.2*	*0.7*	*0.6*
1:32	*6.8*	*0.7*	*0.5*

and a sample of supernatant was removed for counting. Percent lysis was calculated according to the same formula used in the natural killer assay.

II. COMPARISON OF NATURAL KILLER ACTIVITY AND SPECIFIC IMMUNOLOGIC CYTOTOXICITY

A. *Specific Immunologic Reactivity of Normal Females towards MTV Antigenicity Expressed on Mammary Tumor Target Cells*

Spleen cells from females of several strains have been tested for specific immunity to MTV antigenicity using the 42-hour microcytotoxicity assay. Data for C3H, BALB/c, BALB/-cfC3H and BALB/cfDBA females have been reported (Blair *et al.*, 1974; Blair, in press), and data for two other strains, C57BL and I, and their hybrid are presented in Table II. Females of the three strains or sublines neonatally infected with exogenous MTV (C3H, BALB/cfC3H, and BALB/cfDBA) all possess a moderate spleen cell cytotoxicity for MTV-infected mammary tumor targets which is statistically significant in one-half to three-fourths of the females tested. In the BALB/cfC3H strain this specific T-cell immunity develops within the first month of life and remains relatively constant as long as the

TABLE II. Reactivity of Spleen Cells from Normal Females on MTV-Induced MTV-Expressing Mammary Tumor Target Cells as Measured in the 42-Hour Microcytotoxicity Assay, at an Effector:Target Cell Ratio of 100:1

Strain or Hybrid	Number Tested	Age (Months)	Average Percent Cytotoxicity (Range in Parentheses)	
C57BL	6	2-5	0.5	(0-2)
I	9	2-5	25.3	(18-34)
C57BL × I	10	2-6	0	(0)

females are maintained as virgins (Blair *et al.*, 1974). Mice of the other strains (BALB/c, C57BL, and I) are not neonatally infected with exogenous MTV but they are constantly exposed to MTV antigenicity while residing in the same room with neonatally infected mice; this exposure can be prevented if the cages are covered with filter-tops (Blair, in press). BALB/c females of this age (9-10 weeks) have not yet developed specific and strong immunologic reactivity to MTV antigenicity although they will do so when they are older than three months and will continue to be reactive as long as they are exposed to MTV-infected mice (Blair, in press). The data presented in Table II document the importance of genotype in this response; females of the I strain are highly reactive when exposed to MTV antigenicity even at 8 weeks of age, whereas C57BL females, and the hybrid females resulting from the C57BL x I cross, are not reactive at this age or later.

B. *Natural Killer Activity in Spleens of Normal Females*

Spleen cells from C3H, BALB/c, C57BL, I and (C57BL x I) hybrid females, and from two BALB/c sublines, BALB/cfC3H and BALB/cfDBA, were tested in the 4 hour ^{51}Cr-release assay for reactivity against YAC-1 cells. Cytotoxicity data for the effector:target cell ratios of 100:1 and 50:1 are presented in Table III. Mice of two of the strains, C3H and C57BL, and the (C57BL x I) hybrids were high responders in the assay with an average cytotoxicity at the 100:1 ratio of 23.8%, 21.1%, and 20.4% respectively. The three strains of BALB/c genotype were less reactive, with cytotoxicities of 7.2%, 5.7%, and 6.2% at the 100:1 ratio. The I strain was found to be the lowest responder with only 2.8% cytotoxicity at the 100:1 ratio. As expected, responses at the 50:1 effector:target cell ratio were generally lower (Table III) and responses at the 25:1 ratio were even lower (data not shown).

Comparison of Tables II and III reveals that the ability to make a specific immunologic response to MTV is not an important factor in determining the level of natural killer activity in these 9-10 week old females. There is no positive correlation between the response to MTV in microcytotoxicity assay (Table II) and the response in natural killer assay (Table III). BALB/c females of this age do not respond in microcytotoxicity assay (Blair *et al.*, 1974), and are intermediate responders in natural killer assay. C57BL mice and the (C57BL x I) hybrids also do not respond to MTV in microcytotoxocity assay after horizontal exposure, but nevertheless possess strong natural killer activity. Conversely, spleen cells from females of the I strain react strongly in microcytotoxicity assay but are unreactive in natural killer assay.

Similarly, neonatal infection with MTV does not correlate with the level of natural killer activity. Neonatally infected young virgin females of both the C3H and BALB/cfC3H strains have spleen cells with moderate T-cell and no ADCM cytotoxicity to MTV in microcytotoxicity assay (Blair and Lane, 1975a; Blair, in press). In contrast, similarities in reactivity are not seen in natural killer assay; C3H spleen cells are reactive whereas spleen cells from mice of the BALB/c genotype are comparatively unreactive, regardless of whether or not they have been neonatally infected with MTV. This result agrees with that of Tagliabue and associates, who reported in abstract (1979) that mice of the C3H genotype which differ in neonatal infection with MTV, and therefore in subsequent specific immunologic reactivity to MTV, do not differ in natural killer activity against YAC-1 cells.

TABLE III. Natural Killer Activity Against YAC-1 Target Cells of Spleen Cells from Normal Females Aged 9-10 Weeks

Strain of Spleen Donor	No. Tested	Percent Cytotoxicity 100:1[a]		50:1[a]	
		Average	Range	Average	Range
C3H	7	23.8	17.2-34.7	20.0	14.6-32.0
BALB/cfC3H	4	7.2	5.6 - 7.9	6.5	4.8 - 9.0
BALB/cfDBA	5	5.7	2.8 - 9.2	5.6	4.2 - 8.1
BALB/c	4	6.2	5.2 - 7.0	7.3	5.2-10.2
I	6	2.8	0.8 - 5.1	2.2	1.1 - 5.5
C57BL	4	21.1	11.1-27.9	13.9	8.7-18.3
C57BL × I	4	20.4	14.6-24.3	14.3	10.8-18.4

[a]*Effector:target cell ratio*

III. CHANGES IN REACTIVITIES AFTER SPECIFIC OR NON-SPECIFIC IMMUNOLOGIC MANIPULATION

A. *Search for Altered Natural Killer Activity after Infection or Immunization with MTV*

Females of 5 inbred strains and of one hybrid cross were either neonatally infected by foster-nursing or infected (immunized) at 8 weeks of age with MTV derived from the C3H strain. For the infection-immunization at 8 weeks, the females received a single intraperitoneal 0.4 ml injection of freshly collected C3H milk diluted 1:8 in sterile saline. At 9 weeks of age the females were bled from the tail to provide serum for testing for antibodies to MTV and/or their spleens were harvested for testing in the natural killer assay.

Antibody reactivity to MTV was measured in the double diffusion in agar assay developed by Blair (1965) and modified by Yagi (1974) to increase sensitivity, using a 2 mm layer of 0.65% Noble agar (pH 7.2) in 60 mm plastic Petri dishes. The central well was filled with C3H MTV (obtained from the Office of Program Logistics and Resources, NCI) and 4-6 hours later the surrounding wells received individual serum samples. The dishes were incubated at room temperature and observed for 7 days. Sera, tested in duplicate, were graded positive for MTV if the specific MTV immunoprecipitin line appeared within this period. Antibody reactivity developed within the one week test period in the females of all genotypes which were 8 weeks old when infected-immunized, but was not detectable by immunodiffusion assay in normal females or in neonatally infected females at this age (Table IV).

Spleen cell reactivity of the neonatally or 8-week infected females was tested in natural killer assay and compared with that of uninfected or unimmunized females of the same genotype (Table V). No dramatic increases in reactivity as a consequence of neonatal or later infection were noted, although in 9 of the 11 possible comparisons with normal uninfected unimmunized females, the average percent cytotoxicity of the groups infected either neonatally or later was slightly (but not significantly) higher. We conclude that if adult infection-immunization with MTV has any effect on natural killer activity, it is not evident soon after exposure, even though antibody production has occurred. This is in contrast to the effect of infection with several other viruses (Herberman *et al.*, 1977), which induce natural killer activity within this time period (Welsh, 1978).

TABLE IV. Production of Antibodies to MTV

Strain or Hybrid	Number with Antibody Detectable in Immunodiffusion Assay/Number Tested		
	Not infected with exogenous MTV[a]	Infected (Immunized) with C3H-MTV[b]	Neonatally infected with C3H-MTV[c]
BALB/c	0/4	5/5	ND[d]
I	0	5/5	1/4
C57BL	0/5	3/4	0/4
C57BL × I	0/4	2/2	0/4
ABP-CI	0/3	3/3	0/4
ABDS-BI	0/3	4/4	0/4
BPS-CI	0/3	4/4	0/1
AB-BC	0/4	1/1	0/2

[a]Serum samples were collected from 8-9 week-old females, except for the (C57BL × I) hybrids which were 7 weeks old and the AB-BC females which were 12 weeks old. Sera from the I females were tested as a pool rather than as individual samples.

[b]Females were 8 weeks old at the time of infection-immunization with MTV, and serum samples were collected one week later.

[c]Serum samples were collected from 8-9 week old females.

[d]ND = not done

TABLE V. Effect of Infection or Immunization with C3H-MTV on Natural Killer Activity Against YAC-1 Target Cells[a]

Strain of spleen Donor	Average percent cytotoxicity[b] (Range in parentheses)		
	Not infected with exogenous MTV	Infected (Immunized) with C3H-MTV[c]	Neonatally infected with C3H-MTV
BALB/c	6.2 (5.2 - 7.0)	8.5 (8.0 - 9.3)	7.2 (5.6 - 7.9)
I	2.8 (0.8 - 5.1)	4.3 (1.2 - 6.6)	ND
C57BL	21.1(11.1-27.9)	18.9(14.5-22.4)	ND
C57BL × I	20.4(14.6-24.3)	22.4(13.0-31.3)	ND
ABP-CI	7.8 (6.3-10.3)	8.1 (6.3-10.0)	12.1(10.6-13.9)
ABDS-BI	7.2 (2.8-10.5)	10.0 (8.9-12.1)	7.1 (5.2-10.6)
BPS-CI	2.6 (1.1 - 4.8)	7.6 (5.6 - 9.7)	ND
AB-BC	12.2 (3.3-19.6)	ND[d]	13.8 (7.8-24.0)

[a]Each group consisted of 3 to 7 females.

[b]100:1 effector target cell ratio.

[c]Females were 8 weeks old at the time of infection-immunization.

[d]ND = not done.

B. *Effect of Transient Immunosuppression with Antithymocyte Globulin (ATG) on Specific Natural Immunity to MTV and on Activity in Natural Killer Assay*

We documented previously the dramatic effect of transient immunosuppression with ATG upon reactivity to cell-associated MTV antigens as measured in the microcytotoxicity assay. In BALB/cfC3H females treated with ATG at 3 months of age for a two week period, their normal splenic T-cell cytotoxicity against MTV-expressing mammary target cells is supplemented (after recovery from the immunosuppression) by a strong non-T-cell ADCM cytotoxic activity (Blair and Lane, 1977; Blair, in press). To determine if natural killer activity was similarly affected, we repeated the experiment on another group of 3-month-old BALB/cfC3H females and tested their spleen cells in the natural killer assay two weeks and 6 weeks after the first inoculation of ATG. We sampled more than one time interval after treatment because time following treatment is an important variable in level of natural killer reactivity (Herberman *et al.*, 1977; Hochman *et al.*, 1978; Montovani *et al.*, 1978); the intervals chosen were those which resulted in the most dramatic differences in ADCM cytotoxic reactivity to MTV (Blair and Lane, 1977).

For these experiments, antithymocyte antiserum was prepared by inoculating adult New Zealand rabbits monthly for 4 months in several subcutaneous sites with a suspension of 3×10^8 thymocytes obtained from 3-week-old BALB/c males and emulsified in complete Freund's adjuvant. Sera from each bleeding were frozen and, after the last collection, all samples were unfrozen and pooled. ATG was then prepared by precipitation of globulins in saturated ammonium sulfate. Normal rabbit globulin (NRG) was prepared by the same procedure from serum obtained from unimmunized rabbits. Each ATG-treated or control NRG-treated BALB/cfC3H mouse received 11 intraperitoneal injections, each containing in saline a 0.5 ml equivalent of antiserum. The first injections were given daily and the later ones were given at 2- to 3-day intervals so that the last injection was given 15 days after the first.

The activity in natural killer assay detected in these ATG-treated BALB/cfC3H females is compared with that in the NRG-treated controls in Table VI. The response to MTV-expressing mammary tumor target cells previously reported is also presented. Despite the qualitative and quantitative increase in specific anti-MTV immunity which occurs 6 weeks after the first injection, natural killer activity is not altered, either then or earlier (2 weeks after the first injection) when the females are immunosuppressed and not reacting to MTV antigenicity.

These observations, along with the results just presented on reactivity of normal and specifically immunized mice, provide evidence that natural specific immunity to MTV antigenicity as detected in microcytotoxicity assay does not play a major, if any, role in natural killer activity detected in assays using the YAC-1 target cell line. It should be noted that in neonatally infected BALB/cfC3H mice recovered from transient ATG immunosuppression, the specific immunoreactivity to MTV is ADCM cytotoxicity, mediated by antibody secreted in culture, and that ADCM reactivity can be detected in the microcytotoxicity assay with mammary tumor cell targets in as little as 6 hours, which is the earliest time point we have examined. This strong reactivity should be detectable in the 4-hour ^{51}Cr-release assay; that it is not suggests that the ADCM cytotoxicity of these mice is not directed against group-specific MTV antigenicities expressed on the YAC-1 cells.

TABLE VI. Natural Killer Activity in Manipulated BALB/cfC3H Females[a]

Treatment	Natural killer activity: Age at testing (weeks)	Percent cytotoxicity[b]: Aver.	Range	Relative reactivity on mammary tumor cells[c]
NRG Control, 2 wks PI[d]	14	5.7	(2.8-9.8)	+
NRG Control, 6 wks PI	18	6.4	(6.0-6.8)	+
ATG, 2 wks PI	14	5.3	(1.9-7.3)	0
ATG, 6 wks PI	18	7.5	(4.3-9.9)	+++

[a]*At each age, 3 NRG-injected and 6 ATG-injected females were tested.*

[b]*Effector:target cell ratio of 100:1*

[c]*Data presented in Blair and Lane, 1977.*

[d]*Wks PI = time in weeks since the first injection of the 11 injection series was given.*

VI. SUMMARY

Our studies of natural killer activity against YAC-1 target cells, which express not only MuLV-related but also MTV-related antigenicity, revealed no correlation between this activity and the levels of natural specific T-cell or ADCM cytotoxic immunity to MTV. Neither genetic differences in natural specific immunologic reactivity (measured in microcytotoxicity assay) nor immunomanipulations (specific immunization or non-specific transient immunosuppression) which dramatically increase antibody-mediated reactivity, including ADCM cytotoxicity, had any significant effect on cytotoxicity levels in the natural killer assay, even though MTV antigenicity is expressed on the YAC-1 target cells. Thus, if reactivity in natural killer assay is directed against MTV antigenicity, it does not appear to be related to ADCM cytotoxicity, nor do manipulations which alter immunity to MTV necessarily have a similar affect on the levels of natural killer activity.

ACKNOWLEDGMENT

We are grateful to Clara Else for the preparation of the manuscript.

REFERENCES

Åsjö, B., Kiessling, R., Klein, G. & Povey, S. 1977 Genetic variation in antibody response and natural killer cell activity against a Moloney virus-induced lymphoma (YAC) *Eur. J. Immunol. 8:* 554-558

Becker, S., Kiessling, R., Lee, N. & Klein, G. 1978 Modulation of sensitivity to natural killer cell lysis after *in vitro* explantation of a mouse lymphoma. *J. Natl. Cancer Inst. 61:* 1495-1498

Beverly, P. & Knight, D. 1979 Killing comes naturally. *Nature 278:* 119-120

Blair, P.B. 1965 Immunology of the mouse mammary tumor virus (MTV): a qualitative *in vitro* assay for MTV. *Nature 208:* 165-168

Blair, P.B. 1976 Natural immunity in the oncornavirus-infected mouse. *Cancer Res. 36:* 734-738

Blair, P.B. 1980 Immune responses to MTV-induced mammary tumors. *IN* J.W. Blasecki, ed., "Cellular Immunity to Virus-Induced Tumors," Marcel Dekker, Inc., (in press)

Blair, P.B. & Lane, M.A. 1974 Immunologic evidence for horizontal transmission of MTV. *J. Immunol. 113:*1446-1449

Blair, P.B. & Lane, M.A. 1975a *In vitro* detection of immune responses to MTV-induced mammary tumors: qualitative differences in response detected by time studies. *J. Immunol. 114:* 17-23

Blair, P.B. & Lane, M.A. 1975b Non-T cell killing of mammary tumor cells by spleen cells: secretion of antibody and recruitment of cells. *J. Immunol. 115:* 184-189

Blair, P.B. & Lane, M.A. 1977 Effect of immune manipulation on natural immune responses to murine mammary tumor antigens. *J. Natl. Cancer Inst. 59:* 251-257

Blair, P.B., Lane, M.A. & Yagi, M.J. 1974 *In vitro* detection of immune responses to MTV-induced mammary tumors: activity of spleen cell preparations from both MTV-free and MTV-infected mice. *J. Immunol. 112:* 693-705

Blair, P.B., Lane, M.A. & Yagi, M.J. 1975 Blocking of spleen cell activity against target mammary tumor cells by viral antigens. *J. Immunol. 115:* 190-194

Callahan, R.M., Marx, P.A. & Wheelock, E.F. 1979 Group-specific cytolytic antibody directed against the major glycoprotein (gp70) of murine leukemia viruses in serum of mice with dormant FLV infections. *Virol. 97:* 55-67

de Landazuri, M.O., Silva, A., Alvarez, J. & Herberman, R.B. 1979 Evidence that natural cytotoxicity and antibody-dependent cellular cytotoxicity are mediated in humans by the same effector cell populations. *J. Immunol. 123:* 252

Hatzfeld, A., Koo, G.C. & Boyse, E.A. 1979 Viral gp70 and the specificity of natural killer cells. *Proc. Amer. Assoc. Cancer Res. 20:* 267

Herberman, R.B. & Holden, H.T. 1978 Natural cell-mediated immunity. *Adv. Cancer Res. 27:* 305-377

Herberman, R.B., Nunn, M.E., Holden, H.T., Staal, S. & Djeu, J.Y. 1977 Augmentation of natural cytotoxic reactivity of mouse lymphoid cells against syngeneic and allogeneic target cells. *Int. J. Cancer 19:* 555-564

Herberman, R.B., Djeu, J.Y., Kay, D., Ortaldo, J.R., Riccardi, C., Bonnard, G.D., Holden, H.T., Fagnani, R., Santoni, A. & Puccetti, P. 1979 Natural killer cells: characteristics and regulation of activity. *Immunological Rev. 44:* 43-70

Hirsch, M.E., Kelly, A.P., Proffitt, M.R. & Black, P.H. 1975 Cell-mediated immunity to antigens associated with endogenous murine C-type leukemia viruses. *Science 187:* 959-961

Hochman, P.S. & Cudkowicz, G. 1979 Suppression of natural cytotoxicity by spleen cells of hydrocortisone-treated mice. *J. Immunol. 123:* 968-976

Hochman, P.A., Cudkowicz, G. & Dausset, J. 1978 Decline of natural killer cell activity in sublethally irradiated mice. *J. Natl. Cancer Inst. 61:* 265-268

Kelloff, G.J., Knott, W. & Dobbs, J. 1979 Blocking of natural killer cell mediated cytotoxicity with normal serum-antibody. *Proc. Amer. Assoc. Cancer Res. 20:* 106

Kende, M., Hill, R., Dinowitz, M., Stephenson, J.R. & Kelloff, G.J. 1979 Naturally occurring lymphocyte-mediated immunity to endogenous type-C virus in the mouse. *J. Exper. Med. 149:* 358-371

Koide, Y., Kwok, R. & Takasugi, M. 1978 Studies of effector cell, antibody and target cell interactions in natural cell-mediated cytotoxicity. *Int. J. Cancer 22:* 546-551

Lane, M.A., Roubinian, J., Slomich, M., Trefts, P. & Blair, P.B. 1975 Characterization of cytotoxic effector cells in the mouse mammary tumor system. *J. Immunol. 114:*24-29

Lopez, D.M., Sigel, M.M., Ortiz-Muniz, G. & Parks, W. 1978 Specificity and age of appearance of natural immunity to MTV antigens. *Proc. Soc. Exp. Biol. Med. 158:* 23-27

Mantovani, A., Luini, W., Peri, G., Vecchi, A. & Spreafico, F. 1978 Effect of chemotherapeutic agents on natural cell-mediated cytotoxicity in mice. *J. Natl. Cancer Inst. 61:* 1255-1261

Ojo, E., Haller, O. & Wigzell, H. 1978 *Corynebacterium parvum*-induced peritoneal exudate cells with rapid cytolytic activity against tumour cells are non-phagocytic cells with characteristics of natural killer cells. *Scand. J. Immunol. 8:* 215-222

Pape, G.R., Troye, M., Axelsson, B. & Perlmann, P. 1979 Simultaneous occurrence of immunoglobulin-dependent and immunoglobulin-independent mechanisms in natural cytotoxicity of human lymphocytes. *J. Immunol. 122:* 2251-2260

Perlmann, P. & Holm, G. 1969 Cytotoxic effects of lymphoid cells *in vitro*. *Adv. Immunol. 11:* 117-193

Roder, J.C., Lohmann-Matthes, M.L., Domzig, W. & Wigzell, H. 1979 The beige mutation in the mouse. II. Selectivity of the natural killer (NK) cell defect. *J. Immunol. 123:* 2174-2181

Santoni, A., Herberman, R.B. & Holden, H.T. 1979 Correlation between natural and antibody-dependent cell-mediated cytotoxicity against tumor targets in the mouse. I. Distribution of the reactivity. *J. Natl. Cancer Inst. 62:* 109-116

Schrader, J.W. & Nossal, G.J.V. 1974 Effector cell blockade: a new mechanism of immune hyporeactivity induced by multivalent antigens. *J. Exp. Med. 139:*1582-1598

Stockert, E., DeLeo, A.B., O'Donnell, P.V., Obata, Y. & Old, L.J. 1979 $G_{(AKSL2)}$: A new cell surface antigen of the mouse related to the dualtropic mink cell focus-inducing class of murine leukemia virus detected by naturally occurring antibody. *J. Exp. Med. 149:* 200-215

Tagliabue, A., Herberman, R.B. & McCoy, J.L. 1978 Cellular immunity to mammary tumor virus in normal and tumor-bearing C3H/HeN mice. *Cancer Res. 38:* 2279-2284

Tagliabue, A., Herberman, R.B., Lavrin, D.H. & McCoy, J.L. 1979 Immunological reactivities in normal C3H/HeN mice infected with mouse mammary tumor virus (MTV). *Proc. Amer. Assoc. Cancer Res. 20:* 66

Takasugi, M. & Akira, D. 1979 Role of antibodies in the specificity of natural cell-mediated cytotoxicity. *J. Natl. Cancer Inst. 62:* 1361-1365

Welsh, R.M. 1978 Cytotoxic cells induced during lymphocytic choriomeningitis virus infection of mice. I. Characterization of natural killer cell induction. *J. Exp. Med. 148:* 163-181

Yagi, M.J. 1974 Characteristics of mammary tumor cell lines derived from MTV-infected mice. Ph.D. thesis, University of California, Berkeley

Yagi, M.J., Blair, P.B. & Lane, M.A. 1978 Modulation of mouse mammary tumor virus production in the MJY-alpha cell line. *J. Virol. 28:* 611-623

THE USE OF LYMPHOMA CELL VARIANTS DIFFERING IN THEIR SUSCEPTIBILITY TO NK CELL MEDIATED LYSIS TO ANALYSE NK CELL-TARGET CELL INTERACTIONS

Jeannine M. Durdik
Barbara N. Beck
Christopher S. Henney

Basic Immunology Program
Fred Hutchinson Cancer Research Center
Seattle, Washington

NK cells are characterized by their ability to lyse, in short-term 51-Cr release assays, a wide variety of tumors and long-term cell lines, including those allogeneic and xenogeneic to the effector cell source. Normal cells are, in general, much less susceptible to NK cell mediated lytic attack (1, 2). One possible explanation for the ability of NK cell populations to lyse a wide spectrum of target cell types might be heterogeneity within the effector cell pool. Thus, NK cell populations might be composed of diverse subsets of cells, each with a restricted lytic specificity.

We have carried out three sets of related experiments to seek evidence for such a possibility. In the first, we asked whether NK cell populations could be adsorbed onto monolayers of susceptible cells, and, if so, whether such interactions removed NK reactivity against other susceptible target cells. In one experiment typical of this approach, murine NK cell populations (BCG-induced peritoneal exudate cells of C57BL/6 mice (see 3)) were incubated (40 min, 37°) on a monolayer of susceptible lymphoma cells, L5178Y. The cell population used in these studies was a clone of L5178Y, designated cl 27v, which was selected for its particular susceptibility to NK cell-mediated lysis. Later in the chapter these cells are discussed further. Cells nonadherent to the cl 27v cell monolayer were harvested and their cytotoxic activity to cl 27v and to Chang cells, a human liver cell line susceptible to the action of NK cells, was assessed. Incubation on cl 27v cells largely removed cytotoxic activity, not only to this cell but also to Chang cells. Indeed, NK cell adsorption onto cl 27v cells removed cytotoxic activity against all NK susceptible target cells tested. In contrast, parallel adsorption of NK cell populations on NK-insusceptible cell monolayers (e.g. on normal DBA/2 spleen cells), did not remove NK reactivity (1).

Thus, experiments of this nature established: a) that NK cells bind to monolayers of NK-susceptible, but not to monolayers of NK-insusceptible cells, and b) that adsorption on susceptible cell

ISBN 0-12-341350-8

monolayers removed NK reactivity not only against this cell, but also against other NK-susceptible targets.

It proved technically difficult to deplete NK cells totally on cell monolayers and furthermore, the non-adsorbed cell population was often contaminated with cells that detached from the monolayer. To overcome such difficulties, a different approach, based on the interaction of effector and target cells in suspension, was employed. Susceptible or insusceptible target cells were treated with dichlorotriazinyl amino fluorescein and the resulting fluoresceinated cells were incubated with NK cell suspensions under conditions allowing target-effector cell complexes to form. The resulting mixture was fractionated into fluorescent and non-fluorescent populations using a fluorescence-activated cell sorter (Becton and Dickinson FACS II). The NK reactivity of the non-fluorescent population was then assessed, both against the target cell with which it had been incubated and with a series of other target cells comprising both susceptible and insusceptible phenotypes. It was argued that NK cell interaction with a fluorescent target cell would result in a cell-cell complex which would fractionate with the fluorescent compartment and thus, the non-fluorescent population would be selectively depleted of binding cells. Results of three experiments of this type are shown in Table I. As can be seen, incubation with susceptible, cl 27v, target cells was in each case associated with a decline in lytic reactivity in the non-fluorescent fraction. A decline in lytic activity was noted not only using cl 27v but also using other susceptible target cells (e.g. SL3 Expt. I and YAC-I Expt. 3). In contrast, incubation with fluorescent insusceptible cells (EL4 Expt. 2 and L5178Y cl 27av Expt. 3) was not associated with a decline in NK reactivity.

Results compatible with these binding experiments were also obtained in "cold" target inhibition experiments, in which the lysis of 51-Cr-labelled susceptible cells was inhibited by the addition of unlabelled competitors. In the series of experiments shown in Table II, cl 27v was used as the prototype 51-Cr-labelled target cell. The number of competitor cells required to inhibit lysis of cl 27v by 50% is reported in Table II. As can be seen, NK susceptible target cells were all effective inhibitors of the lysis of cl 27v. Indeed, the number of such cells required for 50% inhibition was not significantly different from the number of homologous cells required. Cells susceptible to the action of NK cells included: cl 27v; YAC-I, a Moloney virus induced lymphoma of A/Sn mice; BALB/c 3T3 (clone A31); NSI/I-Ag-4-I of the BALB/c myeloma cell line MOPC 21; Chang cells, a human derived liver cell line and clone K234 of 3T3 Ki MSV, which were cells from the above 3T3 line infected by a nonproductive Kirsten strain of murine sarcoma virus.

In contrast, a series of NK insusceptible target cells were very poor inhibitors. These included: cl 27av, an in vitro adapted NK resistant subline of L5178Y lymphoma and three ascites tumors, P815-X2, a methyl cholanthrene-induced mastocytoma of DBA/2 mice;

TABLE I. Removal of NK activity following binding to fluoresceinated target cells

Effector Cell	Incubation with fluoresceinated target:	% Specific Lysis of: Expt. 1 cl 27v	Expt. 1 SL3	Expt. 2 cl 27v	Expt. 2 EL4	Expt. 3 YAC-1	Expt. 3 cl 27v	Expt. 3 cl 27av
BCG induced C57BL/6 pec	none	45.2	21.9	21.4	2.3	23.9	12.7	4.1
	cl 27v (susceptible)	32.4	12.7	10.3	--	14.5	6.9	4.1
	EL4 (insusceptible)			23.1	1.9			
	cl 27av (insusceptible)					28.6	15.7	3.7

Ten million target cells/ml were chemically derivatized with fluorescein (5-10 μg/ml dichlorotriazinyl amino fluorescein di HCl at pH 9, 20°C for 30 min) and then washed three times. Equal numbers of fluorescent target cells and NK cells (BCG induced peritoneal exudates) were mixed, pelleted and allowed to incubate at 37°C for 30 minutes. Just prior to placing on the FACS II, the cells were gently resuspended and filtered through a Nytex mesh. Criteria for separations were established from independent FACS II analysis of each population. Both low angle scatter and fluorescence parameters were utilized to separate the effector population from the "larger" fluorescent target cell population. After sorting, the non-fluorescent population was tested for its residual NK activity against a variety of 51Cr-labelled targets at an E:T of 13:1. NK cells incubated without targets had been subjected to identical conditions to those NK cells mixed with fluorescent targets. Contamination of the fluorescent-negative NK cell populations with fluorescent positive cells was less than 0.3%.

TABLE II. Inhibition Studies Demonstrating Cross-Reactivity of NK Susceptible Target Cells

Phenotype		Relative susceptibility to NK cell lysis	No. cells ($X 10^{-4}$) required to inhibit lysis of cl 27v by 50%	No. cl 27v cells ($X 10^{-4}$) required to inhibit NK mediated lysis by 50%
NK susceptible	cl 27v	1.0	8	8
	YAC-1	1.7	10	7
	3T3	1.1	9	10
	NS1	1.0	8	--
	Chang	0.9	12	12
	K234	0.5	9	10
NK insusceptible	cl 27av	0.3	25	3
	P815	0.2	35	3
	cl 27a	0.2	50	2
	EL4	0.1	>100	3
	normal spleen cells	0	>>100	--

Values shown are compiled from several experiments in which cells were tested for their ability to be directly lysed by BCG induced NK cells (relative susceptibility = lysis of target/lysis of cl 27v). Additionally, 10^4 51-Cr-labelled cl 27v cells were lysed by BCG-induced C57BL/6 NK cells in the presence of increasing numbers of unlabelled competitor cells. The number of such cells required to inhibit lysis by 50% was enumerated. In reciprocal experiments, cells were 51-Cr-labelled and the number of cl 27v cells necessary to inhibit lysis by 50% was evaluated. Lysis of cl 27v cells in the absence of competitor cells was 20-40%, while the lysis of other targets varied between 10 and 90%.

cl 27a the ascites maintained L5178Y clone 27 subline and EL4, a chemically induced thymoma of C57BL/6 mice. A clear positive correlation was observed between the susceptibility of the cells to NK attack (recorded in Table II in relation to the susceptibility of cl 27v cells) and their ability to inhibit the NK mediated lysis of cl 27v. The one exception to this rule was K234 cells which were good competitive inhibitors but only moderately susceptible to NK cell mediated lysis (Table II). Interestingly, K234 cells were also relatively resistant to lysis by cytotoxic T cells (unpublished observations).

One final point can be made from the data shown in Table II: the small amount of NK cell mediated lysis observed in some of the insusceptible targets (e.g. cl 27av, cl 27a, P815 and EL4) was easily inhibited by the addition of NK susceptible targets (e.g. cl 27v). Indeed, cl 27v cells were more effective inhibitors in these situations than were homologous unlabelled cells (data not shown).

Collectively, these results were incompatible with the concept that distinct subpopulations of NK cells lyse different target cells. We thus found no evidence that NK "specificities" were poly-clonally distributed. Rather, our findings were consistent with the proposition that susceptibility of target cells to NK attack reflected a shared membrane characteristic. Other investigators have reached similar conclusions (2). Furthermore, the fact that some target cells were lysed to only a small extent by NK cells and that such lysis was more readily inhibited by NK susceptible cells than by homologous cells, suggested that heterogeneity in susceptibility to NK cell attack might reflect quantitative differences in the display of a common macro-molecule.

In this context, there have been several attempts to associate NK cell susceptibility with the display of a common target cell "antigen". Suggestion has been made that murine NK cells react with structures associated with endogenous C-type viruses (4, 5). Other investigators have found that expression of viral antigens did not correlate with susceptibility to NK cell attack (6, 7). Recently, Roder et al (8) have used biochemical techniques in a search for cell surface macro-molecules against which NK cells might be directed. They isolated target cell structures from susceptible cells which could inhibit the binding of NK cells to susceptible targets. These surface structures were not present on cells which were insusceptible to NK cell mediated lysis (8).

In the search for a potential molecular basis for NK cell mediated lysis of target cells, our approach has been to seek variants from a given tumor which differ in their susceptibility to NK cell mediated lysis.

To this end, L5178Y lymphoma cells were cloned by limiting dilutions in RPMI 1640 containing 10% fetal calf serum. Samples from each of the resulting clones, approximately 30 in number, were internally labelled by incubation (30 min, 37°C) with 100 μC sodium 51-chromate (Amersham-Searle, Chicago, Ill.) and tested for sensitivity to BCG-induced NK activity in a 4 hr 51-Cr release assay (3). As a result of this initial screening, one clone, L5178Y clone 27 (cl 27v), was selected as a population particularly susceptible to NK cell mediated lysis. This cell population has been cultured for a period exceeding 3 years and has retained its susceptibility phenotype throughout this period.

After in vitro cloning, a portion of cl 27v cells was transferred to syngeneic mice and passaged as ascites. In contrast to the in vitro line, the ascites cells (cl 27a) were very poorly lysed by NK cells (see Table II). The ascites cells remained as susceptible to anti-H-2d serum and complement and to alloimmune cytotoxic T cells (C57BL/6 anti-P815 mastocytoma) as were the in vitro population from which they were derived. Thus, the ascites cells had not simply become resistant to cell-mediated cytolysis. During the tenth month of in vivo passage, the ascites cells were adapted in vitro and were termed cl 27av. As of December 1979, these cells have been cultured for approximately 11 months and have maintained the insusceptible phenotype of the ascites. They were compared to cl 27v cells by a number of criteria. Serological analysis using anti-H-2d antisera in the presence of rabbit complement revealed minimal differences. The following antisera were employed in these characterizations: B10 anti B10.D2; (B10 x A)F1 anti B10.D2 (anti H-2Kd) obtained as NIH serum D-31(2); (B10.AKM x 129)F1 anti B10.A (anti H-2Dd) obtained as NIH serum D-4(2). With each serum, using dilutions between 1:50 and 1:6400, less than a two-fold difference in surface alloantigen display on the two cell lines was demonstrable. Indeed, quantitative adsorption studies using the same sera revealed no differences between cl 27v and cl 27av cells.

In keeping with the serological analysis, cl 27v and the adapted variant were equivalently susceptible to alloimmune cytotoxic T cells (Table III) and were indistinguishable in their ability to inhibit the T cell mediated lysis of cl 27v cells (Fig. 1). Despite identity as targets for cytotoxic T cells, there was a large and striking difference in the abilities of the two cell lines to serve as targets for NK cell mediated lysis (Table III). This distinction was true not only in direct cytotoxic assays, employing 51-Cr-labelled targets, but was observed also when unlabelled cells were used to inhibit the NK cell mediated lysis of cl 27v cells (Fig. 1). As can be seen, cl 27v, the homologous cell type, effectively inhibited NK cell mediated lysis, whereas cl 27av failed to inhibit lysis at any cell concentration tested. This finding suggests that only the susceptible variant binds to NK cells. Two other points are worthy of emphasis: (i) cl 27av has remained insusceptible to NK cells throughout its eleven month culture. This is in contrast to a previous report (9) that YAC cells grown as ascites were resistant to NK attack, but reverted to an NK susceptible phenotype when adapted in vitro, and (ii) cl 27 ascites cells have been recloned without finding susceptible cells within the population, indicating that this population was homogeneous with respect to NK insusceptibility.

TABLE III. Susceptibility of L5178Y Clone 27 Cell Lines to T and NK Mediated Cytolysis

Effector Cell	L5178Y target cell	% Specific Lysis 20:1	40:1	80:1
T	cl 27v	39.4	52.3	58.1
	cl 27av	54.9	63.2	68.2
NK	cl 27v	28.3	37.5	49.4
	cl 27av	7.4	11.0	13.2

Cytotoxic T cells were raised in 7 day primary cultures of C57BL/6 spleen cells with X-irradiated P815 cells at a responder: stimulator ratio of 50:1. NK cells were obtained as peritoneal exudates from BCG-stimulated C57BL/6 mice. The cytotoxic assay was carried out using 10^4 51Cr-labelled targets per well and a 4 hr assay.

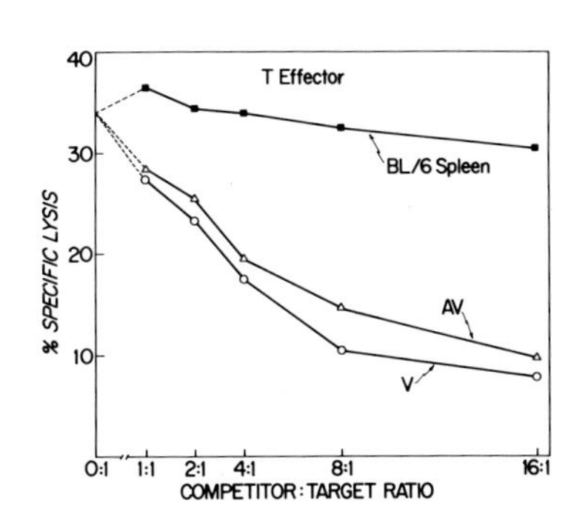

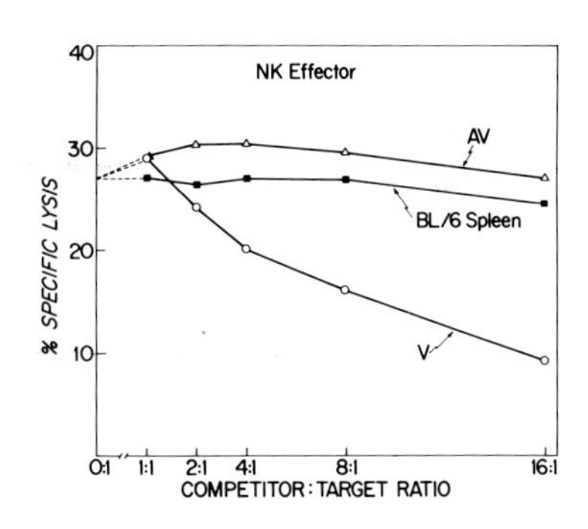

FIGURE 1. Inhibition of lysis of L5178 clone 27v cells by homologous cells, by cl 27av and by C57BL/6 (B6) normal spleen cells. In the left hand figure, lysis was effected by cytotoxic T cells at an effector:target cell ratio of 10:1. Cytotoxic T cells were generated following 2 day in vitro restimulation with X-irradiated P815 cells (at a responder:stimulator ratio of 50:1) of C57BL/6 spleen cells from animals injected 19 days earlier with 10^7 P815 cells. In the right hand figure, lysis was effected by NK cells at an effector:target cell ratio of 40:1. NK cells were obtained from peritoneal exudates from C57BL/6 mice injected with 10^8 BCG i.p. 5 days previously. In both cases a 4 hr lytic assay was employed.

The two in vitro cell lines derived from L5178Y lymphoma behaved as variants only with respect to their susceptibility to the action of NK cells. Interestingly, NK cell populations from a variety of sources were all capable of distinguishing between cl 27v and cl 27av. In tests of direct lysis, cl 27v was killed by normal (and BCG-induced) NK cells from CBA spleen and by NK cell populations from human and non-human primate (pigtail macaques) peripheral blood. Cl 27av was resistant to all of these effector populations.

Collectively, these findings are most compatible with the proposition that cl 27av cells lack a membrane macromolecule present on cl 27v cells which dictates, or is associated with, susceptibility to NK cells. These observations suggested to us that the variants of L5178Y might serve as useful tools in a search for a molecular basis for NK susceptibility. To this end, we have begun treating NK-susceptible and insusceptible target cells with a series of proteolytic and glycosidic enzymes, hoping to change the susceptibility phenotype of the target cells. To date, only papain has been extensively examined. Both YAC-1 and cl 27v cells treated with papain and then tested as targets in a cytotoxic assay in the presence of an inhibitor of protein synthesis, showed significant reductions in their susceptibility both to NK and T effector cell populations (Table IV). Target cells which were insusceptible to NK cells, (e.g. cl 27av) remained insusceptible to NK mediated cytotoxicity and showed considerable diminution in their susceptibility to T effector cells (Table IV). These observations suggest that the susceptibility of a target cell to NK mediated lysis might be associated with the display of a cell surface protein. The concomittant decline in the susceptibility of papain-treated targets to attack by T and NK effector cells does not, of course, necessarily imply that the same target cell structures are involved in both sets of lytic interactions. Presumably, the decrease in susceptibility to alloimmune cytotoxic T cells reflects the removal of surface H-2 alloantigens. On the other hand, H-2 appears not to play a role in NK target cell interaction for antibody against target cell H-2 specificities affects neither the rate nor the extent of NK cell mediated lysis.

Recently, in collaboration with Drs. W. Young, D. Urdal and S-I. Hakomori of the Biochemical Oncology Program at the Fred Hutchinson Cancer Research Center, we have begun an extensive and systematic biochemical analysis of membrane extracts from the cl 27v and cl 27av cells.

Following a number of observations that implicated glycoconjugates as cell surface receptor molecules (10, 11), we examined the glycolipids of cl 27v and cl 27av cells. Total neutral glycolipid and ganglioside fractions are shown in Figure 2. Clone 27av cells (NK insusceptible) displayed a simple neutral glycolipid and ganglioside pattern with ceramide monohexoside (CMH), ceramide dihexoside (CDH), and hematoside (GM3) as the predominant glycolipids. Clone 27v (NK susceptible) cells on the other hand, showed a strikingly

TABLE IV. The Effect of Papain Treatment on Target Cell Susceptibility

Effector Cell	Target Cell	E:T	% Specific Lysis Untreated	Papain treated
BCG induced NK	YAC-1	100:1	30.4	11.8
NK		200:1	14.8	2.3
T		50:1	14.9	-0.9
BCG induced NK	cl 27v	100:1	9.1	0.7
NK		200:1	5.1	-1.2
T		50:1	45.3	0.3
BCG induced NK	cl 27av	100:1	4.8	1.1
NK		200:1	2.4	0.8
T		50:1	43.9	5.2

NK cell populations were either from normal CBA spleens (NK) or from the peritoneal exudates of C57BL/6 mice 6 days after injection i.p. with 10^8 BCG (BCG-induced NK). Alloimmune T cells were generated in 6 day cultures utilizing L5178Y cells as alloantigen and normal C57BL/6 spleen cells as responders. For papain treatment, 1.5 X 10^7 cells/ml were treated for 30 min at 37° with 6 mg papain activated with 1 mM cysteine at pH 6.9 in 2 mM Hepes buffered saline. The lytic assay in each case was for 2 hrs and was carried out in the presence of 10^{-4}M cyclohexamide. This concentration of drug inhibited protein synthesis completely but did not affect the function of NK or T cells.

TABLE V. Immunochemical Detection of Asialo GM2 on L5178Y Cell Variants

L5178Y cell line	anti-asialo GM2 antibody	% Specific cytolysis at ab dilns. of: 1:540	1:180	1:60	1:20
cl 27v	IgG hybridoma	26.0	35.4	35.5	42.2
cl 27av		-1.0	-1.0	-0.4	-0.5
cl 27v	IgM hybridoma	57.4	60.5	60.6	59.8
cl 27av		-0.4	-0.4	-0.5	-0.4

BALB/c monoclonal antibodies specific for asialo GM2 were prepared by the hybridoma procedure (14) and were a kind gift of Drs. Young and Hakomori. The ascites fluid from hybridoma-bearing mice was used without further purification. 10^4 51-Cr- labelled target cells were incubated for 15 min at room temperature with the indicated antibody diluted in Basal Medium, Eagle's in a total volume of 100 µl in a microliter plate. 100 µl of rabbit serum (preabsorbed with cl 27v cells) diluted 1:15 in medium was added to each well as a source of complement and the plates incubated at 37°C for 45 min in a humidified atmosphere of 5% CO_2, 95% air. Lysis in the presence of complement alone was 6.1% for cl 27v and 0.3% for cl 27av.

different glycolipid profile. The neutral glycolipid fraction, in addition to CMH and CDH, displayed three prominent glycolipid bands, all of which were not detectable on the NK insusceptible variant. One of these migrated at the position of asialo GM2 and another corresponded to globoside. On acetylation, the three bands migrated as two bands with mobilities equivalent to acetylated asialo GM2 and acetylated globoside. The identity of one of the bands as asialo GM2 was substantiated immunochemically: clone 27v cells, but not cl 27av, were lysed by asialo GM2 specific hybridoma antibodies in the presence of complement (Table V).

The ganglioside pattern of membrane extracts was also more complex in cl 27v cells than in cl 27av: GM3 was absent and 3-4 resorcinol- positive bands were seen migrating between GM1 and GD1a. Preliminary results indicate that in addition to the differences seen in the glycolipid profiles of the two cells, there are also differences in cell surface glycoproteins (Urdal and Hakomori, unpublished observations).

In sum, to date, we have isolated two cell variants of L5178Y lymphoma cells which differ markedly in their susceptibility to NK cell mediated lysis. These cells showed distinctive neutral glycolipid and ganglioside profiles (Fig. 2). We have addressed the possibility that one marked difference associated exclusively with the NK susceptible cell, asialo GM2, might be the target cell structure against which NK cells are directed. Three lines of evidence suggest that it is not: (i) the susceptibility of target cells to NK cells is papain sensitive (Table IV); (ii) we have not been able to interfere with the NK mediated lysis of cl 27v cells by the addition of anti-asialo GM2 serum and (iii) some susceptible target cells (e.g. BALB/c 3T3 and YAC-1) lack demonstrable asialo GM2.

Nevertheless, it remains possible that the association between NK cell susceptibility and an altered membrane glycolipid profile in cl 27v and cl 27av cells is causually related. We are currently engaged in directly addressing the general hypothesis that NK cell populations may "recognize" membrane glycoconjugates.

ACKNOWLEDGMENTS

This work was supported by grants AI 15384 and CA 24537 from the National Institute of Health. The biochemical analysis of cl 27v and cl 27av cells was carried out by Drs. D. Urdal, W. Young and S-I. Hakomori of the Biochemical Oncology Program of the Fred Hutchinson Cancer Research Center. Dr. E. Clark, of the Regional Primate Center of the University of Washington, provided us with information concerning the susceptibility of cl 27v and cl 27av cells to primate NK cell populations. We are grateful to Dr. D. Tracey, Department of Medicine, Johns Hopkins University, for the original cloning of L5178Y cells.

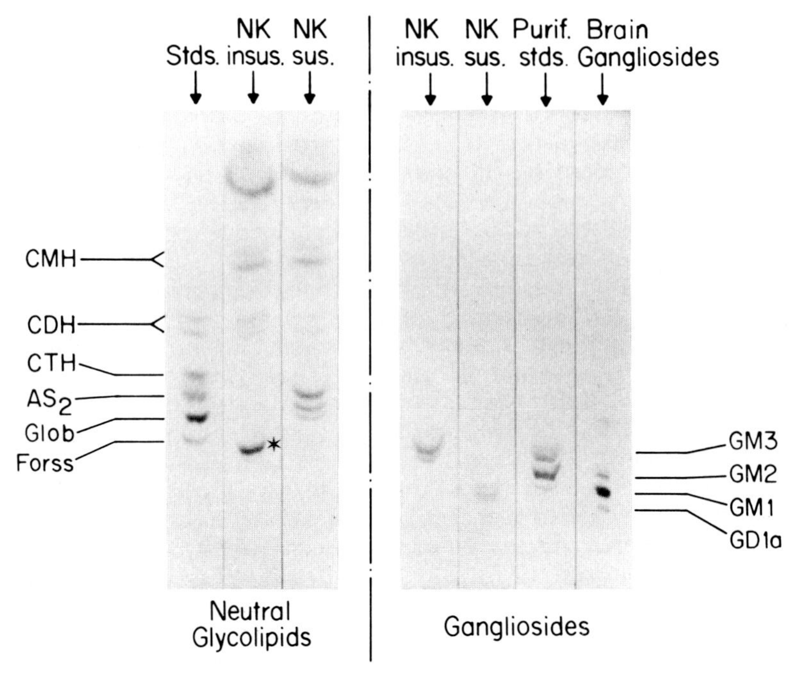

GLYCOLIPID PATTERNS OF NK SUSCEPTIBILITY VARIANTS OF L5178

FIGURE 2. Thin-layer chromatography (TLC) patterns of glycolipids isolated from L5178Y cl 27v (NK susceptible) and cl 27av (NK insusceptible) cells. Cell pellets were extracted with chloroform: methanol (2:1 v/v) and partitioned according to the method of Folch et al (12). The neutral glycolipid fraction was purified from the Folch lower phase by the acetylation procedure (13). Purified neutral glycolipids and the Folch upper phase (containing gangliosides) were analyzed by TLC on Silica gel G plates (Analtech) in the solvent chloroform: methanol: water (60:35:8 v/v). Gangliosides were detected by spraying with resorcinal and neutral glycolipids with orcinol reagent. Glycolipid standards: CDH, Galβ1-4Glc-Cer; CTH, Galα1-4Galβ1-4Glc-Cer; Asialo-GM2 (As2), GalNAcβ1-4Galβ1-4Glc-Cer; Globoside, GalNAcβ1-3Galα1-4Galβ1-4Glc-Cer; Forssman, GalNAcα1-3GalNAcβ1-3Galα1-4Galβ1-4Glc-Cer; GM3, NAcNeurα2-3Galβ1-4Glc-Cer; GM2, GalNAcβ1-4(NAcNeurα2-3)Galβ1-4Glc-Cer; GM1, Galβ1-3GalNAcβ1 -4(NAcNeurα2-3)Galβ1-4Glc-Cer; GD1a, NAcNeurα2-3Galβ1-3GalNAcβ1-4(NAcNeurα2-3)Galβ1-4Glc-Cer. The star indicates the position of GM3 which remained in the lower phase of the Folch partition.

REFERENCES

1. Henney, C. S., Tracey, D. E., Durdik, J. M. and Klimpel, G. Am. J. Path. 93, 459 (1978)
2. Kiessling, R. and Wigzell, H. Immunologic Rev. 44, 165 (1979)
3. Wolfe, S. A., Tracey, D. E. and Henney, C. S. Nature 262, 584 (1976)
4. Herberman, R. B., Nunn, M. E. and Lavrin, D. H. Int. J. Cancer 16, 216 (1975)
5. Lee, J. C. and Ihle, J. N. J. Immunol. 118, 928 (1977)
6. Becker, S., Fenyo, E. M. and Klein, E. Eur. J. Immunol. 6, 882 (1976)
7. Kiessling, R., Haller, O., Fenyo, E. M., Steinitz, M. and Klein, G. Int. J. Cancer 21, 460 (1978)
8. Roder, J. C., Rosen, A., Fenyo, E. M. and Troy, F. A. Proc. Natl. Acad. Sci. 76, 1405 (1979)
9. Becker, S., Kiessling, R., Lee, N. and Klein, G. J. Natl. Cancer Inst. 61, 1495 (1978)
10. Fishman, P. H. and Brady, O. Science 194, 906 (1976)
11. Hakomori, S-I. and Young, W. W. Jr. Scand. J. Immunol. 7 (Supplement 6), 97 (1978)
12. Folch, J., Lees, M. and Sloane-Stanley, G. H. J. Biol. Chem. 226,497 (1957)
13. Saito, T. and Hakomori, S-I. J. Lipid. Res. 12, 257 (1971)
14. Young, W. W. Jr., MacDonald, E. S., Nowinski, R. C. and Hakomori, S-I. J. Exp. Med. 150, 1008 (1979)

KINETIC ANALYSIS OF SPECIFICITY IN HUMAN NATURAL CELL-MEDIATED CYTOTOXICITY

James T. Forbes
Robert K. Oldham

Division of Oncology
Vanderbilt University
Nashville, Tennessee

I. INTRODUCTION

Since the original description of natural killing (NK) in man in 1972, studies have been designed to clarify the role of these cytotoxic cells in normal and human tumor immunology. (1-6) It is clear that an understanding of NK activity is central to progress in tumor immunology. Natural cell-mediated cytotoxicity (NCMC) may represent an initial line of defense by the mammalian host against spontaneous neoplastic transformation. NCMC is found in several species including man (1), rats (7), mice (8), and guinea pigs (9). It is usually quantitated by the in vitro cell mediated destruction of isotopically labeled tumor cells. Since this activity appears to be ubiquitous in those species thus far studied, any future understanding of specific lymphocyte mediated destruction of tumor cells must rest on a firm foundation of knowledge concerning tumor cell lysis by cells mediating NCMC.

In order to precisely study NCMC and its specificity one must first validate the technical aspects of the assay and determine the standards against which NCMC is to be analyzed. Assay standardization (10,11,12), the use of cryopreserved cells (11,13,14,15) and the analysis of the competitive inhibition assay (16) have all been necessary before further investigation of the specificity of NCMC could be approached. The determination and categorization of specificity in natural cell mediated cytotoxicity has been difficult to approach for a variety of reasons. Comparison by direct testing of labeled tumor cells as targets in cytotoxicity assays is confounded by the variability of lysability of these target cells (17). Even

ISBN 0-12-341350-8

with these limitations, evidence has been produced for selective cytotoxicity when analysed by what is termed by its authors as interaction analysis (18). Most of these studies suggest that NK has specificity but that it is directed towards multiple antigens at least some of which are shared by more than one target cell line (17). There is no evidence to suggest that this specificity is directed at histocompatability antigens and in some studies cytotoxicity has crossed xenogeneic barriers (16,19). There is evidence that the determinants most affected by NK activity are those on transformed cell lines. We have studied the specificity of NK cytotoxicity by competitive inhibition using unlabeled target cells (15,16,18). This technique eliminates some of the problems of differential lysability and allows some quantitation in the case of multiple antigen systems in which the labeled cells and the unlabeled cells share some but not all of the NK target antigens. These tests have supported the idea that NK is directed toward specific antigens but it has thus far been difficult to distinguish between inhibition caused by competitive determinants and that caused by physiologic factors not directly related to receptor-ligand binding (16).

It is necessary to define the specificity of NCMC in order to understand the biology of this phenomenon and its impact on other assays of tumor immunity. Until this specificity can be defined, the use of cytotoxicity assays to investigate tumor-specific immunity will be severely limited. As was discussed above, specificity may be determined either by the direct cytotoxic action of NK cells on target cells or by the competitive inhibition of the lysis of labeled cells by non-labeled cells. The former assay is limited by the differential labeling characteristics of each cell line tested and by the target cell lysability while the latter assay presents certain limitations in the interpretation of the results derived from it. The limitations of the competitive inhibition assay and their partial resolution will be the focus of this discussion.

II. METHODS

The following approach has been applied in preliminary investigations of the specificity of NCMC. Ficoll-hypaque separated mononuclear peripheral blood cells from a number of healthy normal donors have been incubated at 37°C with ^{51}Cr labeled target cells as previously reported (14,16). The amount of released ^{51}Cr at the end of this incubation is determined by gamma counting and the results expressed as:

$$\% \text{ Cytotoxicity} = \frac{\text{Experimental Release-Spontaneous Release}}{\text{Total CPM Incorporated-Spontaneous Release}} \times 100$$

The spontaneous release (no effector cells added) of ^{51}Cr is usually less than 5% and any test in which it is greater than 10% is excluded for technical reasons. Competitive inhibition is tested in a similar manner except that varying concentrations of the inhibitor cells are included in the mixture during the incubation. The percent inhibition is calculated by the following formula:

$$\% \text{ Inhibition} = 1- \frac{\%\text{Specific Release in Presence of Inhibitor Cells}}{\%\text{Specific Release without Inhibitor Cells}} \times 100$$

Several reports have suggested that cell mediated cytotoxicity may be considered in a manner analogous to enzyme-substrate interactions and may be subjected to analysis in terms of saturation kinetics (20-26). If this analogy can be applied to the competitive inhibition of NK activity by unlabeled target cells then an objective rather than the previously used subjective treatment (18) of the results is possible. In this analysis the reaction velocity (v) for cell mediated cytotoxicity may be given by the Michaelis-Menten equation:

$$V = \frac{Vmax}{1 + \frac{Km}{s}} \quad (27)$$

where s is the substrate or target cell concentration (isotopically labeled target cells) and Vmax is a constant equal to the maximal cytotoxicity at infinite cell concentration and is always proportional to the effector cell concentration. Km represents the target cell concentration at which $v=\frac{1}{2}$ Vmax and is a measure of effector-target cell affinity. By using the Lineweaver-Burke transformation of the above equation;

$$1/Vmax = \frac{Km}{Vmax + s} + 1/v \quad (27)$$

Vmax can be obtained and plots of 1/v versus 1/s are linear with Vmax equal to the reciprocal of the y intercept and 1/Km numerically equal to -1/s where 1/v = 0. This latter plot may be used to analyze various inhibitor cell target-cell combinations to determine whether the inhibition is competitive or not. Competitive inhibition is presumed to be the result of the competition between antigenically similar ligands on different target cells for the same receptor on the effector cells. If these 1/v or 1/s plots of the number of cells lysed by a particular set of effector cells when incubated with varying concentrations of labeled target cells with or without varying concentrations of inhibitor cells have the same y intercepts (thus the same Vmax), then the inhibitor is defined as competitive. Those having different values for 1/Vmax (y intercept) will be considered as not competitive. This allows a statistical examination of competition between various cell lines for the same receptor sites on the effector cells. For the purposes of this discussion those inhibitors which give parallel lines in Lineweaver-Burke plots will be termed uncompetitive while those inhibitors which change the Vmax of the reaction while leaving Km unaffected will be termed non-competitive. This terminology is analogous to that used for enzyme kinetics but the mechanisms involved may differ from those operative in the inhibition of the cell mediated lysis. The term not competitive is used to include both uncompetitive and noncompetitive inhibition. Typical plots illustrating competitive inhibition versus the other types are shown in a subsequent section in this discussion.

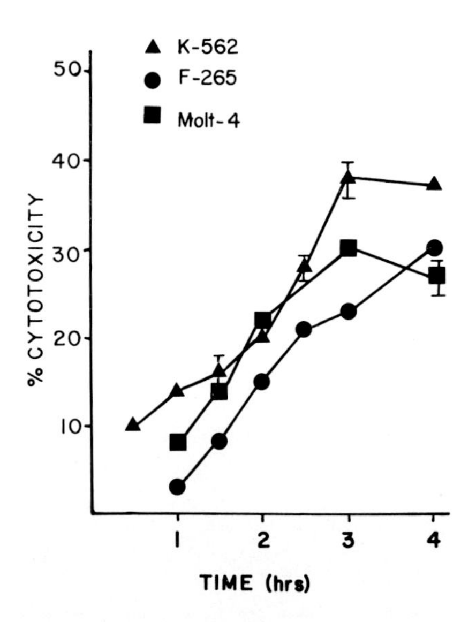

FIGURE 1. NCMC as a function of time of incubation. E:T=50:1.

III. RESULTS

Pollack (28) has shown that care must be taken to ensure that measurements are made during the initial steady state velocity which should be linear throughout the time period used. This linear time period has been found to vary with different target cells. Figure 1 demonstrates that linearity is maintained for three hours when K-562 or Molt-4 are used as target cells but is maintained an additional hour when F-265 is used. Figure 2 represents a typical experiment which demonstrates that changes in effector cell concentrations over the range indicated have little effect on this period of linearity. Changing the target cell concentration from 10^4 to 1.6×10^5 per culture has also been shown to have no effect on this linearity. It is for these reasons, unless otherwise stated, that all experiments are done with effector cell concentrations between 1×10^5 and 1×10^6 per culture. All assays are incubated for a three hour period. If the initial velocity of NCMC is truly linear during this period then

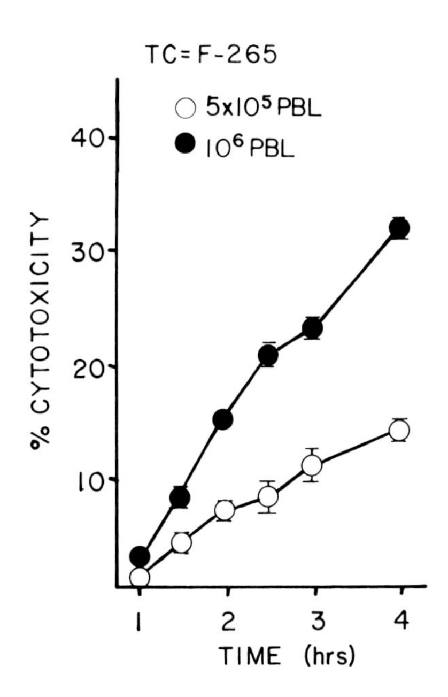

FIGURE 2. NCMC as a function or time of incubation with E:T=50:1 (5×10^5 PBL) or 100:1 (10^6PBL).

TABLE I. Effect of Incubation Time on Kinetics of NCMC[a]

Time of incubation	*Vmax x* 10^4	*Km x* 10^4
60 min	0.19 ± 0.03	0.91 ± 0.08
120 min	0.21 ± 0.08	0.87 ± 0.04
180 min	0.24 ± 0.02	0.90 ± 0.10

[a]*NCMC by 5 x* 10^5 *PBL incubated with 1,2,4 or 8 x* 10^4 ^{51}Cr *K-562 (mean ± SE).*

values obtained at various times during this period for Vmax and Km should be the same. Table I shows the results of an experiment designed to test this. As can be seen, the values obtained for Vmax and Km do not differ significantly when obtained at hourly intervals over a three hour period.

Several testable hypotheses may be formulated using this analogy of NCMC analysis to enzyme-substrate interactions. Km, as an indicator of effector cell-target cell binding affinity, should be characteristic for a given set of effector cells and should therefore not change with a change in effector cell concentration. Vmax, however, is a function of both the killing efficiency or a cell and the concentration of these cells. Callewaert et al (25) found that doubling the number of effector cells in the NCMC assay changed both Vmax and Km whereas our results closely parallel those of Pollack et al (28) in which this doubling produced a two fold increase in Vmax while leaving Km unaffected. Our results (Table II) agree with those of Pollack et al, in that doubling the number of effector cells causes an approximate doubling of Vmax with very little change in Km.

TABLE II. Effect of Effector Cell Concentration on Kinetics of NCMC[a]

Effector cell	*Vmax x* 10^4	*Km x* 10^4
2 x 10^5	0.35 ± 0.11	1.56 ± 0.21
4 x 10^5	0.62 ± 0.04	1.89 ± 0.15
8 x 10^5	1.04 ± 0.07	1.39 ± 0.17

[a]*NCMC incubated 3 hrs. at 37°C with 1,2,4,8 or 16 x* 10^4 ^{51}Cr *K-562 (mean ± SE).*

TABLE III. Kinetic Constants of NCMC with Different Target Cells[a]

^{51}Cr-target cell	Vmax	Km
K-562	0.74 ± 0.12	1.41 ± 0.15
Molt-4	0.32 ± 0.02	0.74 ± 0.03

[a]NCMC by 5 x 10^5 PBL from a single donor incubated 3 hrs. at 37°C with 1,2,4, or 8 x 10^4 ^{51}Cr-Target Cells (mean ± SE).

Table III shows that effector cells from a single donor have different values for Km and Vmax when tested against the two different isotopically labeled target cells K-562 and Molt-4. This suggests that either the receptor for each of these target cells is different for this donor's effector cells or that a different subset of target structures is recognized on each target cell such that the affinity of recognition for each of these target cells differs. The results of a similar experiment, shown in Table IV, demonstrate that effector cells from different donors have different values for Vmax and Km for a single target cell, K-562. This is not surprising as it is known that individuals vary in the expression of NCMC to this target cell.

Data demonstrating different Km values for effector cells from a single individual against K-562 and Molt-4 are especially interesting as it has been previously reported (15, 16) and shown by us (vide infra) using this kinetic analysis that K-562 and Molt-4 are mutually competitive inhibitors. This may mean that the effector cells recognize multiple structures on each cell line and that there is partial (but not complete) identity between these two families of antigens.

TABLE IV. Kinetic Constants of NCMC with Different Effector Cells[a]

Effector cells	Vmax x 10^4	Km x 10^4
Donor 1	1.15 ± 0.17	3.03 ± 0.64
Donor 2	0.55 ± 0.14	1.89 ± 0.10
Donor 3	0.74 ± 0.18	1.41 ± 0.07
Donor 4	0.24 ± 0.05	0.90 ± 0.02

[a]5 x 10^5 PBL incubated for 3 hrs. at 37°C with 1,2,4, or 8 x 10^4 ^{51}Cr K-562 (mean ± SE).

Stated otherwise, there may exist for Molt-4 and K-562 both mutually shared antigens and unique antigens with respect to NCMC. However, care must be taken in making these interpretations because as seen in Table IV effector cells from different individuals may recognize each cell line differently and information regarding mutual specificities between cell lines must be taken from and related to a single donor. Data from different donors can probably not be pooled for analysis of antigenic similarity.

The results of a typical experiment demonstrating competitive and not competitive inhibition of natural cell mediated cytotoxicity are shown in Figure 3. This is a conventional graphic representation of data and shows that the level of inhibition and thus the sensitivity of the assay is affected by the target cell concentration. The addition of either the homologous unlabeled cell line, or a second unlabeled cell line, Molt-4, leads to inhibition of the natural cytotoxicity of human PBL for labeled K-562. This inhibition would be termed competitive by the guidelines we have formulated in earlier publications (16) and would be interpreted as the result of competition by similar determinants on the cell lines K-562 and Molt-4 for the same receptor sites on the effector cells. The low order inhibition effected by the human cell line F-265 would be interpreted as being not competitive and

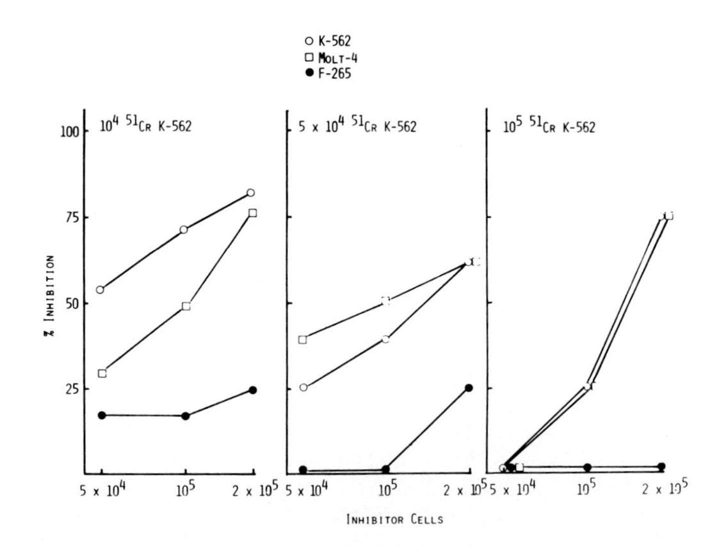

FIGURE 3. Inhibition of NCMC to ^{51}Cr K-562 by unlabeled K-562, Molt-4, or F-265.

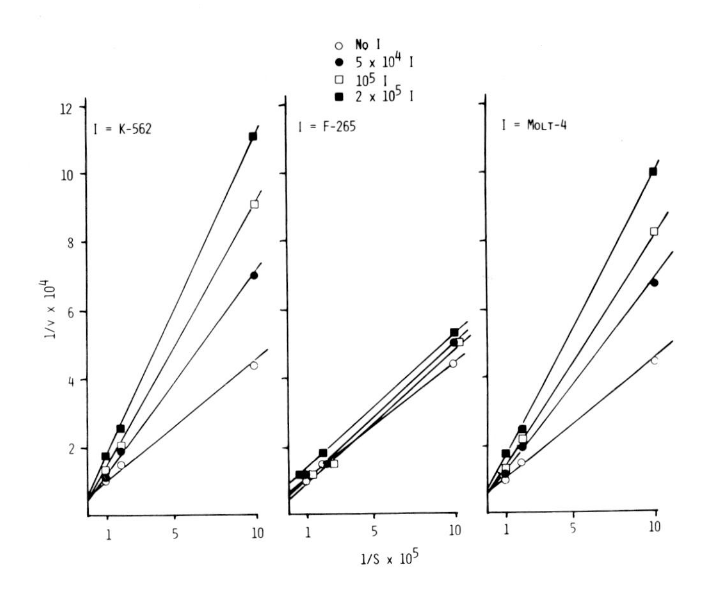

FIGURE 4. Reciprocal plot of velocity (cytotoxicity) as a function of substrate concentration ([51]Cr K-562) of data in Figure 3.

the result of some mechanism other than competition between two cell lines for the same binding sites on the effector cell. When the same data are plotted using the Lineweaver-Burke transformation (Figure 4) both unlabeled K-562 and Molt-4 can clearly be seen to be competitive inhibitors of the natural cytotoxicity toward K-562 (Vmax remains unchanged in the presence of either inhibitor). The inhibition by F-265 which was interpreted as being not competitive by previously used guidelines may now be interpreted more objectively. Close examination of the reciprocal plot of the inhibition of NK lysis of K-562 shows that at the inhibitor cell concentrations tested inhibition is not competitive. Statistical examination of the plots obtained show that they share the same slope and are therefore parallel. This would be interpreted as being an uncompetitive inhibitor by the classical methods of enzyme kinetic analysis.

Data derived from these experiments can be further analysed to give information about the magnitude of the interaction between the target cell surface structure (antigen) and the effector cell receptor sites. If a Dixon plot of the reciprocal of v as a function of the inhibitor concentration is constructed then a Ki (dissociation constant for the inhibitor cell from the effector cell) may be calculated. The point at which the straight line plots obtained at various substrate levels converge is I=Ki for competitive inhibition

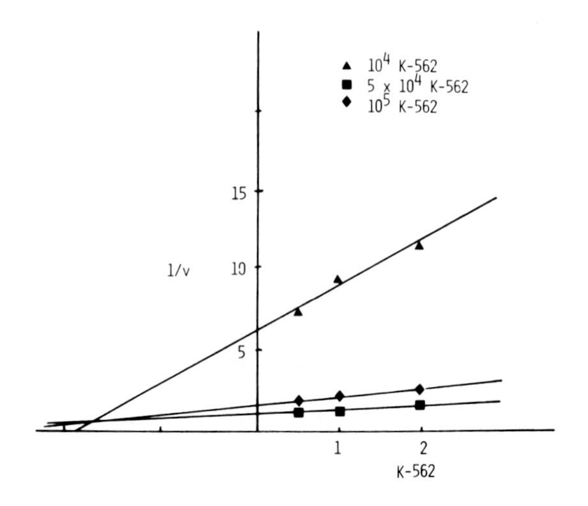

FIGURE 5. Dixon plot of data from Figures 3 and 4 of inhibition of ^{51}Cr K-562 lysis by unlabeled K-562.

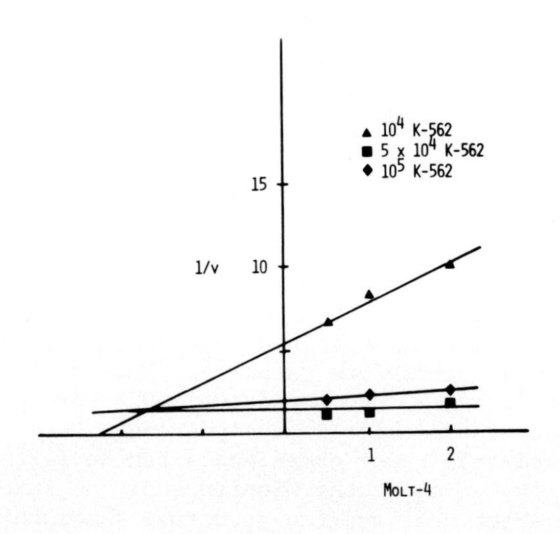

FIGURE 6. Dixon plot of data from Figures 3 and 4 of inhibition of ^{51}Cr K-562 lysis by unlabeled Molt-4.

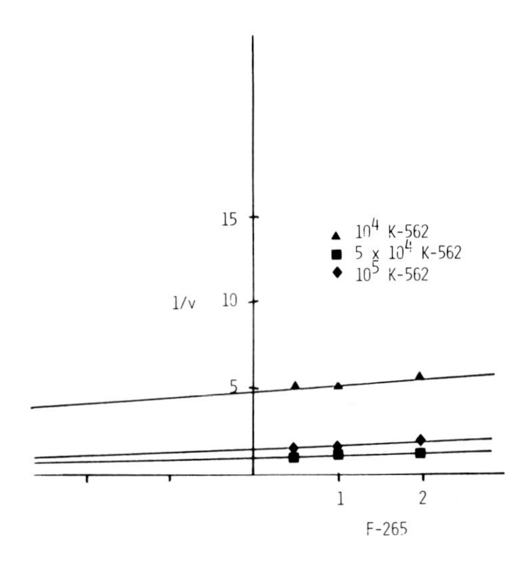

FIGURE 7. Dixon plot of data from Figures 3 and 4 of inhibition of ^{51}Cr K-562 lysis by unlabeled F-265.

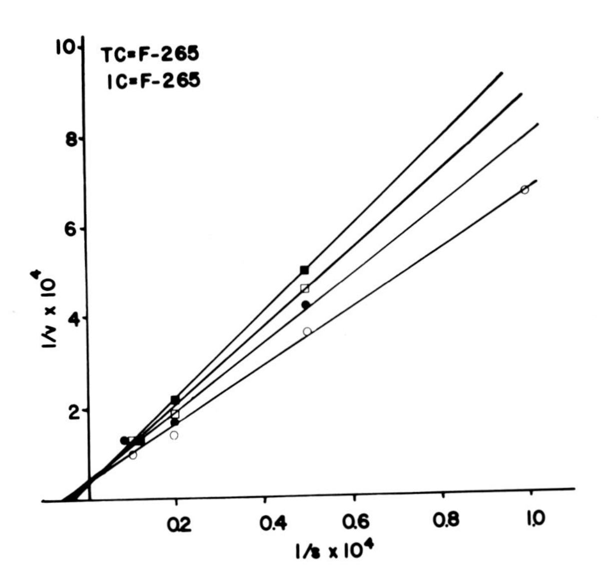

FIGURE 8. Reciprocal plot of velocity (cytotoxicity) as a function of substrate concentration (^{51}Cr F-265) of NCMC incubated with unlabeled F-265.

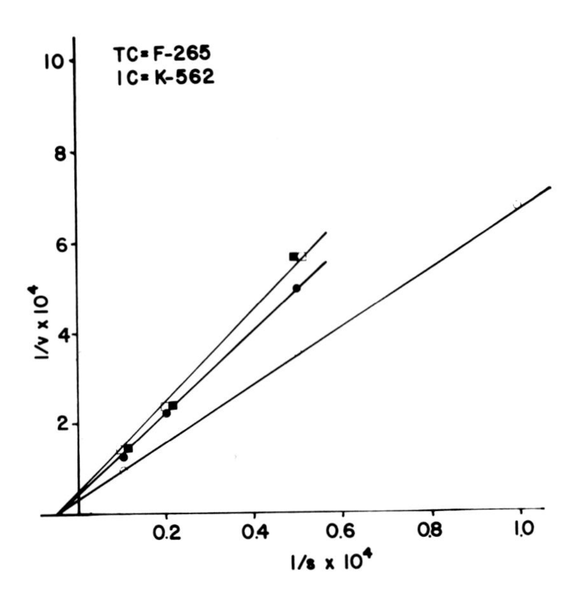

FIGURE 9. Reciprocal plot of velocity (cytotoxicity) as a function of substrate concentration (^{51}Cr F-265) of NCMC incubated with unlabeled K-562.

and is reflective of the affinity between receptor and ligand. Figures 5 and 6 demonstrate Dixon plots of the data presented in Figure 4 for the competitive inhibition of the lysis of labeled K-562 by either unlabeled K-562 or Molt-4. Both cell lines can be seen from these plots to have similar values for Ki and may be interpreted as having similar affinities of binding between themselves and the receptor sites on the effector cells. A Dixon plot of 1/v versus I for the inhibition of cell mediated lysis of K-562 by F-265 (Figure 7) reveals parallel lines which are indicative of uncompetitive inhibition.

Data from reciprocal experiments using labeled F-265 (^{51}Cr F-265) as the target cell are shown in Figures 8-11. The Lineweaver-Burke plot of inhibition of PBL mediated lysis of ^{51}Cr F-265 by various concentrations of non-labeled F-265 are shown in Figure 8. These curves can be seen to have the same Vmax and are indicative of competitive inhibition. Co-incubation of PBL, ^{51}Cr F-265, and unlabeled K-562 yields data shown in Figure 9. These curves do not share the same Vmax and are indicative of inhibition which is not competitive. Dixon plots of the same data (Figure 10 and 11) provide support to this conclusion: K-562 and F-265 are not competitive inhibitors of NCMC of each other and presumably do not

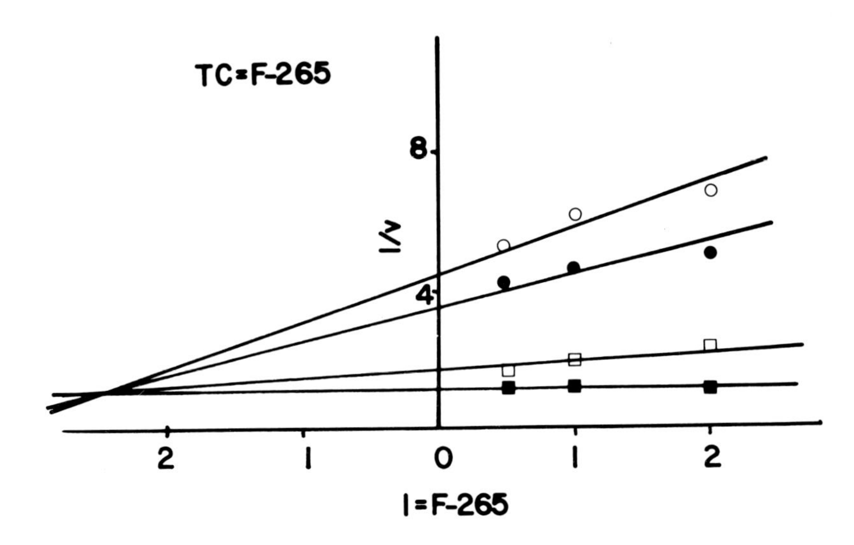

FIGURE 10. Dixon plot of data from Figure 8 of inhibition of ^{51}Cr F-265 lysis by unlabeled F-265.

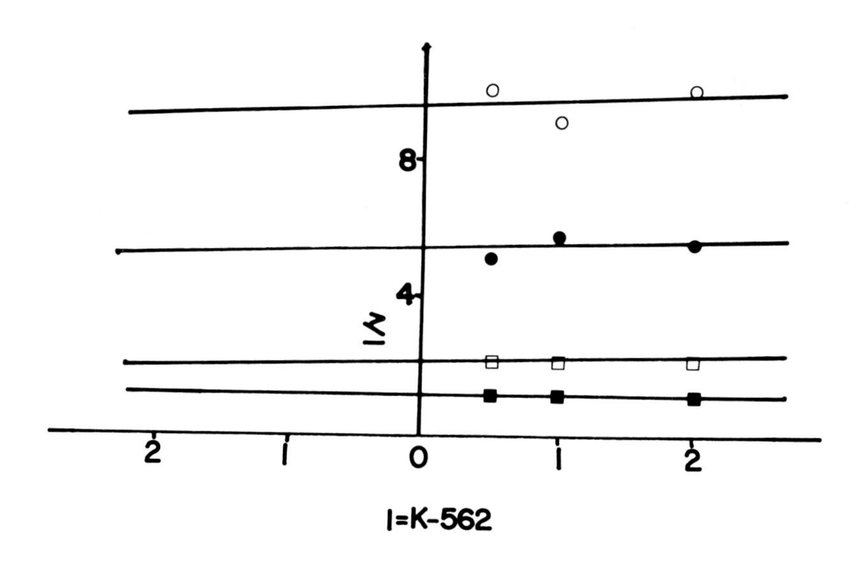

FIGURE 11. Dixon plot of data from Figure 9 of inhibition of ^{51}Cr F-265 lysis by unlabeled K-562.

share the same target structure(s). Similar experiments have shown not competitive inhibition of NCMC to K-562 by the human cell lines 5838, Heidi, Chang, and Raji.

IV. DISCUSSION

Using the enzyme kinetics analogy we have the ability to quantitate certain aspects of NCMC which have previously been expressed in qualitative ways. The Km (and the Ki) are measures of effector - target binding affinity and the Vmax is a measure of both the killing efficiency of the effector and the lysability of the target. This numerical quantitation lends great strength to our ability to investigate and interpret specificity of NCMC when compared to our earlier method of analysis of specificity in the competitive inhibition assay which was only semi-quantitative at best (16). These data, derived from kinetic analysis, demonstrate clearly and objectively that there are at least two nonoverlapping specificities operative in NCMC: one for the cell line K-562 and a distinct set of receptors for the cell line F-265. The data furthermore show that the set of receptors for NCMC against K-562 share a number of specificities with those for Molt-4. These data support but do not prove that these two sets of receptors for F-265 and K-562 are on separate populations of effector cells. If the receptors for K-562 and F-265 were on the same set of effector cells then steric hinderance would be expected cause more notcompetitive inhibition between these two cell lines than was observed. Therefore, we believe two sets of lymphocyte subpopulations are involved in the cytotoxicity toward K-562 and F-265.

The observation that several effector cell donors have similar receptor mechanisms for K-562 and Molt-4 as evidenced by mutually competitive inhibition suggests that these two cell lines have the same target structure array. However, data showing that individual sets of effector cells have distinct values for Km against K-562 and Molt-4 would suggest that only portions of the target structure array are shared by the two target cell lines. Thus, Molt-4 may either have structures all of which are represented on K-562 but make up less than the total target structure complement of K-562 (evidenced by the higher Km for K-562 than for Molt-4). Alternatively Molt-4 and K-562 may have some target structures in common and some structures unique to each cell line. Both of these hypothesis carry the implication that the target cell-effector cell interaction is the result of multiple different receptor-ligand interactions. What is not known and not addressed here is whether each effector cell recognizes the target structure concatenation *in toto* or not. Thus there are no data to determine whether specificity in NCMC is the property of one cell subpopulation with a single receptor array or several different cell subsets each contributing a unique receptor(s) to the total specificity.

In conclusion, it is seen that analysis of cytotoxic reactions in a manner analogous to enzyme kinetics represents a powerful new tool with which to quantitatively catalogue the specificity of NCMC. Data presented herein provide evidence that the specificity for NCMC is similar for at least two separate cell lines, K-562 and Molt-4, with preliminary data to suggest that other unique specificities may exist for other target cell lines. This in turn gives rise to a model consisting of NCMC effector cells composed of many subsets of cells segregated according to their specificities in a manner analogous to other cell mediated immunologic phenomena and confirms the immunologic nature of NCMC.

ACKNOWLEDGMENT

This work supported in part by contracts NCI-CB-64007-31 and BRS6 from the National Cancer Institute.

REFERENCES

1. Oldham, R.K., Siwarski, D., McCoy, J.L., et al, Nat'l Cancer Inst Monogr., 37-49-58, (1973).
2. Rosenberg, E.B., McCoy, J.L., Green, S.S. et al, J. Nat'l Cancer Inst., 52:345, (1974).
3. McCoy, J.L., Herberman, R.B., Rosenberg, E.B., Donnelly, F.C., et al,Nat'l Cancer Inst Monogr., 37:59, (1973).
4. Takasugi, M., Mickey, M.R., Terasaki, P.I., Cancer Res., 33:2898, (1973).
5. Jondal, M., Pross, H., Int J Cancer, 15:596, (1975).
6. Pross, H.F., Jondal, M., Clin Exp Immunol, 21:226, (1975).
7. Holtermann, D.A., Klein, E., Casale, E.P., Cell Immunol., 9:339, (1973).
8. Herberman, R.B., Nunn, M.E., Lavrin, D.H., Asofsky, R.J., Natl Cancer Inst., 51:1509, (1973).
9. Altman, A., Rapp, H.J., J. Immunol. 121:2244, (1978).
10. Oldham, R.K., Djeu, J.V., Cannon, G.B., Siwarski, D., Herberman, R.B., J. Nat'l. Cancer Inst. 55:1305, (1975).
11. Oldham, R.K., Dean, J., Cannon, G.B., Ortaldo, J.R., Dunston, G., Applebaum, F., McCoy, J., Herberman, R.B., Int. J. Cancer 18:145, (1976).

12. Herberman, R.B., Oldham, R.K., J. Natl Cancer Inst. 55:748, (1975).
13. Holden, H.T., Oldham, R.K., Ortaldo, J.R., Herberman, R. B., J. Nat'l Cancer Inst. 58:1061, (1977).
14. Ortaldo, J.R., Oldham, R.K., Holden, H.T., Herberman, R.B., Cell. Immunol. 25:60, (1976).
15. Oldham, R.K., Ortaldo, J.R., Holden, H.T., Herberman, R.B., J. Natl Cancer Inst. 59:1321, (1977).
16. Ortaldo, J.R., Oldham, R.K., Cannon, G.B., Herberman, R.B., J. Na. Cancer Inst. 59:77, (1977).
17. Herberman, R.B., Holden, H.T., Adv. in Cancer Res. 27:305, (1978).
18. Takasugi, M., Mickey, M.R., J. Natl. Cancer Inst. 57:255, (1976).
19. Haller, O., Kiessling, R., Orr, A., Karre, K., Nilsson, K., Wigzell, H. Int. J. Cancer 20:93, (1977).
20. Thoma, J.A., Tonton, M.H., Clark, W.R., J. Immunol. 120:991, (1978).
21. Van Oers, M.H., De Grode, E.Y., Zeijlemaker, W.P., J. Immunol. 121:499, (1978).
22. Zeijlemaker, W.P., Rien, H.J., Van Oers, M.H., De Grode, E.Y., Schellekens, P.T., J. Immunol. 119:1507, (1978).
23. Herrick, M.V., Pollack, S., J. Immunol. 121:1348,(1978).
24. Thorn, R.M., Henney, C.S., J. Immunol. 119:1973, (1977).
25. Callewaert, D.M., Johnson, D.F., Kearney, J., J. Immunol. 121:710, (1978).
26. Forbes, J.T., Oldham, R.K., Fed. Proc., 38:1279, (1979).
27. Wong, J.T., Kinetics of Enzyme Mechanisms, Academic Press, New York, (1975).
28. Pollack, S.B., Emmons, S.L., J. Immunol. 123:160, (1979).

HUMAN NATURAL CELL-MEDIATED CYTOTOXICITY: A POLYSPECIFIC SYSTEM[1]

Jerome Mark Greenberg
Mitsuo Takasugi

Department of Surgery
UCLA School of Medicine
Los Angeles, California

I. BACKGROUND AND HISTORY

A. *Specificity in Early Studies*

Early studies dealing with cell-mediated immunity to human tumors were influenced by the concept that tumors of a similar "histologic" type share antigens. A majority of the studies were primarily aimed at demonstrating this type of specificity (1-6). A study of putative specificity by Hellstrom *et al.*, using the colony inhibition technique and the microcytotoxicity assay, concluded that the antigenic cross-reactivity between tumors of the same "histologic" type did exist (2). In their results, not a single positive reaction was observed by patients against tumors of a different "histologic" type. In spite of the study's emphasis on the reactivity of patients with different cancers, it nevertheless became evident that the study was not investigating specificity. The criterion for specificity was one that prevailed at the time. It was based on a stronger reactivity by a patient than by control individuals against a tumor target derived from the same type of cancer as the patient. When a larger group of individuals was examined later, it was observed that cancer patients were not stronger

[1]*This work was supported in part by contracts N01-CB 74133 from the Tumor Immunology Section and N01-CP43211 from the Biological Carcinogenesis Branch, Division of Cancer Cause and Prevention, National Cancer Institute.*

ISBN 0-12-341350-8

reactors than healthy individuals against the same "histologic" type of tumor target cells (7,8). These studies underscored the weaknesses of the prevailing definition of specificity. Although the studies did not deal directly with specificity, they did demonstrate clearly that most individuals reacted against cultured cells in a reaction now known as natural cell-mediated cytotoxicity (NCMC).

B. *Emergence of Natural Cell-Mediated Cytotoxicity*

In an extensive study employing both short-term and established target tumor cells, the mean reactivity of cancer patients was not greater against their own type of tumor (7). Upon closer examination of the results, the average score was usually lower for cancer patients against most target cells. Most persons normally possessed effector cells in their circulation which were cytotoxic for cultured cells. Thus many questions were raised to challenge the methods employed in studies on specificity which based their conclusions on a greater reactivity by patients over controls. As a result of large-scale testing, it became evident that wide variability in reactivity existed among patients and healthy individuals. The detection of tumor specificity previously reported depended upon the persons selected for controls as well as upon the patients. The possibility of various effects other than tumor-associated reactivity, causing reduction of target cells, had to be considered. These effects included specific immunological factors such as previous sensitization to other target cell antigens (viral, fetal calf serum, etc.) and nonspecific factors (e.g., granulocyte contamination and cell crowding). All of these possibilities had to be investigated before progress could be achieved in the understanding of NCMC.

In a subsequent report, we extended the previous study and demonstrated that lymphocytes from patients with tumors of "histologic" types different from the target tumor cells reacted at least as strongly as lymphocytes from patients with the same "histologic" type (8). Along with comparisons of average reactivity by patients with different cancers, the study applied the Terry-Hoeffding statistical analysis (9) to exclude daily variations in testing which affect most cell-mediated tests. This analysis limited the comparisons to the results obtained on a single plate.

Findings from these two studies (7,8) indicated that improved methods of determining specificity were needed and that reactions to other than tumor-associated antigens were the dominating factors in these tests. Rather than disprove the existence of "histologic" type specificity, we demonstrated that a phenomenon other than reactivity to "histologic" type specificity accounted for what was previously interpreted as tumor-associated reactions.

Most studies concluding that tumor-associated specificity did exist employed a one-dimensional test design with several effector cells tested on a single target. When two-dimensional testing was employed, varying effector and target cells, the number of reactants was small and provided only slight improvement in viewing specificity. Fibroblasts were frequently used as a second target cell, but their low sensitivity to cytotoxicity reverted the tests to the equivalent of a one-dimensional study. With the recognition that normal individuals react in cytotoxic tests against cultured cells, emphasis shifted from tumor-associated antigens to the role of natural cell-mediated cytotoxicity.

II. DEFINING SPECIFICITY IN NATURAL CELL-MEDIATED SYSTEMS

A. *Selectivity and Nonselectivity*

In the search for specificity of natural cell-mediated cytotoxicity, the need for a better understanding of what constitutes specificity became apparent. At the Second Workshop on Cell-Mediated Cytotoxicity held at Sloan-Kettering Memorial Institute for Cancer Research in 1974, Dr. Eva Klein proposed the terms "selective" and "nonselective" cytotoxicity of target cells in place of "specificity" (10). With slight modification, this terminology has proved useful in our search for specificity (11). Selective cytotoxicity has been defined as that part of the cytotoxic reaction caused by a special interaction between the effector and target cell. Nonselective cytotoxicity, which may be considered part of the background, is essentially a reaction against all target cells. The differences in reactivity between target cells are accounted for by differences in the sensitivity of each target cell. It became clear that selective cytotoxic effects must be differentiated from nonselective cytotoxic effects in studies of specificity. In the original studies of specificity, this distinction between selective and nonselective cytotoxicity was attempted by comparing reactivity of patients with healthy individuals. This comparison became invalid when the reactivity among healthy individuals was observed to vary. Later, we will see that NCMC reactivity by healthy persons is partly selective and should not be totally regarded as background.

TABLE IA. Nonselectivity in the Interaction Analysis

Effector cell	Percent cytotoxicity	Target cells 1	2	3	Effector average (E_A)
A	Observed[a]	10	20	30	20
	Nonselective	10	20	30	
	Selective	0	0	0	
B	Observed	20	30	40	30
	Nonselective	20	30	40	
	Selective	0	0	0	
C	Observed	30	40	50	40
	Nonselective	30	40	50	
	Selective	0	0	0	
	Target average (T_A)	20	30	40	30[b]

TABLE IB. Selectivity in the Interaction Analysis

Effector cell	Percent cytotoxicity	Target cells 1	2	3	Effector average (E_A)
A	Observed[a]	10	20	30	20
	Nonselective	9	19	32	
	Selective	1	1	-2	
B	Observed	20	30	40	30
	Nonselective	19	29	42	
	Selective	1	1	-2	
F	Observed	30	40	60	43
	Nonselective	32	42	55	
	Selective	-2	-2	5	
	Target average (T_A)	20	30	43	31[b]

[a]Observed score is T in Eq. (2) of text
[b]Overall average (O_A)

B. Development of the Interaction Analysis

The recognition that effector cells differ in their cytotoxic capabilities and that target cells differ in their sensitivity makes it imperative that studies of specificity in cell-mediated cytotoxic systems be tested in a two-dimensional matrix varying effector and target cells. The implementation of such a design allows application of the interaction analysis to the results. The interaction analysis (11) was modified from the two-way analysis of variance for the purpose of differentiating selective from nonselective reactions. The two-way analysis of variance uses the average reactivity of the effector and target cells to estimate an expected nonselective score for each effector-target combination. It predicts the cytotoxic score based on the mean reactivity of each effector cell, the mean sensitivity of each target cell, and the average overall result. From these general properties of each reactant, the interaction analysis identifies that part of the reaction which does not reflect any special relationship and emphasizes the variation from the estimated scores as selective. It is this part of the reaction that reflects specificity.

Table I illustrates the application of the interaction analysis. In Table IA, three effector cells, A, B, and C, are tested against target cells 1, 2, and 3. Effectors A, B, and C react with target 1 for 10, 20, and 30% cytotoxicity. If only target 1 is tested, one might conclude that C is specific for target 1. However, one can see the fallacy of this conclusion when targets 2 and 3 are included, for the same pattern is observed. It is apparent from the observed and average scores that target cells 2 and 3 are more sensitive than target 1, just as effectors B and C are more reactive than effector A. The observed score in Table 1A, as in most tests, reflects the reactivity of the effector cells and the sensitivity of the target cells.

The nonselective cytotoxicity is calculated by application of the two-way analysis of variance. It is estimated for each combination of effector and target cell by adding the effector and target cell averages and subtracting the average for all tests, as in Eq. (1).

$$\text{Nonselective cytotoxicity} = E_A + T_A - O_A \qquad (1)$$

The effector cell results averaged against all target cells are represented by E_A; the target cell results averaged with all effector cells by T_A; and the average results from all tests by O_A. In the example of Table 1A, the nonselective score is the same as the observed score. The results are thus nonselective. The selective score is the difference between the observed score (T) and the nonselective score, as in Eq. (2).

$$\text{Selective cytotoxicity} = T - (E_A + T_A - O_A) \tag{2}$$

$$= \text{Observed cytotoxicity} - \text{Nonselective cytotoxicity}$$

The selective score was zero for this set of results.

In Table IB, we show approximately the same results except that effector F reacts with target 3 at 60% cytotoxicity, 10% more than effector C reacts with the same target. We introduce this special interaction to illustrate the use of the interaction analysis in distinguishing selective cytotoxicity. The nonselective score was estimated and a selective score of 5% was calculated for effector F against target 3. This is half of the observed 10% difference between effectors F and C against target 3. Thus the selective score is only a minimal estimate of selectivity.

As experience was gained in the application of the interaction analysis and as our understanding of selective scores improved, it became apparent that the analysis introduced certain problems. An awareness of these potential problems was needed to avoid misinterpretation of the results. When a particularly strong or weak interaction occurs, the selective scores of other tests in the same column or row are also affected, since they are compared with the average. For example, in Table IB a strong positive effect by effector F on target 3 drives the other results with F or target 3 to the negative side. This in turn causes the results by effectors A and B on targets 1 and 2 to become weakly positive. Whether these weak positive scores represent true selectivity may be confirmed by reexamining the observed scores, which have not been averaged. The problem is also diminished by expanding the two-dimensional test array.

C. Cold Target Inhibition and the Cross-Competition Assay

There are at least three alternate ways to explain nonselective reactions in direct cytotoxic tests (12). They include: 1) a nonspecific effect against all target cells, 2) a specific reaction by effector cells against antigens present on all target cells, and 3) a polyspecific effect against different antigens on each of the target cells. The use of the cross-competition assay (12,13) allows one to determine which of the above alternatives best describes the actual phenomenon.

TABLE II. Interaction Analysis Applied to Results of NCMC Against Lymphoblastoid Lines

Competitor cells	Percentage ^{51}Cr release by effector against target cells: CEM	8402	8382	NC37
None	43	24	54	46
CEM	0	4	30	9
8402	2	6	37	18
8382	1	5	25	5
NC37	6	5	27	4

Application of interaction analysis to percentage inhibition[a]

Competitor cells	Percent inhibition	Target cells: CEM	8402	8382	NC37	Average observed
CEM	Observed	100	83	44	80	77
	Nonselective	97	81	47	82	
	Selective	3	2	-3	-2	
8402	Observed	95	75	31	61	66
	Nonselective	86	70	36	71	
	Selective	9	5	-5	-10	
8382	Observed	98	79	54	89	80
	Nonselective	100	84	50	85	
	Selective	-2	-5	4	4	
NC37	Observed	86	79	50	91	77
	Nonselective	97	81	47	82	
	Selective	-11	-2	3	9	
	Average observed	95	79	45	80	75[b]

[a] Percentage inhibition is derived from Eq. (3) of text
[b] Overall average (O_A)

If a nonspecific cytotoxic effect is involved, the addition of an unlabeled competitor cell would not cause any selective inhibition (any physical interference would be nonselective). If, however, antigens shared by every target cell are specifically recognized by the effector cell, cytotoxicity for all target cells would be inhibited by any unlabeled competitor cell (this is again nonselective). Finally, if the effector cell suspension reacts specifically with different antigens on each target cell, the presence of a competitor with the same antigens would cause selective inhibition of cytotoxicity for that target cell.

Results of the cross-competition assay testing the same four target and competitor cells supported the third alternative as best describing the cell interactions in NCMC (Table II). Each cell line selectively inhibited cytotoxicity when competing with itself, indicating that the effector cells recognized some antigens unique for that cell. Thus the experimental results support the existence of a polyspecific system which has the appearance of nonselectivity in direct testing.

Nonselective results, even if specific, cannot be distinguished from nonspecific effects and provide no information on specificity. Only selective effects provide such information. The interaction analysis allows distinction of selective from nonselective inhibition and has improved our understanding of NCMC. There is a tendency among investigators to employ a one-dimensional test design with one target cell and several competitors in the cold target inhibition assay. Specificity must be viewed as a two-dimensional problem and tests should be performed in an array using several target cells and several competitors.

D. Rules to Determine Specificity in Polyspecific Systems

Some rules have been suggested which are helpful in defining specificity in a polyspecific system such as NCMC (12). We have already discussed the first rule (Sections II,A and II,C), namely that selective reactivity must be differentiated from nonselective effects. This can be accomplished by two-dimensional testing and by application of the interaction analysis.

The second rule is that the antigen(s) responsible for the selectivity must be identified. This is accomplished by detecting the specificity with two or more target cells. It can also be achieved by selective inhibition of cytotoxicity against a target cell. Selective inhibition identifies the sharing of antigens between the target and competitor cell. We have stated that specificity is determined by identification of an antigen present on at least two target cells; if more target

TABLE III. *Application of Interaction Analysis to Cytotoxicity Results*

Effector cell no.	Cytotoxicity	Mean reduction in titer scores for target cells: 497	548	696	917	372	G11	OG	MeWo	H894	T24	Effector average
112524	Observed	62	47	75	59	79	91	75	68	86	52	69
	Nonselective	71	59	76	61	65	76	69	77	98	40	
	Selective	-9	-12	-1	-2	14	15	6	-9	-12	12	
112525	Observed	65	52	67	53	59	78	76	68	92	32	64
	Nonselective	66	54	71	56	60	71	64	72	93	35	
	Selective	-1	-2	-4	-3	-1	7	12	-4	-1	-3	
112537	Observed	58	51	60	45	29	31	28	67	88	8	47
	Nonselective	49	37	54	39	43	54	47	55	76	18	
	Selective	9	14	6	6	-14	-23	-19	12	12	-10	
	Target average (T_A)	62	50	67	52	56	67	60	68	89	31	60[a]

[a]Overall average (O_A)

cells have the antigen, the specificity is more clearly defined. Reactivity identified at the target cell level may thus be categorized as selective or nonselective. Once the antigen is identified, specificity can then be considered.

The third rule is that the antigen(s) identified above needs to be associated with some causative element (e.g., viruses, disease, or genetic factors). This can be accomplished by associating the antigen(s) with an identifiable class of effectors or with a class of target cells having a known derivation (see chapter by Kamiyama and Takasugi).

III. DETECTING SPECIFICITY IN NATURAL CELL-MEDIATED SYSTEMS

We have discussed the background of NCMC and a new approach toward determining specificity. Having introduced the interaction analysis and having applied it to the direct and cross-competition assay, we now turn to the actual detection of specificity. We will then move to the level of the effector cell and discuss its role in the mediation of specificity.

A. *Direct Testing*

Identification of the target antigens for NCMC was attempted in a study by Takasugi *et al.* (14) using the microassay for cell-mediated immunity (15). The study examined the reactions by effector cells from 240 cancer patients and healthy individuals against 10 cultured cell lines. Four effector suspensions were tested simultaneously against the 10 target cells. Representative results are shown in Table III. Certain cell lines appear to share common target specificities when the selective scores are compared. Since the interaction analysis emphasizes relative differences, the signs of the selective scores may be used to identify similarities and dissimilarities. Target cells 372, G11, and OG react alike. Target cells 497, 548, 696, and 917 also show similarities as do MeWo and H894.

To test whether these groupings do exist, the results obtained for the 240 individuals were analyzed for selectivity in sets of four tested on the same plate. The selective scores were further analyzed for similarity in reactivity against target cells by the regression analysis and the chi-square test. The rationale was that target cells which share antigens behave in a more similar manner than target cells which do not. Employing the selective results for the 240 effector suspensions, coefficients of correlation for the target cells

TABLE IV. Inhibition in the Cross-Competition Assay

Competitor cells	Percent inhibition	Target cells								Average
		548	696	917	372	G11	OG	MeWo	H894	
696	Observed	79	82	100	28	10	73	75	44	63
	Nonselective	44	51	70	27	39	93	84	91	
	Selective	35	31	30	1	-29	-20	-9	-47	
917	Observed	100	87	99	17	39	85	72	90	74
	Nonselective	55	62	81	38	50	104	95	102	
	Selective	45	25	18	-21	-11	-19	-23	-12	
G11	Observed	33	58	54	7	34	93	59	86	53
	Nonselective	34	41	60	17	29	83	74	81	
	Selective	-1	17	-6	-10	5	10	-15	5	
OG	Observed	-51	-15	25	30	34	90	82	90	36
	Nonselective	17	24	43	0	12	66	57	64	
	Selective	-68	-39	-18	30	22	24	25	26	
H894	Observed	13	-2	25	8	32	80	89	100	43
	Nonselective	24	31	50	7	19	73	64	71	
	Selective	-11	-33	-25	1	13	7	25	29	
	Average	35	42	61	18	30	84	75	82	54[a]

[a]Overall average (O_A)

were obtained. Significant positive correlations between target cells confirmed the existence of the groups above. These same similarities existed in experiments testing effector cells from healthy individuals as well as from cancer patients and patients with other diseases.

On the basis of these results, the target cells were tentatively grouped into TA 1 (targets 497, 548, 696, 917), TA 2 (G11, OG, 372), and TA 3 (MeWo, H894). It was becoming more evident that what originally appeared to be nonselective reactivity in NCMC was in fact rather specific.

B. Cross-Competition and Inhibition Studies

In view of the polyspecificity of the reactions, the cross-competition assay provides a more straightforward demonstration of specificity than the direct cytotoxicity assay. The cross-competition assay employs several ^{51}Chromium-labeled (^{51}Cr) target cells and the same unlabeled competitor cells. The interaction analysis is then applied to the inhibition results to obtain selective scores. The percent inhibition is derived from Eq. (3).

$$\%\ \text{inhibition} = 1 - \frac{\%\ \text{cytotoxicity with competitor}}{\%\ \text{cytotoxicity without competitor}} \qquad (3)$$

Stronger inhibition by one competitor cell over another does not by itself provide information on specificity. Cytotoxicity against other target cells may be inhibited in the same way, which is again nonselective. For information on specificity, selective inhibition involving a special relationship of shared antigens between competitor and target cells needs to be differentiated from nonselective inhibition. Thus, the interaction analysis is as applicable to inhibition as it is to cytotoxicity. The analysis applied to the results from the cross-competition assay has aided in the detection of specificity of NCMC in a variety of systems (14,16).

1. Target Antigens (TA) 1, 2, 3. We have already seen as a result of direct NCMC testing that certain tumor-derived target cells could be classified into groups, based on their similar reactivity. Ten target cells were tentatively classified into groups designated TA 1, 2, and 3. We will see that their existence is confirmed by the cross-competition assay. The results from one representative study (14) are presented in Table IV. Positive selective scores indicate an observed inhibition greater than that predicted by overall nonselectivity. It is apparent from Table IV that a target cell in competition with itself displays a positive selective score. This is a prerequisite for demonstrating the sharing of antigens by two or more different cells in the cross-competition assay. Before an assessment of cross-reactivity between target cells can be made, selective inhibition must be observed against a target cell by the same competitor cell.

The similarity of reactivity within the previously designated groups TA 1, 2, and 3 can also be seen in Table IV. Furthermore, when composite selective scores were derived from the results of different tests, selective inhibition by competition was observed among TA 1 cells, i.e., TA 1 cells competed with other TA 1 cells but not with cells from TA 2 and 3. Some cross-reactivity was observed between TA 2 and TA 3 cells. This further emphasizes that we are dealing with a complex polyspecific system involving the recognition of multiple antigens on target cells.

2. *Lymphoblastoid Cell Lines.* The cross-competition assay has also been useful in detecting the specificity of natural cytotoxicity against lymphoblastoid cell lines. In a study of inhibition of NCMC against lymphoblastoid lines, four ^{51}Cr-labeled target cells were tested with the same four unlabeled competitor cells (12). Table II shows representative results from this study in which percent cytotoxicity was converted to percent inhibition (see Eq. (3), this section) and then investigated with the interaction analysis. It is evident from Table II that each cell line establishes its individuality by selective inhibition (positive selective scores) across the diagonal. Furthermore, it can be seen that the two T-cell lines (CEM and 8402) react alike as do the two B-cell lines (8382 and NC37). This is apparent from the similarity in the signs of the selective scores, implying the recognition of antigens specific for B-cell lines and for T-cell lines.

C. Arming in NCMC with Specific Antibodies

Although the reactivity of most normal individuals against target cells is largely nonselective, there exist cells within the effector suspensions which react in a specific manner against different target cell antigens. Specific inhibition by competitor cells supported this hypothesis and served to direct efforts toward further detection of specificity at the level of the effector cell.

When it was observed that pretreating effector cells with trypsin and other proteolytic enzymes decreased NCMC activity against lymphoblastoid cell lines, but had little effect on and in some cases enhanced ADCC (17), it became apparent that the specificity of the natural cytotoxic reaction was mediated by some protein on the effector cell surface. Previously it had been shown that IgG could be dissociated from some IgG-positive cells by exposure to low pH (18). After this treatment was found to decrease NCMC activity (17), it seemed evident that the protein on the NK cell surface was immunoglobulin. Results from the same study demonstrated that, when trypsin treated effector cells were incubated with autologous or allogeneic serum, NCMC activity was recovered. Any selective reactivity which was present before trypsin treatment, was recovered after reconstitution of the effector cells with serum.

In order to confirm that serum antibodies were mediating the specificity of the reaction, the serum used to reconstitute the effector cells was first absorbed with different cultured cells and then tested on these same cells (19). The reasoning behind this procedure was that, by removing antibodies against a target cell, cytotoxicity for that target cell should be selectively abolished. Representative results are shown in Table V. A selective loss of cytotoxicity against a

TABLE V. Selective Loss of Inhibition by Absorption of Natural Antibodies from Serum

Serum absorbed with	Loss	Percent cytotoxicity loss by absorption				Effector average
		497	OG	H894	G11	
497	Observed	45	4	6	11	17
	Nonselective	31	7	12	18	
	Selective	14	-3	-6	-7	
OG	Observed	12	6	2	14	9
	Nonselective	23	-1	4	10	
	Selective	-11	7	-2	4	
H894	Observed	14	2	15	10	10
	Nonselective	24	0	5	11	
	Selective	-10	2	10	-1	
G11	Observed	45	6	15	29	24
	Nonselective	38	14	19	25	
	Selective	7	-8	-4	4	
	Target average	29	5	10	16	15

target cell upon reconstitution with absorbed serum substantiated the important role of antibodies in mediating NCMC. Sharing of specificities or cross-reactivity was observed again (Table V). For example, absorption with target G11 caused selective loss of cytotoxicity for target 497. Natural cytotoxic activity specific for a target cell may also be achieved by eluting specific antibodies from the absorbing cells and reconstituting the effector cells in the neutralized eluate. Reconstitution of effector cells with eluates from a target cell results in selective cytotoxicity for that cell. These results suggest that a major part of NCMC is mediated by a cell that is nonselective with polyspecific natural antibodies directing its specificity.

The arming of effector cells with antibodies has also been useful in revealing specificity against human leukocyte antigens (HLA). In a study by J. Takasugi *et al.*, natural antibodies were partially removed from HLA-specific sera through preabsorption with lymphoblastoid lines which lacked the HLA

TABLE VI. Selective Cytotoxicity by Specifically Reconstituted Effector Cells

Effector cell incubated in anti-HLA:	Percent cytotoxicity	Target cells: CEM[a]	Raji[b]	HSB-2[c]	Average
A1	Observed	44	32	37	38
	Nonselective	36	41	38	
	Selective	8	-9	-1[d]	
A3	Observed	8	38	3	16
	Nonselective	14	19	16	
	Selective	-6	19	-13	
B12	Observed	7	5	25	12
	Nonselective	10	15	12	
	Selective	-3	-10	13	
	Average	20	25	22	22

[a]A1, Aw30, B8, Bw40
[b]A3, A10, Bw18, Bw35
[c]A1, A2, B12, Bw17
[d]False negative

specificity detected by the sera (20). Effector cells were then reconstituted with the absorbed anti-HLA sera. Representative results appear in Table VI. The HLA specificities of the lymphoblastoid lines are shown at the bottom of the table. When the interaction analysis was applied to the results, selective reactivity associated with HLA was observed. A false negative result was obtained with HSB-2 because two of the three target cells carried HLA-1. If all of the target cells carried the A-1 antigen, specific reactivity for this antigen would have the appearance of nonselectivity. When average reactivity is used as a reference, only the stronger reactions are discerned. In total, 8 of 9 combinations in Table VI showed the predicted selective reactivity.

IV. A MODEL FOR THE MEDIATION OF SPECIFICITY BY ANTIBODIES

The mechanism of NCMC is presently involved in controversy and discussion (21-26). Our interest in the mechanism of cell-mediated cytotoxicity was first aroused when we observed a strong similarity between NCMC and ADCC (27). The activity by effector cells from different individuals tested in NCMC and ADCC was observed to correlate. Furthermore, when effector cells were fractionated by a variety of methods, activity for both assays appeared in the same fractions. We felt that the similarity between NCMC and ADCC represented a common element. An important component of each reaction may indeed involve the same class of effector cells.

A majority of the cells that mediate NCMC and ADCC bear Fc receptors (23,28-30). We envisioned a model system, involving antibodies specific for target cells, mediated by cells with Fc receptors. The site and temporal order of antibody-cell interaction differentiated NCMC and ADCC. In NCMC, circulating natural IgG antibodies become loosely attached to the effector cells through Fc-Fc receptor interaction and direct the specificity of the reaction. Polyspecific natural antibodies recognize antigens on most cultured cells giving the overall appearance of nonselectivity. ADCC involves the same effector cells as NCMC but the antibodies in ADCC react first with the target cell. Then the Fc and Fc receptor interact to initiate the cytotoxic reaction.

Two procedures have provided noteworthy exceptions to the parallelism between NCMC and ADCC: the treatment of effector cells with proteases and the addition of protein A to the reaction. Both are compatible with the model outlined above. Trypsin treatment of the effector cells decreases NCMC but has little effect on ADCC and may even increase it (17,23,31). The antibodies held loosely on effector cells may be removed with trypsin, reducing NCMC and at the same time freeing Fc receptors for a slight increase in ADCC. It has been reported that protein A decreases ADCC but does not affect NCMC (23). Protein A blocks ADCC since the Fc-Fc receptor interaction is inhibited. NCMC is unaffected since the Fc-Fc receptor interaction is already completed when protein A is introduced.

The model we proposed has been questioned in two respects: 1) whether antibodies are involved in NCMC and 2) whether the same effector cell mediates both NCMC and ADCC. The model has been useful in initiating studies but is probably an oversimplification of the real phenomenon. NCMC and ADCC are heterogeneous reactions, involving several subclasses of effector cells (see chapter by Kamiyama and Takasugi). Moreover, immunoglobulin dependent and independent reactions have been reported in NCMC (21,24). However, we still hold that there is at least one subclass of effector cells which mediates both NCMC and ADCC and that antibodies are an integral part of NCMC.

The most effective criticisms of our model are based on the inability of some investigators to recover reactivity after trypsin-treatment by incubation in serum (22,23,25) and the observation that effector cells which react in NCMC do not in ADCC (32). In our opinion, the specificity of NCMC is a better indicator of the role of antibodies than is the level of reactivity by itself. Manipulation of the available antibodies in the reconstituting serum or the use of specific antibodies such as those directed to HLA antigens influence the specificity of the reconstituted cytotoxicity. To demonstrate specificity, it is necessary to employ a two-dimensional test design using several reconstituted effector cells against several target cells with analysis for selectivity. Most workers have used a single target cell and have measured reactivity rather than specificity.

When the same effector suspension is tested in NCMC and ADCC and reactivity is observed in one test but not in the other, it appears as if different effector cells are active in the two tests. This is true if NCMC and ADCC are equal in sensitivity. However, ADCC is generally more sensitive than NCMC. Also differences in sensitivity for target cells within each system are observed. These differences need to be considered before reaching the conclusion that separate effector cells react in the two assays. To conclude that different cells are involved, effector cells from other individuals should be tested too. If these control individuals also show a stronger effect in NCMC than in ADCC, it is likely that the results reflect only the sensitivity of the target systems.

In conclusion, we have seen that early studies attempting to deal with specificity of cell-mediated immunity did not really examine specificity. With the emergence of NCMC and the recognition that normal individuals react against cultured tumor cells, it became evident that further investigations would require a better understanding of specificity. We have seen how the use of two-dimensional testing and application of the interaction analysis have aided in distinguishing selective from nonselective reactivity, which is a necessary step toward determining specificity. Results from the cross-competition assay indicated that what appeared to be nonselectivity in direct testing of NCMC was in fact specific and that within the effector suspension were subpopulations which reacted specifically with different antigens on each target cell. We also saw how direct testing and inhibition studies were applied to the detection of specificity in various target systems and how arming of effector cells with specific antibodies supported the polyspecific nature of NCMC. Finally, we discussed a model for the mediation of specificity in which ADCC and NCMC involve a common subclass of effector cells, with the antibody-cell interaction site differentiating the two, and in which antibodies are also an integral part of NCMC. While the mechanism of NCMC continues to be debated, the available evidence appears to support NCMC being a polyspecific system whose nature is indeed complex.

REFERENCES

1. Hellstrom, I., Hellstrom, K. E., Pierce, G. E., and Yang, J. P. S., *Nature (London) 220,* 1352 (1968).
2. Hellstrom, I., Hellstrom, K. E., Sjogren, H. O., and Warner, G. A., *Int. J. Cancer 7,* 1 (1971).
3. Bubenik, J., Perlmann, P., Helmstein, K., and Moberger, G., *Int. J. Cancer 5,* 39 (1970).
4. Bubenik, J., Perlmann, P., Helmstein, K., and Moberger, G., *Int. J. Cancer 5,* 310 (1970).
5. O'Toole, C., Perlmann, P., Unsgaard, B., Moberger, G., and Edsmyr, F., *Int. J. Cancer 10,* 77 (1972).
6. O'Toole, C., Perlmann, P., Unsgaard, B., Moberger, G., and Edsmyr, F., *Int. J. Cancer 10,* 92 (1972).
7. Takasugi, M., Mickey, M. R., and Terasaki, P. I., *Cancer Res. 33,* 2898 (1973).
8. Takasugi, M., Mickey, M. R., and Terasaki, P. I., *J. Natl. Cancer Inst. 53,* 1527 (1974).
9. Gibbons, J. D., "Nonparametric Statistical Inference", McGraw-Hill, New York, (1971).
10. Bean, M. A., Bloom, B. R., Herberman, R. B., Old, L. J., Oettgen, H. F., Klein, G., and Terry, W. D., *Cancer Res. 35,* 2902 (1975).

11. Takasugi, M., and Mickey, M. R., *J. Natl. Cancer Inst. 57,* 255 (1976).
12. Takasugi, M., Koide, Y., Akira, D., and Ramseyer, A., *Int. J. Cancer 19,* 291 (1977).
13. Ortiz de Landazuri, M., and Herberman, R. B., *Nature (London), New Biol. 238,* 18 (1973).
14. Takasugi, M., Akira, D., Takasugi, J., and Mickey, M. R., *J. Natl. Cancer Inst. 59,* 69 (1977).
15. Takasugi, M., and Klein, E., *Transplantation 9,* 219 (1970).
16. Koide, Y., and Takasugi, M., *Eur. J. Immunol. 8,* 818 (1978).
17. Koide, Y., and Takasugi, M., *J. Natl. Cancer Inst. 59,* 1099 (1977).
18. Kumagai, K., Abo, T., Sekizawa, T., and Sasaki, M., *J. Immunol. 115,* 982 (1976).
19. Akira, D., and Takasugi, M., *Int. J. Cancer 19,* 747 (1977).
20. Takasugi, J., Koide, Y., and Takasugi, M., *Eur. J. Immunol. 7,* 887 (1977).
21. Pape, G. R., Troye, M., and Perlmann, P., *J. Immunol. 118,* 1925 (1977).
22. Kay, H. D., Bonnard, G. D., and Herberman, R.B., *J. Immunol. 122,* 675 (1979).
23. Kay, H. D., Bonnard, G. D., West, W. W., and Herberman, R. B., *J. Immunol. 118,* 2058 (1977).
24. Troye, M., Perlmann, P., Pape, G. R., Spiegelberg, H. L., Naslund, I., and Gidlof, A., *J. Immunol. 119,* 1061 (1977)
25. Perussia, B., Trinchieri, G., and Cerottini, J. C., *J. Immunol. 123,* 681 (1979).
26. Herberman, R. B., Djeu, J. Y., Kay, H. D., Ortaldo, J. R., Riccardi, C., Bonnard, G. D., Holden, H. T., Fagnani, R., Santoni, A., and Puccetti, P., *Immunological Rev. 44,* 43 (1979).
27. Ting, A., and Terasaki, P. I., *Cancer Res. 34,* 2694 (1974).
28. Kiuchi, M., and Takasugi, M., *J. Natl. Cancer Inst. 56,* 575 (1976).
29. Bolhuis, R. L. H., Shuit, H. R. E., Nooyen, A. M., and Ronteltap, C. P. M., *Eur. J. Immunol. 8,* 731 (1978).
30. Bakacs, T., Gergely, P., Cornain, S., and Klein, E., *Int. J. Cancer 19,* 441 (1977).
31. Kall, M. A., and Koren, H. S., *Cell. Immunol. 47,* 57 (1979).
32. Koren, H. S., Amos, D. B., and Buckley, R. H., *J. Immunol. 120,* 796 (1978).

INTERACTION BETWEEN NK CELLS AND NORMAL TISSUE: DEFINITION OF A NK-SENSITIVE THYMOCYTE POPULATION

Mona Hansson
Rolf Kiessling

Department of Tumor Biology
Karolinska Institutet
Stockholm, Sweden

Raymond Welsh

Department of Immunopathology
Scripps Clinic and Research Foundation
La Jolla, California

I. INTRODUCTION

Several lines of evidence from murine experiment systems now strongly suggest that NK cells are involved in rejection of tumor cells (for review see ref. 1). The topic of this chapter will, however, be related to the entirely different finding that NK cells, apart from being able to destroy neoplastic cells, also may interact with and lyse certain normal cell types, thymocytes in particular.

Experimental evidence supporting the notion that NK cells may be of importance in rejecting non-transformed hematopoietic tissue stems from two different sets of information. The more indirect approach has been to compare the NK system with the mechanism of rejection of normal bone-marrow grafts, mostly studied in parental to F_1-hybrid grafting ("hybrid resistance"). This resistance to bone-marrow grafts, as studied by Cudkowicz (2), has a quite peculiar immunobiology which sets it apart from "classical" immunological rejection mechanisms of *e. g.*

ISBN 0-12-341350-8

skin grafts. Comparative studies between the mechanism behind bone marrow graft resistance and that of mouse NK activity have pointed to a number of striking similarities (3, 4, 5) such as T-cell independence, sensitivity to in vivo treatment of certain anti-macrophage drugs, relative radiation resistance, and several other common features. These similarities suggest that a common or at least very similar mechanism is operative in both these experimental systems. Recent studies by Hochman and Cudkowicz (6), however, demonstrated a difference in susceptibility to treatment with hydrocortisone between these two systems indicating that this relationship is not a simple one and probably involves a great deal of complexity. Also in regards to the genetic regulation of these two systems, there are some similarities such as a dominance of high reactivity in F_1 hybrid crosses between high and low NK-reactive genotypes and an influence of H-2 linked factors (7, 8). When compared more in detail, however, certain fundamental differences appear (for discussion on this point see ref. 1), also indicating that the relationship between the genetic controls of the two systems, if any, is of a complex nature.

II. ASSAY SYSTEM

While the above mentioned data have provided some indirect evidence for the involvement of the NK system in rejection of non-malignant hematopoietic tissue, more direct evidence in support of this concept stems from experiments using cells from normal tissue as targets in conventional NK assays.

Although earlier experiments in this field almost exclusively used T-cell lymphomas as NK targets, it has since been demonstrated that NK cells are less restricted in their target cell range than originally thought, and that they also can lyse non-lymphoid tumors and primary cells from normal tissues (9, 10, 11).

The range of normal tissue which can be lysed depends very much on the source of NK effector cells used. Thus, when the most efficient source of NK cells, obtained from lymphocytic choriomeningitis virus (LCMV) infected mice are used as effectors, a broad range of different primary tissues can be lysed. These include peritoneal macrophages (9, 10), primary mouse fetal fibroblasts (12) and thymocytes and bone marrow cells. The biological significance of the fact that normal tissues are lysed by virus induced NK cells may be related to the role of NK cells in host resistance against virus infections. However, in this chapter we are mainly concerned with the intriguing finding that in spleens of normal, non-boosted mice there exist NK cells with the capacity to lyse a subpopulation of immature thymocytes. This was initially found in studies where various lymphoid organs from young (1 - 3 week old) mice were tested as target cells in short term (3 - 4 h) NK assays, using normal nylon wool column enriched spleen cells from NK high reactive genotypes (mostly CBA) as effector cells. The results invariably showed that only with thymocytes as targets was it possible to obtain significant sensitivity for lysis (10 - 30%), while cells from lymph nodes, spleens and bone marrow were almost totally resistant to lysis (11). Because thymocytes were unique in their relative high sensitivity, we have mainly concentrated our studies of primary lymphoid targets on this organ. Investigations are, however, in progress to further analyze and enrich for the very low degree of sensitivity seen in bone marrow, since this organ is of particular interest when considering NK cells in relation to the above discussed bone marrow graft resistance system.

We will here briefly review the findings relating to the nature of the NK sensitive thymocyte, the distribution of this thymocyte in mice of various ages and genotypes, the regulation of the thymocyte sensitivity by factors in vivo and in vitro also known to regulate NK activity, and, finally, speculate on the possible in vivo significance of our data.

III. CHARACTERIZATION OF THE NK SENSITIVE THYMOCYTE POPULATION IN THE THYMUS OF YOUNG MICE

Clearly, only a subpopulation of thymocytes are sensitive for NK lysis, since even when the most active NK population is used (obtained from LCMV-infected animals) there is usually not more than 20 - 30% lysis (11). In a series of experiments we have analyzed the nature of this natural killer sensitive thymocyte target (hereafter abbreviated NAT for natural killer sensitive thymocyte) and the main goal of this study has been to determine where in the thymocyte differentiation pathway the NK sensitive population belongs. The results from these studies are summarized in Table I. A standard method for distinguishing the majority (90 - 95%) of immature cortical cells from the small (5 - 10%) mature medullary population is by their sensitivity to in vivo injection with cortisone (13). Injection of young A/Sn mice with cortisone drastically decreased sensitivity of the remaining

TABLE I. Characteristics of NK sensitive thymocytes

	NK-target	Cortical	Medullary
Cortisone sensitivity	+	++	-
RNS, GPC sensitivity	+	+	-
PNA receptors	+	+	-
Size	large	small	medium-sized, large
Rate of division	high	fast	slow

medullary thymus cells for NK lysis, while sensitivity for lysis by anti-H-2 educated CTL blasts was enhanced (14). This demonstrated that the NAT belonged to the cortisone-sensitive cortical cells.

The NK-sensitive population repopulated the thymus following cortisone treatment 2 - 4 days earlier (on day 4 - 6 after cortisone administration) than the majority of the cortical thymocytes. Three other characteristics also classified the NAT population among the cortical thymocytes; their sensitivity for treatment with normal rabbit or guinea pig serum, their expression of receptor for the peanut agglutinin (PNA), and their sensitivity for radiation (14) properties all known to be confined to cortical thymocytes (15, 16).

The most efficient method for enriching for NAT has been by size fractionation on 1-g velocity sedimentation gradients or by the Beckman elutriator centrifuge (14, 17). These methods have clearly demonstrated that NAT are among a population of large thymocytes. Morphological studies of NAT-enriched populations have also confirmed that the majority of the NAT are large and rapidly dividing since a high rate of spontaneous incorporation of ^{3}H thymidine into these NK-sensitive fractions also demonstrates the high mitotic activity among NAT (14).

Although belonging to the cortisone-sensitive cortical population, NAT can clearly be separated from the majority of cortical cells by: 1) a larger size than the bulk of cortical cells, 2) a higher net cell surface charge than the majority of cortical thymocytes, distributing between them and the rapidly migrating medullary population as determined by free flow electrophoresis (14), 3) a more rapid repopulation of thymus following cortisone treatment or irradiation than the majority of cortical cells (14).

Taken together, these results show that the NAT is a subpopulation of thymocytes, clearly distinguishable from the majority of the cortical as well as medullary thymocytes.

IV. AGE- AND GENOTYPE-RELATED VARIATION OF NAT

Mouse NK activity can be influenced by a variety of factors of which the age and genotype of the donor animal play important roles (8, 18, 19). It was therefore natural to ask to what extent the age and genotype also would exert an influence on levels of NAT. The results from these studies were intriguing, since they demonstrated an inverse relationship between the age- and genotype-determined NK reactivity and the thymocyte sensitivity in the same individuals (11). In general, thymocytes from very young mice (1 - 3 weeks) showed highest NK sensitivity, while thymocytes from mice at "peak" NK activity (6 - 8 weeks) were less sensitive (Fig. 1).

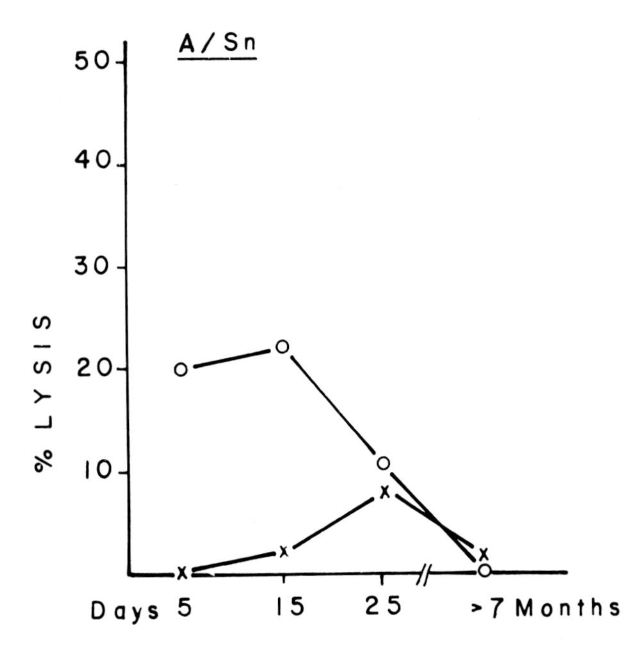

FIGURE 1. Inverse correlation between the age dependence of splenic NK activity and the sensitivity of thymocytes to NK-mediated lysis. Thymocytes from A/Sn mice at different ages were used as target cells, with CBA spleen cells as effector cells. o —— o. Splenic NK-activity in the same mice was determined using YAC-1 as target cell. x——x

A similar inverse relationship between levels of NAT and host NK reactivity was also seen when analyzing the strain distribution of thymocyte NK sensitivity. A clear pattern emerged: thymocytes from NK low reactive genotypes (for further details of genetic classification see ref. 1), such as the A/Sn, AKR, SWR/J, A.CA, A.BY and 129, were invariably more NK-sensitive than thymocytes from NK intermediate or high reactive genotypes (CBA, C3H/St, C57Bl, (DBA/2 x C57Bl) F1 hybrids). It should be mentioned that the differences in levels of NAT between various strains only become clear by comparing age matched thymocytes in the same experiment, and a considerable variation in levels of sensitivity of thymocytes from the same strain was apparent between different experiments. Nevertheless, these experiments have demonstrated that the genetics of the mouse influence the NK reactivity and the levels of NAT in a seemingly inverse manner.

We have recently proceeded with these studies, asking whether levels of NAT were directly related to the genotype-related NK reactivity due to a direct elimination of NAT by NK cells, or whether an indirect relationship between the two phenomena was at hand. For this purpose the mouse mutant beige (bg) was used, carried on C57Bl background. This mutant was recently found to have a deficient NK activity, in contrast to heterozygous bg/+ littermates (20). This is therefore an ideal model to analyze the selective absence of cytotoxic NK cells on an otherwise NK-reactive genetic background. Here, the NK-deficient beige mice were found to have the same levels of NAT as the bg/+ littermates (17) (Fig. 2). Hence, we can conclude that the strain dependent variation in levels of NAT is not directly related to variations in levels of NK activity *per se*.

V. IS THERE AN UNIQUE GENETIC PATTERN OF NORMAL CELL LYSIS DEPENDING ON THE TARGET CELL GENOTYPE?

NK cells can lyse a broad range of syngeneic, allogeneic and xenogeneic tumor targets (19, 21, 22). Since mouse strains can be divided into high- and low-reactive strains, one important question is to what extent the target cell genotype influences the genetic "pattern" of high- and low-reactivity of the effector strain. In other words, is it possible to detect a unique genetic pattern of high- *versus* low-reactive strains on targets depending on their genotypes? This question would be important to resolve when

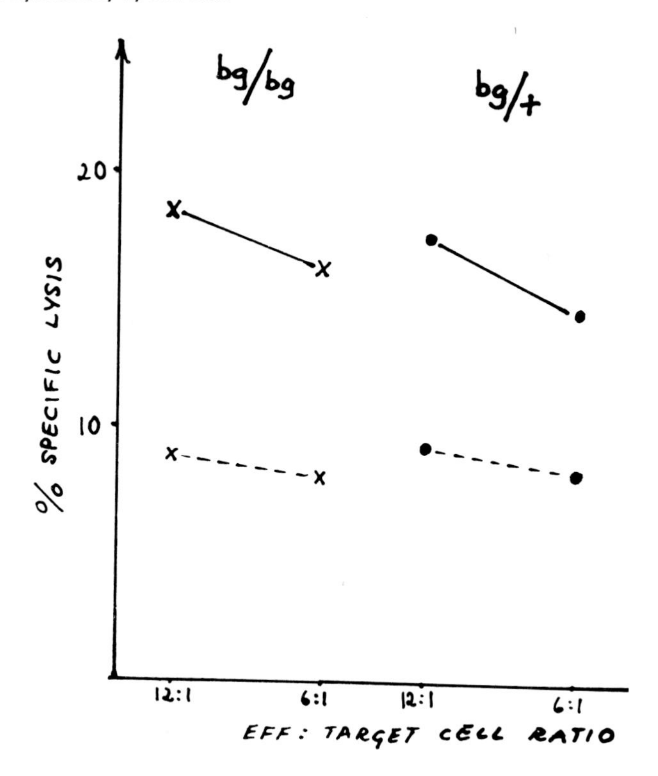

FIGURE 2. Sensitivity of bg/bg and bg/+ thymocytes to NK mediated lysis. Thymocytes from untreated (——) or poly I:C injected (----) 10 day old mice.

discussing the NK system in relation to the resistance to bone marrow grafts ("hybrid resistance"), where it has been postulated that the rejection is directed against Hh-1 determined antigens expressed on bone marrow grafts of certain genotypes only (7).

Previous results from our group using a variety of mouse and human lymphoma targets demonstrated a similar strain distribution and H-2 linkage regardless of the tumor genotype (23), but, results from others have pointed to a unique genetic regulation of NK cells at the "target cell level" (24, 25). To pursue the analysis of this question, we have in a recent genetic study used primary thymocytes and peritoneal macrophages as NK targets. The advantage of using normal tissue as targets for this type of analysis would be to avoid the "individuality" that each tumor line possesses, apart from their genetically determined cell surface antigens.

Figure 3 shows the results from this study, in which

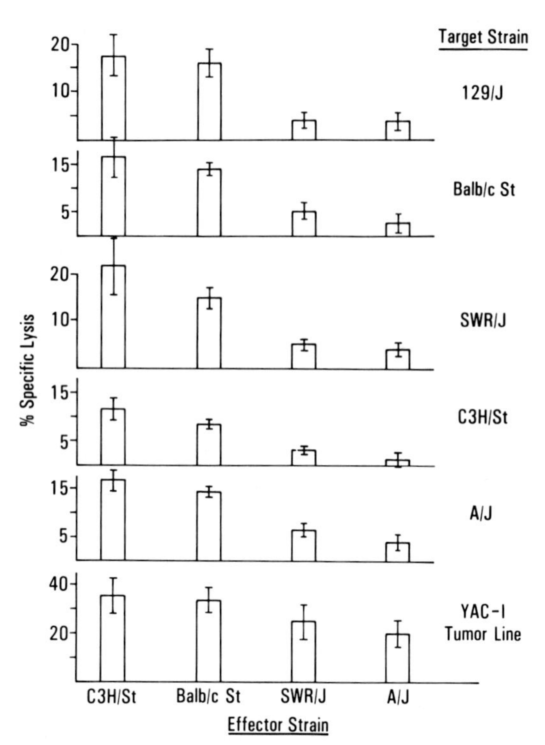

FIGURE 3A. Genotype dependent sensitivity to NK-lysis in the thymocyte target assay. Mean % lysis ± S.E. from four separate experiments.

LCMV-induced NK effector cells from 4 different mouse strains (C3H/St, Balb/c, SWR/J and A/J) were tested against thymocytes (Fig. 3A) or peritoneal (Fig. 3B) cell targets from the same mouse strains. The YAC-1 tumor line was included in these experiments as well. The important point to be made from these experiments is that the same genetic pattern of high or low reactive strains was seen regardless of the genotype of the target cell (thymocyte) donor. Thus, the C3H/St strain invariably showed highest activity against thymocytes of all genotypes, closely followed by the BALB/c strain. The SWR/J and the A/J strains were both considerably less reactive against all five target genotypes. The same genetic pattern was also seen against the YAC-1 lymphoma target (Fig. 3A).

In sharp contrast to the thymocyte-YAC-1 assay, an entirely different genetic regulation seems to be active in the lysis of adherent peritoneal cells. Here, a unique pattern of reactivity is seen for each effector cell genotype, dependent on the strain origin of the target cell (Fig. 3B). In line with previous findings (10), syngeneic combinations of

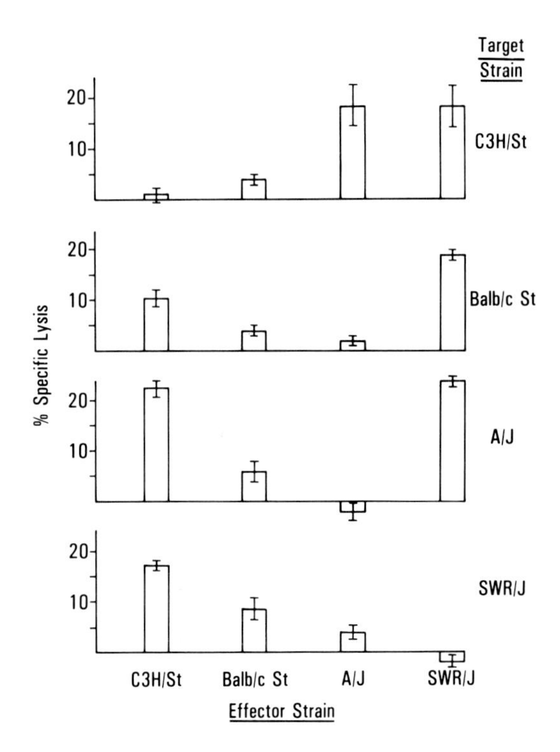

Fig. 3B. Genotype dependent sensitive to NK-lysis in the peritoneal cell assay. Mean % lysis ± S. E. from three separate experiments.

effector-target cells yielded little, if any, reactivity while various allogeneic combinations showed considerable levels of activities. Taken together, these two NK systems can clearly be distinguished by differences in their genetic pattern of lysis. One crucial question is whether the same effector cells, active against thymocytes and YAC-1 cells, are active against PC cells. Cell fractionation experiments and experiments with the mouse mutants nude (normal or enriched in NK) and beige (deficient in NK) clearly indicate that the effector cells active in the thymocyte as well as in the PC system are natural killer cells. There is, however, evidence that various "subtypes" of NK-like cells may exist (24, 26, 27). It is therefore possible that also in regards to lysing normal cells we may be demonstrating various subpopulations of NK cells.

VI. DECREASED NK SENSITIVITY IN THYMOCYTES FROM MICE INJECTED WITH INTERFERON INDUCERS *IN VIVO*

A more direct and "manipulated" way of analyzing the above mentioned inverse relationship between host NK reactivity and levels of NAT has been the injection of mice with agents known to induce interferon production *in vivo* and recently also shown to augment NK reactivity (28, 29, 30, 31). For this purpose we initially used as interferon inducers, *i.e.* synthetical polynucleotides, poly I:C and tilorone. The results revealed that a drastic decrease in levels of NAT was seen 14 hours after injections of these agents into young mice, while NK reactivity of the same mice markedly increased (11).

Recently, the same treatment was performed also in the NK-deficient beige mutant. Here, an identical decrease in levels of NAT in NK-deficient bg/bg mice compared to the NK-reactive bg/+ control was seen (Fig. 2). These experiments therefore argue against NK cells directly eliminating NAT in poly I:C boosted animals. The use of beige mice after activation as a model lacking NK cells is, however, not entirely conclusive, since after optimal activation they can develop considerable levels of NK activity (32).

In another series of experiments we used LCMV infection as the method for inducing NK reactivity. It was previously shown in this model that adult or young mice infected with LCMV developed an acute infection associated with high levels of interferon synthesis in lymphoid organs (33), NK cell activation (34) and a strong virus-specific immune response associated with cytotoxic T-cells (35). In contrast, mice infected congenitally or at birth with LCMV develop a persistent infection and become life-long virus carriers without a detectable interferon or cytotoxic T-cell response (36, 37). It was thought that this model may be useful to monitor the sensitivity of thymocyte targets during the course of infections associated with markedly different levels of interferon production.

Figure 4 demonstrates that the acute infection of LCMV in young mice of 3 strains results in a marked enhancement of spleen NK cell activity on the third day after infection concomitant with a reduction in thymocyte sensitivity.

On the seventh day after infection, the spleen NK activity is only marginally elevated, as reported previously (34), but, their thymocytes remained resistant to killing. It has been shown (30) that in the acute infection, spleen interferon levels peak on the 2nd or 3rd day after infection and there-

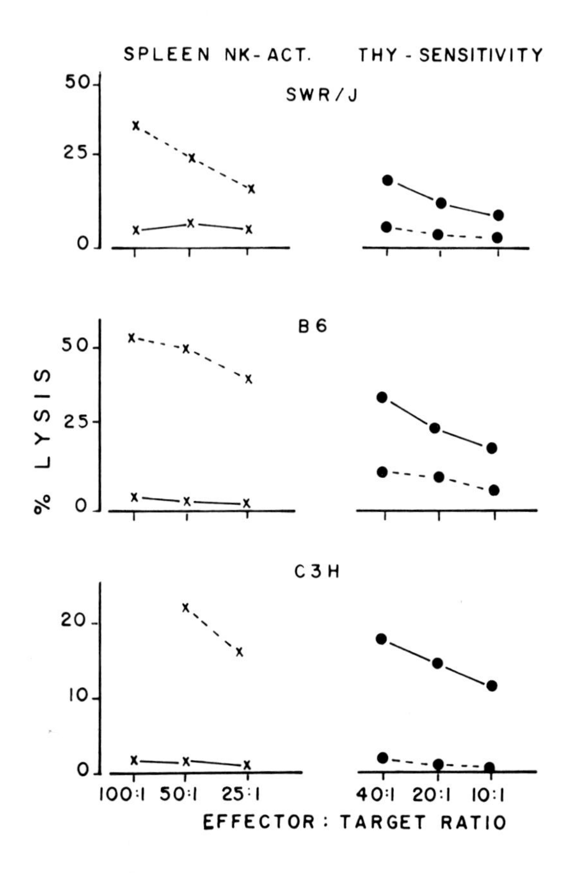

FIGURE 4. Splenic NK activity against YAC-1 and susceptibility of NAT to NK-lysis in mice on the third day after LCMV infection.(——) age-matched control mice, (----) LCMV-infected mice.

fore gradually decline. Interferon levels on the seventh day after infection are low, but still above levels in control mice.

LCMV-carrier SWR/J mice did not have higher levels of NK cells than controls. Correspondingly, the sensitivity of their thymocytes to natural killing also failed to deviate significantly from controls. While in both types of viral infections (persistent and acute) there is virus replication in the spleen and thymus, only in the acute infection are significant levels of interferon produced, and only in the acute infection at these time points can one detect NK cell activation and thymocyte protection.

VII. INTERFERON TREATMENT OF THYMOCYTES *IN VITRO* DECREASES THEIR SENSITIVITY FOR NK LYSIS

Since both poly I:C and LCMV are potent interferon inducers, the above mentioned experiments suggested that IF was responsible not only for the augmenting effect on NK activity of these agents, but also for their ability to reduce levels of NAT.

In line with this interpretation, Trinchieri *et al.* (38) have shown in a human NK system using human fibroblasts as targets, that IF protects target cells from lysis by NK cells. We have recently also confirmed this observation in the mouse system using fetal fibroblasts, peritoneal cells or tumor cells as targets (39).

In a recent series of experiments we investigated the effect that *in vitro* incubation of thymocytes in purified mouse interferon type I (Calbiochem) had on their levels of NAT (17). The results, as depicted in Fig. 5, clearly demonstrated a dose-dependent decrease in NK sensitivity of thymocytes from young strain SWR/J mice as a result of interferon incubation. While 10 u of IF resulted in some protection, 10^3 - 10^4 u was required to reduce levels of sensitivity to NK lysis by ≥ 75% as compared to thymocytes incubated in interferon only. No toxic effect was associated with IF treatment at these concentrations, during this time period, why the decrease in NAT appears to be due to protecting rather than killing the sensitive thymocyte population.

In confirmation of the results of Geeseer *et al.*, we have found that the IF-treated, NK-resistant thymocytes expressed higher levels of cell surface H-2 antigens (17), as measured by complement dependent anti-H-2 serum mediated cytotoxicity assays. Also in line with these findings, an increased sensitivity to allo-antibody-mediated ADCC among the IF-treated, NK-resistant, thymocytes was seen (17, Fig. 5). This finding is interesting, since it suggests an inverse relationship between the expression of H-2 antigens and the NK sensitivity on cells. A similar inverse relationship was previously described by us when the YAC ascites lymphoma was explanted to grow *in vitro*.

Here, the NK sensitivity increased on the YAC tumor during *in vitro* culture concomitantly with a decrease of serologically defined H-2 antigens (40).

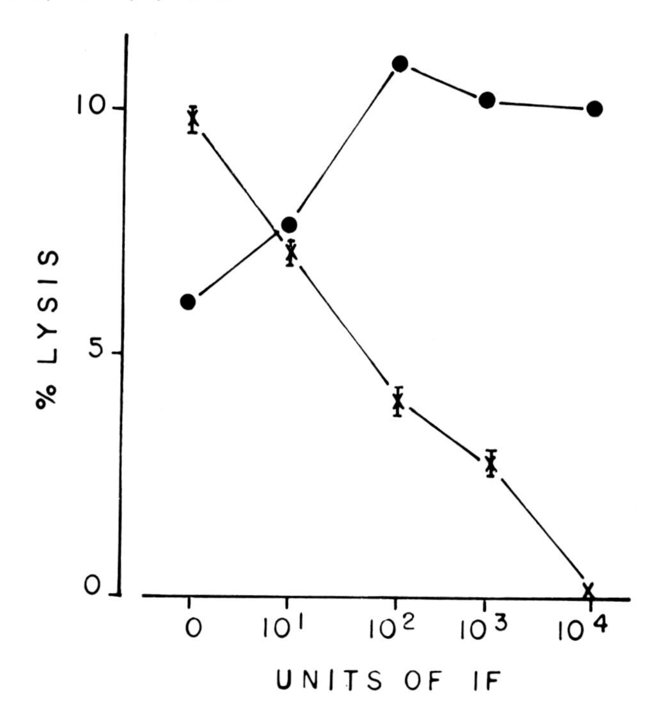

FIGURE 5. In vitro treatment of SWR/J thymocytes with varying doses of mouse interferon. NK-sensitivity (x —— x) and susceptibility to ADCC-mediated lysis (● —— ●) was determined using NK cells from LCMV-activated C3H/St mice.

VIII. INTERFERON-TREATED THYMOCYTES ARE LESS EFFICIENT INHIBITORS IN COLD TARGET COMPETITION ASSAYS AGAINST ISOTOPE-LABELED THYMOCYTES AND YAC-1 TARGETS

It was of interest to determine whether the IF-treated thymocytes would also express less of the "NK target structure" as measured by the cold target inhibition assay. By this assay we would also be able to determine if NAT shared target structures with NK-sensitive lymphoma targets, such as the YAC-1 target. For this purpose, IF-treated thymocytes were used as competitors in cross-competition assays with both YAC-1 and thymocytes as target cells. As can be seen from two representative experiments in Table II, the decreased sensitivity to lysis by IF-treated thymocytes correlated well with a decreased ability of the same thymocytes

TABLE II.

Cold target[1)]		% Inhibition of		% Lysis as target [4)]
		YAC-1 lysis [2)]	NAT lysis [3)]	
Experiment 1				
Contr.-Thy	$2x10^6$	26.7	57.7	20.3 ± 0.6
	$1x10^6$	12.8	35.0	
	$0.5x10^6$	6.4	39.9	
	$0.25x10^6$	5.0	23.2	
IF-Thy	$2x10^6$	13.0	17.2	5.1 ± 0.2
	$1x10^6$	1.8	17.8	
	$0.5x10^6$	5.6	± 0	
	$0.25x10^6$	±0	±0	
Experiment 2				
Contr.-Thy	$2x10^6$	45.6	41.8	22.5 ± 0.3
	$1x10^6$	21.3	33.1	
	$0.5x10^6$	17.5	18.8	
	$0.25x10^6$	±0	16.9	
IF-Thy	$2x10^6$	18.2	37.5	9.6 ± 0.4
	$1x10^6$	10.5	17.8	
	$0.5x10^6$	±0	5.1	
	$0.25x10^6$	±0	±0	

1) Varying numbers of non-labeled SWR/J thymocytes were allowed to a constant number LCMV-activated C3H/St spleen cells and allowed to incubate for 30 min before radio-labeled target cells were added. In each experiment the number of spleen cells giving an effector:target ratio of 20:1 was used.

2) 2×10^4 labeled YAC-1 cells were used, giving competitor:target ratios 100:1, 50:1, 25:1 and 12:1.

3) 4×10^4 labeled SWR/J thymocytes were added giving competitor:target ratios 50:1, 25:1, 12:1 and 6:1.

4) NAT sensitivity of the SWR/J thymocytes used as competitors was determined by using them as targets with effector cells from LCMV-activated C3H/St mice at effector:target ratio 20:1.

to act as competitors against the YAC-1 or thymocyte targets. Since NAT consists of a subpopulation, a relatively high competitor to target ratios had to be used to see inhibition. One cannot rule out that part of the inhibition is due to non-specific crowding effects. However, the fact that an IF-treated, but otherwise comparable thymocyte population competes less than the untreated control thymocytes argues against this explanation. We therefore conclude that the decreased sensitivity to NK lysis observed among IF-treated thymocytes must be due to a decreased ability of NAT to bind NK cells.

The indication from these experiments that a common NK target structure may exist on immature thymocytes and on NK-sensitive T-cell lymphomas has recently also been supported by serological studies. Natural antibodies in rabbit serum were found to recognize NK-associated specificities expressed on young thymocytes and on T-cell lymphomas (41). It is an exciting possibility that this NK target structure may represent some highly conserved differentiation antigen, also expressed across the species barrier on certain human T-cell lymphomas (42). The demonstration that interferon plays a crucial role in modulating the expression of this NK target structure on a subclass of immature thymocytes may be of profound importance in understanding the interaction between NK cells and normal or transformed cell targets.

SUMMARY AND CONCLUSION

In the thymus of young mice there exists a subpopulation of cells which can be lysed by endogenous natural killer cells. The thymus is unique in this respect, since other lymphoid organs show little or no sensitivity for NK lysis. The sensitive thymocyte resided within the cortisone sensitive, radiation sensitive and PNA positive population, and could therefore be classified as cortical. It could, however, be separated from the rest of the cortical cells by its larger size and its higher electrophoretic mobility, and by the fact that it repopulated the thymus faster after cortisone treatment than the majority of cortical cells. Young mice of NK low reactive genotypes have thymocytes of higher NK sensitivity than older mice or than mice of NK high reactive genotypes. The reason for this inverse relationship between NK reactivity and thymocyte NK sensitivity appears not to be due to a direct elimination of the NK-sensitive thymocyte by NK cells since 1) NK-deficient beige mice have thymocytes of normal NK sensitivity and 2) thymocytes from beige mice and control mice after administration of the interferon inducer poly I:C show the same strong reduction of NK sensitivity. Administration of poly I:C to beige mice leads only to a very slight increase of NK activity in these animals, while NK activity in control mice is markedly enhanced. Furthermore, acute infection of young mice with lymphocytic choriomeningitis virus (LCMV), which induces high levels of interferon and activated NK cells, leads to almost total decrease in NK sensitivity of thymocytes. In contrast, mice infected congenitally with LCMV, which develop persistent infection without a detectable interferon response, do not show decreased levels of thymocyte sensitivity. *In vitro* experiments revealed that direct treatment of thymocytes with non-toxic doses of interferon (IF) in concentrations of 10^3 units/μl almost totally abrogated their NK sensitivity, while their expression of H-2 antigen was enhanced. For strong protection,more than 7 hours treatment was necessary and 1 hour was not enough. IF-treated thymocytes were also less efficient than untreated ones in cold target inhibition assays against isotope-labeled thymocytes or YAC-1 target cells.

From these experiments we conclude that interferon plays an important role in modulating levels of NK sensitivity in a population of immature, large thymocytes. The possibility that age- and genotype-related levels of "endogenous" interferon in normal mice may act as a common modulator on both thymocyte sensitivity and NK activity and explain the inverse relationship observed between these two activities, must therefore be entertained. Further studies must be directed towards understanding the biological significance of the NK-sensitive thymocyte population and how it is related to the host NK system.

ACKNOWLEDGEMENTS

This work was supported by U.S. Public Health Grant CA26782 and by the Swedish Cancer Society. This is publication No. 1988 from the Department of Immunopathology, Scripps Clinic and Research Foundation, La Jolla, California.

REFERENCES

1. Kiessling, R., and Wigzell, H., Immunol. Rev. 44, 165 (1979).
2. Cudkowicz, G., in "The Proliferation and Spread of Neoplastic Cells", p. 661. The Williams and Wilkins Co., Baltimore (1968).
3. Kiessling, R., Hochman, P.S., Haller, O., Shearer, G.M., Wigzell, H., and Cudkowicz, G., Eur. J. Immunol. 7, 655 (1977).
4. Trentin, J., Kiessling, R., Wigzell, H., Gallagher, M., Datta, S., and Kulkarni, S., in "Experimental Today" (S. Baum, and D. Ledney, eds.). Springer Verlag, New York, (1977).
5. Lotzova, E., and Savary, C., Biomed. 27, 341 (1977).
6. Hochman, P., and Cudkowicz, G., J. Immunol. 119, 2013 (1978).
7. Cudkowicz, G., and Bennett, M., J. Exp. Med. 134, 1513 (1971).
8. Petrányi, G., Kiessling, R., and Klein, G., Immunogenetics 2, 53 (1975).
9. Nunn, M.E., Herberman, R.B., and Holden, H.T., Int. J. Cancer 20, 381 (1977).
10. Welsh, R.M., Zinkernagel, R.M., and Hallenbeck, L., J. Immunol. 122, 475 (1979).
11. Hansson, M., Kiessling, R., Andersson, B., Kärre, K., and Roder, J., Nature 278, 174 (1979).
12. Kiessling, R., and Welsh, R.M., submitted for publication.
13. Blomgren, H., and Andersson, B., Cell. Immunol. 1, 545 (1970).
14. Hansson, M., Kärre, K., Kiessling, R., Roder, J., Andersson, B., and Häyry, P., J. Immunol. 123, 765 (1979).
15. Reisner, Y., Linker-Israeli, M., and Sharon, N., Cell. Immunol. 25, 129 (1976).
16. Kierszenbaum, F., and Budzko, B., Cell. Immunol. 29, 137 (1977).
17. Hansson, M. Kiessling, R., Welsh, R. subm. for publ.
18. Kiessling, R., Petrányi, G., Klein, G., and Wigzell, H., Int. J. Cancer 15, 933 (1975).
19. Herberman, R.B., Nunn, M.E., and Lavrin, D.H., Int. J. Cancer 16, 216 (1975).
20. Roder, J., and Duwe, A., Nature 278, 451 (1979).
21. Kiessling, R., Haller, O., Fenyö, E.M., Steinitz, M., and Klein, G., Int. J. Cancer 21, 460 (1978).

22. Haller, O., Kiessling, R., Orn, A., Kärre, K., Nilsson, K., and Wigzell, H., Int. J. Cancer 20, 93 (1977).
23. Klein, G., Klein, G., Kiessling, R., and Kärre, K., Immunogenetics 6, 561 (1978).
24. Kumar, V., Luevano, E., and Bennet, M., J. Exp. Med. 150, 531 (1979).
25. Herberman, R.B., and Holden, H.T., Adv. Cancer Res. 27, 305 (1978).
26. Burton, R.C., and Winn, H.J., submitted for publication.
27. Stutman, O., Paige, C.J., and Feo Figarella, E., J. Immunol. 121, 1819 (1978).
28. Gidlund, M., Örn, A., Wigzell, H., Senik, A., and Cresser, I., Nature 273, 759 (1978).
29. Herberman, R.B., Nunn, M.E., Holden, H.T., Staal, S., and Djeu, J.Y., Int. J. Cancer 19, 555 (1977).
30. Welsh, R.M., J. Exp. Med. 148, 163 (1978).
31. Wolfe, S.A., Tracey, D.E., and Henney, C.S., J. Immunol. 119, 1152 (1977).
32. Welsh, R.M., and Kiessling, R., submitted for publication.
33. Merigan, T.C., Oldstone, M.B.A., and Welsh, R.M., Nature 268, 67 (1977).
34. Welsh, R.M., and Zinkernagel, R.M., Nature 268, 646 (1977).
35. Zinkernagel, R.M., and Doherty, P.C., Nature 248, 791 (1974).
36. Volkert, M., Larsen, J.H., and Pfau, C.J., Acta Pathol. Microbiol. Scand. 61, 268 (1964).
37. Welsh, R.M., and Oldstone, M.B.A., J. Exp. Med. 145, 1449 (1977).
38. Trinchieri, G., and Santoli, D. J. Exp. Med. 147, 1314 (1978).
39. Welsh, R.M., and Kiessling, R., in this volume (1980).
40. Becker, S., Kiessling, R., Lee, N., and Klein, G., J. Nat. Cancer Inst. 61, 1495 (1978).
41. Grönberg, A., Hansson, M., Kiessling, R., Andersson, B., Kärre, K., and Roder, J., J. Nat. Cancer Inst., in press.
42. Hansson, M., Kärre, K., Bakacs, T., Kiessling, R., and Klein, G., J. Immunol. 121, 6 (1978).

SPECIFICITY OF NK CELLS

Ronald B. Herberman
John R. Ortaldo

Laboratory of Immunodiagnosis
National Cancer Institute
Bethesda, Maryland

I. INTRODUCTION

Concepts about the specificity of NK cells have gradually evolved as experience in this area has increased and new experimental approaches have been applied to this issue. Although many investigators initially considered the cytotoxic activity of NK cells to be nonspecific, increased evidence has accumulated for a selective pattern of reactivity and for multiple antigenic specificities on susceptible target cells. Recently, a major question has been whether each NK cell can recognize the full range of susceptible targets or whether there are subpopulations of NK cells, each reactive with a more limited number of targets. In this chapter, we will briefly summarize our evidence on each of these points.

II. SELECTIVITY OF NK CELLS

In contrast to the apparent nonspecificity of the cytotoxicity by normal or activated macrophages, which can lyse most if not all transformed cells (see chapter by Keller), NK cells have been found to be rather selective in their effects. In the mouse, *in vitro* cell lines have usually been more susceptible to lysis by NK cells, but some *in vivo* tumor cells have also been susceptible (Herberman *et al.*, 1975). Sublines of the same tumor have often varied widely in their

ISBN 0-12-341350-8

sensitivity. Yet a wide range of types of target cells have been found to be susceptible to NK activity. Most of the early studies of rodent NK cells utilized leukemia or lymphoma target cells and it was initially thought that only those cells were sensitive to NK activity. However, many of the initial observations on human NK were made with monolayer cell lines derived from carcinomas. Such data would suggest that NK cells might actually have a wide range of reactivity. This has been confirmed by extensive studies of the susceptibility of a wide variety of cells to NK activity. Rodent and human NK cells can lyse some sarcoma and carcinoma cell lines as well as cell lines growing in suspension. It has been clear from the outset that NK activity was not restricted to histocompatible target cells, with strong reactivity against a variety of allogeneic target cells. Although it initially appeared that NK reactivity was restricted to target cells of the same species, this was also found not to hold, with mouse, rat, and guinea pig NK reacting against human and other xenogeneic cell lines (Haller *et al.*, 1977; Nunn and Herberman, 1979; Arnaud-Battandier *et al.*, 1978). However, we have failed to detect substantial reactivity of human NK cells in short term ^{51}Cr release cytotoxicity assays against rodent target cells (Nunn and Herberman, 1979). Our observations are at variance with those of other investigators, who have detected rather strong activity of human lymphoid cells against some mouse tumor lines. The reasons for this discrepancy are not clear, but it can not be attributed to a general lack of sensitivity of the mouse targets to lysis by NK cells.

Although most studies on NK activity have used transplantable tumors or cell lines, some primary tumor cells have also been lysed by normal effector cells. In fact, the initial observation of human natural cell-mediated cytotoxicity was made with fresh blast cells from patients with acute leukemia (Rosenberg *et al.*, 1972). Similarly, mouse NK cells have been found to react against some primary AKR thymomas (Nunn *et al.*, 1977).

NK activity has also been shown not to be restricted to tumor cells, with some types of normal cells having at least a low degree of sensitivity to lysis. Mouse NK cells were found to react with peritoneal cells after adherence to plastic for 18 hours (Nunn *et al.*, 1977; Welsh *et al.*, 1979) and also to a lower but significant extent with bone marrow and thymus cells (Nunn *et al.*, 1977). It is of interest that Hansson, Kiessling and their associates have shown that the sensitivity of thymocytes is restricted to a particular subpopulation of cells (see chapter by Hansson *et al.*). In view of the strong parallels between mouse NK cells and the cells mediating *in vivo* bone marrow resistance (Kiessling *et al.*, 1977; Harmon et al., 1977; Riccardi *et al.*, 1978), it seems likely that NK cells can specifically recognize the genetically determined Hh histocompatibility antigens on bone marrow cells as well as on tumor cells. We have also found that human bone marrow cells have a low degree of sensitivity to lysis by NK cells. In contrast, other normal cells that have been tested, including PHA-stimulated peripheral blood lymphocytes and T cells maintained in culture with T cell growth factor, have been resistant to lysis by NK cells.

III. RECOGNITION OF MULTIPLE ANTIGENIC SPECIFICITIES BY NK CELLS

Given this rather wide spectrum of reactivity by NK cells, an important issue is whether a single NK receptor reacts against all of the susceptible target cells or whether there is a variety of NK receptors, each with specificity for one of multiple antigenic specificities on target cells. There are several lines of evidence to support the latter possibility, of recognition by NK cells of at least several antigenic specificities, some of which may be broadly distributed: 1) Some of the above data obtained by direct cytotoxicity testing have pointed to heterogeneity in target cell structures. The susceptibility of targets to lysis by heterologous NK cells has been found to vary considerably from susceptibility to lysis by NK cells of the same species (Haller *et al.*, 1977; Nunn and Herberman, 1979). For example, K562 is highly sensitive to lysis by human NK cells but is substantially less sensitive to lysis by mouse NK cells than are some other human cell lines. Even more striking has been our consistent observation that human NK cells have no effect on YAC-1, which is highly sensitive to lysis by mouse NK cells. Thus, mouse and human NK cells appear to recognize quite distinct specificities on target cells. 2) There have also been some major differences in the patterns of reactivity among different mouse strains or among normal human donors (Herberman *et al.*, 1979). One example is the lack of reactivity of BALB/c mice against RL♂1 ascites cells, whereas these cells are quite susceptible to lysis by NK cells of other strains. 3) Much further support for the multiplicity of antigenic specificities has come from cold target inhibition assays, in which various unlabeled target cells have been tested for their ability to inhibit lysis of

^{51}Cr-labeled target cells. As initially reported (Herberman *et al.*, 1975) and subsequently documented quite extensively by our group and several others (reviewed by Herberman and Holden, 1978, and Herberman *et al.*, 1979), patterns of inhibition by various cells have varied with the labeled target cell. Some cells which could strongly inhibit lysis of one target had little or no inhibitory activity for other target cells. In most instances, the greatest inhibition of lysis has been obtained with the same cells used as labeled target cells. In an extensive cold target inhibition study with K562 target cells, most but not all human cell lines inhibited, and some carcinoma biopsy cells were also positive (Ortaldo *et al.*, 1977). Leukemia blast cells, normal lymphocytes, and heterologous tumor cells did not inhibit the anti-K562 reactivity.

The differences in reactivity patterns among donors have been found to be quite consistent and appear to be intrinsic properties of the effector cells. For example, we have found that the NK cells developing during *in vitro* culture, and thus removed from the usual environmental factors and in the apparent absence of B cells, retain the same specificity pattern as that of the fresh lymphocytes of the particular donor (Ortaldo *et al.*, 1979). In addition, after augmentation of NK activity by interferon, the patterns of reactivity remain similar to those seen with spontaneous NK cells. Some target cells that are resistant to lysis by spontaneous NK cells may become sensitive to IF-boosted NK cells, but this probably just represents a shift from below to above the threshold of sensitivity to lysis. However, a more detailed analysis of the specificity patterns of IF-boosted cells is needed.

IV. CLONALITY OF NK CELLS

Recognition of multiple antigenic specificities by NK cells could be accounted for in either of two ways: 1) Each NK cell of an individual could have a series of different receptors on its surface, providing it with the ability to recognize a wide variety of target cells. The variation in reactivity patterns among individuals or strains would be consistent with this, since only some individuals might have certain receptors on their NK cells. 2) Alternatively, the NK cells within an individual could be heterogeneous, with each clone having the ability to react with only one, or a few, of the wide variety of target cell specificities recognized by the whole population. None of the experimental approaches described above can adequately discriminate between these possibilities. To do this, one has to attempt physical separation of subpopulations of NK cells and examine their specificity. We have utilized monolayers of target cells for specific removal of NK cells. Unadsorbed cells were then tested for residual NK activity against several susceptible target cells. If the adsorption was successful in removing most or all activity against the target cell used for adsorption, it was possible to determine whether other NK cells remained, which were capable of recognizing other target cells.

Several technical points had an important influence on the results. First, it was necessary to have fully confluent monolayers of target cells, to ensure sufficient antigens for contact with most or all of the added effector cells. Second, it was essential to have the target cells remain adherent throughout the procedure, since admixture of nonadherent target cells with unadsorbed effector cells could produce cold target inhibition of cytotoxicity. We have found that a recently developed technique has been satisfactory in both regards (Silva *et al.*, 1978) and this has allowed us to obtain some answers to this important issue.

A. *Mouse NK Cells*

A summary of our results with selective adsorption of mouse NK cells is given in Table I. Monolayers of YAC-1 cells have been consistently able to deplete virtually all NK activity against YAC-1. The unadsorbed cells have also been unreactive against RL♂1, another NK-sensitive mouse lymphoma, and against MOLT, a human lymphoblastoid T cell line derived from a patient with acute lymphocytic leukemia. These data indicate that the same NK cells that recognize YAC-1 also are needed for reactivity against the other targets. In contrast, the cells nonadherent to YAC-1 were still able to react with adherent PEC and also, to some degree, with thymus cells. These data suggest some heterogeneity of mouse NK cells, with separate subpopulations involved in recognition of neoplastic and normal target cells. However, it has not been possible to fully document this heterogeneity in the other direction, by adsorptions on normal target cells. The affinity of binding of NK cells to these targets appears to be weak and this adsorption procedure has been unsuccessful in depleting reactivity against the adsorbing cell. Thus, we have not been able to meaningfully examine residual activity of the unadsorbed cells against YAC-1 or other neoplastic targets.

TABLE I. Cytotoxic Activity of Mouse Lymphocytes after Adsorption on Various Monolayers

Monolayers used for adsorption	*Target Cells*				
	YAC-1	*RL♂1*	*MOLT*	*Adher. PEC*[a]	*Thymus*
YAC-1	--[c]	--	--	++	+
MOLT[b]	--		--		
Adher. PEC	++	++		++	
Thymus	+				+

[a]*Plastic-adherent peritoneal exudate cells*
[b]*Three sequential adsorptions on monolayers needed to remove activity against MOLT.*
[c]*Residual activity after adsorption: -, no activity; +, significant activity but reduced; ++, activity same as unadsorbed control*

Henney and his associates have also examined this question, using a similar monolayer adsorption approach (Henney *et al.*, 1978; Durdick *et al.*, 1979). They failed to detect any heterogeneity, but they only used two neoplastic target cells, one mouse lymphoma and the human Chang cell line. These two lines also appeared to share the same specificities by cold target inhibition.

B. Human NK Cells

Our studies with human NK cells have given more clearcut indications of heterogeneity (Phillips *et al.*, 1980) and Jensen and Koren (see their chapter) have obtained similar results. Peripheral blood mononuclear cells were incubated on monolayers of 5 different NK-susceptible cell lines and nonadherent cells were then tested for residual cytotoxicity against each of the targets. We found that virtually all reactivity could be removed against each of the adsorbing cell lines. However, with 4 of 7 donors tested, the selectively adsorbed cells still had considerable reactivity against one or more of the other target cells. A representative example of such data is shown in Table II. With this donor, adsorption on a monolayer of MOLT cells left substantial activity against the breast cancer-derived cell line, ALab. Even more strikingly, adsorption on G11, another cell line derived from a patient with breast cancer, left the majority of the reactivity against three of the other cell lines. Other normal donors showed similar degrees of

TABLE II. Cytotoxic Activity of Lymphocytes of a Normal Human Donor after Adsorption on Various Monolayers

Monolayers used for adsorption	Target Cells				
	K562	MOLT	F265	G11	ALab
K562	7[a]	18	4	23	1
MOLT	27	3	2	1	48
F265	16	1	1	14	1
G11	63	57	4	1	55
ALab	3	2	40	11	1

[a]% of original cytotoxic activity remaining after adsorption

heterogeneity, but the patterns of reactivity after selective adsorptions varied among them. To account for all of the data, it has been necessary to postulate a minimum of seven antigenic specificities on the five target cells, with at least three subsets of NK cells in each of the donors showing heterogeneity (Table III). Thus, human NK cells in some individuals appear to be heterogeneous and may be clonally distributed. To obtain an adequate estimate of the degree of heterogeneity, it would be necessary to perform selective adsorptions with a wider array of target cells. It should be noted that three donors failed to show any heterogeneity in the tests with the five cell lines. Adsorptions on one target cell removed almost all reactivity against the other target cells. However, it seems likely that retesting of these donors with other targets would also reveal some heterogeneity.

V. NATURE OF ANTIGENS ON NK-SUSCEPTIBLE TARGET CELLS

There is little clear information about the nature of the antigens recognized by NK cells. Based on our early specificity studies with mouse and rat NK cells (Herberman *et al.*, 1975; Nunn *et al.*, 1976), we postulated that NK cells recognized antigens associated with endogenous type C viruses. Since then, others have obtained evidence that such antigens (Lee and Ihle, 1977) and also antigens associated with other viruses (e.g. see chapters by Bloom *et al.* and by Lane) could be recognized by NK cells. With accumulating evidence on the wide diversity of target cells recognized by NK cells,

TABLE III. Summary of Antigenic Specificities on the Target Cells and of the Antigens Recognized by the NK Cells of the Donors

Antigens	*Distribution*
1	common to all of the tested NK susceptible targets
2	G11 and MOLT
2'	G11
3	ALab, G11, weakly on F265
4	K562 and F265
5	K562, MOLT and ALab
6	K562 and ALab
Targets	*Antigens Detected by Adsorption*
K562	1,4,5,6
MOLT	1,2,5
F265	1,3,4
G11	1,2,2',3
ALab	1,3,5,6
Donor	*Subsets of NK Cells reactive against antigen(s)*
1	1,2,3
2	1,2',4
3	1,5,6
4	1
5	1

including xenogeneic cell lines and some normal cells, it seems unlikely that viral specificities account for all of the reactivity of NK cells. It seems more likely that viral antigens, and also a variety of other antigens, possibly including differentiation antigens and Hh histocompatibility antigens, may be recognized by NK cells.

One further issue of some interest is the degree of heterogeneity within a target cell line in susceptibility to lysis by NK cells. Even with the most susceptible cell lines, an appreciable portion of the targets in an assay are not lysed by NK cells. Rather, with increasing effector:target cell ratios, the percent lysis reaches a plateau, rarely exceeding 50-60% of the total isotope incorporated into the cells. The resistance to lysis by a portion of the target cells could be due to reversible variations in the physiological state of the target cells. Expression of cell surface antigens has been shown to vary with the stage in the cell cycle (Cikes *et al.*, 1973) and susceptibility to lysis by antibody plus complement also has been shown to vary with the level of lipid metabolism (Schlager *et al.*, 1978). Consistent with this have been the observations of Becker *et al.* (1978) that the differences in susceptibility to NK cells of *in vitro* and *in vivo* grown YAC cells was reversible in both directions. On the other hand, as mentioned earlier, some sublines of tumors have been found to vary in a stable fashion in their susceptilibity to lysis by NK cells. This has suggested some clonality to the susceptibility, with some cells in an uncloned cell line containing, and others lacking, the needed antigens. To investigate this, N. Navarro in our laboratory has cloned the K562 cell line and at various times examined the clones for their susceptibility to NK cells. In the initial screening, some clones were highly sensitive and others appeared rather resistant. However, with further culture, and particularly when all clones were handled identically and passaged at the same concentration, they all were indistinguishable from the uncloned parental line in their sensitivity to lysis by human or mouse NK cells (Navarro *et al.*, 1980). Thus, we have failed to document a stable heterogeneity in expression on target cells of antigens recognized by NK cells.

REFERENCES

Arnaud-Battandier, F., Bundy, B. M., and Nelson, D.L. (1978). *Eur. J. Immunol 8*, 400

Becker, S., Kiessling, R., Lee, N., and Klein, G. (1978). *J. Natl. Cancer Inst. 61*, 1495.

Cikes, M., Friberg, J. R., and Klein, G. (1973). J. *Nat. Cancer Inst. 50*, 347.

Durdik, J. M., Beck, B. N., and Henney, C. S. (1979). In "Immunobiology and Immunotherapy of Cancer" (W. D. Terry and Y. Yamamura, eds.), p. 105. Elsevier North Holland, New York.

Haller, O., Kiessling, R., Orn, A., Karre, K., Nilsson, K., and Wigzell, H. (1977). *Int. J. Cancer 20*, 93.

Harmon, R. C., Clark, E. A., O'Toole, C., and Wicker, L. S. (1977). *Immunogenetics 4*, 601.

Henney, C. S., Tracey, D., Durdik, J. M., and Klimpel, G. (1978). *Am. J. Pathol. 93,* 459.

Herberman, R. B., Djeu, J. Y., Kay, H. D., Ortaldo, J. R., Riccardi, C., Bonnard, G. D., Holden, H. T., Fagnani, R., Santoni, A., and Puccetti, P. (1979). *Immunol. Rev. 44,* 43.

Herberman, R. B., and Holden, H. T. (1978). *Adv. Cancer Res. 27,* 305-377.

Herberman, R. B., Nunn, M. E., and Lavrin, D. H. (1975). *Int. J. Cancer 16, 216-229.*

Herberman, R. B., Nunn, M. E., and Lavrin, D. H. (1975). Natural cytotoxic reactivity of mouse lymphoid cells against syngeneic and allogenic tumors. I. Distribution of reactivity and specificity. *Int. J. Cancer 16,* 216-229.

Kiessling, R., Hochman, P. S., Haller, O., Shearer, G. M., Wigzell, H., and Cudkowicz, G. (1977). *Eur. J. Immunol. 7,* 655.

Landazuri, M. O., Silva, A., Alvarez, J., and Herberman, R. B. (1979). *J. Immunol. 123,* 252.

Lee, J. C., and Ihle, J. N. (1977). *J. Immunol.* 118, 928.

Navarro, N. J., Nunn, M. E., and Herberman, R. B. (1980). Submitted for publication.

Nunn, M. E., Herberman, R. B., and Holden, H. T. (1977). *Int. J. Cancer 20,* 381.

Nunn, M. E., and Herberman, R. B. (1979). *J. Natl. Cancer Inst. 62,* 765.

Ortaldo, J. R., Bonnard, G. D., Kind, P. D., and Herberman, R. B. (1979). *J. Immunol. 122,* 1489-1494.

Ortaldo, J. R., Oldham, R. K., Cannon, G. B., and Herberman, R. B. (1977). *J. Natl. Cancer Inst. 59,* 77.

Phillips, W. H., Ortaldo, J. R., and Herberman, R. B. (1980). Submitted for publication.

Riccardi, C., Fioretti, M. C., Giampietri, A., Pucetti, P., Goldin, A., and Bonmassar, E. (1978). *J. Natl. Cancer Inst. 60,* 1083.

Rosenberg, E. B., Herberman, R. B., Levine, P. H. Halterman, R. H., McCoy, J. L., and Wunderlich, J. R. (1972). *Int. J. Cancer 9,* 648.

Schlager, S. I., Ohanian, S. H., and Borsos, T. (1978). *J. Immunol.* 120, 463.

Silva, A., Landazuri, M. O., Alvarez, J., and Kreisler, J. M. (1978). *J. Immunol. Methods 23,* 303.

Welsh, R. M. J. R., Zinkernagel, R. M., and Hallenbeck, L. A. (1979). *J. Immunol. 122,* 475.

HETEROGENEITY IN NATURAL KILLING

Pamela J. Jensen
Hillel S. Koren

Division of Immunology
Department of Microbiology and Immunology
Duke University Medical Center
Durham, North Carolina

I. INTRODUCTION

A. Background

Although it appears that the lysis of a cell by the mechanism known as natural killing (NK) requires cell-cell contact, little is known about the complementary membrane structures which must exist on the effector and target cells if effective contact is to be made. A variety of cell types, including some tumor lines (1-4), virally infected lines (5,6), and thymocytes (4) have been shown to be sensitive to NK. What type of membrane structure is recognized on these diverse targets and whether the various targets share common determinants or bear unique ones are questions which only recently have been experimentally examined.

Preliminary evidence in support of the concept of heterogeneity in the NK recognition process has come from unlabelled target cell competitive inhibition experiments. Several laboratories (7-9) have shown that the lysis of ^{51}Cr-labelled tumor

This work was supported by United States Public Health Service Grants T32-CA-09058, CA-14049, and CA-23354. Hillel S. Koren is a recipient of a Research Career Development Award CA-00581

ISBN 0-12-341350-8

cell lines is inhibited in the presence of other, unlabelled cell lines; however, the greatest inhibition is frequently seen when inhibitor and target cells are identical. These findings are consistent with the presence of a variety of NK determinants, some unique and some shared between cell lines.

More recent data (10-12) from two laboratories provides further evidence for NK heterogeneity. A study applying Michaelis-Menten enzyme kinetics to cytotoxicity data (10) has suggested the presence of subpopulations of human NK effector cells, capable of recognizing different determinants on different target cells.

In another study, several glycoproteins termed NK target structures (11,12) have been isolated from the surface of NK-sensitive targets of human and mouse origin. These molecules have been shown to inhibit the target binding cell assay devised by Roder et al. (13,14) which generally correlates with NK activity. Each target cell examined appears to bear several glycoproteins of different molecular weight, and cross-reactivity is noted between glycoproteins from different cells.

B. Experimental Approach

Our approach to the study of human NK heterogeneity has involved the use of two complementary techniques and the repeated testing of a panel of donors. The experimental techniques employed are unlabelled target cell competitive inhibition (15) and selective depletion of NK effector cells by adsorption onto target cell monolayers (16,17).

The former technique, originally employed for the study of cytotoxic T cells (15), has been used to suggest common antigens on different target cells when the lysis of a labelled target can be blocked by the addition of a second, unlabelled target.

Target cell monolayer adsorption was also initially employed in the study of cytotoxic T cells (16,17). A preparation of cells containing the effectors of interest is incubated on an immobilized monolayer of target cells. Effectors which bear the appropriate recognition sites will adhere to the monolayer through interaction with the corresponding membrane determinants of the targets. Therefore, the population of cells non-adherent to the monolayer will be at least partially depleted of cytotoxic activity against the targets which comprise the adsorbing monolayer.

Data which we have generated using each of these techniques provide further evidence in support of heterogeneity both within the population of NK effector cells as well as with regard to NK determinants on different target cells.

II. METHODS

A. Lymphocyte Preparation

Lymphocytes were prepared from the blood of healthy adult volunteers according to the method of Boyum (18), followed by macrophage depletion on plastic as previously described (8,19).

B. ^{51}Cr-Release Assay for NK

Target cells were labelled with $Na_2{}^{51}CrO_4$ (8). All assays were carried out in triplicate in round-bottom microtiter plates in a total volume of 0.2 ml of minimal essential medium (MEM) with 10% fetal calf serum (FCS). In all assays $1x10^4$ targets were added to each well; lymphocyte effector cells were then added to give final effector cell:target cell (EC:TC) ratios of 0.3:1 to 20:1. The plates were centrifuged at 80xg for 3 min and then incubated 1½ to 3 hours at 37° in a humidified 7% CO_2 incubator. To harvest, plates were centrifuged at 500xg for 5 min and 100 μl of supernatant was removed for counting.

C. Tumor cell Monolayer Preparation

Monolayers of K562 or HSB were made on poly-L-lysine coated 60mm polystyrene tissue culture plates as previously described (19). Briefly, tumor cells ($9-12x10^6$) were allowed to adhere to the plates and then fixed with 0.2% formaldehyde for 1 hr at 4°C. The plates were used after gentle washing.

D. Separation on Tumor Cell MOnolayers

Human peripheral blood lymphocytes (PBL)($12x10^6$) in MEM with 10% FCS were allowed to adhere to each tumor cell monolayer for 1 hr at 37°C. The non-adherent PBL were removed by gentle agitation of the plates, decanting, and washing one time (19). The nonadherent PBL suspension was centrifuged, and the pellet resuspended in MEM with 10% FCS, counted, and adjusted to the appropriate concentration for assay.

III. EXPERIMENTAL FINDINGS

A. Monolayer Adsorption Experiments

1. Depletion of NK Effector Cells. PBL which were nonadherent to either K562 or HSB monolayers were assayed for NK activity against NK-sensitive target cells (K562, HSB, or MOLT4). As previously shown (19) the NK activity of nonadherent PBL was depressed relative to that of control, unfractionated lymphocytes (figure 1).

Several control experiments (data not shown, see reference 19) supported the hypothesis that NK effector cells had been selectively removed from the PBL population by adsorption onto the target cell monolayer. Firstly, adsorption of PBL onto a monolayer of SB cells, which are relatively insensitive to NK, did not result in depressed NK activity against HSB, a T cell line originally from the same donor as SB. Secondly, supernatant from a K562 monolayer had no effect when added to an NK assay. Thirdly, using two independent techniques, the level of contamination of the nonadherent fractions with detached tumor cells was found to be very low and could not account for the observed decrease in NK activity.

2. Quantitative Evaluation of NK Depletion. The extent of depletion of NK activity by adsorbing monolayers was quantified using the slope ratio method. Data generated over a 13 month period with several donors are summarized in Table 1.

When PBL from five out of seven donors (Table 1, MQ, HK, LU, AK, and JD) were fractionated on K562 monolayers, it was found that within a given experiment the extent of NK depletion against each

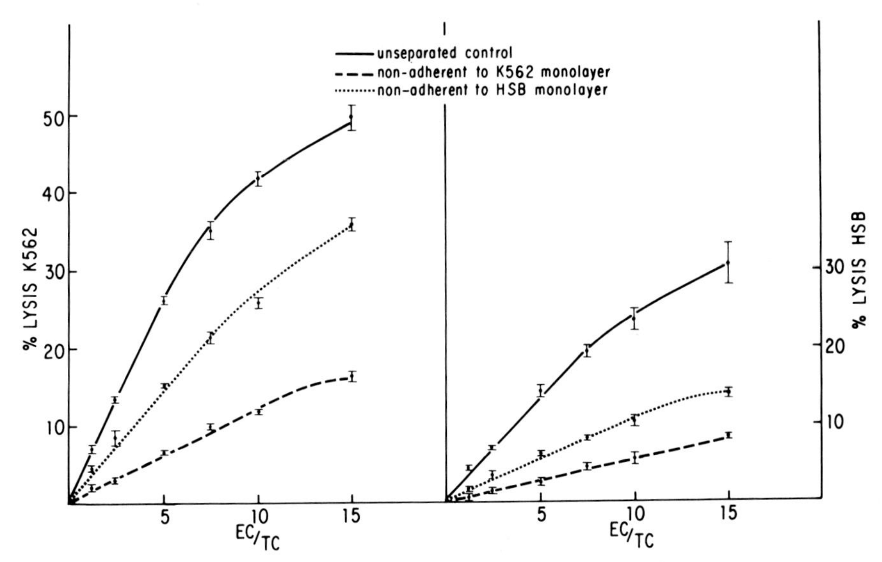

FIGURE 1. NK activity of PBL nonadherent to a K562 or HSB monolayer. Untreated control PBL (——), PBL nonadherent to a K562 monolayer (---), or PBL nonadherent to an HSB monolayer (···) were assayed for NK activity at the indicated EC/TC ratios. After Jensen, et al., see reference 19.

TABLE I: Relative Depletion of NK Activity Against Several Targets

		K562 Monolayer				HSB Monolayer		
	Target:	K562	HSB	MOLT4		K562	HSB	MOLT4
Donor	Date	Slope Ratios			Date	Slope Ratios		
MQ	10/19/78	.20	.21		10/19/78	.49	.14	
	11/14/78	.24	.17		11/14/78	.72	.09	
HK	10/31/78	.26	.23		10/31/78	.55	.40	
	11/19/78	.33	.34		11/19/78	.64	.46	
	7/18/78	.39	.35	.43	9/14/79	.68	.33	
LU	11/7/78	.21	.24		11/07/78	.61	.27	
AK	7/23/78	.41	.37	.35	8/01/79	.59	.39	.66
JD	7/04/79	.17	.15		7/04/79	.52	.13	
					8/28/79	.64	.31	.48
PJ	6/30/78	.23	.98		6/30/78	.51	.17	
	7/25/78	.07	.85		7/25/78	.41	.17	
	7/16/79	.33	1.05	.89	7/17/79	.53	.13	.17
					9/24/79	.57	.35	.47
HW	12/04/78	.32	.67		12/04/78	.57	.37	
	8/30/79	.22	.36	.23	8/31/79	.25	.06	.15

Control PBL and PBL non-adherent to either K562 or HSB monolayers were tested for NK activity against ^{51}Cr-labeled K562, HSB and/or MOLT4 at four or more effector cell concentrations. The data from each labeled target were expressed as slope of activity of non-adherent PBL ÷ slope of activity of unseparated control PBL (i.e. slope ratios).

of the target cells tested was remarkably similar. In contrast, the pattern seen with the other two donors tested (Table 1, PJ, HW) was qualitatively different. With both of these donors, K562 monolayers were able to deplete anti-K562 activity to a greater extent than anti-HSB activity. Donors PJ and HW differed, however, when NK activity against MOLT4 was considered. A K562 monolayer was able to deplete only very little NK activity against MOLT4 when PJ lymphocytes were tested; but when donor HW was tested, a K562 monolayer was found to deplete NK activity against K562 and against MOLT4 to an equivalent extent.

When PBL nonadherent to HSB monolayers were tested, it was found that with all donors NK against HSB was depleted to a greater extent than NK against K562 (or usually MOLT4).

B. Unlabelled Cell Competitive Inhibition Experiments

As a complementary approach to the study of NK heterogeneity, competitive inhibition experiments were performed using both K562 and HSB as labelled targets and unlabelled inhibitors. Similar to the monolayer adsorption experiments, the data obtained using competitive inhibition protocols varied qualitatively with the choice of PBL donor.

With donor HK (figure 2A&B), NK activity against both K562 and HSB was inhibited to a greater extent by unlabelled K562 than by HSB. On the other hand with donor PJ (figure 2C&D) the NK activity against each target was inhibited best by the addition of homologous inhibitor cells. It should be noted that the data from both donors shown in figure 2 were generated on the same day using the same preparations of target and inhibitor cells.

IV. INTERPRETATION

A. General Comments

Two complementary approaches have been employed in our study of NK recognition sites. Both cold cell competitive inhibition experiments and target cell monolayer adsorption data argue that the

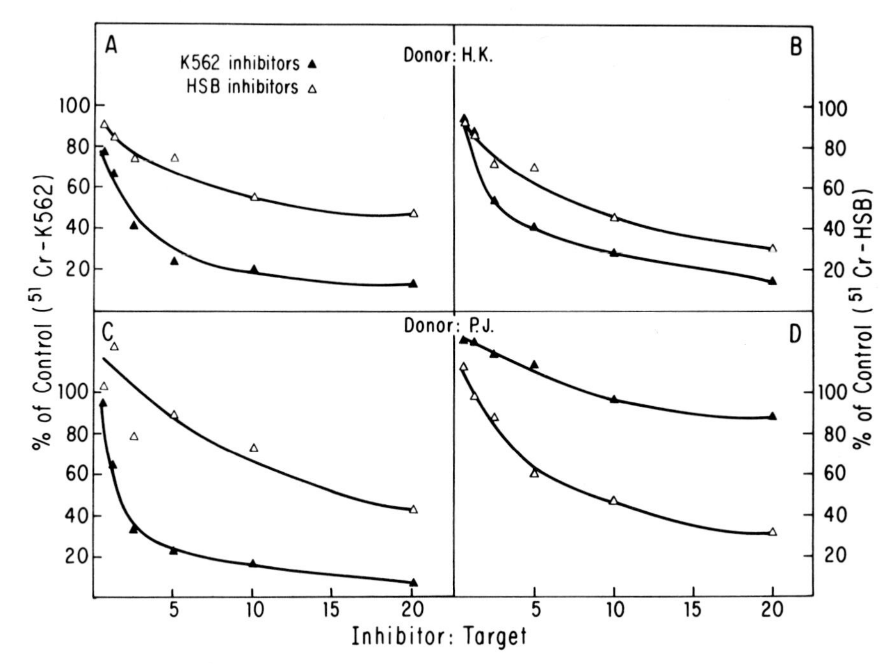

FIGURE 2. Cold Cell Competitive Inhibition. The ability of K562 inhibitor cells (▲) or HSB inhibitor cells (△) to block lysis of ^{51}Cr-labelled K562 or HSB targets was examined using PBL from two different donors. For ^{51}Cr-K562 assays the EC:TC ratio was 10:1, and for ^{51}CR-HSB assays it was 20:1. Percent lysis in the absence of any inhibitors was 48.9±2.2% for panel A, 31.3±0.5% for panel B, 13.6±1.4% for panel C, and 27.5±1.5% for panel D.

process of NK recognition involves both heterogeneous and shared components. Different NK effector cells appear to bear their own repetoire of NK-relevant surface determinants, some of which are overlapping and some unique. Similarly, different NK targets may have one or more types of NK sites which allow them to be recognized by the NK cells. Both experimental approaches which we have employed also reveal a reproducible difference in the nature of effector cells present in different donors.

B. Effector Cell Heterogeneity

With most of the donors tested (Table 1, MQ, HK, LU, AK, and JD), the K562 monolayer adsorption data imply the presence of an effector cell which is capable of lysing all three targets tested since K562 monolayers deplete NK activity to an equivalent extent against each target. The competitive inhibition experiments with donor HK (figure 2A&B) are consistent with the hypothesis that K562 and HSB are lysed by common effector cells. In addition, the HSB monolayer experiments with these same donors (Table 1, MQ, HK, LU, AK, and JD) suggest that there is also a subpopulation of NK effector cells which recognizes K562 (and also MOLT4 when tested), but not HSB, since anti-HSB activity is depleted to a greater extent than NK activity against the other targets on HSB monolayers.

The two other donors tested in this study (PJ, HW) show a qualitatively different pattern from that described above. The findings from donors PJ and HW are consistent with the presence of several types of NK effector cells in the PBL of these individuals: one which can lyse both K562 and HSB and two others which can lyse either K562 or HSB, but not both targets. The relative number of each type of NK cell in the total population is a contributing factor to the extent of NK depletion observed on the target cell monolayers. The competitive inhibition experiments with donor PJ (figure 2C&D) are also consistent with the presence of both shared and unique effector cells to lyse K562 and HSB, since each target is inhibited to a greater extent by the addition of homologous inhibitor cells than by the addition of the other cell type.

C. Target Cell Heterogeneity

The findings from donors PJ and HW also imply that K562 and HSB each have a unique NK determinant, not found on the other, although they may share additional NK determinants as well.

With regard to the possibility of shared NK determinants on target cells it is necessary to point out that the experimental techniques employed here do not allow us to make definitive statements regarding this possibility. The data generated imply that in many cases a single effector cell can kill several different types of targets. Two possibilities are compatible with this finding: 1) A common NK determinant may be present on the targets in question; 2) Multiple NK recognition sites, each specific for a particular target, may be present on a single effector cell. With regard to the second possibility, it would be expected that NK cells with multiple recognition structures could be adsorbed by different target cell monolayers; and it is not unreasonable to imagine that the binding of an inhibitor cell to one NK site on an effector cell might sterically or otherwise prevent the binding of a different, labelled target, resulting in competitive inhibition.

D. Variability Between Donors

A most interesting conclusion from the work described above is that the types of NK effector cells and their relative frequencies differ from one individual to another. Several experimental observations support the concept of individual variability. Repeated testing of the same donor in monolayer adsorption experiments shows qualitatively the same pattern of NK depletion, even when the experiments are carried out over periods of several months or a year (Table I). Also, unlabelled target cell competitive inhibition experiments done concurrently with different donors (figure 1) give qualitatively different results for each donor. Finally, the interpretations of data from two different types of experiments (monolayer adsorption and competitive inhibition) for a single individual are compatible.

E. Summary

Our conclusions, derived from the repeating testing of a panel of donors using two techniques, are compatible with results from other groups (9,10) using very different methods. We suggest that NK recognition sites are heterogeneous, that different types of NK cells with different specificities exist, and that individuals differ with regard to their NK cell repertoire.

REFERENCES

1. Rosenburg, E.B., McCoy, J.L., Green, S.S., Donnelly, F.C., Siwarsky, D.F., Levine, P.H., and Herberman, R.B., J. Natl. Cancer Inst. 52, 345 (1974).
2. Jondal, M., and Pross, H.F., Int. J. Cancer 15, 596 (1975).
3. Haller, O., Kiessling, R., Örn, A., Kärre, K., Nilsson, K., and Wigzell, H., Int. J. Cancer 20, 93 (1977).
4. Ono, A., Amos, D.B., and Koren, H.S., Nature 266, 5602 (1977).
5. Santoli, D., Trinchieri, G., and Lief, F.S., J. Immunol. 121, 526 (1978).
6. Ault, K.A., and Weiner, H.L., J. Immunol. 122, 2611 (1979).
7. Ortaldo, J.R., Oldham, R.K., Cannon, G.C., and Herberman, R.B., J. Natl. Cancer Inst. 59, 77 (1977).
8. Koren, H., and Williams, M.J., Immunol. 121, 1956 (1978).
9. Callewaert, D.M., Kaplan, J., Johnson, D.F., and Peterson, Jr., W.D., Cell Immunol. 42, 103 (1979).
10. Pollack, S.B., and Emmons, S.L., J. Immunol. 123, 160 (1979).
11. Roder, J.C., Rosen, A., Fenyo, E.M., and Troy, F.A., Proc. Natl. Acad. Sci. 76, 1405 (1979).
12. Roder, J.C., Ahrlund-Richter, L., and Jondal, M., J. Exp. Med. 150, 471 (1979).
13. Roder, J.C., and Kiessling, R., Scand. J. Immunol. 8, 135 (1978).
14. Roder, J.C., Kiessling, R., Biberfeld, P., and Andersson, B., J. Immunol. 212, 2509 (1978).
15. deLandazuri, M.O., and Herberman, R.B., Nature (New Biol.) 238, 18 (1972).
16. Stulting, R.D., and Berke, G., J. Exp. Med. 137, 932 (1973).
17. Stulting, R.D., Todd, III, R.F., and Amos, D.B., Cell Immunol. 20, 54 (1975).
18. Boyum, A., Scand. J. Clin. Lab. Invest. 97, (suppl. 21), 77 (1968).
19. Jensen, P.J., Amos, D.B., and Koren, H.S., J. Immunol. 123, 1127 (1979).

ARE NATURAL KILLER CELLS GERM-LINE V-GENE-ENCODED PROTHYMOCYTES SPECIFIC FOR SELF AND NONSELF HISTOCOMPATIBILITY ANTIGENS

Joseph Kaplan[1]

Department of Pediatrics
Wayne State University School of Medicine
Detroit, Michigan

Denis M. Callewaert[2]

Department of Chemistry
Oakland University
Rochester, Michigan

I. INTRODUCTION

This paper summarizes evidence we have obtained that natural killer (NK) cells belong to the T cell lineage, and comprise multiple clones each specific for one of many distinct antigens distributed as overlapping but unique sets on different target cells. Based on consideration of these findings in the light of the work of others, we put forth the hypothesis that NK cells are germ-line V-gene-encoded prothymocytes specifically directed against "self" and "non-self" histocompatibility (H) antigens.

[1] *Supported by NIH grant CA17534 and Research Career Development Award CA00188*
[2] *Supported by NIH grant AI12766 and a Special Fellowship from The Leukemia Society of America*

ISBN 0-12-341350-8

II. NATURAL KILLER CELLS BELONG TO THE T CELL LINEAGE

A. *Conventional T and B Cell Markers*

There is general agreement that human NK cells are lymphocytes, and that most have Fc receptors for IgG. However, their relationship to previously well defined T or B cell populations has been a matter of ongoing controversy. Using such T and B cell-separation procedures as nylon wool filtration, anti-Fab immunoabsorbent columns, and sheep erythrocyte (E)-rosette sedimentation, many investigators have found that NK cells fail to consistently co-purify with surface Ig-positive B lymphocytes or E-rosetting T lymphocytes. Rather, they tend to be concentrated in fractions enriched in "null" cells - lymphoid cells which are simultaneously E rosette-negative and surface Ig-negative (Jondal et al, 1975; Peter et al, 1975; Kiuchi et al, 1976; Cooper et al, 1977; and Nelson et al, 1977). By contrast, West et al (1976) have reported that a considerable proportion of NK cells, like T cells, bind sheep erythrocytes, but only under optimal conditions which permit low-avidity E-binding to be detected. They suggest that the failure of others to detect E-binding by NK cells is due to use of sub-optimal separation conditions. Indeed, it is well known that as a T cell marker and method of T cell purification, T cell binding of sheep erythrocyte varies greatly with minor changes in methodology.

B. *Development and Specificity of Anti-HTLA and Anti-HBLA*

Using antisera specific for human T and B lymphocyte antigens (HTLA and HBLA) it is possible to examine the T or B cell-relatedness of NK cells by a method which avoids the vagaries of rosette sedimentation technics. The antisera are raised by injecting rabbits with one of two autologous human lymphoblast cell lines - HSB-2 and SB. HSB-2 is an E-rosette-positive, Epstein-Barr-virus-negative T cell line, whereas SB is a typical EBV-positive, surface Ig-positive B cell line (Kaplan et al, 1974). Sera obtained from rabbits immunized with one or the other of these autologous T and B cell lines, after reciprocal absorption with the other cell line, specifically react with either E-rosette-positive T cells (anti-HTLA) or surface Ig-positive B cells (anti-HBLA) as shown in Table I.

TABLE I. Specificity of Anti-HTLA and ANTI-HBLA[a]

Cells	%E-RFC	%SIg	%Reactive With[b] Anti-HTLA	Anti-HBLA
T Cell Line MOLT	72	0	100	0
B Cell Line DAUDI	0	100	0	100
Thymocytes	95	5	99	2
Peripheral Blood Mononuclear Cells Unseparated	73	7	69	17
E-RFC-Depleted	5	65	23	77
Nylon Wool-Filtered	74	2	77	22
E-Depleted + Nylon Wool Filtered	9	4	59	39

[a]*For references see Kaplan et al, 1977 a,b.*
[b]*As measured by indirect immunofluorescence.*

The results in Table 1 also demonstrate that anti-HTLA and anti-HBLA react with E-negative surface Ig-negative null cells prepared by sequential E rosette-depletion and nylon wool filtration. Two distinct null cell subsets can be identified with these antisera: one $HTLA^+ HBLA^-$, and the other $HTLA^- HBLA^+$. This is reflected a) by the observation (Kaplan et al, 1977a) that children with "non-T non-B" or "null" cell acute lymphoblastic leukemia (ALL) fall into two distinct groups when their leukemic cells are tested with anti-HTLA and anti-HBLA: $HTLA^+ HBLA^-$ ALL and $HTLA^- HBLA^+$ ALL, and b) more directly, by the fact that complement lysis of normal peripheral blood null cells reactive with anti-HTLA results in reciprocal enrichment of null cells reactive with anti-HBLA, and vice versa (Kaplan et al, 1977b).

The $HTLA^+$ null cell subset contains immature T cells which form E rosettes after in-vitro incubation with thymosin, a thymic hormone (Kaplan et al, 1978a). The $HBLA^+$ null cell subset, on the other hand, contains myeloid and erythroid precursors. Anti-HBLA but not anti-HTLA induces the complement lysis of myeloid colony forming cells (Kaplan et al, 1978b) and erythroid colony-forming cells (Inoue et al, unpublished data).

C. Human NK Cells Express HTLA But Not HBLA

The null cell reactivity of anti-HTLA and anti-HBLA is particularly helpful in clarifying the nature of NK cells since such cells are found in both the E rosette-positive T cell population and in the null cell population. As shown in Table II, treatment with anti-HTLA + C but not with anti-HBLA + C reduces NK activity of peripheral blood mononuclear cells. This is due to lysis of NK cells rather than to formation of non-specifically inhibitory antibody-coated cold targets since no NK inhibition occurs when cells are treated with anti-HTLA in the absence of complement. Thymocytes, cells which consist almost entirely of E^+ T cells lacking NK activity, completely absorb the NK-reactivity of anti-HTLA. Therefore, NK cells express the same HTLA antigens expressed by E^+ T cells, not NK-specific antigens recognized by a minor population of antibodies present in anti-HTLA. Furthermore, since nearly all NK activity is removed by C-lysis of $HTLA^+$ cells, and since HTLA antigens occur on both E^+ T cells and some null cells, it would appear that even if there are two subsets of NK cells- one E^+ and the other E^- - both types express HTLA antigens, - and thus both belong to the T cell lineage.

TABLE II. NK Cells Express T But Not B Cell Antigens[a]

Effector Cell Treatment	*% Reduction NK Activity*[b]
None	*0*
Anti-HTLA + C	*78*
Anti-HBLA + C	*0*
Anti-HTLA	*0*
Anti-HBLA	*0*
Thymus-Absorbed Anti-HTLA + C	*0*

[a] *For references see Kaplan et al (1978 a,b).*

[b] *Ficoll-Hypaque-separated peripheral blood mononuclear cells were treated with anti-HTLA or anti-HBLA in the presence or absence of complement prior to testing for NK activity against 51-Chromium-labelled K562 cells. E:T ratio= 100:1.*

D. *Murine NK Cells Express T Cell-Associated Alloantigens*

The conclusion that NK cells belong to the T cell lineage is strongly supported by recent detection of the following T cell-associated alloantigens on murine NK cells: Thy-1 (Herberman et al, 1978; and Pollack et al, 1979), Ly5 (Cantor et al, 1979; and Pollack et al, 1979), Ly6 (Pollack et al, 1979), and Qa5(Chun et al, 1979).

E. *Resemblance of NK Cells to Pre-Thymic T Cell Precursors*

Because natural killer cell activity is even higher in congenitally athymic nu/nu mice than in normal mice, it is clear that if NK cells are of the T cell lineage they are not thymic or post-thymic T cells. Rather, as pointed out by Herberman et al (1978), they more closely resemble committed pre-thymic T cell precursors. Such cells are known to be present in nude mice, are produced in the bone marrow (Roelants et al, 1976), migrate to the thymus (Basch et al, 1977), and can be induced by thymic hormones to acquire phenotypic markers of mature T cells (Komuro et al, 1975). Like NK cells (Herberman et al, 1978; and Waksal et al, 1979), pre-thymic T cell precursors express a low density of Thy-1 antigen (Roelants et al, 1976), and BAT, a brain-associated T cell antigen (Basch et al, 1977). Furthermore, as described above, many human NK cells are found in the HTLA$^+$ null cell subpopulation, a subset which contains thymosin-inducible precursors of E rosette-positive T cells (Kaplan et al, 1977b).

The implications of the possibility that NK cells are pre-thymic T cell precursors will later be discussed in light of the following evidence concerning NK specificity.

III. NATURAL KILLER CELL SPECIFICITY

A. *Three Models*

We and others have investigated NK specificity by analyzing patterns of direct lysis and cold target inhibition. The results of these studies, summarized below, will be interpreted in the context of the following three divergent models of NK specificity (Figure 1): *A) NK-mediated lysis is nonspecific, and dependent only on target cell sensitivity to lysis and cytotoxic efficiency of effector cells. B) NK cells are nonspecific killer (K) cells which acquire immunological specificity by in vivo or in vitro absorption of antibodies via cell-surface Fc receptors. C) NK cells, like cytolytic T cells, produce their own antibody-like receptors which allow them to specifically bind and kill antigen-bearing target cells.*

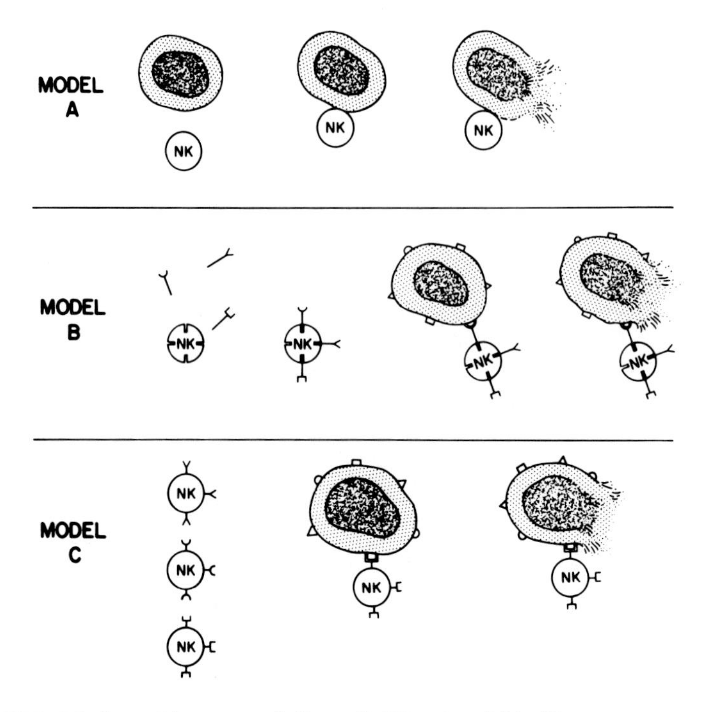

FIGURE 1. Three models of NK specificity.

B. How Do Results of NK Specificity Tests Fit With Each Model.

Each of these models presents different predictions for the results of experiments in which multiple effector cell populations are tested by direct cytotoxicity or cold target inhibition against a panel of target cells. Model A predicts that if NK cells from one donor lyse target X more than target Y, then NK cells from all other donors should do the same. This pattern is obtained when effector cells from many donors are tested against T cell line HSB-2 and autologous B cell line SB (Callewaert et al, 1979). Virtually all donors lyse HSB-2 more efficiently than they lyse SB. However, when the same donors are tested in parallel for lysis of B cell line SB and B cell line Raji, a different pattern emerges. Some donors kill SB but not Raji, whereas others kill Raji but not SB. This pattern of NK lysis is incompatible with model A but fits with either model B or model C. These latter results suggest that antigenic differences exist between certain target cells, and that donors differ in their ability to recognize different NK target antigens. That virtually all donors tested manifest the same relative levels of NK lysis against HSB-2 and SB can then be attributed to these two cells lines sharing a number of widely recognized NK target antigens, with cell line HSB-2 expressing either a higher density or a wider variety of these antigens than cell line SB.

More convincing evidence for the existence and unequal distribution of multiple NK target antigens on different target cells is obtained by cold target inhibition analysis. In this assay, which measure the effect of adding unlabelled cells of different types to mixtures of effector cells and labelled target cells, cross-inhibition by unrelated cell types is frequently observed. Generally, the level of inhibition produced by a given cell line is proportional to its susceptibility to direct NK lysis. However, regardless of the nature of the labelled target, maximal cold target inhibition nearly always occurs when unlabelled cells and labelled target cells are identical (Fig. 2,3).

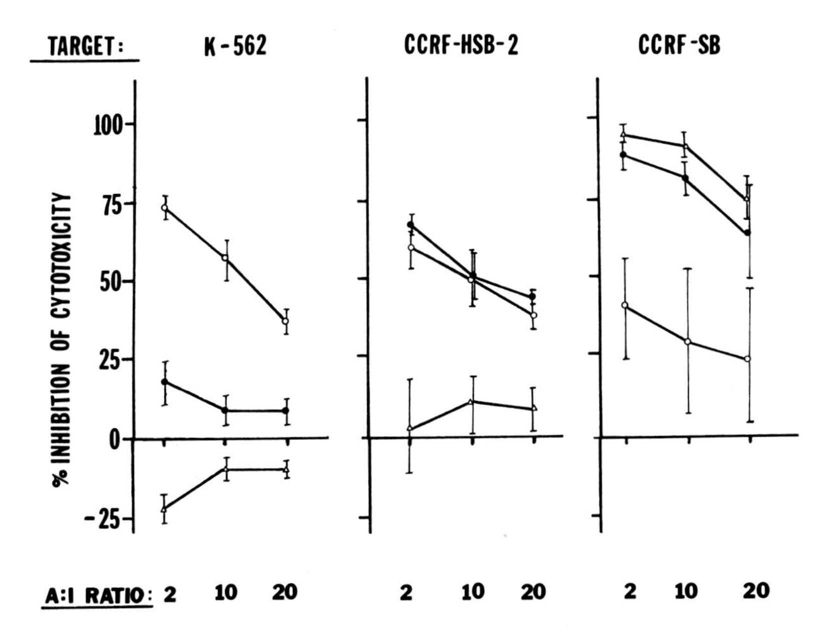

FIGURE 2. The inhibition of NK lysis of cell lines K562, HSB-2, and SB is plotted as the percentage inhibition of cytotoxicity as a function of the concentration of inhibitor cells added to the assay, expressed as attacker: inhibitor ratios. The concentrations of inhibitor cells used were $5X10^4$ *(A:I=20),* 10^5 *(A:I=10), and* $5X10^5$ *(A:I=2). Inhibitor cells are represented by the symbols: K562, open circles, HSB-2, closed circles, and SB, triangles. Effector cells (*10^6*/well) and 51-Cr-labelled target cells (*10^4*) were held constant. For reference, see Callewaert et al (1979).*

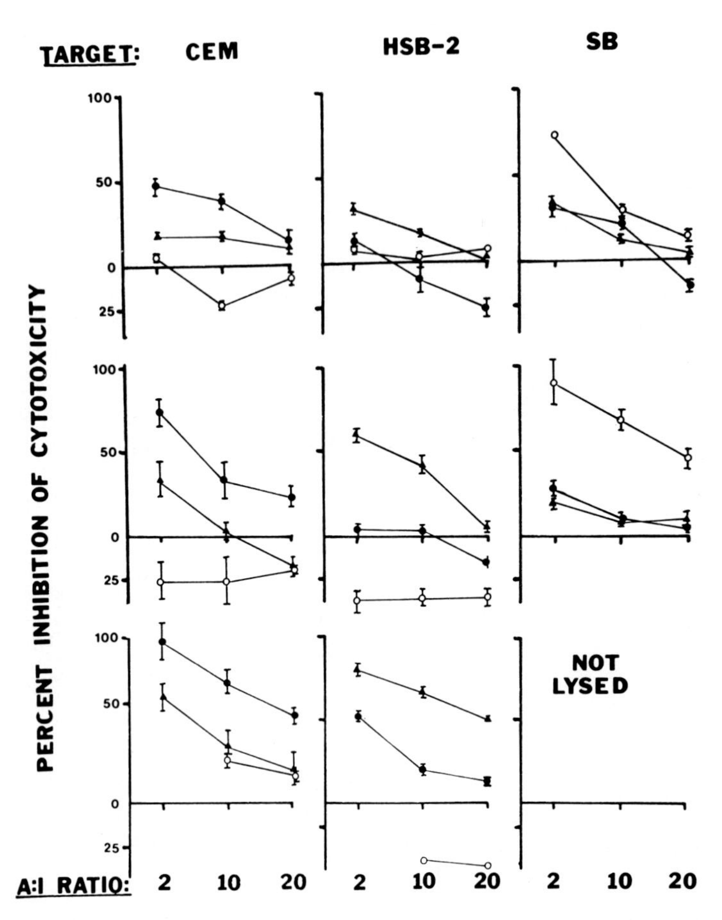

FIGURE 3. The inhibition of NK lysis of the cell lines CEM, HSB-2, and SB, effected by three individual donors, A(top), B(center), and C(bottom), is plotted as the percentage of inhibition of cytotoxicity as a function of the concentration of inhibitor cells added to the assay. The concentration of inhibitor cells is expressed as in Fig. 2. Inhibitor cells are represented by the symbols: CEM, closed circles, HSB-2, triangles, and SB, open circles. Effector cells (10^6/well) and 51-Cr-labelled target cells (10^4/well) were held constant. Uninhibited cytotoxicities for these effector/target mixtures were; A/CEM=14.9%, A/HSB-2=22.3%, A/SB=8.6%, B/CEM=25.6%, B/HSB-2=32.0%, B/SB=16.9%, C/CEM=24.4%, C/HSB-2=15.1%, C/SB=0%. For reference, see Callewaert et al (1979).

For example, as shown in Figures 2 and 3, highly NK-susceptible cell lines K562, CEM, and HSB-2 inhibit lysis of each other and of relatively insusceptible cell line SB far better than cell line SB inhibits NK lysis of K562, CEM, or HSB-2. However, the inhibition produced by unlabelled SB is equal to or better than unlabelled HSB-2, CEM, or K562 when labelled SB is the NK target. These findings imply that although multiple NK target antigens exist, many of which are shared by different cell lines, each cell line must express a unique set. A particularly wide variety and high density of these antigens should be expressed by cell lines such as K562 which are extremely NK-susceptible and show broad cross-inhibition.

C. NK Cells Are Polyclonal

In addition to shedding light on the multiplicity and distribution of NK target antigens, the phenomenon of maximal cold target inhibition by homologous cells, also observed by others in both human and murine systems (Haller et al, 1977; Herberman et al, 1975; and Takasugi et al, 1977) has important implications regarding the possible mechanisms by which NK cells specifically recognize target cells. As analyzed below, it strongly favors the existence, as portrayed in model C, of multiple clones of monospecific NK cells each expressing an intrinsically produced cell-surface receptor with unique specificity, and is inconsistent with both models A and B. The latter predict that for any given effector cell population the level of cold target inhibition produced by given cell should correlate with its susceptibility to NK lysis by that effector population, *regardless* of the identity of the labelled target cell.

In model A, the susceptibility of a target cell to NK lysis is an intrinsic cell property not specifically related to any surface antigen, and this intrinsic property should also determine its ability to compete with other target cells for interaction with and lysis by NK cell. In model B, each NK cell, is rendered capable of recognizing target cells by IgG antibodies adsorbed either *in vivo* or *in vitro* via Fc-receptors. According to this model, antibodies with diverse specificities should absorb to any given NK cell rendering each NK cell functionally multispecific. Only target cells expressing antigens recognized by at least one or more of these antibodies could be lysed by NK cells, or act as cold target inhibitors. Presumably, the relative susceptibility of a given target cell to NK lysis by a given effector population, and its relative ability to act as a cold target inhibitor, would be directly related to the number and/or density of NK-target antigens expressed by the target cell which were complementary to specific antibodies adsorbed to

NK cells in the effector population. Using this model, one would therefore predict that the target cell most susceptible to NK lysis by a given effector population should also be the best cold target inhibitor of that effector population-*regardless* of the of the identity of the labelled target cell.

In order to clarify differences between these models, let us consider a hypothetical example. Assume that cell line "X" expresses 2,500 molecules/cell of NK target-antigens 1,2, 3, and 4, (total of 10,000 NK antigens/cell), whereas cell line "Y" expresses 5,000 molecules/cell of NK target antigen 4 and 5,000 molecules/cell of NK target antigen 5. To consider model B, let us also assume that plasma cells from a given individual synthesize and secrete roughly equivalent numbers of IgG antibodies to NK Target antigens 1,2,3,4, and 5. In this model, each NK cell from this individual should non-specifically absorb equivalent amounts of all 5 antibody specificities. Therefore, if 10 antibody molecules of each specificity absorbed to each NK cell, the total number of antibody-antigen interactions possible between one NK cell and one target "X" cell would be 40, (i.e. 10 for each of the 4 specifically recognized target antigens 1,2,3, and 4), whereas only 20 such interactions would be possible between one NK cell and one target "Y" cell. If, as seems likely, the probability of lysis increases with the strength of binding between effector and target, cell line "X" should be lysed to a greater extent than cell line "Y". Furthermore, by this reasoning, unlabelled cell line "X" should be superior to unlabelled cell line "Y" as a cold target inhibitor of NK lysis of both labelled target "X" and labelled target "Y".

According to model C, on the other hand, a given population of NK cells consists of multiple monospecific clones. Now assume that a given individual possesses roughly equivalent numbers of each of the 5 relevant NK clones specific for NK-target antigens 1,2,3,4, and 5. This individual should possess twice as many NK cells reactive with cell line "X" (expressing antigens 1,2,3, and 4) as compared to NK cells that are reactive for cell line "Y" (expressing antigens 4 and 5). NK cells from this individual might be expected, therefore, to lyse cell line "X" twice as efficiently as they would lyse cell line "Y". Because both cell lines "X" and "Y" express NK-target antigen 4, there should be a certain degree of cross-reactivity between them in cold target inhibition assays. When tested using labelled "X" cells as targets, unlabelled cell line "Y" should compete for the NK cells bearing receptors specific for antigen 4 but not for NK cells bearing receptors for the other target "X" antigens (i.e. 1,2,and 3), and thus might give 25% inhibition. Using labelled "X" cells as targets, unlabelled cell line "X", possessing *all four* of the relevant antigens, should give 100% inhibition. On the other hand, if labelled "Y" cells are used as targets, unlabelled cell line "X" should compete for anti-4 but not anti-5-specific NK cells, and thus might give 50% inhibition. However, unlabelled cell line "Y", possessing both of the relevant antigens, should give 100% inhibition in this case. Thus, in model C (polyclonal NK cells), cells identical to the labelled target cells should, as observed, be the best cold target inhibitors, regardless of their overall susceptibility to NK lysis. Exceptions to this rule should only occur when unlabelled cells express the same set of NK target antigens as the labelled target cells, but in higher density.

IV. THE NATURE OF ANTIGENS RECOGNIZED BY NK CELLS

Although the precise nature of antigens recognized by NK cells remains to be determined, several general trends seem apparent. Firstly, they are widely distributed on both malignant and normal cells from many different tissues (Herberman et al, 1979). Malignant cells probably express a relatively high density of these antigens compared to normal cells since they are, in general, more susceptible than their normal counterparts to NK lysis (Callewaert et al, 1977). Secondly, the antigens belong to both the "self" and "non-self" category since NK cells lyse autologous, allogeneic, and, in some cases, xenogeneic cells (Kiessling et al, 1979). Thirdly, some of the "self" antigens recognized by NK cells appear to be related or identical to histocompatibility antigens. Harmon et al (1977) have shown that in certain strains of mice heterozygous at H-$2D^b$, natural killer cell activity, like F_1 hybrid resistance to parental bone marrow grafts and *in vitro* F_1 anti-parent cytotoxicity, is directed at antigens mapping at the D end of the H-2 complex. Such antigens have been termed hybrid histocompatibility (Hh) antigens, in this case Hh-1^b antigens. Unlike classical histocompatibility antigens, they seem to be inherited as non-codominants. Thus it has been assumed that Hh-1^b antigens are distinct from H-$2D^b$. However, they have yet to be separated from H-$2D^b$ by genetic analysis raising the possibility that the two are, in fact, identical. This possibility is strengthened by the recent finding of O'Neill and Blanden (1979) that some F_1 hybrids express parental antigens in a non-codominant fashion.

V. CONCLUSIONS

A. *NK Cell Characteristics and Specificity*

The evidence summarized above suggests that natural killer cells are pre-thymic committed T cell-precursors comprised of multiple clones of monospecific cells expressing receptors for antigens which, in their pattern of distribution closely resemble self and non-self histocompatibility antigens. Jerne (1971)postulated the existence of cells with precisely these properties in a hypothesis which links "the generation of antibody diversity with the genetic determination of specific immune responsiveness and the alloagressive properties of the immune system".

B. *Jerne's Theory of Generation of Diversity*

Jerne has proposed that the germ cells of an animal contain a set of genes encoding the combing sites of lymphocyte receptors (germ-line variable or v-genes), and these germ-line v-gene-encoded combining sites are specifically directed against a complete set of major histocompatibility complex (MHC)-encoded antigens of the species to which the animal belongs. One pair of these germ-line v-genes is expressed on a lymphocyte at an early stage of differentiation. Mutants that recognize foreign antigens arise in lymphocyte clones expressing germ-line v-genes coding for receptors directed against self-MHC gene products.

For the generation of T cell diversity, this somatic mutation (somatic v-gene recombination also fits with the hypothesis) is proposed to take place in the thymus by the following mechanism: germ-line v-gene-encoded prothymocytes expressing receptors for self (S) or allo (A)- species H antigens migrate to the thymus. Those expressing v-genes of subset S are driven to proliferate by interaction with self-H antigens, and are eliminated. Others undergo a spontaneous v-gene mutation such that they express receptors which have a lower affinity for self-H antigens. Some of these S subset mutants survive, and escape the thymus as mature antigen-sensitive T cells expressing altered receptors which now fit one of a multitude of foreign antigens. By contrast, prothymocytes of the A-subset, because they lack receptors which interact with thymic H-antigens, escape both thymic elimination and somatic mutation, and emerge as mature alloreactive cells which then constitute a sizeable proportion of the post-thymic T cell population. According to this hypothesis, the inherited histocompatibility antigen pattern of an individual influences immune responsiveness by determing the subset S of v-genes available for modification by mutation which, in turn, restricts the range of antibody diversity.

Jerne's hypothesis has received substantial support from experiments which demonstrate that, in the mouse, post-thymic T cells specific for foreign antigens are derived from pre-thymic cells bearing receptors for H-2 antigens expressed by elements of the thymus in which they mature (for review see Zinkernagel, 1979).

C. Hypothesis

We now propose that NK cells belong to the population of pre-thmyic cells postulated by Jerne to express germ-line v-gene-encoded receptors specific for self and non-self histocompatibility antigens. Just as germ-line v-gene-encoded receptors specific for self-cell surface components may have evolved early during phylogeny as cell-cell recognition structures important in the development of specialized tissues, (Jerne, 1971), NK cells expressing such structures may originally have evolved as regulators of hematopoietic stem cells, as proposed by Cudkowicz and Hochman (1979). Subsequently, they may have been adopted by the host as a relatively unsophisticated defense system directed against tumors and intracellular parasites. With development of the thymus, NK cells may then have begun to serve as precursors of the vastly more diverse and specific post-thymic T cell populations.

The present hypothesis is a unifying concept linking the T cell lineage properties of natural killer cells with the pattern of specificity they exhibit. A number of predictions arise from this hypothesis which can be tested. For example, the hypothesis postulates that NK cells are prothymocytes. In mice, such cells can be induced *in vitro* by thymic hormones to express increased amounts of Thy-1 antigen (Komuro et al, 1975). Thymic hormone-treated murine NK cells should, therefore, manifest enhanced susceptibility to complement lysis by anti-Thy-1 antibody. Furthermore, NK cells, isolated by methods such as those described by Roder et al (1978), should migrate to the thymus on adoptive transfer. The postulate that some NK cells are specific for self-H antigens whereas others are specific for non-self-H antigens might be tested by inhibition analysis of NK lysis by H-2D^{b} heterozygotes against H-2D$^{b/b}$ homozygous cell line EL-4, much of which appears to be directed at H-2D^{b}-associated antigens (Harmon et al, 1977). Pretreatment of H-2D^{b} heterozygotes with H-2D$^{b/b}$ homozygous parental spleen cells should partially but specifically inhibit NK activity against EL-4 (Clark et al, 1977) but not NK activity against YAC, which is H-2D$^{d/d}$.

D. Summary

We have presented evidence that NK cells belong to the T cell lineage, resemble pre-thymic T cell precursors, are polyclonal, and specific for antigens which resemble histocompatibility antigens. This has led us to propose that NK cells belong to the germ-line v-gene-encoded prothymocyte population specific for histocompatibility antigens from which, as Jerne has proposed, T cell diversity is generated. Experiments designed to test this hypothesis will hopefully lead to a clearer understanding of the role of natural killer cells in cell-mediated immunity against tumors.

REFERENCES

Basch, R.S., And Kadish, J.L. (1977). *J. Exp. Med. 145,* 405.

Callewaert, D.M., Kaplan, J., Peterson, W.D. Jr., and Lightbody, J.J. (1977). *Cell Immunol. 33.* 11.

Callewaert, D.M., Kaplan, J., Johnson, D.F., and Peterson, W.D. Jr., (1979). *Cell Immunol. 42,* 103.

Cantor, H., Kasai, M., Shen, F.W., Leclerc, J.C., and Glimcher, L. (1979). *Immunol. Rev.44,* 3.

Chun, M., Pasanen, V., Hammerling, U., Hammerling, G.F., and Hoffman, M.K. (1979). *J. Exp.Med. 150,* 426.

Clark, E.A., Harmon, R.C., and Wichker, L.S. (1977). *J. Immunol. 119,* 648.

Cooper, S.M., Hirsen, D.J., and Friou, G.J. (1977). *Cell. Immunol. 32,* 135.

Cudkowicz, G., and Hochman, P.S. (1979). *Immunol. Rev.44,* 13.

Haller, O., Kieslling, R., Orn, A., Karre, K. Nillson, K., and Wigzell, H. (1977). *Int. J. Cancer 20,* 93.

Harmon, R.C., Clark, E.A., O'Toole, C., and Wicker, L.S. *Immunogenetics 4,* 601.

Herberman, R.B., Nunn, M.E. and Lavrin, D.H. (1975) *Int. J. Cancer 16,* 216.

Herberman, R.B., Nunn, M.E., and Holden, H.J. (1978). *J. Immunol. 121,* 304.

Herberman, R.B., Dieu, J.Y., Kay, H.D., Ortaldo, J.R., Riccardi, C., Bonnard, G.D., Holden, H.T., Fagnani, R., Santoni, A., And Puccetti, P. (1979), *Immunol. Rev. 44,*43.

Jerne, N.K. (1971). *Eur. J. Immunol. 1,*1.

Jondal, M., and Pross, H. (1975). *Int. J.Cancer 15,* 596.

Kaplan, J., Shope, T.C., and Peterson, W.D. Jr. (1974). *J. Exp. Med. 139,* 1070.

Kaplan, J., Ravindranath, Y., and Peterson, W.D. Jr. (1977a). *Blood 49,* 371.

Kaplan, J., and Peterson, W.D. Jr. (1977b). *Clin. Immunol. Immunopathol. 8,* 530.

Kaplan, J., and Peterson, W.D. Jr. (1978a). *Clin. Immunol. Immunopathol. 9,* 436.

Kaplan, J. Inoue, S., and Ottenbreit, M.J. (1978b). *Nature 271,* 458.

Kaplan, J., and Callewaert, D.M. (1978c). *J. Nat. Cancer.Inst. 60,* 961.

Kaplan, J. Callewaert, D.M., and Peterson, W.D., Jr. (1978d). *J. Immuno. 121,* 1366.

Keissling, R. and Wigzell, H. (1979). *Immunol. Rev. 44,* 165.

Kiuchi, M. and Takasugi, M. (1976). *J. Nat.Cancer Inst. 56,* 575.

Komuro, K. Goldstein, G., and Boyse, E.A. (1975). *J. Immunol. 115,* 195.

Nelson, D.L., Bundy, B.M. and Strober, W. (1977) *J. Immunol. 119,* 1401.

O'Neill, H.C., and Blanden, R.V. (1979). *J. Exp. Med. 149, 724.*

Peter, H.H., Pavie-Fischer, J., Fridman, W.H., Aubert, C. Cesarini, J-P., Roubin, R., and Kourilsky, F.M. (1975). *J. Immunol. 115,* 539.

Pollack, S.B., Tam, M.R., Nowinski, R.C., and Emmons, S.L. (1979. *J. Immunol. 123,* 1818.

Roder, J.C., Kieslling, R., Biberfeld, P., and Andersson, B. (1978). *J. Immunol. 121,* 2509.

Roelants, G.E., Mayor, K.S., Hagg, L-B, and Loor, F. (1976) *Eur. J. Immunol. 6,* 75.

Takasugi, M., Koide, Y., Akira, D., and Ramseyer, A., (1977). *Int. J. Cancer 19,* 291.

Waksal, S.D., Robert, N., Parkinson, D.R., and Morrissey, P.J. (1979). *In* "Cell Biology and Immunology of Leukocyte Function. Proceedings of the Twelfth Leukocyte Culture Conference" (M.R. Quastel, ed.) p. 935. Academic Press, N.Y.

West W.H., Cannon, G.B., Kay, H.D., Bonnard, G.D., and Herberman, R.B. (1976). *J. Immunol. 18,* 355.

Zinkernagel, R.M. (1979). *Immunol. Rev. 44,* 224.

NATURAL AND ACTIVATED LYMPHOCYTE KILLERS WHICH AFFECT TUMOR CELLS[1]

Eva Klein
Maria G. Masucci[2]
Giuseppe Masucci
Farkas Vanky[3]

Department of Tumor Biology
Karolinska Institutet
Stockholm, Sweden

In the initial studies of lymphocyte mediated cytotoxicity the phenomenon was considered to be the consequence of target cell recognition due to the presence of plasma membrane antigens for which the attacking lymphocyte carried specific receptors. The classical rules of immunology concerning specificity, and memory were shown to be valid for the generation of killer lymphocytes. Assays demonstrating lymphocyte cytotoxicity were used in several systems for demonstration of cellular immunity. In the course of these studies it was discovered that in addition to the effects expected on the basis of the sensitization history other, apparently nonspecific cytotoxicities often occur against some, but not against other targets. Also, certain targets were affected by lymphocytes derived from individuals without previous history of sensitization. This latter phenomenon was regarded as a disturbing factor in search for antigen specific effects, but

[1] *The work of the authors referred to was supported by Grant Number 1 R01 CA25250-01, awarded by the National Cancer Institute, DHEW and by the Swedish Cancer Society.*
[2] *Recipient of a fellowship from the Blancefort-Bon-Compagni-Ludovisi Foundation, Stockholm, Sweden.*
[3] *Recipient of a fellowship from the Stanley Thomas Johnson Foundation, Bern, Switzerland.*

ISBN 0-12-341350-8

some workers proposed that it may be a manifestation of a mechanism operating in immune surveillance (1). This view was strengthened by the fact that among lymphoblastoid cell lines the highly sensitive ones were derived from tumors (2).

I. CHARACTERISTICS OF THE NK SYSTEM

It was thus considered that the NK system (natural killing - one of the designations given to this operational phenomenon i.e. cytotoxicity observed with lymphocytes from donors with no known immunisation history to the particular target used) is important in the rejection of tumor cells. Indeed it was found in mice that the rules which emerged in the *in vitro* studies with regard to genetics (there is a genetically governed difference in the NK activity of mice) age of the donor of the effector cells (NK efficiency peaks at 2-4 months) and the sensitivity of the target cells are reflected *in vivo* in transplantation experiments (3). However there is as yet no evidence to validate the assumption that cytotoxic cells which could be defined as NK effectors would operate in tumor defense in primary induction systems.

The majority of NK studies utilise selected, highly sensitive, targets i.e. those killed in short term tests with low effector target ratios, showing that the proportion of lymphocytes capable of killing these particular targets is high.

The work of Trinchieri et al. (4) and Saksela et al. (5) revealed that in the long term cytotoxicity assays, activation of effectors has to be taken into account as a consequence of their interaction with the target cells. Interferon may be produced by certain lymphocyte subsets which in turn can promptly activate the killer lymphocytes for enhanced activity.

High sensitivity is the property of cultured cells (6). This may indicate that the NK sensitive cells are eliminated *in vivo* and survive only if in the culture condition the cell population is released from the effect of killer lymphocytes. But it may also mean that the conditions prevailing *in vitro* alter the plasma membrane of the target and effects, due to such alterations, are not likely to occur *in vivo*. Freshly harvested targets are usually not affected in short term cytotoxic assays. Human tumor cells derived from biopsies were rarely killed by lymphocytes of healthy donors. Killing occurred only with effector populations which had an exceptionally high proportion of active cells as indicated by their effect on the standard NK targets such as K562 and Molt-4 (7).

In a study aimed at clarifying the conditions influencing NK susceptibility of the target it was shown that the sensitivity of the same mouse tumor line changed depending on whether it was derived from cultures or after retransplantation from animals (8).

The characteristics determining the degree of NK sensitivity of a given cell is unknown. Cell lines can be divided into three categories: 1. Sensitive in short term assays, i.e., within the range of the effector/target ratios used, usually up to 50:1, considerable target cell damage occurring with low ratios. 2. Sensitive only in long term assays. 3. Insensitive. The difference between the first and second categories is probably quantitative. It seems that the threshold level of activity displayed by the effector lymphocyte which is necessary to inflict damage varies for the different cell lines. This is manifested in the assays as a variable number of effector cells necessary to kill a given number of targets. During prolonged interaction the lymphocytes with cytotoxic potential are activated for higher level of activity. As mentioned above it has been shown that interferon is involved in this event (4, 9).

A certain regularity appears when lymphoblastoid lines are used as targets in the human system. In short term tests T cell derived lines are more sensitive than those derived from B cells (10). It is with the B lymphoblastoid lines that the rule emerged that tumor-derived lines are more sensitive than those derived from normal cells (2). Two types of B lines can be distinguished: 1. derived from B cell malignancies, and 2. transformed for infinite growth *in vitro* from normal B cells by infection with Epstein Barr Virus (EBV). In this connection it may be noted that the presence of EBV genome in the cell does not seem to influence NK sensitivity. EBV negative B tumor lines and their EBV converted sublines (derived by superinfection of the EBV negative line with the virus) displayed no difference in sensitivity (to be published).

Human lymphocytes with cytotoxic potential belong to the T subset but are heterogeneous with regard to plasma membrane characteristics (6, 11, 12). Blood lymphocytes separated on the basis of adherence to nylon wool, presence of SIg, E and Fc receptors yielded more than one active subset. The strongest "specific" activity, i.e., activity on a per cell basis, was found in the operational "null" population obtained after elimination of SIg positive B cells by filtration through nylon wool, and removal of those T cells which rosette readily with SRBC (13, 14). In the SRBC rosetting T subset the proportion of killers was high among those which had relatively low avidity E receptors and expressed concomitantly Fc receptors (15). It seems that Fc receptors do not participate in the killing mechanism (16, 17). They are, however, useful markers which can be exploited for separation of the majority of active cells from the SRBC rosetting T subset. Thus, with regard to the functional involvement of the FcR the mechanism of NK differs from that of ADCC which requires this receptor.

II. KILLER CELLS GENERATED IN CULTURE

The NK potential gradually disappears in culture (18). If, however, the conditions are such that the lymphocytes become activated in the culture, they will exert cytotoxicity also against some cultured lines without known antigenic relationship to the stimulus. The seemingly unspecific cytotoxicity accompanying the allospecific killing in the mixed lymphocyte cultures was designated as (AK) "Anomalous Killing" (19).

Cytotoxic populations emerge only if the culture conditions involve activation. Hence we used the term Activated Lymphocyte Killing (ALK).

The characteristics of the killer populations in the natural and the activated systems are slightly different (19). In the latter a relatively higher proportion of cytotoxic cells was found to adhere to nylon wool. ALK also affected targets which were resistant to NK in short term tests. The fresh and cultured populations were similar in that the subsets with high affinity E receptors were the least active. The proportion of active cells with FcR expression was found to be lower in the ALK than in the NK (19). An important similarity is that the histocompatibility restriction phenomenon is not operative either in NK or ALK.

ALK does not represent the survival of active NK cells but is newly generated in the cultures because it appears when lymphocyte subsets depleted of NK activity are exposed to antigen (19). In addition, lymphocytes kept *in vitro* (in medium supported with autologous plasma) for several days and having lost NK activity could be induced again for killing in the condition of mixed cultures (18). There is a quantitative correlation between the extent of activation as indicated by blastogenesis and the efficiency of ALK (20).

Appearance of ALK in mixed lymphocyte culture did not require cell division and thus is not dependent on the enlargement of the alloreactive clone. Precursor cells present at the initiation of the culture are triggered to ALK concomitant with the specific recognition step (21). In accordance with this finding when restimulation with the specific target gave a secondary response, the accompanying ALK was not elevated to a similar extent (19).

We attempted to separate the CTL which affect the specific alloblasts and the ALK cells on the basis of E rosetting and

and expression of Fc receptors. The alloblasts were killed more efficiently by the E rosetting cells, which sedimented in Ficoll whereas the anti-K562 effect (ALK) was enriched in the interphase (22). Absorption to an immunocomplex coated plastic surface was used to separate the population according to the expression of FcR. The allospecificity resided in the FcR negative while ALK (anti-K562) was present both in the FcR negative and positive subsets (19).

III. ENHANCEMENT OF THE KILLER POTENTIAL BY INTERFERON

Short term exposure of lymphocytes *in vitro* to IF results in considerably enhanced cytotoxic activity (4, 9). We will refer to the effect of such lymphocytes as Interferon Activated Killing (IAK). The mechanism by which IF imposes the elevated function on the cells is unknown. It occurs *in vivo* also, administration of interferon inducing substances or viruses to experimental animals and man were shown to result in elevation of the NK activity of their spleen or blood lymphocytes (23).

It is important to note that IAK was shown to be exerted by the same subsets of lymphocytes as NK, the ranking orders were similar but IAK functioned at higher levels (24, 25). As discussed above, we assume a heterogeneity of the killer lymphocytes with regard to the level of function. IF probably elevates the level of activity, and therefore IAK affects also those targets which can be damaged only by effectors operating with higher intensity (26). The observed enhancement depends on the efficacy of the test without the influence of IF. The number of effectors necessary to lyse a given number of K562 or Molt-4 cells was only slightly altered by IF pretreatment (in one experiment calculated for 15% target lysis this increase was 2-fold for K562 and 3-fold for Molt-4). This suggests that the target cells can be killed by a high proportion of lymphocytes without the necessity of elevating their activity. In contrast, the impact of IF treatment on the effects against cell lines with relatively lower sensitivity such as Daudi and Raji was more substantial (in the experiment mentioned above the IF-induced change was about 11-fold for Daudi). The efficiency of killing with the IF-treated cells was similar whether K562 or Daudi were used as targets (25).

Two sets of experiments provide evidence that the elevated IAK compared to NK in a given system is due to recruitment of further effectors, rather than stimulation of cells already active against the particular target in such a way that each cell is capable of killing a higher number of targets. These experiments were 1) Comparative limiting dilutions of effectors in NK and IAK against Daudi as target; increased number - about 10-fold - of active samples were obtained in IAK (26); 2) Elimination of NK cells by pre-exposure of the lymphocyte population to the fibroblast monolayer left potentially active cells in the supernatant inducible by IF treatment (5). In addition, results with an *in vivo* system also pointed to this mechanism. When rats were depleted of NK activity by radiation or drug treatment and injected with IF inducers, cytotoxic cells were found to reappear after a short time (27).

The short term NK and IAK systems differ only in the technical aspects in that the latter involves pretreatment of the effector cells. The two systems overlap, however, because lymphocytes of an individual exhibiting high activity would function similarly to the lymphocytes of another donor with inherent low activity after exposure to IF. Thus, what can be achieved artificially *in vitro* with the lymphocytes of one individual can be a genuine level in another individual. The reason for the different levels of activation in various individuals is unknown. Because of this feature of the two systems, rules emerging from IAK experiments are likely to be valid for the NK system.

Tumor patients have been found to have relatively low activity, though this was not an absolute rule. Whether the patients belonged to the "high" or "low" NK catagory, did not relate to their clinical status (28, 29). "Low" NK active tumor patients lymphocytes can be enhanced by IF showing that the potentially active cells are not absent (7). With all individuals tested IF treatment of the lymphocytes abolished the difference between the efficiencies of killing K562 and Daudi. Fractionation of the lymphocytes into subsets showed a certain selectivity inasmuch as separation on the basis of Fc receptor expression gave populations which functioned differently against K562 and Daudi after IF treatment. K562 was killed by both the Fc receptor positive and negative subsets, whereas Daudi was preferentially affected by the Fc receptor negative cells (25).

The implication of the findings with activated cells is that results with effector populations fractionated on the basis of Fc receptor expression may differ according to the target cell type used. Previously Fc receptor positive cells were considered as being mainly responsible for the NK effect and specific cytotoxicity was searched for after their removal. Since FcR negative killers are more abundant in activated lymphocyte populations and targets may vary in their relative sensitivity to effectors according to the expression of this receptor, removal of FcR positive cells may not guarantee the elimination of a non-disease related, non-selective cytotoxicity.

It is possible that the cytotoxic characteristics of the blood lymphocyte population during the acute phase of EBV- and Cytomegalo Virus-induced mononucleosis is the consequence of its activated state. The lymphocytosis in the blood is due to proliferation of T lymphocytes (31). It was proposed that the lymphocytosis in the EBV-induced disease is a response against the EBV genome-carrying B cells. During the acute phase, when blasts are present in the blood, short term cytotoxicity is not restricted to NK sensitive targets (31). The sensitive target panel suggested that killing is due to the recognition of EBV-determined surface antigens. In order to remove disturbing NK effects EBV mononucleosis lymphocytes were assayed for cytotoxicity after elimination of FcR positive cells since these were known to be mainly responsible for the NK activity in healthy blood donors. Since FcR does not serve as marker for the total killer cell population especially when the lymphocytes are activated, depletion of FcR positive T cells cannot ensure elimination of the nondiscriminative cytotoxicity. In view of the above mentioned difference between K562 and Daudi (and other B lymphoblastoid lines) with regard to sensitivity to FcR positive and negative effectors, the interpretation of the results may be altered. It is likely that the broadening of the sensitive target panel in the mononucleosis syndrome is the consequence of T cell activation rather than representing an EBV specific cytotoxicity.

IV. THE ROLE OF ALLOANTIGENS IN THE NK EFFECT

As mentioned above, in studies concerning the characteristics of the NK phenomenon mainly cultured cells were used as targets. In our studies, primarily concerned with search for tumor specific reactivity in patients with solid tumors (sarcomas and carcinomas) we have seen that tumor cells freshly isolated from biopsies were rarely affected by lymphocytes of healthy donors, i.e., their sensitivity to the NK effect was low. However, when the lymphocytes were activated with IF and thereafter used as effectors against the biopsy-derived tumor cells, killing occurred in 49% of the cases. Using the patient's own lymphocytes, however, no IF-induced cytotoxicity occurred. The blood lymphocytes of other tumor patients, i.e. in tests with allogeneic combinations, were activated to the same extent as seen with the healthy donor's lymphocytes (7).

A likely explanation for the allogeneic killing induced by IF in our experiments with human tumor cells is a polyclonal activation of the cytotoxic potential which is then manifested by the lymphocytes committed to the alloantigen specificities expressed on the particular target cells. The role of the specific receptors may be the establishment of contact between the interacting cells.

Experiments concerning the nature of NK and IAK have not yet been interpreted to reveal the recognition of alloantigens though it may be the cause of the specificity, often detectable superimposed on cross reactivities as seen in cold target competition experiments.

Indications for the recognition of alloantigens in the NK system were seen when *in vivo* activated murine killer cells were tested on macrophage targets in a 16 h assay. The effect was weaker on syngeneic, as compared to on allogeneic targets (32).

It seems that the conditions required to reveal the alloantigen-determined killing have to be strict in the sense that cultured target cells have to be avoided.

The activation of cytotoxic precursors by IF and the manifestation of cytotoxicity toward cells carrying alien histocompatibility antigens are similar to the findings with mitogen-activated murine cells. Spleen cells treated *in vitro* with Concavalin A (Con-A) exerted cytotoxicity only toward targets which expressed alien major histocompatibility locus-determined antigens. This type of cytotoxicity was different from that obtained in the presence of lectin which also affected histocompatible cells. The interpretation proposed was that Con-A activates precursors for expression of cytotoxic potential and in a particular test the clone, which was committed to the MHC antigens present on the target, exerted the killing. Since it is known that the frequency of lymphocytes which recognize MHC antigens is high, such cytotoxicities can often be measurable without the enlargement of the reactive clone (33, 34).

An indication of the contribution of the histocompatibility antigens in the interaction with the targets in the NK system can be seen when analysing the results presented by Callewearth et al. (35). Two lines derived from the same individual, thus expressing the same histocompatibility antigens showed different NK sensitivity. The T line HSB-2 was more sensitive than the B cell derived line SB. The HSB-2 line was almost as sensitive as K562, the standard NK sensitive line. Analysing their cold target competition experiments it can be seen that the HSB-2 and SB lines share target structures recognized by the effectors since the extent of competition when these two lines are involved is stronger than what would be expected on the basis of the direct killing of the cells. Thus, SB competes better the anti-HSB-2 effect than the anti-K562 effect, and HSB-2 competes better the anti-SB effect than K562 does. These results can be interpreted to show that in addition to the recognition mechanism - yet unknown - which is responsible for the killing of the cell lines, a subset of the killing lymphocytes recognize the histocompatibility antigens. This specific recognition may be the cause of the individual differences which were seen in the effects against 5 target cells exhibited by 69 donors as reported in the same paper. Donors showing relatively strong killing against one cell line often showed a strong effect against the other line, though there were individuals which reacted with a certain selectivity.

In another system a similar phenomenon was encountered. When low NK sensitive B lines are superinfected with EBV, the virus cycle is induced in a certain proportion of cells. This measure was shown to elevate NK sensitivity. In cold target competition experiments the standard NK sensitive lines (K562 and Molt-4) cross reacted with the EBV superinfected B lines. The homologous, noninduced and thus low NK sensitive cells also showed a certain extent of competition which suggests that a proportion of lymphocytes may recognize alloantigens (36).

The search for a particular antigen expressed on the culture lines which is responsible for the NK sensitivity did not give support for the existence of a well-defined entity. It is likely that certain membrane properties of the cell lines contribute to the interaction with the killer cells (37). Similar to the cytotoxicity of mitogen activated cells such interactions have a certain specificity inasmuch as targets from the same species are affected with considerably higher efficiency than xenogeneic targets even if they are sensitive to the killing by the lymphocytes of their own species (38, 39). In understanding killing mechanisms it should be noted that the number of lymphocytes recognizing cell surface antigens of an alien species is relatively low compared to those recognizing alloantigens. A species-specific recognition on the cell membrane level has been indicated when T cells or thymocytes were admixed to various target cells. They attached to cells in a species-specific pattern showing the recognition of their own and closely related species (40).

On the basis of the discussed facts the NK (and IAK) effect, when assayed on fresh targets, should be viewed as fundamentally similar to CTL. On the other hand, with some cultured cell lines in the short term assays, due to yet undefined properties of their plasma membrane, events similar to cytotoxicity in the presence of lectins could occur.

The question as to whether the "NK phenomenon" is relevant in tumor surveillance should therefore be raised in more specific terms, such as: Are there lymphocytes which recognize tumor-associated cell surface antigens present in the lymphocyte population? Can these be activated by nonspecific means for cytotoxicity and can such cytotoxicity give an adequate protection? Is the malignant transformation accompanied by changes of the plasma membrane which can interact with T lymphocytes similar to what is seen with cultured lines?

REFERENCES

1. Haller, O., Hansson, M., Kiessling, R., and Wigzell, H. Nature 270, 609 (1977).
2. Jondal, M., Spina, C., and Targan, S. Nature 272, 62 (1978).
3. Kiessling, R., Petranyi, G., Klein, G., and Wigzell, H. Int. J. Cancer 15, 933 (1975).
4. Trinchieri, G., Santoli, D., and Koprowski, H. J. Immunol. 120, 1849 (1978).
5. Saksela, E., Timonen, T., and Cantell, K. Scand. J. Immunol. 10, 257 (1979).
6. De Vries, J.E., Meyering, M., Van Dongren, A., and Rümke, P. Int. J. Cancer 15, 391 (1975).
7. Vanky, F.T., Argov, S.A., Einhorn, S.A.,and Klein, E. J. Exp. Med. (in press).
8. Becker, S., Kiessling, R., Lee, N., and Klein, G. J. Natl. Cancer Inst. 61, 1495 (1978).
9. Santoli, D., and Koprowski, H. Immunol. Rev. 44, 125 (1979).
10. Ono, A., Amos, D.B., and Koren, H.S. Nature 266, 546 (1977).
11. Bakacs, T., Gergely, P., Cornain, S., and Klein, E. Int. J. Cancer 19, 441 (1977).
12. West, W.H., Cannon, G.B., Kay, H.D., Bonnard, G.D., and Herberman, R.B. J. Immunol. 48, 355 (1977).
13. Hersey, P., Edwards, A., Edwards, J., Milton, G.W., and Nelson, O. Int. J. Cancer 16, 173 (1975).
14. Bakacs, T., Klein, E., Yefenof, E., Gergely, P. and Steinitz, M. Z. Immunitatsforsch.-Immunobiol. 154, 121 (1978).
15. Bakacs, T., Gergely, P., and Klein, E. Cell. Immunol. 32, 317 (1977).
16. Kalden, J.R., Peter, H.H., Roubin, R., and Cesarini, J.P. Eur. J. Immunol. 8, 537 (1977).
17. Bolhuis, R.L.H., Schuit, H.R.E., Nooy, A.M., and Ronteltap, C.P.M. Eur. J. Immunol. 8, 732 (1978).
18. Poros, A., and Klein, E. Cell. Immunol. 41, 240 (1978).
19. Seeley, J.K., Masucci, G., Poros, A., Klein, E., and Golub, S.H. J. Immunol. 123, 1301 (1979).
20. Masucci, M.G., Klein, E., and Argov, S. J. Immunol. (in press).
21. Calleweart, D.M., Lightbody, J.J., Kaplan, J., Joroszewski, J., Peterson, W.D., and Rosemberg, J.C. J. Immunol. 121, 81 (1978).
22. Poros, A., and Klein, E. Cell. Immunol. 46, 57 (1979).

23. Herberman, R.B., Nunn, M.E., Holden, H.T., Staal, S., and Djou, J.Y. Int. J. Cancer 19, 555 (1977).
24. Trinchieri, G., Santoli, D., Dee, R.R., and Knowles, B. J. Exp. Med. 147, 1299 (1978).
25. Masucci, M.G., Masucci, G., Klein, E., and Berthold, W. Proc. Natl. Acad. Sci. (in press) (1980).
26. Masucci, M.G., Masucci, G., Klein, E., Berthold, W. *in* "New Trends in Human Immunology and Cancer Immunotherapy," Symposium Montpellier (in press) (1980).
27. Oehler, J.R., Lindsay, R.L., Nunn, M.L., Holden, H.T., and Herberman, R.B. Int. J. Cancer 21, 210 (1978).
28. Pross, H.F., and Baines, M.C. Int. J. Cancer 18, 593 (1976).
29. Vose, B., Vanky, F., Argov, S., and Klein, E. Eur. J. Immunol. 7, 753 (1977).
30. Enberg, R.N., Eberle, B.J., Williams, R.C. J. Infect. Dis. 130, 104 (1974).
31. Svedmyr, E.A., and Jondal, M. Proc. Nat. Acad. Sci. USA 72, 1622 (1975).
32. Welsh, R.M., Zinkernagel, R.E., and Hallenbeck, L.A. J. Immunol. 122, 475 (1979).
33. Bevan, M.J., Langman, R.E., and Cohn, M. Eur. J. Immunol. 6, 150 (1976).
34. Waterfield, D.J., Waterfield, E.M., and Möller, G. Cell. Immunol. 17, 392 (1974).
35. Callewaert, D.M., Kaplan, J., Johnson, D.F., and Peterson, Jr., W.D. Cell. Immunol. 42, 103 (1979).
36. Blazar, B., Patarroyo, M., Klein, E., and Klein, G. J. Exp. Med. (in press).
37. Ährlund-Richter, L., Masucci, G., and Klein, E. Somatic Cell Gen. (in press).
38. Stejskal, V., Holm, G., and Perlmann, P. Cell. Immunol. 8, 71 (1973).
39. Hansson, M., Kärre, K., Bakacs, T., Kiessling, R., and Klein, G. J. Immunol. 121, 6 (1978).
40. Galili, U, Galili, N, Vanky, F., and Klein, E. Proc. Natl. Acad. Sci. 75, 2396 (1978).

MURINE RETROVIRUS - SPECIFIC NATURAL KILLER CELL ACTIVITY[1]

Mary-Ann Lane

Division of Tumor Immunology
Sidney Farber Cancer Institute
Harvard Medical School
Boston, Massachusetts

Neonatal exposure to retrovirus antigens occurs in many strains of laboratory mice. These viruses can be passed maternally, via the milk, to offspring (Nandi and McGrath, 1973), or may be expressed from endogeneous viral genomes during cell differentiation (Meier et al., 1973; Strand et al., 1974). Following long latent periods, these viruses produce neoplasms which grow progressively and ultimately kill the host. Immunologic responses to retroviruses occur early; long before tumors have developed (Blair and Lane, 1975; Lane et al., 1975; Blair and Lane, 1978; Nowinski and Kaehler, 1974; Ihle and Hanna, 1977). The immune reactivity generated against retroviral antigens appears however, in many strains, to provide insufficient protection to prevent neoplasms.

Considerable interest has been expressed recently in the natural killer (NK) cell, which has been proposed by many as a first line of defense against neoplasms (Kiessling et al., 1975; Herberman et al., 1977; Haller et al., 1977). Reactivity of these cells can be detected as early as three weeks of age, and persists late in life (Haller et al., 1977). In this chapter, I will discuss NK cell activity detected in mice which appears to be directed against specific retroviral glycoproteins and proteins expressed on target cell surfaces.

Humoral and cellular immune responses to murine mammary tumor virus (MMTV) and murine leukemia virus (MuLV) have been previously described (Blair and Lane, 1974a; Lane et al., 1975; Ihle et al., 1976; Lavrin et al., 1973; Nowinski and Kaehler, 1974). Lee and Ihle, 1977 were first to report

[1] *This work was supported by Public Health Service Grant CA-26825, and by a grant from the Massachusetts Division of the American Cancer Society.*

ISBN 0-12-341350-8

that in some, but not all strains tested, NK reactivity could be blocked *in vitro* by the addition of whole MuLV virions or by gp71, the major envelope glycoprotein of this virus. This intriguing observation led us to speculate that at least in some cases NK reactivity might also be detected which was specifically directed against proteins and glycoproteins of MMTV. Both MMTV and MuLV are relatively ubiquitous in laboratory mouse strains, both virus groups are present early in life, and both produce neoplasms in mice.

DEFINITION OF TARGET CELL EXPRESSED ANTIGEN

We have made extensive use of three cell lines in these studies. The YAC-1 and the YAC-H, a substrain of this line, were derived from a T-lymphoma which originated in A/SN mice. YAC-1 has been continuously maintained as an *in vitro* cell line while YAC-H was carried for a number of passages *in vivo*, then returned to *in vitro* passage. Both have identical growth characteristics in culture. The RL♂ cell line was derived from a BALB/c mouse with radiation induced leukemia and has been maintained *in vitro*. Both the YAC-1 and the RL cell lines are commonly used as targets to measure NK reactivity in the murine system. In Table I, cell surface expression of MMTV and MuLV antigens in these lines is described. We have found the YAC-1 cell line to express the major envelope glycoprotein of MMTV, gp52, and an internal protein of MMTV, p28. Gp36, another envelope glycoprotein of MMTV, is minimally represented. On this line MuLV expression was also detected with antisera to the whole virion, which recognized predominantly gp71. Interestingly, the YAC-H line which does express theta antigen on its surface characterizing it as a T-lymphycyte, did not possess detectable antigens of either MMTV or MuLV. The RL cell line possesses on its surface no antigens of MMTV but does possess MuLV as characterized by the above mentioned antisera (Lane et al., 1980a). This definition of cell surface expressed antigen on commonly used NK target cells has allowed us to characterize reactivity directed against both MMTV and MuLV. The YAC-H subline has proved useful in providing a control for target cell antigen specificity.

Table I. Complement Mediated Lysis of Nonadherent Cell Lines in the Presence of Antisera Prepared Against MMTV GP52, P28, and P10 or MuLV

	MMTV									
	Anti gp52		Anti gp36		Anti p28		Anti p10		Anti MuLV	
Cell Line	Dilution	% Lysis	Dilution	% Lysis	Dilution	% Lysis	Dilution	% Lysis	Dilution	% Lysis
YAC-1[a] T-lymphoma A/Sn strain	1:10	50	1:10	5	1:10	15	1:10	0	1:10	55
	1:20	25	1:20	0	1:20	5	1:20	0	1:20	30
	1:40	10	1:40	0	1:40	0	1:30	0	1:40	10
	1:60	0	1:60	0	1:60	0			1:60	0
YAC-H Variant of YAC-1	1:10	0	1:10	0	1:10	0	1:10	0	1:10	0
	1:20	0	1:20	0	1:20	0	1:20	0	1:20	0
	1:40	0	1:40	0	1:40	0	1:30	0	1:40	0
									1:60	0
RL Male[a] Radiation induced leukemia, BALB/c strain	1:10	0	1:10	0	1:10	0	1:10	0	1:10	60
	1:20	0	1:20	0	1:20	0	1:20	0	1:20	35
	1:40	0	1:40	0	1:40	0	1:30	0	1:40	20
									1:60	5

[a] *Complement mediated lysis using heat inactivated antisera was carried out in the following manner. Target cells were labelled with ^{51}Cr for 45 minutes, washed two times, counted, diluted and aliquoted to test plates at $2.5X10^5$ cells per well, in RPMI1640 without additions. Test serum was added at the appropriate concentrations, and cells were incubated for 30 minutes at 37°C. Following this incubation, absorbed guinea pig serum was added at a final concentration of 1:16 and cells were incubated for an additional 3 hours. At this time, plates were centrifuged at 1500 rpm, and aliquots of supernate were counted in a gamma spectrometer.*

ASSAY SYSTEM, MOUSE STRAINS AND EFFECTOR CELLS

Target cells used in the NK assay were maintained as serially passaged tissue culture cell lines. One hundred microcuries of ^{51}Cr were added to $4X10^6$ target cells in 0.1 ml and incubated at 37^oC for 45 minutes. Cells were washed three times and suspended to a concentration of $1X10^6$ cells per ml in Eagles minimum essential media plus 10% heat-inactivated FCS. $2.5X10^4$ cells/25 ul were added to the effector cells in a total volume of 200 1 in Linbro microtest plates. The plates were centrifuged at 4^oC for 8 minutes at 1000 rpm and incubated for 4 hours at 37^oC in a humidified atmosphere containing 5% CO_2. At the end of 4 hours, plates were centrifuged at 4° for 10 minutes at 1200 rpm, whereafter 100 1 supernatant media per well was collected and counted in a gammaspectrometer. Spontaneous release of ^{51}Cr was determined by adding target cells to medium alone. As a rule, spontaneous release did not exceed 5-10%.

The percentage of lysis was calculated by the following formula:

$$\% \text{ lysis} = \frac{\text{cpm(test population)} - \text{cpm(control)}}{\text{cpm maximum release}} \times 100$$

The C3H/HeJ strain was chosen for initial characterization of antigenic specificity of NK reactivity. A small colony of these females has been maintained here, and all mice are routinely tested for the presence of exogenous mouse infectious agents such as Sendai virus, polyoma virus and murine hepatitis virus, which can significantly interfere with immune response testing. All mice used in these studies were negative for these agents during the entire period of observation. Multiparous C3H/HeJ females in this colony produce mammary tumors between 10-13 months of age and the incidence of tumor production is 90%.

C3H/HeN nude (thymusless) mice tested in this study were obtained from our nude mouse colony established with the help of Dr. Carl Hansen of the National Institutes of Health. BALB/c nude mice were obtained from Dr. Charles Stiles at the Sidney Farber Cancer Institute. Nude mice were maintained in isolation from conventional mice and were supplied with autoclaved food, water, and bedding. C3H/HeN conventional mice were obtained from Dr. Ronald Herberman. All other strains described in these studies were obtained from Jackson Laboratories.

Effector cells were obtained from the spleens of mice killed by cervical dislocation. Single cell suspensions were obtained by forcing spleens through fine wire mesh screens and filtration through a single layer of nylon gauze. NK reactivity was not reduced by treatment with anti mouse brain (theta) antisera plus complement (single treatment), nor was it abolished by treatment with heat-aggregated human gamma globulin (Lane et al., 1975). Treatment with Ly5.1 antisera plus complement (Kasai et al., 1979) completely removed NK reactivity.

CORRELATION OF NK REACTIVITY WITH CELL SURFACE ANTIGEN EXPRESSION

Testing of spleen cells from C3H/HeJ females (Table 2) against the three targets previously described demonstrated that reactivity could readily be detected against the YAC-1 and RL target cells, but not against the YAC-H target previously demonstrated to express no antigens of MMTV and MuLV. This experiment suggested that the spleens of C3H females possessed NK cells capable of lysing target cells presenting surface retroviral antigens, but that, in the absence of these antigens, no reactivity could be detected.

TABLE II. Levels of NK Reactivity in C3H Females

Cell Source		*Targets (% Lysis)*		
	Target:	*YAC-1*	*RL male*	*YAC-H*
Effectors	*Antigens*[a]:	$52^+28^+71^+$	$52^-28^-71^+$	$52^-28^-71^-$
50:1 E:T ratio				
C3H/HeJ Females				
8 weeks		*40-50%*	*20-25%*	*0.1-0.5%*
12 weeks		*35-40%*	*18-22%*	*0.1-0.5%*
16 weeks		*30-35%*	*15-18%*	*0.1-0.5%*

[a] *Presence or absence of MMTV gp52, p28, and the major envelope glycoprotein of MuLV, pg71 on target cell surface is indicated by + or -.*

It was also observed that lytic activity of C3H/HeJ cells was always approximately 50% less against the RL♂ target than that observed against the YAC-1 target.

These observed patterns of NK reactivity against our three target cell types were suggestive of a possible NK effector cell population capable of recognizing target cell surface expressed retroviral antigens. We concluded that if this were the case, we should be able to block NK lytic activity directly, by preincubation of NK effector cells with whole virus or purified viral proteins and glycoproteins.

C3H MMTV virions, proteins and glycoproteins were prepared as previously described (Teramoto et al., 1974; Teramoto et al., 1977; Teramoto and Schlom, 1978). Purified Rauscher leukemia virus and AKR leukemia virus were obtained through the Office of Logistics and Resources, National

TABLE III. Viral Antigen Blocking of NK Reactivity of C3H/HeJ Females[a]

Virus Range Tested (μg)	*Saturation Level of Blocking (μg) on Target Cells*	
	YAC-1	*RL♂*
C3H MMTV virion		
1-30	*20*	*No Blocking*
C3H MMTV pg52		
1-20	*10*	*No Blocking*
C3H MMTV p28		
1-20	*10*	*No Blocking*
RLV virion		
1-35	*30*	*20*
AKR virion		
1-35	*No Blocking*	*No Blocking*

[a] *Complete blocking of NK activity against the YAC-1 target could be achieved in the presence of 20 μg each of C3H virion, p28, and RLV. RLV virion alone at 20 μg was sufficient to block all NK activity of this strain against the RL♂ target.*

Table IV. Summary of Blocking of NK Lysis of Target Cells

Effector Cells	Target Cell Lysis			Blocked by			
	Yac-1	RL		C3H MTV Virion	MMTV gp52	MMTV p28	RLV Virion
	50:1 E:T						
C3H under 16 weeks	40-50%	20-25%	Yac-1	P[a] (23-29)[b]	P[a] (28-32)[b]	0 (40-50)[b]	P[a] (21-30)[b]
			RL ♂	0 (20-25)[b]	0 (20-25)[b]	0 (20-25)[b]	+[a] (0-2)[b]
C3H over 16 weeks	30-35%	10-15%	Yac-1	P[a] (16-21)[b]	P[a] (18-23)[b]	P[a] (22.5-27)[b]	P[a] (16-20)[b]
			RL ♂	0 (10-15)[b]	0 (10-15)[b]	0 (10-15)[b]	+[a] 0-.9)[b]

[a] Indicates no overlap with control values in the absence of blocking reagents P=.005 by students T test. Blocking is rated P for partial, 0 for no effect, and + for total blocking. Reduction of lysis was carried out with 20 μg of each reagent tested; results expressed here represent value.

[b] Indicates range of % lysis after blocking.

Cancer Institute, Bethesda, Maryland. Antigen was added to effector cells and media in wells and incubated for 30 minutes and 37°C prior to the addition of target cells in the ^{51}Cr release assay. No reduction in NK reactivity was observed in cells preincubated in the absence of virus or virus components. Whole virions or purified viral components were tested for their ability to block NK activity as ranges of 0-35 μg per well. Table 3 describes blocking by antigens of MMTV and RLV against YAC-1 and RL♂ targets in the C3H/HeJ strain. Blocking observed here was both linear and saturable, suggesting the presence on NK cells, of specific receptors for retroviral antigens. These findings confirm our observation of the expression of antigens of both MMTV and MuLV on YAC-1 targets, and confirm the presence of only MuLV, and no MMTV antigens, on the RL♂ target cell line. These findings are summarized in Table 4.

Complete blocking of NK reactivity in the C3H/HeJ strain against the YAC-1 target could be achieved by the addition of 20 μg each of MMTV gp52 and p28, and RLV virion. Complete blocking against the RL♂ target could be achieved by the addition of 20 μg RLV virion alone. No blocking against either target was observed in the presence of up to 35 μg AKR leukemia virus (Lane et al., 1980b).

A difference was observed between females over and under 16 weeks of age. Reactivity of females under 16 weeks of age against the YAC-1 target could be blocked completely by the addition of only MMTV gp52 and RLV virion. To block completely the reactivity of females over 16 weeks, MMTV p28 was also necessary. Blocking patterns in females aged 8-24 weeks are shown in Table 5. P28 is an internal protein of MMTV and is not present on the surface of the virion. Significant exposure to this antigen may first occur during the development of preneoplastic nodules in the mammary gland. We speculate that this antigen, expressed on the surface of cells in developing nodules, is recognized by NK cells at this time. Exposure to p28 as it is released from ruptured virions may generate minimal NK responsiveness in females prior to 16 weeks of age, but this low level of reactivity may fall below that detectable in our assay system. We are currently working to pinpoint precisely, in individual females, the occurrance of this response, and to correlate this with p28 expression on cells in preneoplastic nodules.

TABLE V. Age Dependent Ability of C3H/HeJ Females To Be Blocked By MMTV P28

Age at testing: C3H/HeJ females	*Partial blocking by[a]:* gp52	p28
8 weeks (4)[b]	+	0
10 weeks (2)	+	0
12 weeks (3)	+	0
14 weeks (3)	+	0
16 weeks (6)	+	4/6
17 weeks (4)	+	+
18 weeks (4)	+	+
20 weeks (4)	+	+
24 weeks (4)	+	+

[a] *Presence of partial blocking to indicated antigens is represented by +. Absence of blocking is indicated by 0.*
[b] *Indicates number of females tested at each age.*

A significant difference was noted in patterns of NK reactivity in older multiparous tumor-free and tumor-bearing females. As seen in Table 6, although the ages of both sets were comparable, reactivity against YAC-1 targets was significantly lower in tumor bearing females than in those who remained tumor-free. The reactivity in both groups against the RL ♂ target, however, appeared to remain the same. Viral antigen blocking studies with these females (Table 7) demonstrated that while reactivity patterns in the tumor-free females remained similar to those observed in younger females, patterns in tumor-bearing females altered significantly. Most surprisingly, in the mammary tumor bearing females, no reactivity was blocked by MMTV against either target. Reactivity against both targets was completely blocked by the addition of RLV virion. Tumor bearing females appeared no longer to possess NK reactivity directed against antigens of MMTV.

We favor two possible explanations for this loss of MMTV - specific NK reactivity in tumor bearing females. First, it is possible that, during tumor growth, accompanied by shedding of large quantities of viral antigens, specific NK cells capable of recognizing MMTV antigens may become blocked *in vivo* by antigen. Second, it is equally possible that cells exist which are capable of suppression of NK reactivity. If these cells are functional in this system, one must postulate that the suppression is specific, as MMTV reactivity but not MuLV reactivity has been removed. Experiments are in progress to determine whether one or both of these mechanisms can explain the observed patterns of reactivity.

ANTIGEN SPECIFIC NK REACTIVITY PATTERNS IN OTHER MOUSE STRAINS

In the previous section, we defined NK reactivity of an antigen specific nature in a single strain of mice, C3H/HeJ. The reactivity detected appeared to recognize C3H MMTV virions, the major glycoprotein of this virus, gp52, and an internal protein, p28. We also detected reactivity directed against MuLV which could be blocked by Rauscher MuLV virions (RLV), but not by AKR MuLV virions, suggesting that the MuLV recognized was more closely related to RLV than to AKR-MuLV.

To test whether retroviral-specific NK reactivity was expressed in other mouse strains and substrains, we screened several of these, including two strains of nude mice. Screening for blocking reactivity was carried out using a single concentration of virus per well (25 μg), shown to produce significant reduction of NK activity in the C3H/HeJ strain. Effector cells from all mice tested were used at an E:T ratio of 50:1, and the YAC-1 cells which express antigens of both MMTV and MuLV were used as targets. Females tested in this study were between eight and ten weeks of age.

The greatest reduction in NK lysis by C3H MMTV was observed in the CBA/J strain, which is also an MMTV-positive strain. These females have a substantially lower incidence of mammary tumors (Jackson Laboratories is currently recalculating mammary tumor incidence in this strain. This incidence has dropped significantly over the past 10 years), and these occur later in life than those observed in the C3H/HeJ strain. The CBA strain has been demonstrated by other investigators to be a high NK responder. The BALB/cJ and BALB^{+}/c nu^{+}/nu^{+} strains were intermediate in response and level of blocking. I have also tested NK reactivity in the BALB/cCRGL strain and have found NK reactivity in that substrain to be substantially lower (see Blair and Lane, this edition). BALB/c females do not get mammary tumors except when fostered on MMTV-positive strains. They do, however, possess several copies of endogenous MMTV sequences in their DNA. It is not known

Table VI. Levels of Reactivity in Tumor Bearing and Tumor Free C3H/HeJ Females

Cell Source	*Targets (% Lysis)*		
Effectors 50:1 E:T ratio	*YAC-1*	*RL♂*	*YAC-H*
48-53 weeks (multiparous)	*20-25%*	*10-15%*	*0.1-0.5%*
52-55 weeks multiparous - tumor 15x15 or greater	*10%*	*10%*	*0.1-0.5%*

whether these sequences are transcribed at any phases of cell differentiation. It has previously been reported that BALB/c mice, following horizontal exposure to MMTV-positive strains develop antibody-dependent cell mediated (ADCM) reactivity (Blair and Lane, 1974b) and macrophage migratory reactivity (Tagliabue et al., 1978) specific for MMTV. Some or all of these factors may be important in explaining the presence of antigen-specific NK activity to MMTV in this strain.

The AKR strain possessed virtually no detectable NK specific reactivity directed against MMTV. There exists controversy as to whether this strain is truly MMTV-negative. The AKR/J strain possesses endogenous MMTV but is currently thought not to possess the milk-borne form of the virus (personal communication, Dr. Hans Meier, Jackson Laboratories).

Reactivity to murine leukemia viruses was screened on the same target cell line with the use of both Rauscher and AKR MuLV virions. Rauscher MuLV is a laboratory strain of virus and was originally isolated from a mouse bearing an erythroid leukemia (Rauscher, 1962). This virus is related, but not identical to, Friend (Friend, 1957) and Moloney (Moloney, 1966) leukemia viruses. The AKR leukemia virus is an endogenous ecotropic virus isolated from the AKR mouse strain. Reactivity detected to these viruses may indicate either that exposure to these viruses has previously occurred or that the strains tested may express endogenous leukemia viruses which have antigens crossreactive with these viruses and cell surface expressed antigens.

Table VII. Blocking of NK Lysis in Tumor Bearing and Tumor Free Females

Effector Cells	Target Cell Lysis			Blocked by			
	YAC-1 50:1 E:T	RL ♂		C3H MTV Virion	MMTV gp52	MMTV p28	RLV Virion
C3H multiparous tumor-free females	20-25%	10-15%	Yac-1	P (18)	P[a] (17)	P[a] (17)	P[a] (12)
			RL ♂	0 (20-25)	0 (20-25)	0 (20-25)	+ (0-.5%)
C3H bearing spontaneous mammary tumor	10%	10%	YAC-1	0 (10)[b]	0 (9-10)[b]	0 (9-10)[b]	+[a] (0-.5)[b]
			RL ♂	0 (10)[b]	0 (10)[b]	0 (10)[b]	+[a] (0-.5)[b]

[a] Indicates no overlap with control valves in the absence of blocking reagents. P=.005 by students T test. Blocking is rated P for partial, 0 for no effect, and + for total blocking. Blocking was carried out with 20 g of each reagent.
[b] Indicates % lysis after blocking.

Similar levels of reactivity were detected in both C3H substrains and in C3H/HeN nu^{+}/nu^{+} females against RLV, but no reactivity was detected against AKR-LV. Reactivity to both viruses in both BALB/c strains tested was of an insignificant level. This strain possesses endogenous leukemia viruses, but either no reactivity is directed toward these, or the reactivity is not crossreactive with either virus tested. The CBA/J strain exhibited moderate ability to be blocked by the RLV virion, but again, no blocking was detected with the AKR-LV. Moderate reactivity was detected in the AKR strain against its own endogenous virus. Tumor development in the AKR strain may result from a recombinational event involving this virus. Very low levels of reactivity were also detectable to the RLV virion, again, possibly suggesting either exposure or crossreactivity (Lane et al., 1980c).

What emerges from these studies (summarized in Table 8) is that patterns within substrains are similar, while patterns of reactivity in different strains vary. Variation in levels of NK reactivity has been proposed to be genetically controlled (Kiessling et al., 1975). The mechanism by which this apparent genetic control is exerted could relate to the degree and diversity of strain exposure to either endogenous or exogenous retroviruses. Lee and Ihle (1977) have examined NK responsiveness in the NIH Swiss mouse which differs from the above strains in that it is not inbred and is relatively free of both MMTV and MuLV. Intermediate levels of NK reactivity were present in these mice, but no blocking was detected in Ihle's study using RLV and AKR-MuLV. This population does possess a xenotropic form of MuLV, and antigens of this virus are occasionally expressed during certian phases of cell differentiation. It is interesting to speculate that blocking of NK reactivity against an appropriate target, with xenotropic MuLV from this strain might prove successful.

FACTORS INVOLVED IN MEASUREMENT OF ANTIGEN SPECIFIC NK REACTIVITY

It is important to remember that measurement of this reactivity is based upon three essential elements: target cell expression of antigen; capacity for antigen recognition of effector cells; and relatedness of the virus antigen used in blocking to both target cell expressed antigens and antigens recognized by the effector cells. An effector cell must be capable of recognizing some antigen on the target

Table VIII. *Screening for Murine Retroviral NK Specificity*

Strain	% Lysis (E:T = 50:1) YAC-1 Targets	% Reduction of Lysis in The Presence of 25 μg Virus		
		MMTV	RLV	AKR
C_3H/HeJ	40 - 45%	40 - 48%	41 - 47%	0 - 2%
C_3H/HeN	40 - 45%	34 - 40%	42 - 50%	0 - 2%
C_3H/HeN Nu+/Nu+	40 - 50%	20 - 29%	32 - 40%	0 - 2%
BALB/cJ	22 - 26%	15 - 30%	1 - 6%	0 - 5%
BALB/c Nu+/Nu+	25 - 30%	30 - 35%	4 - 6%	0 - 5%
CBA/J	42 - 51%	41 - 64%	10 - 20%	2 - 5%
AKR/J	19 - 25%	5 - 7%	5 - 10%	25 - 32%

cell in order for NK lysis to occur. Following establishment of the effector's ability to lyse the target, blocking of direct NK lysis can occur only if the antigen used in blocking is sufficiently crossreactive with or identical to the antigen recognized in the lytic event. This implies that in the total spleen population, NK specificities of many types may be present, but only those represented on target cells used to measure the reactivity will be detected. In the studies presented here, it is not implied that retroviral antigens are the only antigens to which NK cells can respond. To test for reactivities to other antigens, it will be useful to examine NK activity against a wide variety of virally infected cells, normal cells, and normal cells during various phases of differentiation. Complete characterization of antigens expressed on target cell surfaces, isolation of these antigens, and use of purified antigens in direct blocking of NK lysis will be most productive.

In conclusion, we are left with several interesting questions and speculations. What is the lineage of the NK cell? Is this an immature form of T-lymphocyte as suggested by the presence of very low levels of theta on its surface (Herberman et al., 1979), and by the presence of a marker expressed on T-cells, Ly 5 (Kasai et al., 1979a; Kasai et al., 1979b)? If, as shown here, this cell is antigen committed, does this same commitment persist in maturity? NK mediated lysis is not H-2 restricted. Does this imply that development of H-2 restriction occurs following cell commitment to antigen specificity? Does this imply that a mature class of T-cells exists, which exhibits antigen commitment and is not H-2 restricted in lysing target cells? T-lymphocytes capable of recognizing retroviral antigens have been previously described. It will be interesting to follow antigen commitment of NK cells and T-killer cells to determine whether a direct relationship exists between NK cells and mature T-lymphocytes.

These studies also raise serious questions as to the role of NK cells in preventing spontaneously arising neoplasms. NK cells can be detected during the first 2½-3 weeks of life in the mouse. Viruses such as MMTV, introduced from day zero in milk, may establish early infections and may, in this fashion, circumvent NK cells. Constantly shed viral antigens may also block NK activity *in vivo*, preventing significant lysis of cells in developing tumor nodules. Do cells exist which are capable of regulating NK activity (Cudkowicz and Hochman, 1979)? In females bearing mammary tumors, we demonstrated an apparent loss of NK activity toward antigens of MMTV. Levels of NK reactivity to MuLV antigens remained comparable to those observed in females of similar ages who were tumor free. Does this constitute a specific suppression of MMTV-committed NK cells? Perhaps the arisal of the neoplasm occurs following actual depletion of NK cells capable of recognizing antigens expressed on the tumor cell. To establish the role of the NK cell in prevention of neoplasms, these questions must be answered.

Finally, if specific NK reactivity against retroviral antigens can be detected in the mouse, what is the spcificity of NK reactivity in humans? There exist tumor virus candidates in humans, but none of these have evolved beyond the candidate stage as yet. Herpesviruses, Hepatitis B virus, a virus possibly bearing a relation to MMTV, and others have been implicated. Screening of human NK targets for expression of these viruses, combined with antigen blocking of NK lysis in humans may prove useful in defining the role of NK cells in relation to human neoplasms.

ACKNOWLEDGMENTS

I would like to thank my collaborators in these studies, in particular, Dr. Jeffrey Schlom, and Dr. Yoshio Teramoto, Laboratory of Viral Carcinogenesis, N.I.H. and Dr. Robert Cardiff, Dept. of Pathology, U.C. Davis for providing viral reagents and antisera. I thank also Drs. Donald W. Kufe, Harvey Cantor and Geoffrey Cooper of the Sidney Farber Cancer Institute, Dr. James Ihle of the Frederick Cancer Research Center, Dr. Phyllis B. Blair, U.C. Berkeley, and Dr. Ronald Herberman, Laboratory of Immunodiagnostics, N.I.H., for useful discussions.

REFERENCES

Blair, P.B., and Lane, M.A. (1974a). J. Immunol. 112, 443.

Blair, P.B., and Lane, M.A. (1974b). J. Immunol. 113, 1446.

Blair, P.B., and Lane, M.A. (1975). J. Immunol. 115, 184.

Blair, P.B., and Lane, M.A. (1978). Int. J. Cancer 21, 476.

Cudkowicz, G., and Hochman, P.S. (1979). Immunol. Rev. 44, 37.

Friend, C. (1957). J. Exp. Med. 105, 307.

Haller, O., Hansson, M., Kiessling, R., and Wigzell, H. (1977). Nature 270, 609.

Herberman, R.B., DJeu, J., Kay, H., Ortaldo, J., Riccardi, C., Bonnard, G., Holden, H., Fagnani, R., Santoni, A., and Puccetti, P. (1979). Immunol. Rev. 44, 43.

Herberman, R.B., Holden, H.T., West, W.H., Bonnard, G.D., Santoni, A., Nunn, M.E., Kay, H.D., and Ortaldo, J.R. (1977). In "Proceedings of International Symposium on Tunour-associated Antigens and Their Specific Immune Response. Academic Press, London.

Ihle, J.N., Collins, J.J., Lee, J.C., Fischinger, P.J., Moennig, V., Shafer, W., Hanna, M.G., and Bolognesi, D.P. (1976). Virology 75, 74.

Ihle, J.N., and Hanna, M.G. (1977). In "Contemporary Topics in Immunobiology" (M.G. Hanna, F. Rapp, eds.) Plenum Press, New York.

Kasai, M., Leclerc, J.C., Shen, F.W., and Cantor, H. (1979a). Immunogenetics 8, 153.

Kasai, M., Leclerc, J.C., McVay-Boudreu, L., Shen, F.W., and Cantor, H. (1979b). J. Exp. Med. 149, 1260.

Kiessling, R., Petranyi, G., Klein, G., and Wigzell, H. (1975). Int. J. Cancer 15, 933.

Lane, M.A., Kufe, D.W., Mahoney, R., Watson, A., Pitman, T., Teramoto, Y., and Schlom, J. (1980a) Submitted to Cancer Immunol. and Immunotherapy.

Lane, M.A., Kufe, D.W., Mahoney, R.J., Watson, A., Pitman, T., and Yunis, E. (1980b). Submitted to J. Immunol.

Lane, M.A., Kufe, D.W., Teramoto, Y.A., and Schlom, J. (1980c). Submitted to Nature.

Lane, M.A., Roubinian, J., Slomich, M., Trefts, P., and Blair, P.B. (1975). J. Immunol. 114, 24.

Lavrin, D.H., Herberman, R.B., Nunn, M., and Soares, N. (1973). J. Natl. Cancer Inst. 51, 1497.

Lee, J.C. and Ihle, J.N. (1977). J. Immunol. 118, 928.

Meier, H., Taylor, B.A., Cheney, M., and Huebner, R.J. (1973). Proc. Natl. Acad. Sci. 70, 1450.

Moloney, J.B. (1966). J. Natl. Cancer Inst. Monogr. 22, 139.

Nandi, S., and McGrath, C.M. (1973). Adv. Cancer Res. 17, 353.

Nowinski, R.C., and Kaehler, S.L. (1974). Science 185, 869.

Rauscher, F.J. (1962). J. Natl. Cancer Inst. 29, 515.

Strand, M., Lilly, F., and August, J.T. (1974). Proc. Natl. Acad. Sci. 71, 3682.

Tagliabue, A., Herberman, R.B., and McCoy, J.L. (1978). Ca. Res. 38, 2279.

Teramoto, Y.A., Kufe, D.W., and Schlom, J. (1977). J. Virology 24, 525.

Teramoto, Y.A., Puentes, M., Young, L. and Cardiff, R. (1974). J. Virology 13, 411.

Teramoto, Y.A., and Schlom, J. (1978). Cancer Res. 38, 1990.

THE SPECIFICITY OF NK CELLS AT THE LEVEL OF TARGET ANTIGENS AND RECOGNITION RECEPTORS[1]

John C. Roder

Department of Microbiology and Immunology
Queen's University
Kingston, Ontario
Canada K7L 3N6

I. INTRODUCTION

A number of criteria must be fulfilled in order to designate a cytolytic phenomenon as specific. Most investigators would agree that NK cells are at least selective since some target cell types are highly sensitive to cytolysis whereas others are not (1,2). NK resistant targets were sensitive to alloimmune T cells thereby demonstrating that they were not simply more resistant to cytolysis in general. The concept of specificity in the context of an immune surveillance system requires that (i) a lock and key, or enzyme substrate model is appropriate to describe the target-effector interactions, and (ii) the system is sufficiently polymorphic to deal with the wide range of target cells sensitive to NK mediated lysis. The list of NK sensitive targets now includes cells of xenogeneic, allogeneic or syngeneic origin which may be transformed or non-transformed and derive from normal tissues or tumours from diverse histogenic origins (melanocytes, lymphocytes, mast cells, fibroblasts, macrophages, nerve cells and others). A priori it would seem highly unlikely that this plethora of diverse targets would share a common determinant and hence the requirement for a polymorphic recognition system if NK cells are to be of general significance in a surveillance system.

II. COMPETITIVE INHIBITION OF NK CYTOLYSIS BY UNLABELLED TARGET CELLS

Previous work has shown that various unlabelled competi-

[1] *Supported by the MRC and NCI of Canada*

ISBN 0-12-341350-8

tor cells could inhibit isotope release from labelled target cells (3) and similar observations in the NK system were used to infer that the target and competitor shared common determinants which were recognised by surface receptors on the NK cell (1,2). Those cells most sensitive to NK lysis proved to be the best competitors and a good correlation was found between susceptibility to direct lysis and competition among a wide variety of targets (1,2,4,5,6). However, simple competition tests alone are not enough to designate an NK interaction as specific. What are the non-specific effects that could occur during a lytic reaction in a competitive inhibition assay? When examining real data one sometimes observes that potent effectors against a given target also give higher background levels against target cells that are usually insensitive. Likewise, highly sensitive targets are usually sensitive to a broader range of effectors. This general susceptibility of targets to lysis could represent a membrane property (possibly) and is therefore a threshold event, unrelated to the presence or absence of particular antigens. Similarly, high levels of effector activity could reflect (i) their degree of activation over a more specific resting state, if activation of NK cells causes non-specific lysis as occurs in the macrophage system, or (ii) some general membrane property (charge, hydrophobicity, fluidity, cell size, motility, glycocalyx, microvilli) that allows more intimate contact with certain targets regardless of the target antigens they carry (7).

Recently a powerful statistical method, called interaction analysis, has become available to help distinguish the underlying specificities involved in NK mediated lysis (8-10). Interaction analysis starts from the premise that both specific and non-specific reactions occur during NK mediated lysis. Testing one effector against a target panel is not very informative and says nothing about specificity except how broad the reactions are. Likewise testing many effectors against one target says nothing about specificity. However, if effectors from different donors show different patterns against a panel of targets then different recognition receptors and target antigens are involved in the system. Therefore in the Takasugi system a panel of effectors and targets are measured for the degree of lysis and then a two-way analysis of variance is set up to test the hypothesis that no specific reactions have occurred.

The analysis is rigorous because it tends to underestimate specific effects. In addition, if "non-selective" lysis really represents (i) a sum of many specificities shared between targets, or (ii) one antigen shared on many targets which is equally recognised by all the effectors, then interaction analysis in reality will only pick out interactions involving very unique and infrequent antigens. The method is probably an underestimate of the real number of specificities involved. If the analysis indicates significant selective reactions by one effector on different targets this could be interpreted as a sharing of antigens or as one heterogeneous effector suspension reacting to two different antigens. The only method for distinguishing these possibilities is a cross competition assay in which unlabelled targets are added to the reaction mixture of effectors and ^{51}Cr labelled targets. The ability of different cell lines to compete infers the existence of cross reacting target antigens and a complementary receptor on the effector cell. The data obtained can also be analysed by interaction analysis to distinguish specific from non-specific inhibitory effects (11).

The discovery that certain target cells can induce interferon (12) which can subsequently enhance the cytolytic activity of NK cells (13-15), and at the same time protect certain targets from cytolysis (16) will require a re-evaluation of all the competition experiments reported to date. Trinchieri has shown (14) that when target cells and competitor cells are both interferon inducers, target cells are less efficiently lysed than in systems in which target and competitor cells differed in their ability to induce interferon. Interaction analysis of this data revealed two classes of target cells most likely on the basis of interferon inducing activity rather than the presence or absence of antigens recognised by NK cells. The problem becomes more apparent in comparing intraspecies NK restrictions (4) since both the NK augmenting and target protecting actions of interferon are species specific, whereas interferon induction itself is not. Some of these complications could be resolved (i) using tumour derived targets rather than fibroblasts since the former appear refractory to the inhibitory effects of interferon, (ii) using short competition assays (stopped with EDTA and cytochalasin B) in the presence of anti-interferon antibody.

III. COMPETITIVE INHIBITION OF EFFECTOR-TARGET BINDING WITH SOLUBILIZED TARGET STRUCTURES

The most direct approach to elucidating NK specificity will lie in the isolation of target "antigens" and recognition structures. The recognition receptor on the NK cell, which is necessary for target-effector binding, was found to be a de novo synthesised, cell surface protein based on trypsin sensitivity and the inability to regenerate in the presence of cycloheximide or at 0° (17). It is not yet known if the receptors are coded by the V region genes or if they represent remnants of a more primitive surveillance mechanism. At the target cell level an attempt was made to isolate the target antigens recognised by NK cells.

Pre-incubation of NK cells with detergent solubilised, cell surface proteins of YAC lymphoma cells prevented subsequent binding to intact YAC targets (18). The inhibitory material bound to Con A-Sepharose columns and could be eluted with the specific sugar suggesting that the target structures may be glycosylated. The target structures consisted of 3 molecular species tentatively assigned molecular weights of 130, 160, and 240 x 10^3 ± 10 x 10^3 based on electrophetic mobility in SDS-polyacrylamide gels. These molecules could not be detected in gels of NK insensitive target cells such as P815, A9HT, or YWA and the quantity obtained from the gels varied directly with the NK sensitivity of YAC (18) which, like other tumour cells, is more NK sensitive when grown in vitro than in vivo (19). The NK target structures from YAC were selective since they inhibited the binding of NK cells but not alloimmune T cells to their appropriate targets. Conversely, H-2 antigens specifically inhibited alloimmune T cells, but not NK cells, from binding to targets expressing the appropriate H-2 haplotype (20). Therefore the receptors on NK cells have a specificity distinct from the receptors on T cells. This conclusion is also supported by the observation that interferon protects fibroblast targets from lysis by NK cells but not CTL (16) presumably by shutting off synthesis of the NK-TS. Immune T cells therefore must recognise a different determinant. Additional cell lines (F9, K562) which completely lack MHC related structures are also sensitive to NK cells which further argues that MHC products are not the target of NK cells. In addition, NK sensitive targets have been found which lack Fc, C3 and SRBC receptors as well as surface Ig (6), thereby suggesting that none of these surface entities serve as the NK target structure.

Additional NK sensitive tumour cells also expressed some or all of the target molecules exhibited by YAC and some of these structures shared specificities in the case of MPC-11, 136-6 and X-63 or were unique in the case of MOLT-4 and K562 as shown by cross inhibition studies (18).

When the three NK-TS molecules were compared in a number

of different cell lines, the large 240K molecule most often carried the unique NK specificity whereas the smaller 140K molecule always cross-reacted in all the cell lines tested (21).

This is in agreement with recent NK depletion studies on target cell monolayers which show that most tumour cell lines share one specificity and maintain others which are unique (Ortaldo, J.; to be published). These results together suggest that NK cells recognise more than one specificity. In addition murine NK cells recognised a different spectrum of NK-TS molecules than human NK cells (21).

IV. THE NATURE OF THE TARGET STRUCTURES

Although the nature of the NK-TS is not fully understood, it does not possess determinants common to gp71, Moloney cell surface antigen, p30, p15E or H-2 (18). This provides the first direct evidence that in some instances, the NK-TS may not be related to murine leukaemia virus products. Several lines of indirect evidence also support the conclusion. Hence, there was no correlation in 11 different cell lines between expression of virion gp71, p30, p15 or p12 and sensitivity to NK cell mediated lysis by CBA spleen cells (22). In addition, immunoresistant sublines of YAC selected for low expression of MCSA are equally sensitive to NK cells (22). In further studies, NK sensitive human cell lines were superinfected with xenotropic murine leukaemia virus and were shown to express virion gp71, p30 and p12. The sensitivity of these cells to NK mediated lysis, however, was not influenced (23). These data taken together, strongly argue against the involvemnet of endogenous virus products in the target cell specificity of NK cells from some strains of mice such as CBA. In different strains, however, gp71 was shown to inhibit NK cell mediated cytolysis of an AKR tumour by C57BL x C3H, F_1 mice but not NIH Swiss mice (24). In addition pre-treatment of targets with anti-gp71 partially blocked NK cytolysis (25). It is likely therefore that different strains of mice possess unique specificity repertoires with respect to the endogenous viruses. The response to exogenous virus may be a more generalized phenomenon.

It has recently been shown that NK cells in nude mice possess a remarkable degree of virus specificity against a variety of exogenous RNA viruses (26). NK insensitive, xenogeneic tumour cells (HeLa) became susceptible to lysis by NK cells when infected with measles, VSV or mumps virus. In cold target competition experiments, NK mediated lysis of isotope labelled Hela-measles was inhibited only by unlabelled HeLa-measles targets and not HeLa-mumps or HeLa-VSV which were equally susceptible to cytolysis. Reciprocal combinations of targets and competitors were not reported. In view of the possible interferon induction in these cultures and the limitations of competition assays (above) it will be important to determine if target-effector conjugates are specifically inhibited by virus or virus containing membranes from infected targets.

The widespread nature of common NK-TS might suggest that the NK-TS are (i) de-repressed foetal antigens of a highly conserved nature, (ii) differentiation antigens, or (iii) environmentally determined antigens. Although it is not possible to distinguish between these alternatives at present it is interesting to note that normal unimmunised rabbits have naturally occurring IgG in their serum with similar specificity as mouse NK cells which suggests the possibility that an infectious agent common to rabbit and mouse may generate antibody in the rabbit and NK cells in the mouse (27). The NK-like specificity of the rabbit antibody was shown by (i) a positive correlation between those targets in a panel which were lysed both by NK cells and natural rabbit antibody plus complement, (ii) a correlation between NK sensitivity and the ability of a given target to absorb the rabbit antibody and (iii) target cells pre-treated with natural rabbit antibody were less sensitive (blocked) to NK mediated lysis in a short-term ^{51}Cr release assay, whereas anti-H-2 or anti-gp71 antibody had no effect.

It has also been shown that immature cells in the normal thymus are sensitive to lysis by NK cells (5,28). Therefore the NK-TS may be an autoantigen which is not directly dependent on neoplastic transformation for expression, although it may be expressed more abundantly on transformed cells, which are often more sensitive to NK cytolysis. Finally, it cannot be ruled out that NK-TS represents a lectin like substance or glycosyltransferases since models of cell-cell contact involving at least a few specificities are possible under these circumstances (29,30

V. REGULATION OF TARGET-STRUCTURE EXPRESSION

Factors which may be important in the expression of NK-

TS have also been examined. A somatic cell hybrid between NK sensitive and NK insensitive parental cell lines did not express the NK-TS and consequently was not bound or lysed by NK cells (21). Several additional hybrids in NK high/low combinations were also low in NK sensitivity (31). Since alloantigens are usually codominantly expressed in somatic hybrids, whereas differentiation states or markers are usually suppressed, the low NK sensitivity in this and other similar hybrids had led to the suggestion that NK sensitivity is related to differentiation (31). The finding that NK-TS is not expressed on the YAC-IR/A9HT hybrid further suggests that the NK-TS itself may be expressed according to differentiation regulatory mechanisms, thus leading to low NK sensitivity in the YAC-IR/A9HT hybrid (21).

A different form of NK-TS modulation is also shown to occur. YAC cells, when removed from the selective pressures of an NK containing milieu in vivo and grown in vitro gradually exhibit increasing sensitivity to NK mediated lysis over a period of weeks (19). We have previously shown a concomitant increase in the quantitative expression of NK-TS in these in vitro explanted cells (18). Cell cycle effects may not be important in the expression of NK-TS since NK cells bind to targets equally well which are at various stages in the cell cycle (unpublished observation).

VI. THE RECOGNITION RECEPTOR

The available evidence supports the concept of limited heterogeneity in the putative NK "recognition" receptor. Hence, NK cells from high (CBA) and low (A/Sn) NK reactive strains exhibited identical avidities for NK-TS from YAC cells (32). That some heterogeneity in the receptor exists is suggested by the observation that receptor avidity increases in early post-natal development in CBA mice (32). In addition NK cells from mice recognised different patterns of NK-TS than did human NK cells (21). Since several unique NK-TS specificities have also been found (18,21) then these observations taken together suggest that the NK cell pool is polyspecific and has some heterogeneity in the recognition structure, albeit much less than would be expected of an antibody combining site. Cross depletion studies on target cell monolayers would suggest that NK specificities are polyclonally distributed (Ortaldo, J., to be published).

REFERENCES

1. Kiessling, R., Klein, E. and Wigzell, H., *Eur. J. Immunol.* *5*, 112 (1975).
2. Herberman, R.B., Nunn, M.E. and Lavrin, D.H., *Int. J. Cancer* *16*, 216 (1975).
3. Ortiz de Landazuri, M. and Herberman, R.B., *Nature New Biol.* *238*, 546 (1972).
4. Hansson, M., Karre, K., Bakacs, T., Kiessling, R. and Klein, G., *J. Immunol.* *121*, 6 (1978).
5. Hansson, M., Kiessling, R., Andersson, B., Karre, K. and Roder, J., Nature *278*, 174 (1979).
6. Haller, O., Kiessling, R., Orn, A., Karre, K., Nilsson, K. and Wigzell, H., *Int. J. Cancer* *20*, 93 (1977).
7. Becker, S., Magnusson, K. and Stendahl, O., *Immunol. Comm.* In Press.
8. Takasugi, M. and Mickey, M.R., *J. Natl. Cancer Inst.* *57*, 255 (1976).
9. Takasugi, M., Akira, D., Takasugi, J. and Mickey, M., *J. Natl. Cancer Inst.* *59*, 69 (1977).
10. Koide, Y. and Takasugi, M., *J. Natl. Cancer Inst.* *59*, 1009 (1977).
11. Takesugi, M., Koide, Y., Akina, D. and Ramseyer, A., *Int. J. Cander* *19*, 291 (1977).
12. Trinchieri, G., Santoli, D. and Knowles, B., Nature *270*, 611 (1977).
13. Gidlung, M., Orn, A., Wigzell, H., Senik, A. and Gresser, I. Nature *273*, 759 (1978).
14. Trinchieri, G., Santoli, D. and Koprowski, H., *J. Immunol.* *120*, 1849 (1978).
15. Trinchieri, G., Santoli, D. Dee, R. and Knowles, B., *J. Exp. Med.* *147*, 1299 (1978).
16. Trinchieri, G. and Santoli, D., *J. Exp. Med.* *147*, 1314 (1978).
17. Roder, J.C., Kiessling, R., Biberfeld, P. and Andersson, B., *J. Immunol.* *121*, 2509 (1978).
18. Roder, J.C., Rosen, A., Fenyo, E.M. and Troy, F.A., *Proc. Natl. Acad. Sci.* *76*, 1405 (1979).
19. Becker, S., Kiessling, R., Lee, N. and Klein, G., *Int. J. Cancer* In Press.
20. Roder, J. and Karre, K. Submitted.
21. Roder, J.C., Ahrlund-Richter, L. and Jondal, M., *J. Exp. Med.* *150*, 471 (1979).
22. Becker, S., Fenyo, E.M. and Klein, E., *Eur. J. Immunol.* *6*, 882 (1976).

23. Kiessling, R., Haller, O., Fenyo, E.M., Steinitz, M. and Klein, G., *Int. J. Cancer 21*, 460 (1978).
24. Lee, J.C. and Ihle, J.N., *J. Immunol. 118*, 928 (1977).
25. Kende, M., Hill, R., Dinowitz, M., Stephenson, J. and Kelloff, G., *J. Exp. Med. 149*, 358 (1979).
26. Minato, N., Bloom, B., Jones, C., Holland, J., Reid, L. *J. Exp. Med. 149*, 1117 (1979).
27. Gronberg, A., Hansson, M., Kiessling, R., Andersson, B., Karre, K. and Roder, J.C., *J. Natl. Cancer Institute*, In Press.
28. Hansson, M., Karre, K., Kiessling, R., Roder, J., Andersson, B. and Hayry, P., *J. Immunol. 123*, 765 (1979).
29. Marchase, R.B., Vosbeck, K. and Roth, S., *Biochim. Biophys. Acta. 457*, 385 (1976).
30. Shur, B.D. and Roth, S., *Biochim. Biophys. Acta. 415*, 473 (1975).
31. Ahrlund-Richter, L. and Klein, E., *Som. Cell Genet.* In Press.
32. Roder, J.C. Submitted.

NATURAL CYTOTOXIC (NC) CELLS AGAINST SOLID TUMORS IN MICE: SOME TARGET CELL CHARACTERISTICS AND BLOCKING OF CYTOTOXICITY BY D-MANNOSE[1]

Osias Stutman
Philip Dien
Roberta Wisun
Gene Pecoraro
Edmund C. Lattime

Cellular Immunobiology Section
Memorial Sloan-Kettering Cancer Center
New York, New York

I. INTRODUCTION

Although there has been extensive characterization of many features of natural cell-mediated cytotoxicity (CMC) in mice and other species, especially of the NK (natural killer) type (1,2), little is known or agreed upon about the specificity of the reactions and on the recognition structures or target sites involved in the effector-target cell interaction leading to target cell death. NK-susceptible and resistant targets have been described, as well as high and low reactors against a certain target (1,2). In addition, when other targets besides lymphomas were studied, sub-types such as the natural cytotoxic (NC) cells which are cytotoxic for target cells derived from non-lymphoid tumors, were described (3). In the NC system, targets may also be susceptible or resistant to lysis by effector cells of a given mouse strain (3), and

[1] *Supported by National Institute of Health Grants CA-08748, CA-17818, and CA-15988 and American Cancer Society Grant IM-188.*

ISBN 0-12-341350-8

different strains may be high or low reactors for a given target, although the genetic patterns appear as different from those governing NK-activity against YAC-1 cells (see our Chapter in the Immunogenetics Section). In this chapter, we will present some new studies on competitive inhibition showing that NC-susceptible targets can successfully interfere with lysis of YAC-1 cells by NK effectors, as well as some other studies on NC targets. In addition, we will present evidence that some simple sugars can block NC and NK-mediated in vitro CMC, with a preferential effect for D-mannose in the NC system. These results suggest that simple sugars, probably as part of complex membrane glycoproteins or glycolipids, may act as recognition sites for NC and NK cytotoxic cells.

As in our other entries in this Volume, we will mainly describe our studies with NC cells, as well as some comparisons with the NK system.

II. SOME TARGET CELL PROPERTIES

In our Chapter on "Characterization" of NC cells, we described some basic properties of the NC assay using adherent target cells (3). We showed differences in mouse strain distribution of high reactivity with different targets (see also our Chapter in the Immunogenetics Section). We also discussed the role of mycoplasma infection as a complicating factor increasing target susceptibility to lysis and showed differences in susceptibility to natural CMC depending on whether the same target cells were grown in suspension or as adherent monolayers. This last property is rather interesting since Meth A, for example, which is the prototype susceptible NC target when grown as monolayer, is a resistant target to NK when in suspension and tested in short term assays (however, it can be lysed in suspension in short assays by specifically allosensitized cytotoxic T cells, unpublished). Thus, it may well be that the target sites in Meth A for natural CMC may only be properly displayed when the cells grow as monolayers. On the other hand, other adherent targets which are sensitive to NC-mediated CMC are also good targets when tested in suspension.

A wide variety of lymphoma and other tumor cell lines from mice, rats or humans (4-10) as well as xenogenic persistently infected lines (11), or even normal tissues such as fibroblasts (10), thymocytes (12, 13), bone marrow cells or macrophages (12) have been used as targets for NK cytotoxicity. On the other hand, chemically induced fibrosarcomas, virus induced mammary tumors and Moloney-sarcoma virus-induced tumors (3, 14), but not normal fibroblasts (3) have shown susceptibility to NC cells in vitro.

A. *Cold-target Inhibition*

Competition by unlabelled target or cold-target inhibition of CMC (15), has been extensively used in determining the possible specificity of NK-mediated CMC (4-10), and in general, it has been shown that susceptible targets, even from other species (although there is some intraspecies preference, 8, 9), will be the most effective competitors for lysis of YAC-1 or other susceptible targets by NK cells. Conversely, resistant targets will tend to be less inhibitory (4-9), although some exceptions to the above rules have been observed (4-9).

Table I shows that Meth A and Meth 113 cells, which are both NC-susceptible targets, although showing a different spectrum of strain distribution of reactivity (3), produce excellent cold-target inhibition of cytotoxicity of YAC-1 cells mediated by NK cells. This would indicate that NC-

TABLE I. Cold-target Inhibition of NK-mediated CMC Against YAC-1 Targets by Meth A and Meth 113

Competing cells[a]	*Percent CMC (inhibition*[b]*)*
None	*24*
YAC-1	*8 (67%)*
Meth A	*2 (92%)*
Meth 113	*5 (79%)*
BALB/c thymocytes	*22 (8%)*

[a]*At 10:1 cold-to-labelled ratios. Five, 2 and 1:1 ratios were also tested. Competition was observed for the YAC at 5 and 2:1, while 1:1 competing ratios were also inhibitory for Meth A and Meth 113. Thymocytes had no effect at any ratio.*

[b]*CMC given for 100:1 effector:target ratios. Similar effects were observed for 50 and 10:1 ratios. Effector cells were from 5-9 week old BALB/c mice, tested against* ^{51}*Cr-labelled YAC-1 cells in a 4 hr assay. Percent inhibition of CMC in parentheses.*

susceptible targets share "determinants" with NK-susceptible targets. It is interesting to note that the BALB/c strain used in the experiment in Table I is a good NC-killer of Meth A targets but a poor killer of Meth 113 (3), suggesting that, although both cells have the recognition sites for lysis by NC cells (since Meth 113 is killed by NC cells from other strains) the BALB/c effector may not be able to produce lysis against one of the targets, although both appear to compete equally well against YAC-1 targets. Perhaps these differences are due to concentration or other aspects of surface display of the recognition sites.

Due to the long-term assay and especially to the geometry of the effector:target interaction when adherent pre-labelled targets are used, cold-target inhibitions are not easy to test in the NC system. For example, when mixtures of labelled and unlabelled target cells are made, keeping the total number of target cells per well constant, the results shown in Table II, suggesting cold -target inhibition, can be only obtained when

TABLE II. Cold-target Inhibition of NC-mediated CMC

Labelled/unlabelled cells[a]	*Ratio*	*Percent Inhibition of CMC*[b]
A + A	*1:7*	*45**
A + A	*1:1*	*11*
A + 113	*1:7*	*11*
A + 113	*1:1*	*6*
113 + 113	*1:7*	*38**
113 + 113	*1:1*	*13*
113 + A	*1:7*	*72**
113 + A	*1:1*	*60**
113 + Fibroblasts	*1:7*	*3*

[a]*Two thousand target cells/well in all experiments at the indicated ratios of labelled/unlabelled cells. For further details on Meth A and Meth 113 see ref. 3. Both are chemically induced BALB/c fibrosarcomas. "Fibroblasts" were derived from BALB/c embryos (3).*

[b]*Percent inhibition of CMC by the mixtures. CMC measured against 3H-proline pre-labelled cells using 5-8 week old BALB/c spleen cells as NC-effectors at 100:1 effector:target ratios in a 24 hr assay. The % CMC for the unmixed targets was 65-77% for Meth A and 18-22 % for Meth 113. (*) indicates a* $p <$ *0.05 or 0.91 using a Student t test.*

2000 target cells are tested, and not with lower or higher total number of targets (unpublished). In addition, due to the dilution of the labelled cells, it is very difficult to go beyond a 1:7 ratio of labelled-unlabelled cells. On the other hand, if a constant amount of labelled cells is used, and the unlabelled cells are just added, the experiment becomes uncontrollable, since each set of wells will have different total amounts of cells.

As part of our studies to determine the mechanism of resistance of the BALB/c fibrosarcoma Meth 113 to NC-mediated CMC by syngeneic spleen cells (3), we did mixing experiments to see if the resistant cells would inhibit NC activity against the susceptible Meth A target, or, conversely, if lysis of Meth A produced any "bystander" effects on Meth 113. Table II shows that neither "inhibition" nor "bystander" effects were observed. In addition, Table II shows studies on cold-target inhibition. Firstly, unlabelled Meth A cells could inhibit Meth A killing at the 1:7 labelled/unlabelled (L/U) ratio, but not at the lower L/U ratio. Secondly, unlabelled Meth 113 did not inhibit NK killing of Meth A by BALB/c spleen cells, although they could inhibit killing of Meth 113 cells at 1:7 L/U ratio. Thirdly, Meth A was a powerful inhibitor of NC killing of Meth 113 targets, even at 1;1 L/U ratios. These results suggest, as was discussed previously, that both targets may be sharing the same recognition sites for NC, although due to display or concentration of such sites on the cell surface, both BALB/c tumors differ in susceptibility to syngeneic NC killing. Thus, the BALB/c effector cells would be competitively inhibited by the susceptible (Meth A) but not the "resistant" (Meth 113) tumor. That this may be a problem of "recognition" by the effector cells, is supported by our preliminary observations that using NC-effector cells from A/J or NZB mice, which are high reactors against both targets, both targets produce reciprocal cold-target inhibition. Similarly, the presence of the appropriate recognition sites in Meth 113 is also supported by the fact that BCG or similar agents, can augment NC reactivity against Meth 113 targets even in BALB/c mice (3, see also our Chapter on "Characteristics").

B. Resistant Targets

As we have indicated in our Chapter on "Characteristics" of NC cells, when different adherent tumor targets are studied, two patterns arise: 1) targets like Meth A which are killed by NC cells from all the mouse strains tested and 2) targets, like Meth 113 and others, that are killed by NC cells of only certain strains, which may or may not include that syngeneic for the tumor. So far we have not been able to find a target that is "absolutely" resistant, that is, not affected by NC cells from any mouse strain. On the other hand, NC cells do not react with normal fibroblasts (3). As was observed with the NK system (4-6), culture lines are more susceptible to lysis than the same tumors after in vivo passage (3). The F9 teratocarcinoma cell line (kindly provided by Dr. K. Artz, Sloan-Kettering Institute) proved to be consistently resistant to NC-killing by BALB/c spleen cells (unpublished). Whether this is due to the absence of H2 surface antigens on that tumor (16), deserves further study.

Although some authors may feel differently (17-19), the same comments may be made concerning NK-resistant targets. Thus, the "absolutely" NK-resistant target has still to be described. For example, P815, which for some is a prototype resistant target to which NK cells do not bind and seems to lack the membrane "recognition structures" for NK lysis (17-19), may not belong to that category. For example, P815 is killed by NK cells from certain strains, especially NZB and NZW (20, 21), as well as by BCG activated (22) or other types of activated NK cells from a variety of mouse strains (10, 21). In addition, contradictory results for cold-target inhibition have been reported, describing either no effect on YAC-1 killing (6) or positive inhibition of YAC-1 and other targets (5). Thus, it is probable that the target sites for NK lysis are present in P815, but either at low concentration or improperly displayed. Otherwise, we may need to accept at least two different recognition sites for NK cells: one for resting NK cells which is expressed by targets like YAC-1 and one for "activated" NK cells, which is expressed by cells like P815. Such type of dual recognition mechanisms, one being "non-specific" and resulting in lysis of continuous or transformed lines by LCM-activated NK cells, while another is "specific" resulting in a more selective lysis of primary cells, has been proposed (10). Whether the recognition and the lytic signal are given by the same or different structures remains open to investigation. Whether concentration or proper display of the *same* structure may give either a recognition of a lytic signal, is also a possibility. Whether different structures or just reorganization of the same structure may present different "antigenicities" or recognition sites to the NK-NC systems, also remains as an open area of research.

Based on our studies described in Section III of this paper, in which simple sugars are capable of blocking NC and NK-mediated cytotoxicity, it is expected that true resistant lines may be rare or nonexistent. Thus, susceptibility-resistance may be more a matter of appropriate display and concentrations of glycoproteins and/or glycolipids, which are more probably either normal constituents of the cell membrane or expressed in all transformed cells (23), exposing the appropriate structures (sugars) which permit the successful lytic interaction. Since recognition (binding) and lysis of NK-susceptible targets are related but different events (18), the type of results just discussed are not surprising.

C. MuLV Antigens?

Although some of the initial studies with NK cells suggested (based mostly on cold-target inhibition studies) that cytotoxic activity was directed against either M-MuLV (6) or some type of endogenous MuLV (4, 6, 7), later studies showed that susceptibility or resistance to NK-killing did not correlate with the expression of either serologically defined MuLV antigens or group-specific antigenic determinants of MuLV 24). Similarly, resistance or susceptibility to NC-killing did not correlate with expression of MuLV defined antigens (3) or with the serologically defined private antigens of Meth A (3, 25). Thus, it is generally accepted that MuLV antigens are probably not involved in either NK (1, 2) or NC (3) reactivity.

However, some exceptions in the NK system have been described (26, 27). One study showed that direct addition of either AKR intact MuLV or the gp71 from that virus (and to a lesser extent R-MuLV or its gp71), could inhibit an NK-like killing of AKR lymphoma targets (26). That report indicated also, that such inhibition could be observed when effector cells from normal mice were used, but *not* with effector cells from nude mice (26). Another study showed that a variety of antisera with MuLV reactivity, such as anti-R-MuLV, anti-gp70 or p12, etc. could block the cytotoxicity of an NK-like cell against MuLV infected targets (27). This study showed a remarkable MuLV specificity of the cytotoxic response (27). Although these studies suggest that a sub-class of NK-like cells can show strict specificity for MuLV proteins or glycoproteins, based on blocking studies (26, 27), some alternative hypotheses cannot be excluded. For example, a T cell with low or "undetectable" levels of Thy 1 may be mediating both virus specific reactions, thus the response is absent in nudes (26). Especially since a T response to gp71 has been described (28) and "low Thy 1" mature T cells are not unusual (29). Thus, a better definition of the T properties of these responses with Lyt 1, 2 and 3 sera would be of interest. Conversely, the culture-induced T cells with "promiscuous cytotoxicity" (30), as well as other responses showing "non-specific" T cell cytotoxicity (31-33), may well be mediated by NK-like cells expressing surface Thy 1 (34). Another possibility could be that these blocking agents are doing so through some form of steric hindrance at effector or target cell level, and are not directly involved in the lytic event. A third possibility may be related to the results discussed in Section III.

III. BLOCKING OF NC AND NK CYTOTOXICITY BY SIMPLE SUGARS

The cold-target inhibition (4-10) as well as the assays measuring target-binding of effector NK cells (17-19) have suggested a certain degree of specificity for the NK recognition event. In addition, crude cell extracts of probable glycoprotein nature have been isolated from some NK susceptible targets, which can inhibit or block the binding of NK cells to the appropriate susceptible target (19, 35).

In this section we will briefly present results showing that some simple sugars can block NC and NK-mediated in vitro CMC, with a preferential effect for D-mannose in the NC system. On the other hand, none of the sugars tested, even at higher concentrations, had any effect on CMC mediated by allosensitized T cells. These results suggest that simple sugars, probably as the exposed parts of complex membrane glycoproteins or glycolipids, may act as recognition sites for NC and NK cytotoxic cells.

Table III shows the results. D-mannose at all concentrations tested from 100 mM to 10 mM, significantly blocked NC killing of Meth A targets, while the other sugars (as well as N-acetyl glucosamine and N-acetyl galactosamine) produced blocking only at 100 mM. D-galactose showed significant blocking at 50 mM in one of five experiments. These results were observed in five different experiments. Pre-incubation of the NC effector cells for 24 hrs with the different sugars at 100 or 50 mM concentration, followed by extensive washing, and subsequent use of the cells in a CMC assay against Meth A targets, showed no effect on activity (data not shown). Thus, the sugars are not acting via some form of toxicity for the effector cells. It is obvious that due to the length of the assay, these pre-treatment experiments cannot be considered as arguing against a recognition unit for D-mannose on the effector cells.

On the other hand, Table III also shows that a different picture appears for NK cells: D-mannose, D-galactose and D-glucose (as well as N-acetyl-glucosamine, not shown) all had the capacity to block NK cytotoxicity at almost all concentrations tested from 100 to 10 mM. This was observed in four

TABLE III. Effect of Simple Sugars on NC and NK-Mediated CMC

Sugar[a]	*% Inhibition of CMC at Different Concentrations*[b]							
	NC				*NK*			
	100mM	*50mM*	*20mM*	*10mM*	*100mM*	*50mM*	*20mM*	*10mM*
D-Mannose	*98*[+]	*56**	*49**	*43**	*100**	*47**	*31**	*28**
D-Galactose	*51**	*44**	*0*	*0*	*65**	*31**	*25**	*25**
D-Glucose	*69**	*18*	*15*	*10*	*65**	*44**	*28**	*0*
L-Fucose	*69**	*10*	*0*	*0*	-	-	-	-

[a]*All sugars from Sigma Chemicals (St. Louis, MO) at indicated final concentrations per well. Also tested, N-acetyl glucosamine and N-acetyl galactosamine, which show inhibition of NC activity at 100 mM but not at lower concentrations, and also inhibited NK activity at 100, 50 and 20 mM concentrations.*

[b]*Inhibition compared to control CMC values without sugars. CMC control values for NC activity ranged from 32 to 41 at 100:1 effector:target ratios. NK control activity at 100:1 ranged from 23 to 32%. Similar results were observed at 50 and 10 E:T ratios (not shown). NK activity tested against* ^{51}*Cr pre-labelled YAC-1 cells in a 4 hr assay. Five to 8 week old BALB/c mice used as spleen donors. (*) indicates* $p > 0$*, 0.05 or 0.91 by Student* t *test. (+) Significantly different from other sugars. The effects of D-mannose in the NC system were observed in five experiments. D-galactose showed inhibition in one of five experiments. The effects of the sugars on NK activity were observed in 4 experiments.*

experiments.

Conversely, when in vitro allosensitized T cells were tested for CMC against the appropriate targets (this was either a BALB/c anti-C57Bl/6 response tested on EL4 targets or a C57Bl/6 anti-BALB/c tested on P815 targets, generated as described in ref. 36) in the presence of sugars, no blocking was observed in a 4 hr assay using ^{51}Cr labelled targets, even at 100 mM concentrations. For example, at 1:1 E:T ratios in the BALB-anti-C57Bl response, the control CMC was 47%, while the "inhibition" at 100 mM for D-mannose, D-galactose and D-glucose respectively was 7, 7 and 13%, which have no statistical significance. Similarly, no effects were observed at 50 mM. In some experiments an actual increase in CMC, especially at the lower E:T ratios was observed, a phenomenon presently under study. The lack of effect of sugars on CMC-mediated by allosensitized T cells was observed in three experiments. A more detailed manuscript on these observations has been submitted for publication.

Four possible interpretations of these results can be proposed: 1) The NC effector cells have a "lectin-like" receptor which recognizes sugars (D-mannose) on the surface of the targets (the sugars are part of the complex glycoproteins or glycolipids of the membrane, 23, 37). Saturation of the binding sites in the effector cells by the sugars prevents the appropriate effector-target interaction to occur and lysis is inhibited. Whether the effect is on the binding or on the lytic process itself requires further study. For the NK cells, a similar lectin-like structure but with less specificity for a determined sugar can be postulated. Variation in sugar specificity and avidity of binding between different lectins has been described (38). In addition, the sugar concentrations used in the study agree with those used in lectin-sugar binding studies (38).

2) The lectin-like sugar receptors are on the target cells. Thus, the target cell would bind the NC or NK cell via a lectin-like structure recognizing sugars on the effector, and such binding, under the appropriate conditions would lead to killing of the target.

3) A variation of (2). The lectin-like structure is on the target but the effector is actually recognizing such structure (i.e. the effector NC or NK cells have "receptors" for the lectin-like structure). The binding of the appropriate sugar to the lectin-like structure on the target would interfere with the recognition of the structure by the effector cell.

4) Also a variation of (2), although a similar argument may be made for (1). The lectin-like receptor on the target (or on the effector NC or NK cell) is not the relevant determinant, but, once reacted with the appropriate sugar, it would block cytotoxicity via steric hindrance or a similar mechanism.

A wilder fifth possibility could hinge on the role of interferon on NK (1, 2) and probably NC (see our Chapter on "Characterization") cells. Thus, since interferon activity (at least its antiviral activity) can be inhibited by the interaction with the carbohydrate moiety of some membrane gangliosides (39), it is tempting to assume, that even in the short term assays, constant interferon activation of NK activity is present, and that the sugars may be reducing NK kill by inhibiting such activation. However, I have to accept that at present, this seems a far fetched interpretation.

Obviously, none of these speculations apply to the specific T cell-mediated cytotoxicity to allogeneic targets. Further studies with NC and NK cells are required to elucidate the mechanism of sugar blocking of cytotoxicity. Our present working hypothesis, without dismissing any of the other possibilities, is that the sugars are acting by saturation of a lectin-like recognition unit on the effector NC and NK cells.

The role of surface sugars in cell sociology (40) is well accepted. Interactions between lectin-like structures and either simple sugars or the sugar moieties of complex glycoproteins or glycolipids from the cell membrane are well established biological phenomena (41-56). These interactions appear important in cell adhesion and aggregation (41-44), platelet activation (43), cell differentiation (41, 45, 46), binding of virus and bacteria to host cells (47-52), viral induced malignant transformation (40, 53), phagocytosis (54) or binding of lymphokines by macrophages (55), interferon function (39) and fertilization (56). All but the last reference deal with systems using mammalian cells. Interactions involving selectively D-mannose or mannose-containing glycoproteins have been described for teratocarcinoma cellular adhesion (44), attachment of E. coli to epithelial cells (49) or macrophages (50),murine sarcoma virus transformation (53) and phagocytosis (54). In almost all of these systems, the concentrations are either higher or similar to those used in the present studies.

Thus, it is tempting to postulate that a similar type of "lectin-sugar" interaction as described above may be involved in the "natural" cell-mediated cytotoxicity against tumor cells (1-10), virus-infected targets (10, 11), certain normal tissues (12, 13) or some other mechanisms of defense against viral or bacterial infections which appear to be mediated by NK-like effector mechanisms (57).

ACKNOWLEDGMENTS

We would like to thank Ms. Linda Stevenson for her help in preparing this manuscript.

REFERENCES

1. Herberman, R.B., Djeu, J.Y., Kay, H.D., Ortaldo, J.R., Riccardi, C., Bonnard, G.D., Holden, H.T., Fagnani, R., Santoni, A. and Puccetti, P., Immunol. Rev. 44, 43 (1979).
2. Kiessling, R. and Wigzell, H., Immunol. Rev. 44, 165 (1979).
3. Stutman, O., Paige, C.J. and Feo Figarella, E., J. Immunol. 121, 1819 (1978).
4. Sendo, F., Aoki, T., Boyse, E.A. and Buafo, C.K., J.

Natl. Cancer Inst. 55, 603 (1975).
5. Herberman, R.B., Nunn, M.E. and Lavrin, D.H., Int. J. Cancer 16, 216 (1975).
6. Kiessling, R., Klein, E. and Wigzell, H., Eur. J. Immunol. 5, 112 (1975).
7. Zarling, J.M., Nowinski, R.C. and Bach, F.H., Proc. Natl. Acad. Sci. USA 72, 2780 (1975).
8. Hansson, M., Karre, K., Bakacs, T., Kiessling, R. and Klein, G., J. Immunol. 121, 6 (1978).
9. Nunn, M.E. and Herberman, R.B., J. Natl. Cancer Inst. 62, 765 (1979).
10. Welsh, R.M., Zinkernagel, R.M. and Hallenbeck, L.A., J. Immunol. 122, 465 (1979).
11. Minato, N., Bloom, B.R., Jones, C., Holland, J. and Reid, L.M., J. Exp. Med. 149, 1117 (1979).
12. Nunn, M.E., Herberman, R.B. and Holden, H.T., Int. J. Cancer 20, 381 (1977).
13. Hansson, M., Kiessling, R., Andersson, B., Karre, K. and Roder, J., Nature 278, 174 (1979).
14. Heinin, Y., Gomard, E., Gisselbrecht, S. and Levy, J.P., Brit. J. Cancer 39, 51 (1979).
15. Ortiz de Landazuri, M.D. and Herberman, R.B., Nature (New Biol.) 238, 18 (1972).
16. Artz, K. and Jacob, F., Transplantation 17, 632 (1974).
17. Roder, J.C. and Kiessling, R., Scand. J. Immunol. 8, 135, (1978).
18. Roder, J.C., Kiessling, R., Biberfeld, P. and Andersson, B., J. Immunol. 121, 2509 (1978).
19. Roder, J.C., Rosen, A., Fenyo, E.M. and Troy, F.A., Proc. Natl. Acad. Sci. USA 76, 1405 (1979).
20. Greenberg, A.H. and Playfair, J.H.L., Clin. Exp. Immunol. 10, 99 (1974).
21. Croker, B.P., Zinkernagel, R.M. and Dixon, F.J., Clin. Immunol. Immunopath. 12, 410 (1979).
22. Wolfe, S.A., Tracey, D.E. and Henney, C.S., Nature 262, 584 (1976).
23. Hakomori, S.I., Adv. Cancer Res. 18, 265 (1973).
24. Becker, S., Fenyo, E.M. and Klein, E., Eur. J. Immunol. 6, 882 (1976).
25. DeLeo, A.B., Shiku, H., Takahashi, T., John, M. and Old, L.J., J. Exp. Med. 146, 720 (1977).
26. Lee, J.C. and Ihle, J.N., J. Immunol. 118, 928 (1977).
27. Kende, M., Hill, R., Dinowitz, M., Stephenson, J.R. and Kelloff, G.J., J. Exp. Med. 149, 358 (1979).
28. Enjuanes, L., Lee, J.C. and Ihle, J.N., J. Immunol. 122, 665 (1979).
29. Cantor, H. and Weissman, I.L., Progr. Allergy 20, 1 (1976).

30. Shustick, C., Cohen, I. R., Schwartz, R.S., Latham-Griffin, E. and Waksal, S.D., Nature 263, 699 (1976).
31. Pfizenmaier, K., Trostmann, H., Rollinghoff, M. and Wagner, H., Nature 258, 238 (1975).
32. Komatsu, Y., Nawa, Y., Bellamy, A.R. and Marbrook, J., Nature 274, 802 (1978).
33. Simpson, E., Mobraaten, L., Chandler, P., Hetherington, M., Hurme, M., Brunner, C. and Bailey, D., J. Exp. Med. 148, 1478 (1978).
34. Mattes, J.M., Sharrow, S.O., Herberman, R.B. and Holden, H.T., J. Immunol. 123, 2851 (1979).
35. Roder, J.C., Ahrlund-Richter, L. and Jondal, M., J. Exp. Med. 150, 471 (1979).
36. Lattime, E.C., Gershon, H.E. and Stutman, O., J. Immunol. 124, 274 (1980).
37. Nicholson, G.L., Biochem. Biophy. Acta 458, 1 (1976).
38. Lis, H. and Sharon, N., Ann. Rev. Biochem. 42, 541 (1973).
39. Besancon, F., Ankel, H. and Baus, S. Nature 259, 576 (1976).
40. Kalckar, H.M., Science 150, 305 (1965).
41. Balsamo, J. and Lilien, J., Biochemistry 14, 167 (1975).
42. Vicker, M.G., J. Cell. Sci. 21, 161 (1976).
43. Gartner, T.K., Williams, D.C., Minion, F.C. and Phillips, D.R., Science 200, 1281 (1978).
44. Grabel, L.B., Rosen, S. D. and Martin, G.R., Cell 17, 477 (1979).
45. Hausman, R.E. and Moscona, A.A., Proc. Natl. Acad. Sci. USA 72, 916 (1975).
46. Muramatsu, T., Gachelin, G., Damonville, M., Dalarbre, C. and Jacob, F., Cell 18, 183 (1979).
47. Gelb, L.D. and Lerner, A.M., Science 147, 404 (1965).
48. Gesner, B. and Thomas, L., Science 151, 590 (1966).
49. Laver, W.G., Adv. Virus Res. 18, 57 (1973).
50. Ofek, I., Mirelman, D. and Sharon, N., Nature 265, 623 (1977).
51. Bar-Shavit, Z., Ofek, I., Goldman, R., Mirelman, D. and Sharon, N., Biochem. Biophys. Res. Commun. 78, 455 (1977).
52. Levy, N.J., Infec. Immun. 25, 946 (1979).
53. Hatanaka, M., Proc. Natl. Acad. Sci. USA 70, 1364 (1973).
54. Brown, R., Bass, H. and Coombs, J., Nature 254, 434 (1975).
55. Remold, H.G., J. Exp. Med. 138, 1065 (1973).
56. Vacquier, V. and Moy, G., Proc. Natl. Acad. Sci. USA, 74, 2456 (1977).
57. Cudkowicz, G., Landy, M. and Shearer, G. (eds). Natural resistance systems against foreign cells, tumors and microbes. Academic Press, New York (1978).

MODIFICATION OF TARGET SUSCEPTIBILITY TO ACTIVATED MOUSE NK CELLS BY INTERFERON AND VIRUS INFECTIONS

Raymond M. Welsh, Jr.

Department of Immunopathology
Scripps Clinic and Research Foundation
La Jolla, California

Rolf W. Kiessling

Department of Tumor Biology
Karolinska Institute
Stockholm, Sweden

I. INTRODUCTION

Natural killer (NK) cells can be activated in mice by biological and chemical interferon-inducing agents (1-4) and by interferon, itself (5,6). The activation results in increased lysis of target cells sensitive to "endogenous" NK cells as well as *de novo* lysis against otherwise resistant cells. This suggests that the activation of NK cells results in a decrease of their lytic specificity. In our hands the most efficient way to activate NK cells is by infecting mice with lymphocytic choriomeningitis virus (LCMV) and using the spleen as an NK source 2 to 3 days after infection (3,6,7). In this report we will review our work concerning the target range of the LCMV-induced activated NK cell and the effects of interferon and viral infections on target cell susceptibility to lysis.

II. TARGET CELLS SENSITIVE TO LCMV-INDUCED ACTIVATED NK CELLS

Virtually every continuous cell line which we have tested is sensitive to lysis by LCMV-induced activated NK cells, though the sensitivities vary markedly from target to target (7). Target cells sensitive to endogenous NK cells, such as

ISBN 0-12-341350-8

YAC-1 lymphomas, are generally more sensitive to the activated cells than are targets resistant to endogenous NK killing. Although the activated NK cells appear to have reduced specificity in regards to lysing targets, there is no evidence that they recognize new antigenic determinants. Thus, YAC-1 cells compete very well in cold target inhibition assays with the killing of L-929 cells, which are resistant to endogenous NK cell killing. Furthermore, L-929 cell monolayers absorb compatable levels of activated and endogenous NK cells, as assayed on YAC-1 targets. No H-2 or species preferences in regards to lysis was found between activated NK cells and continuous cell lines in our studies (7).

Using activated NK cells against comparably NK-sensitive target cells in cold target inhibition assays, Welsh and Zinkernagel (3) showed preferential competition by homologous cells, though considerable heterologous competition was also noted. While these results can be taken as evidence for NK cell heterogeneity, other types of experiments must be done to definitively prove this point.

With the exception of a subpopulation of cortical thymocytes found predominantly in young (less than 3 weeks old) mice, endogenous NK cells usually do not lyse normal primary mouse cells (8). Many normal primary cells are lysed by LCMV-induced activated NK cells, however (7,9,10). The same distribution in high versus low reactive mouse strains in regard to lysing targets with endogenous NK cells (11) is seen against YAC-1 cells, thymocytes, and fibroblasts when activated NK cells are the effectors (10,12). The lysis of primary macrophages contrasts markedly with this pattern of lysis, however. In this system, lysis is usually low against isologous macrophages and high against allogeneic macrophages (7,10,12). These results also may be interpreted as evidence for heterogeneity within the mouse NK cell population. Alternatively, NK activator or suppressor factors in these mixed leukocyte cultures may play some role in this apparent selective lysis of macrophages, though we have no evidence for these as yet (7).

III. MODIFICATION OF TARGET CELL SUSCEPTIBILITY BY INTERFERON

An elegant study in the human system by Trinchiari and Santoli (13), showed that, in addition to activating NK cells, interferon paradoxically could protect target cells from NK cell-mediated lysis. Nontransformed fibroblasts were more sensitive than tumor cells to this interferon-induced protection, leading the authors to speculate this as a mechanism for directing NK cells to lyse only tumor cells *in vivo*.

We have examined this phenomenon in the mouse system, which allows for more experimental manipulation. Table I shows that the activated NK cell-mediated lysis of primary thymocytes, macrophages, and fibroblasts, and of a number of continuous cell tumor lines was markedly inhibited by interferon treatment. Only Vero cells of xenogeneic monkey origin, were not protected by mouse interferon. While there were differences in interferon sensitivity from cell to cell, normal cells on the whole did not appear appreciably more or less sensitive than tumor cells to the interferon treatment.

Because L-929 cells were among the most sensitive targets to interferon-mediated protection, mechanistic and kinetic studies were done using that cell line. Treatment of L-929 cells with cycloheximide (25 μg/ml) before interferon exposure prevented the interferon-mediated protection (data not shown). This indicates that protein synthesis is required for the protective effect, a result also found by Trinchiari and Santoli (13). Treatment of L-929 cells with 500 units/ml interferon for 2 H before radiolabeling (1 H) and exposure to activated NK cells in a 4 H cytotoxicity assay was sufficient to protect cells by about 30% (Table II). In a number of experiments about 50% protection was seen after 4 H treatment and maximum protection after 12 H. The interferon-mediated protection, at least in part, resulted from the removal of the expression of the functional NK target antigen from the L-929 cell surface. In cold target competition experiments, interferon-treated L-929 cells competed poorly against the lysis of control L-929 cells (Table II).

While interferon markedly protected L-929 cells from killing by NK cells, it failed to protect them from anti-H-2 antibody dependent cell cytotoxicity (ADCC) mechanisms and from allospecific cytotoxic T cells (Table IIIA). Under conditions where L-929 cells were protected from activated NK cell killing it was clear that the activated effector cell population was more efficient at ADCC than endogenous effectors. This activation of ADCC mechanisms adds further support to theories linking NK and K cell functions.

TABLE I. Protection of Target Cells from NK Cell-Mediated Lysis by Interferon

Target	H-2	IF[1] units/ml	E:T[2] ratio	% Lysis
L-929	k	0	100	26
		20		14
		200		5.8
		2000		5.6
P-52	b	0	100	38
		100		27
		1000		14
		10000		9
P-815	d	0	100	14
		100		8
		1000		4
		10000		3
RBL-5	b	0	100	38
		100		27
		1000		5
		10000		4
Vero	xeno-geneic	0	50	15
		4000		12
YAC-1	a	0	25	39
		100		31
		1000		24
		10000		26
YWA	s	0	100	39
		100		28
		1000		26
		10000		21
SWR/J fetal fibroblasts	q	0	50	29
		1000		1.6
SWR/J macrophages	q	0	100	25
		1000		13
SWR/J thymocytes	q	0	20	10
		1000		2.5
		10000		0

[1] *Interferon units* [2] *Effector to target ratio*

Target cells were incubated with various doses of interferon for 12 to 16 H before assay against LCMV or Pichinde virus-induced activated C3H/St (H-2^k) mouse NK cells. Interferon was purified fibroblast (Type I) interferon purchased from Calbiochem, Inc., La Jolla, CA.

TABLE II. Interferon-Mediated Resistance of L-929 Cells To Bind and Be Lysed By Activated NK Cells

Exp. A.		Time of interferon treatment (H)				
		0	2	4	8	20
Direct cytotoxicity on these targets	100:1	20.	14.	12.	4.3	2.7
	25:1	7.5	5.6	5.7	1.4	0.40
Exp. B.						
Cold target competition by these targets	10:1	3.5	3.0	4.9	5.9	10.
	5:1	6.8	6.8	7.6	11.	12.
	2.5:1	10.	9.1	10.	14.	15.
	0:1	20.	(20)	(20)	(20)	(20)

Results tabulated are % lysis in 4 H cytotoxicity assays. L-929 cells treated with 500 units per ml interferon for different time periods were tested directly for sensitivity to activated NK cells (Exp. A) or for their ability to to cold target inhibit the lysis of normal (time = 0) L-929 cells. (Exp. B). In Exp. A the ratios are effector to target ratios. In Exp. B the ratios given are cold target to labeled target ratios; the effector to target ratio in Exp. B is 100:1.

TABLE III. NK Cell-Mediated Lysis of Interferon-Virus- and Antibody-Modified Targets

Target	Treatment	Effector	E:T[1]	% Lysis
Exp. A	-	Endogenous S.C.[2]	100	5.1
L-929	-	Activated S.C.	100	27.
	AB[3]	Endogenous S.C.	100	23.
	AB	Activated S.C.	100	45.
	-	Anti-H-2^k MLC[4]	50	38.
	IF[5]	Endogenous S.C.	100	0.30
	IF	Activated S.C.	100	5.6
	IF + AB	Endogenous S.C.	100	8.8
	IF + AB	Activated S.C.	100	21.
	IF	Anti-H-2^k MLC	50	45.
Exp. B	-	Activated S.C.	150	13.
	HSV	Activated S.C.	150	8.6
	Sindbis virus	Activated S.C.	150	10.
	VSV	Activated S.C.	150	10.
Exp. C	-	Endogenous S.C.	200	-0.45
	-	Activated S.C.	200	18.
	AB	Endogenous S.C.	200	6.6
	AB	Activated S.C.	200	34.
	Sendai virus	Endogenous S.C.	200	-0.30
	Sendai virus	Activated S.C.	200	1.7
	Sendai + AB	Endogenous S.C.	200	1.7
	Sendai + AB	Activated S.C.	200	11.
Exp. D	-	Activated S.C.	150	20.
	HSV	Activated S.C.	150	2.9
Vero	Sendai virus	Activated S.C.	150	34.

These are results from cytotoxicity assays run for 16 H (Exp. A) or about 4 H (Exp. B,C,D). [1]Effector to target cell ratio. [2]Spleen cells from C3H/St mice uninfected or infected with LCMV (similar results in Exp. A and C were also obtained with spleen cells from C57Bl6 x DBA/2 mice). [3]Anti-H-2^k antiserum. [4]Mixed leukocyte cultures of SWR/J (H-2^q) leukocytes responding to C3H/St (H-2^k) cells. [5]Plat were treated for 16 H with 2000 units interferon (IF) per m

IV. MODIFICATIONS OF TARGET CELL SUSCEPTIBILITY BY VIRUS INFECTIONS

Several reports have claimed that NK cells may preferentially lyse virus-infected target cells (14-19). In theory, this could be due to an NK cell interaction with a virus-modified cell membrane. It has been shown in a number of systems that the addition of endogenous human or mouse NK cells to uninfected and virus-infected cultures has resulted in substantially more lysis of the infected ones (14-19). In one human NK cell study, Santoli *et al.*(20), concluded that this apparent preferential lysis was actually a nonspecific lysis due to the virus-induced interferon-mediated activation of NK cells in the virus-infected cultures. Using Herpes simplex Type I (HSV), Sendai, Sindbis, and vesicular stomatitis (VSV) viruses, we have confirmed Santoli's results and conclusions in the mouse system (21). However, the question remained open whether NK cells could selectively interact with virus-infected cells. To examine this, LCMV-activated spleen (NK) cell populations were exposed to virus-infected or uninfected targets in short (4 H) assays to prevent any secondary *in vitro* NK cell activation. Table III B,C shows that virus-infected L-929 cells actually tended to be *less* sensitive than uninfected controls to activated NK cells. Sendai virus-infected L-929 cells were markedly resistant to cell-mediated lysis, even though nylon wool-passed spleen cells rosetted (2 to 10 per cell) around Sendai virus-infected targets (data not shown). Sendai virus-infected L-929 cells competed as well or better than uninfected cells in cold target competition assays which used activated NK cells and L-929 cell targets or endogenous NK cells and YAC-1 cell targets (Table IV).

TABLE IV. Effect of Virus Infections on Cold Target Competition

	C:L[1]	% Lysis Competitors	
		L-929	L-929 + Sendai
Exp. A. Target cell: YAC-1	20:1	20	15
Effector cell: Endogenous NK	10:1	27	20
% Lysis, control: 27	5:1	28	23
Exp. B. Target cell: L-929	10:1	5.7	1.7
Effector cell: Activated NK	5:1	12.	7.4
% Lysis, control: 29	2.5:1	19.	15.
		Vero	Vero + HSV
Exp. C. Target cell: Vero	10:1	5.9	18.
Effector cell: Activated NK	5:1	8.9	19.
% Lysis, control: 20	2.5:1	13.	19.

[1] *Cold target to labeled target ratio.*

This indicates that these NK-resistant Sendai virus-infected L-929 cells could bind both endogenous and activated NK cells but still not be lysed. These same cells, however, were sensitive to ADCC (Table IIIC). Our interpretation of these results is that an NK/K cell must bind to target cells in a particular way in order to confer lysis. Perhaps the interferon induced in these cultures by Sendai virus renders the required (interferon-sensitive) NK target antigens unavailable for binding NK cells in a way which promotes cytotoxicity. The presence of an antibody could substitute for those antigens. Supporting this concept is the fact that Sendai virus-infected Vero cells are more sensitive than controls to lysis by activated NK cells (Table IIID). Vero cells neither produce interferon themselves nor are sensitive to mouse interferon. Possibly the combination of available NK target antigens and "sticky" viral membrane proteins render these cells more sensitive to lysis.

HSV-infected Vero cells were markedly resistant to lysis by LCMV-induced activated NK cells (Table IIID). These targets failed to bind lymphocytes in target binding cell assays (21,22) and failed to compete against uninfected Vero cell targets in competition assays (Table IV). Thus, the HSV infection, by altering the Vero cell membrane, removed the expression of the functional NK target antigen and rendered the cells resistant to NK cell-mediated lysis by an interferon-independent mechanism. This virus-mediated protection of cells could presumably be due to virus-induced alterations in the cell's metabolic process.

V. SUMMARY AND CONCLUSIONS

Mouse NK cells activated *in vivo* by virus infection lyse a broad range of continuous cell lines and primary "normal" tissue. Interferon plays a dual role by activating NK cells and protecting target cells. The latter phenomenon is at least in part due to the removal of the functional expression of the NK target antigen. Interferon did not significantly protect target cells from ADCC or cytotoxic T cells. Thus, this protection phenomenon may help prevent indiscriminate NK cell cytotoxicity *in vivo* while allowing specific effector mechanisms to function.

In most studied virus-target cell combinations, the virus infections reduced the cell's susceptibility to NK cell-mediated lysis by interferon-independent and possibly interferon-dependent mechanisms. In one system (Sendai virus-infected Vero cells), the virus infection enhanced the NK sensitivity of the targets. The resistance of the virus-infected targets did not necessarily correlate with their ability to bind NK cells. Sendai virus-infected L-929 cells bound NK cells but were only lysed in the presence of anti-H-2 antibody. While much needs to be resolved concerning the target antigens on NK-sensitive cells, it is clear that infection with agents capable either of inducing interferon or of directly causing cell membrane changes may alter the NK target antigens. It is further clear that NK cells must bind to target cells in a specified manner in order to confer lysis.

ACKNOWLEDGMENTS

This is publication number 1993 from the Department of Immunopathology, Scripps Clinic and Research Foundation, La Jolla, CA. We thank Ms. Lori Kunkel for technical assistance, Ms. Mona Hansson for helpful discussions and providing us with the thymocyte data, Ms. Laura Taxel for preparation of the manuscript, and Dr. M.B.A. Oldstone for support.

REFERENCES

1. Wolfe, S.A., Tracey, D.E., and Henney, C.S., *J. Immunol. 119*, 1152 (1977).
2. Herberman, R.B., Nunn, M.E., Holden, H.T., Staal, S., and Djeu, J.V., *Int. J. Cancer 19*, 555 (1977).
3. Welsh, R.M., and Zinkernagel, R.M., *Nature 268*, 646 (1977).
4. MacFarland, R.I., Burns, W.H., and White, D.O., *J. Immunol. 119*, 1569 (1977).
5. Gidlund, M., Orn, A., Wigzell, H., Senik, A., and Gresser, I., *Nature 273*, 759 (1978).
6. Welsh, R.M., *J. Exp. Med. 148*, 163 (1978).
7. Welsh, R.M., Zinkernagel, R.M., and Hallenbeck, L.A., *J. Immunol. 122*, 475 (1979).
8. Hansson, M., Kiessling, R., Andersson, B., Karre, K., and Roder, J., *Nature 278*, 174 (1979).
9. Nunn, M.E., Herberman, R.B., and Holden, H.T., *Int. J. Cancer 20*, 381 (1977).
10. Kiessling, R., and Welsh, R.M., manuscript submitted for publication, (1979).
11. Petranyi, G., Kiessling, R., Povey, S., Klein, G., Herzenberg, L., and Wigzell, H., *Immunogenetics 3*, 15 (1976).
12. Hansson, M., Kiessling, R., and Welsh, R.M. This volume in press (1980).
13. Trinchiari, G., and Santoli, D., *J. Exp. Med. 147*, 1314 (1978).
14. Anderson, M.J., *Infect. Immun. 20*, 608 (1978).
15. Harfast, B., Andersson, T., and Perlmann, P., *J. Immunol. 121*, 755 (1978).
16. Minato, N., Bloom, B.R., Jones, C., Holland, J., and Reid, L.M., *J. Exp. Med. 149*, 1117 (1979).
17. Blazer, B., Patarroyo, M., Klein, E., and Klein, G., *J. Exp. Med., in press.*
18. Santoli, D., Trinchiari, G., and Lief, F.S., J. Immunol. 121, 526 (1978).
19. Ault, K.A., and Weiner, H.L., *J. Immunol. 122*, 2611 (1979).
20. Santoli, D., Trinchiari, G., and Koprowski, H., *J. Immunol. 121*, 532 (1978).
21. Welsh, R.M., and Hallenbeck, L.A., manuscript submitted for publication.
22. Roder, J.C., Kiessling, R., Biberfield, P., and Andersson, B., *J. Immunol. 121*, 2509 (1978).

SUMMARY: SPECIFICITY OF CYTOTOXICITY BY NK CELLS AND NATURE OF RECOGNITION STRUCTURES ON EFFECTOR AND TARGET CELLS

Much recent information has been obtained regarding the specificity of cytotoxicity by NK cells, and these efforts have been aided by the development of a variety of experimental approaches. Most investigators now agree that NK cells can specifically recognize their target cells and current attention is focused on the multiplicity of the antigens recognized and their nature, and on the characteristics and distribution of the recognition structures on NK cells.

I. TARGET CELLS RECOGNIZED BY NK CELLS

NK cells have been found to react with a wide variety of target cells. *In vitro* passaged leukemia lines are particularly susceptible to lysis but some carcinoma and sarcoma lines, and some *in vivo* transplanted tumors, are also quite susceptible to rapid lysis. NK reactivity can be seen against syngeneic tumors and also against allogeneic and some xenogeneic lines. It has also become clear that a limited assortment of normal cells may also be lysed by NK cells. These are mainly subpopulations of thymocytes, bone marrow cells and macrophages and cultured fetal fibroblasts. Despite the broad range of susceptible targets, clear selectivity is seen, with many tumor cells and normal cells being quite resistant to lysis.

When augmented NK cells are tested, lysis may be seen against some targets that usually resist the action of spontaneous NK cells. This might be attributed to an alteration in the specificity of the effector cells or to the ability of more highly active effector cells to induce detectable lysis of resistant target cells. The available evidence favors the latter possibility. For example, Trinchieri *et al* noted that target cells showed the same rank order of susceptibility to lysis by spontaneous and interferon (IF)- boosted NK cells,

ISBN 0-12-341350-8

although the range of susceptibility was narrower with the augmented effector cells. This issue needs to be examined more carefully, especially by the more discriminatory techniques that have become available, i.e. cold target inhibition and monolayer adsorptions. Comparisons of the biochemical nature of antigens recognized by spontaneous and boosted NK cells should also be useful.

It should be noted that prolongation of the cytotoxicity assay, from the usual 4 hrs. to overnight, also broadens the range of target cells susceptible to NK lysis. Some of this change in the pattern of reactivity may be due to augmentation of NK cells by IF produced in response to the stimulation by some targets. However, other target cells, e.g. human fetal fibroblasts, become susceptible to NK lysis in prolonged assays yet do not stimulate detectable amounts of IF.

An important issue is whether primary tumor cells, as well as transplanted or cultured cell lines, are susceptible to lysis by NK cells. Limited information is available but it is becoming clear that at least some primary tumor cells are susceptible. Only infrequent and low levels of lysis have usually been seen with spontaneous NK cells, but after augmentation with IF or IF-inducers, appreciable activity was observed. Zarling reports reactivity of IF-treated human NK cells against an appreciable proportion of allogeneic leukemia target cells (acute myelogenous leukemia, chronic myelogenous leukemia in blast crisis, and chronic lymphocytic leukemia). Furthermore, Vose observed frequent reactivity of IF-boosted NK cells from normal donors against most solid tumor cells tested.

II. EVIDENCE FOR RECOGNITION BY NK CELLS OF MULTIPLE ANTIGENIC SPECIFICITIES

Initially, most investigators felt that NK cells recognized one common structure on target cells, and this view is still held by some. However, evidence for recognition of multiple specificities has accumulated. With such data have also come indications for subsets of NK cells, each recognizing a more limited number of target cells. As summarized below, this issue has been approached by a variety of experimental procedures.

A. *Patterns of Reactivity Seen with Direct Testing of Different Target Cells*

If all NK cells recognized the same structure on all susceptible target cells, one would expect that the same patterns of reactivity would be seen, regardless of the donor of the effector cells. Several contributors provide evidence that this is not the case. For example, some target cells are susceptible to lysis by NK cells from only certain strains of mice (Hansson et al, Herberman and Ortaldo, Tai and Warner). Similarly, normal human donors have been found to vary in their patterns of reactivity against various target cells (Greenberg and Takasugi; Herberman and Ortaldo; Kaplan and Callewaert), and by the statistical method of interactional analysis, Greenberg and Takasugi defined three groups of antigens on target cells, TA1, 2 and 3.

B. *Cold Target Inhibition*

The results by this procedure have confirmed the suggestions provided by direct testing. For example, Greenberg and Takasugi obtained further support for the above mentioned three antigens and in addition defined one antigen shared by T cell lines and another shared by B cells lines. A further observation, made by several groups (Greenberg and Takasugi; Herberman and Ortaldo; Kaplan and Callewaert) was that the homologous target cell usually gave the greatest cold target inhibition, pointing out some individual or restricted specificities on the targets. It should be noted that much sharing of specificities, even by cells from different species, has also been seen. Evidence for multiple specificities has come only from tests with large numbers of different inhibitor cells. This probably accounts for the failure of Durdik et al to discern any differences since they only tested a few target cells. Tai and Warner on the one hand provide evidence for multiple specificities but also demonstrate that when only three targets were compared, no heterogeneity was identified.

C. *Enzyme Kinetics Analysis*

Several groups have analyzed their data according to the model of enzyme kinetics. Forbes and Oldham confirmed the observation of Pollack that different binding constants, Km, are seen when the same donor is tested against various target cells, thus pointing to different recognition structures. It should be noted, however, that Callewaert found a similar or identical Km for each target reacted with by a given donor. The reasons for this difference are not clear. Based on their analysis, Forbes and Oldham further conclude that cold target inhibition by only some cells is competitive, whereas that by others is not competitive. This is an interesting point but the example given does not well support the conclusion since only minimal inhibition was seen with the so-called noncompetitive target.

D. Physical Separation of Subsets of NK Cells

To determine whether each NK cell can recognize the whole array of antigens or whether there are subsets of NK cells, each recognizing one or a few of the multiple specificities, various cell separation procedures have been used. Several groups have utilized monolayers of target cells to selectively adsorb out the NK cells recognizing antigens on those cells and to then examine the residual activity in the unadsorbed effector cell population. With human NK cells, this procedure readily defined several subsets of NK cells that recognized various shared and restricted antigens on target cells with variation in the specificity patterns among donors (Herberman and Ortaldo, Jensen and Koren). In comparable studies with mouse NK cells, less heterogeneity was seen (Herberman et al). All tumor targets examined, including xenogeneic lines, appeared to share the same specificities. Similarly, Durdik et al, who only examined two tumor targets, found no heterogeneity by this or another separation procedure. However, a separate subpopulation seemed to be involved in reactivity against normal adherent peritoneal cells (Herberman and Ortaldo). This observation fits well with the data of Hansson et al, who also obtained indications for a different subset of NK cells reactive with peritoneal targets.

Evidence for heterogeneity in specificity among NK cells also has come from separation of cells according to size. Tai and Warner and also Lotzova observed that larger cells had a different pattern of reactivity than did smaller NK cells.

The relationship of the different NK subsets with each other is not clear. One hypothesis, favored by most groups, is that the heterogeneity is an indication of clonality of NK cells, with each clone reacting against only one or a few specificities, and the broad pattern of reactivity of the whole NK cell population due to a mixture of multiple clones. An alternative possibility, that presently can not be ruled out, is that the different subsets represent different stages of differentiation or activation of NK cells. However, the consistency of results for each donor but the major differences among donors is difficult to reconcile with this possibility. To further elucidate this point, it will be important to characterize the cell surface and other characteristics of each subset. The apparent recent ability to propagate NK cells in vitro by the use of T cell growth factor, and the possibility of cloning these cultured NK cells, should be particularly helpful to resolve the question of clonal heterogeneity of NK cells.

III. NATURE OF RECOGNITION STRUCTURES ON NK CELLS

This is an important and interesting issue, for which very little information is available. Greenberg and Takasugi, who favor the armed K cell hypothesis for NK activity (see section IB), believe that natural antibodies bound to the Fc receptors on NK cells account for the specificity. This is a simple and attractive hypothesis, that would easily account for the ability of NK cells to recognize multiple target cell antigens. However, as discussed in section IB, there are several lines of evidence against this hypothesis. In addition, as pointed out by Kaplan and Callewaert, this hypothesis is difficult to reconcile with the indications for heterogeneity within the NK cell population. One would expect to have random binding of the range of antibodies to each NK cell, rather than segregation of certain antibodies to subsets of NK cells.

Kaplan and Callewaert put forward another hypothesis, raised by other contributors as well, that the receptors on NK cells are similar to those on cytotoxic T lymphocytes and are immunoglobulin V gene products. Although this is an intriguing possibility, there is no direct evidence available to support it. There are, in fact, reasons to believe that the nature of recognition by NK cells is substantially different from that of CTL. In addition to the disparities in specificity summarized below, there appear to be fundamental differences in the processes known to induce or activate these effector cells. Induction of CTL is usually dependent on sensitization with a given antigen, the resultant CTL have specific reactivity limited mainly to the immunogen, and later re-exposure to the same antigen evokes a rapid and specific memory response. In contrast, NK cells appear without known antigenic stimulation and as soon as they are detectable, have reactivity against the full array of specificities that are associated with this effector system. In addition, NK cells have not been demonstrated to undergo a specific memory response but rather, upon stimulation with cells bearing NK related antigens or with IF, rapidly develop augmented reactivity against a wide range of specificities.

One characteristic of the NK receptor that is widely believed in is its trypsin sensitivity. This is based on the finding that trypsin treatment of NK cells diminishes or eliminates their activity. However, even this point requires better documentation, by directly examining the effect of trypsin on formation of conjugates with target cells.

The conjugate technique appears to be the most promising one for obtaining concrete information on the nature of the recognition receptors on NK cells. As Roder has done for analysis of target cell structures, one would expect that solubilized NK recognition structures would inhibit conjugate formation and this would provide an assay for monitoring purification procedures.

IV. NATURE OF ANTIGENS ON NK-SUSCEPTIBLE TARGET CELLS

Since the initial studies on NK cells, there has been much speculation on the nature of the antigens that are recognized on the target cells. The evidence for multiple antigens has complicated this question and as yet little is known about them. Most evidence is rather indirect and circumstantial. The following is a summary of the various possibilities that are being considered.

A. *Role of Major Histocompatibility Complex (MHC) and Comparison with Cytotoxic T Lymphocytes (CTL)*

There are several reasons for serious consideration of the role of MHC antigens in the specificity of NK cells: a) evidence that NK cells belong to the T cell lineage and the possibility that they may be early cells along pathway of differentiation of CTL (e.g. see Kaplan and Callewaert, Ortaldo and Herberman); b) NK activity is generated during mouse and human mixed lymphocyte cultures (Seeley); c) some association between levels of NK activity among donors and their H2 or HLA loci; and d) with certain targets, e.g. adherent mouse peritoneal cells, reactivity is largely resticted to allogeneic cells (Welsh and Kiessling). However, there is a number of features that distinguish NK cells from CTL. In addition to the differences in cell surface and other characteristics that are discussed in section IA, there are some major differences in their specificity (summarized in Table

TABLE I. Specificity of NK Cells as Compared to Cytotoxic T Lymphocytes (CTL)

Characteristic or treatment	*CTL*	*NK cells*
MHC restriction	*at least some (usually complete in 4 hr assay)*	*none*
Reactivity against targets lacking MHC	*none*	*strong against some*
Inhibition by antibody to MHC antigens on targets	*yes*	*no*
Reactivity against normal or mitogen-activated lymphocytes	*strong against those with relevant MHC antigens*	*none*
Genetic regions in mouse MHC influencing reactivity	*H2D and K*	*some linkage to H2D*

I). One important characteristic feature of the specificity of CTL is the at least partial restriction of their reactivity to targets that are MHC compatible with the effector cells. In a 4 hr cytotoxic assay, this restriction appears to usually be absolute, particularly in the mouse. In contrast, NK cells can display strong reactivity against a variety of allogeneic and even xenogeneic target cells. Of course, the complete MHC restriction for CTL does not apply to alloimmune CTL and one could argue that MHC antigens themselves are the targets for NK activity (see Kaplan and Callewaert). Against this possibility are the observations that NK cells can react strongly against some target cells lacking detectable MHC antigens. Gidlund et al (section IA) found that some mouse teratoma cells are very sensitive to lysis by NK cells, and similarly, K-562 and Daudi, human cell lines very sensitive to cytotoxicity by NK cells, have been shown to be deficient in MHC determinants. Gidlund et al have also found that Fab fragments of antibodies to MHC determinants, which effectively block CTL activity, had no effect on lysis by NK cells. Another strong argument against much of the specificity of NK cells being directed against MHC determinants is that PHA- or Con A-blasts, that are excellent targets for alloimmune CTL, are consistently resistant to lysis by NK cells and are unable to act as cold target inhibitors of NK-susceptible targets (e.g. Seeley et al).

The findings that levels of NK reactivity among different mice was linked to the H2D region of the mouse MHC pointed toward some type of association. However, although alloimmune CTL can react well against differences at the H2D region, they also can recognize and be immunized strongly against H2K region differences. It seems more likely that the associations of NK rectivity with the H2D region is related to the nearby Hh locus that has the major influence on resistance to bone marrow allografts. As discussed by Cudkowicz and by Lotzova, NK cells appear to be the principal effector cells for this phenomenon and antigens determined by the Hh gene may be among the specificities recognized by mouse NK cells.

B. Antigens of Viruses or Other Microbial Agents

Much consideration has been given to the role of endogenous type C viruses in the specficity of mouse and rat NK cells. Initial studies, by direct testing and cold target inhibitions, showed some correlation between susceptibility of targets to lysis by NK cells and their expression of endogenous type C viruses (Herberman et al, 1975; Nunn et al, 1976). The findings since then of NK reactivity against xenogeneic target cells and some normal target cells have indicated that other, non-virus associated antigens are probably recognized by rodent NK cells. However, since NK cells appear able to recognize multiple specificities, it seems possible that viruses are responsible for some of the antigens that NK cells react with. The observations of Lee and Ihle (1977) that the gp71 envelope antigen of AKR endogenous viruses could inhibit NK reactivity of one NK cell-target combination but not another, and the partial inhibition of NK activity by antibodies to gp71 (Kende et al, 1979), are consistent with this hypothesis.

Despite these indications for a possible recognition of type C viral antigens by mouse or rat NK cells, substantial negative evidence has also been presented. As summarized by Roder, some studies found no correlation between susceptibility to lysis and expression of various type C virus associated antigens. Superinfection of a human cell line with a mouse xenotropic endogenous virus did not increase susceptibility to lysis by mouse NK cells, and similarly, Tai and Werner noted that a virus positive mouse tumor was resistant to lysis by NK cells. However, these observations don't rule out an involvement of endogenous type C viral antigens in natural killing since the relevant virus(es) might be other than those detected or worked with. Since there is a variety of endogenous murine type C viruses, negative findings with some can not be generalized to eliminate the recognition by NK cells of all such viral antigens.

The recent finding that YAC-1, the widely used target cell for studies of mouse NK activity, expressed antigens of mouse mammary tumor virus (MTV) (Blair et al, Lane) raises the question of a role of these viral antigens in natural cytotoxicity. Lane has observed at least partial inhibition by MTV of NK activity against YAC-1 and has also seen blocking by gp71 of Rauscher leukemia virus. If confirmed, such findings would provide important insight into the nature of mouse NK activity. However, several lines of evidence raise questions about the specificity of the inhibition by these viruses or their soluble antigens. In general, it has been very difficult to demonstrate antigen-specific inhibition of cell-mediated cytotoxicity in short term assays by materials other than intact cells. Experiments in my laboratory have indicated that MTV can produce some, although not appreciable or consistent, inhibition of NK activity against YAC-1. However, MTV also partially inhibited lysis of K562 by human NK cells, strongly suggesting that such blocking can be nonspecific. In addition, Blair et al have noted a general lack of correlation between levels of mouse NK activity and specific reactivity against MTV. Neonatal infection with MTV or specific immunization against MTV did not affect reactivity against YAC-1.

The studies of Bloom et al indicate that mouse NK cells may specifically recognize antigens associated with other RNA viruses. It is difficult to dissociate specific recognition from the ability of virus-infected target cells to induce interferon, but the lack of cross cold-target inhibition by targets infected by measles and mumps virus is quite suggestive of reactivity against separate specificities. Welsh and Kiessling also considered the possibility of mouse NK cells reacting against antigens associated with lymphocytic choriomeningitis virus. However, they drew negative conclusions, since uninfected target cells were actually more sensitive to lysis than virus-infected targets and competed as well or better in cold target inhibition tests.

Roder suggests that antigens of some infectious agent(s) common to mice and rabbits may be involved in NK activity. This argument is based on the similarity in reactivity of mouse NK cells and rabbit natural antibodies. However, this association is equally compatible with the natural recognition by both species of common differentiation or other non-microbial antigens.

C. Differentiation Antigens

There are increasing indications that differentiation antigens may comprise some of the major specificities recognized by NK cells. Fetal fibroblasts are sensitive to lysis by NK cells, and the susceptible thymocytes appear to be a small subpopulation of immature cortical cells (Hansson et al). Among a series of mouse teratomas, the least differentiated cells were most sensitive to lysis, and induction of maturation or differentiation in various NK-susceptible mouse and human cell lines made them resistant to cytotoxicity (Wigzell, 1980). S. Gupta (personal communication) has observed that human NK cells inhibited colony formation by bone marrow stem cells, although Zarling reports negative results in similar studies.

Several investigators have raised the intriguing possibility that NK cells may play an important role in regulating the differentiation of certain hematopoietic or other normal cells. Lysis or cytostasis of cells at some early stage of differentiation may prevent excessive accumulation of nonfunctional precursors.

D. Biochemical Nature of Target Cell Antigens

Roder has reported that soluble extracts of target cells could not inhibit cytotoxicity by NK cells but could interfere with conjugate formation with NK-susceptible target cells. This provided the basis for monitoring the separation of antigens by column chromatography and polyacrylamide gel electrophoresis. The results indicated that the antigens recognized by NK cells were glycosylated and polydisperse, occurring in three molecular weight ranges. Furthermore, these separated antigens appeared to have both cross-reactive and individual specificities.

These studies appear to represent an important new approach for the understanding of the antigens recognized by NK cells. Efforts are underway in other laboratories to confirm and extend these observations.

Durdik et al have taken another approach to the biochemical identification of target cell structures associated with susceptibility to lysis. They have compared the glycolipids on NK susceptible and resistant sublines of a mouse lymphoma.

Although some major differences in some glycolipids were found, none of these could be incriminated as NK antigens.

E. REGULATION OF EXPRESSION OF ANTIGENS ON TARGET CELLS

In addition to the induction of decreased susceptibility to lysis by interferon (see section IC3), other factors have also been reported to affect expression of NK-related antigens on target cells. Roder summarizes data indicating that expression of antigens is under genetic control, with all somatic cell hybrids between NK-susceptible and resistant mouse target cells being resistant to lysis. These data are taken as indirect support for the involvement of differentiation antigens. Durdik _et al_ also provide evidence that susceptibility to NK cells is a stable genetic trait, with two different clones of the same lymphoma varying markedly in their sensitivity to lysis. Similarly, Lane describes a resistant variant of YAC-1. It is not clear how the resistant sublines or clones arose. The one of Durdik _et al_ was found after repeated _in vivo_ passage of cultured lymphoma cells. However, since this process was not re-examined, it remains to be determined whether this is a reproducible procedure for selecting NK-resistant clones. A few direct efforts to identify clonal variation in susceptibility to NK cells of other target cell lines have meet with negative results. Repeated _in vitro_ culture of YAC-1 cells in the presence of highly reactive mouse NK cells did not select for a resistant subline (E. Gorelik and R. Herberman, unpublished observations). Similarly, examination of many clones of K562 for susceptibility to lysis by human or mouse NK cells did not reveal any stable clonal variation (Navarro _et al_, 1980). As summarized by Roder, susceptibility or resistance of a cell line to lysis by NK cells may be altered reversibly, depending on the growth conditions. Passage of YAC-1 for a brief time _in vivo_ resulted in resistance to lysis by NK cells. Such alteration in YAC-1 cells was correlated with changes in the levels of expression of NK-related antigens. The mechanism for these reversible changes has not been elucidated and appears not to be dependent on the stage of the cell cycle. It will be of interest to determine whether this is related to the protective effects of IF on target cells. Growth of YAC-1 _in vivo_ may expose the cells to IF produced by the host and reculturing of the cells might allow them to recover from such effects. Against this possibility are the observations mentioned above that prolonged culture of YAC-1 with spleen cells, where interferon production would be expected, didn't induce resistance to lysis. Similarly, Welsh and Kiessling found that direct treatment of YAC-1 with interferon caused only a modest decrease in susceptibility to lysis by NK cells.

REFERENCES

Herberman, R.B., Nunn, M.E., and Lavrin, D.H., Int. J. Cancer 16, 216 (1975).

Kende, M., Hill, R., Dinowitz, M., Stephenson, J.R., and Kelloff, G.J. J. Exp. Med. 149, 358 (1979).

Lee, J.C. and Ihle, J.N., J. Immunol. 118, 928 (1977).

Navarro, N.J., Nunn, M.E., and Herberman, R.B., submitted for publication.

Nunn, M.E., Djeu, J.Y., Glaser, M., Lavrin, D.H., and Herberman, R.B., J. Natl. Cancer Inst. 56, 393 (1976).

Wigzell, H., "Thymus, Thymic Hormones and T Lymphocytes" (F. Aiuti, ed.), Academic Press, New York, in press.

INTRATUMOR NK REACTIVITY[1]

Susanne Becker

Department of Obstetrics & Gynecology
University of North Carolina
Chapel Hill, North Carolina

INTRODUCTION

The evidence for NK cells as a contributing *in vivo* mechanism in tumor surveillance comes from experiments where high and low NK reactive mice have been compared for tumor development following challenge with small inocula of lymphoma lines of different NK sensitivities. Nude mice, lowreactive mice with bone marrow grafts from highreactive mice, T-cell and B-cell depressed mice of highreactive strains are more resistant to syngeneic lymphoma transplants than strains with low NK reactivity. Further evidence for an *in vivo* role for NK cells comes from experiments described by Kasai *et al* (1). Using an anti-NK serum, they reported that only cells of Ly 5^+ NK phenotype conferred *in vivo* protection against two NK sensitive lymphomas; effector and target cells, however, were co-inoculated subcutaneously and thus it is questionable if this represents an *in vivo* model for NK surveillance.

If NK cells are relevant in tumor regression, they should be present *in situ*. This communication describes two experimental models where the possible *in vivo* role for NK cells has been investigated by testing the cells isolated from the site of tumor induction. In the first experiments to be described, the highly NK sensitive YAC-1 lymphoma has been injected intra peritoneally (i.p.) and subcutaneously (s.c.) into syngeneic mice. The second model is the primary Moloney sarcoma virus-induced lesion which previously has been described to contain NK active cells (2).

[1]*This work supported by NIH Contract No. 1-CB-64023, ACS Grant IM-84 and USPHS Grant CA-17694.*

ISBN 0-12-341350-8

I. *IN SITU* NK ACTIVITY IN MICE INOCULATED WITH YAC-1 LYMPHOMA

In a series of experiments we have investigated whether inflammatory cells with NK characteristics can be isolated from the site of an i.p. or a s.c. injection of the highly NK sensitive YAC-1 lymphoma line (tissue culture of the NK insensitive YAC-*vivo*).

A. *Composition of Cells Recovered from the Peritoneal Cavity after Inoculation of YAC Cells*

The NK lowreactive strain A/Sn syngeneic with the tumor cells and the NK highreactive F_1 hybrid A/Sn x C57Bl were injected i.p. with 2 x 10^6 YAC-1. This cell number was rejected in the F_1 mice while A/Sn mice developed detectable ascites within 14 days. The same dose of the NK insensitive YAC-*vivo* line produced tumors also in the F_1 mice (10/14 mice developed YAC ascites). We chose to study the peritoneal cells in mice injected five days earlier, as we found that at this time a maximal inflammatory response was recoved from mice that rejected the tumor. A follow-up was done by day 8 on another set of mice to document further changes. Table I shows the total number and the composition of cells harvested from the peritoneum by flushing with 10 mls of PBS. The types of cells present were determined on cytocentrifuge preparations by morphology or by immunofluorescence. At day 5 the YAC-*vivo* cells had proliferated in the lowreactive mice, and the inflammatory component constituted only a minor part (10%) of the cells recovered. The differential and cell recovery data from the YAC-1 injected A/Sn mice indicated that a reduction of tumor cells had occurred. The day 8 time point on both groups of mice showed that both YAC lines now proliferated rapidly.

In A x C57Bl F_1, one of the two mice shown in Table I had rejected the YAC-*vivo*, while the other mouse presumably was a progressor. In none of the mice injected with YAC-1 could any tumor cells be detected. Thus the *in vivo* growth of YAC and YAC-1 correlated with the NK sensitivity of the target cells and the NK reactivity of the hosts.

B. *NK Activity of Cells Recovered from the Peritoneum*

Lymphocytes rather than macrophages composed the bulk of the inflammatory response following injection with YAC-1. In order to test the activity of the lymphoid population, macrophages were removed by adherence or when YAC cells also were present by 1xg velocity sedimentation in 50 ml plastic

TABLE I. *Yield of Inflammatory and Tumor Cells from Peritoneum Following Injection of 2 x 10^6 Lymphoma Cells*

	Cells injected	Animal #	DAY 5 Total cell recovery x 10^6	DAY 5 % tumor cells	DAY 5 % lymphoid cells	DAY 8 Total cell recovery x 10^6	DAY 8 % tumor cells[a]
A/Sn							
	YAC	1	16.0	90	N.D.	96.0	95
		2	20.0	92	N.D.	100.0	96
	YAC-1	1	3.2	23	60	15.0	80
		2	2.1	25	45	10.0	75
	-		1.5	0	62	1.8	0
A/Sn x C57Bl F_1							
	YAC	1	3.0	0	70	50.0	98
		2	4.8	50	30	2.2	0
	YAC-1	1	3.1	0	75	2.5	0
		2	4.0	0	68	2.8	0
		3	4.8	0	73	2.1	0
	-		2.0	0	58	1.5	0

[a]*Measured by immunofluorescence with anti-MCSA serum.*

centrifuge tubes. This proceedure gave an effector cell population containing less than 1% macrophages and less than 5% tumor cells. The tumor cell contamination was further reduced by treatment with anti-MCSA (Moloney cell surface antigen) serum and complement.

In Table II, the NK activities of the tumor-associated lymphoid populations, as well as the spleen activities, are shown. In A/Sn mice, increased anti-YAC-1 activity could be detected neither in spleen nor peritoneum, despite the apparent *in vivo* reduction of YAC-1 cells. Preliminary results suggest that the decrease in YAC-1 cells occurs very rapidly, and only 20% of the cells injected can be recovered 1 hr after inoculation. In A/Sn x C57Bl F_1, elevated anti-YAC-1 activity was detected both in spleen and peritoneum. The evidence for the effect being mediated by NK cells comes from experiments where overnight incubation in 37°C abolished the activity, while spleens containing cytotoxic T-cells were still as active. Also, these effector cells are not sensitive to anti-Thy 1.2 serum dilutions which abolish cytotoxic T-cell activities.

TABLE II. NK Activity in Spleen and Peritoneum Five Days after YAC or YAC-1 Injection

	Cells injected	Animal #	Spleen 50:1	Spleen 15:1	Peritoneum 20:1
A/Sn					
	YAC	1	2	6	N.D.
		2	5	4	N.D.
	YAC-1	1	1	0	0
		2	5	1	0
	-		8	2	4
A/Sn x C57Bl F_1					
	YAC	1	45	23	0
		2	53	25	N.D.
	YAC-1	1	40	16	28
		2	68	31	40
		3	54	46	41
	-		18	10	12

C. NK Activity Recovered From Subcutaneously Induced YAC-1 Tumors

A subcutaneous injection of 5 x 10^5 YAC-1 cells gives 100% tumors in A/Sn mice. In A/Sn x C57Bl F_1 this dose also resulted in tumors, some of which later regressed. Since the site of injection 5 days after injection could not be visually determined, and thus too few cells could be recovered to perform an experiment, the inflammatory response at the site of lymphoma injection was investigated 8 days after injection. Tumors from two groups of 5 mice were pooled and cut into small pieces before treatment with 0.15% collagenase to obtain a single cell suspension of tumor cells and inflammatory cells. Cytocentrifuge preparations of the suspension revealed a very low number of host cells in the A/Sn tumors, while in A/Sn x C57Bl F_1 more than 50% of the cells recovered were cells with lymphocyte morphology, only few macrophages were observed (Table III). The lymphoid inflammatory cells in the A/Sn x C57Bl F_1 were purified by 1xg sedimentation and the activity tested against YAC-1. The anti-YAC-1 activity was mediated by NK cells, as the effect was not influenced by anti-Thy 1.2 and complement treatment. Too few inflammatory cells could be obtained from the A/Sn tumors to perform experiments.

TABLE III. NK Activity of Cells Isolated from Subcutaneous YAC-1 Tumors

	Tumor pool #	% tumor cells	Lymphoid cells[a]	% Cytotoxicity[b]
A/Sn	*1*	*80*	*10*	*N.D.*
	2	*92*	*5*	*N.D.*
A/Sn x C57Bl F_1	*1*	*42*	*55*	*45*
	2	*36*	*59*	*52*
	spleen			*12*

[a] *Determined by morphology on cytocentrifuge preps.*

[b] *The lymphoid cells isolated by 1g velocity sedimentation and tested against YAC-1 cells at an effector:target cell ratio of 10:1. Spleen cells were also tested 10:1.*

D. Summary

These experiments strongly suggest that in the NK high-reactive A/Sn x C57Bl F_1 the *in vivo* rejection of YAC-1 cells both i.p. and s.c. depends on NK cells and thus confirms the conclusions by Kiessling *et al* from their *in vivo* studies (3). In A/Sn mice there is no direct evidence for NK mediated YAC-1 rejection; however the data comparing recovery of YAC-*vivo* versus YAC-1 cells suggests that NK cells might be of importance, as the two cells differ in susceptibility to NK activity *in vitro*, as well as in their capacity to induce tumors *in vivo* (4).

II. NK CELL ACTIVITY AND REGRESSION OF MOLONEY SARCOMA VIRUS (MSV)-INDUCED TUMORS

MSV injection results in an increase in spleen NK activity reaching a peak 3 days after injection and then rapidly declining to levels lower than normal (5). At maximum tumor size (10-12 days after virus injection), NK activity is decreased in both spleen and blood (2). NK activity, however, can be recovered from the tumor, suggesting that NK cells could add to the complexity of effector mechanisms identified in MSV tumors (6-8).

TABLE IV. NK Activity in MSV Tumors Induced in NK High and Low Reactive Strains[a]

	Spleen		Tumor
	50:1	15:1	
A/Sn	5	2	2
C57Bl	22	12	36
CBA	56	42	49
DBA	28	16	25
A/Sn x C57Bl	32	15	42

[a]Data collected from separate experiments.

A. NK Activity in MSV Tumors in High and Low Reactive Strains

Testing mice with different NK reactivities, it was found that activity recovered from the MSV tumor reflects the NK status of the mice (Table IV).

The NK activity in the lowreactive A/Sn mice is also low in the tumor. Despite this, the lesion regresses faster than in the highreactive strains CBA and C57Bl. Stutman *et al* described A/J mice ($H-2^a$ identical with A/Sn) as a NC (natural cytotoxic cell) highreactive strain against certain solid tumor lines (9). The possibility thus existed that the A/Sn mice, although NK lowreactive against the YAC-1 lymphoma line, might have reactivity against the MSV sarcoma cells

B. Isolation and Characterization of MSV Sarcoma Cells

In the collagenase-dispersed MSV tumor suspension, 85-90% of the cells were inflammatory macrophages, granulocytes and lymphocytes, but around 10% of the cells could be classified as atypical cells and presumably the MSV-sarcoma cells. These cells were purified from the inflammatory cells by 1xg sedimentation and EA rosetting which removed the same size macrophages. A closer characterization of the cells (Table V) showed that they are virus-infected and actively producing MSV-MLV virus. They induced new regressing lesions with the same characteristics as the primary lesion, that is, a high inflammatory response and around 10% atypical cells at peak tumor size. These properties clearly demonstrated their importance in propagation of the MSV-lesion and qualified them as target cells for host defense mechanisms against MSV.

TABLE V. Some Characteristics of the MSV Sarcoma Cells

Latex ingestion	-
Fc receptors	-
Morphology	fibroblastoid
Virus antigen expression	
gp70	+
p30	+
p12	+
Produces infectious C-type particles	+
Produces new MSV sarcoma lesions	+

C. Anti-YAC-1 versus Anti-MSV Target Cell Activity in A/Sn MSV Tumors

In spleen (10) and within the MSV tumor, NK cells against lymphoma lines have been shown to peak at a 1xg sedimentation velocity of 4-5 mm/hr (Fig. 1). The same sedimentation rate

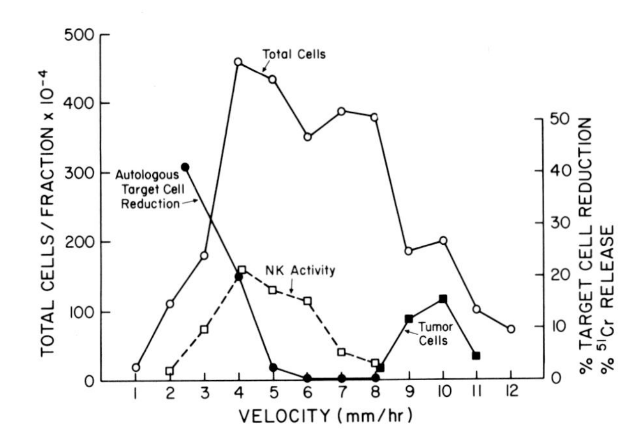

FIGURE 1. Sedimentation velocity profile of both natural killer (NK) and autologous activity induced with various fractions of infiltrating cells present in regressor MSV tumors (Day 11).

has been shown for the NC cell (11). When inflammatory cells from A/Sn MSV tumors were tested against the autochthonous MSV target cells, or autologous target cells isolated the day before and kept in culture overnight, the peak reactivity was confined to cells sedimenting 3 mm/hr (Fig. 1). The active cells were non-T as anti-Thy 1.2 + complement did not remove the activity and they were neither B-cells (immunofluorescence) nor macrophages (morphology). A high proportion (~ 40%) of the active population, however, consisted of granulocytes.

D. Characterization of the Effector Cells Against MSV Target Cells

Further characterization of the active cells revealed many similarities with the "induced" NK cell described by Welsh *et al* (12), but also several discrepancies (Table VI). Two different cell populations of small non-T-cell character might be active against the autochthonous target cells, thus explaining the partial loss of activity by Ficoll-Hypaque and nylon wool separations. However, the cytocentrifuge preparations revealed that no satisfactory separation of the MSV infiltrating cells into lymphoid versus granulocytic fractions was obtained with any of these methods. Not until

Table VI. Properties of Endogenous and Induced NK Cells Compared with the MSV in Situ *Killer Cell*

	Endogenous NK	*Induced NK*	In situ *killer cells*
Adherence			
Plastic	–	–	–
Nylon wool	+–	+–	+–
Fc receptor	– or weak	weak	weak
Loss of activity			
37°C 6 h	+	+	+
4°C 16 h	–		+
Ficoll-Hypaque separation (interphase)	–	–	+–
Passage through nylon wool	–	–	+–
Specificity of killing			
H-2 restriction	–	–	–
Normal fibroblast	–	+	+
Syngeneic macrophages	–	+	–

a BSA density gradient separation was done, activity of the different fractions tested for cytotoxicity and the active cells characterized by both morphology and myeloperoxidase marker, could the effector cells be identified as granulocytes (Fig. II).

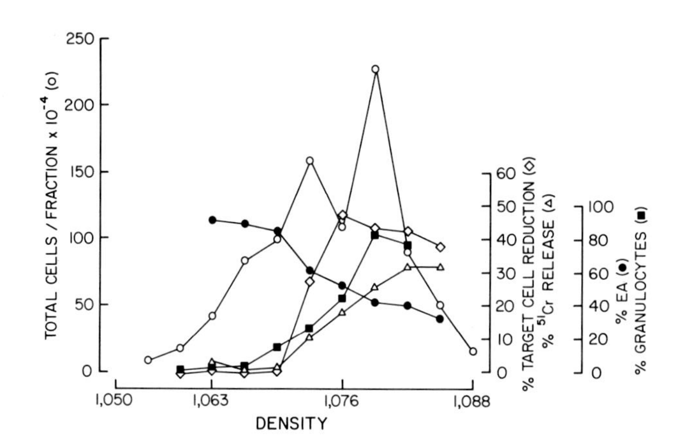

FIGURE 2. BSA density separation of MSV tumor infiltration cell (1xg sedimentation rate 2-4 mm/hr). Cytotoxic activity against the autochthonous MSV-"target" cells was determined by the microcytotoxicity test (◇) and by ^{51}Cr release (△). The granulocyte content (■) in each fraction was determined by morphology.

E. Splenic Activity Against MSV Target Cells

In the A/Sn tumor bearer spleen, the anti-MSV target cell activity also is non-T-cell mediated and appears not to be a conventional NK cell. As spleen cells from ALG treated MSV tumor-bearing mice are more active against autologous MSV cells than spleen cells from nontreated mice, we decided to further characterize the autochthonous killer cells in the ALG spleens. The active cells were myeloperoxidase positive cells in earlier stages of granulopoiesis (myelocytes and neutrophils with doughnut-shaped nuclei). This spleen activity differed from the *in situ* activity by not being eliminated by overnight storage in 4°C, probably because of the immature stage of the cell. A similar killer cell has recently been identified in *in vitro* bone marrow cultures by Lohmann-Mathes *et al* (13). They showed that promonocytes had the functional characteristics of NK cells. Also the A/J strain produced similar levels of activity as NK highreactive C57Bl/10 mice.

F. Summary

In A/Sn mice NK cells apparently are not necessary for MSV rejection. Other cell types (myeloid and monocytic) with similar functional characteristics might instead promote rejection.

In NK highreactive strains, MSV tumors are infiltrated by NK cells. In order to establish the role of NK cells in highreactive strains, it has to be investigated if these cells that kill YAC-1 also kill MSV autochthonous target cells.

III. DISCUSSION

Although NK cells are speculated to be of importance in tumor defence, there is little evidence to support this in primary tumors. In human tumors, the only spontaneous tumors that have been investigated, NK activity cannot be found *in situ* despite the normal levels of NK activity demonstrated in the blood (14, 15, H. Koren, S. Haskill and S. Becker, in preparation).

The two mouse tumor models investigated in this paper have been chosen because of two properties, neither of which is associated with spontaneous tumors. First, the YAC-1 tumor is highly sensitive to NK mediated effects. Second, the MSV tumor regresses spontaneously in a low NK reactive strain. Thus, although neither is representative of a spontaneous malignancy, both provide convenient test systems for the analysis of intratumor defense mechanisms.

The A/Sn mice are NK low reactive but still the NK cells are believed to be of importance in the rejection of YAC cells, as the *in vitro* demonstrated difference between the NK sensitivity of YAC-1 and YAC-*vivo* also can be demonstrated *in vivo* (4). In the experiments described above, we could demonstrate this difference by the difference in tumor cell yield from peritoneum. However, no NK reactivity could be demonstrated among the inflammatory cells.

The kinds of inflammatory cells in MSV lesions vary with

the strain of the mouse; in some strains lymphoid cells constitute the majority of the inflammatory populations, in others macrophage and granulocytic infiltration predominates, supporting the concept that different mechanisms fight the same stimuli depending on genetic background. MSV tumor bearing A/Sn mice reject their tumors despite the low or usually undetectable *in situ* NK activity. The regressor kinetics is even faster in these mice than in strains from which highly active intratumor NK cells can be isolated. A/Sn MSV tumors contained another population of non-T, non-B, non-macrophage cells with NK-like activity against the autochthonous MSV target cells, different from the anti-YAC-1 activity by 1xg velocity sedimentation. This activity was characterized as mediated by myeloperoxidase positive granulocytes in the tumor and by less mature myelopoietic cells in the spleen. This suggests that mice deficient in one mechanism, in this case NK cells, might compensate for this with another nonspecific mechanism.

In the highreactive A/Sn x C57Bl F_1 mice, *in situ* NK activity was demonstrated both after i.p. and s.c. YAC-1 inoculation, but rather than representing an antitumor response this could be a demonstration of the very similar hybrid resistance mechanism (16). As the specificity of the NK cells from MSV tumors in highreactive mice has not yet been investigated, in these mice NK cells might be active also against the autochthonous targets.

REFERENCES

1. Kasai, J., Leclerc, L., McVay-Boudreau, F. and H. Cantor. *J. Exp. Med. 149*, 1260 (1979).
2. Becker, S. and Klein, E. *Eur. J. Immunol. 6*, 892 (1976).
3. Kiessling, R., Petranyi, G., Klein, G. and Wigzell, H. *Int. J. Cancer 17*, 1 (1976a).
4. Kiessling, R., Petranyi, G., Klein, G. and Wigzell, H. *Int. J. Cancer 15*, 933 (1975c).
5. Herberman, R., Nunn, M., Holden, H., Staal, S. and Djeu, J. *Int. J. Cancer 19*, 555 (1977b)
6. Holden, H.T., Haskill, J.S., Kirchner, H., and Herberman, R.B. *J. Immunol. 117*, 440-446 (1976).
7. Plata, F., MacDonald, H.R., and Sordat, B. *Bibl. Haematol. 43*, 274-277 (1976).
8. Puccetti, P., and Holden, H.T. *Int. J. Cancer 23*, 123-133 (1979).
9. Stutman, O., Paige, C., and Figarella, E. *J. Immunol. 121*, 1819-1825 (1978).

10. Karre, K., Haller, O., Becker, S., Kiessling, R., Rank, A.M., Anderson, L.C. and Hayry, P. Submitted for publication (1978).
11. Paige, C., Figarella, E., Cuttito, M., Cahan, A., and Stutman, O. *J. Immunol. 121,* 1827-1835 (1978).
12. Welsh, R.M. *J. Exp. Med. 148,* 163 (1978).
13. Lohmann-Matthes, M., Domzig, W., and Roder, J. *J. Immunol. 123,* 1883-1886 (1979)
14. Vose, B.M., Vanky, F., Argov, S., and Klein, E. *Eur. J. Immunol. 7,* 753-757 (1977).
15. Herberman, R.B., and Holden, H.T. *J. Natl. Cancer Inst. 62,* 441-444 (1979).
16. Kiessling, R., Hochman, P.S., Haller, O., Shearer, G.M., Wigzell, H. and Cudkowiez, G. *Eur. J. Immunol. 7,* 655 (1977).

CYTOTOXICITY AND CYTOSTASIS MEDIATED BY SPLENOCYTES OF MICE SUBJECTED TO CHEMICAL CARCINOGENS AND OF MICE-BEARING PRIMARY TUMORS

Rachel Ehrlich
Margalit Efrati
Isaac P. Witz[1]

Department of Microbiology
The George S. Wise Faculty of Life Sciences
Tel-Aviv University
Tel-Aviv, Israel

I. INTORDUCTION

Some of the contributors to this volume as well as other investigators hold the opinion that mechanisms inhibiting nascent aberrant cells from developing into malignant tumors operate or should be operating in healthy individuals. Natural anti-tumor immunity mediated by cellular (Herberman and Holden, 1978) or humoral (Menard et al, 1977)components may, most likely, constitute one of these mechanisms. Some information is available on a deficient NK activity of cancer patients (Heppner et al, 1975; Cannon et al, 1977; Takasugi et al, 1977) and of animals bearing transplanted tumors (Becker and Klein, 1976). Aiming to analyse natural immune effector mechanisms in mice subjected to various oncogenic stimuli we report in the present study on alterations in naturally occuring cellular effector functions in tumor bearers and in clinically normal animals that had been exposed to 2 chemical carcinogens.

[1]*This investigation was supported by Contract number NO1-CB-74134 awarded by the National Cancer Institute DHEW.*

ISBN 0-12-341350-8

II. EXPERIMENTAL

A. *Early Effects of Carcinogen Treatment on Natural Cell Mediated Cytotoxicity*

In this series of experiments we studied the early effects of carcinogen administration on cell-mediated natural cytotoxic (NK) activity.

BALB/C mice were treated with 3 weekly i.p injections of urethan (10mg/injection). About 60% of mice treated with such a dose develop within 2-4 months 1-10 lung foci diagnosed as adenomas (unpublished observations). These tumors are relatively benign in as much as the mice bearing them have essentially a normal life span. Two mice were sacrificed every week after the last urethan injection and their spleens were tested for NK activity utilizing the ^{51}Cr release assay with labeled YAC-1 cells as targets. The data are summarized in Fig. 1. A slight elevation of activity was measured in urethan-treated mice three weeks after the last injection, and the increased activity continued for the next 5 weeks.

Another group of BALB/C mice was treated with dimethylbenzanthracene (DMBA). The treatment consisted of 6 weekly intragastric feedings of 1 mg DMBA per feeding. Ninety-five percent of the mice treated with such a dose developed solid malignant mammary tumors mostly adenocarcinomas and adenoacanthomas. The first tumors appeared about 2 months after the last feeding while the last tumors appeared up to 6 months later.

A decrease in NK activity was already seen 2 weeks after the last DMBA treatment (Fig. 1). The suppressed NK activity which continued for 6 weeks occured concomittantly with a 40-80% decrease in the number of cells per spleen. During the seventh week after the last DMBA treatment both NK activity as well as the number of cells per spleen began to increase to normal levels, and at the eighth week the NK activity and the number of cells per spleen reached the levels of normal controls.

It should be of great importance to determine whether or not the different biological behaviour of the urethan and the DMBA-induced tumors (benign and malignant tumors respectively) is related to the different response of the NK cells to treatment with the 2 carcinogens.

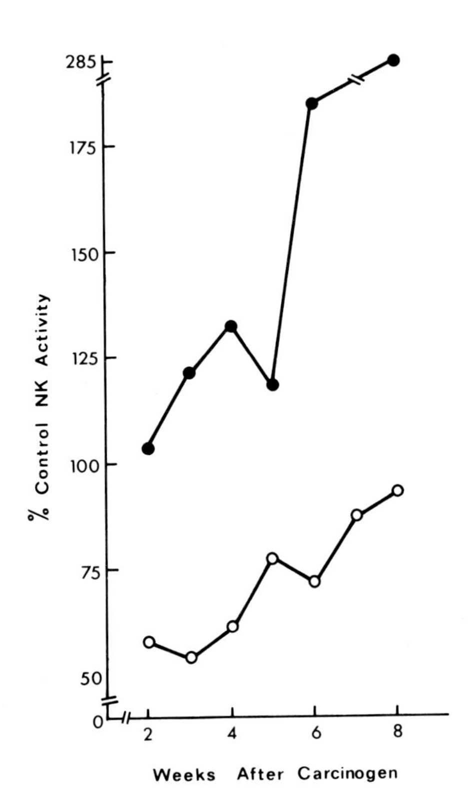

FIGURE 1. % of control NK activity of splenocytes from mice treated with urethan (●) or DMBA (o); 100% activity is that of untreated controls. The actual NK values of controls were 20-30% ^{51}Cr release at an effector: target ratio of 100:1

B. *Cytotoxic and Cytostatic Activities Mediated by Splenocytes from Mice Bearing Primary Urethan-Induced Lung Adenomas*

BALB/C mice were treated with 1-5 injections of urethan (see above). Four months after the last injection the mice were sacrificed and their lungs checked for adenomas. All mice receiving 4 or 5 urethan treatments had 1-10 pulmonary adenoma foci per mouse. Among the mice receiving

1-3 urethan injections, there were some which did not develop adenomas, while the others presented with various tumor loads. All of these mice regardless of their tumor-bearing status expressed cytostatic (measured by the ^{125}IUDR I-I assay described elsewhere in this volume) and cytotoxic NK activities similar to untreated controls.

C. *Cytotoxic and Cytostatic Activities Mediated by Splenocytes from Mice Bearing Primary DMBA-induced tumors*

BALB/C mice were hormonally-stimulated by a pituitary isograft and then treated with DMBA as described above. Splenocytes from adenocarcinoma and adenoacanthoma-bearing mice were assayed for their ability to lyse ^{51}Cr-labeled YAC-1 cells and to inhibit ^{125}IUDR incorporation into B16-F10 cells.

The results presented in Fig. 2 show that compared to sex and age-matched controls tumor-bearer splenocytes expressed a sharp decrease in NK activity, especially at high ratios of effector to targets. On the other hand, the same splenocytes showed a considerable increase in cytostatic activity compared to normal controls. It would be highly interesting to determine whether or not this negative correlation is causally related. One could ask, for example, if the strong cytostatic activity in tumor-bearing mice was directed against determinants expressed both on the tumor targets as well as on NK cells.

A depressed NK activity in spleens from primary tumor-bearing mice can be attributed to at least 4 non-mutually exclusive factors:

(1) Killing or inactivation of NK cells by the carcinogen or by tumor-derived materials.

(2) Emigration of NK cells from the spleen to other locations for example to the tumor site.

(3) Infiltration of tumor cells into the spleens of the tumor-bearers. The infiltrating cells could conceivably compete against the labeled YAC-1 target cells for NK cells.

(4) Spleens of tumor-bearing mice contain suppressor cells for NK cells.

As a first attempt to distinguish between these possibilities we separated between adherent and non-adherent splenocytes from tumor-bearing mice by depleting the adherent population. The rationale for performing these experiments was that certain types of tumor cells (Moore and Moore, 1979) as well as some suppressor cells (Jerrels *et al*, 1979) were

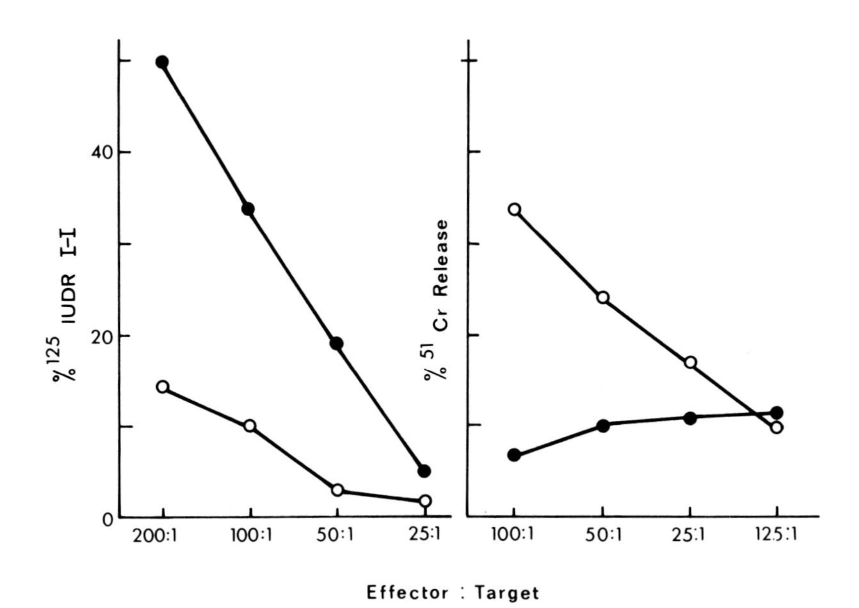

FIGURE 2. Cytostasis (^{125}IUDR I-I) and NK (^{51}Cr release) activities mediated by splenocytes from normal (o)and DMBA-induced tumor bearing mice (●).

found to be adherent. Depletion of splenocytes which adhere to plastic surfaces did neither change the NK activity nor the cytostatic activity of the non-adherent splenocyte population which expressed activity patterns similar to the unfractionated suspension i.e. a higher cytostatic activity and a lower cytotoxic activity than normal controls (results not shown). On the other hand, depletion of cells adherent to G-10 sephadex columns (Fig. 3) caused an increase in NK activity in the non-adherent population while lowering only slightly the cytostatic activity. The fact that the NK activity of the non-adherent population reached almost control levels essentially rules out the first two possibilities mentioned above namely, that the spleens of the tumor-bearing mice were devoid of potentially functional NK cells. Although we are not yet in the position to state with certainty which of the remaining possibilities (presence of infiltrating tumor cells or of suppressor cells in the spleen) caused the depressed NK activity in tumor-bearers, the

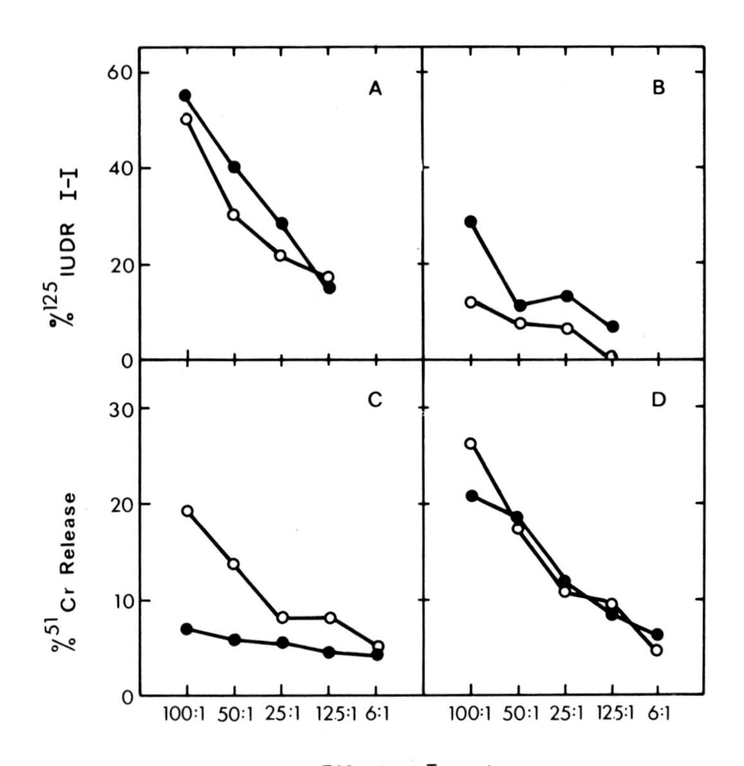

FIGURE 3. Cytostasis (A,B) and NK (C,D) activities mediated by splenocytes from tumor bearing (A,C) and normal (B,D) mice. The reactivity of the unfractionated cell population (●) and that of the sephadex G-10-non-adherent population (o) are compared.

available evidence supports the latter possibility. An injection of cells from tumor-bearer spleens into normal mice did not cause tumor development. Furthermore, histopathological examinations of tumor-bearer spleens did not reveal the presence of tumor cells within them. It is thus not unlikely that spleens from mice bearing primary DMBA-induced tumors contain sephadex G-10-adherent suppressor cells which inhibit NK activity. The results of preliminary NK assays in which tumor-bearing splenocytes were mixed with normal splenocytes support this hypothesis.

Table I summarizes the results of experiments measuring cytotoxic activities of splenocytes from BALB/C mice bearing early (2nd-5th)transplant passages of primary DMBA induced tumors. The results show that similarly to splenocytes from mice-bearing primary tumors, splenocytes from the transplanted tumor-bearing mice express a reduced NK activity. As found in another study (Ehrlich et al this volume) the activity of normal splenocytes was significantly higher in an 18 hour assay than in a 4 hour assay. However, in contrast to the situation with normal splenocytes the NK activity of most tumor bearers did not increase during the 18 hour incubation period.

These results indicate that a depressed NK activity is caused either by the lack of active NK cells in spleens of tumor-bearing mice or that suppressor cells reside in these spleens. Depletion of G-10 sephadex-adherent-cells caused in two out of four tumor-bearer spleens tested, an increase in NK activity. However, the increase occured only in the 18 and not in the 4 hour ^{51}Cr release assay (results not shown). This indicates that the activity of the suppressor cells persists in-vitro and prevents (unless removed by sephadex G-10) the activation of existing NK cells even during a prolonged incubation period. The results also showed that recovery from suppression following the depletion of suppressors takes at least 4 hours.

The fact that early transplant passages of primary DMBA induced tumors maintain some of the biological characteristics of the corresponding primary tumors provides the opportunity to examine the exact nature of the active and suppresive cell populations in the spleens of tumor-bearing mice.

D. *Cytotoxic and Cytostatic Activities Mediated by Splenocytes from Mice Bearing Primary Mammary Carcinomas*

In a previous report (Ehrlich et al, submitted for publication) we showed that splenocytes from 60% of C3HeB mice bearing mammary carcinomas induced by forced-breeding (but otherwise untreated) had a significantly lower NK activity than control tumor-free mice having had a similar number of pregnancies. The remaining 40% of the tumor-bearing mice had the same levels of activity as control mice. Further experiments suggested that splenocytes from mice which had a large and necrotic tumor, and which presented with splenomegaly had a depressed NK activity compared to controls while their ^{125}IUDR I-I activity was higher than that of the tumor-free mice. Examples of such cases are summarized in Table II.

TABLE I. NK Activity Mediated by Splenocytes from BALB/C Mice Bearing Early Passages of Primary DMBA-Induced Tumors

Cell Ratio	Mouse	Appearance of Spleen	% ^{51}Cr-Release[a] Duration of Assay 4 hrs	18 hrs
100:1	Normal Control	Normal	22	48
50:1			19	38
25:1			13	19
100:1	Tumor[b] Bearer	Splenomegaly[c]	-1	6
50:1			0	9
25:1			0	5
100:1	Tumor Bearer	Splenomegaly	16	-2
50:1			12	-1
25:1			10	-1
100:1	Tumor Bearer	Normal[d]	6	9
50:1			13	12
25:1			6	13
100:1	Tumor Bearer	Normal	6	2
50:1			13	5
25:1			12	4
100:1	Tumor Bearer	Normal	8	22
50:1			8	16
25:1			1	14
100:1	Tumor Bearer	Normal	13	38
50:1			13	27
25:1			9	15

[a]A 4 or 18 hr ^{51}Cr release assay was performed with cultured YAC-1 lymphoma cells as targets.

[b]The weight of the tumors was about 300mg and there were no signs of necrosis.

[c]The weight of spleens with splenomegaly was 2.5 times higher than the weight of control spleens. The number of splenocytes was 5-7 times higher and there was a very high percent of lymphoblasts in those spleens.

[d]The weight of normally appearing spleens of tumor bearers was the same or 1.5 times higher than of normal controls. The number of splenocytes and their morphological appearance was similar to control mice.

TABLE II. Cytostasis and NK Activity Mediated by Splenocytes from Mice Bearing Primary Mammary Tumors Induced by Forced-Breeding

E/T Cell Ratio	Appearance Tumor and Spleen	% ^{125}IUDR I-I		% ^{51}Cr Release[a]			
		Unfractionated	Non-Adherent[b]	Unfractionated		Non-Adherent[b]	
		Exp. 1	Exp. 1	Exp. 1	Exp. 2	Exp. 1	Exp. 2
200 :1		43	21				
100 :1	Tumor free	41	6	36	79	32	39
50 :1	Control. Spleen	32	11	30	57	21	38
25 :1	macroscopically	17	5	25	41	17	22
12.5:1	normal			14	45	11	17
200 :1		38	45				
100 :1	Relatively	36	36	49	43	32	23
50 :1	small tumor.	17	30	43	30	29	30
25 :1	Spleen macros-	26	4	28	15	18	26
12.5:1	copically normal	10	3	15	11	12	18
200 :1		91	80				
100 :1	Relatively	83	52	4	18	10	15
50 :1	large and	62	32	14	9	18	14
25 :1	necrotic tumor.	28	20	13	9	11	0
12.5:1	Splenomegaly	13	5	8	0	8	0

[a]The 18 hr assay was used.
[b]Depletion of adherent cells was performed by sephadex G-10 columns.

Normal NK activity could not be restored by removal of cells adhering to sephadex G-10 columns from the splenocyte suspensions. This indicates that several mechanisms for the suppression of NK cells may operate in mice bearing primary tumors.

E. Differences Between Young and Aging Mice in Resistance against a Transplanted Tumor Inoculum and the Cytotoxic Activities of Splenocytes from Normal Mice and Mice Bearing Transplanted Tumors

It is known that NK activity declines with age (Herberman et al, 1975). The results presented elsewhere in this volume (Ehrlich et al) confirmed this and indicated that while 12 month-old mice showed a decreased NK activity compared to young mice, they expressed sometimes a slightly higher cytostatic activity than 3 month-old mice. It was also shown that the cytostatic splenocyte population of the aging mice differed in its adherence properties from that of the young

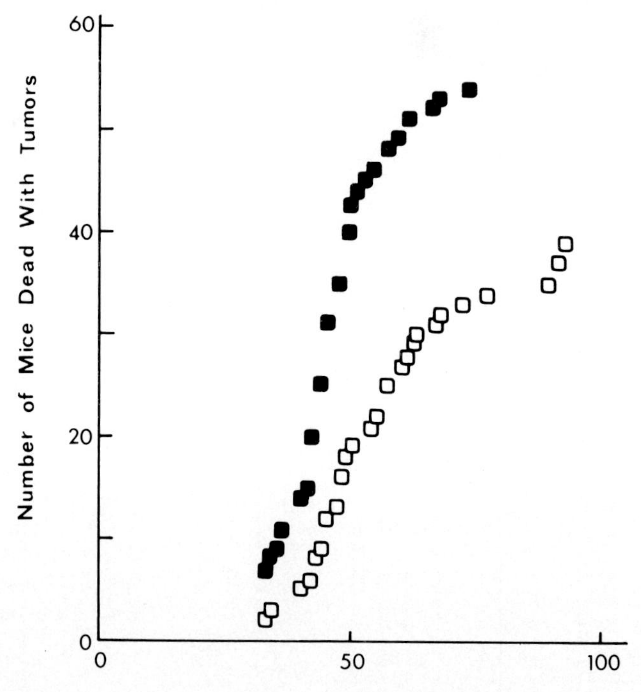

FIGURE 4. Mortality of 3 month (■) and 12 month old (□) mice after a s.c. inoculation in the footpad of 10^4 B16-F10 (F10) melanoma cells.

mice. These data as well as the results of Stutman (1979) on differences in succeptibility to methylchotanthrene carcinogenesis between old and young mice prompted us to study tumor incidence in young (3 month) and aging (12 month) C57BL/6 mice inoculated with a lethal dose (for young mice) of syngeneic B-16 melanoma cells. Fig. 4 represents the mortality curve from transplanted tumors of 54 young and 54 aging mice. It can be seen that aging mice were significantly ($P<0.001$ as determined by the Log rank test) more resistant than the young mice to this tumor transplant. Similar results were obtained in other experiments of the same kind.

These data may suggest that in this system of transplanted melanoma tumors a depressed NK activity of aging mice does not increase their succeptibility to a tumor inoculum. In fact, it seems that a depressed NK activity is associated with a hightened resistance to the transplanted tumor. It would be interesting to find out if the non-adherent cytostatic splenocytes whose activity increases in aging mice (Ehrlich _et al_, this volume) are involved in the hightened resistance of these mice to the melanoma challenge. We did not detect any differences in NK or cytostatic activities between young normal and young tumor-bearing mice and between aging normal and aging tumor-bearers.

III.DISCUSSION AND CONCLUDING REMARKS

The results of this study as well as those published elsewhere by other investigators behoove us to consider the following points:

(1) The heterogeneity of naturally-occuring immune effector mechanisms reacting with tumor cells and the validity of generalizations and of conclusions on the biological roles of such mechanisms when based on a single system.

(2) The possibility of the occurence of cells with the potential to suppress naturally-occuring immune effector cells or their activity.

(3) The usefulness of transplanted tumor systems in studies on naturally-occuring immune effector mechanisms.

It is clear from previously published results that numerous effector mechanisms exist in tumor-free individuals that are able to interact in one way or another with one or more of arbitrarilly-chosen tumor targets. NK cells (Herberman and Holden, 1978) Macrophages (Puccetti and Holden, 1979; Mantovani _et al_, 1979; Adams and Snyderman, 1979) NC cells

(Stutman, 1978) and antibodies (Pierotti and Colnaghi, 1976; Menard et al, 1977) are documented examples. In-vitro these immune effector mechanisms are able to kill or to prevent the multiplication of the target cells. No-one has so far the slightest clue whether or not these mechanisms play any significant role in the fact that some individuals, during their earlier life do not show evidence for clinical cancer. Below we will attempt to raise some arguments as to why the answer to this question is extremely hard to obtain and why the utilization of only certain experimental cancer systems could, possibly, answer it. In any event, and as is evident from the 3 primary and 2 transplanted tumors investigated in this study, a direct or an indirect evidence on the involvement or lack of involvement of a particular type of immune effector mechanism in a certain tumor system does not indicate a similar situation in other tumor systems. Moreover, different effector mechanisms could be involved in different tumor systems.

The results obtained in this study reaised the possibility that cells which adhere to sephadex G-10 columns and which express the ability to suppress NK activity of normal splenocytes reside in spleens of BALB/C mice bearing primary and early transplant passages of primary DMBA-induced tumors. Although this finding awaits rigorous experimental confirmation, the occurence of an active suppressive mechanism involved in lowering natural immune effector reactivities should be borne in mind. Again, and as stressed above, no generalization is possible also in this suppressive system. So far we were unable to demonstrate any involvement of sephadex G-10 adhering suppressor cells in the declined NK activity of splenocytes from C3HeB mice bearing primary mammary tumors.

Most of the available information on the biological role of naturally-occuring immune effector mechanisms was obtained from work with transplanted tumors. We feel that such tumors may be the wrong system in studies of this type. Primary experimental tumors develop usually after a relatively prolonged latency period. During this period and concomitantly with tumor progression the individuals subjected to the oncogenic stimuli undergo, most probably, a series of alterations, adaptations and responses to signals emitted by the oncogenic stimulus; the transformed cells; and/or by the nascent tumor. Thus, a potential primary tumor-bearer much before a tumor is visible or otherwise demonstrable, is most likely a conditioned individual different in certain functions, properties and capabilities from normal individuals. It is not unlikely that among the altered functions of the tumor-bearer to be, are a few connected with natural anti-tumor immunity. It would be of extreme theoretical and practical importance to identify each alteration or adaptation step involving natural immune effectors. The achievement of this goal is obviously an extremely difficult task as it involves the analysis of the progression of nascent primary tumors, a field which is largely terra incognita.

Transplanted tumors, useful as they are in numerous research areas are unsuitable for this purpose since upon inoculation they encounter a normal, unconditioned host, and the cells comprising the final tumor are essentially replicas of the inoculated ones.

The altered expressions of naturally-occuring immunity observed sometimes in animals bearing transplanted tumors are thus, probably, secondary responses to the growth of a finally "shaped" malignant product rather than primary responses to the progression of a nascent tumor.

REFERENCES

Adams, D.O. and Snyderman, R. (1979). J. Natl. Cancer Inst., 62, 1341-1345.

Becker, S. and Klein, E. (1976). Eur. J. Immunol. 6, 882-885.

Cannon, G.B., Bonnard, G.D., Djeu, J., West, W.H. and Herberman, R.B. (1977). Int. J. Cancer, 19, 487-497.

Herberman, R.B., Nunn, M.E. and Larvin, O.H. (1975). Int. J. Cancer, 16, 230-239.

Herberman, R.B. and Holden, H.T., (1978). Adv. Cancer Res., 27, 305-375.

Heppner, G.H., Henry, E., Stolbach, L., Cummings, F.J., McDonough, E. and Calabresi, D. (1975). Cancer, Res., 35, 1931-1937.

Jerrels, T.R., Dean, J.H., Richardson, G., Cannon, G.B. and Herberman, R.B. (1979). Int. J. Cancer, 23, 768-776.

Mantovani, A., Peri, G., Polentarutti, N., Bolis, G., Mangioni, C. and Spreafico, F. (1979). Int. J. Cancer, 23, 157-164.

Menard, S., Colnaghi, H.T. and Della Porta, G. (1977). Int. J. Cancer, 19, 267-274.

Moore, K. and Moore, M. (1979). Br. J. Cancer, 39, 636-647.

Pierotti, M.A. and Colnaghi, M.I. (1976). Int. J. Cancer, 18, 223-229.

Puccetti, P. and Holden, H.T. (1979). Int. J. Cancer, 23, 123-133.

Stutman, O., Paige, C.T. and Figarella, E.F. (1978). J. Immunol., 121, 1819-1826.

Stutman, O. (1979). J. Natl. Cancer Inst. 62, 353-358.

Takasugi, M., Ramseyer, A. and Takasugi, J. (1977). Cancer Res., 37, 413-418.

NK CELL ACTIVITY IN THE BLOOD, TUMOUR-DRAINING LYMPH NODES AND PRIMARY TUMOURS OF WOMEN WITH MAMMARY CARCINOMA

Oleg Eremin

Division of Immunology
Department of Pathology
University of Cambridge
Cambridge

I. INTRODUCTION

A variety of cellular effector mechanisms (macrophage cytotoxicity and cytostasis, antibody-dependent cellular cytotoxicity, antigen-specific T lymphocyte cytotoxicity and natural cell-mediated immunity) have been postulated to be operative in humans with malignant disease and to play an important role in host resistance to initiation and growth of solid tumours (Cerrotini and Brunner, 1974; Hëllstrom, 1974; Fink, 1976; Henney, 1977; James et al., 1977; Herberman and Holden, 1979).

The precise biological significance of natural cell-mediated immunity or natural cytotoxicity is at present unclear and the relevance of the effector cell, the natural killer (NK) cell, to tumour growth or regression is rather speculative. Data accumulated from athymic nude mice and various rodent tumour-bearing models, however, suggests a possible anti-tumour role for the NK cell in such animals.

Athymic nude mice, lacking thymus-dependent lymphocytes and therefore unable to generate immune cytotoxic T lymphocytes, have a normal or diminished incidence of spontaneous tumours (Stutman, 1974; Rygaard and Povlsen, 1976; Stutman, 1978; Sharky and Fogh, 1979). Tumour induction by chemical carcinogens in athymic nude mice shows a longer latent period and a slower growth rate of the induced tumour,

ISBN 0-12-341350-8

compared to normal thymus-bearing animals of the same background strain (Stutman, 1974; Gillette and Fox, 1975; Outzen, 1975; Stutman, 1978). Several authors have also reported an inhibition of growth of both syngeneic and allogeneic lymphoid tumours in nude mice (Campanile et al., 1977; Warner et al., 1977). Carcinoma and sarcoma, on the other hand, are said to grow as well as in the normal background strain (Warner et al., 1977). Thymectomised, irradiated and bone-marrow reconstituted mice behave similarly to athymic nude mice and normal mice of the same background strain in their tumour susceptibility to chemical carcinogens and incidence of spontaneous tumours (Gillette and Fox, 1975; Dawson et al., 1978). Such findings in thymusless mice imply that non-T lymphoid cells, such as the NK cells, could be important host defense effectors.

Prominent NK cell activity has been described in the various lymphoid compartments of athymic nude mice, in particular in mononuclear cell preparations from the spleen (Herberman et al., 1975; Kiessling et al., 1975a; Warner et al., 1977; Santoni et al., 1979). In several studies a good correlation was found between the lytic capacity *in vitro* of murine spleen cells against target cells of a particular tumour type and the ability of an inoculum (defined tumour cell dose) of the same tumour to initiate growth *in vivo*. Such a correlation has been described both in athymic nude mice (Kiessling et al., 1975b; Warner et al., 1977) and in normal mice (Sendo et al., 1975; Haller et al., 1977; Henney et al., 1978).

Adoptive transfer of lymphoid cells, possessing prominent NK cell activity, into irradiated rats (Shellam and Hogg, 1977), and Winn type *in vivo* transfer experiments in mice (Kiessling et al., 1976) and rats (Harmon et al., 1977) induced resistance to tumour take and growth in the host animals. These results further suggest a possible anti-tumour role for the NK cell in rodents.

The association between defective cellular immunity (mediated by thymus-dependent lymphocytes) and the development of malignancy in humans has not been satisfactorily resolved (for review see Stutman, 1975). Clinical evidence from children with primary immunodeficiency disease suggests that the incidence of the common childhood solid tumours is not increased in such children, the malignancies which develop being primarily lymphoreticular in nature (Kersey et al., 1974). In adults with lepromatous leprosy (where severe defects of thymus-dependent immunity have been described) there is no evidence of an increased incidence of solid tumours (Oleinick, 1969). The data from various transplantation centres indicate that, apart from atypical lymphomas, most of the common solid tumours are not more prevelant in transplanted patients with the possible exception of carcinoma of the cervix and skin (Stutman, 1975; Penn, 1977).

These findings imply that immunological surveillance against most solid tumours in man, if operative, is probably not exerted exclusively by a thymus-dependent cellular response. Other effector mechanisms such as natural cell-mediated immunity could have an important anti-tumour role to play.

The aim of this communication is to explore and evaluate the possible beneficial role of the natural killer cell in the general circulation, regional tumour-draining lymph nodes and in the tumour lymphoreticular infiltrate in patients with malignant tumours, and in particular in women with clinically localised mammary carcinoma.

II. NK CELL ACTIVITY IN THE BLOOD OF PATIENTS WITH CANCER

In man, natural killer cell activity has been well documented (particularly in the mononuclear cell preparations from blood) but the NK cell has not been precisely characterized nor the nature of the target cell antigen(s) elucidated (for review see Herberman and Holden, 1978; Moller, 1979). Difficulties have also arisen in past studies in the interpretation of the different *in vitro* assays used, especially where the target cells employed were originally derived from the same type of tumour as borne by the patient. Tumour antigen specific and disease associated or related cytotoxicity (which may possibly be tumour specific) may contribute in varying degrees to target cell damage in such *in vitro* assays, and the contribution by the NK cell is then less readily measured (Bean et al., 1975; Herberman and Oldham, 1975; Oldham et al., 1975; Takasugi and Mickey, 1976; Baldwin and Embleton, 1977). To obviate such problems and lessen the complexicity of interpretation of the assays, in the studies reported here, the two target cells employed were (1) CLA4 - a lymphoblastoid cell line (Epstein-Barr virus positive) growing as a suspension culture and (2) Detroit 6 (D6) - a Hela subline growing as a monolayer. In the *in vitro* assays used to measure NK cell activity, lymphocytes were incubated with ^{51}Cr labelled target cells (CLA4, D6) at $37^{o}C$ for 16 to 24 hrs at various lymphocyte to target cell ratios (5:1 to 200:1) and target cell lysis (and hence NK cell activity) assessed by ^{51}Cr released (Eremin et al., 1978a). The patients investigated were women, aged between 30 and 70 yrs with a clinical stage I or stage II mammary carcinoma (clinically confined to the breast and axilla) and who had a mastectomy and axillary clearance carried out as a potentially curative procedure.

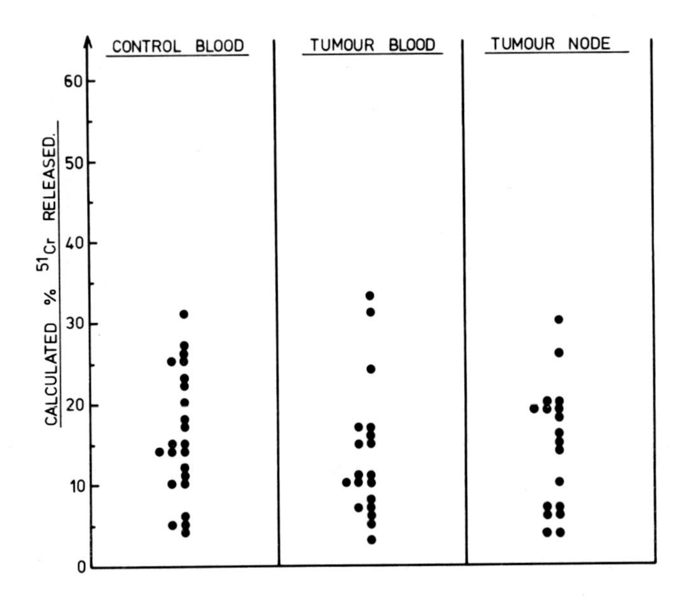

FIGURE 1. Levels of NK cell activity found in the blood and regional lymph nodes of women with clinically localized mammary carcinoma are within normal limits. Lymphocytes from the blood of patients with mammary carcinoma (clinically localized to the breast and axilla) and from axillary lymph nodes removed at mastectomy (where spread of tumour to axilla had occurred, tumour-free nodes only used), were added to ^{51}Cr labelled D6 target cells and incubated at 37°C for 16 to 24 hrs. ^{51}Cr release was calculated by subtracting the background release (in the absence of lymphocytes) from the obtained experimental release. Maximal lymphocyte to target cell ratios (40:1) only shown.

Figures 1 and 2 show that the NK cell activity of blood lymphocytes from women with mammary carcinoma, clinically localized to the breast and axilla, has a wide biological spectrum but the pattern of reactivity was comparable to that detected in normal healthy controls, irrespective of the target cell used. Competitive inhibition studies

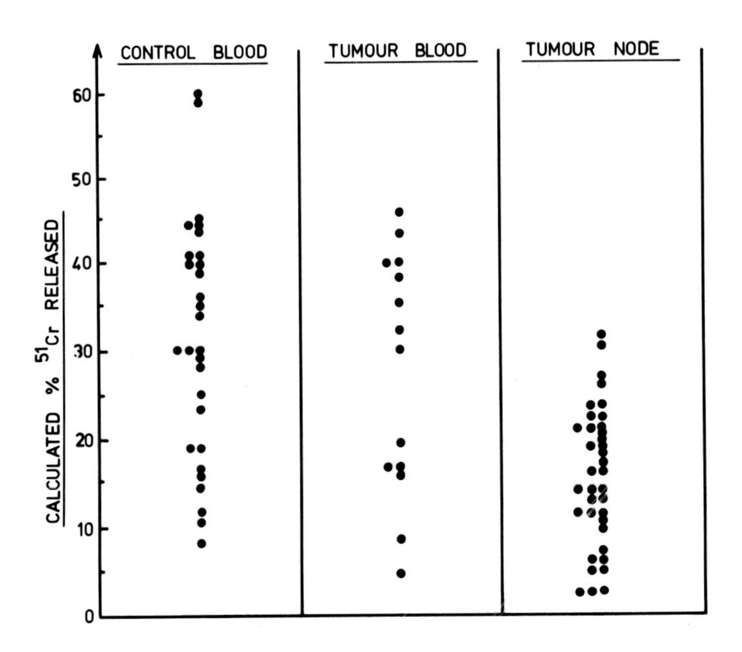

FIGURE 2. Prominent levels of NK cell activity found in the blood (carcinoma of breast) and significant levels found in the regional lymph nodes draining various solid tumours (carcinoma of colon, lung and breast). Lymphocytes from the blood of patients with mammary carcinoma (clinically localized to the breast and axilla) and from regional lymph nodes removed at operation (draining a variety of clinically localized solid tumours - colon, lung and breast) were added to ^{51}Cr labelled CLA4 target cells and incubated at 37°C for 16 to 24 hrs. Where tumour spread to regional lymph nodes had occurred, tumour-free nodes only used. ^{51}Cr release was calculated by subtracting the background release (in the absence of lymphocytes) from the obtained experimental release. Maximal lymphocyte to target cell ratios only shown - blood at 50:1 and lymph node at 100:1.

revealed that the same killer cell was responsible for cell damage against both types of target cell. No obvious correlation was found between the level of NK cell activity detected in a given patient and such clinical parameters as age and hormonal status of the patient; or various pathological parameters such as the tumour size, histological type or degree of inflammatory infiltrate. Tumour invasion of the regional draining axillary lymph nodes similarly did not affect the natural cytotoxicity detected in the blood of tumour bearers (Eremin et al., 1978a).

Prominent natural cytotoxicity, comparable to the levels detected in healthy controls, has been found in the blood of patients bearing various types of solid tumours (Oldham et al., 1975; Pross and Baines, 1976; Cannon et al., 1977; Takasugi et al., 1977; Vose et al., 1977; Töttermann et al., 1978). In agreement with our findings in patients with breast carcinoma, Cannon et al. (1977) with breast tumours and Vose et al. (1978) with lung neoplasms found no correlation between the level of natural cytotoxicity in the blood and tumour spread to the regional draining lymph nodes. In the same study, patients with benign breast disease (fibrocystic disease, fibroadenoma) were reported as having prominent levels of NK cell activity in blood, comparable to healthy controls (Cannon et al., 1977). Thus most patients bearing different pathological types of solid tumours appear to possess a normal range of natural killer cells in their general circulation.

Extensive metastatic spread of cancer, on the other hand, does appear in some cases to modify this normal pattern of NK cell activity. Reduced natural cytotoxicity has been described in patients showing widespread tumour involvement (McCoy et al., 1973; Pross and Baines,1976; Takasugi et al., 1977). Vose et al. (1977), on the other hand, were unable to find such an association and Levin et al. (1976) found no correlation between the level of natural cell-mediated immunity and the clinical status of the patients.

Studies in animals have similarly shown reduced NK cell activity in tumour-bearing mice, particularly with progressively growing tumours and consequently a large tumour load (Herberman et al., 1975a; Becker and Klein, 1976).

The reduction of generalised natural cytotoxicity in some patients with widespread metastases may possibly signify a further breakdown of host defense mechanisms, but whether this is a cause or an effect of the progressively increasing tumour load is uncertain.

III. NK CELL ACTIVITY IN THE REGIONAL TUMOUR-DRAINING LYMPH NODE

Significant NK cell activity in lymph nodes, from different anatomical sites, has been described in both mice (Greenberg and Playfair, 1974; Herberman et al., 1975a; Kiessling et al., 1975b; Santoni et al., 1979) and rats (Nunn et al., 1976; Shellam and Hogg, 1977; Oehler et al., 1978). Very few studies have been done in man to determine the natural cytotoxicity of lymph nodes. Although Herberman and Holden (1978) found minimal NK cell activity in human

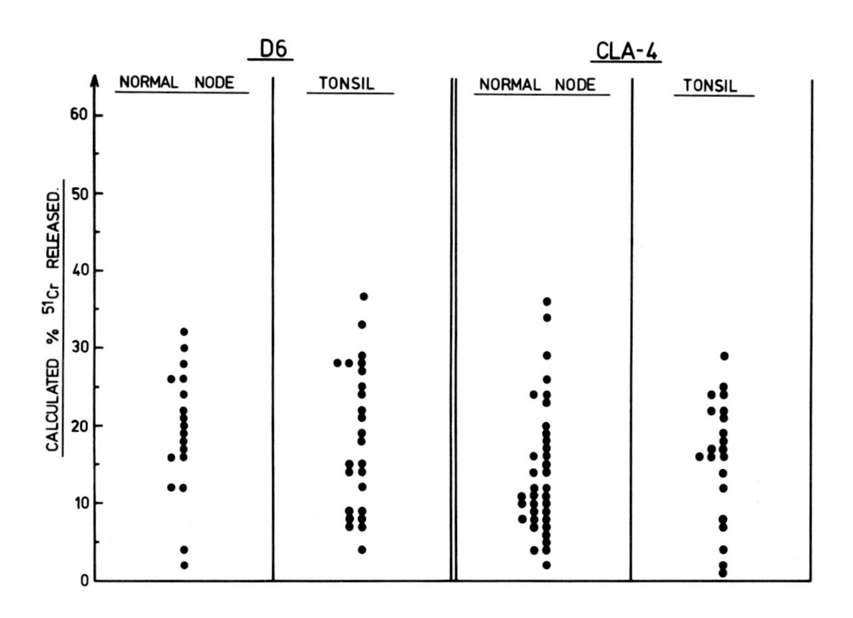

FIGURE 3. NK cell activity of lymphocyte preparations from normal lymph nodes and tonsils. Lymphocytes from normal lymph nodes (cervical area, thorax, abdominal cavity, inguinal area) and from tonsils (removed for recurrent or chronic tonsillitis but in a quiescent phase), were added to ^{51}Cr labelled D6 and CLA4 target cells and incubated at 37°C for 16 to 24 hrs. ^{51}Cr release was calculated by subtracting the background release (in the absence of lymphocytes) from the obtained experimental release. Maximal lymphocyte to target cell ratios only shown - D6 at 50:1 and CLA4 at 100:1.

lymph nodes and tonsils, we (Eremin et al., 1978a) detected a variable but significant level of NK cell activity in lymphocyte preparations from both tonsil and lymph node (Figure 3). There was no difference in natural cytotoxicity detected in normal lymph nodes from different anatomical areas (cervical, thoracic, abdominal) and in lymph nodes draining areas of subacute or chronic inflammation (compared to normal nodes) irrespective of the target cell used. As in the case of blood, competitive inhibition assays showed the same cell lysing both target cells (Eremin et al., 1978a).

Human regional lymph nodes draining mammary carcinoma and other pathological types of solid tumours (stomach, colon, lung) (Figures 1 and 2) similarly showed variable but significant levels of NK cell activity, the pattern of reactivities being similar to that found in normal lymph nodes (Figure 3). As with blood, there was no obvious association between NK cell activity detected and various parameters such as tumour size, histological type or evidence of prominent inflammatory cell infiltrate. Proximity of the draining lymph node to the various solid tumours or metastatic spread to the lymph node did not alter the pattern of natural cytotoxicity elicited. Also, prolonged washing, incubation at 37°C for 24 hrs, or pre-treatment with trypsin, had no effect either on normal or tumour-draining lymph node lymphocytes (Eremin et al., 1978a).

Vose et al. (1977), on the other hand, found absent or very low levels of NK cell activity in tumour-draining lymph nodes, but did not present data relating to NK cell activity in normal lymph nodes. What we are seeing, with virtually all human solid tumours, is a particular stage of a long and continuing biological process and the level of NK cell activity detected may not be representative of killer activity in the early phase of tumour initiation and growth. Such a hypothesis is given some credence by certain animal tumour models where inoculation of tumour cells (or viruses) does lead to a very rapid, but not necessarily prolonged augmentation of NK cell activity within lymph nodes, comparable to the activity found in the spleen (Herberman et al., 1977).

The lack of alteration of natural cytotoxicity in lymphocyte suspensions from lymph nodes and tonsils following trypsin treatment, contrasts sharply to the significant fall of cytotoxicity in lymphocyte suspensions from blood (Peter et al., 1975; Pross & Jondal, 1975; Eremin et al., 1978a). The differential susceptibility to pre-treatment with ammonium chloride (used as a red blood cell lytic agent) (Eremin et al., 1978c) also suggests that the NK cell in blood is different to the NK cell in lymph node and tonsil. This was confirmed by selective lymphocyte subpopulation depletion and enrichment studies (Eremin et al., 1978b; see relevant section in this volume). This could imply a differential target cell susceptibility by the two different killer cells (although not the case in our studies) and possibly explain the lack of NK cell activity detected by some workers (Vose et al., 1977; Herberman and Holden, 1978).

IV. NK CELL ACTIVITY IN THE TUMOUR-INFILTRATING LYMPHOCYTES

Lymphoreticular infiltration of various human solid tumours has been extensively documented in the literature (for review see Underwood, 1974). Such lymphocyte infiltrates, particularly if prominent, have been invoked as an important host defense mechanism and reported to be associated with an improved patient survival, e.g. in carcinoma of the head and neck (Bennett et al., 1971; Sala and Ferlito, 1976), carcinoma of the stomach (Inokuchi et al., 1967; Hawley et al., 1970), carcinoma of the colon (Murray et al., 1975; Watt and House, 1978) and carcinoma of the breast (Moore and Foote, 1948; Hamlin, 1968; Cutler et al., 1969; DiPaola et al., 1974; Fisher et al., 1975).

Recently, various workers have isolated and begun to investigate the properties of these tumour-infiltrating lymphocytes (Nind et al., 1973; Yata et al., 1974; Jondal and Klein, 1975; Claudy et al., 1976; Vose et al., 1977; Häyry and Tötterman, 1978; Svennevig et al., 1978; Tötterman et al., 1978). The natural killer cell activity of lymphocytes isolated from different human solid tumours has not been extensively investigated, but the few studies done to date have reported absent or minimal levels of killer cell activity (Vose et al., 1977; Tötterman et al., 1978; Gerson et al., 1979).

Our studies (Eremin et al., 1980a) reveal (Figure 4) that the lymphocytes isolated from primary mammary carcinomas show minimal or low levels of natural cytotoxicity. The NK cell activity in the blood of these patients, on the other hand, was variable but quite prominent. The method of tumour cell preparation (mechanical disaggregation or enzymic digestion with collagenase) or lymphocyte isolation from the tumour cells and macrophages (passage on Sephadex G-10 columns) had no effect on the level of NK cell activity detected. Various clinical parameters (age and hormone status) or pathological parameters (size and type of tumour, degree of

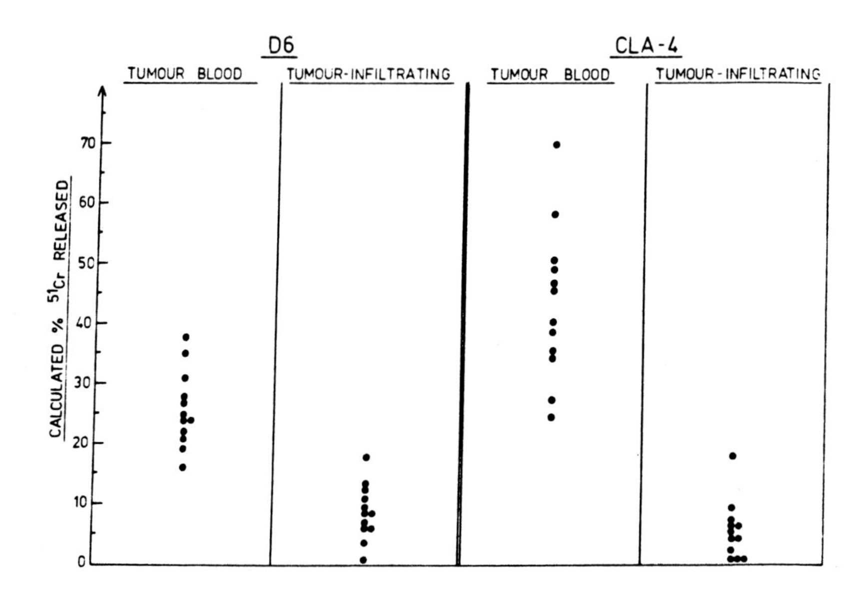

FIGURE 4. Tumour-infiltrating lymphocytes show a reduced level of NK cell activity. Lymphocytes from the blood of patients with mammary carcinoma (clinically localized to the breast and axilla) and isolated from the tumour (mechanical disaggregation; collagenase digestion and passage on Sephadex G-10 column), were added to ^{51}Cr labelled D6 and CLA4 target cells and incubated at 37°C for 24 hrs. ^{51}Cr release was calculated by subtracting the background release (in the absence of lymphocytes) from the obtained experimental release. Maximal lymphocyte to target cell ratio (40:1) only shown.

tumour-lymphocyte infiltration, tumour spread to regional nodes) had no obvious bearing on the level of natural cytotoxicity detected. Antibody-dependent cellular-cytotoxicity (data not shown) was similarly minimal or totally absent.

Lymphocytes isolated from animal tumours induced by Moloney sarcoma virus, on the other hand, appear to possess significant killer cell activity (Becker and Klein, 1977; Gerson et al., 1979). Should this prove to be a consistent discrepancy, it may suggest further differences in host responses to "spontaneous" tumours (humans) and chemically or virally induced tumours (animals).

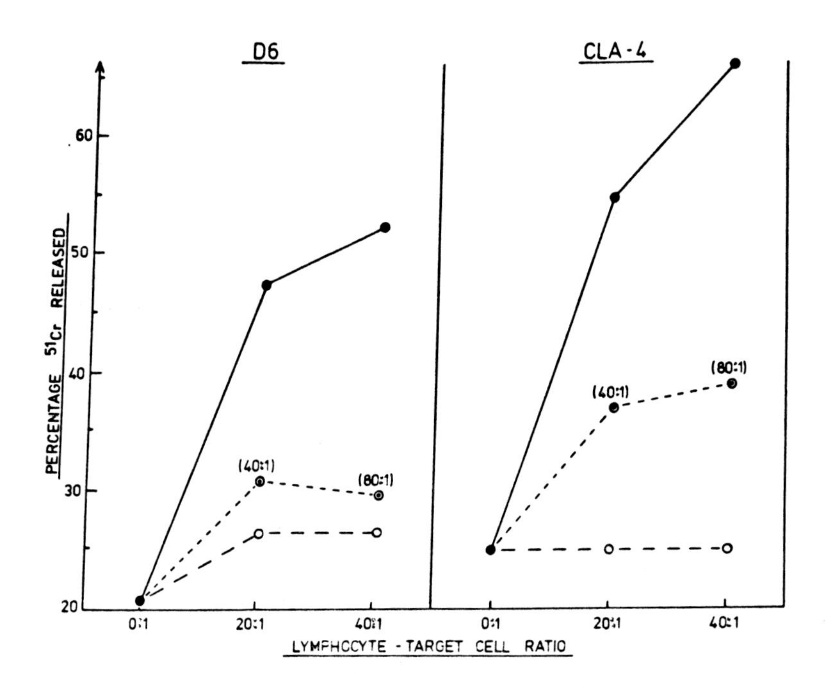

FIGURE 5 Tumour-infiltrating lymphocytes can suppress blood lymphocyte NK cell activity. Lymphocytes from [(●) tumour bearer's blood; (o) tumour (collagenase digested); (⊙) tumour bearer's blood mixed with lymphocytes from tumour (collagenase digested) in a 1 to 1 ratio], were added to ^{51}Cr labelled D6 and CLA4 target cells and incubated at 37°C for 24 hrs. Percentage ^{51}Cr release was the measured experimental release. Lymphocyte to target cell ratios were 0:1, 20:1 and 40:1, in the mixed lymphocyte preparations (⊙),the ratios were 0:1, 40:1 and 80:1. Statistical analysis : statistically significant reduction of NK cell activity (against D6 and CLA4) occurred when tumour-infiltrating lymphocyte preparations were added to patient's autochthonous blood lymphocyte suspensions ($p < 0.001$).

Figure 5 shows that tumour-infiltrating lymphocytes not only show low levels of natural cell-mediated immunity, but suppress the prominent natural cytotoxicity of blood lymphocytes (autochthonous and control). The mechanism of this suppression is uncertain, but reduction of killer cell activity by competitive inhibitor or suppressor lymphocytes has been described recently (Parkman and Rosen, 1976; Eremin et al., 1978b; Osband and Parkman, 1978).

Hence, the lymphocytes infiltrating solid primary mammary carcinomas show an absent or low level of killer cell activity, even though the circulating blood lymphocytes possess significant levels of cytotoxicity. This suggests that selective migration into the tumour, in situ phenotypic modification or retention of different lymphocyte subpopulations may occur. The signal(s) for selective cellular migration into a growing tumour are poorly defined (Haskill and Parthenais, 1978; Radov et al., 1979). Boetcher and Leonard (1974) and Snyderman et al. (1978) have described defective blood monocyte chemotactic function in patients bearing different types of solid cancers. Norman et al. (1979) have also found evidence of defective monocyte migration into inflammatory sites in rats bearing sarcomas and this defect was abolished following tumour removal. It is possible that similar defects of lymphocyte subset migration may be operative within the tumour environment. The factors responsible for possible phenotypic modification or selective retention in situ are as yet unknown.

V. LYMPHOCYTE SUBPOPULATIONS IN THE BLOOD, TUMOUR-DRAINING LYMPH NODES AND PRIMARY TUMOURS OF WOMEN WITH MAMMARY CARCINOMA

The lymphocyte subpopulations found in the blood and regional tumour-draining lymph nodes in women with stage I or II mammary carcinoma are shown in Table 1. The data reveals that the Fc receptor-bearing (Fc^+) lymphocyte subset is larger than the C3 receptor-bearing ($C3^+$) lymphocyte subset in blood (controls, patients) but that the pattern is reversed in lymph nodes (normal, tumour-draining). Mixed rosetting reactions confirmed a prominent (Fc^+ $C3^-$) lymphocyte subpopulation in blood and selective lymphocyte subpopulation depletion studies established that the NK cell in blood was a sIg-bearing (Fc^+ $C3^-$) lymphocyte. The (Fc^+ $C3^+$) lymphocytes, although unable to kill *in vitro*, could function as competitive inhibitor or suppressor lymphocytes (Eremin et al., 1976; Eremin et al., 1978a).

TABLE 1. Lymphocyte Subpopulations in the Blood and Tumour-Draining Lymph Nodes of Women with Mammary Carcinoma[a]

Lymphocyte source	*Percentage lymphocyte subpopulations*[b]			
	T-rosettes	*Fc-rosettes*	*C3-rosettes*	*sIg-rosettes*
Normal blood (n = 30)	*69 ± 4*	*33 ± 8*	*25 ± 9*	*29 ± 6*
Tumour blood (n = 30)	*72 ± 6*	*30 ± 7*	*19 ± 8*	*26 ± 6*
Normal lymph node (n = 27)	*71 ± 6*	*23 ± 4*	*33 ± 6*[c]	*26 ± 5*
Tumour lymph node[d] *(n = 30)*	*58 ± 12*	*31 ± 7*	*46 ± 11*[c]	*41 ± 11*

[a]*The patients were women, aged between 30 and 70 yrs, presenting with stage I or II mammary carcinoma (confined to the breast and axilla), and who had a mastectomy and axillary clearance carried out as a potentially curative procedure.*

[b]*Lymphocyte subpopulations determined by rosetting reactions. The immunoglobulin-bearing lymphocytes detected by the mixed antiglobulin rosetting reaction (Eremin et al., 1976). Values are expressed as means ± standard deviations.*

[c]*The C3-receptor-bearing lymphocyte counts are higher than the Fc-receptor-bearing lymphocyte counts in lymph nodes (normal, tumour-draining).*

[d]*Statistically significant alterations in the percentages of the different lymphocyte subsets found in tumour-draining axillary lymph nodes ($p<0.005$). Where metastatic spread to axilla had occurred, tumour free nodes only used.*

Table 2 shows the type of lymphocyte subsets detected in tumour-infiltrating lymphocytes (Eremin et al., 1980b). Both T and B lymphocytes were found in lymphocyte suspensions prepared from primary breast tumour specimens, irrespective of the method used for lymphocyte isolation-mechanical disaggregation, collagenase digestion with or without Sephadex G-10 column passage.

TABLE 2. Tumour-infiltrating lymphocyte subpopulations isolated from human breast carcinoma[a]

Method of lymphocyte isolation	Percentage lymphocyte subpopulations[b]			
	T-rosettes	Fc-rosettes	C3-rosettes	sIg-rosettes
Mechanical[c] disaggregation	62	25	27	40
	51	35	55	49
	50	30	30	38
Collagenase[d] digestion	65	20	10	25
	43	12	1[f]	47
	70	25	8	27
Collagenase digestion[e] + Sephadex G-10 column passage	60	18	3[f]	44
	41	24	9	54
	63	15	12	30

[a]The breast tumour specimens were obtained in a sterile manner at operation from the excisional biopsy sent for frozen section.

[b]Values given are for individual tumour specimens.

[c]The tumour specimens were cleared of fat and fascia, washed in medium (RPMI 1640 + 10% foetal calf serum) and carefully sliced into small thin slices. Spill out of cells occurred during this procedure.

[d]The small, thin tumour slices were incubated with collagenase [300 units (Sigma, type 1) per ml of RPMI 1640] at 37°C for 12 to 16 hrs.

[e]Sephadex G-10 columns (Eremin et al., 1980a) were used to isolate lymphocytes from enzymatically digested tumour cell preparations. The much larger macrophages and tumour cells being entrapped on the columns.

[f]The low C3-rosetting percentage following collagenase digestion was due to the enzymatic removal from the cell surface of the receptor for the third component of complement. Resynthesis of the C3 receptor occurs following incubation at 37°C for 36 - 48 hrs (Eremin et al., 1980b).

The low percentage of C3 receptor-bearing lymphocytes detected after collagenase treatment was due to enzymatic removal from the cell surface of the receptor for the third component of complement. Resynthesis of the C3 receptor occurred following incubation at 37°C for 48 hrs and reappearance of the predominance of the ($C3^+$) lymphocyte subset (Eremin et al., 1980b). The sIg-bearing lymphocyte subpopulations detected in the mammary tumours appear to be predominantly (Fc^+ $C3^+$) cells, that is lymphocytes which have been shown previously to both lack any NK cell activity and to competitively inhibit or suppress blood natural cytotoxicity.

VI SUMMARY

Our studies in women with mammary carcinoma, clinically localized to the breast and axilla, showed different levels of NK cell activity in the various compartments examined. Natural cytotoxicity in the general circulation, although variable, was prominent and comparable to the spectrum found in healthy controls. Regional draining axillary lymph nodes, whether tumour-free or invaded by metastases, also possessed significant levels of NK cell activity. Tumour-infiltrating lymphocytes, obtained by mechanical disaggregation or collagenase digestion and isolated from the tumour cell preparations on Sephadex G-10 columns, showed minimal or low levels of natural cytotoxicity - even though the corresponding autochthonous blood lymphocytes had a high lytic capacity. The tumour-infiltrating lymphocytes not only lacked significant cytotoxicity, but could suppress the prominent killer cell activity of blood. These findings suggest that selective migration into, in situ cell surface modulation or retention of different lymphocyte subsets occurs in the primary mammary tumours by some, as yet undefined, process.

The results presented do not necessarily support the hypothesis that natural cytotoxicity is an important host defense mechanism in humans with malignant growths. The data does suggest, however, that if the NK cell in man did possess an anti-tumour activity *in vivo* (as yet unproven), then its paucity in the tumour-host cell milieu, as well as the intra-tumour presence of suppressor cells, offers a possible explanation for the persistent and progressive growth of solid tumours in man.

ACKNOWLEDGMENTS

The data presented was obtained in collaboration with Professor R.R.A. Coombs, J. Ashby and D. Plumb. The work was supported by the Cancer Research Campaign (U.K.). Figures 1, 2 and 3 are reproduced, by kind permission, from the International Journal of Cancer, *21*, 35-41, 1978. Table 1 is reproduced, by kind permission, from the International Archives of Allergy and Applied Immunology, *52*, 277-290, 1976. I gratefully acknowledge the encouragement and help provided by Professor R.R.A. Coombs, Head of the Immunology Division, Department of Pathology, University of Cambridge.

REFERENCES

Baldwin, R.W., and Embleton, M.J., *Int. Rev. Exp. Path. 17*, 49 (1977).
Bean, M.A., Bloom, B.R., Herberman, R.B., Old, L.J., Oettgen, H.F., Klein, G., and Terry, W.D., *Cancer Res. 35*, 2902 (1975).
Becker, S., and Klein, E., *Eur. J. Immunol. 6*, 892 (1976).
Bennett, S.H., Futrell, J., Roth, J.A., Hoye, R.C., and Ketcham, A.S., *Cancer 28*, 1255 (1971).
Boetcher, D.A., and Leonard, E.J., *J. Natl. Cancer Inst. 52*, 1091 (1974).
Campanile, F., Crino, L., Bonmassar, E., Houchens, D., and Goldin, A., *Cancer Res. 37*, 394, (1977).
Cannon, G.B., Bonnard, G.D., Dieu, J., West, W.H., and Herberman, R.B., *Int. J. Cancer 19*, 487 (1977).
Cerottini, J.C., and Brunner, K.T. In "Advances in Immunology", (F. Dixon and H.G. Kunkel, eds.), Academic Press, New York. (1974).
Claudy, A.L., Schmitt, D., Viac, J., Alario, A., Staquet, M.J., and Thwolet, J., *Clin. exp. Immunol. 23*, 61 (1976).
Coombs, R.R.A., Wilson, A.B., Eremin, O., Gurner, B.W., Haegert, D.G., Lawson, Y.A., Bright, S., Munro, A.J. *J. Immunol. Methods 18*, 45 (1977).
Cutler, S.J., Black, M.M., Mock, T., Harvei, S., and Freeman, C., *Cancer 24*, 653 (1969).
Dawson, P.J., Fieldsteil, H.A., and McCusker, J. *Br. J. Cancer 38*, 476 (1978).
Di Paola, M., Angelini, L., Bertolotti, A., and Colizza, S. *Br. Med. J. (IV)*, 268 (1974).

Eremin, O., Plumb, D., and Coombs, R.R.A. *Int. Arch. Allergy appl. Immunol. 52,* 277 (1976).
Eremin, O., Ashby, J., Stephens, J.P., *Int. J. Cancer 21,* 35 (1978a).
Eremin, O., Coombs, R.R.A., Ashby, J., and Plumb, D., *Int. J. Cancer 21,* 42 (1978b).
Eremin, O., Ashby, J., and Plumb, D., *J. Immunol. Methods 24,* 257, (1978c).
Eremin, O., Coombs, R.R.A., and Ashby, J. Submitted for publication (1980a).
Eremin, O., Coombs, R.R.A., Plumb, D., and Spencer, J. Submitted for publication (1980b).
Fisher, E.R., Gregorio, R.M., Fisher, B., Redmond, C., Vellios, F., and Sommers, S.C. *Cancer 36,* 1 (1975).
Fink, M.A. The Macrophage in Neoplasia, Academic Press, New York (1976).
Gerson, J.M., Holden, H.T., Bonnard, G.D., and Herberman, R.B. *Proc. American Assoc. Cancer Res 20,* 238 (1979).
Gillette, R.W. and Fox, A. *Cellular Immunol. 19,* 328 (1975).
Greenberg, A.H., and Playfair, J.H.L. *Clin. exp. Immunol. 16,* 99 (1974).
Haller, O., Hansson, M., Kiessling, R., and Wigzell, H. *Nature 270,* 604, (1977).
Hamlin, I.M.E. *Br. J. Cancer 22,* 383 (1968).
Harmon, R.C., Clark, E.C., Reddy, A.L., Hildermann, W.H., and Miller, Y. *Int. J. Cancer 20,* 748 (1977).
Haskill, J.S., and Parthenais, E. *J. Immunol. 120,* 1813 (1978).
Hawley, P.R., Westerholm, P., and Morston, B.C. *Br. J. Surg. 57,* 876 (1970).
Häyry, P., and Tötterman, *Eur. J. Immunol. 8,* 866 (1978).
Hellström, K.E., Hellström, I. In "Advances in Immunology", (F.J. Dixon and H.G. Kunkel, eds), 18, 209-277, Academic Press, New York (1974).
Henney, C.S. In "Mechanisms of Tumour Immunity", (J. Green, S. Cohen, R.T. Clusky, eds.), p. 55-86, John Wiley and Sons. Inc. (1977).
Henney, C.S., Tracey, D., Durdik, M., and Klimpel, G. *Am. J. Pathol 93,* 459 (1978).
Herberman, R.B., and Oldham, R.K. *J. Natl. Cancer Inst. 55,* 749 (1975).
Herberman, R.B., Nunn, M.E., and Lavrin, D.H. *Int. J. Cancer 16,* 216 (1975).
Herberman, R.B., Nunn, M.E., Holden, H.T., Staal, S., and Dieu, J.Y. *Int. J. Cancer 19,* 555 (1977).

Herberman, R.B., and Holden, H.T. In "Advances in Cancer Research" (G. Klein and S. Weinhouse, eds.), 27, p. 305, Academic Press, New York.
Herberman, R.B. and Holden, H.T. *J. Natl. Cancer Inst. 62,* 441 (1979).
Inokuchi, K., Inutsuka, S., Purusawa, M., Soejema, K., and Ikeda, T. *Cancer 20,* 1924 (1967).
Jondal, M., and Klein, G. *Biomedicine 23,* 163 (1975).
Kersey, J.H., Spector, B.D. and Good, R.A. *J. Paediatrics 84,* 263 (1974).
Kiessling, R., Klein, E., Pross, H., and Wigzell, H. *Eur. J. Immunol. 5,* 117 (1975a).
Kiessling, R., Petranyi, G., Klein, G., Wigzell, H. *Int. J. Cancer 15,* 933 (1975b).
Kiessling, R., Petranyi, G., Klein, G., and Wigzell, H. *Int. J. Cancer 17,* 275 (1976).
Levin, A.G., Massey, E.J., Wolter, J., Schauf, V., and Deinhardt, F. *Proc. American Assoc. Cancer Res. 17,* 65 (1976).
The Macrophage and Cancer "Proceedings of the EURES Symposium", (K. James, W. McBridge and A. Stuart, eds.), Edinburgh Sept. 12-14th, 1977.
McCoy, J., Herberman, R.B., Perlin, E., Levine, P., and Alford, C., *Proc. American Assoc. Cancer Res 14,* 107 (1973).
Moller, G. (ed.) Natural killer cells, Immunological Reviews, 44, Munksgaard, Copenhagen.
Moore, Jr., P.S. and Foote, Jr., F.W. *Cancer 2,* 635 (1948).
Murray, D., Hreno, A., Dutton, J. and Hampson, L.G. *Arch. Surg. 110,* 908 (1975).
Nind, A.P.P., Nairn, R.C., Rolland, R.C., Guli, E.P.G., and Hughes, E.S.R. *Br. J. Cancer 28,* 108 (1973).
Norman, S.J., Schardt, M. and Sorkin, E. *Int. J. Cancer 23,* 110 (1979).
Nunn, M.E., Dieu, J.Y., Glaser, M., Lavrin, D.H. and Herberman, R.B. *J. Natl. Cancer Inst. 56,* 393 (1977).
Oehler, J.R., Lindsay, L.R., Nunn, M.R. and Herberman, R.B. *Int. J. Cancer 21,* 204 (1978).
Oleinick, A. *J. Natl. Cancer Inst. 43,* 775 (1969).
Oldham, R.K., Djeu, J.Y., Cannon, G.B., Swarski, D., and Herberman, R.B. *J. Natl. Cancer Inst. 55,* 1305-1318.
Osband, M. and Parkman, R. *J. Immunol. 121,* 179 (1978).
Outzen, H.E., Custer, R.Ph., Eaton, G.-J. and Prehn, R.T. *J. Retic. Soc 18,* 1 (1975).
Parkman, R. and Rosen, F.S. *J. Exp. Med 144,* 1520 (1976).
Penn, I. *Transpl. Proc. 9,* 1121 (1977).
Peter, H.H., Pavie-Fischer, J., Fridman, W.H., Aubert, C., Césarini, J-P., Roubin, R. and Kourilsky, F.M. *J. Immunol. 115,* 539 (1975).

Pross, H.F., and Jondal, M. *Clin. exp. Immunol.* *21,* 226 (1975).
Pross, H.F., and Baines, M.G. *Int. J. Cancer* *18,* 593 (1976).
Radov, L.A., Haskill, J.S., Korn, J.H., Fett, J.W. *J. Natl. Cancer Inst.,* *62,* 103 (1979).
Rygaard, J., and Povlsen, C.U. *Transplantation Rev.* (G. Möller ed.) *28,* 43, Munsgaard, Copenhagen.
Sala, O., and Ferlito, A. *Otolaryngol* *81,* 353 (1976).
Santoni, A., Herberman, R.B. and Holden, T.H. *J. Natl. Cancer Inst.* *62,* (1979).
Sendo, F., Aoki, T., Boyse, E.A. and Buafo, C.K. *J. Natl. Cancer Inst.* *55,* 603 (1975).
Sharky, F.E. and Fogh, J. *Cancer Res.* *39,* 833 (1979).
Shellam, G.R. and Hogg, N. *Int. J. Cancer* *19,* 212 (1977).
Snyderman, R., Meadows, L., Holden, W. and Wells, S. *J. Natl. Cancer Inst.* *60,* 737 (1978).
Stutman, O. *Science* *183,* 534 (1974).
Stutman, O. "Advances in Cancer Research", 22, 261, (Ed. G. Klein & S. Weinhouse), Academic Press (1975).
Stutman, O. in "The nude mouse in experimental and clinical research", (J. Fogh and B.C. Giovanella, eds.), p. 414, Academic Press, New York. (1978).
Svennevig, J.L., Closs, O., Harboe, M., and Svaar, H. *Scand J. Immunol.* *7,* 487 (1978).
Takasugi, M., and Mickey, M.R. *J. Natl. Cancer Inst.* *57,* 255 (1976).
Takasugi, M., Ramseyer, A., and Takusugi, J. *Cancer Res.* *37,* 413, (1977).
Tötterman, T.H., Häyry, P., Saksela, E., Timonen, R. and Eklund, B. *Eur. J. Immunol.* *8,* 872 (1978).
Underwood, J.C.E. *Br. J. Cancer* *30,* 538 (1974).
Vose, B.M., Vanky, F., Fopp, M. and Klein, E. *Br. J. Cancer* *38* , 375 (1978).
Warner, N.L., Woodruff, M.F.A. and Burton, R.C. *Int. J. Cancer,* *20,* 146, (1977).
Watt, A.G. and House, A.K. *Cancer,* *41,* 279 (1978).
Yata, J., Desgianges, C., De-Thé, G., Mourali, N., Ellouz, R., Tachibana, T. and Brugere, J. *Biomedicine* *21,* 244 (1974).

NATURAL CELL-MEDIATED CYTOTOXICITY IN HUMAN TUMOR PATIENTS

James T. Forbes
F. Anthony Greco
Robert K. Oldham

Division of Oncology
Vanderbilt University
Nashville, Tennessee

I. INTRODUCTION

Natural cell-mediated cytotoxicity (NCMC) was originally described as a complicating factor in the in vitro demonstration of tumor-specific immunity (1,2,3). Initially the existance of NCMC as a phenomenon was disputed (4) then considered an artifact of the cytotoxicity assay and finally it was recognized as a distinct and reproducible form of cytotoxicity mediated by a definable sub-class of effector cells (4). Since these observations NCMC has become the focus of much research interest and has been implicated as being an integral part of the tumor-host interelationship rather than an impediment to the understanding of this relationship. The results of this extensive research effort from many laboratories into the nature of NCMC have suggested that NCMC may play an acitve role in the in vitro resistance to tumor development and growth (5,6,7,8). This has been supported by the demonstration of both high levels of NCMC and resistance to tumors in nude and neonatally thymectomized mice in which resistance to tumor growth by the traditional cytotoxic T-lymphocyte effector cell is greatly diminished or absent altogether. These observations along with increased knowledge of the nature of NCMC have prompted a re-examination of this phenomenon in human cancer patients. It is of interest to ascertain whether there is any correlation of NCMC activity with the clinical course of cancer patients.

ISBN 0-12-341350-8

II. METHODS

In order to determine the existence of such correlations, NCMC against a single target cell line was tested in the following manner. Briefly, heparinized whole venous blood from normal donors or tumor patients was seperated by centrifugation on discontinous ficoll-hypaque gradients. The interface, rich in mononuclear cells, was washed with balanced salt solution and adjusted to the appropriate cell concentration in RPMI-1640 containing 10 percent fetal calf serum. Various concentrations of these cells were incubated with 10^4 Na $^{51}CrO4$ labeled K-562 target cells for four hours at 37°C. After this incubation the cell free supernatant of each culture was counted in a gamma scintillation counter to determine the levels of released ^{51}Cr and this was related to the cytotoxicity by the following formula:

$$\% \text{ Cytotoxicity} = \frac{\text{lymphocyte mediated release - spontaneous release}}{\text{total incorporation - spontaneous release}} \times 100$$

K-562, a cell line derived from the pleural effusion of a patient with myelogenous leukemia, was chosen as the target cell because of its widespread use on a standard target cell line for human NCMC (4). All data presented are the result of cytolysis at an effector cell: target cell ratio of 50:1. These results were taken from a linear dose-response curve determined for each set of effector cells. Statistical differences between sets of data were tested using the student's t test.

III. RESULTS

A. Reproducibility of NCMC

Central to any discussion of the population dynamics of NCMC is the reproducibility of results in the measurement of this phenomenon. That NCMC is serially reproducible in healthy normal donors has been demonstrated previously by ourselves (9), Levin et al., (10) and confirmed and extended here. Table I demonstrates the high degree of reproducibility of this assay with multiple measurements from the same donors over a nine month interval. The data show only minor variation and suggest that the values for NCMC for the same donor collected at various times may be directly compared. Further evidence for the reproducibility of NCMC is found in Table II which tests the possibility that target cells may represent a

TABLE I. Serial NCMC Values by Healthy Donors on K-562

Donor	Mean percent NCMC on 2-6 occasions over nine months					
T.S.	9±0.4[a]	14±1.0	12±0.6	15±1.7	11±0.7	16±1.0
F.J.	20±0.7	19±1.1	18±1.8	19±1.0		
H.C.	25±2.6	21±2.5	20±1.3			
L.W.	31±1.1	33±1.4	34±1.9			
C.D.	37±1.9	33±2.0				
J.J.	25±2.3	31±1.1				
C.K.	19±0.9	18±0.8				

[a]*Mean percent NCMC ± S.E.*

source of variability in this assay. K-562 seeded at 1 x 10^5 cell/ml and harvested at 24 hour intervals were tested as ^{51}Cr labeled target cells for NCMC by cryopreserved effector cells from a single donor (11). The data indicate that changes in culture kinetics during this period are not a major source of variation in NCMC. These data demonstrate the reproducibility of this assay.

TABLE II. Effect of K-562 Culture Time on NCMC

	Days in culture			
	1	2	3	4
[a]*K-562 in culture (x10^5/ml)*	2.5	5.0	6.8	7.3
Spontaneous release of ^{51}Cr (x ± S.E.)	10±0.4	8±0.3	6±0.5	7±0.2
[b]*NCMC by cryopreserved effector cells*	40±2.1	35±1.6	35±1.1	40±1.8

[a]*Initial cultures seeded at 1 x 10^5/ml.*

[b]*Effector cells from single donor cryopreserved and tested at effector: target ratio of 50:1.*

B. *NCMC by Normal Donors*

Having established that NCMC can be reproduced on a day to day basis it became necessary to establish the baselines for NCMC in normal populations. These data, which are reported elsewhere (9,12) and summarized here in Table III, represent a total sample of over 250 normal non-pregnant individuals who have been screened to exclude those on medication, those with a history of viral infection less than two weeks prior to testing, and those with a personal history of neoplastic or other serious disorders. Further analysis of the normals in Table III shows that among older age groups, males were slightly more reactive than females, but there were no statistically significant differences (at the $p < .05$ level) in cytotoxicity associated with gender. When considered alone, young males (age 11-20) were more reactive than males between the ages of 21 and 50 ($.01 > p > .001$). Males above 50 years of age were also more reactive than those between 21 and 50 ($p < .05$). There were no significant age related differences in the females tested. This study also demonstrated that neither pregnancy nor parity significantly altered the NCMC among the populations tested. These data (Table III) serve as the baseline values with which to compare the NCMC of cancer patients.

TABLE III. NCMC Values in the Normal Population

Age-Group	*Number tested*	*NCMC*[a]
11-20	*29*	*31.50 ± 2.31*
21-30	*89*	*21.10 ± 1.93*
31-40	*35*	*24.94 ± 2.86*
41-50	*38*	*23.19 ± 1.73*
51-60	*23*	*24.99 ± 2.94*
>60	*49*	*27.08 ± 2.30*

[a]*Mean percent ± S.E. at effector: target = 50:1*

C. Patients with Small Cell Carcinoma of the Lung.

Studies were designed to evaluate the NCMC of peripheral blood lymphocytes from patients being treated for small cell carcinoma of the lung (SCC), an extremely anaplastic and rapidly growing tumor (13). This disease has been demonstrated to be remarkably responsive to chemotherapy (14) and as such represents a good model to assess NCMC in relationship to tumor burden. Patients with this disease may be initially classified according to the extent of their disease as either limited (disease limited to one hemithorax) or extensive (disease in both lungs or outside of the chest). The values for NCMC from patients with either limited or extensive SCC are shown in Figure 1. These data demonstrate that among those patients with limited disease the NCMC values are not significantly different from normal (Table III) prior to chemotherapy but fall during and after chemotherapy. Those patients with extensive stage SCC show a similar low NCMC when on chemotherapy ($p<.05$). There are currently too few pretherapy values for analysis of change with treatment.

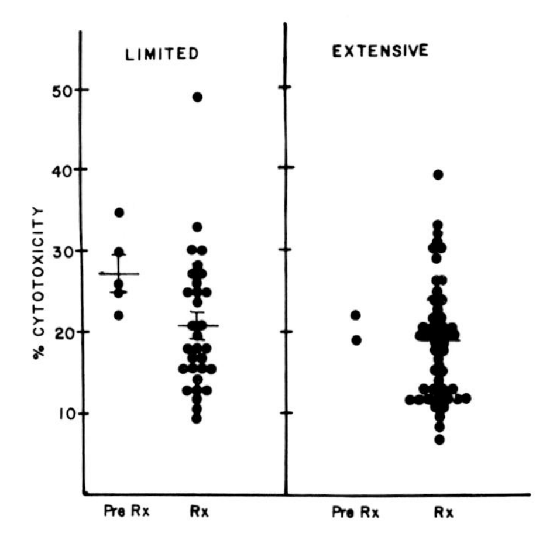

FIGURE 1. NCMC from patients with limited or extensive small cell carcinoma tested prior to and during therapy.

Initial examination of these data would suggest that the decrease in levels of NCMC associated with patients being treated is due to the treatment. These limited stage patients were treated as described by Greco et al (14) and received induction therapy consisting of radiation therapy in association with cyclophosphamide, adriamycin, and vincristine every three weeks for six cycles followed by consolidation therapy with VP-16-213 and hexamethylmelamine for 3 cycles. Those patients in complete remission at this time were randomized to methotrexate alone or with Corynebacterium parvum for seven months. Almost all (90%) of these patients initially showed a complete clinical response to this treatment. The NCMC of patients receiving such therapy is shown in Figure 2. The data in Figure 2 are divided according to those patients who are receiving chemotherapy and those patients who are disease free and not receiving chemotherapy. The data indicate that both groups are below normal but that the group receiving chemotherapy is the lowest. Those patients receiving

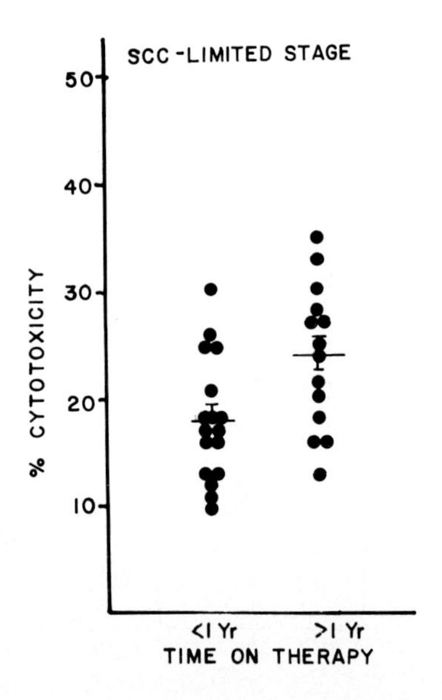

FIGURE 2. NCMC for patients with limited stage small cell carcinoma receiving chemotherapy (< 1 yr.) or those having finished chemotherapy (> 1 yr.).

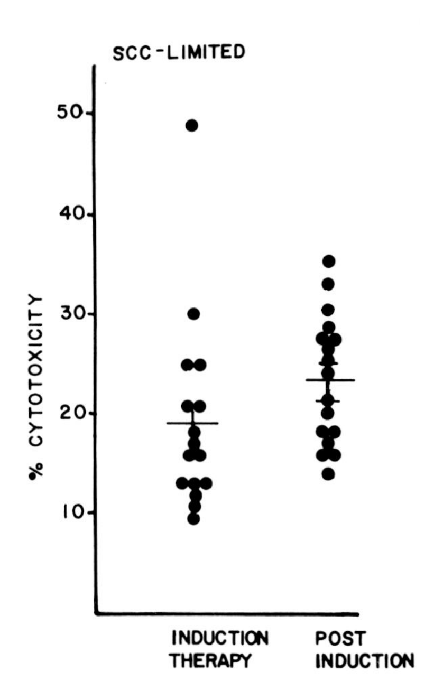

FIGURE 3. NCMC for patients with limited stage small cell carcinoma during induction therapy or following induction therapy.

induction therapy (cyclophosphamide, adriamycin, and vincristine), the most intense phase of the treatment, are only slightly less reactive in NCMC (Figure 3) than those receiving consolidation or maintainence therapy. These data suggest that perhaps chemotherapy regimen can affect levels of NCMC. The difference between these groups is not statistically significant ($p>0.1$).

That chemotherapy is not solely responsible for the decrease in NCMC in these patients is supported by the data in Figure 4. These data are NCMC values of blood from patients with extensive small cell carcinoma (disease outside of one lung). These patients were all being treated with chemotherapy (cyclophosphamide, adriamycin, vincristine, and methotrexate) and prophylactic radiation (10 x 300 rads) to the brain. Those patients not in remission are generally sicker, protein depleted and have a lower performance status than those whose disease is in remission. As seen in Figure 4 those patients in remission have lower NCMC than those patients in relapse. These data would suggest that NCMC levels are related to tumor burden and that when the tumor

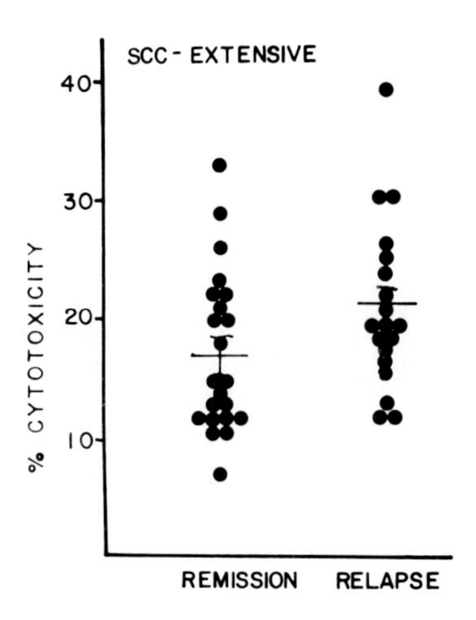

FIGURE 4. NCMC for patients with extensive stage small cell carcinoma either in clinical remission or relapse.

burden is high the NCMC is elevated and this value is decreased when the tumor burden is decreased. Re-examination of the data in Figures 1-3 would also support this hypothesis as tumor burden would be highest in the pretreatment population and would be lowest in those patients undergoing intensive treatment (Figure 1).

This interpretation of these data is further supported when serial values for NCMC from each of three selected individuals are compared with the clinical history of each of those patients (Figure 5). All three of these patients (C.S., W.H., and R.C.) had limited stage small cell carcinoma and demonstrated complete responses to chemotherapy (cyclophosphamide, adriamycin, and vincristine) and radiotherapy with complete disappearance of all clinical signs and symptoms of disease. Two of these patients (C.S. and W.H.) were tested for NCMC against K-562 prior to the initiation of therapy and this value was the highest obtained for these patients. Subsequent values obtained when the tumor burden of these patients was greatly reduced were also reduced. Patient R.C. who had demonstrated a complete response and clinical remission following therapy suffered a recurrence of disease at 16 months after beginning treatment. This clinical recurrence was predated and accompanied by an increase in the levels of

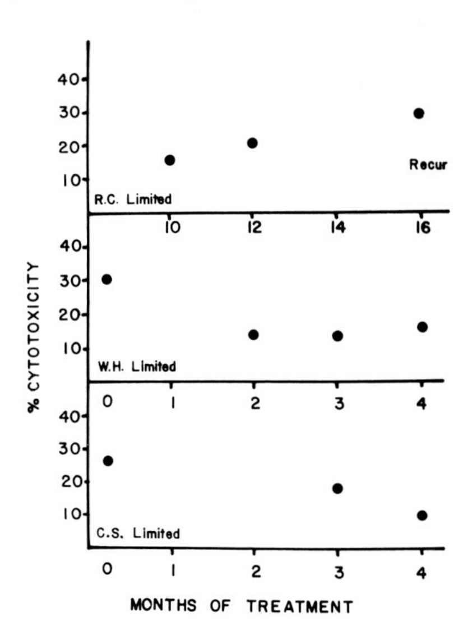

FIGURE 5. NCMC serial values for three patients with limited stage small cell carcinoma.

NCMC against K-562. These data are preliminary and no attempt has yet been made to assess the accuracy of the serial measurement of NCMC for predicting tumor burden.

D. *NCMC in Patients with Resectable Non-Small Cell Carcinoma of the Lung*

Tests of NCMC from patients suffering from resectable non small cell carcinoma of the lung are shown in Figure 6. These patients were tested preoperatively and from 3 to 24 months postoperatively. All were $T_1N_0M_0$ or $T_2N_0M_0$ at the time of surgery. Those patients consenting were randomized and treated with intrapleural BCG plus isoniazid or intrapleural saline plus placebo ten days after surgery. These patients are part of a large study effort in resectable lung cancer (Lung Cancer Study Group) and are coded according to treatment. The code has not yet been broken so NCMC values from both the BCG and placebo groups are lumped together. These data are also consistent with the above interpretation that NCMC is directly related to tumor burden as patients who are clinically tumor-free following surgery have lower average NCMC values than patients tested prior to resection.

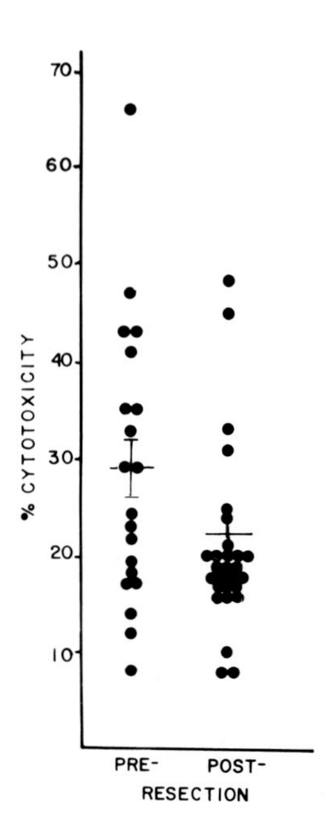

FIGURE 6. NCMC from patients with resectable non small cell carcinoma of the lung pre and post surgery.

E. NCMC in Patients with Melanoma

Similar results may be observed with melanoma patients receiving adjuvant therapy following surgery (Figure 7). These patients are about equally divided between resected stage one and two and were randomized to adjuvant therapy with BCG plus either Me CCNU or DTIC. Those patients remaining clinically disease-free have substantially lower values for NCMC than those patients which demonstrated a recurrence of their disease.

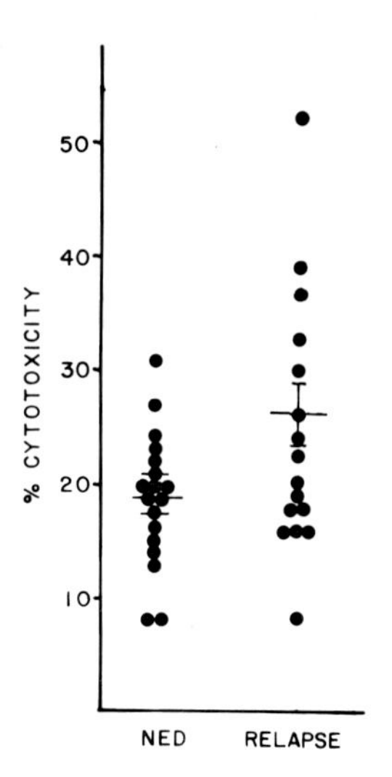

FIGURE 7. NCMC from stage one and stage two resected melanoma patients who are either clinically disease free or have suffered a relapse.

TABLE IV. Summary of NCMC in Cancer Patients

		Stage of treatment		
Disease	Pre-therapy	Chemotherapy	Post-Therapy	Recurence
A. Small Cell Carcinoma of the Lung				
1. Limited	27.6±2.3[a]	18.0±1.5	23.8±1.8	24.3±1.8
2. Extensive	20[b]	17.3±1.4	16.1±1.4	21.2±1.6
B. Non-Small Cell Carcinoma of the Lung (Resectable $T_1N_0M_0$ or $T_2N_0M_0$)	28.8±3.2		22.3±1.9	19.0±3.8
C. Melanoma (Stage I and II)	37.6±5.1	13.3±3.2	19.8±1.5	23.5±2.2

[a]Mean % NCMC ± SE

[b]Too few entries for evaluation

F. Summary of NCMC in Cancer Patients

A summary of the NCMC values for all cancer patients tested is presented in Table IV. This summary shows data in agreement with the hypothesis that the level of NCMC is in direct proportion to the tumor burden. This is in opposition to the results of another immunologic assay: the high affinity T-cell rosette tested on these same individuals and summarized here (Figure 8). We have previously reported (15) that this parameter is inversely proportioned to tumor burden.

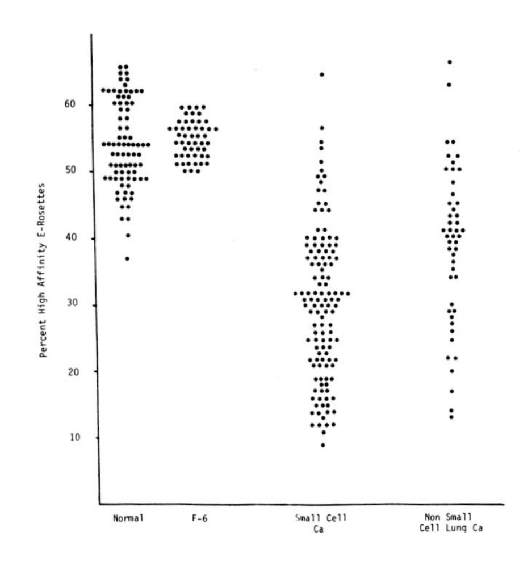

FIGURE 8. High affinity (29 C) T-cell rosette forming cells in the peripheral blood of normal individuals as compared with those having small cell carcinoma of the lung or resectable non small cell carcinoma of the lung. Cryopreserved normal standards (F-6) are run as technical controls.

IV. DISCUSSION

Early studies demonstrated that lymphocytes from cancer patients or animals bearing experimental tumors were cytotoxic in a specific manner for target cells cultured from the same tumor (16,17,18,19). More rigorous testing lead to the observation that lymphocytes from normal donors were often equally as cytotoxic as lymphocytes from tumor patients for these cells (1). This observation provided difficulty for using cytotoxicity as a means of assessing the anti-tumor immunoreactivity of a tumor patient as it was reasoned that this natural cytotoxicity might co-exist with any tumor related cytotoxicity (4,5,6,7,8). Since the specificities of this natural cell-mediated cytotoxicity and the disease induced cytotoxicity were unknown and could be distinct or overlapping then further use of cytotoxicity as an assay of tumor-specific immunity was obviated until more was learned of the nature and specificity of NCMC.

The *in vivo* significance of NCMC is, as yet, unclear. However, the presence of active NCMC in nude mice and neonatally thymectomized mice provides a potential mechanism for the resistance of these T cell immunologically deficient mice to *in vivo* carcinogenesis (4). Further evidence includes the nude mice (these mice have very high levels of NCMC)(20,21,22). Tumors that do arise in nude mice are resistant to NCMC and those tumors known to be sensitive to NCMC demonstrate poor growth when transplanted to nude mice (4). Kiessling (23,24) has shown a strong correlation between the levels of NCMC in several mouse strains and the transplantation resistance of F_1 hybrids between these strains and parental strain mice to parental strain lymphoma. NCMC has also been suggested as a mechanism for the rejection of Hh loci incompatible bone marrow grafts (8,25). Indeed, a number of similarities between natural cytotoxicity and hybrid resistance have been noted.

All previous studies of the level of NCMC in tumor-bearing mice and patients have shown depression of this function (26, 27,28,29,30). Most of these models have dealt with hosts which support a large tumor burden and this may be responsible for their depression. The results of our studies, shown above, have been in basic agreement with this prior observation that NCMC is depressed in tumor patients ($P<.05$). These studies, however, differ from those previously reported in one significant point. Some attempt has been made to correlate NCMC with tumor burden by using models in which the disease responds dramatically to chemotherapy or is potentially curable by surgery. These models include small cell carcinoma of the lung which is remarkably susceptible to chemotherapy which can induce rapid changes in tumor-burden as well as resectable non small cell lung cancer and locally resectable melanoma in which surgical ablation is potentially curable. This categorization by tumor burden is not exact since this assessment is clinical in nature and is subject to limitations of detection. Thus, in a real sense, a patient who suffers a recurrence of previously undetectable tumor has never truly been tumor-free. However, for the purpose of this study those patients without detectable clinical signs or symptoms are considered clinically tumor-free and probably have a smaller tumor burden.

Our studies have shown that almost all tumor patients have depressed levels of NCMC when compared to age-matched normal controls, as has been previously reported. Those patients with recurrent tumors tend to have higher levels of NCMC than their disease-free counterparts. When patients with small cell carcinoma of the lung are studied carefully, it can be seen that those patients being treated for limited disease have lower levels of NCMC than patients from the same category prior to treatment. Among those patients treated for limited disease, NCMC levels are higher prior to completion of therapy than after completion of therapy. During therapy NCMC is lowest during the most agressive phase of chemotherapy and rises during less intense treatment. The most reasonable alternative interpretations of these data are that NCMC is depressed by chemotherapy or that the increased NCMC is correlated with an increased tumor burden. When NCMC is assessed in patients with extensive small cell carcinoma of the lung, all of whom receive chemotherapy, those patients whose disease is in remission have lower values for NCMC than those patients in relapse. This observation would favor the hypothesis that NCMC is correlated more with tumor burden than with chemotherapy.

When the levels of NCMC are determined for patients with non-small cell carcinoma of the lung further support for the above hypothesis is found. Those patients tested prior to surgery, who have known disease, have higher levels of NCMC than those post-surgery patients that are clinically disease free. Since none of these patients are being treated with immunosuppressive chemotherapy then the observed difference cannot be interpreted to be due to drug effects. A similar interpretation can be applied to the data on NCMC levels in melanoma patients receiving adjuvant chemotherapy following surgery for their disease. Since all of these patients are receiving chemotherapy for their disease then this cannot explain the higher NCMC in those patients with recurrent disease as compared to clinically tumor-free patients.

Serial observations of NCMC levels in individual patients with small cell carcinoma of the lung provide further evidence for the direct relationship between tumor-burden and NCMC.

These preliminary data suggest that NCMC against K-562 rises or falls with increases or decreases in the amount of clinically detectable tumor. These data suggest that NCMC may be useful or a marker for tumor recurrence although the reliability and sensitivity of this assay is as yet unknown.

The direct relationship of the level of NCMC to tumor burden would suggest that this reaction is part of the host's defense against neoplastic growth in human disease. Further knowledge concerning their relationship awaits more understanding of the specificity and dynamics of this reaction.

ACKNOWLEDGMENTS

This study supported in part by contract NCI-CB-64007-31 from the National Cancer Institute.

REFERENCES

1. Oldham, R.K., Siwarski, A., McCoy, J., Plata, E., and Herberman, R., Natl Cancer Inst Monogr 37;49, (1973).
2. Herberman, R., Nunn, M., Lavrin, D.H., and Asofsky, R. J Natl Cancer Inst 51:1509, (1973).
3. Rosenberg, E.B., McCoy, J.L., Green, S.S., Donnelly, F.C., Siwarski, D.R., Lerine,P.H., and Herberman, R.B., J Natl Cancer Inst 52:345, (1974).
4. Herberman, R.B. and Holden, H.T. Adv in Cancer Res 27:505, (1978).
5. Skov, C.B., Holland, J.M., and Perkins, E.H., J Natl Cancer Inst 56:193, (1976).
6. Fidler, I.J., Caines, S., and Dolan, Z. Transplantation 22:208, (1976).
7. Gillete, R.W., and Fox, A. Cell Immunol 19:328, (1975).
8. Bonmassar, E., Campanile, F., Houchens, D., Crino, L., and Goldin, A. Transplantation 20:343, (1975).
9. Forbes, J.T., and Oldham, R.K. Fed. Proc. 37:1591, (1978).
10. Levin, A.C., Massey, R.J., and Deinhardt, F. J Natl. Cancer Inst. 60:1283, (1978).
11. Oldham, R.K., Dean, J.H., Cannon, G.B., Ortaldo, J.R., Dunstan, G., Applebaum, F., McCoy, J.L., Djeu, J., and Herberman, R.B., Int J Cancer, 18:145, (1976).
12. Forbes, J.T., Niblack, G.D., Fuchs, R., Richie, R.E., Johnson, H.K., and Oldham, R.K. Submitted for publication.
13. Muggia, R.M., Krezoski, S.K., and Hansen, H.H. Cancer, 34:1683, (1969).

14. Greco, F.A., Richardson, R.L., Snell, J.D., Stroup, S.L., and Oldham, R.K., Amer J Med. 66:1979.
15. Oldham, R.K., Neese, J.L., Herberman, R.B., Perlin, E., Mills, M., Heims, W., Blom,J., Green,D., Reid, J., Bellinger, S., Law,I., McCoy, J.L., Dean,J.H., Cannon, G.B., and Djeu, J. Int J Cancer 18:739, (1976).
16. Hellstrom, I. Int J Cancer 2:65, (1967).
17. Hellstrom, K.E., and Hellstrom, I. Adv Immunol. 18:209, (1974).
18. Takasugi, M., and Klein, E. Transplant Rev. 9:219, (1970).
19. Bubenik, J., Perlmann, P., Helmstein, K., and Moberger, G. Int J Cancer 5:39. (1970).
20. Ruggard, J., and Povlsen, C.O. Transplant. Rev. 28:43, (1976).
21. Stutman, O. Science 183:534, (1974).
22. Outzen, H.C., Custer, R.P., Easton, G.J., and Prehn, R.T. J Reticuloendothel. Soc 17:1, (1975).
23. Kiessling, R., Petranyi, G., Klien, G., and Wigzell, H. Int. J. Cancer 15:933, (1975).
24. Petranyi, G., Kiessling, R., Povey, S., Klein, G., Herzenberg, E., and Wigzell, H. Immunogenetics 3:15, (1976).
25. Gallagher, M.T., Lotzova, E., and Trentin, J.J., Biomedicine 25:1, (1976).
26. Herberman, R.B., Nunn, M.E., and Lavrin, D.H., Int J Cancer 16:216, (1975).
27. Becker, S., and Klein, E. Eur J Immunol. 6:892, (1977).
28. McCoy, J., Herberman, R., Perlin, E., Levine, P., and Alford, C. Proc Amer Assoc Cancer Res. 14:107, (1973).
29. Pross, H.F., and Baines, M.G., Inst. J. Cancer 18:593, (1976).
30. Takasugi, M., Ramseyer, A., and Takasugi, J. Cancer Res. 37:413, (1977).

SYSTEMIC AND IN SITU NATURAL KILLER ACTIVITY IN TUMOR-BEARING MICE AND PATIENTS WITH CANCER

James M. Gerson[1]

Laboratory of Immunodiagnosis
National Cancer Institute
Bethesda, Maryland

I. INTRODUCTION

Natural killer (NK) cells are attracting considerable interest for their possible role in host defenses against cancer, and have been proposed as contributors to immunosurveillance against neoplastic transformation (1). Both murine and human NK cells are nonadherent, nonphagocytic, have receptors for the Fc portion of IgG, and contain markers characteristic of the T-cell lineage (1). A recent important finding has been that the activity of rat, mouse, and human NK cells is augmented by interferon or interferon inducers (2,3,4).

In mice, levels of NK activity have been shown to vary according to the strain and age of the mice tested (5,6), to be inherited as an autosomal dominant trait (7), and numerous studies have provided indirect evidence that NK cells have a role in tumor rejection in vivo (8). Studies of splenic NK activity in mice bearing primary virus-induced or transplantable tumors have shown NK activity to be decreased (5,9,10). However, systemic immune reactivity may not reflect immunologic events at the tumor site (11).

[1]*present address: The Milton S. Hershey Medical Center, Hershey, Pennsylvania*

ISBN 0-12-341350-8

In man, only limited information on the genetics of expression on NK activity is available (12), the levels of activity remain fairly stable over prolonged periods of time and thus appear to be independent of age (13,14), and evidence for the role of NK cells in vivo is lacking. There have been few studies of NK activity in cancer patients and these have focused on systemic or peripheral blood leukocyte (PBL) activity. NK activity of the patients studied appeared to be inversely correlated with stage of disease, but not necessarily tumor burden, for patients with large, localized primary tumors had significant levels of NK activity (15,16,17). The few studies of in situ NK activity have reported low or absent activity (17,18,19).

There are many crucial questions to be answered: 1) why are NK cells ineffective in preventing the initiation of tumor growth at the onset? 2) does decreased systemic activity reflect a selective recruitment or entrapment of NK cells at the tumor site? or 3) the influence of specific or nonspecific suppressor cells or factors? 4) can NK cells enter and persist in tumors? and 5) do NK cells play a role during the growth of established tumors? In an attempt to clarify some of these questions we have studied systemic and in situ NK activity in murine and human tumors of different origins.

II. MATERIALS AND METHODS

Animal Experiments

All animals were obtained from the Division of Research Services, National Institutes of Health, Bethesda, Maryland.

A. Murine-Sarcoma Virus (MSV) Induced Regressor Tumors. Male C57BL/6N and CBA/N mice at 5-8 weeks of age or greater than 10 weeks of age were inoculated intramuscularly in the right hind leg with 0.05 ml of regressor strain M-MUSV as previously described (20). Tumors were first detected at about 7 days, reached peak size at 12-15 days; and consistently regressed after 21 days. Specimens were obtained at peak tumor size.

B. Murine-Sarcoma Virus (MSV) Induced Progressor Tumors. CBA male and female mice at 2-3 weeks of age were inoculated intramuscularly in the right hind leg with 0.05 ml of progressor strain M-MUSV. Nearly all mice had palpable tumors at 5 days after inoculation, and all mice had tumor at 10 days, the time of peak tumor size. The tumors killed 94% of the mice by 49 days. Specimens were obtained at peak tumor size.

C. Spontaneous Mammary Tumors. Primary autochthonous mammary tumors which arose spontaneously in C3H/HeN MTV + mice at approximately one year of age were used. Primary tumors of varying sizes were excised and tested.

Tissue Culture Target Cells: YAC-1, a cell line derived from an A-strain lymphoma, was maintained in suspension culture in RPMI-1640 medium containing 20% heat inactivated fetal calf serum (FCS) (Grand Island Biological Co., Grand Island, New York), 100 units/ml penicillin, 100 ug/ml streptomycin and 1 mM glutamine (complete medium). This line has previously been shown to be a very sensitive target for NK activity, and was used as the target cell for all NK assays. Cells were washed with complete medium and prepared at a concentration of 10^7 per ml and labelled with ^{51}Cr for 45 minutes at 37°C.

Preparation of Effector Cells.

Spleen cells. Spleen cell suspensions were prepared from tumor-bearers (TB-SC) and from age matched controls (NSC). In all instances except for experiments with spontaneous mammary tumor bearing mice, spleens from 3-5 mice were pooled. For the latter, individual mice were tested.

Tumor cell suspensions. Tumors were aseptically excised at the time intervals mentioned above, weighed, disaggregated with a scalpel to 2-3 mm fragments, and then sequentially digested with enzymes to obtain a single cell suspension (CfT). The enzyme treatments were done with 125 mg % collagenase (Sigma, Type I, St. Louis, Missouri) and DNAse and consisted of three - 30 minute digests with stirring at 37°C in a 5% CO_2 atmosphere. The resultant single cell suspensions were pooled, washed with complete medium, and filtered through double layered gauze to remove clumps. It should be noted that enzyme lots were pre-screened to insure no effect on NSC NK activity. Tumors from 3-5 mice were pooled for each experiment with the exception of the spontaneous mammary tumors which were tested individually.

Separation of CfT by adherence. CfT were incubated for 1 hour at 37°C in a 5% CO_2 atmosphere in plastic petri dishes (Corning Glass Works, Corning, New York) at a concentration of ~2 x 10^6 cells/ml. The dishes were vigorously washed twice with complete medium to obtain the non-adherent cell fraction (CfT-NA). The cells adherent to the petri dishes were removed with a rubber policeman (CfT-ADH).

Removal of phagocytic cells from CfT. 20 x 10^7 CfT in 20 ml complete medium were incubated with 2 mg of carbonyl iron at a concentration of 10 mg/ml FCS in a 50 ml conical tube. The mixture was incubated at 37°C in a 5% CO_2 atmosphere on a rocker for 1 hour. Then to yield the non-phagocytic CfT (CfT-NP), the iron ingesting cells were removed by magnet. The percent of macrophages was determined by latex ingestion.

Assay for NK activity. Effector cells were mixed with 5 x 10^3 ^{51}Cr labelled target cells at effector to target ratios of 100:1, 30:1, and 10:1 in 35 mm petri dishes (Corning Glass Works, Corning, New York). The cells were incubated for 4 hours at 37°C in a 5% CO_2 atmosphere on a rocker platform. Unlabelled autologous target cells in place of effector cells served as baseline control to determine spontaneous release. Results are expressed as % cytotoxicity =

$$\left[\frac{(A-B) - (C-B)}{T - B}\right] \times 100$$

where A = mean counts per minute (cpm) released in the test combination, B = mean cpm of machine background, C = mean cpm of autologous control, and T = mean cpm of total ^{51}Cr incorporated into 5 x 10^3 target cells. Significance of cytotoxicity was assessed by two-tailed students' t-test.

Suppression of NK activity. CfT and their subpopulations were tested for their ability to inhibit the NK activity of NSC of 6 week-old CBA mice. The details of the inhibition assay have been described previously (21). Briefly, NSC at an attacker to target cell ratio of 50:1 were used to assess NK activity against 5 x 10^3 ^{51}Cr labelled YAC-1 target cells. The CfT and subpopulations were added as inhibitor ratios. The assay was set up in triplicate in 35mm petri dishes and incubated for 4 hours at 37°C on a rocker platform. The percent inhibition of cytotoxicity was calculated by the formula

$$\left[\frac{1-E}{C}\right] \times 100$$

where E = experimental % cytotoxicity and C = control %

cytotoxicity without inhibitors percent. YAC-1 served as the positive control inhibitor cells and thymus cells as the negative control.

Human Experiments

Systemic (PBL) NK activity was tested on 27 patients with cancer prior to treatment. Of this group 18 were also tested for in situ NK activity.

Peripheral Blood Leukocytes (PBL). PBL were obtained by centrifugation of heparinized whole blood on Ficoll-Hypague (22). The PBL were washed and suspended in complete media plus 10 mM HEPES buffer.

Tumor Cell Suspensions. Biopsy specimens were received on wet ice in complete medium within 4 hours of surgery. Necrotic tissue was debrided, the specimen was dissociated into 2-3 mm fragments with scalpels, and then sequentially digested with 125 mg% collagenase (Sigma, Type I, St. Louis, Missouri) and DNAse. The cell-rich supernatants were pooled, washed with complete media and passed through double layered gauze to remove clumps. The cells from the tumor (CfT) were then either incubated overnight in plastic flasks (Corning Glass Works, Corning, New York) at a concentration of 2 x 10^6 cells/ml in 37°C - 5% CO_2 atmosphere or cryopreserved. The following day, the cells were vigorously washed twice to obtain CfT-NA. The CfT or CfT-NA was then separated by several procedures in an attempt to obtain an enriched or pure lymphocyte population.

Discontinuous Sucrose Gradient. We adopted the method developed by Fauci et al. (23) to obtain lymphocytes from human bone marrow. Sucrose was layered by pipet in 2 ml aliquots at 5% increments from 15-35% sucrose in a 17 x 100 Falcon plastic tube. Two milliliters CfT or CfT-NA was overlayed by pipet at a concentration of 25-30 x 10^6 cells per ml and the gradient was centrifuged for 7 minutes at 100 g at 24°C. The fractions were removed by pipet from above, washed, and tested for NK activity.

Linear Density Gradient (LDG) of Ficoll. A linear isokinetic gradient of Ficoll, ranging from 2.7 to 5.5%, has been shown by Pretlow et al. (24) to be effective in separating lymphocytes from tumor cells and stromal cells. We have previously characterized PBL separated by this method for NK activity (25). In brief, the LDG was made utilizing a

2-chambered gradient maker (Lido Glass, Sterling, New Jersey) and a peristaltic pump with a flow rate of 1 ml/min. The gradient was layered over a 5.5 ml cushion of 43% Ficoll (Pharmacia, Piscataway, New Jersey) in a siliconized 100 ml polycarbonate tube and ranged from 2.7% at the sample gradient interface to 5.5% at the gradient cushion interface. Linearity was monitored by refractive index determination. Thirty to 50 x 10^6 viable cells in 7.0 ml were layered onto the gradient and spun at 97g at 4°C for 17 min. Twenty-four fractions were then collected by displacement with 40% sucrose via a tapping cap (Halpro, Rockville, Maryland). The cells were washed in complete medium and fractions tested for NK activity.

Nylon Column Passage. CfT or CfT-NA were passed through a nylon column according to the method of Julius et al. (26) to remove loosely adherent cells and to enrich for T-lymphocytes.

Cytotoxicity. NK activity was assayed in a 4 hour ^{51}Chromium release assay (CRA) using the human myeloid line, K-562, as target cells. The assay was run in microplates (Linbro, Hamden, Connecticut), in triplicate, and at attacker to target ratios of 100:1, 50:1, and 25:1. Percent cytotoxicity was calculated as shown above.

Competitive Inhibition Assay. This assay has been previously described in detail (21). Briefly, tumor cell suspensions were tested for their ability to inhibit or suppress the cytotoxicity of normal PBL against ^{51}Cr-labelled K-562 target cells in a 4 hour assay. The assay was run in triplicate, in 12 x 75 mm glass tubes in a 1.0 ml volume. The effector to target ratio was kept constant at 50:1 and the number of inhibitors added was varied from 4-fold excess to 6% of the normal PBL. Results are expressed as % inhibition =

$$[1 - \frac{E}{C}] \times 100$$

where E = experimental and C = control % cytotoxicity without inhibitors present.

III. RESULTS

Animal Experiments

A. MSV - Induced Regressor Tumors in C57BL/6N and CBA Mice.

Systemic NK activity. (Table I) Tumor-bearing animals had depressed levels of NK activity relative to age matched controls tested in the same experiment. The level of activity was influenced by the age of the mice tested.

In situ NK activity. (Table I) NK activity was detectable in mice 5-8 weeks of age with the level of activity paralleling that found in the TB-SC. No significant activity was detected in the CfT from mice >10 weeks. Depletion of adherent cells in preliminary experiments resulted in enhanced activity.

B. MSV - Induced Progressor Tumors in CBA Mice.

Systemic and in situ NK activity. (Table II) TB-SC had significantly decreased levels of NK activity compared to age matched normal controls. In situ NK activity, however was very low or undetectable.

TABLE I. Systemic and In Situ NK Activity in Mice Bearing MSV-Induced Regressor Tumors

			Mean % Cytotoxicity[a]			
Strain	*Age*	*# Expt.*	*NSC*	*TB-SC*	*CfT*	*CfT-NA*
C57BL/6N	*5-8 wks.*	*4*	*29.7*	*10.5*[b]	*10.9*	*23.4*[c]
	>10 wks.	*2*	*4.4*	*5.2*	*2.3*	*nt*[d]
CBA	*5-8 wks.*	*3*	*45.3*	*34.2*	*30.9*	*nt*
	>10 wks.	*3*	*5.7*	*4.4*	*1.8*	*nt*

[a] *Effector: Target Ratio - 100:1*
[b] $p \leq .05$
[c] $p \leq .05$
[d] *nt = not tested*

TABLE II. Systemic and In Situ NK Activity in 3-4 Week CBA Mice Bearing MSV - Induced Progressor Tumors

		% Cytotoxicity[a]	
Expt. #	*NSC*	*TB-SC*	*CfT*
1	20.8	10.4	7.0
2	19.3	17.4	1.4
3	27.3	19.8	4.2
4	36.5	9.4	2.2
5	24.0	15.9	3.2
Mean ±S.D.	25.6 ±8.3	14.6 ±4.7[b]	3.6 ±2.3[c]

[a] *Effector: Target Cell Ratio - 100:1*
[b] $p \leq .05$
[c] $p \leq .05$

NK activity after removal of adherent or phagocytic cells. It seemed possible that the very low or negative cytotoxicity results with CfT were due to inhibition or suppression of reactivity rather than to the absence of NK cells. We therefore fractionated the CfT to obtain Cft-NA and CfT-NP. Removal of plastic adherent cells or of phagocytic cells by carbonyl iron ingestion resulted in a marked increase in NK activity (Table III).

Suppression of NK activity by CfT. The finding that removal of adherent or phagocytic cells resulted in enhanced NK activity suggested that the low activity seen in CfT was due to suppression by macrophages. CfT and the various subpopulations were therefore tested for their ability to inhibit the activity of NSC from 4 week old CBA mice. The CfT were found to strongly depress NSC NK activity and their suppressor activity was enriched in the adherent cell fraction. CfT-NA or CfT-NP had substantially less suppressor activity (Table IV). The suppressor activity was not eliminated by treatment with anti-Thy 1.2 plus complement indicating that an adherent, phagocytic cell is most likely responsible for the suppression of NK activity.

TABLE III. Effect of Removal of Adherent and Phagocytic Cells on In Situ NK Activity

		% Cytotoxicity[a]	
Expt. #	CfT	CfT-NA	CfT-NP
1	7.0	18.4	16.0
2	1.4	13.4	8.4
3	4.2	7.7	10.2
4	2.2	6.9	4.3
5	3.2	6.3	7.3
Mean ±S.D.	3.6 ±2.3	10.5 ±5.0[b]	9.2 ±4.5[c]

[a] Effector: Target Cell Ratio - 100:1
[b] $p \leq .05$
[c] $p \leq .05$

C. Systemic and In Situ NK Activity in C3H/HeN Mice with Spontaneous Mammary Tumors. TB-SC NK activity was very low as was that of the normal age matched (approximately 1 year) controls. However, animals with single tumors <2 grams had appreciable in situ activity (Table V). There was an apparent inverse relationship between the primary tumor size and NK activity. In 2 experiments small primary tumors were removed from mice bearing multiple tumors. In both instances in situ NK activity was negligible suggesting that expression of NK activity is influenced by the total tumor burden.

Human Experiments

Systemic (PBL) NK Activity. PBL NK activity was tested in 27 patients with various cancers prior to treatment. Nearly all patients had local or regional disease. In comparing results from the cancer group with the normal controls, there were significant differences, with the patient group having lower activity (Table VI). However, in analyzing the data by histologic groups with neuroblastoma patients comprising the largest group, it became apparent that the significant difference seen was due to this histologic group, for the remaining patients' NK activity were not significantly different from the controls (Table VI).

TABLE IV. Inhibition of NSC - NK Activity Against YAC-1 Target Cells by CfT and CfT Subpopulations Obtained in CBA Mice

Inhibitor	*Inhibition*[a] *Attacker: Inhibitor Ratio*				
	1/4	*1/2*	*4/1*	*8/1*	*16/1*
YAC	*88*	*82*	*61*	*42*	*20*
Thymus	*5*	*4*	*1*	*0*	*0*
CfT-ADH	*67*	*52*	*28*	*7.5*	*nt*[b]
CfT	*51*	*40*	*30*	*10*	*nt*
CfT[c]	*53*	*32*	*9*	*2*	*nt*
CfT-NA	*24*	*18*	*3*	*2*	*nt*
CfT-NP	*16*	*13*	*2*	*nt*	*nt*

[a] *Mean % Inhibition From 4 Experiments*
[b] *nt = not tested*
[c] *Anti-Thy 1.2 Plus Complement Treated*

In Situ NK Activity. By the methods utilized, in situ NK activity was not detected (Figure 1). It is important to note that the "enriched" effector populations never contained <5% contaminating tumor cells, making competitive inhibition of NK activity by cold target inhibitors a possible explanation.

Competitive Inhibition of NK Activity. Freshly prepared CfT were utilized to test for possible cold target inhibition of NK activity. Inhibition was present at higher inhibitor to attacker ratios (Figure 2).

TABLE V. Systemic and In Situ NK Activity Against YAC-1 on C3H/HeN MTV+ Mice with Spontaneous Mammary Tumors

Tumor Weight (grams)	# Expt.	Mean % Cytotoxicity ± S.D.[a]		
		CfT	TB-SC	NSC
<2	3	15.6 ±4.0[b]	7.1 ±1.6	
<2[c]	2	1.3	nt	
>2	6	4.8 ±2.2[d]	7.6 ±2.6	
	9		6.2 ±3.8	3.9 ±2.2

[a] Effector: Target 100:1
[b] $p \leq .01$
[c] small tumors from mice with multiple tumors
[d] $p \leq .01$

TABLE VI. Systemic NK Activity in Patients and Controls Against K-562 at an Effector: Target Ratio of 100:1

Effector PBL	n	% Cytotoxicity
A. Normal	15	34.8 ±12.9
Cancer	27	22.9 ±14.5[a]
B. Neuroblastoma	11	14.9 ±10.8[b]
Cancer	16	26.6 ±15.3[c]

[a] $p \leq .05$
[b] $p \leq .001$
[c] no significant difference

FIGURE 1. Systemic vs. in situ natural killer activity against K-562 in patients with cancer.

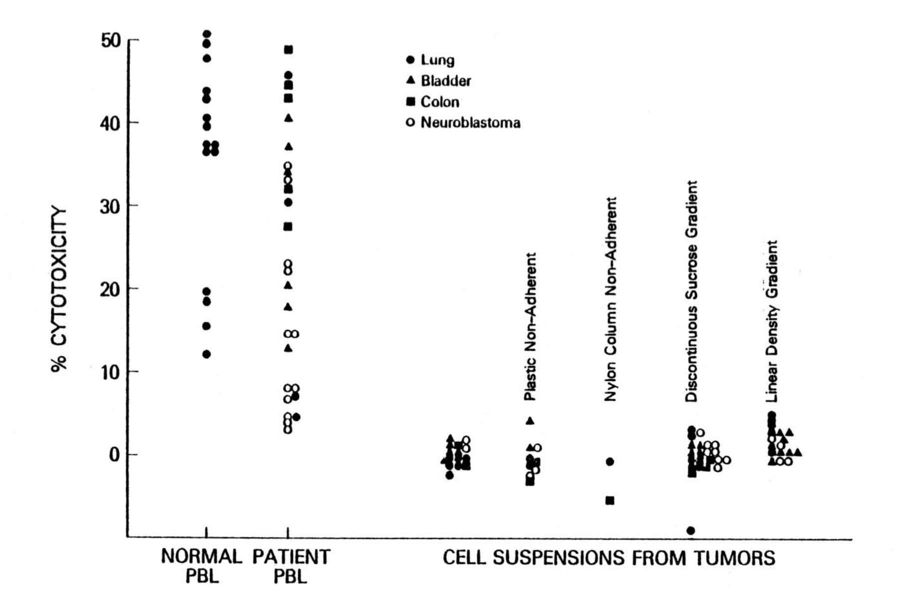

FIGURE 2. Inhibition of natural killer activity against K-562 by single cell suspensions from human solid tumors.

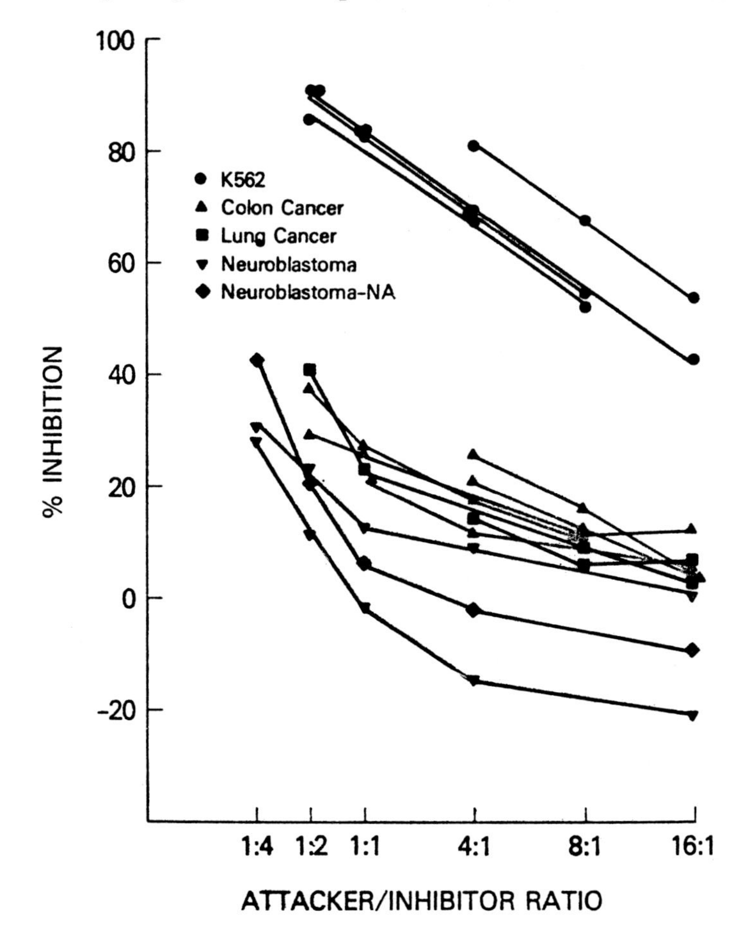

DISCUSSION

The animal experiments demonstrated that NK cells can migrate to or differentiate at the tumor site, and can enter and persist, at least for some time within the tumor. The lack of in situ NK activity seems to reflect the effects of suppressor cells or factors rather than a deficit of NK cells. It is unclear whether the depressed systemic NK activity is secondary to a selective emigration of NK cells to the tumor site, systemic immune suppression or both.

In the MSV regressor and progressor tumor systems, systemic NK activity was depressed and differences were observed in the degree of in situ NK activity. In the former, the level of activity paralleled that present in the spleen, and there was some evidence for an adherent in situ suppressor cell. In the latter, the level of NK activity in situ was much lower than splenic NK activity, and suppressor cells in the CfT were shown to be adherent, phagocytic and resistant to anti-Thy 1.2 plus complement. The causal relation between suppression and the failure of the host to reject his tumor needs further clarification. More direct comparative studies in this system may demonstrate quantitative differences in suppressor cells or different subpopulations of suppressor cells to be present.

Spontaneous mammary tumors in mice is perhaps a better model system to study because of the many similarities that have been made with human breast cancer (27). The results in this system provided strong evidence that NK cells or precursors in older mice are selectively recruited to the tumor site, can possibly differentiate there and be activated. The inverse relationship of tumor burden to the presence of in situ NK activity indirectly suggests that suppressor cells or factors or cold target inhibition by tumor cells can mask expression of activity.

The results of the cancer patient studies showed that PBL-NK activity may be depressed depending on the histology of the tumor. The finding that patients with large primary tumors may have normal systemic NK activity implies that other factors besides tumor burden should be considered in explaining decreased levels of NK activity in patients with more advanced disease.

The in situ studies with human cancer showed that by the methods used, NK activity could not be detected. In that the effector cells never had <5% contaminating tumor cells, the lack of activity may be attributed to possible cold target inhibition by tumor cells. Using CfT, competitive inhibition experiments showed inhibition of normal PBL-NK activity at higher inhibitor to attacker cell ratios. Further studies employing purer CfT subpopulations are necessary to further clarify this observation. In discussing in situ studies it is important to emphasize several technical and methodologic variables. First, the tumor specimen must be representative. Often the mononuclear infiltrate will be around the tumor periphery, and will be missed if a deep biopsy is used. Second, the time interval between surgery and the preparation of the specimen is crucial, for cell degeneration and enzyme release may occur if this interval is too long, thus contributing to an already metabolically toxic milieu. Third, the role of enzymes used to digest the tumor, the length and conditions of the reaction, and the possible effect on normal

NK activity must be considered. Fourth, the cell separation prodecures utilizing gradients separating cells by size and/or density may not differentiate between the blastic tumor cell or lymphoblast and the small tumor cell or mature lymphocyte. Accurate identification of the cell subpopulation is important.

It is apparent that there may not be correlations between systemic and in situ NK activity and that it is essential to consider the tumor milieu as a source of suppressor cells or factors before concluding that the absence of NK activity reflects a deficit of NK cells in situ.

ACKNOWLEDGMENTS

The author wishes to thank Drs. Luigi Varesio, Howard Holden and Ronald Herberman for their expert advise and comments, and Mrs. Nancy Nelson for her help in preparing the manuscript.

REFERENCES

1. Herberman, R. and Holden, H., *in* "Advances in Cancer Research" (G. Klein and S. Weinhouse, eds.), *Vol. 27*, pp. 305-377, Academic Press, New York and London, (1978).
2. Djeu, J.Y., Heinbaugh, J.A., Holden, H.T., and Herberman, R.B., *J. Immunol. 122,* 175 (1979).
3. Einhorn, S., Blomgren, H. and Strander H., *Int. J. Cancer 22,* 405 (1978).
4. Herberman, R.B., Ortaldo, J.R., and Bonnard, G.D., Nature, *277,* 221 (1979).
5. Herberman, R.B., Nunn, M.E., and Lavrin, D.H., *Int. J. Cancer 16,* 216 (1975).
6. Kiessling, R., Klein, E., and Wigzell, H., *Eur. J. Immunol. 5,* 112 (1975).
7. Petramyi, G.G., Kiessling, R., and Klein, G., Immunogenetics *2,* 53 (1975).
8. Herberman, R.B., and Holden, H.T., *J. Natl. Cancer Inst. 62,* 441 (1979).
9. Becker, S., and Klein, E., *Eur. J. Immunol. 6,* 892 (1976).
10. Gerson, J.M., Holden, H.T., Bonnard, G.D., and Herberman, R.B., *Proc. Amer. Assn. Cancer Res. 20,* 238 (1979).

11. Haskill, J.S., Hayry, P., Radov, L.A., *in* "Contemporary Topics in Immunobiology, *8*,107 (1978).
12. Trinchieri, G, Santoli, D., Zmijewski, C.M., and Koprowski, H., *Transpl. Proc. 9*, 881 (1977).
13. Jondal, M. and Pross, H., *Int. J. Cancer 15*, 596 (1975).
14. Takasugi, M., Mackey, M.R. and Terasaki, P.I., *Cancer Res. 33*, 2898 (1973).
15. Pross, H.F. and Baines, M.G., *Int. J. Cancer 18*, 593 (1976).
16. Takasugi, M., Ranseyer, A. and Takasugi, J., *Cancer Res. 37*, 413 (1977).
17. Gerson, J.M. and Herberman, R.B., *in* "Advances in Neuroblastoma Research", Raven Press, New York, New York, in press, (1979).
18. Vose, M.M., Vanky, F., Argov, S. and Klein, E., *Eur. J. Immunol. 7*, 353 (1977).
19. Totterman, T.H., Hayry, P., Saksela, E., Temonen, T. and Eklund, B., *Eur. J. Immunol. 8*, 872 (1978).
20. Lavrin, D.H., Herberman, R.B., Nunn, M. and Soares, N., *J. Natl. Cancer Inst. 41*, 1497 (1973).
21. Herberman, R.B., Nunn, M.E. and Holden, H.T., *in* "In Vitro Methods of Cell Mediated and Tumor Immunity" (R.B. Bloom and J.R. David, eds.), pp. 489-495, Academic Press, New York, NY, (1953).
22. Boyum, A., *Scan. J. Clin. Invest. 21*, 1 (1968).
23. Fauci, A.S., *J. Clin. Invest. 56*, 98 (1975).
24. Pretlow, II,T.G., *Biophys. Chem. 5*, 99 (1976).
25. Gerson, J.M., Chiapella, C. and Ortaldo, J., *Fed. Proc. 38(3)*, 1278 (1979).
26. Julius, M.H., Simpson, E. and Herzenberg, L.A., *Eur. J. Immunol. 3*, 645 (1973).
27. Martin, D.S., Fugman, R.A., Stolfi, R.L. and Hayworth, P., *Cancer Chemother. Rep. 5(2)*, 89 (1975).

NATURAL KILLER CELLS IN TUMOUR-BEARING PATIENTS[1]

Hugh F. Pross[2]

Departments of
Radiation Oncology and Microbiology & Immunology
Queen's University
Kingston, Ontario, Canada

Malcolm G. Baines

Departments of
Obstetrics & Gynecology and Microbiology & Immunology
Queen's University
Kingston, Ontario, Canada

I. INTRODUCTION

The phenomenon of "natural" killer cell activity against tumour target cells was first observed by investigators interested in the ability of lymphocytes from patients with malignant disease to specifically lyse cell line targets derived from tumours similar to that borne by the patient (1-3). Since that time, spontaneous lymphocyte-mediated cytotoxicity (SLMC) (4,5) has progressed from being an annoying incidental observation to being the subject of intense research on the part of virtually every laboratory involved in tumour immunology. Although there are several reasons for this development, two of them relate particularly to cancer. These are, first, the peculiar target cell

[1]*Support for this work was received from the Ontario Cancer Treatment and Research Foundation (HFP) and the Medical Research Council of Canada (MGB).*

[2]*Research Associate of the Ontario Cancer Treatment and Research Foundation.*

ISBN 0-12-341350-8

selectivity of the killer cells, and second, the almost universal occurrence of these cells in human peripheral blood. It is hard to believe that a cell type which is found in virtually every donor, from the neonate (6) to the elderly (7), does not have some important function *in vivo*. Since the *in vitro* activity of these lymphocytes is directed against tumour cells, the obvious inference is that this may be their role *in vivo*, either as a form of surveillance against newly arising malignant clones, or as a mechanism by which the accessible cells of established tumours are destroyed. As is discussed elsewhere in this volume, the evidence from animal models that such a role exists is very compelling. In man, however, the attempt to prove a cause and effect relationship between natural killer cell function and malignant disease has proven to be considerably more difficult. Our own studies on the NK phenomenon, in so far as it relates to cancer, have dealt largely with the effect of malignancy on NK function, on the one hand, and the way in which cytotoxicity is affected by cytoreductive therapy on the other. In this chapter, we will discuss our research on the NK phenomenon as follows: (a) the K562 assay, its advantages and disadvantages; (b) the effect of a specific malignancy, adenocarcinoma of the ovary, on NK function and (c) the sequential analysis of NK activity over the long term.

II. THE K562 ASSAY

Certain characteristics make the K562 line the target of choice for NK experiments, and these are itemized in Table I. Although high NK sensitivity and low spontaneous release are of obvious importance, the combination of these characteristics with HLA-A,B,C and Epstein-Barr nuclear antigen negativity make this line unique. The hoped-for advantage of the latter characteristics was that in a given population of normal or patient donors, the level of cytotoxicity observed against K562 would be uninfluenced by relative differences in HLA between the target and effectors, or by donors' reactivity against EBV antigens. This is indeed the case with respect to reactivity against EBV antigens (8), but extensive studies have not been done comparing NK activity against K562 with HLA typing. This type of study has been done in other systems, in which the target cells express HLA or H2 antigens, and it has been shown that donors with HLA-B7 or HLA-A3, B7 are depressed in spontaneous cytotoxicity (9,10). Whether this is the case using K562

TABLE I. K562 - Target of Choice for NK Assays[a]

1. *Highly sensitive in both 5 hour and overnight assays.*
2. *Low spontaneous release (15% in overnight assays)*
3. *HLA-A,B,C negative (11)*
4. *Epstein-Barr nuclear antigen negative (12)*
5. *Easily maintained suspension culture*
6. *Comparatively insensitive to spontaneous monocyte and granulocyte-mediated lysis.*

[a]*K562 is a continuous cell line derived by Lozzio and Lozzio from the pleural effusion of a patient with chronic myelogenous leukemia in blast cell crisis (13). The NK assay referred to is a ^{51}Chromium release assay using granulocyte-monocyte depleted peripheral blood lymphocytes in various ratios of lymphocyte to labelled K562. The assay is done in V-bottomed microtiter plates and the supernatants are harvested for gamma counting at 5 or 16 hours (5,7).*

has not been reported, although in our own pool of normal donors who have been assessed repeatedly over the last 7 years, at least one of the consistently high donors is HLA-B7.

Another advantage to using the K562 assay is that there is at present considerable interest in the K562 line on the part of cell biologists in general, especially with respect to whether the line is of granulocytic or erythroid origin (12, 14). The wealth of knowledge which is thus accumulating concerning the K562 line can only be of benefit to its use in NK assays. Whatever the exact origin of the line may be, the fact that it is not derived from a common tumour such as carcinoma of the lung or breast is also useful. Although the statement may be controversial, it could be said that the target cell in NK assays should be as different antigenically and developmentally from the common tumours as possible. In this way, "tumour-specific" reactivity on the part of cancer patient lymphocytes would not influence the standard NK assay. By the same reasoning, K562 would presumably be inappropriate for studies of the NK activity of patients with myelogenous leukemia.

There are several disadvantages to the use of K562 for assessing spontaneous cytotoxicity, but most of these apply to cell lines in general. A frequent criticism of our own work is that we usually only employ the one cell line, i.e. K562, and that this may not reflect the true status of patient cell-mediated cytotoxic function. From time to time, we have assessed many different cell lines in comparison with K562 and in none of these experiments did we detect higher NK activity against the other cells than was seen against K562. For several years we assessed NK routinely against the murine mastocytoma line P815 (4), as well as against K562. The rationale behind this was that the xenogeneic assay may give different information from that obtained using the allogeneic assay. Again, in terms of absolute cytotoxicity, K562 was always more sensitive. Furthermore, when the data was expressed as cytotoxicity relative to the normal control, in the majority of patients, the conclusion as to whether NK activity was low or normal was the same irrespective of the assay used (Fig 1). It should be pointed out that the use of certain targets may result in the detection of other types of cell-mediated cytotoxicity. For instance, leukocyte-mediated cytotoxicity against rabbit red blood cells is mediated by granulocytes and monocytes, while NK lymphocytes are ineffective against them (15). In terms of assessing NK (lymphocyte) activity, there appears to be no advantage to using a large battery of targets, whereas the additional cells which are required for these assays could well be used for better things.

A second criticism of the use of K562 as the target involves the fact that these cells are Fc receptor positive. This presents a problem when experiments involving NK inhibition by immune complexes are performed since inhibition may be due to target cell binding of the complexes instead of effector cell binding. It is also possible that NK cytotoxicity is caused by Fc receptor binding between the target and effector by antigen-antibody complexes. To examine this question we have developed a subline of K562 which has a very low proportion of Fc receptors (1-8%), and we have shown no difference between the sensitivity of this line and the parent, Fc receptor-positive K562. Similar results were obtained if Fc-rosette depletion was done to eliminate the last remaining Fc receptor positive K562 cells from the line, presumably ruling out Fc receptor binding as a mechanism of cytotoxicity in this case (unpublished data).

Another problem with the K562 assay is the variability in the apparent sensitivity of the line from assay to assay. This seems to be common to most lines, but it is more obvious with K562 because of the high levels of cytotoxicity which are obtained. As is discussed below, expression of

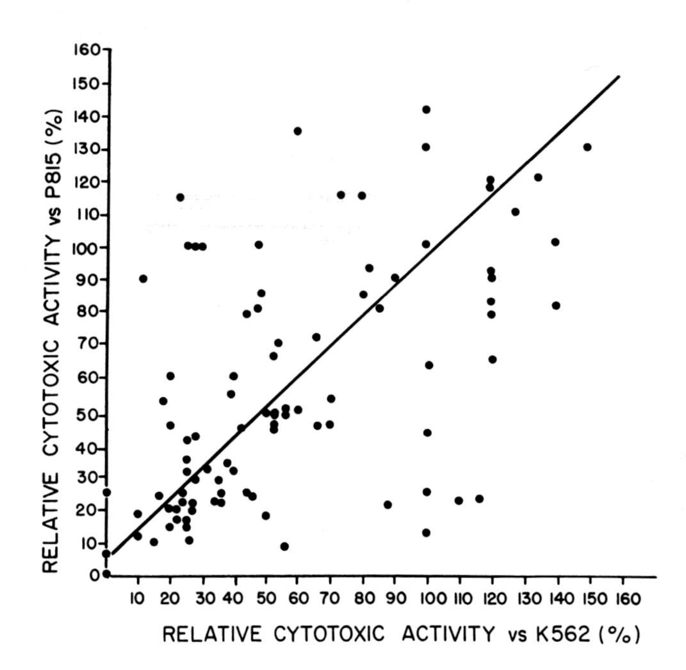

FIGURE 1. Comparison of the relative NK activity of 92 cancer patients using two different target cells, P815 (xenogeneic) and K562 (allogeneic). The solid line is the major axis of the scattergram. The r value for this data is 0.56, with an F variance ratio of 40.59, indicating a positive correlation between the two assays at a level of significance of $p < 0.001$. The relative NK activity was calculated from the patient's lymphocyte dose response curve in comparison with that of the normal control and is the ratio of the number of normal control effector cells to the number of patient effector cells producing the same level of cytotoxicity (7).

the data as relative cytotoxicity in comparison to control values compensates for this variability to some extent.

III. NK ACTIVITY IN PATIENTS WITH ADENOCARCINOMA OF THE OVARY

As with several other immunological functions, natural killer cell activity is reduced in patients with advanced metastatic malignant disease (7). Similar results have been reported in leukemic patients and in patients with solid tumours, especially melanoma (16-20), and have led to a number of interesting speculations as to the role of NK cells in human cancer, especially with respect to their possible function, or lack of it (20), in delaying the onset of metastatic or recurrent disease. At present we are in the process of assessing several different methods of expressing NK function, prior to reporting our accumulated data on several hundred patients. In the meantime, however, we are presenting a portion of this data, obtained from patients with ovarian carcinoma (Table II), and analyzed as described in the legend to Fig 1 (7).

The most striking observation in this table is that relative NK cytotoxicity diminished with the stage of the disease, going from 120% at diagnosis in stage I disease to 18% in stage IV. There was relatively little change in cytotoxicity with treatment and follow-up within each stage, and, if the results prove to be similar after more patients have been entered, the data would suggest that malignant disease *per se* has a more profound effect on NK function than pelvic irradiation and chemotherapy. Although the number of patients with stage IV disease was too minute to allow comparisons between the different follow-up groups, it is tempting to speculate that the patients who did survive longer than three years in spite of their disease, have done so because of their higher levels of relative NK activity.

Table II also points out several problems associated with studying NK in cancer patients. As with all studies on patients with cancer, the necessity of dividing the patients into disease stages, different therapy regimes, or long and short term survivors, results in such small groups that meaningful comparisons are difficult to make. This is compounded by the variability in the assay from time to time, especially in a situation where one is interested in data collected over several years. This is partly overcome by expressing the data in comparison with controls, but some variation is attributable to variability from time to time on the part of an individual donor; which may also include the controls (see below).

IV. SEQUENTIAL ANALYSIS OF NK ACTIVITY

The majority of published data on NK activity in cancer patients has involved comparing the mean cytotoxicity of

TABLE II. Relative Natural Killer Activity in Patients with Ovarian Carcinoma

Stage at diagnosis	Duration of follow-up (years)			
	0	< 1	1-3	> 3
I (9)[a]	120[b] (3) [2.08 ± .08]	77 (7)* [1.89 ± .05]	89 (6) [1.95 ± .12]	84 (6) [1.92 ± .12]
II (5)	74 (4) [1.87 ± .15]	64 (4)* [1.80 ± .06]	59 (4)* [1.78 ± .07]	67 (1) [1.82 ± .11]
III (14)	51 (11)* [1.71 ± .10]	43 (11)*** [1.64 ± .06]	53 (4)* [1.72 ± .12]	54 (2)** [1.73 ± .08]
IV (4)	18 (2)** [1.25 ± .09]	19 (2)** [1.29 ± .10]	40 (2)* [1.60 ± .17]	41 (2)* [1.61 ± .11]

[a]Total patients per group, staged by the FIGO classification. Treatment during follow-up consisted of conventional radiotherapy and chemotherapy. Each patient was assessed on first admission and every 4-6 weeks thereafter (to be reported).

[b]Geometric mean percent NK. Square brackets indicate the log geometric mean percent NK ± standard error, $*p < 0.05$, $**p < 0.01$, $***p < 0.005$, by Student's "t" test, compared with normal controls.

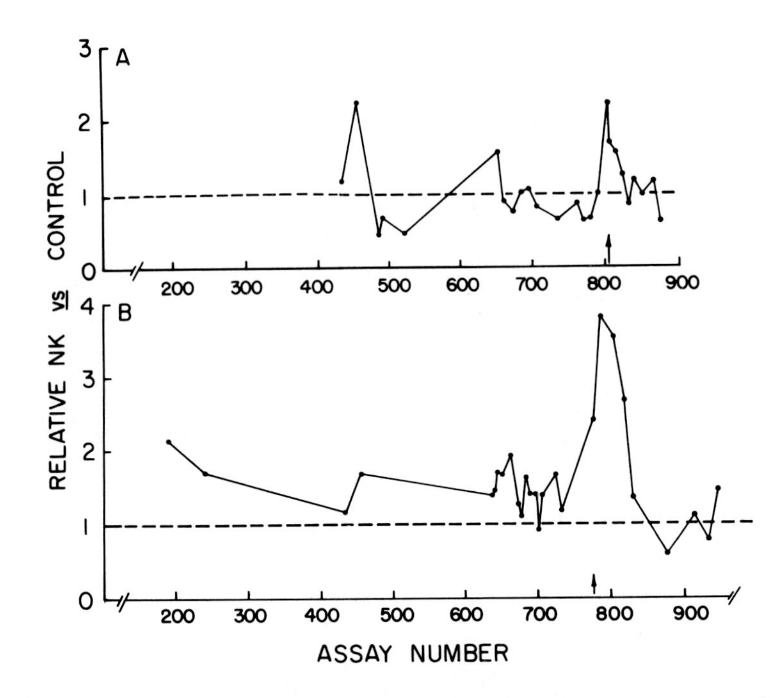

FIGURE 2. Relative NK activity of 2 donors compared to the same normal control donor tested over 5 years. A - Donor MB. The arrow indicates the first "post-diagnosis" assay, done 3 weeks after the onset of severe viral (?) pneumonia. Sputum culture showed mixed bacterial flora. The pneumonia was treated with Bactrim and Erythromycin, and the donor was asymptomatic when the assay was done. B - Donor HR. The arrow indicates the first "post-diagnosis" assay, done 2 days after the onset of a severe viral (?) upper respiratory tract infection with bronchitis and laryngitis lasting 10 days. In this Figure, 100 assays is approximately 30 weeks.

groups of patients in comparison with normals. The sequential analysis of NK activity in individual patients is more difficult primarily because of the difficulty in determining whether a change in cytotoxicity is related to the disease process, its treatment, or is merely a reflection of coincidental minor illness. For the most part we have not observed clear-cut changes in SLMC with minor viral infections. More serious infections can have a definite systemic effect, however. Figure 2 illustrates results obtained from two normal persons who have been regularly tested for 5 years. Over this time it was established that each donor had a level of cytotoxicity characteristic for that person, MB fluctuating at about the same level as the control and HR being consistently higher. In the spring of 1979, each donor had a severe viral infection resulting in pneumonia (Fig 2A) and bronchitis/laryngitis (Fig 2B). In both cases, the disease resulted in a profound increase in NK activity, which returned to normal over the 2 or 3 weeks after symptoms had ceased. These results were interesting in that a systemic illness was seen to have a definite effect on the donors' NK activity. The cytotoxic activity was, of course, unrelated to cancer, further illustrating the difficult task which lies ahead for those who wish to accurately define the effect of malignant disease on NK lymphocyte function.

V. CONCLUSION

Using the K562 assay, it can be shown that natural killer cells are found in the peripheral blood of virtually every normal human being. This killer cell activity was diminished in patients with stage III and IV ovarian carcinoma and was found to be markedly enhanced in 2 normal donors who had severe viral infections. These observations suggest that NK cells respond to systemic illness and may play a role in response to disease. In terms of the *in vivo* relevance of NK cells, the hypothesis that the cells are responsible for anti-tumour surveillance is obviously attractive. Whatever the relevance of the NK lymphocyte *in vivo*, however, there is no doubt that these cells are a very real phenomenon *in vitro*, and must be understood more thoroughly if progress is to be made in the field of human cell-mediated cytotoxicity against tumour target cells.

ACKNOWLEDGMENTS

We are grateful to Mrs. M. Chau, Mrs. J. Tremblay, Mrs. V. Masters and Mrs. B. Milgrom for excellent technical assistance, to Miss J. Milian for chart review, to Miss Helen Roughton for drawing bloods, and to Mrs. Nancy Wainman for typing the manuscript. We would also like to thank Dr. John Carmichael, Department of Obstetrics & Gynecology, and the Cancer Clinic staff for their co-operation in performing these studies.

REFERENCES

1. Oldham, R.K., Siwarski, O., McCoy, J.L., Plata, E.J., and Herberman, R.B., *Natl. Cancer Inst. Monogr. 37*, 49 (1973).
2. Takasugi, M., Mickey, M.R., and Terasaki, P.I., *Cancer Res. 33*, 2898 (1973).
3. Hellstrom, K.E., and Hellstrom, I., *Adv. Immunol. 18*, 209 (1974).
4. Pross, H.F., and Jondal, M., *Clin. Exp. Immunol. 21*, 226 (1975).
5. Jondal, M., and Pross, H.F., *Int. J. Cancer 15*, 596 (1975).
6. Baines, M.G., Pross, H.F., and Millar, K.G., *Am. J. Obstet. Gynecol. 130*, 741 (1978).
7. Pross, H.F., and Baines, M.G., *Int. J. Cancer 18*, 593 (1976).
8. Svedmyr, E., and Jondal, M., *Proc. Natl. Acad. Sci. (Wash.) 72*, 1622 (1975).
9. Petranyi, G., Ivanyi, P., and Hollan, S.R., *Vox. Sang. (Basel) 26*, 470 (1974).
10. Trinchieri, G., Santoli, D., Zmijewski, C.M., and Koprowski, H., *Transplant. Proc. 9*, 881 (1977).
11. Klein, E., Ben Bassat, H., Neumann, H., Ralph, P., Zeuthen, J., Polliack, A., Vanky, F., *Int. J. Cancer 18*, 421 (1976).
12. Lozzio, C.B., and Lozzio, B.B., *Blood 45*, 321 (1975).
13. Lozzio, C.B., and Lozzio, B.B., *J. Natl. Cancer Inst. 50*, 535 (1973).
14. Andersson, L.C., Nilsson, K., Jokinen, M., and Gahmberg, C.G., *Int. J. Cancer 23*, 143 (1979).
15. Banerjee, D., Fernando, L., Sklar, S., and Richter, M., *Submitted for publication.*
16. Takasugi, M., Ramseyer, A., and Takasugi, J., *Cancer Res. 37*, 413 (1977).
17. Menon, M., and Stefani, S.S., *Oncology 35*, 3 (1978).
18. Peter, H.H., Pavie-Fischer, J., Fridman, W.H., Aubert, C., Cesarini, J.P., Rougin, R., and Kourilsky, K.M., *J. Immunol. 115*, 539 (1975).
19. Behelak, Y., Banerjee, D., and Richter, M., *Cancer 38*, 2274 (1976).
20. Livnat, S., Seigneuret, M., Storb, R., and Prentice, R.L., *J. Immunol., in press.*

NATURAL CYTOTOXIC (NC) CELLS IN TUMOR-BEARING MICE[1]

Osias Stutman
Elizabeth Feo Figarella
Roberta Wisun

Cellular Immunobiology Section
Memorial Sloan-Kettering Cancer Center
New York, New York

I. INTRODUCTION

A decrease in natural killer (NK) activity in spleen and blood, was described in mice bearing either transplanted tumors or after development of local tumors induced by the Moloney sarcoma virus (1-3). On the other hand, studies in man showed some decline of NK activity in blood of tumor-bearing patients (4-6), although in many instances, NK levels were comparable to those in normal controls (6-18). No clear correlation with tumor type or tumor load was observed (6-18), athough NK activity tended to be decreased in patients with metastatic disease (6, 8). In the present report we will describe studies with tumor-bearing (TB) mice, showing that natural cytotoxic (NC) cells (19, 20) are well preserved, while NK activity is decreased, especially in spleen of such animals.

II. NC AND NK ACTIVITY IN TUMOR-BEARING MICE

Tables I and II show some of our results. For details on tumors and procedures see our Chapter on "Characterization," as well as references 19 and 20.

[1]*This work was supported by grants CA-08748, CA-15988, and CA-17818 of the National Institutes of Health and grant IM-188 from the American Cancer Society.*

ISBN 0-12-341350-8

TABLE I. NC and NK Cells in Tissue of Tumor-bearing Mice

Tumor Graft[a]	Effector cells[b]	Percent Cytotoxicity[c]			
		NC		NK	
		TB	C	TB	C
Meth A	Spleen	72	75	10	48
Meth A	L. Nodes	81	17	20	12
Meth 113	Spleen	70	76	12	43
Meth 113	L. Nodes	68	14	ND	ND
Meth 113	L. Nodes[d]	70	19	ND	ND

[a]BALB/c hosts were grafted subcutaneously with the syngeneic fibrosarcomas Meth A or Meth 113 (10^6 cells), and tested after 4-6 weeks of tumor growth.

[b]Effector cells for NC or NK assays obtained from tumor bearing and age-matched controls. L. Nodes, represents the pooled peripheral lymph nodes.

[c]NC activity tested against 3H-prelabelled Meth A targets in a 24 hr assay. NK activity measured against 51Cr-labelled YAC-1 cells in a 4 hr assay. The results presented are from cytotoxicity produced by 100:1 effector:target ratios.

[d]The recipients of the tumor graft were splenectomized 3 weeks before tumor grafting.

Table I shows that in mice bearing two different types of transplanted syngeneic chemically-induced fibrosarcomas, NC activity in the pooled peripheral lymph nodes was increased four-fold above the control levels. NC activity in peripheral lymph nodes is usually quite low in normal mice, representing approximately 30% of the activity in spleen (19). Since the tumors were implanted in the nape of the neck, the pooled nodes included those draining the site (i.e. brachial, axillary and cervical) as well as distant nodes. A more detailed study of the lymph node reactivity of TB mice is presently under way. In addition, line 5 in Table I shows that the increase in NC activity in the nodes is not due to a mobilization of NC cells from spleen, since the same type of increase was observed in TB animals which were previously splenectomized. On the other hand, since Meth A and Meth 113, the tumors used as targets and grafts respectively in the experiments, do not have cross-reacting tumor associated antigens (21, 22), the increased lymph node responses are probably not due to specific immune mechanisms.

In contrast with the NC results, Table I shows that NK activity (tested against YAC-1 targets) was consistently depressed in spleens and nodes of those same animals, supporting the published results with NK cells (1-3).

Table II shows a summary of experiments using 4 different types of TB mice: BALB/c mice grafted with the syngeneic tumors; Meth A and Meth 113, as in Table I; DBA/2 mice grafted with the syngeneic P815 mastocytoma and C3H/HeJ females which had developed spontaneous mammary adenocarcinomas (MT). The NC activity of spleen cells was tested against Meth A targets (as in refs. 19,20 & Table I) at different times after tumor grafting or tumor appearance, ranging from 1 to 9 weeks. Again, no significant decline in spleen NC activity was observed in any of the groups when compared to age-matched controls. It should be indicated that at 6-9 weeks Meth A and Meth 113 usually grow as large tumors representing approximately 10% of the body weight of the TB mouse. The same type of results, not shown in the table, were observed at lower effector:target ratios.

TABLE II. NC Activity in Spleen of Different Types of Tumor-bearing Mice

Weeks after tumor graft[a]	*Percent NC Activity of Age-matched Controls*[b]			
	Meth A (BALB/c)	*Meth 113 (BALB/c)*	*P815 (DBA/2)*	*MT (C3H/HeJ)*
1	106	100	98	98
2	125	100	-	100
3	100	98	-	108
4	100	111	-	100
5	98	100	-	97
6	99	97	-	95
7	104	98	-	100
8	96	100	-	-
9	-	96	-	-

[a]*Meth A, Meth 113 and P815 were all transplanted. MT (mammary adenocarcinomas) were the spontaneous tumors appearing in C3H/HeJ females, and the time indicates macroscopic tumor appearance.*

[b]*The indicated tumors (mouse strains in parentheses) were grafted to syngeneic recipients, except the MT which were spontaneous. Meth A and Meth 113 were grafted subcutaneously (10^6 cells) and P815 was grafted intraperitoneally (10^5 cells). All recipients of tumor grafts were 4-6 week old mice. The mean age of appearance for MT in C3H/HeJ virgin females was 270 days of age. Spleen cells from tumor-bearing and age-*

Table II footnotes continued.

matched syngeneic controls were obtained at the indicated times after tumor grafting and tested against 3H-proline prelabelled Meth A target cells in a 24 hr assay (19). The percent cytotoxicity was calculated as in ref. 19 and the presented results were calculated for 100:1 effector:target ratios. Similar results, not shown, were observed at 50 and 10:1 effector:target ratios.

In summary, it is apparent that NC activity in spleen is unchanged in TB mice, while NK activity is usually markedly depressed in those same animals. Since NC activity is measured in a 24 hr assay and NK in a 4 hr, we also tested NK activity of spleens from TB mice in 18 hr assays against RBL-5 targets (3), which also showed low activity (i.e. 19% cytotoxicity for cells from TB mice versus 48% in controls, to cite just one example). Thus, even in longer assays, the NK defect in TB mice can be observed.

The NC activity in spleens of TB mice was mediated by cells that had the same characteristics as NC cells from normal animals (i.e. low adherence to nylon wool, Thy 1-, NK.1-, Ig-, FcR- and non-phagocytic, see our Chapter on "Characteristics" and refs. 19, 20), although due to space limitations we are not presenting those results (this fact also argues against any form of specific immune response explaining the cytotoxic activity of nodes or spleen in the TB animals). Characterization of the NC cells in nodes of TB mice is presently under study.

III. NC ACTIVITY WITHIN GRAFTED TUMORS

Using velocity sedimentation at unit gravity as described in ref. 20, we tested cell suspensions obtained from grafted Meth A or Meth 113 tumors to determine if the NC compartment could be recovered from the local tumor. Our preliminary studies indicate that, indeed, NC cells could be detected in the grafted tumors at 3-4 weeks after transplantation. For example, when the teased tumor cells were separated by velocity sedimentation and the samples divided into two fractions, one with the large fast-migrating tumor cells (i.e. larger than 5 mm/hr) and one with the slow migrating smaller cells, presumably containing the NC cells (i.e. with a velocity of less than 5 mm/hr, as supported by our previous studies for NC activity in spleen, ref. 20), we found cytotoxic activity in both. fractions. For example, 43% cytotoxicity at 100:1 effector:

target ratios for the "large cell" fraction and 82% for the "small cell" fraction, while the spleen from the same animal had 66% cytotoxicity at the same E:T ratio, with comparable results observed with Meth A or Meth 113, which differ in susceptibility in vitro to NC killing (19). These results suggest that NC cells can be detected within tumors, although the fractionation procedure seems not to be ideal. The NC activity in the "large cell"fraction may be explained by some form of "rosette" formation or entrapment of the smaller NC cells in the "large cell" fraction. Further studies on this subject appear mandatory. Recovery of NK activity from tumors has been obtained in mice (3, 16, 18) and man (6, 15, 17), although not regularly in all tumors tested.

IV. CONCLUSIONS

The present studies show yet another difference between NC and NK cells, exemplified by the present studies with tumor-bearing animals. However, we still ignore so many details of the mechanisms of development, maintenance and regulation of NC-NK levels of activity at a given site, that generalizations are not easy to make. It is quite possible that different tumors may affect NC or NK levels, either increasing or decreasing them, via different mechanisms. For example, just to cite a few possibilities, tumors may produce prostaglandins (23) which in turn may affect NK activity either directly or indirectly (24), certain tumors may induce augmentation of regulatory cells that suppress NK activity (25) or certain tumors may produce excess antigen or other cell products with formation of antigen-antibody complexes which may selectively affect the FcR+ NK cells (6, 16, 18, 26), etc. Thus, we would not be surprised if even with the NK systems, which have shown consistent decline of activity in TB animals, variations in levels of NK activity depending on the different tumor-bearing models will be described that somewhat mimic the situation with NK activity in patients with tumors (4-18).

ACKNOWLEDGMENTS

We would like to thank Linda Stevenson for preparation of this manuscript.

REFERENCES

1. Herberman, R.B., Nunn, M.E. and Lavrin, D.H., Int. J. Cancer 16, 216 (1975).
2. Becker, S. and Klein, E., Eur. J. Immunol. 6, 892 (1976).
3. Santoni, A., Herberman, R.B. and Holden, H.T., J. Natl Cancer Inst. 62, 109 (1979).
4. Pross, H.F. and Baines, M.G., Int. J. Cancer 18, 593 (1976).
5. Takasugi, M., Ramseyer, A. and Takasugi, J., Cancer Res. 37, 413, 1977.
6. Pross, H.F. and Baines, M.G., Cancer Immunol. Immunother. 3, 75 (1977).
7. Takasugi, M., Mickey, M.R. and Terasaki, P.I., J. Natl. Cancer Inst. 53, 1527 (1974).
8. Pavie-Fischer, J., Kourilsky, F.M., Picard, F., Banzet, P. and Puissant, A., Clin. Exp. Immunol. 21, 430 (1975).
9. Mukherji, B., Vassos, D., Flowers, A., Binder, S.C. and Nathanson, L., Int. J. Cancer 16, 971 (1975).
10. Bean, M.A., Bloom, B.R., Herberman, R.B., Old, L.J., Oettgen, H.F., Klein, G. and Terry, W.D., Cancer 35, 2902 (1975).
11. deVries, J.E. and Rumke, P., Int. J. Cancer 17, 182 (1976).
12. Bloom, E.T. and Seeger, R.C., Cancer Res. 36, 1361 (1976).
13. Behalak, Y, Banerjee, D. and Richter, M., Cancer 38, 2274 (1976).
14. Peter, H.H., Knoop, F. and Kalden, J.R., Z. Immunitatforsch. 151, 263 (1976).
15. Vose, B.M., Vanky, F., Argov, S. and Klein, E., Eur. J. Immunol. 7, 753 (1977).
16. Herberman, R.B. and Holden, H.T., Adv. Cancer Res. 27, 305 (1978).
17. Sakasala, E., Timonen, T., Ranki, A. and Hayry, P., Immunol. Rev. 44, 125 (1979).
18. Herberman, R.B., Holden, H.T., Wesr, W. H., Bonnard, G., Santoni, A., Nunn, M.E., Kay, H.D. and Ortaldo, J.R. in Tumor-associated Antigens and their Specific Immune Responses" (F. Spreafico and R. Arnon, eds), p. 129, Academic Press, New York (1979).
19. Stutman, O., Paige, C.J. and Feo Figarella, E., J. Immunol 121, 1819 (1978).
20. Paige, C.J., Feo Figarella, E., Cuttito, M.J., Cahan, A., and Stutman, O., J. Immunol. 121, 1827 (1978).
21. DeLeo, A.B., Shiku, H., Takahashi, T., John, M. and Old, L.J., J. Exp. Med. 146, 270 (1977).
22. Shiku, H., Bean, M.A., Old, L.J. and Oettgen, H.F., J. Natl. Cancer Inst. 54, 415 (1975).
23. Jaffe, B.M., Prostaglandins 6, 453 (1974).

24. Droller, M.J., Schneider, M.U. and Perlmann, P., Cell Immunol. 39, 165 (1978).
25. Cudkowicz, G. and Hochman, P.S., Immunol. Rev. 44, 13 (1979).
26. Herberman, R.B., Bartram, S.J., Haskill, J.S., Nunn, M., Holden, H.T. and West, W.H., J. Immunol. 119, 322 (1977).

NATURAL KILLERS IN HUMAN CANCER: ACTIVITY OF TUMOR-INFILTRATING AND DRAINING NODE LYMPHOCYTES[a]

by

B M Vose

Department of Immunology
Paterson Laboratories
Christie Hospital and Holt Radium Institute
Manchester
ENGLAND

I. INTRODUCTION

Allograft rejection can be accelerated by transfer of suitably sensitised lymphoid cells to graft recipients (1). Several studies have suggested that cellular infiltration of the graft may be a critical factor in rejection with the accumulation of heterogeneous cytotoxic effectors at the antigenic site (2-4). Early reports indicated that lymphoid accumulation in the graft was non specific (5) being largely attributable to increased blood flow through antigen challenged sites. More recently the development of double isotope assays in which labelled sensitised lymphocytes can be transferred and their migration pattern monitored has established that accumulation at the antigenic site is not random but includes a selective trapping of specific effectors (6-8). It has been stressed that this selective local recruitment can lead to a depletion of sensitised cells in the blood and non-draining nodes (7). If such a situation were to apply in the

[a]*This study was supported by grants from the Medical Research Council and Cancer Research Campaign of Great Britain.*

ISBN 0-12-341350-8

tumor host relationship, killer cells may be concentrated in the tumor and draining nodes and blood could be a poor source of lymphocytes for assays of anti-tumor cytotoxic reactions. The infiltration of some human tumors by mononuclear cells is now firmly established and several authors have suggested that this reflects the consequences of an ongoing immune reaction at the tumor site (9-12). The enumeration, isolation and characterisation of these mononuclear cells has been actively pursued in many centers. The cellular infiltrate varies in different tumors and is heterogeneous with macrophages, T cells, B cells and null lymphocytes as well as some polymorphonuclear cells all detectable (13-19). In at least some cases specific killer T lymphocytes have been found within the tumor (17, 20, 21) and macrophages from solid tumors or ovarian ascites are frequently lytic for tumor targets (22, 23). Animal model studies suggest that a further effector mechanism may operate within the tumor mass - the natural killer (NK) system (24, 25). The observation in man that NK levels in the blood lymphocytes declines with advancing disease (26) might indicate depletion of effectors in the periphery by concentration at the tumor site, as described above. The objective of this present report was to detail the NK potential of tumor infiltrating lymphocytes against the K562 cell line and to examine the effect of admixture of various tumor components on the NK levels of previously reactive blood lymphocytes from healthy individuals.

II. MATERIALS AND METHODS

A. *Blood Lymphocytes (PBL)*

Heparinised peripheral blood samples (20 mls) were taken from healthy laboratory personnel and from patients with pulmonary and colonic malignancies prior to any treatment. Mononuclear cell preparations were prepared by centrifugation (900g, 15 minutes, 20°C) on Ficoll-Triosil (F-T) gradient as previously described (17). Cells were collected from the interface, washed 3 times in RPMI 1640 and adherent components depleted by incubation in Corning 25 cm^2 tissue culture flasks (30 minutes, 37°C, in RPMI 1640 + 10% fetal calf serum (FCS)). Non-adherent cells were incubated overnight (37°C in RPMI + 10% FCS) before use in cytotoxicity assays.

B. Lymph Node Cells (LNC)

Lymph nodes draining pulmonary and colonic tumors were taken at surgery. They were finely chopped with scissors in RPMI 1640 and passed through 120 mesh stainless steel grids. Adherent cells were depleted as detailed above and non adherent cells centrifuged on Ficoll-Triosil gradients. Mononuclear cells were washed three times and incubated overnight in RPMI 1640 + 10% FCS before use in cytotoxicity assays. Nodes were carefully monitored to determine whether they contained macroscopic metastatic deposits and one half of the node subjected to histological examination. Only studies on non involved nodes are reported here unless indicated otherwise in the text.

C. Tumor-Infiltrating Lymphocytes (TIL)

Lung tumor infiltrating lymphocytes were prepared from specimens obtained from surgery within 3 hours of removal. Tumors were received in sterile containers filled with RPMI. They were freed of necrotic and fatty material and as much stroma and capsule as possible. Tissue was finely minced with scissors and passed through a 60-mesh stainless steel grid into RPMI. The cell suspension was washed twice in RPMI and dead cells removed by treatment with 0.1% trypsin for 1 minute at $4^{o}C$ in the presence of DNAase which prevented clumping. TIL were also prepared from a small number of breast tumors. The tissues were minced and stirred for 2-3 hours in the presence of 0.1% collagenase, 0.01% hyaluronidase and 0.01% DNAase (all enzymes from Sigma Chemical Co.). The viable cell suspensions obtained by the two procedures were washed a further twice and centrifuged (900 g, 10 minutes) on F-T gradients as used for the preparation of blood lymphocytes. Cells were collected from the interface, washed once and adherent cells removed by incubation (30 minutes, $37^{o}C$ in RPMI + 20% FCS) on microexudate-coated plastic culture flasks, as described below. Non adherent cells were applied to gradients comprising 6 mls F-T density 1.077 overlaid with 6 mls F-T corresponding to 3:4 dilution of this with normal saline. Following centrifugation tumor enriched fractions could be removed from the top of the interface and lymphocyte enriched populations from the second. The latter was washed once and laid onto a bovine serum gradient and allowed to sediment at 1G for 2 hours at room temperature. The top fraction contained lymphocytes and contaminating tumor cells appeared further in the bovine serum. Cells were washed twice and stained cytocentrifuge preparations prepared. Populations were used as TIL only if they contained more than 95% lymphocytes. TIL were incubated overnight in RPMI + 10% FCS before use in cytotoxicity assays.

D. *Tumor Cells*

Tumor enriched populations from the F-T gradient described above were examined. If necessary the two stage F-T gradient step was repeated and adherent cells further depleted by overnight incubation at 37°C in Corning culture flasks in RPMI + 20% FCS. Only rarely did tumor cells adhere in large numbers. Cytological examination of the preparations revealed that the major component was tumor cells with some low level contamination with columnar epithelial cells and degenerate macrophage-like cells. Some specimens were received from tumor free areas of lung from patients with pulmonary neoplasms. These were processed in an identical manner to the lung tumors to prepare 'normal lung' suspensions.

E. *Adherent Cells*

Adherent cells were prepared from blood, lung tumors and normal lung tissue by incubation on microexudate coated plastic flasks (27). Chang liver cells were grown to confluence in 25 cm^2 Corning culture flasks and removed by treatment (10 minutes, 37°C) with 1mM EDTA in PBS. Blood or tissue cell suspensions taken from the initial F-T gradients were allowed to adhere to the plastic (30 minutes, 37°C in RPMI + 20% FCS) and non adherent cell removed by vigorous washing. Adherent cells were kept overnight in RPMI + 10% FCS and could be removed by treatment (10 minutes, 37°C) with 1 mM EDTA in PBS. Cells were washed twice and resuspended in RPMI + 10% FCS for counting. These cells comprised 92-97% NSE positive cells with 87% showing uptake of latex particles.

F. *Cytotoxicity Tests*

One million cells of the erythroleukemic line K562 or of freshly isolated tumor cells were labelled in RPMI + 10% FCS with ^{51}Cr Sodium Chromate and used as targets in 4 hr ^{51}Cr release assays as described previously (17). Effector:target ratios were 50:1 unless otherwise stated. Results are expressed as % cytotoxicity =

$$\frac{\%\ ^{51}\text{Cr release test} - \text{spontaneous}\ ^{51}\text{Cr release}}{\text{maximum}\ ^{51}\text{Cr release} - \text{spontaneous}\ ^{51}\text{Cr release}} \times 100$$

Significance of cytotoxicity was assessed by Mann Whitney U Test.

G. Cold Inhibition Assays

The capacity of cells to interfere with killing of K562 was assessed by addition of unlabelled inhibitor cells to give blocker:target ratios of 20:1 - 5:1 in the presence of a constant number of effectors (generally 25:1). Similar experiments were performed using adherent cells from blood, tumor and normal lung as inhibitors. These cells were added to give inhibitor:effector ratios of 1:3 - 1:12. Inhibition was considered positive when a significant reduction of cytotoxicity was seen and a dose dependency of inhibition was apparent.

H. Stimulation Assays

Blood lymphocytes were dispensed into Sterilin round-bottomed microtest plates M24 ARTLS in 0.2ml RPMI 1640 + 10% FCS. They were cultured for 6 days in the presence of PHA (2 μg/ml Wellcome purified grade) or mitomycin-C-treated (25 μg/ml, 30 minutes, 37°C) autologous tumor cells at a responder: stimulator ratio of 2:1 (28). Mitomycin-C-treated PBL, TIL or LNC were added at an inhibitor:responder ratio of 1:1 or 1:2. Samples were pulsed for 6 hours with 1 μCi/well [(^{3}H)] thymidine specific activity 2.5 Ci/m mole and harvested onto paper discs using a SAM2 multiple culture harvester. Discs were counted using a toluene scintillator and results expressed as mean counts per minute.

I. Boosting of NK by Interferon

Effector cells (3 x 10^{6}/ml) were treated with 'Nomalva' leukocyte interferon (a gift from Dr K H Fantes, Wellcome Laboratories, Beckenham, Kent) by overnight incubation with 250 units/ml interferon at 37°C. Cells were washed twice prior to use in cytotoxicity assays.

III. RESULTS

A. *Cytotoxic Activity of Lymphocytes from Different Sources*

Blood lymphocytes from all 16 healthy donors and 43 of 49 cancer patients had significant cytotoxic activity against the K562 cell line. There was considerable variation of reactivity between individuals (Table 1) and with the extremes of reactivity shared by both groups. Taken as a group, however, patients with lung cancer showed significantly lower cytotoxic potential than the healthy donor group ($P<0.01$). Subdivision of the cancer group into those with and without nodal metastases did not reveal any further discrimination of lytic activity. Similar patterns of reactivity were apparent against other cell lines (CCRF/CEF, Molt 4, Chang) although the levels of cytotoxicity were considerably lower than those recorded against K562. The Raji cell line was insusceptible to killing and significant lysis was only rarely found against this line.

TABLE I. Cytotoxic Potential of Peripheral Blood Lymphocytes Against the K562 Cell Line

	Healthy donor lymphocytes	*Cancer patients no metastases*	*Cancer patients node metastasis*
Mean % cytotoxicity ± SD	*46.7[a]±16.8*	*32.2±15.9*	*28.1±23.8*
Range	*27-81*	*10-73*	*1-73*
No. Tested	*16*	*30*	*19*

[a] *Effector:Target Ratio 50:1*

Lymph node populations were obtained from patients undergoing surgery for colonic and lung malignancies. Tumor-infiltrating lymphocytes were also so prepared from a proportion of the lung carcinoma group. This was not generally possible in the colon cancer group for technical reasons although lymphocytes were present in the tumor cell suspensions. Different isolation procedures are currently under investigation in an attempt to overcome these problems. The yield of TIL was variable but when isolation was possible some $1 - 8 \times 10^5$ lymphocytes/gram tumor was obtained. In all but two preparations T cells were the major component of TIL (mean 49% cells forming rosettes with sheep erythrocytes) with 6 - 24% cells forming rosettes with antibody-coated ox erythrocytes. Blood and lymph node lymphocytes showed 65% E rosettes and 16% EA rosettes. In agreement with earlier studies (17, 18, 21, 29) LNC and TIL were only rarely reactive against the K562 cell line (Table 2). Forty LNC preparations were examined including 5 which were involved. Of the node preparations, 7 showed significant cytotoxicity (3 mecentric 13%, 21%, 35% and 4 hilar 15%, 17%, 31%, 37%). None of the involved nodes showed reactivity and cytotoxicity was not related to the levels of NK found in PBL. The cytotoxic potential in LNC could be removed by passage of the effectors through nylon columns and therefore showed different characteristics to blood NK, which were unaffected or often concentrated in the nylon column passed fraction (Vose *et al* in preparation).

TABLE II. Cytotoxic Reactivity of Lymphocytes from Different Sites Against the K562 Cell Line

	Effector cells from		
	Blood	*Lymph node*	*Tumor*
Colon carcinoma			
No. tested	*11*	*19*	*1*
Mean cytotoxicity ± SD	*19.5[a]±15.3*	*5.2±7.2*	*0.2*
No. significant	*9*	*3*	*0*
Lung carcinoma			
No. tested	*38*	*21*	*23*
Mean cytotoxicity ± SD	*33.9±19.1*	*7.0±10.1*	*5.3±7.4*
No. significant	*34*	*4*	*5*

[a] *Effector:Target Ratio 50:1*

Lung TIL showed low but significant reactivity in 5 of 23 samples (% cytotoxicity 10%, 11%, 13%, 23%, 27%). Again this was not related to the levels of reactivity in blood lymphocytes i.e. was not associated with unusually high levels of reactivity in PBL nor to contamination of the tumor specimen with blood (erythrocyte:leukocyte ratio was of the order of 1:1 - 5:1 prior to separation). Similar low NK activities were found with TIL prepared from breast neoplasms.

B. *Possible Factors Inhibiting Cytotoxicity*

The possibility existed that active cells were present in LNC and TIL preparations but that their lytic activity was inhibited by factors released from the tumor or the local milieu. Experiments were therefore initiated to investigate the capacity of different preparations of cells obtained from the tumor to inhibit NK activity in blood lymphocytes. Initial experiments established that suppressor cells were indeed present in both TIL and tumor-draining LNC (Table 3).

TABLE III. Effect of Addition of Tumor Infiltrating Lymphocytes (TIL) or Tumor-Draining LNC on Mitogen and MLTI Responses of Blood Lymphocytes.

Responder	*Inhibitor*	*R:I*	^3H *Thymidine incorporation after stimulation with*		
			-	*PHA*	*Autologous tumor*
PBL	PBL[a]	1:1	474[b]	6883	4749
	TIL	1:1	672	5630	1953
PBL	PBL	1:1	408	25678	958
	TIL	1:1	1539	15863	1474
PBL	PBL	1:1	235	3772	2230
	TIL	1:1	187	1051	1073
PBL	PBL	2:1	486	6250	
	LNC	2:1	461	4053	-
	LNC RF[c]	2:1	154	1732	
PBL	PBL	2:1	581	191	
	LNC	2:1	887	4176	-
	LNC RF[c]	2:1	490	640	

[a] *MMC-treated PBL were used as control but did not significantly alter the responses of blood lymphocytes to PHA and tumor.* [b] *Counts per minute.* [c] *SRBC rosette forming cells.*

Admixture of mitomycin C treated lymphocytes from tumor or node inhibited [(^{3}H)] thymidine incorporation of blood lymphocytes following stimulation with PHA or autologous tumor. Preliminary studies suggested that the suppressor passed nylon wool filtration (28) and could be concentrated in LNC by formation of SRBC rosettes (Table 3). Comparable experiments in which TIL or LNC were added to blood lymphocytes and cytotoxicity against K562 assayed failed to show any suppression of lytic potential (Table 4). LNC and TIL which themselves showed no NK activity were mixed at different ratios with autologous blood lymphocytes and tested against K562.

TABLE IV. Effect of Addition of TIL or LNC on Killing of K562 by Blood Lymphocytes.

		% Cytotoxicity against K562 at effector:target ratio of		
		50:1	25:1	12:1
Blood lymphocytes		17.7*	8.6*	2.2
LNC		1.8	0.1	0.1
Blood lymphocytes + LNC	1:1	18.4*	9.8*	6.1
	1:2	21.4*	14.7*	8.1*
	1:4	23.3*	13.8*	7.6*
Blood lymphocytes		43.0*	23.4*	9.6*
TIL		4.4	0	0
Blood lymphocytes + TIL	1:1	45.1*	22.6*	10.4*
	25:1	41.7*	22.9*	16.7*
	5:1	41.3*	21.6*	12.6*

$P<0.05$ of killing of K562.

In no case was a significant reduction of cytotoxicity found, and in some experiments a slight increase in cytotoxicity was apparent.

Further experiments of this type used adherent monocyte/macrophage populations from blood, tumor or normal lung as inhibitors. These adherent cells were mixed with autologous blood lymphocytes at different ratios and cytotoxicity tested against K562. The adherent cells *per se* showed no cytotoxic potential against K562 but were effective in reducing the lytic activity of blood lymphocytes (Table 5). Cells from normal lung had the greater reactivity in this respect with tumor derived adherents being more frequently inhibitory and effective at lower blocker:effector ratios than those from blood. A limited number of assays suggest that lymphocytes derived from normal lung tissue show a level NK activity comparable to that of TIL.

A further potentially inhibitory cell type was the tumor itself or soluble factors released by it. Tumor cell preparations were therefore used in cold inhibition assays with K562 as target. Blood lymphocytes from healthy donors were used as effectors since in approximately 30% of cases killing of autologous tumor targets was found. Unlabelled K562 and Raji acted as positive and negative controls. K562 gave a dose dependent inhibition of cytotoxicity while Raji was ineffective giving significantly reduced lysis only at the highest blocker:target ratio (20:1). Unlabelled tumor and normal lung cells showed the latter pattern in the majority of cases, i.e. significant inhibition was demonstrable only at 20:1 and no dose dependency was apparent (Table 6).

TABLE V. Effect of Addition of Adherent Cells on the Cytototxicity of Blood Lymphocytes for K562

Expt. no.	*Lymphocyte: adherent ratio*	*% Cytotoxicity[a] in the presence of adherent cells from:-*		
		Blood	*Tumor*	*Normal lung*
1	-	38.5		
	3:1	25.9*[b]	25.9*	22.3*
	6:1	27.6*	32.0*	25.3*
	10:1	31.3	35.9	33.3
2	-	17.1		
	3:1	14.7	18.3	8.0*
	6:1	16.2	17.1	10.3*
3	-	23.4		
	3:1	20.2	13.4*	15.4*
	6:1	23.1	25.3	14.2*
4	-	30.3		
	1:1	20:1*	13.0*	10.7*
	3:1	24.9	17.8*	14.7*
	6:1	27.5	21.6*	18.0*
5	-	19.5		
	6:1	16.6	9.0*	13.0*
	12:1	14.8	13.0*	14.0
6	-	16.6		
	3:1	9.7*	10.7*	10.7*
	6:1	11.6*	10.2*	-

[a] *Effector:Target Ratio 40:1.*

[b] *Significant reduction of cytotoxic reactivity.*

In a total of 14 cold inhibition assays with freshly isolated tumor cells only 2 showed dose dependent blocking. None of the normal lung preparations tested showed inhibition of K562 lysis.

TABLE VI. Inhibition of Lymphocyte Killing of ^{51}Cr Labelled K562 by Addition of Unlabelled Cells.

		% Cytotoxicity[a] against K562 in the presence of unlabelled		
Expt.	*Blocker:target ratio*	*K562*	*Lung tumor*	*Normal lung*
1	-	*33.3*		
	10:1	*11.4**	*35.6*	*29.4*
	1:1	*39.8*	*32.9*	*35.4*
	1:5	*35.5*	*34.6*	*31.5*
2	-	*34.9*		
	20:1	*6.1**	*18.8**	*18.2**
	10:1	*10.3**	*27.4*	*34.1*
3	-	*38.5*		
	20:1	*14.2**	*47.0*	*37.9*
	10:1	*22.0**	*46.5*	*44.2*
4	-	*25.3*		
	20:1	*11.4**	*17.5**	-
	10:1	*15.3**	*25.3*	-
	5:1	*21.2*	*22.2*	-

[a] *Effector:Target Ratio 25:1*

* *Significant reduction of killing of K562.*

C. *Susceptibility of Fresh Tumor Cells to Lysis*

The failure of the majority of freshly isolated tumor preparations to interfere with killing of K562 by healthy donor lymphocytes suggested that they did not express the relevant NK binding structure. In a series of assays ^{51}Cr labelled tumor cells were used as targets with healthy donor effectors (*Figure* 1). Significant lysis was seen with only 4 of 17 samples under conditions where the majority of donors showed high reactivity against K562. Increasing the attacker: target ratio did not increase the number of positive cases. However, treatment of effectors with purified interferon

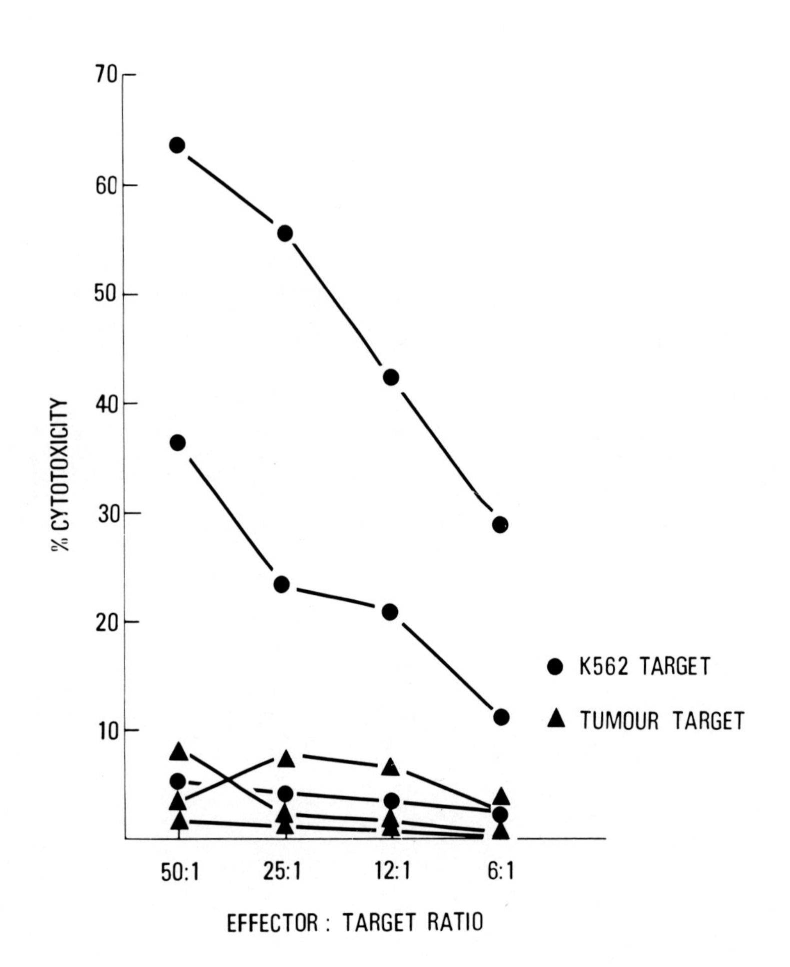

FIGURE I. Cytotoxicity of 3 healthy donor lymphocyte preparations for K562 and freshly isolated lung tumor targets in a 4 hour ^{51}Cr release assay. One sample did not show killing of K562 and none lysed tumor targets. Spontaneous release from K562 10.3% tumor 19.1%.

preparations increased cytotoxicity against K562 and killing of fresh tumor cells was then apparent (Table 7).

TABLE VII. *Effect of Interferon on Killing of Tumor and K562 by Healthy Donor Lymphocytes.*

Target cells	Spontaneous ^{51}Cr release	Treatment of effectors	% Cytototxicity at E:T of 50:1	25:1
Experiment 1				
K562	8.7	-	48.5*	32.2*
		250 Units IF	57.2*	44.5*
Lung tumor 11	19.5	-	4.3	5.8
		250 Units IF	1.8	4.7
Colon tumor 14	17.4	-	13.5	2.7
		250 Units IF	24.5*	14.7*
Raji	7.5	-	2.2	1.5
		250 Units IF	17.8*	16.4*
Experiment 2				
K562	25.6	-	81.2*	73.7*
		250 Units IF	91.1*	85.6*
Lung tumor 35	30.2	-	14.9*	10.1*
		250 Units IF	25.8*	26.1*
Lung tumor 36	43.9	-	11.5	9.5
		250 Units IF	3.8*	28.7*
Lung tumor 37	32.7	-	2.4	1.8
		250 Units IF	28.5*	30.8*
Experiment 3				
K562	24.6	-	42.3*	35.4*
		250 Units IF	57.4*	41.4*
Lung tumor 42	24.6	-	0	0
		250 Units IF	14.3*	9.2*
Normal lung 42	17.6	-	5.5	3.1
		250 Units IF	12.7*	9.1*

* $P<0.05$

Following interferon treatment killing was also demonstrable against the previously resistant Raji cell line. Significant cytotoxicity was found against 5 of 6 tumors after interferon boosting. Treatment of effectors with interferon also induced killing of normal lung cell preparations which comprised predominantly columnar epithelial cells (Table 7, Expt. 3). The degree of boosting depended upon the interferon dose and time of exposure as described by Moore and Potter (30).

IV. DISCUSSION

This study reveals that lymphocytes infiltrating human tumors or found in tumor-draining lymph nodes have low NK activity: Two explanations of the data can be considered. 1). That NK effectors are present in negligible numbers in the majority of solid neoplasms or 2). That they enter the tumor where activity is depressed in the local milieu by factors released from the tumor or by suppressor cells of NK such as those which have been demonstrated in the spleens of C. Parvum treated mice (31). In order to investigate these possibilities TIL, macrophages and tumor cells have been admixed with effectors from peripheral blood and cytotoxicity against the K562 cell line determined.

Initial experiments revealed that tumor infiltrating lymphocytes had the capacity to reduce thymidine incorporation in mitogen stimulated blood lymphocytes (28 and Table 3); a characteristic shared by at least some lymph node preparations from patients with colonic malignancies. However, TIL and LNC did not appear to contain suppressors of NK since they did not depress the cytotoxicity of blood lymphocytes against K562. Similar data has been described in animal models where admixture of inactive LNC and active blood effectors showed no diminution where admixture of inactive LNC and active blood effectors showed no diminution of cytotoxic potential (32). By contrast, addition of cells isolated by adherence and composed almost exclusively of cells of the monocyte-macrophage series did reduce lytic activity. The effect was dependent upon the effector:macrophage ratio with adherents from tumor, normal lung and blood all showing significant suppressive activity. It was not clear if this inhibition of killing was attributable to cold inhibition by macrophage which can function as NK targets (33) or alternatively to inhibition of killing by release of, for example, prostaglandins. These substances have a potent depressive action on NK (34), can be released by monocytes, and inhibit PHA stimulation (35). Preliminary experiments in which Indomethacin (an inhibitor of prostaglandin synthetase) was present throughout the assay with adherent cells have not revealed any lowering of inhibitory activity.

Similar experiments in which freshly isolated tumor cells were used in inhibition experiments showed that positive blocking of killing was rare. In only 2 of 14 tumor cell preparations was dose dependent reduction of lysis apparent although several showed significant interference at the highest blocker:target ratios used. These data may contrast to those of Ortaldo et al (36) in whose experiments inhibition of NK by freshly isolated lung and breast tumor preparations was apparent although the frequency of blocking was not given. The finding of low inhibitory activity in tumor cells is in accord with their low sensitivity to NK lysis in direct assays. In only a minority of cases was low but significant killing demonstrable at the limits of detection. Several studies have shown the capacity of different targets to block NK largely, parallels susceptibility to lysis (37). It should be stressed that the low levels of lysis of tumor cells by natural killers would not be incompatible with the view that these effectors might have an immunosurveillance role (38, 39). The appearance of tumors of low susceptibility to killing as a result of immunoselective pressure against sensitive targets can be considered. Boosting of NK by interferon as described by many groups in this book markedly increased killing of K562 and in the present study induced reactivity in previously non-reactive combinations with tumor cells as targets. Similar data were obtained with the non reactive cell line Raji and cells isolated from normal lung tissue. The implication of this observation is that differences in NK sensitivity are quantitative rather than qualitative with highly active preparations revealing previously non detectable killing. Since such boosting can be achieved, the susceptibility of fresh tumor cells to NK may not be so low as to be biologically insignificant, although the appearance of killing of normal lung cells is difficult to explain and suggests a totally non specific activity in such boosted populations.

The low levels of NK activity in the majority of TIL preparations may thus indicate that these effectors upon entering the local environment are exposed to the high concentrations of monocyte/macrophages which can inhibit effector function. The alternative view that NK cells do not enter the tumor is difficult to reconcile with the clear evidence of their presence during at least some stages of growth of experimental animal tumors (24, 25). Treatment of TIL with interferon preparations or their maintenance in vitro to release from putative suppression may help to further understanding of this phenomenon and to establish if NK effectors are capable of extravasation in large numbers other than in a few sites such as the peritoneal cavity in the presence of ovarian carcinoma ascites (Mantovani - personal communication). Studies suggest that tissue derived lymphocytes from normal lung (Vose, unpublished finding) and lamina propria (40) from individuals with malignancy are also inactive against K562.

ACKNOWLEDGMENTS

The author is grateful to M Moore for help and discussion, Mr W. K. Douglas, R. A. M. Lawson, P. F. S. Schofield and P. Gallagher for the provision of material and Roger Ferguson for technical assistance and Miss E Mercer for preparation of the manuscript.

REFERENCES

1. Billingham, R. A., Brent, L. and Medawar, P.B., *Proc. R. Soc. Lond., 143,* 58 (1955).
2. Tilney, N. L., Strom, T. B., Macpherson, S. G. and Carpenter, C. B., *Transplantation, 20,* 323 (1975).
3. Roberts, P. J. and Häyry, P., *Cellular Immunol., 30,* 236 (1977).
4. Häyry, P., Soots, A., v. Willebrand, E. and Wiktorowitz, K., *Transplant Proc., XI,* 785 (1979).
5. Hall, J. G., *J. Exp. Med., 125,* 737 (1967).
6. Tilney, N. L. and Ford, W. L., *Transplantation, 17,* 12 (1974).
7. Emeson, E. E., *J. Exp. Med., 147,* 13 (1978).
8. Chang, A. E. and Sugarbaker, P. H., *Transplantation, 28,* 247 (1979).
9. Cochran, A. J., *J. Path., 97,* 459 (1969).
10. Elston, C. W. and Bagshawe, K. D., *Br. J. Cancer, 28,* 245 (1973).
11. Ioachim, H. L., Dorsett, B. H. and Paluck, E., *Cancer, 38,* 2296 (1976).
12. Di Paola, M., Bertolotti, A., Colizza, S. and Coli, M., *J. Thoracic Cardiovasc., Surg., 73,* 531 (1977).
13. Jondal, M. and Klein, G., *Biomedicine, 23,* 163 (1975).
14. Gauci, C. L. and Alexander, P., *Cancer Letters, 1,* 29 (1975).
15. Husby, G., Hoagland, P. M., Strickland, R. G. and Williams, R. C., *J. Clin. Invest., 57,* 1471 (1976).
16. Wood, G. W. and Gallahon, K. A., *J. Natl. Cancer Inst., 59,* 1081 (1977).
17. Vose, B. M., Vánky, F. and Klein, E., *Inst. J. Cancer, 20,* 895 (1977).
18. Vose, B. M., Vánky, F., Argov, S. and Klein, E., *Eur. J. Immunol., 7,* 753 (1977).

19. Svennevig, J-L., Lövik, M. and Svaar, H., *Int. J. Cancer, 23,* 626 (1979).
20. Jondal, M., Svedmyr, E., Klein, E. and Singh, S., *Nature, 255,* 405, (1975).
21. Klein, E., Vánky, F., Galili, U., Vose, B. M. and Fopp, M. *Contemp. Topics Immunobiol., 8,* (1980 in press).
22. Vose, B. M., *Cancer Immunol. Immunother., 5,* 173 (1978).
23. Mantovani, A., Peri, G., Polentarutti, N., Bolis, G., Mangioni, C. and Spreafico, F., *Int. J. Cancer, 23,* 153 (1979).
24. Becker, S. and Klein, E., *Eur. J. Immunol., 6,* 892 (1976).
25. Moore, K. and Moore, M. *Br. J. Cancer, 39,* 636 (1979).
26. Pross, H. F. and Baines, M. G., *Int. J. Cancer, 18,* 593 (1976).
27. Mantovani, A. in "Manual of Macrophage Methodology" (H. B. Herscawitz., H. T. Holden., J. A. Bellanti and A. Ghaffar, Eds.) Marcel Dekker, Inc., New York (1980 in press).
28. Vose, B. M. and Moore, M., *Int. J. Cancer, 24,* 579 (1979).
29. Tötterman, T. H., Hayry, P., Saksela, E., Timonen, T. and Eklund, B., *Eur. J. Immunol., 8,* 872 (1978).
30. Moore, M. and Potter, M. R., *Br. J. Cancer, 41,* (1980 in press).
31. Savary, C. A. and Lotzova, E., *J. Immunol., 120,* 239 (1978).
32. Potter, M. R. and Moore, M., *Clin. Exp. Immunol., 37,* 78 (1978).
33. Nunn, M. E., Herberman, R. B. and Holden, H. T., *Int. J. Cancer, 20,* 381 (1977).
34. Droller, M. J., Lindgren, J. A., Claessen, H. E. and Perlmann, P., *Cell Immunol., 47,* 261 (1979).
35. Goodwin, J. S., Bankhurst, A. D. and Messner, R. P., *J. Exp. Med., 146,* 1719 (1977).
36. Ortaldo, J. R., Oldham, R. K., Cannon, G. C. and Herberman R. B., *J. Natl. Cancer Inst., 59,* 77 (1977).
37. Becker, S., Kiessling, R., Lee, N. and Klein, G., *J. Natl. Cancer Inst., 61,* 1495 (1978).
38. Haller, O., Hansson, M., Kiessling, R. and Wigzell, H., *Nature, 270,* 609 (1977).
39. Kiessling, R. and Haller, O., *Contemp. Topics in Immunobiol., 8,* 171 (1978).
40. Bland, P. W., Lloyd, J. V., Richens, E. R. and Britton, D. C., *Proc. British Society Immunol.,* (Nov., 1979).

SUMMARY: NK ACTIVITY DURING CARCINOGENESIS AND TUMOR GROWTH AND ITS EXPRESSION WITHIN TUMORS

An important issue in regard to the possible involvement of NK cells in resistance to tumors is how their activity might be affected during the course of tumor development and growth. If NK cells play a major role in immune surveillance, one would predict that successful induction of tumors by carcinogenic agents might be dependent on depression of NK activity during a critical period during carcinogenesis. Likewise, the tumor-bearing state might be expected to be associated with depressed NK activity. As a further, more direct indication of a possible involvement of NK cells in resisting primary tumor growth, one would expect to find some evidence that NK cells have the capacity to migrate into the site of tumor growth but, on the other hand, find deficient NK activity in well established tumors that had managed to escape from host control. Evidence on each of these points is accumulating and the main findings are summarized below.

I. NK ACTIVITY DURING CARCINOGENESIS

In the past, much effort was expended to determine the extent of immune depression associated with carcinogenesis (reviewed by Stutman, 1975). The focus of most studies was on T cell-mediated immunity and humoral immunity. The results have been difficult to evaluate, with similar experiments with the same carcinogens giving apparently contradictory data. The observations that T cell deficient mice did not have a clear increase in tumor incidence after treatment with various carcinogens, or after exposure to some viruses (e.g. mouse mammary tumor virus, MTV), raised serious doubts about the validity of immune surveillance. With the current awareness of the possible role of NK cells and other natural immune defense mechanisms, this question needs to be carefully re-evaluated. Unfortunately, to date there have been very few studies on this issue. Most of the limited available data are summarized in the chapters here.

ISBN 0-12-341350-8

Ehrlich et al have obtained data on the effects of two chemical carcinogens, dimethyl benzanthracene (DMBA) and urethane, on NK activity in mice. DMBA produced substantial depression of NK activity, persisting for about 6 weeks. In contrast, they found that treatment with urethane did not depress, but actually appeared to increase, NK activity in BALB/c mice. However, another study in CBA and A/J mice has shown that urethane can produce strong but transient depression of NK activity (E. Gorelik and R.B. Herberman, unpublished observations). The apparent discrepancies are probably due to differences in the time intervals between administration of the carcinogen and testing for NK activity. These studies indicate that two chemical carcinogens can produce early and appreciable effects on NK activity and it will be important to determine whether this is a general property of most carcinogenic agents. In situations in which depressed NK activity is found during the latent period of carcinogenesis, attempts at selective restoration of NK activity can be made as a possible means of interfering with the development of tumors.

Some attention has been directed towards the levels of NK activity in female mice that were infected at birth with MTV and that consequently develop mammary tumors more than 6 months later. Blair et al found that the increases in immune reactivity were due to development of cytotoxic T lymphocytes and to antibody-dependent cell-mediated cytotoxicity, with secretion of antibodies to MTV during culture. In contrast, at various times during the latent period, no shift in levels of NK activity were observed that could be related to infection with MTV. Similarly, Tagliabue et al (1980) have compared levels of NK activity in MTV-infected and uninfected mice, between 6 and 38 weeks of age, and found no significant differences. Thus there is no evidence that NK cells have a role in coping with the development of virus-induced mammary tumors in mice.

II. NK ACTIVITY IN TUMOR-BEARERS

In several studies, tumor-bearing individuals have been shown to have NK activity depressed appreciably below that of normals. However, most of these data have come from studies with only a limited variety of tumors and it will be important to determine how general this association is and the point in tumor development at which depression occurs.

Several studies have demonstrated that mice bearing primary or transplanted murine sarcoma virus (MSV)-induced tumors have depressed levels of splenic NK activity. Brunda and Holden (section IC4) provide evidence that this depression may be due, at least in part, to production of prostaglandins, since administration of inhibitors of prostaglandin synthesis was able to reverse much or all of the depression.

Ehrlich _et al_ found that mice with primary or early transplants of DMBA-induced tumors had depressed NK activity and elevated levels of cytostatic activity. Some suggestion of a role of adherent suppressor cells was obtained, since passage of spleen cells over Sephadex G10 columns resulted in an increase of NK activity. The NK activity of mice bearing primary urthane-induced lung adenomas was not found to be depressed by Ehrlich _et al_, but in another study (E. Gorelik and R.B. Herberman, unpublished observations) substantial depression was observed.

Studies on NK activity in C3H mice bearing primary mammary tumors have also given divergent results. Ehrlich _et al_ observed depressed NK, but no cytostatic activity in mice with large tumors. Lane also found depressed reactivity in tumor-bearers, but only against YAC-1 and not against another target. She attributed the selective depression to a loss in reactivity to MTV-associated antigens. In contrast, Gerson found similar levels of low NK activity in the spleens of both tumor bearers and normal one year-old female mice.

Several investigators have examined NK activity in the blood of tumor patients. Pross and Baines report their results with ovarian cancer patients, with depressed activity appearing to become more profound with advanced stages of disease. Activity was not appreciably affected by therapy, and patients surviving for long periods after therapy tended to have higher levels. This suggested that minimal or no depression of NK activity might be a good prognostic indicator. Gerson studied patients with a variety of tumor types and found depression to be mainly associated with neuroblastomas. Depressed NK activity appeared to be correlated with extent of disease but not with tumor size, since some patients with large local tumors had high levels of NK activity. Eremin studied patients with stage I and II operable breast cancer and found most to be in the normal range.

Two studies on patients with lung cancer have yielded divergent results. Vose found comparable degrees of depressed NK activity in patients with preoperative stage I or II lung cancer. In contrast, Forbes et al observed preoperative activity to be in the normal range and depression occurring after resection of tumors. They attribute the decline in activity to the decrease in tumor burden, but alternative explanations include the possible depressive effects of BCG being received by some patients or the presence of occult metastatic disease. Forbes et al obtained a similar pattern of results in patients with small cell carcinoma of the lung or malignant melanoma, and they suggest that increased tumor burden leads to augmentation of NK activity. However, since these results appear to run counter to those of most other studies and patients had often received chemotherapy, other causes for the observed patterns need to be examined.

III. PRESENCE OF NK CELLS WITHIN TUMORS

From studies with tumors in mice, it seems clear that NK cells can enter the site of tumor growth, especially into early, small tumors. Becker reports her findings with transplants of YAC-1. After subcutaneous or intraperitoneal inoculation of this NK-susceptible cell line, high levels of NK activity could be detected in situ in a strain of hybrid mice with high NK activity but not in A strain mice. In mice bearing regressor MSV-induced tumors, both Becker and Gerson observed levels of NK activity in the tumors that were parallel to those in the spleens of the same mice. However, in A strain mice with low NK reativity, Becker found very little anti-YAC-1 activity at the tumor site but did observe substantial, granulocyte-mediated cytotoxicity against MSV tumor cells. Gerson found that mice bearing progressively growing MSV tumors had low or undetectable activity in situ. This did not appear to be due to an absence of NK cells since removal of adherent or phagocytic cells led to a marked increase in activity. A role for suppressor macrophages within the tumor was supported by mixing experiments, in which cells from the tumor inhibited the activity of normal spleen cells.

Gerson also measured NK activity in cells isolated from primary mouse mammary tumors. Mice with small tumors had appreciable NK activity in situ, whereas those with larger tumor burdens had no detectable activity in situ.

Studies with human tumors have given largely negative results. Vose detected activity in only a small proportion of tumors and Gerson and Eremin obtained uniformly negative results. Activity could not be uncovered by removal of adherent cells or by other fractionation procedures. However, each investigator obtained evidence for the inhibition of NK activity of normal donors by cells from the tumors. Despite the usual lack of NK activity in human tumors, in some situations, appreciable activity has been seen. Mantovani *et al* have found NK cells in peritoneal effusions of patients with ovarian cancer and Eremin has detected NK activity in the region of breast and colon cancers, in lymph nodes without tumor involvement.

The largely negative human data might be taken as indications for a lack of ability of NK cells to enter the tumor site and thereby be involved in resistance against progressive growth. However, the findings of positive results in various types of mouse tumors and of occasional human tumors with NK activity point toward an alternative explanation. As observed with the larger mouse tumors, most clinically detectable human tumors may simply be beyond the point of ready detection of NK cells *in situ*. If NK cells have a role in defense against primary tumor growth, this is likely to be at an early stage and the very presence of clinically detectable tumors may be an indication of the failure of adequate control by this effector mechanism. The escape of tumors from the cytotoxic effects of NK cells may be attributed in part to inhibition by antigen-bearing cells or by suppressor cells. Another point that needs to be kept in mind in these studies is that the real issue is not so much the presence of NK cells reactive with a highly susceptible standard target cell but rather the possible reactivity of a subset of NK cells or other effector cells against the autochthonous tumor cells. The latter should be an important focus for further studies in this area.

REFERENCES

Stutman, O., *Adv. Cancer Res.* 22, 261 (1975).

Tagliabue, A., Boraschi, D., and McCoy, J.L., *J. Immunol.* in press.

IN VIVO ACTIVITY OF MURINE NK CELLS

Otto Haller

Department of Experimental Microbiology
Institute for Medical Microbiology
University of Zürich
Zürich, Switzerland

Anders Örn
Magnus Gidlund
Hans Wigzell

Department of Immunology, Biomedical Center
University of Uppsala
Uppsala, Sweden

INTRODUCTION

Until recently, the immune system, in particular the T cell system, has been thought to specifically prevent development and growth of neoplastic cells *in vivo* (1,2). There is no doubt that T and B cell immunity can be established against subsequently transplanted syngeneic tumors in various tumor-host systems (3). However, there is little evidence to suggest that conventional immune reactions are responsible for resistance against syngeneic tumor cells in normal, unimmunized hosts. Also, immunodeficiencies are frequently not associated with an increased incidence of malignancies (4). For example, athymic nude mice which are incapable of generating T effector cells develop spontaneous tumors at the same low rates as their immunologically fully competent littermates (5,6). Nude or other T-cell-deficient mice have been found to exhibit an unexpectedly high degree of resistance towards transplantation of a variety of syngeneic, allogeneic and xenogeneic tumor cells (7-13). Therefore, alternative non-T-cell dependent mechanisms have been suggested to play a role in protection against tumor growth *in vivo* (14). Most attention in this respect has been focused on macrophages (15,16) and natural killer (NK) cells (17). The potential involvement of macrophages is discussed in

ISBN 0-12-341350-8

detail by other contributors to this volume. Here, we will concentrate on NK cells and their possible relevance in host defense against tumors. As the mouse is a convenient species for *in vivo* experimentation, we have primarily investigated the murine NK system. The present data support the view that, in the normal, unprimed animal, NK cells may function as a first barrier of defense against tumor growth. The role of NK cells in host defense against nonmalignant cells and viruses is reviewed in other chapters of this volume.

PHYSIOLOGY OF MURINE NK CELLS

Some notable features concerning the genetics and the physiology of the murine NK system are summarized here, because they are essential for the proper understanding of the present *in vivo* experiments. Generation of NK cells in the mouse is under polygenic control involving at least 2 different loci on chromosome 17 and probably several other non-H-2 linked genes (18). Mouse strains can be classified as high (CBA, C57BL/6, C57L, B10.A) or low reactive (A and A congenics, AKR, 129/J) with regard to their levels of NK activity as assessed in *in vitro* cytotoxicity assays using spleen effector cells and YAC-1 tumor targets (18). High NK reactivity is dominant in crosses between low reactive A strain and various high reactive strains (19). In congenic resistant strains NK reactivity does not follow the H-2 haplotype but resembles the reactivity of the background strain. Thus, pairs of mouse strains which are identical at their H-2 regions but differ with regard to their NK activity (Table I) are available for chimera experiments as described below.

TABLE I. Classification of Histocompatible Mouse Strains According to their Levels of NK Reactivity

H-2	*High reactive strains*	*Low reactive strains*	*References*
a	*B10.A*	*A/Sn, A/J*	*23*
b	*C57BL/6J, C57L*	*A.BY, 129/J*	*23,31*
k	*CBA/J*	*AKR/J*	*18*

In mice, NK activity shows a distinct organ distribution and characteristic changes with age (17,20). Spontaneous NK activity is first detectable at the end of the third week after birth, rises to maximal levels between 6 to 8 weeks and declines thereafter (21). The mechanisms which govern NK reactivity are still poorly understood but seem to depend on many factors involving intact bone marrow function and interferon. Treatment of mice with radioactive strontium (^{89}Sr) leads to the destruction of the bone marrow and causes a profound depression of NK activity without affecting T cell and macrophage mediated effector mechanisms (22). It is thus conceivable that NK cells may require the microenvironment of the bone marrow for their functional differentiation and that a continuous supply of fresh marrow-derived cells may be necessary for the maintenance of normal NK activities.

Using transfer of bone marrow stem cells into irradiated recipients we have demonstrated that NK cells are indeed derived from precursor cells in the bone marrow (23). When bone marrow or fetal liver cells from mouse strains exhibiting either high or low NK reactivity are allowed to repopulate lethally irradiated H-2 compatible recipients, the levels of eventual NK activity in such chimeras are always of donor type as demonstrated in Table II. This strongly suggests that the regulation of NK activity levels is an autonomous function of bone marrow cells (23). Neither spleen nor thymus are mandatory for normal maturation of NK cells in such chimeras (24).

Recently, Roder and Duwe (25) have reported that the beige mutation (bg) in the mouse, previously proposed as an animal model of the Chediak-Higashi syndrome in man (26), causes a profound impairment of NK cell function. Since other anti-tumor effector mechanisms mediated by T cells or macrophages are apparently undisturbed, this mutant mouse may be extremely useful in delineating the *in vivo* relevance of NK cells as will be discussed later.

TABLE II. Levels of NK Reactivity in Spleens from Bone Marrow Chimeras[a]

Type of chimeras[b]	*% Cytotoxicity*	*Type of chimeras*[b]	*% Cytotoxicity*
A.BY → C57L	*11.7 ± 1.7*	*C57L → A.BY*	*25.6 ± 1.6*
A.BY → A.BY	*12.2 ± 0.7*	*C57L → C57L*	*35.7 ± 1.1*
A.BY controls	*15.8 ± 2.3*	*C57 controls*	*28.8 ± 4.8*

[a]Recipients were irradiated with 800 rad and reconstituted i.v. with 3 x 10^7 viable bone marrow cells of sex-matched histocompatible donors.

[b]Chimeras prepared by transfer of cells from donor A into irradiated B recipients are referred to as A → B mice.

[c]Spleen cells from individual chimeras (7 to 12 per group) were tested 6 wks after bone marrow grafting for NK activity against YAC-1 target cells as described (23). Figures represent mean percent lysis ± standard error of the mean.

POSITIVE CORRELATION BETWEEN LEVELS OF NK ACTIVITY AND TUMOR RESISTANCE IN MICE OF VARIOUS GENOTYPES

A first approach to evaluate activity of NK cells *in vivo* took advantage of the genetically determined differences in NK reactivity among various inbred mouse strains (as measured *in vitro* against YAC-1 tumor target cells). In essence, the degree of *in vivo* resistance against a challenge dose of NK-sensitive tumor cells was compared with the levels of *in vitro* NK reactivity. When small numbers (10^3 - 10^4) of YAC (H-2^a) cells were inoculated in A/Sn F_1 hybrids of high or low NK type, a positive correlation was seen between these two parameters in all genotypes tested (27). With larger tumor doses resistance was no longer detectable. Similar correlations between NK activity and *in vivo* resistance of F_1 hybrids have also been observed in several other tumor systems (28,29).

If NK activity *in vitro* and resistance to NK-sensitive tumors *in vivo* were closely correlated, the two properties should co-segregate in suitable backcrosses. To test this possibility, spleen cells from individual (F_1 x A/Sn) backcross mice were tested for NK activity and the splenectomized mice were then challenged with viable YAC tumor cells (splenectomy does not impair NK cell function (24)). Mice with high *in vitro* NK activity generally also had better tumor growth resistance (30).

The non-T-cell nature of this resistance was confirmed in thymectomized, irradiated and fetal-liver-reconstituted mice which showed similar patterns of *in vivo* resistance as their normal counterparts (9).

INFLUENCE OF AGE ON TUMOR RESISTANCE

A close association of NK activity *in vitro* and tumor resistance *in vivo* was also observed when mice of different ages were tested (31). F_1 hybrids between A/Sn and the high reactive strain CBA/H were used. Table III illustrates that young animals at peak NK activity were more resistant to subcutaneous growth of a low dose of YAC lymphoma cells than old mice in which spontaneous levels of NK activity are notoriously low. Thus, tumor resistance *in vivo* seems to parallel the well known changes with age in spontaneous NK activity. Similar observations in other tumor systems have been reported (20,28). NK activity can be boosted in old age by interferon and interferon inducers (including certain tumor cells) (32, 33). Age related changes in resistance are probably most prominent in situations where the tumor inocula themselves are bad NK inducers. Although the findings described so far are compatible with a tumor protective role of NK cells *in vivo*, the contribution of many other factors can hardly be excluded.

TABLE III. Resistance of (A/Sn x CBA/H)F_1 Mice of Varying Ages towards Transplantation with YAC Cells[a]

Age of animals	*Frequency of tumor takes*[b]			
	day 9	*day 18*	*day 25*	*day 56*
3 weeks	*0/10*	*2/10*	*3/10*	*3/10*
6 weeks	*0/8*	*4/8*	*4/8*	*4/8*
6 months	*0/10*	*7/10*	*9/10*	*9/10*
12 months	*0/9*	*7/9*	*8/9*	*8/9*

[a]*Inoculated with 10^3 YAC cells subcutaneously on day 0. (A/Sn x CBA/H)F_1 hybrids have high in vitro NK activity which drops dramatically between 6 wks and 6 months of age (21).*

[b]*Number of mice with tumour out of total number inoculated.*

TUMOR PROTECTIVE ROLE OF NK CELLS IN T CELL DEFICIENT CHIMERAS

To make the striking correlation between levels of NK activity (measured *in vitro*) and expression of resistance in individual animals more significant we looked for means to minimize the complexity of possible effector mechanisms usually involved in *in vivo* phenomena. Adult A/Sn hybrid mice were lethally irradiated and reconstituted with bone marrow cells from H-2 compatible high or low NK donors (see Table I and IV). Since NK activity is predetermined at the stem cell level (23), the repopulated F_1 hybrids eventually exhibited either high or low NK levels according to the genotype of the bone marrow donor. In order to exclude the participation of the T cell system, some of the recipient animals were thymectomized before irradiation and repopulation with marrow or fetal liver cells. Thus, T-cell deficient mice that were genetically nearly identical but differed dramatically in their levels of NK activity could be tested for their tumor rejection potential. These tests revealed significant differences in resistance to subcutaneous growth of YAC tumor cells. High NK F_1 hybrids displayed far better resistance than the low NK hybrids when transplanted with various low doses of YAC tumor cells as summarized in Table IV. These findings indicated that natural resistance against tumor outgrowth *in vivo* may be exerted via NK cells rather than via conventional cell mediated immune reactions (31).

GROWTH OF NK-SENSITIVE AND NK-INSENSITIVE AKR LYMPHOMAS IN CHIMERAS OF HIGH OR LOW NK TYPE

Our previous experiments were limited to a single NK-sensitive tumor, the A/Sn Moloney lymphoma YAC. We have recently extended these studies to another tumor-host system which allowed us to correlate the *in vivo* growth potential of tumors with their *in vitro* sensitivity to NK cells and with the NK activity of the host (34). Out of several AKR T lymphoma lines recently established by Riesenfeld and collaborators (35) two lines were selected, one sensitive (I-522), the other insensitive (I-51) to lysis by NK cells. Both lines showed similar growth patterns in NK low reactive AKR/J mice and in (AKR/J x CBA/J)F_1 chimeras repopulated with AKR/J bone marrow cells. In contrast, F_1 chimeras reconstituted with marrow cells from the NK high reactive strain CBA/J resisted outgrowth of

TABLE IV. *In vivo Resistance of NK Chimeras towards Challenge with Semisyngeneic Tumor Cells*

Exp.	Type of marrow reconstituted chimeras[a]	NK levels[b]	Tumor takes/total[c]	Mortality[d]
1	(A.BY x A/Sn)F_1 → (C57BL/6J x A/Sn)F_1	low	10/10	100%
	(C57BL/6J x A/Sn)F_1 → (C57BL/6J x A/Sn)F_1	high	6/10	60%
	A/Sn controls	low	5/5	100%
2	(129/J x A/Sn)F_1 → ATX(C57BL/6J x A/Sn)F_1	low	9/15	60%
	(C57BL/6J x A/Sn)F_1 → ATX(C57BL/6J x A/Sn)F_1	high	1/14	7%
3	(129/J x A/Sn)F_1 → ATX(129/J x A/Sn)F_1	low	7/8	88%
	(C57BL/6J x A/Sn)F_1 → ATX(129/J x A/Sn)F_1	high	0/8	0%
	A/Sn controls	low	6/6	100%
	(C57BL/6 x A/Sn)F_1 controls	high	0/6	0%

[a]Recipients were irradiated with 750 rad and immediately reconstituted with anti-Thy-1 + C treated bone marrow cells in Exp. 1 and 3 or with fetal liver cells in Exp. 2 as previously described (23,24). A.BY, C57BL/6 and 129 have the same major histocompatibility complex, $H\text{-}2^b$. ATX indicates thymectomy 3 wks before reconstitution (24). Designation of chimeras as in table II.

[b]NK activity of reconstituted mice as assessed in vitro using spleen effector cells and YAC-1 targets (21).

[c]Animals displaying tumor growth out of total number grafted on day 30 after tumor challenge. Tumor challenge consisted of 10^4 (Exp. 1), 5 x 10^3 (Exp. 2) or 10^3 (Exp. 3) cells of the YAC in vivo line transplanted subcutaneously.

[d]All tumor-bearing animals died with tumors.

the NK-sensitive tumor, but were unable to reject transplanted I-51 tumor cells known for their relative insensitivity to NK cells (Table V). The differences in tumor takes observed between the AKR marrow chimeras (low NK type) and the CBA marrow chimeras (high NK type) upon challenge with 5×10^3 cells of the NK sensitive tumor I-522 were highly significant (p below 0.0005 in Chi-square test). Also, the differences in tumor takes between I-522 (NK sensitive) and I-51 (NK insensitive) in CBA marrow chimeras were statistically significant (p below 0.001 for a challenge dose of 5×10^3 tumor cells). F_1 hybrid mice thymectomized as young adults before bone marrow reconstitution (ATX-F_1) had higher levels of NK activity in their peripheral blood and were equally or even better protected against challenge with the NK-sensitive tumor than their immunologically fully competent counterparts. Again, no protection was detectable in such mice against the NK resistant tumor line I-51.

Our results are in line with the findings of Warner and associates (13). They compared the growth of a range of BALB/c tumors in nude (nu/nu homozygous) and non-nude (nu/+ heterozygous) littermates. Tumors which were lysed *in vitro* by spleen cells from normal nude mice exhibited a reduced growth rate in nu/nu as compared to syngeneic nu/+ mice. However, tumors which were resistant to *in vitro* NK lysis grew as well in nude or normal syngeneic mice.

These results strongly support the suggestion that T cells, normally considered to be important in graft rejection, are of relatively little significance compared to NK cells in resistance against transplantation of certain syngeneic tumor cells.

FURTHER EVIDENCE FOR NK CELL MEDIATED RESISTANCE

If there exists a causal relationship between NK function and resistance to tumors, mice lacking a normal NK cell system should exhibit increased tumor susceptibility. This seems to be the case: NK-defective mice, homozygous for the recessive beige gene (bg/bg) (25) develop progressively growing tumors faster and at higher frequency than phenotypically normal (bg/+) littermates when challenged subcutaneously with low doses of syngeneic NK-sensitive leukemias (Klas Kärre, pers. communication). The NK cell defect in bg/bg mice is predetermed at the level of progenitor cells in the bone marrow (36). It would be interesting in the present context to investigate whether transplantation of high NK bone marrow to lethally ir-

TABLE V. In vivo Resistance of NK Reconstituted Chimeras towards Transplantation with NK-Sensitive (I-522) or Non-sensitive (I-51) Lymphomas

Type of reconstituted $(CBA/J \times AKR/J)F_1$ chimeras[a]	NK activity in blood[b]		Tumor dose[c]	Frequency of tumor takes[d]	
	40:1	10:1		I-522	I-51
AKR/J → F_1	9.1	3.5	5×10^3	11/13 (85%)	13/14 (93%)
			5×10^4	15/15 (100%)	14/14 (100%)
CBA/J → F_1	19.9	11.2	5×10^3	2/14 (14%)	10/13 (77%)
			5×10^4	9/11 (82%)	11/11 (100%)
AKR/J → ATX-F_1	23.5	7.6	5×10^4	11/12 (92%)	12/13 (92%)
CBA/J → ATX-F_1	37.5	15.7	5×10^4	6/11 (55%)	9/9 (100%)

[a] $(CBA/J \times AKR/J)F_1$ hybrids were irradiated with 850 rad and immediately reconstituted i.v. with 7×10^6 parental bone marrow cells as indicated (24). One group of 4 wk old F_1-mice was surgically thymectomized 28 days before reconstitution (= ATX) (24).

[b] Blood samples from 10 mice per group were tested for NK activity against YAC-1 target cells 4 wks after reconstitution. Figures indicate mean percent lysis of pairwise pooled samples at the effector to target cell ratios indicated.

[c] Number of tumor cells inoculated subcutaneously 6 wks after bone marrow reconstitution. The AKR lymphoma I-522 is highly sensitive to lysis by NK cells whereas I-51 is relatively insensitive (34).

[d] Number of mice with tumor on day 60 out of total number of mice inoculated. (Percentages are given in brackets.)

radiated beige recipients could substitute for the low natural resistance to small tumor inocula observed in this mutant mouse.

More direct proof for a functional role of NK cells in tumor rejection was attempted in experiments in which NK rich spleen cell populations were admixed with sensitive tumor cells and inoculated subcutaneously into irradiated syngeneic recipients. It was evident that spleen cell fractions depleted of mature T cells, B cells and macrophages, but highly enriched for NK activity, were most efficient in preventing tumor growth (9,37).

CONCLUDING REMARKS

We have considered here some current evidence for the potential of NK cells in tumor graft rejection. While these data indicate a prominent role of the NK system in natural resistance towards transplantable tumor cell lines *in vivo* they suggest, but by no means prove, the participation of NK cells in surveillance against newly arising tumor cell clones. An argument in favor of a surveillance mechanism mediated by NK cells is the finding that T cell deficient nude mice, known to exhibit high NK levels, do not develop spontaneous tumors at greater rates than normal mice (5,6). In fact, NK cells would seem to be extremely well equipped to serve as effector cells in immune surveillance: They preexist in the normal, unprimed animal, they are generated in an autonomous manner independently of T or B cell functions and they are able to act at early stages of tumor development before an adapative, conventional immune response is established. All evaluations of the *in vivo* activity of NK cells performed so far have used tumor rejection experiments. It should be kept in mind that rejection of grafted tumor cells is probably an inadequate model for immune surveillance. The inoculation of small numbers of syngeneic tumor cells into the subcutaneous space of an unprimed animal seems to be an awkward way of imitating the process of spontaneous tumor development during which autochthonous cells get transformed and start to grow in their own natural microenvironment within discrete anatomical compartments.

Whereas the present data indicate that NK cells most likely provide the host with a rapidly acting first level of defense against transplanted tumor cells, future work will have to clarify the role of NK cells in primary tumor induction and immune surveillance.

ACKNOWLEDGMENTS

We thank Jean Lindenmann for critical reading of the manuscript. This work was supported, in part, by grants from the Swiss National Science Foundation (No. 3.139-0.77), the Swedish Cancer Society and NCI contract NOI-CB 64033.

REFERENCES

1. Cerottini, J.C., and Brunner, K.T., *Adv. Immunol. 18,* 67 (1974).
2. Burnet, F.M., *Progr. Exp. Tumor Res. 13,* 1 (1970).
3. Klein, G., *Harvey Lectures 69,* 71 (1975).
4. Stutman, O., *Adv. Cancer Res. 22,* 261 (1975).
5. Rygaard, J., and Povlsen, C.O., *Transplant. Rev. 28,* 43 (1976).
6. Stutman, O., *Science 183,* 534 (1974).
7. Giovanella, B.C., Stehlin, J.S., and Williams, L.J. jr., *J. Natl. Cancer Inst. 52,* 921 (1974).
8. Bonmassar, E., Campanile, F., Hochens, D., Crino, L., and Goldin, A., *Transplantation 20,* 343 (1975).
9. Kiessling, R., Petranyi, G., Klein, G., and Wigzell, H., *Int. J. Cancer 17,* 1 (1976).
10. Gillette, R.W., and Fox, A., *Cell. Immunol. 19,* 328 (1975).
11. Greenberg, A.H., and Greene, M., *Nature 264,* 356 (1976).
12. Epstein, A.L., Herman, M.M., Kim, H., Dorfman, R.F., and Kaplan, H.S., *Cancer 37,* 2158 (1976).
13. Warner, N.L., Woodruff, M.F.A., and Burton, R.C., *Int. J. Cancer 20,* 146 (1977).
14. Baldwin, R.W., *Nature 270,* 557 (1977).
15. Adams, D.O., and Snyderman, R., *J. Natl. Cancer Inst. 62,* 1341 (1979).
16. James, K., McBride, B., and Stuart, A. (eds.) "The Macrophage and Cancer". Econoprint, Edinburgh (1977).
17. Kiessling, R., and Haller, O., *Contemp. Top. Immunobiol. 8,* 171 (1978).
18. Kiessling, R., and Wigzell, H., *Immunol. Rev. 44,* 165 (1979).
19. Petranyi, G.G., Kiessling, R., and Klein, G., *Immunogenetics 2,* 53 (1975).
20. Herberman, R.B., and Holden, H.T., *Adv. Cancer Res. 27,* 305 (1978).
21. Kiessling, R., Klein, E., and Wigzell, H., *Eur. J. Immuno-*

logy 5, 112 (1975).
22. Haller, O., and Wigzell, H., *J. Immunol. 118*, 1503 (1977).
23. Haller, O., Kiessling, R., Örn, A., and Wigzell, H., *J. Exp. Med. 145*, 1411 (1977).
24. Haller, O., Gidlund, M., Kurnick, J.T., and Wigzell, H., *Scand. J. Immunol. 8*, 207 (1978).
25. Roder, J., and Duwe, A., *Nature 278*, 451 (1979).
26. Windhorst, D.B., and Padgett, G., *J. Invest. Dermatol. 60*, 529 (1973).
27. Kiessling, R., Petranyi, G., Klein, G., and Wigzell, H., *Int. J. Cancer 15*, 933 (1975).
28. Sendo, F., Aoki, T., Boyse, E.A., and Buofo, C.K., *J. Natl. Cancer Inst. 55*, 603 (1975).
29. Harmon, R.C., Clark, E., O'Toole, C., and Wicker, L., *Immunogenetics 4*, 601 (1977).
30. Petranyi, G.G., Kiessling, R., Povey, S., Klein, G., Herzenberg, L., and Wigzell, H., *Immunogenetics 3*, 15 (1976).
31. Haller, O., Hansson, M., Kiessling, R., and Wigzell, H., *Nature 270*, 609 (1977).
32. Gidlund, M., Orn, A., Wigzell, H., Senik, A., and Gresser, I., *Nature 273*, 759 (1978).
33. Djeu, J.Y., Heinbaugh, J.A., Holden, H.T., and Herberman, R.B., *J. Immunol. 122*, 175 (1979).
34. Riesenfeld, I., Örn, A., Gidlund, M., Axberg, I., Alm, G. V., and Wigzell, H., *Int. J. Cancer*, in press (1980).
35. Riesenfeld, I., Tufveson, G., and Alm, G., *Acta Path. Microbiol. Scand. Sect. A 85*, 739 (1977).
36. Roder, J.C., *J. Immunol. 123*, 2168 (1979).

ANALOGY BETWEEN REJECTION OF HEMOPOIETIC TRANSPLANTS AND NATURAL KILLING

Eva Lotzová

Department of Developmental Therapeutics
The University of Texas System Cancer Center
M.D. Anderson Hospital and Tumor Institute
Houston, Texas

For its unusual immunogenetics, rejection (or "take") of bone marrow transplants has represented an arcane and unpredictable phenomenon for more than a decade (see for review 1). It has been difficult for immunogeneticists to conform to the fact that other than classical histocompatibility genes govern marrow rejection and that the cells mediating it have such peculiar characteristics, as radioresistance, thymus independence, late maturation, and capacity to kill rapidly and naturally (i.e. without any previous immunization with target tissue). Prior to the discovery of the phenomenon of natural killing (2-3), cellular mechanism expressing these uncommon characteristics has been unknown. With its revelation, we and other investigators (4-6) began comparative studies on natural killer (NK) cells mediated immunity and anti-bone marrow immunity. We have found that NK cells and bone marrow effector (BM-E) cells share multiple characteristics, most of which are listed in Table I (also see for review 1,4,7).

After this initial observation, we have tested the effect of various cytocidal and immunomodulating agents on NK cell activities and examined whether changes in NK cell cytotoxicity also reflected changes in anti-bone marrow graft reactivity. NK cell cytotoxicity was measured by 16 hrs. chromium-51 cytotoxicity assay as described previously (6) and the growth of bone marrow cells was measured by two different techniques,

This work was supported by Grant CA 21062 from NCI

ISBN 0-12-341350-8

TABLE I. Major Common Characteristics of Natural Killer Cells and Bone Marrow Effector Cells

Natural Occurrence (Without Previous Contact with Antigen)
Rapid Function (Within a Few Hours)
Reactivity to Normal and Malignant Tissues
Thymus Independence
Bone Marrow Dependence
Late Maturation
Partial Declination with Age
Relative Radioresistance
Sensitivity to Tolerance Induction
Sensitivity to Similar Agents

by incorporation of radiolabelled DNA precursor 5-iodo-2' deoxyuridine (^{125}IUdR) (1) and by spleen colony assay (CFU-S) as described by Till and McCulloch (8). As can be seen from Table II, there was a close relation between NK cell levels and bone marrow graft rejection potential, namely high NK cell activities were paralleled by strong anti-bone marrow transplant reactivity and vice versa, low NK cell activities reflected the failure to reject marrow transplants. For instance, agents such as glucan (2mg/mouse, i.v.), *C.parvum* (0.5mg/mouse,i.v.), cytoxan (350mg/kg, i.p.), silica (3-5mg/mouse,i.v.) and carrageenan (2.5mg/mouse,i.v.) caused significant decline in NK cell cytotoxicity and simultaneously promoted the growth of bone marrow cells. On the other hand, piperazinedione (8.3mg/kg, i.v.), interferon (virus-induced, $5x10^4$ units/mouse, i.v.) and levamisole (20mg/kg, i.v.) did not affect either NK cell or BM-E cell functions. This functional and biological similarity between bone marrow effectors and cells mediating natural killing is too evident to be merely coincidental. Thus, it appears that NK cells and BM-E cells may represent the same cell population and consequently NK cells are implicated in bone marrow graft rejection.

One point of discrepancy between BM-E and NK cells which would appear to weaken the hypothesis of NK cell and BM-E cell identity has been published recently. It was reported that whereas splenic NK cell activity decreased after hydrocortisone treatment, splenic rejection potential, directed against parental bone marrow transplants, remained unaltered (9). This observation was based on the failure to detect significant ^{125}IUdR uptake (reflecting the growth of transplanted bone marrow cells) 5 days after transplantation. We have argued, that since cortisone did not cause complete destruction of NK cells (at least 25% of NK cell activity remained in cortisone treated mice- see Table III), the remaining NK cells could still effectively reject significant number of transplanted marrow cells. Consequently, ^{125}IUdR uptake (reflecting the cell growth) may not be appreciable on day 5; however, the cell growth may be detected at later time intervals after transplantation. On the basis of this reasoning, we have transplanted cortisone treated mice and measured the growth of transplanted cells on days 5 and 8 post transplant. As can be seen in Table III, indeed on day 8, expressive cell growth, associated with significant uptake of ^{125}IUdR was obtained. The ^{125} IUdR uptake could be contributed only to the growth of injected marrow cells, and not to endogenous cell proliferation,because the recipients were firstly, lethally irradiated and secondly, there was no uptake in radiation control mice (see legend of Table III). Hence, independently what the mechanism of delayed marrow growth is, it is apparent from these experiments that the effect of cortisone on NK cells and BM-E cells is comparable; both functions were decreased (but not totally abolished) after cortisone treatment.

TABLE II. Analogy Between NK Cell Activities and the Growth of Parental Bone Marrow Transplants in B6DF$_1$ Mice

Type of Treatment	*% Splenic Cytotoxicity*[a,b]	*%Splenic Uptake of ^{125}IUdR*[b,c]	*CFU-S Formation*[c]
None	*41.6±3.4(20)*	*0.04±0.01(17)*	*None*
Piperazinedione	*38.6±2.9(7)*	*0.03±0.01(9)*	*None*
Interferon	*38.7±2.3(6)*	*0.02±0.06(10)*	*None*
Levamisole	*41.0±4.3(10)*	*0.05±0.01(9)*	*None*
Glucan	*10.1±1.2(7)*	*0.75±0.08(20)*	*Confluent*
C.parvum	*7.8±2.0(10)*	*1.30±0.09(10)*	*Confluent*
Cytoxan	*5.5±1.3(7)*	*0.86±0.04(5)*	*Confluent*
Silica	*13.4±3.2(10)*	*0.91±0.09(7)*	*ND*
Carrageenan	*3.7±1.1(10)*	*1.30±0.06(10)*	*Confluent*

[a] *$2x10^4$ YAC-1 target cells were incubated with treated or untreated B6DF$_1$ spleen cells (1:50 T:E ratio) for 16 hrs.*

[b] *Natural killing and splenic uptake are presented as means ± S.E; number of mice is indicated in parenthesis.*

[c] *Mice were given 1100R whole body irradiation and transplanted 24 hrs. later with 10^6 B6 bone marrow cells. ^{125}IUdR was injected 7 days after bone marrow transplantation. ^{125}IUdR in syngeneic controls was 0.97±0.10(20) and in radiation controls 0.01±0.001(20). CFU-S were confluent in syngeneic B6 mice and were not formed in radiation controls.*

Even though the direct evidence for involvement of NK cells in bone marrow transplantation reactivity remains to be furnished, there is currently no resolute discrepancy between natural killer and bone marrow rejection phenomenona.

TABLE III. There is No Discrepancy Between Sensitivity of NK Cell and BM-E Cell to Cortisone

Treatment[a]	*% Splenic Natural Killing*[b]	*% Splenic Uptake of $^{125}IUdR$*[c]	
		5 days	*8 days*
None	*52.3±2.2(13)*	*0.01±0.02(6)*	*0.04±0.01(16)*
Cortisone	*13.0±2.4(9)*	*0.08±0.01(5)*	*0.79±0.11(20)*

[a] *5mg of cortisone acetate was injected i.p., 48 hrs, prior to transplantation.*

[b] *$2x10^4$ YAC-1 target cells were incubated with $B6DF_1$ mice spleen cells (1:50 T:E ratio) for 16 hrs. The values represent the mean ± S.E.*

[c] *$B6DF_1$ were given 1100R whole body irradiation and transplanted 24 hrs. later with 10^6 B6 bone marrow cells. $^{125}IUdR$ in syngeneic controls was 1.20±0.2(10) and that in radiation control mice 0.04±0.008(7). The values represent the mean ± S.E.*

REFERENCES

1. Lotzová, E., *Exp. Hematol*, *5*,215 (1977).
2. Herberman, R., Nunn, M.E., and Lavrin, D.H., *Int. J. Cancer 16*, 216 (1975).
3. Kiessling, R., Klein, E., and Wigzell, H., *Eur. J. Immunol. 5*, 112 (1975).
4. Lotzová, E., and Savary, C.A., *Biomedicine 27*, 341 (1977).
5. Kiessling, R., Hochman, P.S., Haller, O., Shearer, G.M., Wigzell, H., and Cudkowicz, G., *Eur. J. Immunol. 7*, 665, (1977).
6. Savary, C.A., and Lotzová, E., *J. Immunol. 120*, 239 (1978)
7. Lotzová, E., and McCredie, K.B., *Cancer Immunol. & Immunother. 4*, 215 (1978).
8. Till, J.E., and McCulloch, E.A., *Radiat. Res. 14*, 213 (1961).
9. Hochman, P.S., and Cudkowicz, G., *J. Immunol. 119*, 2013 (1977).

ROLE OF NK CELLS IN RAPID *IN VIVO* CLEARANCE OF RADIOLABELED TUMOR CELLS

C. Riccardi[1]
A. Santoni
T. Barlozzari

Institute of Pharmacology
University of Perugia
Perugia, Italy

R. B. Herberman

Laboratory of Immunodiagnosis
National Cancer Institute
Bethesda, Maryland

I. INTRODUCTION

There has been great interest in the role of the immune system in the control of *in vivo* tumor growth and dissemination and in the possible efficacy of immunotherapy of cancer (Salmon, 1977). Different mechanisms have been implicated in tumor resistance. For years, particular attention was focused on cytotoxicity or lymphokine production by T cells and the keyrole of thymus-dependent immunity in immune surveillance was stressed (Burnet, 1970). Recently other kinds of effector mechanisms have been described, especially macrophages and natural killer (NK) cells. The possible involvement of these thymus-independent systems in the control of *in vivo* growth of tumor cells and in immune surveillance must now be considered.

[1]*This work was supported by Progetto Finalizzato "Controllo della crescita neoplastica, no. 79.00668.96, CNR, Italy*

ISBN 0-12-341350-8

Naturally occurring cytotoxicity by NK cells has been detected in various experimental animals and in man (Herberman and Holden, 1978). Reactivity has been detected against malignant cells and also against virus-infected cells, fetal fibroblasts and some thymocytes, macrophages and bone marrow cells. The wide range of NK reactivity suggests their involvement in the regulation of differentiation of normal cells and in the defense against pathogens as well as resistance against neoplastic cells (Cudkowicz *et al.*, 1979; Trischmann *et al.*, 1978; Herberman *et al.*, 1979).

Most available data on NK reactivity was obtained in *in vitro* studies. However, there have been some indirect indications that this spontaneously occurring and rapidly inducible effector mechanism may be one of the first lines of defense against tumors *in vivo*. The correlation between levels of NK activity and resistance to growth of some transplantable NK-sensitive tumor cells, and the transfer of tumor resistance as well as NK reactivity by bone marrow transfer, have provided support for this hypothesis (Haller *et al.*, 1977 a,b; Warner *et al.*, 1977, Harmon *et al.*, 1977). In addition, NK activity has been found to correlate with *in vivo* reactivity of lethally irradiated mice against Hh antigens on bone marrow transplants (Kiessling *et al.*, 1977). However, in all of these studies, *in vivo* results could only be evaluated after several days or weeks, thereby increasing the likelihood for involvement of multiple effector mechanisms and preventing the distinction between cytolytic and cytostatic events. To avoid these problems and to obtain more direct evidence for the *in vivo* role of NK cells, we have recently utilized a rapid *in vivo* assay in which elimination of isotopically labeled tumor cells is measured in various organs and compared to the levels of *in vitro* NK reactivity (Riccardi *et al.*, 1979a). As summarized here, we have found a remarkably good correlation between the *in vivo* and *in vitro* assays, indicating that NK cells play an important role in the rapid *in vivo* elimination of transplantable tumor cells and of some normal cells.

II. KINETICS OF *IN VIVO* AND *IN VITRO* REACTIVITY AGAINST PRE-LABELED TUMOR CELLS

Tumor cells were labeled *in vitro* by culturing them in the presence of ^{125}IUdR and then injected intravenously in groups of 6-8 animals. After different times, mice were killed and the elimination of tumor cells from various organs was estimated by measuring the recovery of radioactivity.

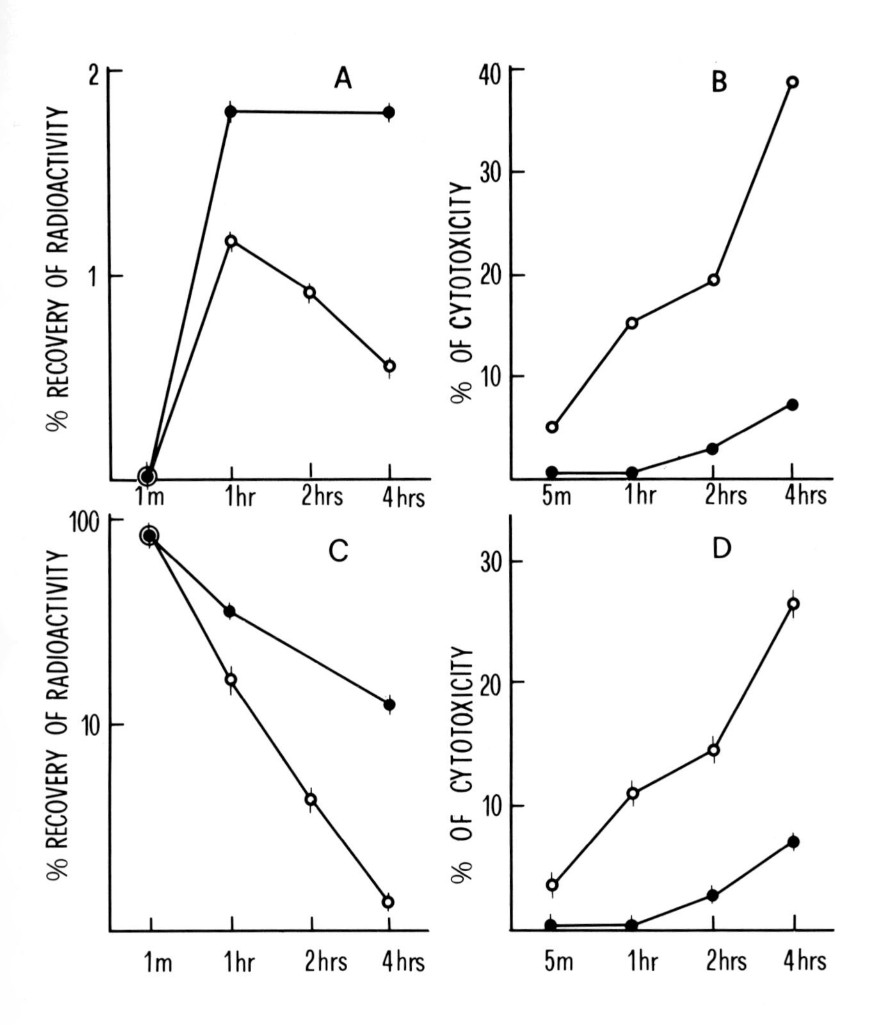

FIGURE 1. Kinetics of in vivo *and* in vitro *cytolysis exhibited by spleen and lungs of age-matched (8 week-old) CBA (o--o) and SJL (●--●) mice.* 10^6 *YAC-1 prelabeled cells were injected intravenously and the radioactivity retained in the spleen (Panel A) and lungs (Panel C) was evaluated at different times. Spleen cells (Panel B) and cells from the lungs (Panel D) were tested for NK activity against YAC-1, (A/T ratio 100:1) and release of* ^{51}Cr *was measured at different times. The* in vivo *data are expressed as geometric means and the vertical bars indicate the range. % recovery of radioactivity in the lungs on log scale and in spleen on arithmetic scale.* In vitro *data: arithmetic means, on arithmetic scale.*

The exact procedure has been previously described (Riccardi *et al.*, 1979). The data were expressed as the geometric mean of the percent recovery of radioactivity. Figure 1 shows the results obtained when high NK-reactive CBA/J and low NK-reactive SJL/J were injected iv with 10^6 prelabeled YAC-1 tumor cells. The kinetics of the *in vivo* clearance in the spleen and in the lungs show an equal distribution of prelabeled neoplastic cells at 1 minute after injection. However, at 1 hour significant ($p < 0.01$) differences in the levels of radioactivity between the two mouse strains were detected. Such differences became more marked at 2 and 4 hours after challenge. Total body counts (data not shown) ruled out the possibility that we were simply measuring redistribution of tumor cells and rather indicated that loss of radioactivity was due to cell destruction. In the same figure, the kinetics or *in vitro* lysis of ^{51}Cr labeled YAC-1 cells by splenic cells or by effector cells obtained from mincing of the lungs (Puccetti *et al.*, 1980) are reported. Similar to the *in vivo* assay, highly significant differences between the strains were observed when the levels of *in vitro* cytolysis were measured at 1, 2 and 4 hours after initial target-effector cell contact.

The characteristic age-dependency of NK reactivity in mice offers another approach to study the correlation between the *in vivo* clearance of tumor cells and natural cytotoxicity *in vitro*. As an example, in Figure 2 the kinetics of *in vivo* reactivity in the spleen, lungs and liver of young and older CBA/J mice are compared to the *in vitro* NK activity of spleen cells. Similar to the difference in NK activity between the groups, lower levels of *in vivo* reactivity at 2-4 hrs have been observed in all the organs of older mice when compared with those in young animals.

III. STRAIN DISTRIBUTION AND AGE-DEPENDENCY OF *IN VIVO* CYTOLYTIC REACTIVITY AND RELATION TO *IN VITRO* CYTOTOXICITY BY NK CELLS OR MACROPHAGES

The above parallels between NK activity and *in vivo* cytolytic reactivity were supported by a study of the distribution of both reactivities among various mouse strains. A total of 25 strains (inbred, F_1 and F_2 hybrids) of different ages has been analyzed in different experiments. Some strains were

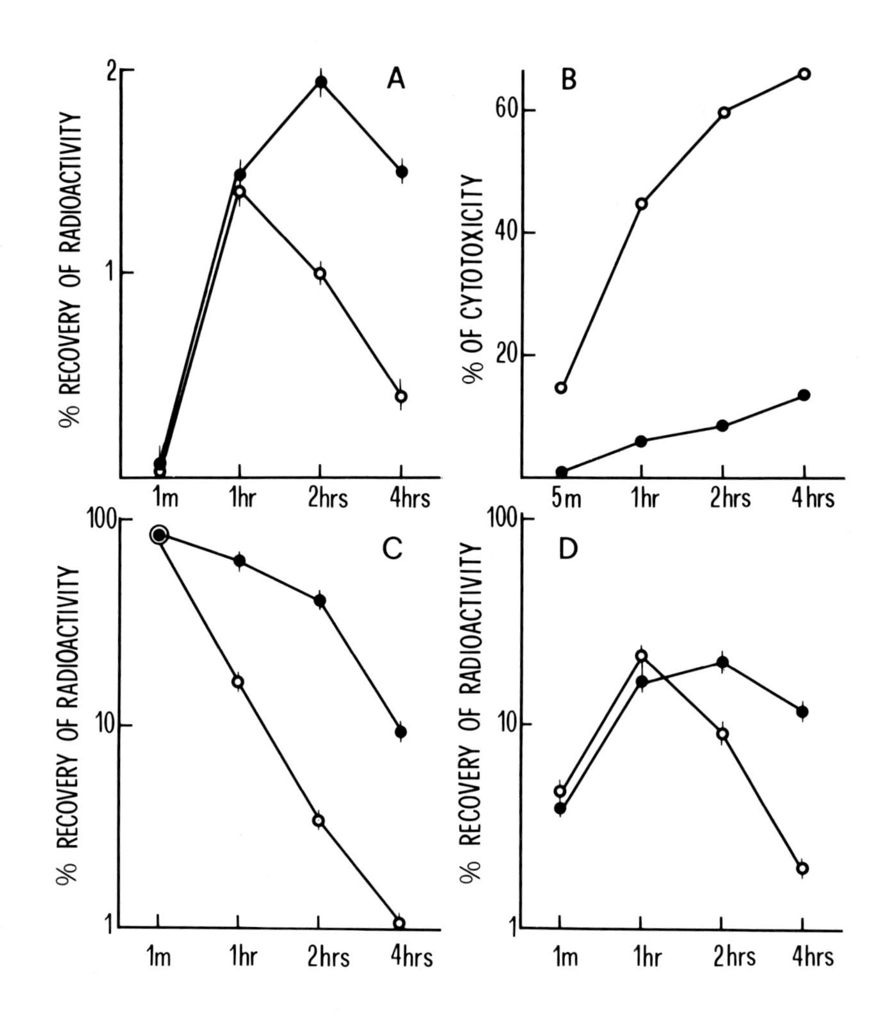

FIGURE 2. Kinetics of in vivo *and* in vitro *cytolytic activity of young (8 week-old, o--o) and old (20 week-old, (●--●) CBA mice.* 10^6 *YAC-1 prelabeled cells were injected intravenously and the radioactivity retained in the spleen (Panel A), lungs (Panel C) and liver (Panel D) was evaluated at different times. Spleen cells (Panel B) were tested for NK activity against YAC-1 (A/T ratio 100:1) and release of* ^{51}Cr *was measured at different times. % radioactivity recovered in the spleen and lungs and %* in vitro *cytotoxicity expressed as in Figure 1. The % recovery of radioactivity in liver, geometric means and scale. Vertical bars indicate the range.*

found to have low reactivity both *in vivo* and in *in vitro* assays of NK activity, and these included SJL/J, DBA/2, ASW, A/J, ABy, and C57BL/6 bg/bg (beige) mice. In contrast, CBA, C57BL/6, $BD2F_1$, $(CBAxB6)F_1$, $(B6xC3H)F_1$, C57Bl/10, $CD2F_1$ and others have been shown to have high reactivity in both assays. Moreover, in all the strains analyzed, both reactivities declined after 10-12 weeks of age. The results of a typical study are presented in Table I. Among young mice of the different strains, SJL, the one strain with low NK activity, also showed less clearance of radiolabeled cells, especially from the lungs and liver. Also, the clearance of radiolabeled tumor cells in older mice of the high NK reactive strains was much reduced compared to younger mice of the same strains. In general, the *in vivo* data are more impressive for the lungs, with often only small differences seen in the spleen. In this Table is also reported the *in vitro* cytotoxic activity of

TABLE I. Strain distribution of in vivo *clearance of radiolabeled tumor cells, NK activity, and macrophage-mediated cytolytic activity*

Strain	*Age (wks)*	*recovery of radioactivity*[a]			*% cytotoxicity vs. YAC-1*[b]	*% cytotoxicity vs. TU5*[c]
		Spleen	*Liver*	*Lungs*		
					100:1[d]	*20:1*
CBA/J	*8*	*0.2*	*1.7*	*0.5*	*47.1*	*24.2*
SJL/J	*8*	*1.2*	*7.9*	*14.6*	*5.0*	*29.5*
$(SJLxCBA)F_1$	*8*	*0.4*	*2.5*	*1.7*	*24.1*	*28.1*
C57BL/6	*6-7*	*0.5*	*1.0*	*0.5*	*59.1*	*26.3*
C3H	*8*	*0.7*	*2.0*	*0.4*	*45.8*	*39.7*
$(B6xC3H)F_1$	*8*	*0.7*	*2.1*	*0.5*	*36.7*	*23.0*
$BD2F_1$	*8*	*0.3*	*0.9*	*0.2*	*47.2*	*33.1*
CBA/J	*20*	*1.8*	*11.3*	*10.8*	*9.5*	*20.8*
C57BL/6	*23*	*1.4*	*10.1*	*10.5*	*8.6*	*21.1*
$(B6xC3H)F_1$	*32*	*1.1*	*6.9*	*3.2*	*23.7*	*20.0*

a) *% recovery of radioactivity at 4 hrs after IV inoculation of YAC-1.*

b) *NK activity was measured in 4 hr-CRA.*

c) *Effector cells were adherent spleen cells tested in a 48hr cytotoxicity assay directed against ^{125}IUdR-labeled TU5 cells.*

d) *E/T = effector/target ratio.*

splenic macrophages, measured in a 48-hr-assay against ^{125}IUdR labeled TU5 tumor cells. As previously described by others (Keller, 1978; Tagliabue *et al.*, 1979), similar levels of cytotoxicity were seen among mice of different ages and genotypes, and no correlation was found between *in vivo* natural reactivity and natural cytotoxic activity mediated by macrophages.

IV. REGULATION OF *IN VIVO* AND *IN VITRO* REACTIVITIES

A variety of biological and synthetic agents such as interferon, *C. parvum*, BCG, lymphocytic choriomeningitis virus, murine sarcoma virus, pyran copolymer, poly I:C and tumor cells, administered at the appropriate time have been shown to augment *in vitro* NK reactivity (Herberman *et al.*, 1977; Djeu *et al.*, 1979a; Santoni *et al.*, 1979), and these treatments also altered *in vivo* clearance of labeled tumor cells. For example, the kinetic study of *in vivo* and *in vitro* reactivity summarized in Figure 3 shows the augmentation of these reactivities following intravenous injection of Poly I:C 18 hours before assay. The finding that strong and rapid augmentation of *in vivo* and *in vitro* natural reactivities in older mice can be obtained by stimulation with a variety of agents (including tumor cells) suggests that NK activity could be relevant in the *in vivo* surveillance against tumors in older mice as well as in young mice exhibiting high levels of spontaneous reactivity.

A general observation which has emerged from studies on regulation of NK activity is that the same agent which is capable of inducing augmentation of reactivity at one time may also be responsible for the depression of reactivity at a different time.

For example, we have found that pyran copolymer may enhance the *in vivo* and *in vitro* reactivities when administered 2-3 days before the assay. (Santoni *et al.*, 1979), but a marked decrease in the levels of NK reactivity may be seen at 7 days. The depression of NK activity has occurred at a time when highly activated macrophages have been detected (Puccetti *et al.*, 1979; Riccardi *et al.*, 1979b) and these macrophages appear to be responsible for inhibiting the *in vitro* lytic function of NK cells. As a further correlation with NK activity, we have found that *in vivo* elimination of tumor cells from the lungs and other organs is reduced during this later period after treatment. For example, we have performed a kinetic study of *in vivo* and NK reactivity of young mice of a

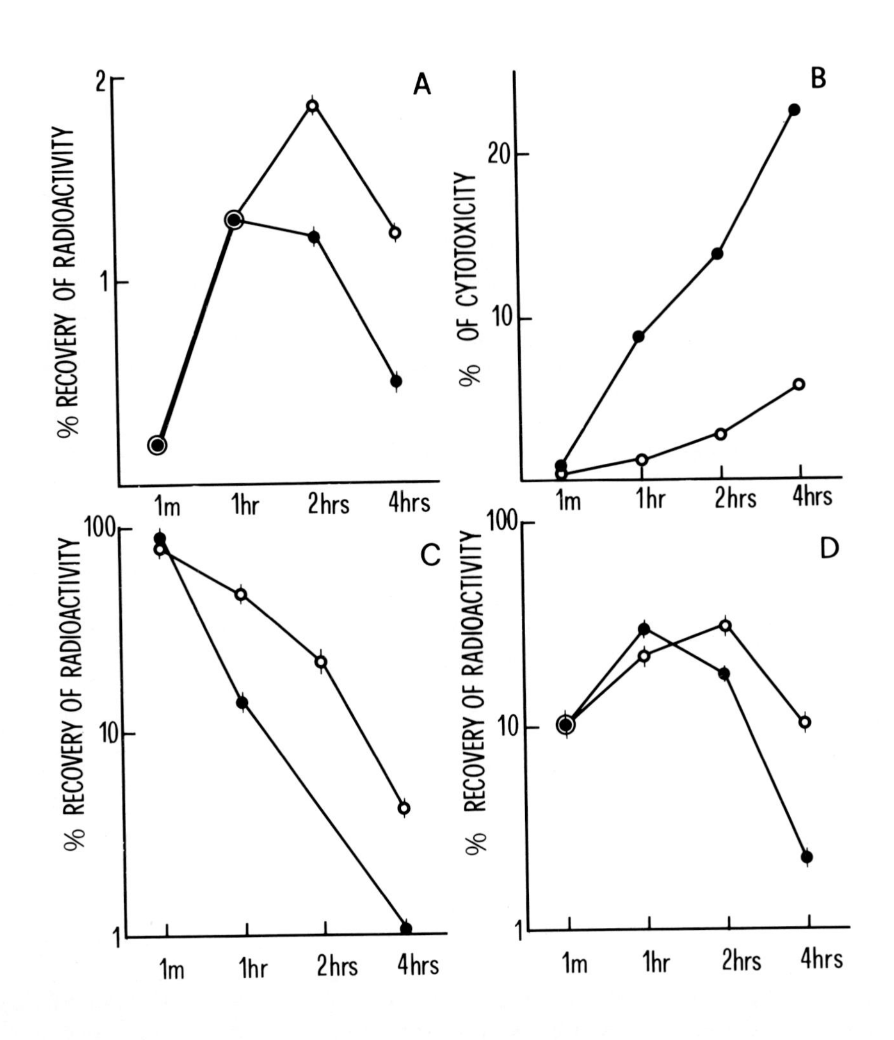

FIGURE 3. Kinetics of in vivo and in vitro cytolytic activity of untreated (o--o) and Poly I:C treated (●--●, 5 mg/kg iv 18 hrs earlier) 20 week-old $CD2F_1$ mice. 10^6 prelabeled YAC-1 cells were injected IV and the radioactivity retained in the spleen (Panel A), lungs (Panel C) and liver (Panel D) was evaluated. Spleen cells (Panel B) were tested for NK vs. YAC-1 (A/T ratio 100:1). Data expressed as in Figs. 1 and 2.

high reactive strain, injected iv 7 days before with pyran copolymer (Fig. 4). In parallel with the severe depression of NK reactivity in the spleen of pyran-treated mice, the efficiency of treated mice in eliminating tumor cells was clearly impaired.

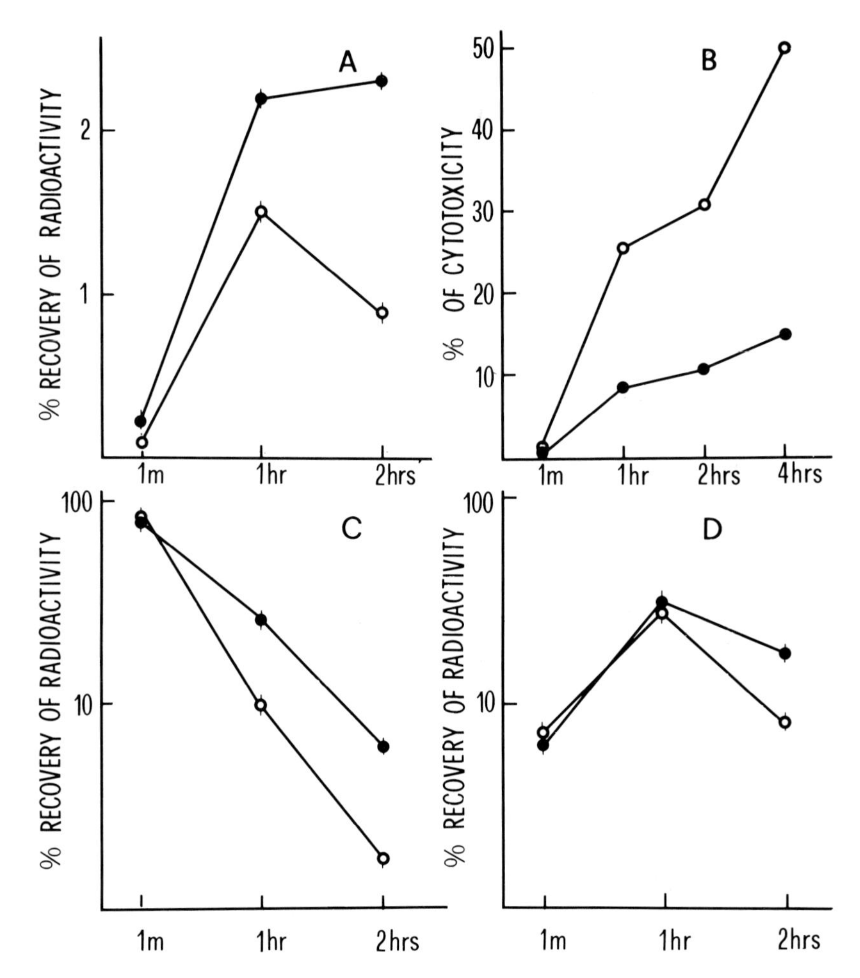

FIGURE 4. Kinetics of in vivo *and* in vitro *cytolytic activity of untreated (o--o) and pyran copolymer-treated (●--●, 75 mg/kg iv 7 days earlier) 8 week-old CBA mice.* 10^6 *YAC-1 prelabeled cells were injected iv and the radioactivity retained in the spleen (Panel A), lungs (Panel C) and liver (Panel D) evaluated. Spleen cells (Panel B) were tested for NK vs. YAC-1 (A/T ratio 100:1). Data expressed as in Fig. 1 and 2.*

Similar marked depressive effects on both *in vivo* and *in vitro* reactivities have also been obtained following other immunopharmacological treatments. Treatment with silica was found to have similar depressive effects on both *in vivo* and NK reactivities (Riccardi et al., 1979a). Another antimacrophage agent, i-carrageenan, given iv 1 day before assay, also caused depression in NK activity and an impairment of *in vivo* reactivity, particularly in the spleen (Fig. 5).

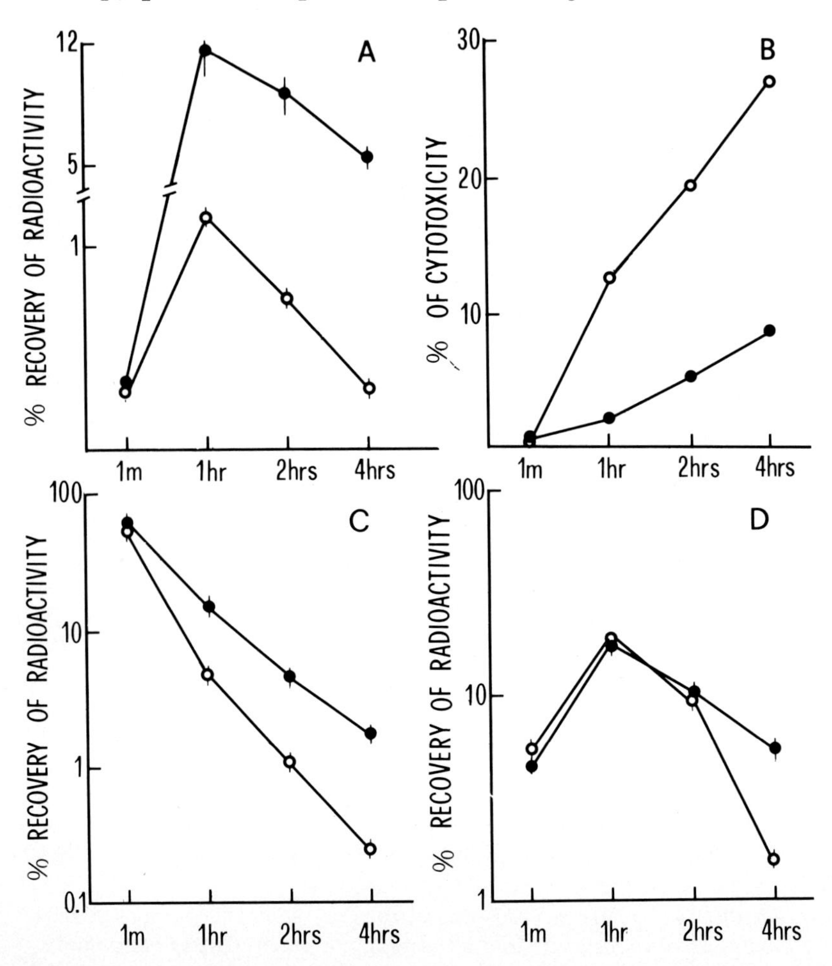

FIGURE 5. Kinetics of in vivo *and* in vitro *cytolytic activity of untreated (o--o) and i-carrageenan-treated (●--●, 1 mg/ mouse iv 1 day earlier) 8 week-old C57BL/6 mice. 10^6 YAC-1 prelabeled cells were injected iv and the radioactivity retained in the spleen (Panel A), lungs (Panel C) and liver (Panel D) was evaluated. Spleen cells (panel B) were tested for NK vs. YAC-1 (A/T ratio 100:1). Data expressed as in Fig. 1 and 2.*

In vivo and *in vitro* cytolytic activity have also been studied 1 day after injection with cyclophosphamide (Fig. 6) or 2, 24 and 72 hours after exposure to lethal doses of

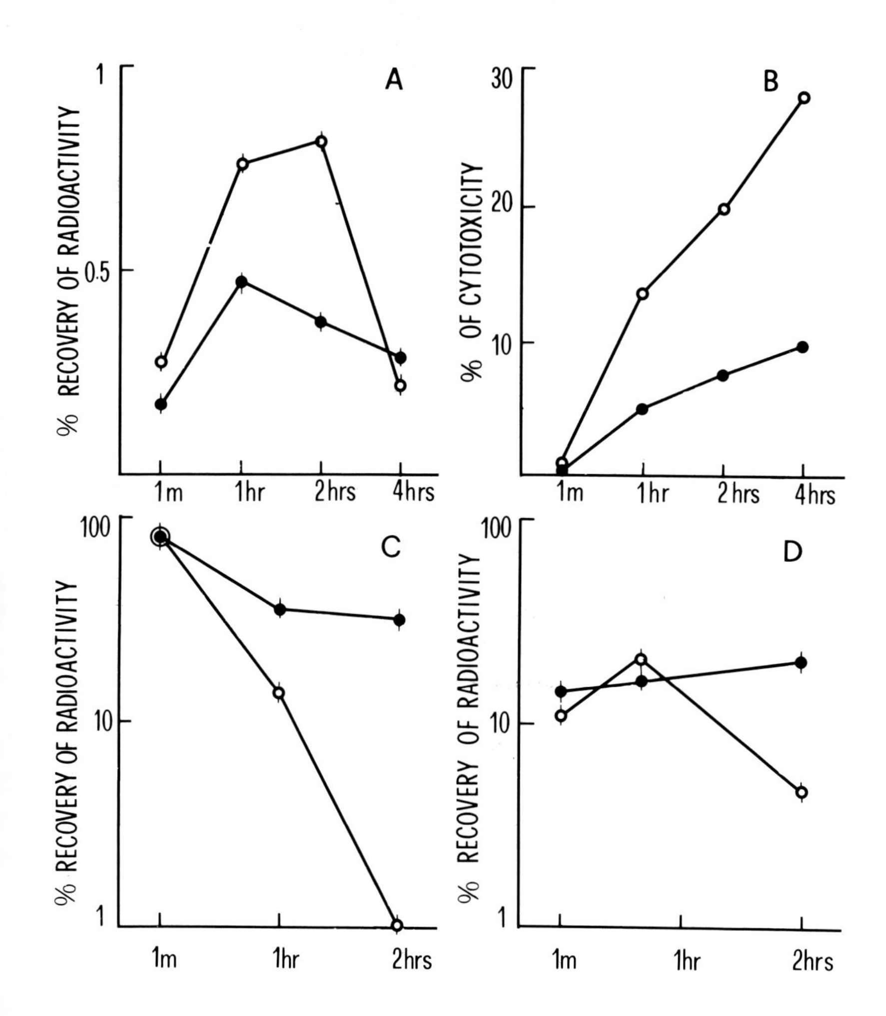

FIGURE 6. Kinetics of in vivo *and* in vitro *cytolytic activity of untreated (o--o) and cyclophosphamide-treated (●--●, 300 mg/kg iv 1 day earlier) 8-week-old C57BL/6 mice. 10^6 YAC-1 prelabeled cells were injected iv and the radioactivity retained in the spleen (Panel A), lungs (Panel C) and liver (Panel D) was evaluated. Spleen cells (Panel B) were tested for NK vs. YAC-1 (A/T ratio 100:1). Data expressed as in Fig. 1 and 2.*

irradiation (850R) (Fig. 7). Treatment with cyclophosphamide or exposure to lethal irradiation 1 or 3 days earlier, resulted in marked depression of NK reactivity. There was an

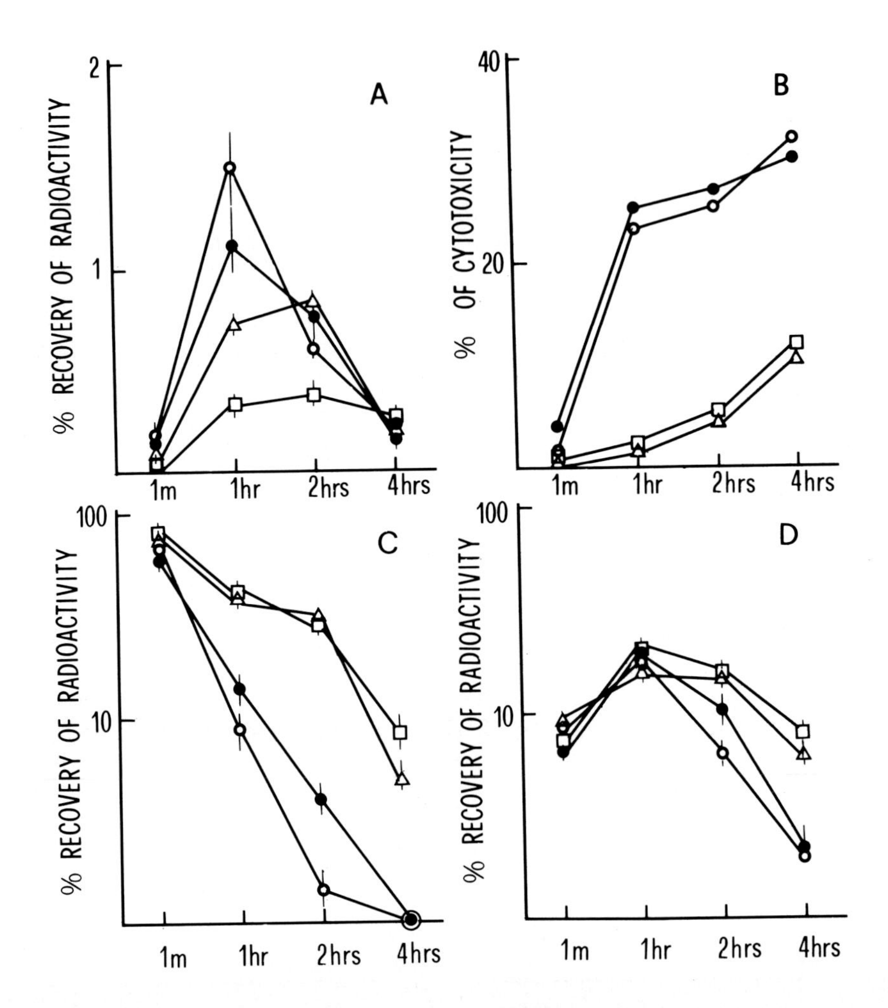

FIGURE 7. Kinetics of in vivo *and* in vitro *cytolytic activity of untreated (o--o) and lethally irradiated (850 Rads γ-rays, ●--● 2 hours, △--△ 1 day, □--□ 3 days earlier) 8 weeks-old CBA mice. 10^6 prelabeled YAC-1 cells were injected iv and the radioactivity retained in the spleen (Panel A), lungs (Panel C) and liver (Panel D) was evaluated. Spleen cells (Panel B) were tested for NK vs. YAC-1 (A/T ratio 100:1) Data expressed as parallel in Fig. 1 and 2*

impairment in elimination of tumor cells *in vivo* from the liver and lungs. A similar *in vivo* impairment was not evident in the spleen. However, the amount of radioactivity, retained in this organ in the treated mice was lower than that detected in the spleen of untreated controls. The marked reduction of spleen cellularity that was produced by the treatments (data not shown) and the diminished surface available for tumor cell seeding may be responsible for the results obtained in the spleen. Indeed, by calculating the level of spleen radioactivity with respect to the splenic cell number, a marked inhibition of *in vivo* cytolytic reactivity also becomes evident in the spleen of animals treated with cyclophosphamide on day-1 or irradiation 1 or 3 days previously (Riccardi *et al.*, 1980). Furthermore, if one calculates the degree of elimination in the spleen at 4 hrs relative to the peak levels seen earlier in that organ, both treatments can also be seen to result in impaired reactivity. In contrast to the depressive effects seen at 1 or 3 days after irradiation, no impairment in *in vivo* or *in vitro* natural reactivities was observed at 2 hours after exposure to 850 rads (Figure 7).

The depression of NK reactivity by i-carrageenan, cyclophosphamide, or x-irradiation may be attributed to a variety of mechanisms. The depression induced by carrageenan on day-1 has been ascribed to elimination of accessory macrophages possibly needed to produce interferon for activation of NK cells (Djeu *et al.*, 1979b). In addition, carrageenan has been shown to induce suppressor cells (Cudkowicz and Hochman, 1979), but their presence has been described only in the spleens of animals treated 5 days earlier. Suppressor cells also have been found in the spleens of irradiated mice, but only at 2 weeks after treatment (Cudkowicz and Hochman, 1979). Thus, it is possible to argue that the depressive effects that we have observed are due to different mechanisms, including induction of suppressor cells or elimination of accessory macrophages. The factors involved in depression of reactivity following treatment with cyclophosphamide on day-1 or lethal irradiation 24 or 72 hours before, remain to be elucidated. However, it appears that, regardless of mechanism, the various treatments cause parallel alterations in *in vivo* and NK activities.

Corresponding depression in *in vivo* elimination of tumor cells has also been observed in mice chronically treated with 17β-estradiol, previously shown to depress NK activity (Seaman *et al.*, 1978). Figure 8 summarizes the results of a study of the *in vivo* and *in vitro* natural reactivity of mice treated with 17β-estradiol. NK activity was significantly lower in estradiol-treated mice, as compared to that of untreated or sham-operated controls. Similarly, in all the organs tested, there was a decrease of *in vivo* reactivity in the hormone-treated mice.

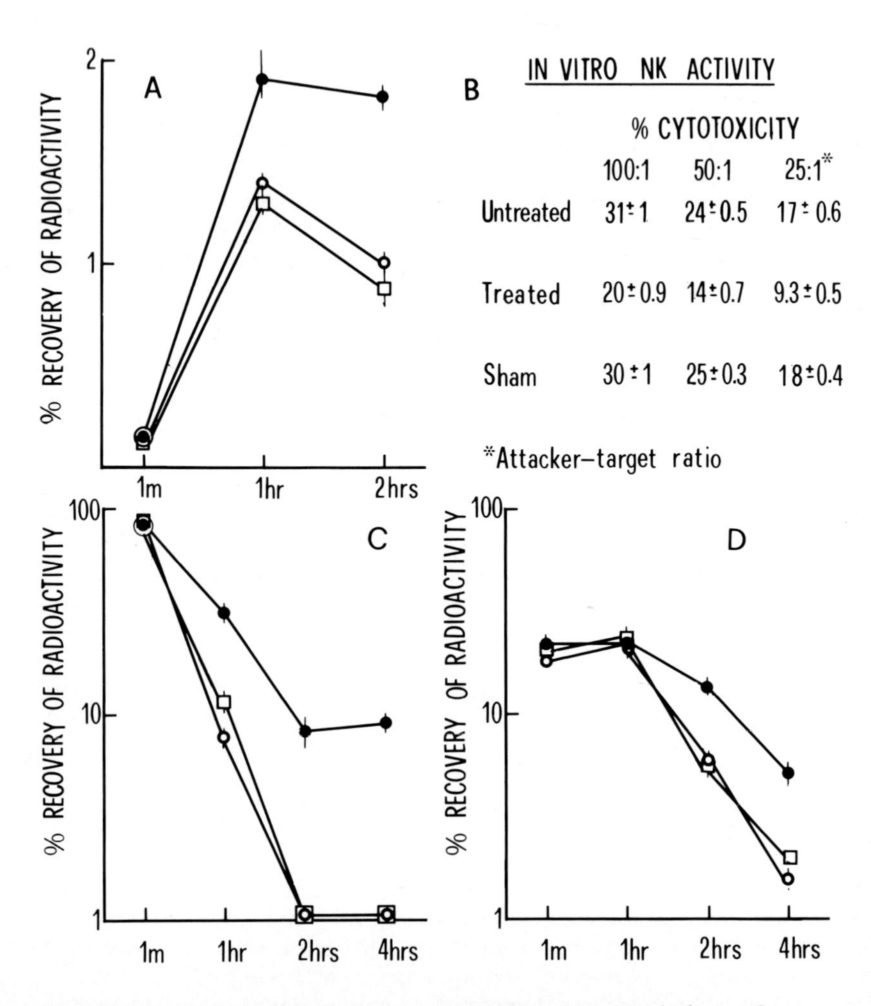

FIGURE 8. Kinetics of in vivo *cytolytic activity of untreated (o--o), sham-operated (□--□) and 17β-estradiol-treated (●--●) 9 weekold $CD2F_1$ mice. 10^6 prelabelled YAC-1 cells were injected iv and the radioactivity retained in the spleen (Panel A), lungs (Panel C) and liver (Panel D) was evaluated. Data expressed as in Fig. 1 and 2. Spleen cells were tested for NK (Panel B) vs. YAC-1. Data expressed as mean % cytotoxicity ± SEM.*

V. *IN VIVO* AND *IN VITRO* REACTIVITIES AGAINST DIFFERENT TUMOR TARGETS

In our previous studies (Riccardi *et al.*, 1979, 1980) we have compared the *in vivo* elimination of a variety of tumors, of different species or histological origin, by high NK-reactive CBA and low NK reactive SJL mice. Differences between the strains were only found with cell lines having some susceptibility to lysis by NK cells. However, the magnitude of the difference in *in vivo* clearance did not correlate with the degree of sensitivity to NK cells *in vitro*. This is illustrated by the results shown in Table II, with three tumor lines that varied considerably in sensitivity to lysis by NK cells. The differences between the susceptibility of tumor lines to *in vivo* and *in vitro* lysis could be due to a variety of factors: there could be differences in kinetics of lysis *in vivo* vs. *in vitro* for some tumors, the dose of cells for detection of optimal *in vivo* elimination may vary among cell lines, different tumor cells have different *in vivo* homing patterns, and there may be a variable background of *in vivo* clearance due to mechanisms other than NK reactivity. In view of these probable complexities, it is rather remarkable that the differences in clearance between the two strains could be so consistently observed.

TABLE 2. In vivo *and* in vitro *cytolytic activity of CBA and SJL mice against tumor targets*

Mouse strain	*Age (wks)*	*Target*	% In vivo *recovery of radioactivity at 4 hrs*			In vitro *cytotoxicity of spleen cells vs YAC - 1 at 100:1*
			Spleen	*Liver*	*Lungs*	
CBA/J	*8*	*YAC-1*	*0.5*	*1.7*	*0.4*	*55.1*
SJL/J	*8*	*YAC-1*	*2.1*	*8.1*	*12.1*	*5.1*
CBA/J	*8*	*MBL-2*	*0.7*	*2.4*	*1.1*	*5.9*
SJL/J	*8*	*MBL-2*	*1.5*	*4.6*	*8.1*	*2.0*
CBA/J	*8*	*TU5*	*0.6*	*1.9*	*1.7*	*16.4*
SJL/J	*8*	*TU5*	*1.3*	*3.1*	*9.2*	*5.1*

VI. *IN VIVO* AND *IN VITRO* REACTIVITY AGAINST NORMAL CELLS

It has been shown that NK cells can also lyse some normal cells such as bone marrow and thymus cells (Nunn *et al.*, 1977; Welsh *et al.*, 1979; Hansson *et al.*, 1979). To determine whether natural reactivity against normal cells could also occur *in vivo* we have tested both *in vivo* and *in vitro* reactivities of normal mice against bone marrow cells and fetal fibroblasts (Table III). As with tumor targets, CBA mice were more reactive than SJL mice against CBA bone marrow cells and (B6xC3H) F_1 fetal fibroblasts, both *in vivo* and *in vitro*. Similar results also have been obtained against thymus cells of CBA and SJL mice (data not shown). Futhermore, *in vivo* reactivity against normal cells was affected in the same manner as NK reactivity or *in vivo* reactivity against tumors. In Table 4 are shown the suppressive effects exerted by i-carrageenan on the *in vivo* reactivity against bone marrow and fetal fibroblasts. *In vivo* and *in vitro* reactivity against these targets also were modulated in parallel by other agents, with stimulation of lysis by poly I:C, and depression by cyclophosphamide.

TABLE 3. In vivo *and* in vitro *cytolytic activity of CBA and SJL mice against normal cells*

Mouse strain	*Age (wks)*	*Target*	% In vivo *recovery of radioactivity at 4 hrs*		In vitro *cytotoxicity*
			Spleen	*Lungs*	
CBA/J	*7*	*CBA bone marrow*	*0.5*	*0.6*	*7.7*[a]
SJL/J	*7*	*CBA bone marrow*	*2.2*	*1.1*	*1.2*[a]
CBA/J	*8*	*(B6xC3H)F_1 fetal fibroblast*	*0.7*	*12.6*	*11.7*[b]
SJL/J	*8*	*(B6xC3H)F_1 fetal fibroblast*	*1.1*	*32.1*	*6.3*[b]

[a] *Effector: target ratio of 20:1*
[b] *Effector: target ratio of 100:1*

VII. CONCLUSIONS

The similarities we have found between *in vitro* and *in vivo* natural reactivities strongly support the hypothesis that rapid elimination *in vivo* of tumor cells and some normal cells can be mediated by NK cells. The possible role of cytotoxic T cells can be ruled out since in this system there was not sufficient time for sensitization and since similar results have been obtained in nude or lethally irradiated mice (Riccardi *et al.*, 1979a). A role for activated macrophages in the *in vivo* assay is also unlikely, since the depression of reactivity by pyran was observed at a time when highly activated macrophages were detected (Fig. 4). Naturally, cytotoxic macrophages also do not appear to be involved in the rapid *in vivo* elimination of the tumor lines that we have studied. As shown in Table 1, the pattern of reactivity of natural macrophages among various strains of mice did not correlate with the results of *in vivo* assay.

In contrast to the lack of correlation between other effector cells and rapid *in vivo* elimination of radiolabeled tumor cells, the *in vivo* results have correlated well with levels of NK reactivity, when evaluated under a wide variety

TABLE 4. Effect of treatment with i-carrageenan on in vivo *natural reactivity against normal tissues.*

Mouse strain	*Age (wks)*	*Treatment*	*Target*	%. In vivo *recovery of radioactivity*	
				Spleen	*Lungs*
CBA/J	*8*	-	*bone marrow CBA/J*	*1.3*	*1.4*
CBA/J	*8*	*i-carrageenan, day - 1*	*bone marrow CBA/J*	*5.6*	*17.5*
(B6xC3H)F$_1$	*8*	-	*(B6xC3H)F$_1$ fetal fibroblast*	*0.7*	*22.6*
(B6xC3H)F$_1$	*8*	*i-carrageenan, day - 1*	*(B6xC3H)F$_1$ fetal fibroblast*	*2.5*	*33.4*

of conditions. *In vivo* clearance of tumor cells, especially from the lungs, varied in parallel with splenic or lung NK activity, in mice of different strains or ages and in mice treated with a variety of immunopharmacological agents. The *in vitro* and *in vivo* kinetics of lysis of YAC-1 tumor cells were similar and NK reactivity appeared to be involved in the elimination of a variety of other mouse and human tumor lines. Although other factors are probably also involved in *in vivo* elimination of tumor cells, other data strongly support the conclusion that NK cells play an important *in vivo* role. The rapidity of this *in vivo* reactivity is consistent with the hypothesis that NK cells represent a first line of defense against growth or dissemination of neoplastic cells.

Our results indicate that NK cells also play a role in the *in vivo* elimination of some normal cells. The results with normal bone marrow cells are consistent with previous indications that NK cells mediate resistance to marrow transplants (Kiessling *et al.*, 1977) but differ in that reactivity has been seen against syngeneic as well as allogeneic cells. Involvement of NK cells in clearance of thymus cells is of interest in view of the recent findings that the targets in the thymus of NK reactivity are within a subpopulation of immature cells (Hansson *et al.*, 1979). The *in vivo* as well as *in vitro* sensitivity of such thymocytes and of fetal fibroblasts to lysis by NK cells is consistent with the hypothesis that NK cells may be involved not only in resistance to tumors but also in control of differentiation of some normal cells.

REFERENCES

Burnet, F. M. (1970) *Prog. Exp. Tumor Res.* 13, 1.

Cudkowicz, G., Hochman, P. S. (1973) *Immunol. Rev. 44,* 13.

Djeu, J.Y., Heinbaugh, J. A., Holden, H. T., and Herberman, R. B. (1979a) *J. Immunol. 122,* 175.

Djeu, J. Y, Heinbaugh, J. A., Vieira, W., Holden, H. T., and Herberman, R. B. (1979b) *Immunopharmacology 1,* 231.

Haller, O., Hansson, M., Kiessling, R., and Wigzell, H. (1977a) *Nature 270,* 609.

Haller, O., Kiessling, R. Orn, A., and Wigzell, H. (1977b) *J. Exp. Med. 145,* 1411.

Hansson, M., Kiessling, R., Andersson, Karre, K., and Roder, J. (1979) *Nature 278,* 174.

Harmon, R. C., Clark, C. A., O'Toole, C., and Wieker, L. S. (1977) *Immunogenetics 41,* 601.

Herberman, R. B., Djeu, J. Y, Kay, D. H., Ortaldo, J. R., Riccardi, C., Bonnard, G. D., Holden, H. T., Fagnani, R., Santoni, A., and Puccetti, P. (1979) *Immuno. Res. 44,* 43.

Herberman, R. B., and Holden, H. T. (1978) *Adv. Cancer Res. 27,* 305.

Herberman, R. B., Nunn, M. E., Holden, H. T., Staal, S., and Djeu, J. Y. (1977) *Int. J. Cancer 19,* 555.

Keller, R. (1978) *Br. J. Cancer 37,* 732.

Kiessling, R., Hochman, P. S., Haller, O., Shearer, G. M, Wigbell, H., and Cudkowicz, G. (1977) *Eur. J. Immunol. 7,* 655.

Nunn, M. E., Herberman, R. B., and Holden, H. T. (1977) *Int. J. Cancer 20,* 381.

SUMMARY: IN VIVO ROLE OF NK CELLS IN HOST DEFENSE

I. ROLE OF NK CELLS IN RESISTANCE TO TUMOR GROWTH

There is increasing evidence for an important role of NK cells in resistance against growth of tumors *in vivo*. The main lines of evidence are summarized in Table I. The growth of YAC and some other NK-sensitive tumor lines has been found to be influenced to an appreciable extent by the levels of NK activity in the recipients (Haller *et al*). In mice with high NK activity (high NK strains, nude mice 5-8 week old mice), a lower proportion of progressively growing tumors occurred than in mice of the same or different strains with low NK activity. Recent studies with beige mice, with a selective deficit in NK activity, have fit this pattern, showing increased tumor growth than in normal C57BL/6 mice. The experiments with chimeras, lethally irradiated mice reconstituted with bone marrow from donors that were high or low in NK, have added further evidence for the cell-mediated nature of the *in vivo* resistance, and since the chimeras developed NK levels characteristic of the cell donors, provided indications for the origin of NK cells from the bone marrow. Even more direct evidence for *in vivo* activity of NK cells has come from local adoptive transfer experiments, in which mixture of NK-sensitive tumor cells with spleen cells positive for Ly5 or NK1.1 antigens resulted in inhibition of tumor growth. A limitation in those experiments is the artificial aspect of *in vitro* mixture before inoculation. One could argue that it is similar to *in vitro* NK assays, the only difference being the end-point used for measurement of cell lysis. The reliance on this same end-point in all the above approaches, i.e. percent survival or tumor growth rate, introduces further potential problems in interpretation. The presence of tumor cells over some period of time could result in activation of macrophages and other natural effector cells, and also of T cells in euthymic mice, and these cells could have an important influence in the results.

ISBN 0-12-341350-8

TABLE I. Evidence for In Vitro Role of NK Cells in Host Defense

---

1. *Correlations between levels of NK activity and resistance of growth of NK-sensitive tumors in various strains of mice.*
2. *Poor growth of NK-sensitive tumors in nude mice as compared to euthymic mice of the same strain.*
3. *More rapid and progressive growth of NK-sensitive tumors in beige mice.*
4. *More resistance to growth of tumors in young mice, at the peak of NK activity, than in older mice.*
5. *T cell deficient chimeras, reconstituted with bone marrow from high NK strain, having high NK activity and increased resistance to growth of NK-sensitive tumors.*
6. *Local adoptive transfer of resistance to tumor growth, by NK cell enriched populations.*
7. *Close correlation between levels of NK activity and degree of rapid clearance, of IV-inoculated, radiolabeled NK-sensitive tumor cells, from the lungs and other organs.*
8. *Close parallels between NK activity and genetically determined (Hh) bone marrow resistance in mice.*

The studies of Riccardi et al have allowed a closer examination of the role of NK cells. Since effects on the clearance of radiolabeled tumor cells from the lungs and other organs were detected in the first 1-2 hrs after IV inoculation, there would not appear to have been sufficient time for activation and cytotoxicity by macrophages or other lymphoid effector cells. This experimental approach has also provided the opportunity to rapidly assess the correlations between in vitro and in vivo activities under a wide range of conditions, in which NK activity was naturally or experimentally-induced to be high or low. In all such situations tested, in vivo clearance of tumor cells, especially from the lungs, paralleled the levels of NK activity. Further weight to the associations was added by the ability to confirm the prediction that the very rapid clearance from the lungs was related to the preexistence of NK cells in that organ. It is also of considerable interest that these correlations have been seen even with tumor lines with low sensitivity to lysis by NK cells.

Hanna and Fidler (1980a,b) have recently confirmed that the clearance of radiolabeled tumor cells correlates with NK activity and have further observed that the tumor resistance of cyclophosphamide-treated mice could be rapidly restored by systemic transfer of spleen or bone marrow cells. Mice treated in this way have been found to have restored NK activity and increased *in vivo* clearance of radiolabeled tumor cells (C. Ricardi and A. Santoni; personal communication). The combination of this procedure for reconstitution of NK activity and the rapid *in vivo* assay appears to offer a powerful method for documenting the *in vivo* role of enriched or purified populations of NK cells.

Based on all of the above evidence on the *in vivo* antitumor activity of NK cells, one may speculate about their role relative to other effector mechanisms. It seems likely that NK cells are more effective in dealing with a small number of tumor cells rather than with a large tumor load. Furthermore, the efficient clearacne of tumor cells from the lungs of mice with high NK activity raises the question of their primary role being to eliminate or at least interfere with metastatic dissemination of tumor cells.

One note of caution needs to be raised regarding the relevance of the above evidence to *in vivo* resistance against autochthonous tumors. All of the studies to date have utilized cell lines that were mainained for long periods in transplant or *in vitro*. There is as yet no conclusive evidence for a role of NK cells in the protection against primary tumors, in the incidence of spontaneous tumors, or in the induction of tumors by known carcinogenic agents. This area will be a major and critical one for future research, to obtain direct evidence for the importance of NK cells for immune surveillance. Some of the procedures that have been recently developed for assessing *in vivo* growth of cell lines should be adaptable to soon obtain the needed data with autochthonous tumors.

II. ROLE OF NK CELLS IN CONTROL OF GROWTH OF NORMAL CELLS

There have been many, detailed studies on natural, radioresistant resistance to tranplantation of bone marrow allografts in mice. When the characteristics of NK cells become known, investigators in this area of bone marrow transplants recognized a number of similarities. As Lotzova summarizes here, direct comparisons between NK activity and resistance to bone marrow transplants have demonstrated a close correlation. Any apparent discrepancies between the two activities have been attributable to technical differences in the assays, particularly in the times at which activity was assessed. The findings that some cells in bone marrow are susceptible to lysis by NK cells provided further support for the conclusion that NK cells are the main effector cells for resistance to bone marrrow transplants. Additional confirmation has now come from the findings that radiolabeled bone marrow cells were cleared more rapidly from mice with high NK activity (Riccardi *et al*). Studies by this same procedure with fetal fibroblasts and thymus cells have indicated that the *in vitro* susceptibility of these cells to NK activity is paralleled by susceptibility *in vivo*.

Taken together, these data raise the intriguing possibility that NK cells may have an important role in controlling the growth of some normal cells, possibility in regulating their rate of differentiation (see section ID) as well as in resistance against growth of neoplastic cells.

REFERENCES

1. Hanna, N. and Fidler, I.J., *J. Natl. Cancer Inst.* in press (1980a).
2. Hanna, N. and Fidler, I.J., *J. Natl. Cancer Inst.* in press (1980b).

NATURAL RESISTANCE OF MICE TOWARD ORTHOMYXOVIRUSES

Otto Haller
Heinz Arnheiter
Jean Lindenmann

Department of Experimental Microbiology
Institute for Medical Microbiology
University of Zürich
Zürich, Switzerland

INTRODUCTION

It is well known that various strains of mice exhibit striking differences in their susceptibility to certain viruses. In most instances, resistance or susceptibility to viral infections is under polygenic control and has a complex mode of inheritance. There are, however, simple situations where a single gene locus determines differences in susceptibility to a group of closely related viruses. Thus, the differences in susceptibility to mouse hepatitis virus between inbred strains of mice are controlled by one single gene locus, susceptibility being dominant (1). Resistance of PRI or C3H/RV mice to flaviviruses is governed by one dominant allele (2). Similarly, in inbred A2G mice, a dominant gene, Mx, confers a high degree of resistance towards infection with various mouse adapted orthomyxoviruses (3).

Here, some of the characteristics of this resistance against influenza viruses will be reviewed and possible resistance mechanisms will be discussed in the light of earlier and more recent findings.

ISBN 0-12-341350-8

RESISTANCE OF A2G MICE TO ORTHOMYXOVIRUSES IS DETERMINED BY THE DOMINANT ALLELE Mx

A high degree of resistance to the lethal action of neurotropic influenza A virus was found by accident when mice of the inbred strain A2G were inoculated intracerebrally with an otherwise very regularly lethal dose of NWS virus (4). The strain A2G originated at Glaxo Laboratories between 1942 and 1950 from an illegitimate mating between A and an unknown mouse. Inbreeding has been strict since 1950 for more than 100 generations (5). Whereas A2G carries many alleles that differ from those in A/J, the major histocompatibility locus appears to be the same ($H\text{-}2^a$, (6)). In crosses between A2G and other strains, resistance is dominant, and backcrosses on many different genetic backgrounds yield 50% resistant animals, indicating the presence of a dominant allele (7 and unpublished observations).

From our previous work, the inborn resistance towards orthomyxoviruses found in mice carrying the dominant resistance allele Mx can be characterized as follows: 1. In homozygous animals resistance develops within 48 hrs of birth, in heterozygous animals within 7 days (7). 2. Resistance is specific for members of the orthomyxo family. Mice bearing the resistance allele Mx are resistant to influenza viruses but are as sensitive as control mice to several other viruses, such as flaviviruses, encephalomyocarditis virus or herpes viruses (3, 8). Although A2G mice have a certain degree of resistance to Sendai virus, it has not been established that this is due to the allele Mx, nor have other paramyxoviruses been extensively studied (8). 3. Resistance is expressed in various organs, namely in lung, in brain and in liver against pneumotropic, neurotropic and hepatotropic strains of influenza virus (3,9). Virus replicates to 100 times higher levels in susceptible as compared to resistant mice (3,9).

A liver adapted variant of influenza A virus, TURH, has proved extremely useful for the analysis of inborn resistance of A2G mice. After intraperitoneal inoculation this hepatotropic virus, originally derived from an avian influenza A virus, grows rapidly in the livers of susceptible mice causing acute liver failure and death within 2-3 days (10). The livers of affected mice become pale-yellow, swollen and necrotic. The histological examination of such livers reveals widespread and severe necrosis of hepatocytes. Resistant, Mx-bearing mice survive up to 10^4 lethal doses (as measured in susceptible mice) of TURH (9). Histological sections of livers from infected resistant mice show only a few focal lesions with cellular infiltrates, which are self-limiting (Fig. 1).

NUDE MICE EXPRESS RESISTANCE

It was therefore conceivable that a particularly early or particularly efficient immune response would be responsible for resistance. If this were the case one would expect the expression of the resistance gene to be impaired in mice immunologically not fully competent. Nude mice homozygous for the gene nu lack a functional T cell system. We have therefore introduced the gene Mx into nu/nu mice, and we have investigated the phenotypic expression of resistance to various influenza A viruses in Mx-bearing nude mice (Table I). Breedings were performed as previously described (11): Brother-sister matings among (nu/nuBALB/c x A2G)F_1 mice yielded an F_2 generation of which approximately 25% were phenotypically nude. Assuming independent segregation of the genes Mx and nu, 75% of these nude F_2 should carry the gene Mx either in homozygous or heterozygous form. If the nude phenotype did not prevent expression of virus resistance 75% of these nude mice should resist an otherwise lethal challenge dose of virus. Table I illustrates that this was indeed the case with all virus strains tested. Nude mice surviving virus challenge had significantly lower antibody titers against the hemagglutinin and the nucleoprotein antigen of influenza A virus than similarly infected non-nude littermates (11). We therefore concluded that expression of resistance was independent of a functional T cell system and of orderly formation of antiviral antibodies.

RESISTANCE OF MICE WITH A GENETICALLY DETERMINED B CELL DEFECT CARRYING THE ALLELE MX

In T cell deficient Mx-bearing nude mice an early IgM response to the hemagglutinin of the challenge virus was regularly detected. The possibility existed that such T cell independent immune responses in the initial phase of the viral infection were important for antiviral resistance. CBA/N mice carry an X-linked recessive B cell defect which prevents them from making antibodies to thymic independent antigens (12). Spleen cells from these animals have an impaired ability to participate in antibody-dependent cell-mediated cytotoxicity

(13). On the other hand, these mice display normal T-lymphocyte functions as measured by T-cell cytotoxicity and skin graft rejection (13) and exhibit high levels of natural killer cell activity (14). We have therefore investigated whether this particular immune unresponsiveness would modulate the expression of the resistance allele Mx. A2G mice were mated with CBA/N females homozygous for the X-linked recessive trait. The F_1 male progeny should express the B cell defect whereas the F_1 female progeny should not, both sexes however would carry the dominant, autosomal gene Mx in heterozygous form. Table II shows that (A2G x CBA/N)F_1 male mice were resistant towards lethal doses of our hepatotropic influenza virus strain.

TABLE I. Resistance of Nude F_2 Mice[a] to Various Influenza A Viruses

Virus strain[b]	Route of inocul.	Total No.	Resistant[c]	Susceptible[d]
NWS	i.c.	40	31 (78%)	9
WS	i.n.	125	93 (74%)	32
HONG-KONG	i.n.	14	11 (78%)	3
TURH	i.p.	25	18 (72%)	7

[a] 75% expected to be Mx-carriers

[b] Human influenza A virus strains were the neurotropic variant NWS (H_oN_1), the pneumotropic variants WS (H_oN_1) and A/Hong-Kong/1/68 (H_3N_2). The hepatotropic avian strain TURH was originally derived from A/Turkey/England/63 (Hav_1Nav_3).

[c] Survived virus challenge with 100 LD_{50} for 4 wks or longer.

[d] Died of viral infection with signs of either neurological disorder, pneumonia or acute liver failure.

TABLE II. Resistance of Mx-Bearing Mice with an X-Linked B Cell Defect to TURH Virus

Mouse strain	*Sex*[a]	*B cell defect*	*Mortality*[b]
(A2GxCBA/N)F$_1$	*f*	-	*0/8*
(A2GxCBA/N)F$_1$	*m*	+	*0/8*
(A2GxCBA/J)F$_1$	*m*	-	*0/8*
CBA/J	*m*	-	*8/8*

[a]*f = females, m = males*
[b]*No. of dead animals on day 7/total no. of mice inoculated. Mice were infected i.p. with 100 LD*$_{50}$ *of hepatotropic influenza A virus, TURH.*

EFFECT OF IMMUNOSUPPRESSION

Immunosuppression has been widely used to delineate the contribution of immune defense mechanisms to recovery from viral infections (15,16). Treatment of mice with cyclophosphamide has been shown to increase neurovirulence of influenza viruses in genetically susceptible animals (17,18). We have therefore tested the effects of cyclophosphamide and other immunosuppressive drugs on the course of hepatotropic infection in resistant A2G mice. Resistance could not be abrogated by these treatments although they prevented inflammatory infiltration by mononuclear cells at the site of viral replication (Fig. 1) and seemed to delay virus clearance (9). Similarly, Fiske and Klein (19) have shown that immunosuppression by cyclophosphamide or X irradiation did not influence the course of neurotropic infection despite the fact that these treatments rendered A2G mice unable to produce specific antiviral antibody or to generate cell-mediated delayed-type hypersensitivity responses.

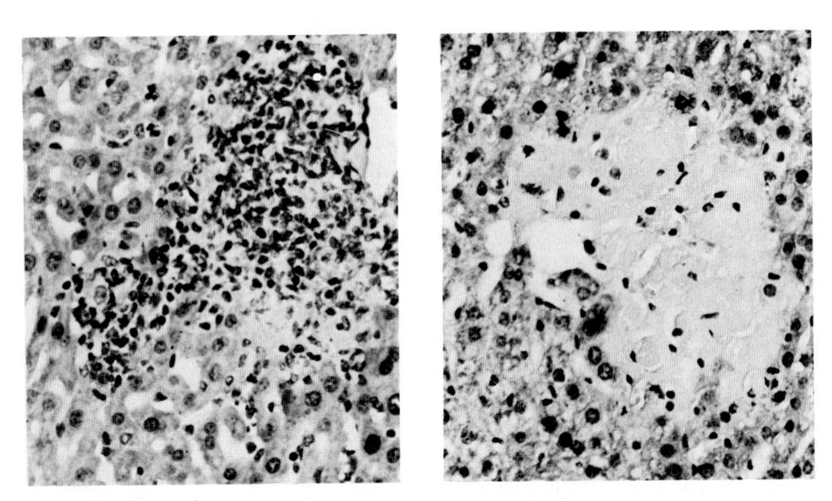

FIGURE 1. Liver sections from adult A2G mice 96 hrs after intraperitoneal infection with 100 LD_{50} of the hepatotropic influenza A strain TURH.
Left side: Focal infiltration by mononuclear cells in normal mice.
Right side: Focal liver cell necrosis without inflammatory infiltrate in A2G mice treated with 150 mg/kg cyclophosphamide 24 hrs before and 24 hrs after infection. These foci represent sites of virus replication as evidenced by immunofluorescence (9). Hematoxylin and eosin. 180x.

NATURAL KILLER CELLS AND ANTIVIRAL RESISTANCE

Viruses have been shown to induce high levels of natural killer (NK) cell activity in infected animals, possibly via induction of interferon (see relevant chapters in this volume). After infection with lymphocytic choriomeningitis virus the increase in NK cell activity in mice correlated with interferon production. It preceeded the appearance of virus specific T killer cells (20). Although the significance of NK cells in acute viral infections is not yet clear, activation or recruitment of NK cells early in the infectious process and at the sites of initial virus replication might be a decisive factor controlling the degree of virus spread. A pertinent finding in this respect is the capacity of T cell deficient nude mice to reject otherwise tumorigenic cell lines when persistently infected with various RNA viruses including measles, vesicular stomatitis virus and influenza (21). There is evidence that NK like cells are involved in natural resistance of certain inbred mouse strains against infection with herpes simplex virus type 1 (22).

Our own investigations have shown that inborn resistance towards influenza viruses is expressed in nude mice known to exhibit high NK cell activity in spleen and blood and that resistance is highly dependent on interferon (see below). Yet, we have failed to reveal a major role for NK cells in this form of resistance. Immunosuppressive treatments with cyclophosphamide, cortisone, whole body irradiation and with silica, previously shown to greatly reduce NK cell activity in mice (23), did not abrogate innate resistance of A2G mice (9, 19). Furthermore, treatment with doses of radioactive strontium (^{89} Sr) that led to drastic impairment of NK cell function (24), to abolishment of marrow allograft reactivity (25) and to abrogation of natural resistance against Friend virus leukemia (26) did not affect A2G resistance (Table III). Moreover, whereas NK cell-mediated resistance to tumors was transferable to lethally irradiated recipients with bone marrow stem cells from donor mice of high NK cell activity (see chapter "In vivo activity of NK cells"), attempts at transferring myxovirus resistance to genetically susceptible mice with marrow stem cells from resistant animals were never successful (Table IV).

TABLE III. Resistance of ^{89}Sr-Treated A2G Mice to Hepatotropic Influenza A Virus

Group	*Animals*	*Mortality*
1	*A2G controls*	*0/6*
2	*^{89}Sr-treated A2G*	*0/6*
3	*CBA controls*	*6/6*
4	*^{89}Sr-treated CBA*	*6/6*

100 μCi ^{89} Sr were injected i.p. on two separate occasions 5 wks apart. Mice were infected intraperitoneally 6 wks after the second injection with 100 LD_{50} of TURH virus. Controls received saline instead of ^{89} Sr.

MACROPHAGES EXPRESS RESISTANCE IN VITRO

Tissue culture experiments had indicated that kidney cells, fibroblasts and nerve cells from resistant and susceptible mice were equally permissive for influenza virus replication *in vitro* (27,28). These cells are usually obtained from embryonal or neonatal animals which themselves do not yet exhibit the full resistance of the adult (7). We thought that cells isolated from adult mice, such as peritoneal macrophages, might be better candidates for the study of resistance *in vitro*. The capacity of macrophages to express virus resistance *in vitro* has been observed both in flavivirus resistance (29) and resistance to mouse hepatitis virus (1). A strain of influenza A virus was adapted to grow in cultures of mouse peritoneal macrophages. This virus strain, called M-TUR, grew to high titers in macrophages from susceptible mice thereby producing a marked cytopathic effect 36 to 48 hrs after infection.

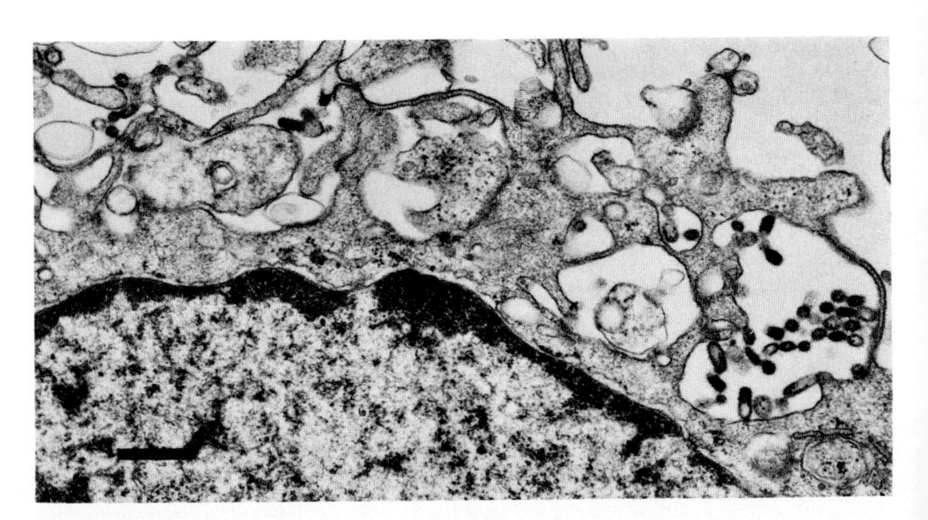

FIGURE 2. Electron microscopic thin section of an A/J macrophage 18 hrs after infection with M-TUR. Note budding of influenza virus particles at the cell surface. (Electron microscopy by Th. Bächi). Bar represents 0,5 μ.

Fig. 2 shows influenza virus particles budding at the plasma membranes of a susceptible A/J macrophage 18 hrs after infection. Freshly cultivated macrophages from resistant animals were resistant to *in vitro* infection with M-TUR (30). Fig. 3 illustrates the difference in susceptibility to M-TUR infection between susceptible A/J and resistant A2G macrophages as evidenced by specific immunofluorescence.

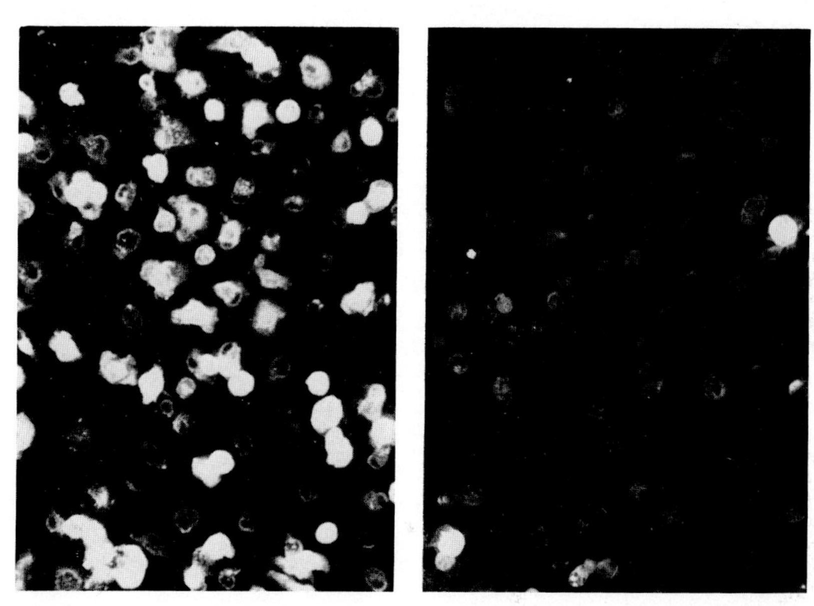

FIGURE 3. Immunofluorescence of peritoneal macrophages from susceptible A/J (left) and resistant A2G mice (right) 18 hrs after infection with the macrophage adapted influenza virus strain M-TUR at high multiplicity. Indirect staining of acetone-fixed cells (using mouse hyperimmune serum specific for M-TUR and FITC coupled rabbit anti-mouse Ig) shows bright nuclear and cytoplasmic fluorescence of infected cells. 160x.

ROLE OF MACROPHAGES FOR IN VIVO RESISTANCE

A clear correlation between *in vivo* resistance of individual mice and *in vitro* resistance of their macrophages was found in segregation analyses using backcrosses between resistant (A/J x A2G)F_1 hybrids and susceptible A/J mice (30). Hence, it seemed quite conceivable that resistant macrophages, by constituting a barrier between the virus and its secondary target cells, might be the real mediators of resistance *in vivo*. To test this possibility transfer experiments were performed in which macrophage precursors were adoptively transferred from resistant to lethally irradiated H-2 identical susceptible mice and *vice versa*. The results from such an experiment are summarized in Table IV. Peritoneal macrophages taken 12 weeks after the transfer had the susceptibility pattern of the donor. The same was true for Kupffer cells in the liver, indicating that not only mobile macrophages, but also tissue macrophages of the liver had been successfully replaced (31). Nevertheless, susceptibility or resistance of individual chimeric mice was according to the macrophage recipient and not according to the macrophage donor (31). We concluded that macrophage resistance and *in vivo* resistance of the animal did not seem to be causally related. The genetic make up of the macrophage population and the capacity of these cells to express resistance was obviously not decisive for *in vivo* resistance.

It is now well established that NK cells are derived from precursor cells in the bone marrow (32). We therefore had to assume that, in the present hemopoietic chimeras, NK cell populations were of donor genotype. Our previous work with similar chimeras has shown that a high degree of *in vivo* resistance towards NK-sensitive tumors could be transferred to irradiated recipients with bone marrow cells from high NK donors (33). Similarly, Lopez has demonstrated that enhanced resistance to herpes simplex virus type 1, possibly mediated by NK cells, was transferable to irradiated susceptible mice by bone marrow cells from genetically resistant donors (22). No such transfer of antiviral resistance with NK precursor cells from genetically resistant animals was detectable in the present system. This, again, indicated that myxovirus resistance was not mediated by NK cells of the appropriate genotype.

TABLE IV. *In Vivo Resistance of Chimeras Repopulated with Resistant or Susceptible Macrophages*

Type of chimeras[a]	*Phenotype of macrophages*[b]	*Mortality*[c]
$(A/JxA2G)F_1 \rightarrow A/J$	resistant	100%
$A/J \rightarrow (A/JxA2G)F_1$	susceptible	0%
$(A/JxA2G)F_1 \rightarrow (A/JxA2G)F_1$	resistant	0%
$A/J \rightarrow A/J$	susceptible	100%

[a]*Recipients were irradiated with 850 rad and reconstituted with* $3x10^7$ *viable bone marrow cells of sex-matched histocompatible donors. Chimeras prepared e.g. by transfer of cells from donor* $(A/JxA2G)F_1$ *into irradiated A/J recipients are referred to as* $(A/JxA2G)F_1 \rightarrow A/J$.

[b]*Macrophage cultures were established 12 wks after marrow grafting and tested for susceptibility to infection with the macrophage-adapted influenza virus strain M-TUR.*

[c]*Macrophage donors were allowed to recover for 14 d and were then challenged i.p. with 100* LD_{50} *of the hepatotropic influenza virus strain TURH. Percentage of animals that died of viral infection was recorded.*

INTERFERON IS AN IMPORTANT FACTOR IN INBORN RESISTANCE

That interferon would be involved in the resistance of A2G mice towards orthomyxoviruses seemed unlikely, mainly because resistance was highly specific for this group of closely related viruses, whereas interferon is thought to protect cells in a virus-nonspecific way. Furthermore, the amount of interferon produced after infection with influenza virus was found to be much lower in Mxbearing mice than in susceptible controls (19,34). However, when potent antiserum prepared against partially purified mouse interferon became available (35), it was found that treatment with this antiserum abolished resistance of A2G mice (34).

Table V shows that treatment with sheep anti-mouse interferon globulin (AIFG) at the time of infection rendered genetically resistant mice fully susceptible to the lethal action of the hepatotropic influenza virus TURH. Virus titers in such mice reached levels similar to those observed in genetically

TABLE V. Abrogation of Inborn Resistance in Anti-Interferon Treated Mice Infected with 100 LD_{50} of Hepatotropic Influenza A Virus TURH

Mouse strain	*Genotype*	*Treatment*[a]	*Mortality*[b]	*Day of death*
A/J	*(+/+)*	*NSG*	*4/4*	*3,3,3,3*
		AIFG	*4/4*	*2,2,2,2*
A2G	*(Mx/Mx)*	*NSG*	*0/4*	*-*
		AIFG	*4/4*	*3,3,3,6*
$(A/JxA2G)F_1$	*(Mx/+)*	*NSG*	*0/4*	*-*
		AIFG	*4/4*	*3,3,3,3*

[a]*Sheep anti-mouse interferon globulin (AIFG), neutralizing titer of 1.2×10^{-6}, or normal sheep serum globulin (NSG) were given i.v. immediately before virus challenge as described (34).*

[b]*No. of dead animals/total no. of mice challenged i.p.*

susceptible animals as demonstrated in Table VI. The same treatment also abrogated *in vivo* resistance to neurotropic and pneumotropic virus strains (34). Peritoneal macrophages taken from Mx-bearing animals treated with AIFG proved fully suscep-

TABLE VI. Growth of TURH Virus in Livers from Resistant Mice Treated with Anti-Interferon Serum

Mouse strain	*Genotype*	*NSG*	*AIFG*
A/J	*(+/+)*	*9.5*[a]	*8.5*
A2G	*(Mx/Mx)*	*2.0*	*8.0*
$(A2GxA/J)F_1$	*(Mx/+)*	*5.0*	*9.0*

[a]*LOG_{10} EID_{50}/ml*

0.1 ml of sheep anti-mouse interferon globulin (AIFG) with a neutralizing titer of 1.2×10^{-6}, or normal sheep serum globulin (NSG) were diluted 1:3 in phosphate-buffered saline and were given i.v. immediately before virus challenge with 100 LD_{50} of hepatotropic TURH virus. A 50% liver extract was prepared 48 hrs after infection and infectivity titers were determined.

tible to M-TUR virus *in vitro* (34). In contrast, freshly cultivated macrophages from untreated resistant mice were resistant even when infected in the presence of AIFG (34). We had to pretreat the donor mouse in order to obtain susceptible Mx-bearing macrophages. This indicated that, in our conventionally reared animals, peritoneal macrophages were exposed to interferon *in vivo*. We then observed that this *in vivo* induced resistance of macrophages was gradually lost during prolonged cultivation *in vitro* in the absence of interferon (36,37). After 2-3 weeks in culture, macrophages from resistant animals were phenotypically susceptible to M-TUR virus (Table VII). We concluded that interferon was an essential factor both for *in vivo* resistance and resistance of macrophages *in vitro*.

THE ALLELE MX INFLUENCES SENSITIVITY TO INTERFERON ACTION SELECTIVELY FOR INFLUENZA VIRUS

If interferon were responsible for resistance, it should be possible to restore the resistance phenotype of Mx-carrying cells by treatment with doses of interferon which would leave non-Mx-bearing cells susceptible. Furthermore, it would be necessary to demonstrate virus specificity of interferon action in such cells. In other words, we had to demonstrate that orthomyxoviruses were more sensitive to the antiviral state induced by interferon in Mx-bearing cells than in control cells and that the antiviral state towards other viruses was not affected by Mx. Such experiments were performed with cultivated peritoneal macrophages (37) and with hepatocytes isolated from adult mice (38). Table VII shows that, in macrophages, increasing doses of interferon markedly inhibited vesicular stomatitis virus (VSV), a rhabdovirus, independently of the Mx genotype. In contrast, 10 units of interferon severly impeded the growth of M-TUR virus in Mx-bearing cells (3 logs difference in virus yields 24 hrs after infection), but affected the same virus much less in control cells (1.2 logs). In hepatocytes essentially the same results were obtained. However, whereas small interferon doses were sufficient to protect macrophages against M-TUR, much larger doses were required for hepatocytes. Preliminary results indicate that mouse kidney cells could hardly be protected by interferon. These differences in interferon sensitivity between various cell types may explain the initial failure to detect expression of resistance in tissue culture.

TABLE VII. Effect of Interferon on Virus Yield in Cultures of Adult +/+ or Mx/Mx Cells

Type of culture[a]	Mouse strain	Interferon[b] units/ml	Log $TCID_{50}$/ml[c] M-TUR	VSV
Macrophages	A/J (+/+)	0	6.2	4.0
		10	5.0	1.5
		20	4.5	1.0
		40	4.0	1.0
	A2G (Mx/Mx)	0	6.5	4.0
		10	3.5	1.8
		20	3.0	1.3
		40	2.0	1.0
Hepatocytes	A/J (+/+)	0	7.5	7.1
		1000	7.3	5.3
	A2G (Mx/Mx)	0	7.2	7.0
		1000	5.0	5.2

[a]Peritoneal macrophages were cultured for 3 wks and were then incubated for 18 hrs with various doses of interferon. Thereafter, cultures were washed and infected at a multiplicity of 5 with either M-TUR or VSV. After an incubation period of 60 min at 37^oC the virus inoculum was removed by repeated washings. Hepatocytes were isolated by a collagenase perfusion technique and primary monolayer cultures were established. They were treated with interferon or normal control medium as described (38) and were infected with either M-TUR or VSV at multiplicities of 10. M-TUR, originally derived from the hepatotropic virus strain TURH, grows equally well in macrophages and hepatocytes.

[b]Induced by NDV in mouse C-243 cells and partially purified to $1x10^7$ reference units/mg protein (39).

[c]Virus yield was determined 24 hrs after infection by titration of VSV virus in monolayer cultures of L_{929} cells and M-TUR virus in chick embryo fibroblasts.

SUMMARY

We have shown here that mice bearing the dominant allele Mx were resistant to infection with influenza viruses, but as sensitive as control mice for several other mouse pathogenic viruses. Resistance developed shortly after birth, was expressed in various organs and was independent of a functioning immune system. This suggested the existance of some systemic factor of non-immunological nature which matured early in life and provided antiviral protection *in vivo.* Since macrophages from resistant mice expressed resistance *in vitro,* we first thought that macrophages might be mediating resistance. However, transfer experiments showed that resistance of macrophages and resistance of the animal, both depending on the presence of the allele Mx, were not causally related. We therefore anticipated that, *in vivo,* a resistance mechanism possibly very similar to that found in macrophages had to be operative in most, if not all, cells throughout the body. This view was compatible with the finding that both *in vivo* resistance and resistance of macrophages *in vitro* depended on interferon. *In vitro* experiments with macrophages and hepatocytes revealed that interferon together with the resistance gene Mx limited influenza virus replication in the actual host cell.

ACKNOWLEDGMENTS

We thank Dr. Th. Bächi for electron microscopy. This work was supported by the Swiss National Science Foundation, grant 3.139-0.77.

1. Bang, F.B., and Warwick, A., *Proc. Natl. Acad. Sci. USA 46*, 1065 (1960).
2. Brinton-Darnell, M., Koprowski, H., and Lagerspetz, K., *J. Infect. Dis. 129*, 240 (1974).
3. Lindenmann, J., Lane, C.A., and Hobson, D., *J. Immunol. 90*, 942 (1963).
4. Lindenmann, J., *Virology 16*, 203 (1962).
5. Staats, J., *Cancer Res. 36*, 4333 (1976).
6. Klein, J., ed. "Biology of the Mouse Histocompatibility-2 Complex", p. 120. Springer-Verlag, New York (1975).
7. Lindenmann, J. *Proc. Soc. Exp. Biol. Med. 116*, 506 (1964).
8. Lindenmann, J., and Klein, P.A., *Arch. Gesamte Virusforsch. 19*, 1 (1966).

9. Haller, O., Arnheiter, H., and Lindenmann, J., *J. Infect. Immun. 13*, 844 (1976).
10. Haller, O., *Arch. Virol. 49*, 99 (1975).
11. Haller, O., and Lindenmann, J., *Nature (Lond.) 250*, 679 (1974).
12. Scher, I., Steinberg, A.D., Berning, A.K., and Paul, W.E., *J. Exp. Med. 142*, 637 (1975).
13. Scher, I., Ahmed, A., Strong, D.M., Steinberg, A.D., and Paul, W.E., *J. Exp. Med. 141*, 788 (1975).
14. Herberman, R.B., and Holden, H.T., *Adv. Cancer Res. 27*, 305 (1978).
15. Allison, A.C., *Transplant. Rev. 19*, 3 (1974).
16. Nathenson, N., and Cole, G.A., *Adv. Virus Res. 16*, 397 (1970).
17. Mayer, V., Schulman, J.L., and Kilbourne, E.D., *J. Virol. 11*, 272 (1973).
18. Miyoshi, K., Gamboa, E.T., Harter, D.H., Wolf, A., and Hsu, K.C., *J. Immunol. 106*, 1119 (1971).
19. Fiske, R.A., and Klein, P.A., *Infect. Immun. 11*, 576 (1975).
20. Welsh, R.M., *J. Exp. Med. 148*, 163 (1978).
21. Minato, N., Bloom, B.R., Jones, C., Holland, J., and Reid, L.M., *J. Exp. Med. 149*, 1117 (1979).
22. Lopez, C. (1978). *In* "Oncogenesis and Herpesviruses III" (G. de The, W. Henle, and F. Rapp, eds.), p. 775. Inter-National Agency for Research on Cancer, Lyon.
23. Kiessling, R., and Haller, O., *Contemp. Top. Immunobiol. 8*, 171 (1978).
24. Haller, O., and Wigzell, H., *J. Immunol. 118*, 1503 (1977).
25. Bennett, M., *J. Immunol. 110*, 510 (1973).
26. Kumar, V., Bennett, M., and Eckner, R.J., *J. Exp. Med. 139*, 1093 (1974).
27. Rusanova, N.A., and Soloview, V.D., *Vopr. Virusol. 11*, 398 (1966).
28. Vallbracht, A. "Neurovirulenz in einem Influenza-A-Rekombinationssystem". Ph.D. Dissertation, University of Tübingen, W. Germany (1977).
29. Goodman, G.T., and Koprowski, H., *Proc. Natl. Acad. Sci. USA 48*, 160 (1961).
30. Lindenmann, J., Deuel, E., Fanconi, S., and Haller, O., *J. Exp. Med. 147*, 531 (1978).
31. Haller, O., Arnheiter, H., and Lindenmann, J., *J. Exp. Med. 150*, 117 (1979).
32. Haller, O., Kiessling, R., Örn, A., and Wigzell, H., *J. Exp. Med. 145*, 1411 (1977).
33. Haller, O., Hansson, M., Kiessling, R., and Wigzell, H.,

Nature 270, 609 (1977).
34. Haller, O., Arnheiter, H., Gresser, I., and Lindenmann, J. *J. Exp. Med. 149,* 601 (1979).
35. Gresser, I., Tovey, M.G., Bandu, M.-T., Maury, C. and Brouty-Boyé, D., *J. Exp. Med. 144,* 1305 (1976).
36. Haller, O., Arnheiter, H., Lindenmann, J., and Gresser, I., *in* "Proceedings of the Second International Lymphokine Workshop, Ermatingen, Switzerland" (A.L. de Weck, ed.) Academic Press, New York, in press.
37. Haller, O., Arnheiter, H., Lindenmann, J., and Gresser, I., *Nature,* in press (1980).
38. Arnheiter, H., Haller, O., and Lindenmann, J., *Virology,* submitted.
39. Tovey, M.G., Begon-Lours, J., and Gresser, I., *Proc. Soc. Exp. Biol. Med. 146,* 809 (1974).

NATURAL MACROPHAGE CYTOTOXICITY AGAINST PROTOZOA[1]

Santo Landolfo
Maria Giovanna Martinotti
Giorgio Cavallo

Institute of Microbiology
University of Torino
Torino, Italy

I. HOST-PARASITE RELATIONSHIP

The host-parasite relationship is a dynamic process in which the parasite's chances of survival depend on its ability to overcome both the natural resistance and the required immunity of the host (Landolfo *et al.*, 1978).

Natural resistance is determined by various non-immunological and immunological factors, that act either singly or sinergically. Examples of metabolic or physiological resistance can be seen in the effect of diet on *Entamoeba histolytica* implant in the large intestine (Balamuth and Siddiqui, 1970) and the influence of ambient pH on the ability of *Trichomonas vaginalis (T. vaginalis)* to survive and multiply (Honigberg, 1978). On the other hand, the inability of some Plasmodia to infect individuals bearing the sickle cell trait or negative for the Duffy blood group determinants, can be regarded as a form of non-immunological resistance under genetic control (Miller and Carter, 1976). As far as it concerns the natural immune defenses, they are closely interconnected even if constituted by mechanisms apparently independent. A distinction between non-adaptive, natural and acquired immunity can thus be retained, even though the community between the mechanisms involved means that these terms are riddled with semantic ambiguity (Varesio *et al.*, 1980). Non-adaptive immunity may depend on various serum

[1]*This work was supported by a research contract with the Italian National Research Council (C.N.R.).*

ISBN 0-12-341350-8

factors, such as complement, lysozime and others, which display intra- or interspecies genetic variations (Playfair, 1978). Examples of this are the resistance of chickens to *Trypanosoma cruzi* infection mediated by C3 activated via the alternative pathway (Kierszenbaum *et al*., 1976), or the resistance of human hosts to *Trypanosoma brucei brucei* infection, due to a factor present in human serum (Desowitz, 1970). Lastly, natural resistance can be mediated by immune mechanisms falling within the definition of "natural immunity" in the strict sense (Cudkowicz *et al*., 1978). This kind of immunity differs from its counterpart "acquired immunity" since it is not the result of the individual's exposure to the infection, but was already present, has not primarily evolved on the principles of adaptability to various pathogens, and displays a smaller variety of specific effector mechanisms than acquired immunity (Herberman and Holden, 1978). Although these features make natural immunity an apparently more primitive and less sophisticated defensive weapon than acquired immunity, nevertheless in some cases it may play a crucial role against an enemy as clever as parasites, which have evolved an extraordinary variety of mechanisms for surviving the immune response of their hosts (Bloom, 1979). Moreover, it should be pointed out that natural immunity can be mediated by natural antibodies, or by lymphoid cells, which appear to be quite heterogeneous in their origins, characteristics and activity against different kinds of pathogens, such as viruses, bacteria and tumors.

This paper presents recent results obtained in our laboratory on the mechanisms of natural cell-mediated immunity against an extracellular protozoon, *Trichomonas vaginalis*, responsible for disturbing and hard-to-eradicate inflammation of the human female and male urogenital apparatus.

II. NATURAL MACROPHAGE CYTOTOXICITY

The procedures used to isolate, culture and label *T. vaginalis* with ^{3}H-thymidine (^{3}H-TdR) have been previously described in detail (Cappuccinelli *et al*., 1972; Martinotti *et al*., 1979).

Briefly, *T. vaginalis*, isolated from human vaginal infection and maintained axenically in Diamond's medium without *t* agar (Diamond, 1957), was seeded in RPMI 1640 supplemented with fetal bovine serum (FBS), antibiotics and ^{3}H-TdR for 24 hour. The natural cytotoxicity of different lymphoid cell populations was measured from the release of ^{3}H-TdR by prelabelled protozoa after 48 hour of interaction with effector cells (Martinotti *et al*., 1979).

The procedures used to deplete or enrich the effector cells for different cell populations have been described in detail elsewhere (Landolfo *et al.*, 1980).

Lymphoid cells from various anatomical sites of normal 8-10 week-old female BALB/c mice were used as effector cells. High cytotoxicity levels were observed when labelled protozoa were mixed with uninduced resident peritoneal cells, harvested by simple washings of the peritoneal cavity (Table I).

TABLE I. Natural Cytotoxicity of Lymphoid Cells from Various Tissues of Normal 8-10 Week-Old Female BALB/c Mice against T.vaginalis.

Source of effector cells	% Cytotoxicity[a]		
	50:1[b]	25:1	12:1
Thymus	3.7 ± 1.3	1.2 ± 0.5	1.4 ± 0.8
Peripheral Blood	3.3 ± 1.2	2.6 ± 1.2	3.8 ± 1.4
Lymphnodes	3.0 ± 1.0	2.5 ± 1.8	3.2 ± 1.3
Spleen	7.7 ± 1.6	6.1 ± 1.7	5.5 ± 1.4
Bone Marrow	13.1 ± 3.8	10.2 ± 3.3	9.8 ± 3.2
Lung	17.8 ± 5.3	20.0 ± 6.3	17.2 ± 4.3
Peritoneum	27.8 ± 3.6	26.1 ± 3.6	20.1 ± 3.1

[a]*Percentage cytotoxicity from three replicates ± S.D.*

Effector:target ratios

Effector cells from lung and bone marrow showed variable but constantly lower cytotoxicity. Lymphoid cells from the other tissues did not display distinct levels of activity at all the ratios tested. Moreover, comparable levels of cytotoxicity by peritoneal cells were observed, in the microcytotoxicity assay, using both 10% septically collected fetal bovine serum or 1% fresh adult mouse serum (Landolfo *et al.*, 1980). These findings indicate the occurrence of natural cytotoxicity against *T. vaginalis* in the peritoneal cavity of normal mice that appears to be independent of environmental factors capable of activating macrophages *in vitro* (Hibbs *et al.*, 1977). Its tissue distribution is quite different from that reported for various tumor systems. The spleen is a consistent source of high natural cytotoxicity against tumor cells, whereas peritoneal cells have low natural reactivity. The activity of other tissues is related to the kind of tumor target used (Herberman and Holden, 1979). Our findings on tissue distribution suggested that different effector cells are responsible for natural cytotoxicity against tumors and protozoa. We therefore sought to characterize the peritoneal effector cells. Resident peritoneal cells from untreated BALB/c mice were depleted of adherent cells by nylon wool columns or plastic surfaces (Landolfo *et al.*, 1980), and tested against *T. vaginalis*. Lymphoid cells not adhering to nylon wool fibers or plastic surfaces did not show any cytotoxicity against labelled protozoa, whereas partial recovery of natural cytotoxicity was observed in the adherent fraction. In further experiments, uninduced peritoneal cells from normal BALB/c mice were treated twice with carbonyl iron powder in order to remove phagocytic cells, and tested against *T. vaginalis*. Table II shows that this treatment completely destroys the ability of peritoneal cells to lyse protozoa, indicating that effector cells cytotoxic against *T. vaginalis* are phagocytic. Taken together, by showing that such natural cytotoxic effector cells are adherent and phagocytic, these results suggest that a macrophage-like cell plays a major role in this activity. By contrast, the natural killer (NK) or natural cytotoxic (NC) cells, responsible for natural cytotoxicity against various tumor lines, do not appear to display any reactivity against *T. vaginalis*. On the other hand, the mechanisms by which the normal macrophage kills *T. vaginalis in vitro* are still obscure, though preliminary experiments indicate that the protozoa might be lysed by direct contact without any evidence of phagocytosis.

Our last set of experiments assessed the possibility of modulating macrophage natural cytotoxicity against *T. vaginalis* by i.p. injection of agents known to affect the activity of these cells. The following agents, injected intraperitoneally, were used: a) Polyinosinic-Polycytidilic acid (Poly I:C) (Boehringer, Mannheim, West Germ.) at 0.1 mg per mouse 48 hour before the assay. b) Lypopolisaccharide (LPS) from *E. coli* 055:B5 (Difco Lab., Detroit, Mich.) at 0.5 mg per mouse 48 hour before the assay. c) Seakem-9 carrageenan (Marine Colloids, Inc., Rockland, Maine) dissolved in phosphate buffer saline (PBS) and injected at a concentration of 1 mg per mouse 24 hour before the assay. d) Light mineral

TABLE II. Natural Cytotoxicity of Peritoneal Cells after Treatment with Different Techniques.

Treatment	*Cell population*	*% Cytotoxicity*[a]	
		25:1[b]	*12:1*
-	*Total*	*30.2 ± 2.6*	*21.4 ± 1.9*
Nylon wool columns	*Non-adherent*	*3.1 ± 2.6*	*1.8 ± 0.7*
	Adherent	*19.9 ± 2.1*	*17.3 ± 2.4*
Plastic surface	*Non-adherent*	*2.5 ± 0.2*	*1.0 ± 0.4*
	Adherent	*16.3 ± 0.8*	*12.3 ± 1.3*
Carbonyl I. + magnet	*Non-phagocyting*	*1.1 ± 0.5*	*0.2 ± 0.2*

[a]*Percentage cytotoxicity from three replicates ± S.D.*

[b]*Effector: target ratios*

oil (LMO) (Marcol 52, Humble Oil and Refining Co., Houston, Tex.), 3 ml per mouse, injected 96 hour before the assay.

As shown in Table III, Poly I:C, LPS, LMO strongly enhanced macrophage natural cytotoxicity against *T. vaginalis*. It will be recalled that Poly I:C and LPS have been shown to induce the production and release of interferon (Stewart II, 1979), and stimulate macrophage activities (Regelson and Munson, 1970; Alexander and Evans, 1971). Yet it is not certain whether interferon is directly involved in the increased cytotoxicity, since this could be due to direct stimulation of macrophage activity by Poly I:C and LPS. LMO, however, is known to increase the number of peritoneal monocyte-macrophage-like cells, without inducing evident levels of activation. The increased natural cytotoxicity observed with peritoneal exudate cells induced with LMO may therefore be due to the relatively higher macrophage percentage in these populations (unpublished observations). Lastly, impairment of peritoneal exudate cells by carrageenan injection could be a consequence of its toxicity against macrophage (Catanzaro *et al.*, 1971).

TABLE III. Natural Cytotoxicity of Peritoneal Cells after Injection In Vivo of Different Agents.

Treatment	% Cytotoxicity at E/T[a]	
	25:1	12:1
-	26.3 ± 1.8	17.8 ± 2.7
Poly I:C	55.1 ± 3.4	40.7 ± 4.5
LPS	41.4 ± 2.5	30.4 ± 2.9
LMO	65.6 ± 3.9	40.6 ± 2.1
Carrageenan	9.1 ± 1.7	5.6 ± 0.9

[a]Percentage cytotoxicity from three replicates ± S.D.

We believe that this is the first demonstration *in vitro* of macrophage natural cytotoxicity against protozoa. It remains to be established if macrophage natural cytotoxicity is a phenomenon related solely to *T. vaginalis* or can be generalized to other protozoan systems. Recent work suggests that macrophages may play an important role in mediating natural resistance to protozoa. Thrischmann *et al.* (1978) and Brooks and Reed (1979) have observed that injection of anti-macrophage agents, namely silica or Tripan blue respectively, decreases the resistance of inbred mice to infection by *panosoma cruzi* or *Trypanosoma musculi*. Furthermore, Behin *et al.* (1979) have demonstrated that macrophages from healer mice can destroy *Leishmania tropica*, whereas those from non-healer mice can not.

The *in vivo* importance of natural macrophage cytotoxicity against *T. vaginalis* remains a matter of speculation. Since this protozoon induces normally an inflammation locally restricted to the urogenital apparatus, cells of the monocyte-macrophage lineage, ubiquitous in organs and tissues, could provide a mechanism of defense that may explain why *T. vaginalis* inflammation is confined to the urogenital tract.

In conclusion, our results indicate that normal "non-activated" macrophages, besides modulating the immune response by presenting antigens to lymphocytes (Nelson, 1976), or suppressing lymphocyte activation (Varesio *et al.*, 1980), may constitute an early surveillance system against growing tumors or protozoan infections.

ACKNOWLEDGMENTS

The author wish to express their appreciation to Dr. Guido Forni for careful review of the manuscript.

REFERENCES

Alexander, P., and Evans, R., *Nature New Biol. 232,* 76, (1971)

Balamuth, W., and Siddiqui, V. A., in "Immunity to Parasitic Animals" (G. J. Jackson, R. Herman, I. Singer, eds.) 2, p. 439, Appleton, New York, (1970)

Behin, M., Mauel, J., and Sordat, B., *Exp. Parasit. 48,* 81, (1979)

Bloom, B. R., *Nature. 279,* 21, (1979)

Brooks, B., and Reed, N., *J. Reticuloendothel. Soc. 22,* 605, (1977)

Cappuccinelli, P., Lattes, C., and Cagliani I., *Proc. XVI Congr. Ital. Soc. Microbiol. 3,* 411, (1972)

Catanzaro, P. J., Schwartz, H. J., and Graham, R. C., *Am. J. Path. 64,* 387, (1971)

Cudkowicz, G., Landy, M., and Shearer, G. M., (eds.) in Natural Resistance Systems against Foreign Cells, Tumors and Microbes, Academic Press, New York (1978)

Desowitz, R. S., in "Immunity to Parasitic Animals" (G.J. Jackson, R. Herman, I. Singer, eds.), 2, p. 551, Appleton, New York, (1970)

Diamond, L. S., *J. Parasit. 43,* 488, (1957)

Herberman, R. B., and Holden, H.T., *Advan. Cancer Res. 27,* 305, (1978)

Hibbs, J. B., Taintor, R. R., Chapman, H. A., and Wieberg, J. B., *Science 197,* 279, (1977)

Honiberg, B. M., in "Parasitic Protozoa" (J. P. Kreier, ed.) 2, p 275, Academic Press, New York, (1978)

Kierszenbaum, F., Ivanyi, J., and Budzko, D. B., *Immunonology, 30,* 1, (1976)

Landolfo, S., Martinetto, R., and Cavallo, G., *Giorn. Batt. Virol. Immunol. 71,* 192, (1978)

Landolfo, S., Martinotti, M. G., Martinetto, P., and Forni, G., *J. Immunol.*, in press, (1980)

Martinotti, M. G., Di Matteo, C., Martinetto, P., Negro Ponzi A., and Landolfo, S., *Microbiologica 2,* 405, (1979)

Miller, L. H., and Carter, R., *Exp. Parasit. 40,* 132, (1976)

Nelson, D. D., (ed.) in "Immunobiology of the Macrophage" Academic Press, New York, (1976)

Playfair, J. H. L., *Current Topics In Microbiol. and Immunol. 80,* 37, (1978)

Regelson, W., and Munson, A. E., *Ann. N. Y. Acad. Sci. 173,* 831, (1970)

Stewart II, W. E., (ed.) in " The Interferon System " Springer Verlag, New York (1979)

Trischmann, T., Tanowitz, H., Wittner, M., and Bloom, B., *Exp. Parasit. 45,* 160, (1978)

Varesio, L., Landolfo, S., Giovarelli, M., and Forni, G., *Dev. Comp. Immunol,* in press (1980)

NATURAL KILLER CELL ACTIVITY AGAINST VIRUS-INFECTED CELLS

Daniela Santoli
Bice Perussia
Giorgio Trinchieri

The Wistar Institute of Anatomy and Biology
Philadelphia, Pennsylvania

Increased natural cytotoxic activity of human lymphocytes against cells infected with viruses.

Peripheral blood lymphocytes from randomly selected healthy donors are significantly more cytotoxic *in vitro* against allogeneic virus-infected fibroblasts than against their uninfected counterparts. This phenomenon has been shown with a variety of viruses in a Cr-release assay: measles virus (Edmonston and Braxator strains), SSPE virus (LEC strain), paramyxovirus-1 (6/94 strain) mumps (MPS), herpes simplex type 1 (HSV-1), influenza viruses A/Hong Kong/107/68 (HK), A/PR/8/34 (PR8), and A/Japan/305/57 (JAP) (Santoli et al., 1978a,b); rabies virus (HEP and ERA strains) (unpublished results). Human fetal skin fibroblasts (FS1) or other human target cells were infected several hours before addition to lymphocytes, and in any instance were lysed more efficiently than uninfected target cells under the same experimental conditions. In the first three hours after addition of lymphocytes, the rate at which virus-infected and uninfected fibroblasts were killed was the same (Fig. 1). At longer incubation times, the rate of cytotoxicity with uninfected cells remained constant whereas it sharply increased with virus-infected targets. After 18 hr the infected cells were lysed several times more efficiently than their uninfected counterparts (Fig. 1). Increased cytotoxicity against infected cells was observed with lymphocyte preparations from all the donors tested, although some variation was seen in the values of relative cytotoxicity obtained with lymphocytes from different donors or with preparations from the same donor tested in separate experiments (Table 1).

**The experimental work described in this paper has been supported by NIH grants CA-20833, CA-10815, CA-43882 and NS-11036 and by the National Multiple Sclerosis Society.*

ISBN 0-12-341350-8

TABLE 1. Cytotoxic Activity and Interferon Production by Lymphocytes Incubated with Virus-Infected FS1 Cells

Virus	Relative cytotoxicity*	Interferon produced† by lymphocytes incubated with infected targets
none	1 ± 0**	≤ 1
6/94	4.3 ± 0.5	658 ± 326
HSV-1	6.3 ± 1.3	362 ± 237
MPS	5.0 ± 0.7	n.d. ‡
HK	8.3 ± 1.1	711 ± 286
PR8	5.6 ± 1.4	1170 ± 389
JAP	4.4 ± 1.0	303 ± 72

*Ratio between cytotoxic activity (LU/10^8 cells) against infected target and cytotoxicity against uninfected target cells (18-hr test).

†Interferon in the supernatants from lymphocytes incubated 18 hr with infected fibroblasts.

**Mean ± S.E. from 4 to 20 donors.

‡Not determined.

Characterization of the effector cell.

Using several different lymphocyte fractionation techniques, it was not possible to separate the effector cells mediating the spontaneous cytotoxicity against uninfected fibroblasts from the effector cells acting against their virus-infected counterparts (Santoli *et al.*, 1978a). Moreover, all the lymphocyte fractions displayed about the same relative cytotoxicity when tested against virus-infected and uninfected cells. The effector cells in both systems are lymphocytes; granulocytes and monocytes are inactive and, when present in large number, exert an inhibitory effect. Both the uninfected cells and the infected fibroblasts were killed by natural killer (NK) cells which are lymphocytes with receptors for the Fc fragment of IgG but with no surface Ig or complement receptors. When lymphocytes were separated on the basis of their ability to form rosettes with either neuraminidase- or AET(2-aminoethylisothiouronium bromide hydrobromide)-treated sheep erythrocytes, the majority of the cytotoxic activity was consistently recovered in the non-rosetting fraction. Some cytotoxic activity, however, was always present in the rosetting fraction and was, again, mediated by lymphocytes carrying receptors for the Fc fragment of IgG.

Mechanism of lysis of virus-infected cells.

The mechanisms by which human NK cells lyse virus-infected fibroblast cultures were analyzed with particular consideration of the role of antiviral antibodies and interferon (Santoli *et al.*, 1978b). As described in more detail by Trinchieri *et al.*, in this book, interferons (IF) react with lymphocytes to rapidly increase the cytotoxic activity of NK cells. IF induced upon exposure of lymphocytes to virus-infected targets, appeared to be responsible for enhancing the cytotoxic efficiency of NK cells against the infected fibroblasts. Uninfected human fibroblast cultures were never able to induce antiviral activity when incubated alone or when mixed with lymphocytes; in contrast, infection of target cells with any one of the viruses tested resulted in both IF induction in the lymphocytes and increased cytotoxicity (Table I). Kinetics studies of cytotoxicity against virus-infected cells and of antiviral activity during the cytotoxic assay showed that the increased rate of cytotoxicity against infected targets, as compared to uninfected cells, was

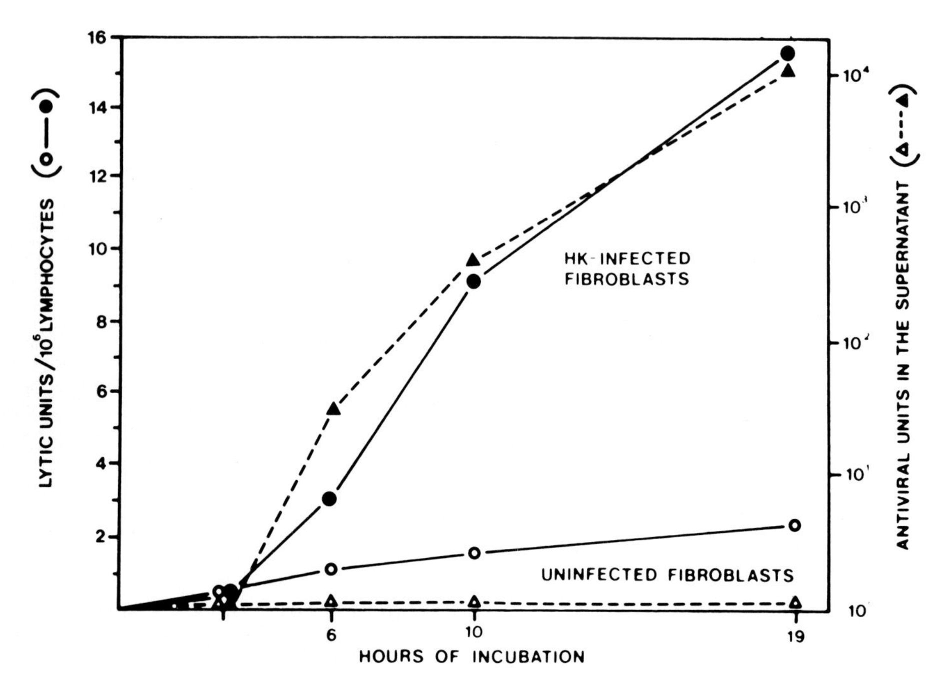

Figure 1. Spontaneous CMC and production of IF by human lymphocytes tested against virus-infected or uninfected cells. Human lymphocytes were added at different concentrations to monolayers of ^{51}*Cr-labeled human skin fibroblasts which were either previously infected with the Hong Kong strain of influenza virus or not. The supernatants were collected after the indicated times of incubation at 37°C; lytic units (number of lymphocytes able to lyse 50% of the target cells in the test time) and the IF antiviral units were determined as described by Trinchieri* <u>*et al.*</u> *(1978). ●——●, cytotoxicity and Δ——Δ, IF released by lymphocytes added to virus-infected target cells; O——O, cytotoxicity and, ▲——▲, IF released by lymphocytes added to uninfected target cells. Reproduced by permission from Trinchieri* <u>*et al.*</u> *(1979).*

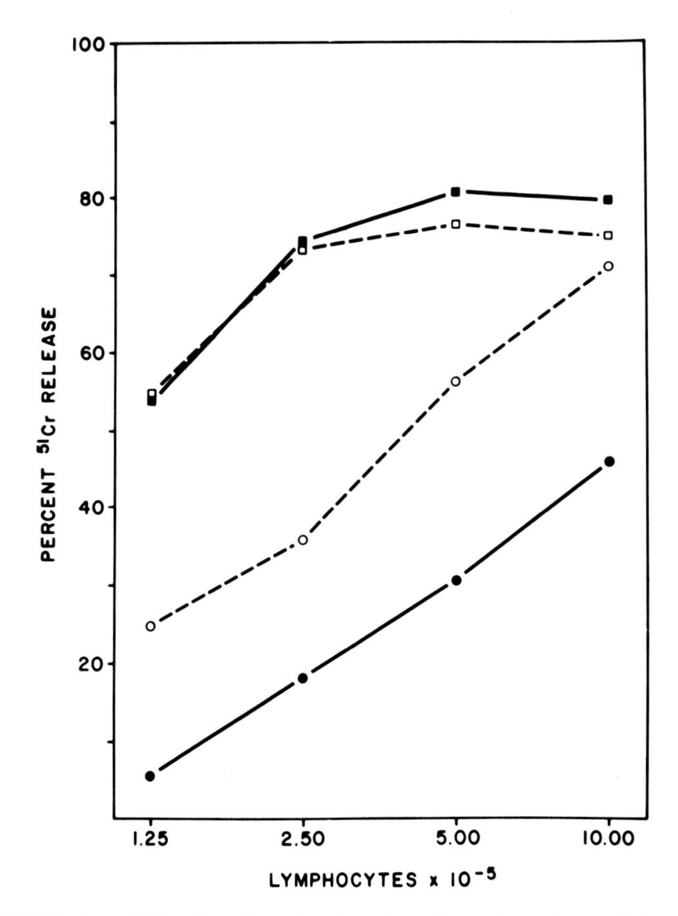

FIGURE 2. Effect of stimulating lymphocytes with exogeneous interferon on CMC against uninfected and HSV-1 infected FS1 cells (4 x 10^4/well). Lymphocytes were washed 3 times before the 18-hr cytotoxic test. ●, fresh lymphocytes against uninfected FS1 cells; 0, fresh lymphocytes against HSV-1-infected FS1 cells; □, lymphocytes stimulated overnight with NDV-induced interferon (NDV-IF) against FS1 cells; ■, lymphocytes stimulated overnight with NDV-IF against HSV-1-infected FS1 cells. Reproduced by permission from Santoli et al. (1978b).

detectable only after the appearance of IF in the supernatants. As shown in Fig. 1, a constant linear rate of cytotoxicity was observed with uninfected fibroblasts, and no antiviral activity was observed in the supernatants at any time. When HK-infected cells were used, IF was present in the supernatants as early as 3 hr after addition of the lymphocytes; the increase in the rate of cytotoxicity against the infected target became apparent only at that time, after which both the titer of antiviral activity in the supernatants and the rate of cytotoxicity increased in parallel up to 18-20 hr (Fig. 1). Preincubation of lymphocytes with an NDV-induced leukocyte IF preparation (NDV-IF) (18 hr at 37°C, 10^3 antiviral units) resulted in a several-fold increase of their cytotoxic activity against uninfected target cells (Fig. 2). The IF-stimulated effector cells lysed virus-infected and uninfected targets with the same efficiency in contrast with the increased cytotoxicity against the infected target observed when fresh lymphocytes were used as effector cells (Fig. 2). This observation argues against the hypothesis that the higher efficiency of NK cells against virus-infected targets may simply be due to the fact that these targets are more fragile and, therefore, more susceptible to NK-lysis. Other arguments against an increased fragility of the virus-infected cells are based on the findings that for the first 3 hr of incubation cytotoxicity against infected cells does not increase, and the spontaneous release of ^{51}Cr from infected targets is not higher than from uninfected cells, regardless of the cytopathic effects observed.

The possible role of antiviral antibodies in the mechanism of NK-lysis of virus-infected cells has also been investigated. No correlation was found between donors' antibody titers to any virus tested and the cytotoxic efficiency of their effector cells (Santoli *et al.*, 1978a): infected targets were lysed by both seropositive and sero-negative individuals. However, antibody-dependent cell-mediated cytotoxicity (AbCMC) against virus-infected target cells could be easily induced when sera from seropositive donors were added. The maximum levels of AbCMC could be detected at 4 hr after incubation (Fig. 3). $F(ab')_2$ fragments of rabbit anti-human IgG completely inhibited AbCMC, whereas they did not affect NK cells at any time during the cytotoxic test whether IF-inducing (virus-infected) or noninducing (uninfected) target cells were used (Fig. 3). Kinetics studies indicated that after 4 hr of incubation AbCMC can no longer be demonstrated even in the presence of antiviral antibodies.

To further investigate the possible importance of humoral antibodies and of specific sensitization in the mechanism of lysis of virus-infected cells, lymphocytes from volunteers who had been immunized with rabies vaccine (Wiktor *et al.*, 1969) were analyzed for their ability to kill rabies virus-infected target cells in the absence of antiviral antibodies. No difference could be detected in the relative cytotoxicity when lymphocytes were obtained before immunization (when donors' sera contained no anti-viral antibodies) as compared to during and after the immunization schedule (when donors' sera presented high anti-rabies antibody titers). It should be emphasized, however, that the experimental protocol of using target cells allogeneic to the effector cells, did not allow the detection of virus-specific cytotoxic T lymphocytes.

In summary, the present data show that the increased cytotoxic activity displayed by lymphocytes from healthy donors against virus-infected cells, as compared to uninfected targets, is not due to an increased fragility of the target cells nor to an enhanced ability of the lymphocytes to recognize virus-infected cells. The phenomenon is due to an increase in the rate of cytotoxicity induced upon co-cultivation of lymphocytes with infected targets and is manifest after a few hours of incubation. Once stimulation of lymphocytes has taken place, the increase in cytotoxicity is not specific for the inducer (virus-infected) target; any other target is also lysed with a high efficiency.

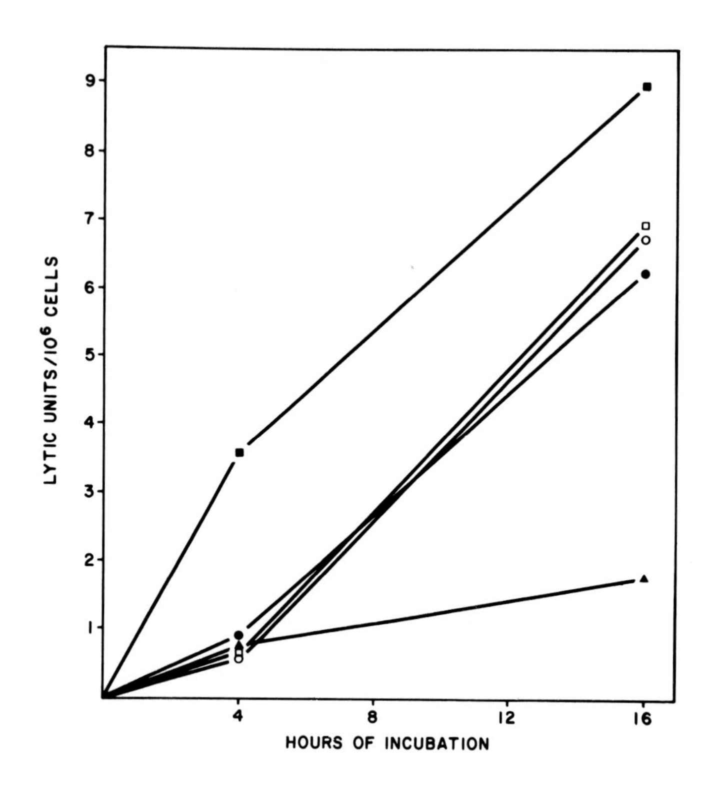

FIGURE 3. Kinetics of SpCMC and AbCMC against HK-infected FS1 in the presence of F(ab')$_2$ anti-human IgG. Samples were harvested at 4 and 16 hr. CMC against; ▲, uninfected FS1; ●, HK-infected FS1; ■, HK-infected FS1 sensitized with anti-HK antibodies; O, HK-infected FS1 in the presence of F(ab')$_2$ anti-human IgG, □, HK-infected FS1 sensitized with anti-HK antibodies, in the presence of F(ab')$_2$ anti-human IgG. Reproduced by permission from Santoli et al. (1978b).

Such an increase in cytotoxic efficiency is induced by IF molecules which are released by lymphocytes upon stimulation with virus-infected cells. If cytophilic antiviral antibodies are bound to the effector cells, they should be able to induce an early lysis of the infected cells, and anti-human IgG reagents should inactivate them. However, no evidence of this type of cytotoxicity could be shown in any experimental systems analyzed even when the donors' sera contained high titers of antiviral antibodies which, if added intentionally to the test, are able to induce an efficient AbCMC.

REFERENCES

Santoli, D., Trinchieri, G., and Lief, F.S. *J. Immunol. 121*, 526-531 (1978a).

Santoli, D., Trinchieri, G., and Koprowski, H. *J. Immunol. 121*, 532-538 (1978b).

Trinchieri, G., Santoli, D., Dee, R., and Knowles, B.B. *J. Exp. Med. 147*, 1299-1313 (1978).

Trinchieri, G., Perussia, B., Santoli, D., and Cerottini, J.C. *Transplant. Proc. XI*, 807-810 (1979).

Wiktor, T.J., Sokol, F., Kuwert, E., and Koprowski, H. *Proc. Soc. Exp. Biol. Med. 131*, 799-805 (1969).

SUMMARY: NATURAL IMMUNITY AND RESISTANCE AGAINST MICROBIAL AGENTS

In addition to a possible role of natural cell-mediated immunity in controlling growth of tumor cells and some normal cells (see section IF), natural resistance mechanisms may make an important contribution to host defenses against microbial agents. Among the chapters represented here are reports of natural cell-mediated immunity against virus-infected cells and protozoa.

I. NATURAL IMMUNITY AGAINST VIRUSES AND VIRUS-INFECTED CELLS

The possibility of reactivity of NK cells against cells expressing oncogenic viruses, type C viruses and mouse mammary tumor virus, or some other viruses (e.g. measles, mumps) has already been discussed in section ID. Here, it seems worthwhile to consider the possible role of NK cells or some other natural resistance mechanisms in the _in vivo_ control of viruses or of virus-infected cells. Bloom _et al_ (section IC3) have shown that hamster tumor cells persistently infected with various RNA viruses (e.g. mumps, measles, influenza) grow less well in nude mice. In addition to the possibiltity that the viruses might introduce additional antigens to be recognized by NK cells, their ability to stimulate interferon (IF) production appears to be very important since resistance to tumor growth was blocked by anti-IF. These authors also raised the question of a similar role of NK cells and IF production in some human diseases in which persistent virus infection may be involved. Patients with systemic lupus erythematosis, multiple sclerosis, and juvenile diabetes had depressed IF production by leukocytes in response to IF, and a portion of the patients had depressed levels of NK activity, which responded poorly to exogenous IF. Bloom _et al_ also discussed the experiments of Schellekens _et al_ (1979), which indicate that protection of mice by IF against infection with vaccinia virus is mediated by host cells, presumably NK cells. Similarly, Lopez

ISBN 0-12-341350-8

found that resistance of mice to herpes simplex virus was conferred by transfer of bone marrow cells from genetically resistant donors, and the data were compatible with a primary role of NK cells.

In contrast to the above positive evidence for a role of NK cells in resistance against viruses, Welsh and Kiessling (section IC3) found no increased NK activity against target cells infected by LCM virus. This might be related to the conditions of their assays, since Santoli _et al_ found that increased lysis by human NK cells of virus-infected fibroblasts was seen only after 6 hrs of incubation and effects became maximal at 18 hrs. Their evidence pointed to the dependence of increased lysis of virus-infected cells on stimulation of IF production, since lymphocytes pretreated with IF had similar activity against infected and uninfected target cells. Even if virus infection does not confer new NK related antigens on target cells, the susceptibility of virus-infected cells to lysis by IF-augmented NK cells might result in some control of virus infections _in vivo_. However, Welsh and Kiessling did not detect such a role for NK cells in limiting persistence of infection by LCM virus.

Haller has performed detailed experiments on the nature of the natural, genetically determined, resistance of some mice to lethal infection by influenza and other orthomyxoviruses. Resistance was observed in nude mice and one might have considered NK cells or macrophages to be responsible. However, resistance was not depressed by cyclophosphamide, lethal irradiation or ^{89}Sr and in contrast to NK activity, it couldn't be transferred with bone marrow cells or macrophage precursors. Despite the apparent lack of involvement of NK cells, IF seemed to play a key role since anti-IF abolished resistance. It appears that cells of the genetically resistant mice are more responsive to the protective effects of IF, but this hyper-responsiveness to IF was not reflected in a general increased resistance to other viruses. This study indicates that genetic factors can influence natural resistance in various ways, including levels of NK activity, degree of IF production in response to viruses or other stimuli, and responsiveness of host cells to IF.

REFERENCES

1. Lopez, C., in "Oncogenesia and Herpesviruses III" (G. de The, W. Henle, and F. Rapp, eds.), p. 775, International Agency for Research on Cancer, Lyon, (1978).

2. Schellekens, H., Weimar, W., Cantell, K., and Stitz, L., _Nature_ 278, 742 (1979).

INTERFERON PRODUCTION IN MURINE SPLEEN CELL CULTURES

Holger Kirchner

Institute of Virus Research
German Cancer Research Center
Heidelberg, FRG

Interferon is an antiviral protein which has been discovered by Isaacs and Lindenmann about 20 years ago (1). However, the antiviral effect is in reality an anticellular effect because interferon doesn't act on the virus itself but renders the cell incapable of virus replication. Subsequently, a great number of additional effects of interferon on cellular functions have been described which have been comprehensively reviewed (2). Initially, there have been objections to these data because pure interferon has not been available. In the meantime, however, it has been established that highly purified interferon also causes these "non-antiviral" effects.

In the context of this book, it is of special interest to mention that interferon has been shown to augment cytotoxicity in test systems of natural killer (NK) cells. This possibility has been first suggested by the results of Oehler and Herberman who have pointed to the parallels between the capacity of certain substances and viruses to induce interferon and to cause augmentation of NK cell killing (3). Lateron, it has been formally shown by two laboratories that interferon causes boosting of NK cell activity, both _in vivo_ and _in vitro_ (4,5). It is not within the scope of this article to discuss the mechanisms by which interferon boosts NK cell activity. Recent data suggest that this occurs by recruitment of pre-NK cells (6,7).

An exciting finding has been reported by Trinchieri et al., who have shown that many of the cells which are commonly used as target cells for NK cell killing themselves induce interferon in lymphocyte cultures (8). This interferon induction occurs relatively fast, so that, at least in long-term assays of NK cell killing, the possibility exists that there is an additional activation of NK cells by the interferon produced in the reaction itself. In short-term assays of NK cell activity killing can obviously occur in the absence of measurable amounts of

ISBN 0-12-341350-8

interferon (Peter et al., this volume). The exact correlation between NK cell activity and autochtonous interferon production remains to be determined.

Our own laboratory has taken a different approach. We have initially found that C. parvum, an immunomodulatory agent widely used in immunotherapy of experimental tumors (9) also very effectively protected mice against infection with Herpes Simplex Virus (HSV) - (10). We have then found that C. parvum represented an interferon inducer in vivo in mice (11) and in vitro in lymphocyte cultures of murine and human origin (11,12). Subsequently, we have performed several extensive series of experiments concerned with interferon production in murine and human lymphocytes. We want to summarize here our data of the murine systems. The experimental details of these, however, will be found in the cited references.

C. PARVUM - INDUCED INTERFERON PRODUCTION

Mice were injected intraperitoneally with 350 μg of C. parvum (strain CN 6134), their spleens were removed at various times, and spleen cells were cultured for 48 hr in vitro. Considerable titers of interferon were found in the spleen cell supernatants. When spleen cells of previously untreated mice were cultured in the presence of C. parvum also high titers of interferon were induced (11). The highest titers of interferon, however, were found when spleen cells of mice injected with C. parvum were cultivated in the presence of additionally added C. parvum. At the moment, conflicting data exist as to the producer cell of C. parvum-induced interferon. Our data using spleen cells from previously untreated mice suggested that B cells were the producer cells of interferon (11). However, Neumann and Sorg have isolated macrophages from spleens of C. parvum-injected mice and have concluded that macrophages were the producers of interferon in this situation (13). There are many differences in the experimental procedures of both laboratories and, obviously, further experiments are needed to clarifiy these points.

MITOGEN - INDUCED INTERFERON

Induction of interferon production in murine spleen cells by the T cell mitogens phytohemagglutinin (PHA) and concanavalin A (Con A) has been shown several years ago by Stobo et al. (14). Similarly to these data, we have found that pretreatment of spleen cells by anti-theta serum plus complement abolished interferon production induced by PHA or Con A, indicating that interferon production was a T cell dependent function. We have also confirmed the very interesting finding of Wietzerbin et al. who have shown that spleen cells from nu/nu mice which did not respond to PHA with lymphoproliferation, produced equal amounts of interferon as spleen cells of their heterozygous littermates when stimulated with PHA (15). In addition to these data, however, we have shown that spleen cells of nu/nu mice did not produce interferon in response to Con A or to allogeneic cells (unpublished data).Interferon production induced by PHA was abolished by pretreatment of nu/nu spleen cells by anti-theta serum plus complement suggesting that the minor population of T cells known to be present in spleen cells of nu/nu mice was responsible for interferon production. The observation that the cell type producing interferon in response to Con A was absent in spleens of nude mice may suggest that subsets of T cells are responding to PHA with interferon production which are different from those subsets that respond to Con A with interferon production. Interestingly, thymocytes of C57BL/6 mice did not react to PHA nor to Con A with interferon production. Interferon production was independent of lymphoproliferation, since mitomycin C-treated spleen cells who did not react with increased incorporation of ^{3}H-thymidine were capable of producing interferon in response to PHA or Con A. Also, fractions of spleen cells collected by a 1 g sedimentation procedure which were incapable of a lymphoproliferative reaction to the T cell mitogens, produced high titers of interferon when stimulated by PHA or Con A.

INTERFERON PRODUCTION IN THE MIXED LYMPHOCYTE CULTURE (MLC)

Measurement of interferon production represents a third parameter of alloantigen recognition besides measurement of lymphoproliferation and of lymphocytotoxicity. Interferon production in the murine MLC has been demonstrated first by Gifford et al. (16) and by Virelizier et al. (17). We have confirmed and extended these findings (18,19). We have found interferon production after one or two days of culture, both in primary and secondary MLC, in the presence of fetal bovine serum or of normal mouse serum. Serum-free conditions usually were not optimal for interferon production in the MLC, whereas for PHA- or Con A-induced interferon production serum-free conditions consistently yielded good results. Interferon production in the MLC was proliferation-independent, since it could be demonstrated in an MLC between two spleen cell populations which were both treated with mitomycin C. Thus, mitomycin C was not useful for performing a One-Way MLC. Puromycin treatment which initially was successfully used for establishing a One-Way MLC, lateron yielded erratic results. Thus, to perform One-Way-MLC in experiments in which interferon production is measured has proven to be a difficult task. However, One-Way-MLC's could be established in parent/F1 combinations. Interferon production in the MLC was T cell-dependent since it was abolished when the parent population was pretreated with anti-theta serum plus complement whereas treatment of the F1 population with anti-theta serum plus complement did not abolish interferon production in the parent/F1 combination. Spleen cells of nu/nu mice did not respond with interferon production to allogeneic spleen cells. Preliminary evidence suggested that the interferon producing cell belonged to the Lyt $1,2,3^+$ subtype of T lymphocytes (unpublished collaborative data with M. Simon).

Interferon production was demonstrated in various combinations of spleen cells differing at the complete H-2 complex and in a few combinations of spleen cells from mice identical at the H-2 complex but differing at minor histocompatibility loci. Interferon production was demonstrable in combinations differing only at the K end or the D end of the H-2 complex. In our laboratory, no interferon production was detected in MLC combinations differing at the M locus or at the I-region of the H-2 complex (18). However, Landolfo et al. have found interferon production in the latter types of combinations (20). The reasons for this discrepancy are not clear. Presently, in a collaborative effort between the two laboratories we are reinvestigating this situation.

The interferon produced in the MLC similarly to the interferons induced by PHA or Con A appeared to represent type II interferon, since it was not neutralized by an antiserum raised against type I interferon and since it was labile at pH 2.

INTERFERON INDUCED BY HSV IN MOUSE SPLEEN CELLS

Because of the interest our laboratory has developed in an *in vivo* model of HSV-infection (21) we have also tested HSV-induced interferon production both *in vivo*, and *in vitro* in different strains of mice. In these studies we have used C57BL/6 mice which are relatively resistant to ip infection with HSV and DBA/2 mice which are quite susceptible. At high doses of HSV, however, resistance of C57BL/6 mice could be broken. Serum interferon could be detected in both strains of mice after ip injection of HSV when virus doses were injected high enough to kill even C57BL/6 mice. However, serum interferon levels were significantly higher in B6 mice than in D2 mice. Lower doses of HSV did not induce serum interferon in either strain. Additionally, we have also tested *in vitro* production of interferon by spleen cells. When a preparation of purified and concentrated HSV virions (kindly provided by Dr. Hilfenhaus, Behringwerke Research Laboratories) was used, high titers of type I interferon were produced by spleen cells of non-immune B6 mice, whereas only moderate titers were produced by D2 spleen cells under the same conditions. We have spent considerable efforts to define the producer cell of HSV-induced type I interferon in mouse spleen cells. This cell was present in spleens of nu/nu mice (22) and was not inactivated by treatment with anti-theta serum plus complement. The latter treatment was done under conditions which reduced NK cell activity against YAC cells by 40-60%. The producer cell of interferon was not removed by several cycles of plastic adherence and it was not destroyed by treatment with high doses of silica. Spleen cells of newborn B6 mice which were inactive in the NK cell assay produced interferon in response to HSV. Treatment of B6 spleen cells by one passage through a nylon wool column did not remove the producer cell of interferon. However, two cycles of nylon wool treatment removed the producer cell of type I interferon. The majority of cells positive for surface immunoglobulin markers was removed by the first passage through the nylon column. Nevertheless, our data do suggest that a subpopulation of B lymphocytes that are less adherent to nylon than the majority of B lymphocytes are the producers of HSV-induced type I interferon in mouse spleen cell cultures. The observation that this cell was inactivated by 1000 R of irradiation is also consistent with this conclusion.

INTERFERON PRODUCTION IN THE MIXED LYMPHOCYTE TUMOR CELL INTERACTION (MLTI)

Trinchieri et al. have shown that human lymphocytes produce interferon when they are cocultivated with allogeneic tumor cells (7). We were interested to investigate this phenomenon in murine lymphocyte cultures. Mouse spleen cells when cocultivated with YAC ($H\text{-}2^a$) or MDAY ($H\text{-}2^d$) lymphoma cells produce considerable titers of interferon. Equal titers were found when DBA/2 or A/J mice were compared in the syngeneic or in the allogeneic MLTI. Although there is no definitive proof for this conclusion as yet we infer that the interferon produced in the MLTI is a product of the spleen cells and not of the tumor cells, since it was produced when the lymphoma cells were irradiated by 4000 R. The interferon produced was not inactivated by an antiserum against type I interferon under controlled conditions, and therefore appear to represent type II interferon. This finding differs from the data obtained in the human MLTI where the interferon produced appeared to be type I interferon. At the time of completion of this article we have not conclusively defined the producer cell of interferon in the murine MLTI (for our data on the human MLTI see the paper by Peter et al. in this volume). It was apparently not a T cell, because there were no differences when spleen cells of nu/nu mice were compared with those of their heterozygous littermates and interferon production was not abolished by pretreatment of spleen cells by anti-theta serum plus complement. The identity of the interferon producing cell, however, remains to be determined.

CONCLUSIONS

Interferon production in mouse spleen cells was investigated after stimulation with C. parvum, PHA, Con A, HSV, allogeneic spleen cells (MLC), or syngeneic tumor cells (MLTI). Attempts were undertaken to define the producer cell of interferon in each of these systems. At present, these attempts have not been fully conclusive in all of the systems studied. We feel that investigating interferon production particularly in the MLC and in the MLTI may serve as a very useful system of recognition of alloantigens or "tumor antigens". The interferon assay may also be useful as a parameter for mitogen-activation where interferon production obviously occurs in the absence of lymphoproliferation.

Previously, it has been shown that exogenously added interferon affected cellular functions in the MLC and in the MLTI (for example T cell killing or NK cell killing). It may be hypothesized that interferon produced in the reaction itself serves an important regulatory role. To prove this hypothesis the subtypes of interferon produced in these reactions will have to be purified that they may be added back to the reactions under various experimental conditions.

REFERENCES

1 Isaacs, A., and Lindenmann, J., (1957). Proc. Royal Roc. B 147, 258.
2 Stewart, W.E. (1979). The Interferon System, Springer Wien New York.
3 Oehler, J.R., and Herberman, R.B. (1978). Int. J. Cancer 21, 221.
4 Gidlund, N., Oern, A., Wigzell, H., Senik, A., and Gresser, I. (1978). Nature 273, 759.
5 Djeu, J.Y., Heinbaugh, J.A., Holden, H.T., and Herberman, R.B. (1978). J. Immunol. 122, 175.
6 Saksela, E., Timonen, T., and Cantell, K. (1979). Scand J. Immunol. 10, 257.
7 Trinchieri, G., Santoli, D., and Knowles, B.B. (1977). Nature 270, 611.
8 Berthold, W., Masucci-Cecchetti, M.G., Klein, E., Strander, H., (1980) Annals of NYAS, in press.
9 Milas, L., and Scott, M.T. (1978). Advances Cancer Res. 26, 257.
10 Kirchner, H., Hirt, H.M., and Munk, K. (1977). Inf. Immun. 16, 9.
11 Hirt, H.M., Becker, H., and Kirchner, H. (1978) Cell. Immunol. 38, 168.
12 Hirt, H.M., Schwenteck, M., Becker, H., and Kirchner, H. (1978). Clin. Exp. Immunol. 32, 471.
13 Neumann, C.H., and Sorg, C. (1979). Immunobiol. 156, 259.
14 Stobo, J., Green, I., Jackson, L., and Baron, S., (1974). J. Immunol. 112, 1589.

15 Wietzerbin, J., Stefanos, S., Falcoff, R., Lucero, M., Catinot, L., and Falcoff, F., (1978) Infect. Immun. 21, 966.
16 Gifford, G.E., Tibor, A., and Peavy, D.L. (1971) Infect.Immun.3,164.
17 Virelizier, J.L., Allison, A.C., and DeMaeyer, E. (1977) Infect. Immun. 17, 282 (1977).
18 Kirchner, H., Zawatzky, R., and Schirrmacher, V. (1979). Eur. J. Immunol. 9, 97.
19 Kirchner, H., Zawatzky, R., Engler, H., Schirrmacher, V., Becker, H., and v. Wussow, P. (1979) Eur. J. Immunol., in press
20 Landolfo, S., Marcucci, F.,Giovarelli, M., Viano, I., and Forni, G. (1979) Immunogenetics. in press.
21 Kirchner, H., Kochen, M., Hirt, H.M., Keyssner, K., and Munk, K. (1978). Z. Immunforsch. 154, 147.
22 Zawatzky, R., Hilfenhaus, J., and Kirchner, H. (1978). Cell. Immunol. 47, 424.

Natural Production of Macrophage-Migration Inhibitory Factor and Human-Leukocyte Inhibitory Factor

Aldo Tagliabue

IRF Mario Negri Institute
Milan, Italy

James L. McCoy

Carcinogenesis Testing Program
National Cancer Institute
Bethesda, Maryland

It was originally felt that lymphokine production was the result of a specific immunological reaction triggered by antigen and its detection in vitro reflected a state of cellular immunity in vivo. Lymphocyte stimulants which can initiate release of lymphokines have subsequently been broadened to include non-specific mitogens and mixed leukocyte cultures. A series of different investigators have also encountered a phenomenon in which normal lymphocytes and cultures of established lymphoid and even non-lymphoid cell lines secrete effector molecules without any stimulus. These effector molecules have mimicked activity characteristic of interferon (IF), lymphotoxin (LT), migration inhibitory factor (MIF), and leukocyte inhibitory factor (LIF). This review presents a brief discussion of the reports of natural MIF and LIF production by lymphoid and non-lymphoid cells and their biological and physicochemical similarity to well characterized MIF and LIF preparations. Although spontaneous LT production has been described by Granger, et al (1) and similar natural IF synthesis has been reported by Kasel et al. (2) these studies will not be discussed here.

Supernatants from continuous cultures of both human lymphoid (1,3,4) and non-lymphoid (1,3-5) cells and animal lymphoid (3,4) and non-lymphoid (3,4,6) cells have been found to contain MIF-like activity. Production of MIF in some of these studies appears to be dependent on cell division, with the greatest quantity being detected in supernatants collected during the S phase after the cells were synchronized in G-1 (3), although other investigators have failed to find such an obvious relation between MIF-like activity and cell cycle.

ISBN 0-12-341350-8

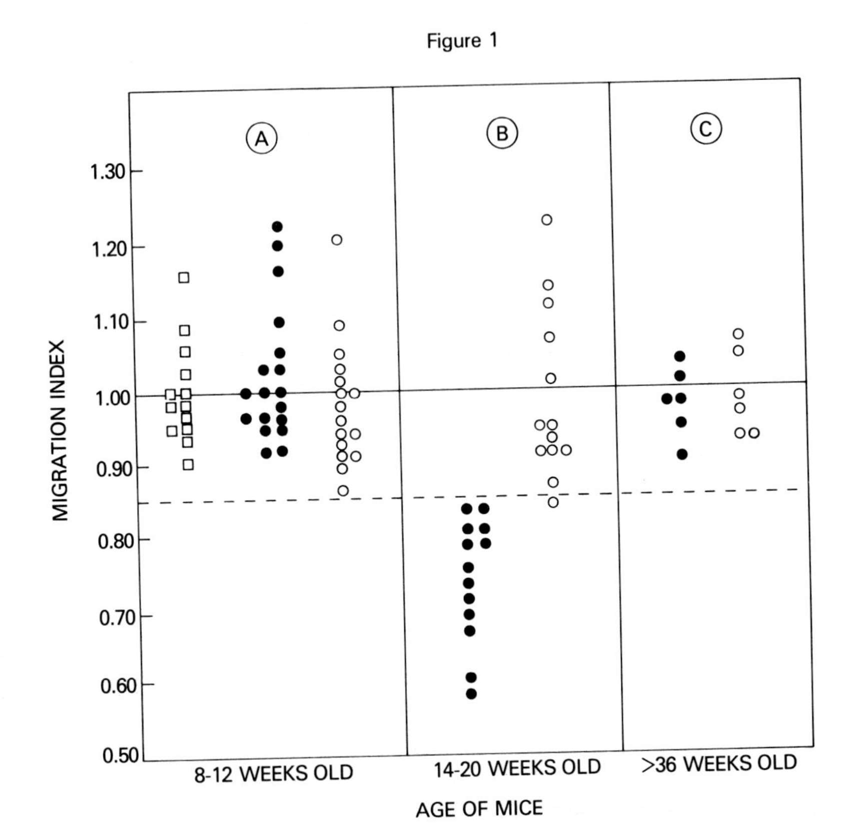

FIGURE 1. Migration inhibition reactivity of spleen cells from C3H+ (o), C3H- (●) and C57BL/6 (□) mice of different ages in response to 1 ug/ml of MTV. Migration inhibition values of less than 0.85 were considered positive.

Spontaneous MIF (7) and LIF (8) production has been obtained by culturing fresh human peripheral blood lymphocytes without any intended stimlus. When T and B lymphocytes were purified by carbonyl iron and sheep red blood cell rosette sedimentation, only B cells produced LIF (8). Other reports have also indicated that normal mouse (9) and rat (10) lymphoid cells produce MIF upon in vitro culture with mouse mammary tumor virus (MTV) or with tumor cells. Cell characterization studies in the rat system revealed that non-adherent, non-T cells devoid of Fc receptors were responsible for MIF production.

Some representative data (Figure 1 and Table 1) from our laboratory depicts how spleen cells from normal C3H mice respond to MTV stimulation in producing MIF as detected by the

TABLE I - Inhibition of Migration of Mouse Peritoneal Cells by Supernatants of Cultures of Unstimulated Spleen Cells from 14-week-old C3H+ and C3H- Mice

DILUTION OF CONDITIONED MEDIUM		AVERAGE MIGRATION INHIBITION AREAS		
		C3H+	C3H-	MI Value[a]
Undiluted		3,218[b]	3,951	
		3,540	4,345	
		3,748	4,278	
	MEAN	3,502	4,191	0.84
1:5		2,961	3,766	
		3,076	3,956	
		3,413	3,803	
	MEAN	3,150	3,842	0.82

[a] $MI = \frac{\text{C3H+ mean areas of migration}}{\text{C3H- mean areas of migration}}$

[b] Each number represents results from an individual mouse

p $\leq$ 0.01 versus C3H- mice

indirect agarose microdroplet macrophage MIF assay that has been previously described (11). Figure 1 presents data of the ability of spleens from individual C3H mice infected with MTV at birth (C3H+) and genetically similar C3H mice free of MTV infection (C3H-) to produce MIF in response to in vitro MTV stimulation. No difference in migration inhibition values was observed when MTV stimulated supernatants were prepared from spleen cells of C3H+, C3H- or C57BL/6 mice less than 12 weeks of age, thus indicating that animals of this age are not naturally producing MIF in response to MTV. Spleen cells from normal C3H+ mice greater than 14 weeks of age produced MIF in response to MTV, whereas only 1 C3H- animal was positive. Reactivity to MTV was no longer detected in 36 week old C3H+ mice nor in C3H- animals, suggesting an immunological eclipse in reactivity in C3H+ mice. It is known that almost all C3H+ mice develop primary mammary tumors with increased age. Presumably most 36 week old C3H+ animals are harboring microscopic or even macroscopic tumors at a time when MIF reactivity against MTV is eclipsed. During the course of these studies we also observed that supernatants of unstimulated cultures of spleen cells from 14 week old C3H+ mice possessed some ability to spontaneously produce MIF (Table 1). Taken together (Figure 1 and Table 1) the results suggest that MTV infection may induce an in vivo activation of lymphocytes in C3H+ mice, resulting in "natural" MIF production in vitro.

Other somewhat related studies with humans have shown a high incidence of indirect leukocyte migration inhibition reactivity of normal donors in contact with lung cancer to a 3M KCl extract from a fresh pleural effusion of a patient with adenocarcinoma of the lung. (Suslov, McCoy, Cannon and Herberman unpublished observations). The fact that the individuals in contact with lung cancer patients or materials have a high level of tumor associated reactivity than the normal population suggests a horizontal transmission of the reactivity associated with lung cancer. Although extensive physicochemical characterization of LIF-like supernatants in the human studies have not yet been performed, the observations (8) that the activities are maintained after heating supernatants at 56°C and can be neutralized by a sugar (i.e., N-acetyl glucosamine) known to inhibit LIF, strengthen the idea that LIF is the responsible molecule in those studies.

Although clear-cut definitive evidence for natural MIF and LIF production has not been proven, it does appear that cells of lymphoid and even non-lymphoid nature can spontaneously produce these molecules, and that their existence is not artifactual. The function as well as the specificity of spontaneously arising MIF and LIF can at best only be speculative at this time. The phenomenon must, however, be a natural event that can occur in vivo (possibly following antigen stimulation) and also in vitro under certain conditions by both lymphoid and non-lymphoid cells undergoing no apparent stimulation.

REFERENCES

1. Granger, G. A., Moore, G. E., White, J. G., Matzinger, P., Sundsmo. J. S., Shupe, S., Kolb, W. P., Kramer, J. and Glade, P. R. J. Immunol 140; 1476 (1970).
2. Kasel, J. A., Haase, A. T., Glade, P. R., and Chessin, L.N., Proc. Soc. Exp. Biol. Med. 128; 351 (1968).
3. Tubergen, D. G., Feldman, J. D., Pollock, E. M., and Lerner, R. A., J. Exp. Med. 135; 255 (1972).
4. Papageorgiou, P.S., Henley, W. L., and Glade, P R., J. Immunol., 108; 494 (1972).

5. Poste, G., Cancer Res. 35; 2558 (1975).
6. Hammond, M. E., Roblin, R. O., Dvorak, A. M., Seluaggio, S. S., Black, P. H., Dvorak, H. F., Science 185; 955 (1974).
7. Arvilommi, H. and Rasanen, L., Nature, 257; 144 (1975).
8. Arvilommi, H., Rasanen, L. Laatikainen, A. and Karhumaki, E., Acta. Path. Microbiol, Scand. 86; 53 (1978).
9. Lopez, D. M., Ortiz-Muniz, G., and Siegel, M. M., Proc. Soc. Exp. Biol. Med. 151; 225 (1976).
10. Sharma. J. M., Herberman, R.B., Djeu, J. Y., and Nunn, M. E., J. Immunol. 123; 222 (1979).
11. Tagliabue, A., Herberman, R. B., and McCoy, J.L., Cancer Res. 38; 2279 (1978).

INTERFERON PRODUCTION IN LYMPHOCYTES CULTURED WITH TUMOR-DERIVED CELLS*

Giorgio Trinchieri
Bice Perussia
Daniela Santoli

The Wistar Institute of Anatomy and Biology
Philadelphia, Pennsylvania

Antiviral activity released in the supernatant of mixed cultures of lymphocytes with cell lines.

Viral inhibitors are released in the supernatant of mixed cultures of lymphocytes and certain tumor-derived or virus-transformed cell lines (Trinchieri et al., 1977, 1978a). The results obtained in a typical experiment using human lymphocytes and a rhabdomyosarcoma-derived cell line (RDMC) are shown in Fig. 1. The supernatants of RDMC cultures or of lymphocytes cultured alone did not display antiviral activity, but the supernatant of a mixed culture of the two did. Antiviral activity was detectable as early as 3 to 4 hr from the time of incubation and reached a maximum level in 18 to 24 hr, though it appeared slightly later than that induced by viruses [Newcastle disease virus (NDV), Fig. 1; influenza virus, Hong Kong strain (HK), Fig. 3]. The levels of antiviral activity at 24 hr were, however, comparable in both the mixed culture and the virus-infected culture. Table I summarizes the results obtained by testing different human cell lines for their ability to induce antiviral activity when cultured with lymphocytes. None of the 15 strains of fibroblasts tested were inducers. In contrast, 21 of 30 tumor-derived cell lines were able to induce IF. Only 2 of 16 SV40-transformed fibroblasts were inducers, whereas the 3 EBV-transformed human B-cell lines tested were all inducers. Similarly, most of the murine transformed fibroblast cell lines were not inducers whereas all of the tumor-derived were (Table I). The human and murine lines that induced

*The experimental work described in this paper was supported by NIH grants CA-20833, CA-10815, CA-43882 and NS-11036 and by the National Multiple Sclerosis Society.

ISBN 0-12-341350-8

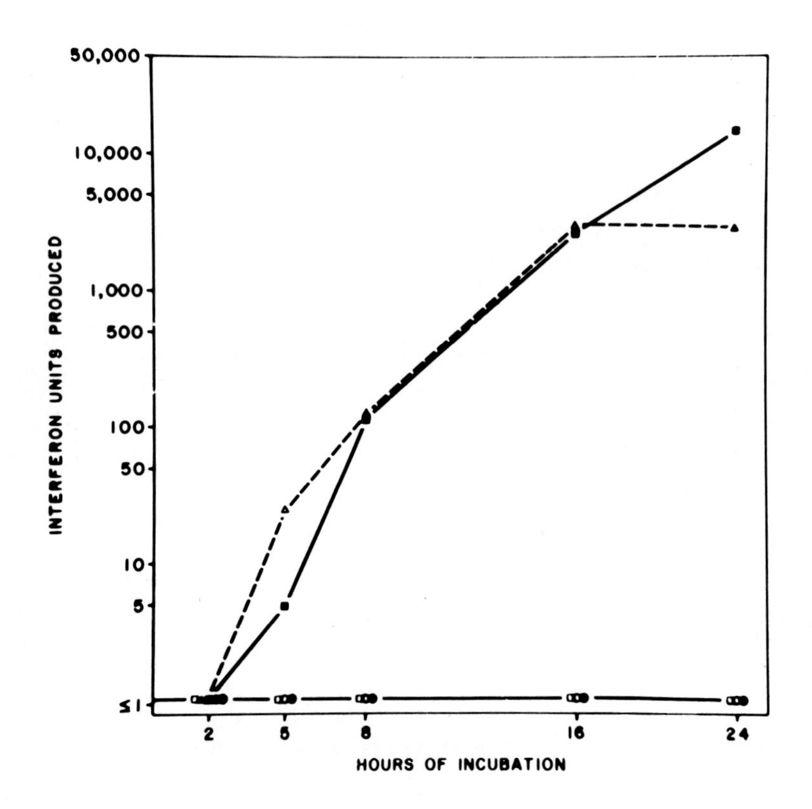

FIGURE 1. Kinetics of interferon production from human lymphocytes infected with Newcastle disease virus or cultured with a human rhabdomyosarcoma-derived cell line (RDMC). Human peripheral blood lymphocytes were isolated on a Ficoll-Hypaque gradient. Adherent cells were removed by two incubations (1 hr each, 37°C) on glass petri dishes. The cells were resuspended at 10^7 ml in RPMI 1640 medium with 10% fetal bovine serum, and 1 ml of medium containing cells was added to 16-mm wells (Linbro Disposo trays FB16-24TC) either empty or containing a monolayer of RDMC. The supernatants were taken at the indicated times, centrifuged at 1,000 g for 30 min and tested for antiviral activity. Supernatants from Newcastle disease virus-infected lymphocytes were treated at

pH 2 for 4 days and then neutralized before testing. The antiviral activity was expressed in terms of the cytopathic effect (50% end-point inhibition test). Serial dilutions (100 μl) of the supernatant were added to the wells of microtiter plates (Microtitre II, Falcon) containing monolayers of human fetal skin fibroblasts. After overnight incubations, the supernatants were removed and 50,000 plaque-forming-units of vesicular stomatitis virus (Indiana strain) were added in a volume of 0.2 ml. The final evaluation of cytopathic effect was done after 48 hr. Each assay included a standard interferon preparation (NIH human reference interferon G-023-901-527 with a titer of 20,000 units). Supernatants from: ●, lymphocytes alone; ◻, RDMC monolayer alone; ■ mixed culture lymphocytes and RDMC; O, mixed culture lymphocytes and RDMC in presence of cycloheximide 100 μg/ml; ▲, lymphocytes infected with Newcastle disease virus at multiplicity of infection of 10. Reproduced with permission from Trinchieri et al. (1977).

antiviral activity in human lymphocytes also induced such activity in mouse spleen cells, although the activity with mouse lymphocytes was always much lower. The ability to produce antiviral activity varied among different mouse strains: much higher titers were consistently observed with BALB/c spleen cells than with C57BL/6 or (BALB/c x C57Bl/6)F spleen cells.

Identification of the antiviral inhibitor as interferon.

The antiviral substance from mixed cultures of human lymphocytes with cell lines meets the criteria established by Lockart (1973) for classifying the viral inhibitor as an interferon (IF): a) it is a protein which is readily digested by trypsin; b) it does not inhibit viral replication through a toxic effect on the cells; c) it is active against a variety of viruses, d) it does not inactivate the virus directly, but rather induces an antiviral status in the cells that persists when the inhibitor is removed from the medium; both RNA and protein synthesis by the cells are required for the induction of the antiviral status. In addition, the viral inhibitor has other properties in common with most IF types: it is more active in homologous than in heterologous cells; it is not released spontaneously but only in the presence of the inducer cell line; and it is stable at pH 2.0. The viral inhibitor is eluted after gel filtration in a main peak corresponding to a mol. wt. approximately 25,000. All

TABLE 1. *Ability of Cell Lines to Induce Antiviral Activity When Cultured with Lymphocytes*

Cell type	No. of cell lines tested	No. of IF-inducing cell lines
<u>Human</u>		
Fibroblasts, fetal skin	6	0
Fibroblasts, skin	7	0
Fibroblasts, brain	2	0
Fibroblasts, skin, SV40-transformed	5	0
Fibroblasts, brain, SV40-transformed	11	2
Melanoma-derived	11	10
Colorectal carcinoma-derived	6	2
Sarcoma-derived	5	2
Lymphoid, tumor-derived	8	7
Lymphoid, EBV-transformed	3	3
<u>Murine</u>		
Fibroblasts, continuous lines	5	3
Fibroblasts, Adenovirus 5-transformed	7	0
Fibroblasts, SV40-transformed	33	6
Lymphoid, tumor-derived	3	3

of these characteristics and the ability to inhibit virus replication in heterologous cow cells (an ability not shared by fibroblast-IF or type II immune leukocyte-IF) identify this IF as type I leukocyte-IF (Youngner and Salvin, 1973). A small part of the activity, however, is eluted in a 45,000 peak, and is sensitive to acid treatment. The possibility that this IF may be analogous to type II immune leukocyte-IF is under investigation.

Allogeneic and syngeneic mixed cultures and identification of the lymphocytes as the producers of antiviral activity.

Production of IF was observed in cultures of lymphocytes with xenogeneic, allogeneic and autologous (syngeneic) cell lines. Allogeneic differences between lymphocytes and the inducing cell lines are, therefore, not required for IF induction. EBV-transformed lymphoid cells from a human donor were cultured with the lymphocytes of the same donor to produce autologous mixed cultures. IF-inducing syngeneic SV40-transformed murine cells were cultured with spleen cells from mice of inbred strains. IF produced in mixed cultures of human lymphocytes with murine cell lines or in cultures of mouse spleen cells with human cell lines inhibited viral replication only in human or in mouse cells, respectively (Table II). These results indicate that the lymphocytes and not the cell lines are the producers of IF in the mixed cultures.

The induction of IF in mixed allogeneic lymphocyte cultures (MLC) differs in many respects from the induction of IF in lymphocyte-cell line cultures (Mangoni *et al*., 1979). Different lymphocyte subpopulations are responsible for IF production in the two systems, as discussed in the next section. The kinetics of induction differ, with the peak of IF production being reached in few hours in the lymphocyte-cell line culture and in 4 to 6 days in MLC. Lymphocyte-cell line cultures produce a "viral" leukocyte type of IF that is resistant to pH 2.0 and to treatment at 56°C and cross-reacts on heterologous cow cells whereas in MLC an "immune" IF is produced sensitive to both pH 2.0 and to 56°C and non-crossreactive on cow cells.

TABLE II. Species-Specificty of the Antiviral Activity in the Supernatant of Mixed Cultures of Lymphocytes and Cell Lines

*Mixed cultures**		*Antiviral units† in supernatant tested on*	
Source of lymphocytes	*Cell line*	*Human FS2*	*Mouse L cells*
Human blood	*RDMC*	*15625*	8
Human blood	*C57SV*	*3125*	2
Mouse spleen	*RDMC*	*< 1*	64
Mouse spleen	*C57SV*	*< 1*	32

**Human rhabdomyosarcoma-derived cells (RDMC) and SV40-transformed C57BL/6 mouse fibroblasts (C57SV) were grown as monolayers in 16-mm plastic wells. Lymphocytes from human peripheral blood or from BALB/c spleens were added to the monolayers (10^7 cells/ml). After 24 hr of incubation at 37°C, the supernatants were collected.*

†Antiviral activity in the supernatants was tested by inhibition of the cytopathic effect of vesicular stomatitis virus (VSV) on monolayers of human fetal skin fibroblast (FS2) or on mouse L cells.

Characterization of the human lymphocyte populations producing IF.

The ability of lymphocytes and their subpopulations to produce IF in culture with cell lines was tested using RDMC cells as inducers (Trinchieri *et al.*, 1978a). Induction with the NDV and HK viruses was also used for comparison in some experiments. Human lymphocytes incubated at 20°C for a period up to 24 hr maintained the ability to produce IF when induced by RDMC cells or by NDV. In contrast, after 17 hr of pre-incubation at 37°C, lymphocytes could not be induced by RDMC cells, but still responded to NDV infection with the level of IF production reduced to 20% of that observed with fresh cells (Fig. 2). Treatment of lymphocytes with trypsin

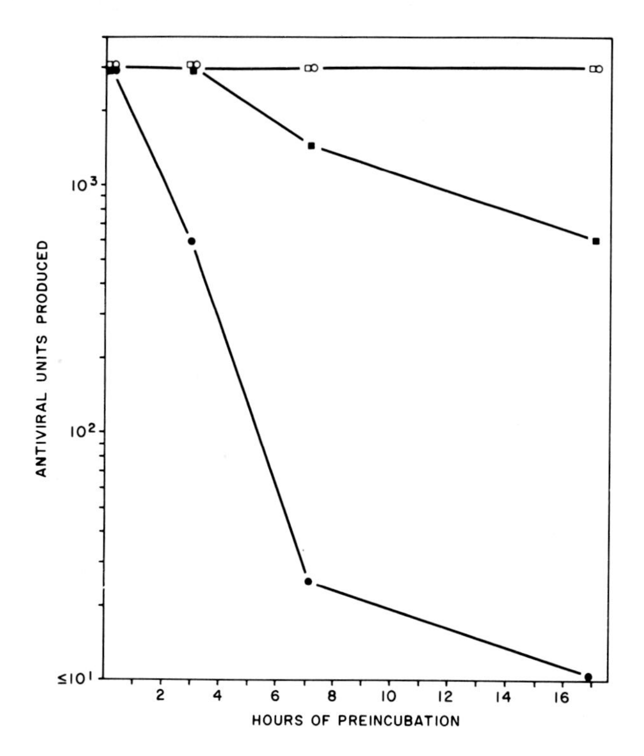

FIGURE 2. Loss of ability to produce IF of human lymphocytes incubated at 37°C. Human peripheral blood lymphocytes were preincubated at 37°C or at 20°C for the indicated time and then tested for IF induction with RDMC cells or NDV. Supernatants for IF-testing were collected 18 hr after the cells were mixed or after infection. ●——● preincubation 37°C, RDMC inducer; ■——■ , preincubation 37°C, NDV inducer; 0——0, preincubation 20°C, RDMC inducer; □——□, preincubation 20°C, NDV inducer.

or pronase (1 mg/ml, 20 min at 37°C) destroyes the ability of lymphocytes to produce IF when induced either by HK virus or by RDMC cells (Fig. 3). However, the cells treated with trypsin regain their ability to produce IF after 3 hr for HK induction and after more than 6 hr for RDMC induction. Cells treated with pronase only partially recover their activity.

The results of the experiments performed with lymphocyte subpopulations are presented in Table III. Depletion of glass-adherent cells from human lymphocytes determines a decrease in the monocyte contamination: monocyte-deprived lymphocyte preparations are better IF producers in response

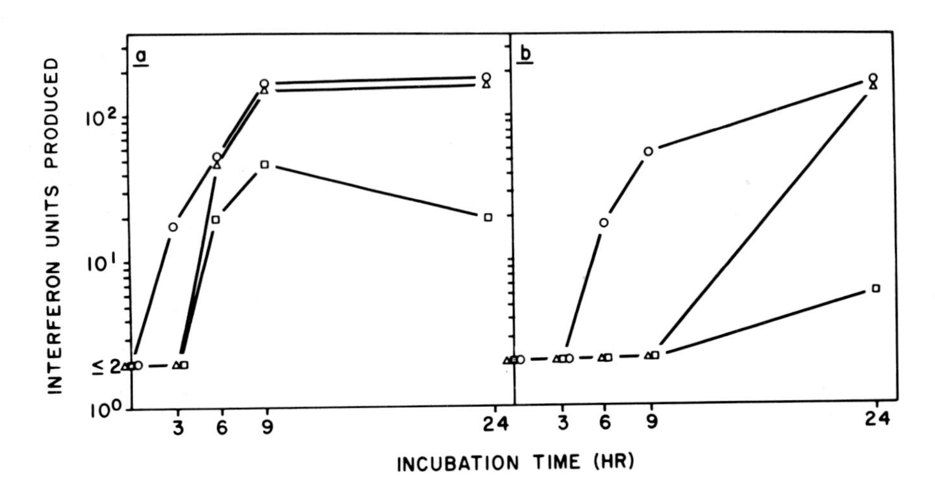

FIGURE 3. Effect of trypsin and pronase on the ability of human lymphocytes to produce IF upon infection with influenza virus, HK strain (a) or in mixed cultures with RDMC cells (b). Human lymphocytes were incubated 20 min at 37°C in the presence of 1 mg/ml trypsin or pronase, washed and tested for IF production. Supernatants for IF-testing were collected at the indicated times. 0——0, untreated lymphocytes; Δ——Δ, trypsin-treated lymphocytes; □——□, pronase-treated lymphocytes.

to RDMC when compared with the Ficoll-Hypaque separated mononuclear cells. On the contrary the induction of IF in response to viruses appears to be monocyte-dependent, and the depletion of glass-adherent cells results in a decreased IF production. The major population responsible for IF production in mixed cultures of lymphocytes and RDMC cells is non-adherent to nylon wool columns. The non-adherent cells, almost completely depleted of monocytes or B cells, are good producers of IF in response to RDMC cells, but poor producers in response to HK virus. The cells that adhere to the nylon wool column, mostly B cells and monocytes, respond to RDMC with either poor production or no production of IF, but are quite responsive to HK virus. When lymphocytes are separated into two subpopulations (T and non-T), on the basis of their ability to form rosettes with AET (2-aminoethyl isothiouronium bromide hydrobromide)-treated sheep erythrocytes, the non-rosetting fraction always produces high levels of IF in culture with RDMC. The cells in the rosetting fraction (T cells), responded by either poor or no production of IF in most of the experiments. The T cells appear to be the producers of "immune" IF in MLC (unpublished results).

When cells with receptors for the Fc fragment of IgG were removed from the total lymphocyte population, the remaining lymphocytes completely lost the ability to produce IF upon induction with both RDMC cells and HK virus. The Fc receptor-bearing cells were removed either by rosetting with ox erythrocytes sensitized with IgG antibodies, or by adherence to a monolayer of sheep erythrocytes sensitized with IgG antibodies, or by adherence to immune complexes coupled to Sepharose beads. When the EA7S monolayer technique was used, cells obtained by trypsinization of the sensitized monolayer were able to produce IF (Table III). The same results have been obtained with Fc receptor-positive and - negative "null" cells (not shown). When Fc-positive cells react with immune complexes, the Fc receptor becomes irreversibly modulated, and the ability to mediate spontaneous (SpCMC) and antibody-dependent (AbCMC) cytotoxicity is lost or greatly reduced (Perussia _et al_., 1979). These lymphocytes did, however, retain a normal ability to produce IF in response to inducing cell lines and viruses (unpublished results). The reaction with immune complexes and the modulation of the IgG-Fc receptor have a differential effect on the production of IF on NK and K activities of the Fc-receptor-positive "null" lymphocytes.

Because the IF produced in mixed cultures of lymphocytes and inducing cell lines is responsible for 80-90% of the total NK cell activity (Trinchieri et al., 1978b), it would be interesting to know whether the cells that are stimulated by IF and actually destroy the target, are also the cells that produce IF. The ability of various

TABLE III Ability of Human Lymphocyte Subpopulations to Produce Interferon in Mixed Culture with RDMC Cells or Upon Infected with Influenza Virus (HK Strain)

Lymphocyte fraction	ANAE* %	sIg† %	E-RFC** %	EAox-RFC‡ %	IF-units induced by RDMC cells	IF-units induced by HK virus
Exp. A Ficoll-Hypaque separated	22.3	ND	ND	ND	125	1200
glass non-adherent	6.7	ND	ND	ND	3000	600
Exp. B Ficoll-Hypaque separated	17.9	22.7	62.9	ND	160	640
Nylon column non-adherent	1.4	2.4	86.4	ND	640	160
Nylon column adherent		55.8	24.2	ND	10	320
Exp. C Nylon column non-adherent	0.9	1.7	88.4	21.7	600	600
AET-E non-rosetting	11.4	32.0	0	49.2	3000	1200
AET-E rosetting	0	0	97.6	8.3	25	80
Exp. D. Ficoll-Hypaque separated	ND	ND	ND	25.0	486	162
E monolayer non-adherent	ND	ND	ND	18.0	486	54
EA7S monolayer adherent	ND	ND	ND	7.8	486	486
EA7S monolayer non-adherent	ND	ND	ND	2.5	< 5	< 5

Table IV Ability of Lymphocyte Subpopulations to Mediate Spontaneous and Antibody-Dependent Cytotoxicity and to Produce IF Upon Induction with RDMC Cells and Influenza Virus (HK Strain)

Cell preparation	Cytotoxicity		IF induction	
	K cells	NK cells	RDMC cells	HK virus
Total lymphocytes (Ficoll-Hypaque)	+++*	+++	+++	+++
Lymphocytes treated with immune complexes	+†	+†	+++	+++
Trypsinized lymphocytes	+++	-	-	-
Monocyte-depleted lymphocytes	+++	+++	++++	++
Nylon-adherent cells (B cells, monocytes)	-	-	-	++
"Null" cells	++++	++++	++++	++++
Fc receptor-negative "null" cells	-	-	-	-
Fc receptor-positive "null" cells treated with immune complexes	+†	+†	++++	++++
T cells	++	++	±	+

*The activity of the different fractions is indicated on the basis of an arbitrary score from - to ++++.
†Inhibition of cytotoxic activity due to modulation of the Fc receptors.

**Staining for non-specific acid esterase, strongly positive cells (monocytes) scored.*
†Positive fluorescence for surface immunoglobulin [fluorescein-rabbit F(ab')$_2$ anti-human F(ab')$_2$].
***Cells forming rosettes with AET-treated sheep erythrocytes (AET-E).*
‡Cells forming rosettes with ox erythrocytes sensitized with rabbit IgG antibodies. E, sheep erythrocytes; EA7S, E sensitized with rabbit IgG; ND, not done.

lymphocyte subpopulations to produce IF and to mediate cytotoxicity is reported in Table IV. The two activities are always found associated with the same lymphocyte subsets, with the exception of T cells. While T cells contain a relevant proportion of the cytotoxic activity, both spontaneous and antibody-dependent, they are unable to produce high levels of IF in response to either viruses or inducer cell lines.

In conclusion, the lymphocytes producing IF when cultured with RDMC cells are Fc receptor-positive "null" lymphocytes. The modulation of Fc receptors in the lymphocytes following interaction with immune complexes results in the inhibition of K and NK activity, but does not preclude the possibility of interaction of the lymphocytes with the RDMC cells and the induction of IF. The data available do not allow a positive identification of the IF-producing cells with the NK cells. The NK cells contained in the "null" fraction have characteristics similar to those of the IF producer cells, and they may also be involved in IF production. The T-cell fraction, however, contains a large proportion of the NK cell activity and produces almost no IF. The results obtained with HK virus are similar, except that monocytes and, perhaps, B cells may be involved in IF production.

REFERENCES

Lockart, R.Z., Jr. *in "Interferons and Interferon Inducers" (N.B. Finter, ed.) pp.11-27.* North Holland, Amsterdam. (1973)
Mangoni, L., Trinchieri, G., Engers, H.D., and Perussia, B., *Proc. 1st Intern. Congr. Interferons. in press* (1979).
Perussia, B., Trinchieri, G., and Cerottini, J.-C., *J. Immunol. 123,* 681-687 (1979).
Trinchieri, G., Santoli, D., and Knowles, B.B., *Nature 270,* 611-612 (1977).

Trinchieri, G., Santoli, D., Dee, R.R., and Knowles, B.B., *J. Exp. Med. 147*, 1299-1313 (1978a).
Trinchieri, G., Santoli, D., and Koprowski, H., *J. Immunol. 120*, 1849-1855 (1978b).
Youngner, J.S., and Salvin, S.B., *J. Immunol. 111*, 1914-1923, (1973).

SUMMARY: NATURAL LYMPHOKINE PRODUCTION

I. NATURAL INTERFERON PRODUCTION

It has been long known that leukocytes can produce interferon (IF) in response to viruses or some other stimuli and that much of this IF is type I, as opposed to the type II IF produced by immune lymphocytes in specific response to the relevant antigens (for review, see Stewart, 1979). This ability of lymphoid cells to rapidly produce a potent soluble factor, which can induce resistance to virus infection and a wide range of other biological activities, may be viewed as an important aspect of natural cell-mediated immunity. As with other components of natural immunity, there are a number of characteristics that set this response apart from antigen-induced immunity. Even the biological product, leukocyte IF, has physicochemical features which distinguish it from fibroblast type I or immune, type II IFs. The interest in IF production and its role in host resistance has been further accentuated by recent indications, as discussed below, of some association of this response with NK cells.

A. *Stimuli for Natural IF Production*

It is clear that a wide range of materials can induce IF production by normal leukocytes. These include viruses, bacteria, poly I:C and other synthetic substance, and some tumor cells and normal cells. The ability of tumors and other cells to stimulate IF production was demonstrated several years ago (Svet-Moldavsky et al, 1975) but only recently has this been explored in depth. Trinchieri et al summarize their findings in this area. About two-thirds of tumor cells, all B lymphoblastoid cell lines and a small proportion of SV40-transformed cell lines were able to induce the production in vitro of IF by human peripheral blood mononuclear cells. IF was detectable at 3-4 hrs. and reached maximal levels at 18-24 hrs. Syngeneic, allogeneic, and xenogeneic cell lines gave positive results. In contrast, normal fibroblasts did not

ISBN 0-12-341350-8

stimulate IF production. The IF produced had the characteristics of type I IF, including stability at pH 2.

As briefly summarized here by Ortaldo et al (section IC3), Djeu et al (1980) obtained similar results by inoculation of various cells into mice. A variety of tumor cells induced very high levels of circulating levels of IF, detectable within 4 hrs and reaching peak levels at 1-3 days. Normal thymus cells, but not syngeniec or allogeneic spleen cells, were also found to induce IF. In contrast to the characteristics of IF produced by human leukocytes in response to tumor cells, the IF in mouse serum was labile at low pH and had some other features distinguishing it from type I IF. However, it was also not typical type II IF, being neutralized by antibodies to type I IF.

The ability of only certain tumor or normal cells to elicit rapid production of IF indicates the need for selective recognition by the responding cells. It is intriguing that the specificity of IF induction has some similarity to the specificity of NK cells. Some of the tumor cells and the thymus cells that induced IF production were sensitive to NK lysis. However, the correlation has not been complete (e.g. see Leibold et al) and further studies are needed to carefully compare the target cell structures that are recognized in each of these reactions.

B. Cells Responsible for Natural IF Production

There have been several recent efforts to characterize the leukocytes that produce IF in response to various stimuli. Macrophages appear to be the predominant cell type producing IF in mice in response to poly I:C (Djeu et al, 1979) and some investigators have favored their involvement in production of IF in response to C. parvum. However, most of the data summarized here point towards lymphocytes as the producer cells in response to various stimuli. An intriguing question is whether the NK cell is responsible for part or all of the IF production upon stimulation with some materials. That is an attractive hypothesis, which would have the same cell responsible for a variety of natural immune responses and would also indicate an aspect of positive self regulation to this system. Despite its appeal, more documentation will be needed to justify firm conclusions about the role of NK cells in producing IF.

In studies with human lymphoid cells, production of IF in response to tumor cells and C. parvum appears to be mediated by similar cells. The producer cells are mainly nonadherent and appear to have Fc_{γ} receptors (Peter *et al*, Trinchieri *et al*). At least some of the IF-producer cells in response to *C. parvum* seem to have lower affinity Fc_{γ} receptors than NK cells, since an additional passage on an anti-immunoglobulin column was needed to deplete them. Both Trinchieri *et al* and Koide and Takasugi found that cells without detectable E receptors produced IF in response to cell lines and E receptor-bearing cells produced little or no IF. Peter *et al* obtained similar results with *C. parvum* as the stimulus. It should be noted, however, that Sugiyama and Epstein (1978) obtained apparently divergent results, concluding that T cells were responsible for IF production in response to *C. parvum*. The reasons for these differences are not clear, but Sugiyama and Epstein separated their cells by a different procedure and also performed their cultures for 2-7 days as opposed to the 1-3 day cultures of Peter *et al*. Overall, the data in these studies showed some overlap between the characteristics of IF-producing cells and NK cells, but also some differences. The study of Saksela *et al* provided the strongest association between these two functions. By immunofluorescence studies with anti-IF, they showed that large granular lymphcotyes in conjugates with K562 targets were positive. Also, IF production in response to tumor cells was localized in the same Percoll fractions that contained large granular lymphocytes.

In studies with mice, a more heterogeneous assortment of lymphoid cells seem to be involved in IF production. Kirchner found that *C. parvum* appeared to stimulate IF production by B cells. The cells responsible for the response to herpes simplex virus were incompletely characterized, but were Thy 1 antigen negative, somewhat adherent to nylon, present in nude and newborn mice and radiosensitive. The relationship between these cells and NK cells is not yet clear. In contrast, Bloom *et al* have studied the production of IF in response to cells infected with various RNA viruses, e.g. measles and mumps, and have observed two important points of similarity between the IF-producer cells and NK cells. The IF-producer cells appeared to express both Ly5 and Qa5 antigens, which have been found on most or all mouse NK cells (see section IA).

The associations between IF-producing cells and NK cells that have been detected, particularly those of Saksela *et al* with human cells and Bloom *et al* with mouse cells, are most intriguing. They point to some relationship between the cell types. However, it remains to be determined whether the same cells can both produce IF and kill target cells. It is possible that different cells within the same subset have each function. Combination of the anti-IF immunofluorescence procedure and the single cell agarose assay should allow visualization of the overlap between these activities.

II. NATURAL PRODUCTION OF OTHER LYMPHOKINES

There is only limited evidence that production of other lymphokines may be a manifestation of natural cell-mediated immunity. Leibold _et al_ (section IC3) report parallel production of lymphotoxin along with IF in cultures of human lymphoid cells with lymphoid cell lines. Sharma _et al_ (1979) found that normal rats produced macrophage migration inhibition factor (MIF) upon culture with rat cell lines. This response did not appear to be dependent on environmental stimuli, since reactivity was seen with germfree rats as well as with conventially reared animals. It is of particular interest that there were several parallels with rat NK activity. The strain and tissue distribution of both effector cells were similar and the specficitiy patterns were indistinguishable. Only rat cell lines with expression of endogenous type C viruses induced MIF production and it was suggested that the reactivity was directed against virus associated antigens. As has been suggested for some IF-producer cells, it seemed possible that NK cells were the MIF-producer cells. Although the cells producing MIF were distinct from mature T cells, they also differed from NK cells in having no detectable Fc_γ receptors. However, as discussed for NK cells (see section IA), some subsets of NK cells or NK cells at certain stages of differentiation may lack Fc_γ receptors.

The studies of Tagliabue and McCoy bear some resemblance to the above report. Normal mice produced MIF in response to antigens associated with mouse mammary tumors virus (MTV). However, in contrast to the rat studies, reactivity appeared to be directly related to vertical or horizontal infection with MTV. Thus, although the observed reactivity was spontaneous, it seems likely that it was induced as an immune response to the natural exposure to virus. Thus, as with the cytotoxic reactivity to MTV antigens observed by Blair _et al_, these responses may not be equivalent to non-antigen induced natural cell-mediated immunity. Similarly, since the reactivity of some normal human donors to lung tumor antigens was associated with contact with lung cancer patients or specimens, it was probably induced by exposure to some antigen.

REFERENCES

Djeu, J.Y., Huang, K-Y., and Herberman, R.B., *J. Exp. Med.* in press.

Sharma, J.M., Herberman, R.B., Djeu, J.Y., and Nunn, M.E., *J. Immunol*. 123, 222 (1979).

Stewart, W.E., II, "The Interferon System" Springer-Verlag, New York, (1979).

Sugiyama, M. and Epstein, L.B., *Cancer* 38, 4467 (1978).

Svet-Moldavsky, G.J., Slavina, E.G., Leipunskaya, I.L., Nemirovaskaya, B.M., Zinzar, S.N., and Morozova, L.F., *Interferon Scientific Memoranda* I-A144 (1975).

REGULATORY CAPACITIES OF MONONUCLEAR PHAGOCYTES WITH PARTICULAR REFERENCE TO NATURAL IMMUNITY AGAINST TUMORS[1]

Robert Keller

Immunobiology Research Group
Institute for Medical Microbiology
University of Zurich
Schönleinstrasse 22
CH-8032 Zurich/Switzerland

TABLE OF CONTENTS

[1]*This work was supported by the Swiss National Science Foundation (grant 3.173.77) and the Canton of Zurich.*

Abbreviations: *ADCC: antibody-dependent cellular cytotoxicity. AM: activated macrophages. CSA: colony stimulating activity. DMBA: dimethylbenz(a)anthracene. LPS: bacterial lipopolysaccharide. MAF: macrophage activating factor. PMA: phorbol myristate acetate. PMN: polymorphonuclear leukocyte.*

ISBN 0-12-341350-8

I. INTRODUCTION

Concepts on the mechanisms involved in antitumor surveillance and on the functional diversity of mononuclear phagocytes have undergone considerable changes during the past decade, reflecting several major developments. First, the notion of a central role for immunospecific (T cell) antitumor surveillance has been challenged by various observations (1-3). In parallel, evidence has been increasing to indicate that innate, natural immunity may prove to be a more important factor in host resistance against tumors. It is becoming appreciated that the outcome of the interaction between the tumor and the host during the early decisive phase of tumor growth is largely determined by the potential of the natural defense mechanisms rather than by immunospecific reactivity (4-14). Natural tumor resistance is likely to represent the cumulative effects of a number of cellular and humoral mechanisms; the involvement of the individual components could vary depending on the type of tumor, the local conditions and still other variables. Among the cellular components involved, only 'natural killer' (NK) cells (7,8,15-17, and references in this issue) and mononuclear phagocytes (4-6,18) have thus far been studied to any considerable extent. Apart from their established role in antimicrobial host defense and tissue repair by phagocytosis, intracellular killing and digestion, mononuclear phagocytes are now perceived to have a number of other important capabilities (19). Among these, the capacity to either promote or suppress proliferation (20-24) and other activities of a variety of cell types and/or tissues (25-32) and to acquire the ability to destroy other cells (33,34), notably tumor cells, are especially relevant in this context. The manifestations of the components involved in innate, natural and/or acquired, specific immunity are closely interwoven rather than expressed separately and sequentially. Interactions between the mononuclear phagocyte and the lymphoid system are particularly intimate and multifarious (4,19,25,27,35-37). It is in the perspective of this background that the array of mononuclear phagocyte functions devolving on tumor resistance is to be discussed.

As the contributions of macrophages to both innate and acquired immunity have been repeatedly reviewed during the past 3 years (4-6,38), the present discussion focusses instead on a number of concurrent developments relevant to their role in the regulation of other cell systems. These developments and their assessment is in part based on work carried out in the author's laboratory.

II. CHARACTERISTICS OF MONONUCLEAR PHAGOCYTES

A. *Origin, Differentiation, Turnover, Heterogeneity*

Mononuclear phagocytes are cells widely distributed in the body; they originate and mature in the bone marrow, then enter the circulation and pass into the tissues. The descendants of the mononuclear phagocyte lineage in the bone marrow (predominantly precursors, promonocytes), blood (monocytes) and other tissues (macrophage, histiocytes, Kupffer cells, osteoclasts, microglia) thus represent different stages in a progressive differentiation process (39,40). Such a conception has been corroborated by the recent finding that various differentiation stages develop sequentially in cell cultures of bone marrow-derived proliferating precursor cells (41-44). Under physiological steady state conditions, the resident macrophage population in peripheral tissues, shows little mitotic activity and is replenished at a low rate from the bone marrow and/or by circulating monocytes (45,46). In keeping with such a conception is the recent finding that selective radiation damage to bone marrow by ^{89}Sr-treatment effectively abolishes spontaneous cytotoxicity expressed by mononuclear phagocytes from the peritoneum and the spleen (47).

In inflamed sites, monocytes emigrate through inter-endothelial gaps and develop into macrophages with enlarged cytoplasms and increased phagocytic activity. After an interval of up to 2 days, they initiate DNA synthesis and begin to divide. Thus, in inflammatory sites both recruitment of blood monocytes and local proliferation may contribute in sustaining the local macrophage population; these processes are likely to be under the control of humoral factors such as CSA (32,48). Another important feature of mononuclear phagocytes is that, even in neonates, they are already competent cells in terms of specific functions and activities (49,50).

Apart from their traditional role in host defense and tissue repair, mononuclear phagocytes have an astonishing array of other important capabilities. Together with the increasing number of functions ascribed to this unique cell type within the past decade, the thesis has been put forward that the diverse functions are likely to be mediated by different subpopulations. There is indeed varied evidence that macrophages are heterogenous with respect to morphologic, biochemical, metabolic, immunologic and functional attributes (51-59). It is not yet clear, but becomes more and more likely that this heterogeneity reflects the existence of clearly separable subpopulations. But it is not yet ruled out that the expression of these changes proceeds with maturation and/or activation. In that event, this could be attributable to the intrinsic reactivity of a pluripotent cell to its environment (cf. sect. II,C).

B. *Biochemistry, Metabolism*

Mononuclear phagocytes have inherent potential to synthesize an exceptionally large array of biologically active agents (60). These agents are not only relevant in processes such as phagocytosis, intracellular killing and digestion but may also be secreted and exert major extracellular functions (61). Whereas some secretory products, such as lysozyme, growth factors, and α_2-macroglobulin are released by nonstimulated macrophages, other agents such as acid hydrolases, neutral proteinases, interferon, prostaglandins, pyrogens, components of the complement system, platelet activating factor, require stimulation for their production and/or release (60,62). The mechanisms by which these biologically active macrophage products interfere with other cell types, are complex and in part opposite. Even under the greatly simplified *in vitro* conditions, we are presently unable to quantitatively follow in parallel synthesis and secretion of the numerous biologically active molecules and to relate them to distinctive cellular functions. Hence, we are still far from comprehending the biological significance of each of the relevant macrophage products, nor can they be properly integrated into the functioning of the immune system. This is of paramount importance in any consideration of the regulatory role of the mononuclear phagocyte.

C. *Macrophage Activation*

The term 'macrophage activation' was introduced by Mackaness (63) to describe morphological changes in mononuclear phagocytes obtained from animals immune to *Listeria monocytogenes*. These cells rapidly adhere to the substratum and show considerable ruffled membrane activity. The terms 'activation' and 'stimulation' have since come into extensive but rather casual use to describe diverse morphologic (spreading, adherence, membrane activity), biochemical (lysosomal hydrolases, neutral proteinases, interferon, prostaglandins, H_2O_2 production, chemotactic factors, colony stimulating factor, membrane 5'-nucleotidase, glucose utilization, glucosamine incorporation), and functional phenomena (pinocytosis, phagocytosis, intracellular killing, digestion, receptor binding capacities, cytostasis, cytotoxicity (64-67). It is important to remember, however, that mononuclear phagocytes produce a different set of responses to many of the numerous materials known to have stimulatory or activating capacity, such as bacteria or their products, immune complexes, products of activated lymphocytes, polyanions, interferon, complement components. As indicated earlier, there is evidence to suggest that mononuclear phagocytes may pass through a sequence of functional stages, representing either different stages of the macrophage differentiation or activation process (41,57,68,69). The possibility should thus be considered that the resting macrophage can be stimulated, eventually by passing through a series of sequential activation steps, to a highly activated cell, and that it subsequently returns to the resting state (19,70.71). The previously discussed concept that a defined kind and/or extent of macrophage activation may be associated with a distinct pattern of effector functions, i.e. that the mononuclear phagocyte represents a pluripotent cell capable of expressing, in a defined functional state, a selected set of associated inherent effector functions, is supported by various recent findings. In particular, the work of Stewart *et al.* (72) has shown that clones of mouse peritoneal exudate macrophages which had grown out *in vitro* from single cells in the presence of growth factor, all acquired cytocidal capacity when exposed to serum rich in MAF. The issue remains unresolved, however, whether CSA triggers *all* mononuclear phagocytes to enter proliferation and to form clones or whether a subpopulation with inherent cytolytic potential is particularly susceptible and thus selectively induced. According to Lohmann-Matthes *et al.* (44), growth factor-induced differentiation of bone marrow-derived stem cells is paralleled by the sequential appearance of cells (promonocytes ?) expressing first spontaneous short-term cytotoxicity against a narrow range of target cells ('natural killer' cell activity) or antibody-dependent, K cell-like killer capacity, and then either ADCC (73,74) or spontaneous long-term cytotoxicity against a wide array of tumor targets (macrophage-like natural cytotoxicity). Further work is required to establish whether these effectors are (1) indeed all descendants of the mononuclear phagocyte lineage, and (2) whether these differing effector potentials are associated with the progeny of one cell type which sequentially passes through various differentiation stages. As the principal requirements for the induction of differentiation and/or activation of mononuclear phagocytes under defined *in vitro* conditions are now available, it should be possible to resolve some of these issues in the near future. Other recent evidence indicates that activation is associated with induction of a special surface antigen (75,76) and with an increase in receptors for Fc, complement and growth factors (51,77,78). This can be taken to indicate that the macrophage activation process is associated with a modulation of its membrane structure and configuration.

D. *Macrophage Cell Lines*

As purification procedures yielding macrophages uncontaminated by other cell types are not available, identification of mononuclear phagocytes and analysis of their diverse roles in the development and manifestation of the various host defense mechanisms is rendered difficult even under greatly simplified *in vitro* conditions. Therefore, the accessibility of a steadily increasing number of well characterized and pure permanent murine and human multifunctional macrophage-like cell lines will facilitate the identification and characterization of the various macrophage-associated effector functions. Such macrophage cell lines mediate effector functions of macrophages such as antibody-dependent phagocytosis and ADCC (79-82).

III. REGULATORY FUNCTIONS OF MONONUCLEAR PHAGOCYTES

After it had been recognized that mononuclear phagocytes contributed to natural host resistance against tumors, interest focussed upon suppressor mechanisms of cell growth such as cytostasis and cytotoxicity. However, evidence is steadily accumulating that the regulatory role of macrophages is by no means restricted to these suppressive effector functions. It rather covers a more general control of differentiation, growth, and functional activity of various cell types and tissues. In particular, present knowledge suggests that under physiological, steady-state conditions, the varied capabilities of the macrophage that promote other cell types, are predominantly expressed. It now seems likely that mononuclear phagocytes affect a variety of cytological, biochemical and functional properties of other cells in multiple fashions utilizing cellular, endocrine, monokine, and humoral mechanisms (19-21,26,83-87). Probably, it is this remarkably diverse regulatory potential of macrophages which can also become operative against transformed cells and may thus result either in promotion or inhibition of tumor growth. In the regulation of the immune response, the operation of a close and multifacetted mutual relationship between mononuclear phagocytes and the lymphoid system is now firmly established (4,25,72,88-94). Whereas the macrophage effect is quite nonspecific in some instances, lymphocytes and macrophages have to share the I region of the H-2 gene complex for effective interaction in other experimental situations. Although the present work focusses on the significance of the macrophage effector functions for other cell types, it should be borne in mind that basic macrophage capabilities such as functional activity and proliferation in tissues remote from bone marrow depend on the microenvironment which is conditioned by other humoral and cellular elements, in particular by lymphocytes and/or their soluble products (87, 95-98). At present, their experimental manipulation is almost entirely empiric. It has to be recognized that the promotion of one particular parameter may well be associated with alterations either up or down in other parameters and functionally related capacities are not necessarily expressed in parallel. Hence, it is not always easy to clearly discriminate between cause and effect. This is best documented by recent evidence that the antiviral effect of interferon can be considerably amplified via its nonspecific macrophage-activating properties. Through this pathway, interferon may affect even the host's management of nonsusceptible viruses (99,100). Other macrophage products such as CSA and complement components, also capable of modulating macrophage functional activity, may also be involved in self-regulation (32,101,102).

In the subsequent sections of this communication, present knowledge on the control of cell differentiation and proliferation is briefly summarized. Spontaneous cytotoxicity mediated by macrophages may be particularly relevant for the maintenance of the integrity of the host and possibly contributes to tumor resistance. This attribute has aroused special interest and is discussed in a separate chapter (sect. IV). As already considered, various other regulatory capacities of mononuclear phagocytes may also be as important for the functioning of the mechanisms involved in natural antitumor resistance.

A. *Control of Lymphoid and Haemopoietic Cell Differentiation*

In vitro interaction between mononuclear phagocytes and other cells may result in enhancement or suppression of a variety of target cell functions, depending on the functional activity of the effectors, the actual ratio of effectors to targets, and as yet undefined characteristics of the target cell. The effector cell may affect differentiation, proliferation, viability, and/or functional ability of the target cell but often, the effects on these different parameters are not clearly separable. Thus, it is generally appreciated by cell biologists that viability of target cells in culture is often promoted by the presence of macrophages as a feeder (103,104).

CSA is a term used to denote any of a variety of materials that can induce the growth and differentiation of stem cells into macrophage and granulocyte colonies *in vitro* (24,32). Blood monocytes and tissue macrophages are potent producers of CSA (105,106). There is now evidence that macrophages are important not only in the regulation of the growth and differentiation of the myeloid cell lineage, but may have multiple influences on the differentiation and proliferation of erythroid cells and thus play a major role in the homoeostatic control of haemopoiesis (48,107,108).

Apart from CSA, the stimulatory and/or regulatory influence of macrophages on cell differentiation is presently best documented by their effects at various stages in the life of the lymphocyte (4,35,36,83,109). Among the few lymphoregulatory activities secreted by macrophages ('monokines') which have thus far been characterized to some extent, is the thymic differentiation factor. This factor induces the antigen-independent differentiation of immature thymocytes into T lymphocytes responsive in mixed leukocyte reaction, as well as the production of molecules which promote the differentiation of functional activity of B lymphocytes (83,85,110,111). Soluble macrophage-derived factors are also essential in T-helper cell induction, a major step in antibody formation (27). The important message from these still limited data is that the various cell promoting capacities of macrophages are mediated by a series of clearly separable effector mechanisms and/or molecules. Macrophage dependence for the differentiation of other cell types has up to now received relatively little attention.

B. *Control of Cell Proliferation*

In vitro interaction of a large array of proliferating cells with macrophages, which do not themselves replicate under conventional culture conditions, may result in enhancement or suppression of target cell proliferation (21,31). The conditions which determine whether proliferation is promoted or inhibited are still poorly defined (67). Variables such as the particular properties of the target cell type, its proliferation rate, the functional activity of macrophages, the ratio of effectors to targets, actual cell density, the source and quality of serum, and the availability of nutrients are all involved in the outcome of the interaction.

1. *Promotion*. Similarly to the differentiation and proliferation of precursors of the mononuclear phagocyte and neutrophil lineages in the bone marrow, the proliferation of macrophages in peripheral tissue is also under the control of growth factors (32,97). L cell-derived growth factor induces macrophages to multiply in culture; after its removal, macrophages enter a resting condition but again reenter the cell cycle when growth factor is provided (112).

It was established some time ago that macrophages are essential for, and markedly facilitate lymphocyte stimulation induced by antigens, allogeneic cells and mitogens (4,29,113). Lymphocyte proliferation was shown to be particularly enhanced when the macrophage:lymphocyte ratio was low (20). Other, still limited evidence indicates that macrophages and/or their products can likewise promote the proliferation of other cell types, such as fibroblasts (23,31,114-116), epidermal cells from normal skin (114), vascular endothelium (24), and tumor cells (23,114,117). Resting rather than activated macrophages, a low effector to target cell ratio and a target cell replicating at a low rate provide conditions favourable for the enhancement of target cell proliferation (23,114,115). Although it is established that some of these effects are mediated by soluble factors, the biochemical basis of the macrophage-mediated promotion of target cell replication and its possible relationship to enhanced target cell viability is only now receiving attention (83). For some of these functions, macrophages can be replaced by 2-mercaptoethanol (29).

2. *Inhibition*. When peritoneal macrophages obtained from rodents a few days after local inoculation of stimulants such as *C. parvum*, BCG or proteose peptone are interacted *in vitro* with rapidly replicating cells at an initial effector to target cell ratio of 5:1 or higher, target cell proliferation is consistently slowed down and usually comes to a complete standstill on prolongation of the culture period (21-23). This phenomenon has been monitored by morphologic, morphometric, impulse cytophotometric and cytofluorimetric means (115). Adherent, predominantly phagocytic mononuclear cells expressing spontaneous cytostasis against diverse target cells *in vitro* are present in the tissues and organs of different strains of rats and mice (114). Manifestations of natural macrophage-mediated cytostasis are fully reversible at least within the first 16-24 h. As the incorporation of both tritiated uridine and thymidine is distinctly reduced already within a few hours, such measurements represent an easy, reproducible way to assess this particular macrophage effector capacity (21,22).

When effector and target cells are seeded at low density and interaction is restricted to a period of 4-8 h before post-labeling, complications such as interference by the various nucleosides synthesized by macrophages with the assay (118, 119), are largely avoided.

Apart from the actual ratio of effectors to targets, the origin (120) and functional activity of effector cells, the extent to which cytostasis is expressed depends to a considerable extent on the type of target cell involved (22,23,117). The macrophage-mediated cytostatic effect is quite nonspecific since a wide array of rapidly replicating cells derived from diverse tissues of syngeneic, allogeneic or xenogeneic origin, and from normal or transformed tissues, are accessible. Nevertheless remarkable differences in target cell susceptibility are apparent. Susceptibility or resistance to cytostasis often remains constant over a period of years and thus appears to reflect a characteristic innate property of a particular target cell type, probably associated with its particular surface structures. It is thus not unexpected that virus infection rendered fibroblasts more prone to cytostasis (121).

Analysis by impulse cytophotometry and cytofluorimetry of the changes occurring in target cell DNA have shown that interaction with macrophages consistently led to a progressive decrease in the number of nuclei exhibiting high DNA content, i.e. most target cells were arrested in the G_1 phase of the cell cycle (115). The mechanism(s) underlying these changes remain unknown. It now seems likely, however, that the ways by which macrophages interfere with other cells and regulate their proliferation, are manifold. Some of the effects are dependent on the presence of live effector cells whereas others can be duplicated by cell-free macrophage culture fluids. In an antibody-dependent system, macrophages have been shown to generate cytostasis in murine lymphoma cells in two sequential processes, a contact-dependent and a contact-independent step (122). It is moreover, not entirely clear whether the cell-mediated capacities absolutely require close effector-to-target cell contact or rather depend on the continuing supply of active molecules released by macrophages. As pointed out earlier, in assessing the role of the diverse mechanisms involved in macrophage-mediated cytostasis, possible interference of a mechanism in question with the assay system has always to be considered. Macrophage products which could be involved in the regulation of proliferation of lymphocytes and other cell types, such as mitogenic protein, T cell activating factor, nucleosides, polyamine oxidase, interferon, prostaglandins, cyclic AMP and/or GMP, have recently been reviewed in some detail (28,30,83,117).

The *in vivo* relevance of macrophage-mediated cytostasis is not easily ascertained (123). It is conceivable, however, that such effects become operative in localized regions of chronic inflammation, such as granulomas, which are characterized by the presence of a high proportion of activated macrophages. The mechanism(s) by which macrophages suppress immune reactivity are not yet elucidated (124).

IV. NATURAL CYTOTOXICITY EXPRESSED BY MONONUCLEAR PHAGOCYTES *IN VITRO*

Under *in vitro* conditions, the presence of macrophages can either promote or impair the viability of target cells. The conditions which determine the outcome of the interaction are still poorly defined. Again, parameters such as the functional activity of the macrophage, the actual ratio of effectors to targets, and the susceptibility of the target cell seem to be important. The few consistent data which indicate that macrophages can be effective in enhancing target cell viability have already been discussed previously and need not to be taken up again.

It is now generally appreciated that macrophages manifest an impressive cytotoxic-cytolytic potential (4-6,125). Extracellular cytotoxicity is expressed either spontaneously, i.e. after infection or activation by lymphokines, interferon, LPS, or after arming with derivatives of the specific immune system such as antibody or products of sensitized T lymphocytes, e.g. specific macrophage arming factor (21,33,126-130). Spontaneous nonspecific cytotoxicity is effective against a wide range of target cells, whereas cytotoxicity mediated by components of the specific immune system, e.g. antibody fixed to the macrophage Fc receptor and exhibiting specificity towards a target cell surface antigen (ADCC), is directed only against that particular antigen (59,73,74,122,126,131-133). It is not yet clear whether the mode by which the macrophage expresses cytotoxicity under these varying conditions is in any way related. A major advantage of the immunospecific interaction between 'armed' macrophages and targets may be that it not only determines the direction but by providing close contact, could also markedly intensify the expression of the macrophage cytolytic potential. This communication focusses on spontaneous cytotoxicity by macrophages, and in particular on recent work performed in the author's laboratory; reference is also made to pertinent papers.

A. *Cytotoxicity Assays*

For the measurement of cytolytic capacities expressed by effector cells involved in cellular immunity, a variety of cytotoxicity assays have been developed (117,134-141). As macrophages are metabolically active cells manifesting spontaneous cytotoxicity after prolonged interaction with targets, securing of nutrient supply and the choice of the cytotoxicity test are of primary importance. The problems already inherent in short-term assays, in particular spontaneous release of label, increase considerably as the time for the interaction is prolonged (134-136,142). Nuclear prelabeling of targets with nucleosides, in particular uridine and thymidine, has the important advantage of being relatively stable (134,143). By the use of prelabeled targets, the possibility that nucleosides produced by macrophages might interfere with the assay (118, 119) are minimized. As alternatives, the ^{3}H-proline assay (134, 139) and the recently introduced ^{75}selenium release assay (144) may prove useful. To minimize artifacts and misinterpretations, the following guidelines are followed in the author's laboratory: (1) low initial cell density (up to 5×10^{6} cells per 35 mm dish; for higher cell densities 60 mm dishes); (2) abundant culture medium (2 ml/35 mm dish); and (3) basic experiments are performed utilizing in parallel both the ^{14}C-thymidine and the ^{3}H-proline release assay (134). The results obtained with these two cytotoxicity tests have thus far been in good agreement, indicating that the results with the thymidine release assay are not substantially affected by macrophage-derived nucleosides and/or their metabolites. When the critical requirements are adequately fulfilled, such cytotoxicity tests are appropriate for accurately reflecting the consequences of effector/target cell interaction manifested after 24-36 h, or even 48 h, as affirmed by parallel morphologic, cytophotometric and cytofluorimetric analysis (115). Postlabeling techniques are clearly more sensitive to possible secondary influences; accordingly it is judged inappropriate that they are utilized alone to monitor cell-mediated cytotoxicity.

Apart from isotope release assays, morphologic methods have been utilized to assess the cytolytic ability of AM *in vitro* (22,115,143,145-149). Among these, the test developed by Hibbs and his coworkers, in which effector and target cells were interacted for 60 h in microtiter plates, stained, and the results read either directly or from low-power photographs, seems particularly useful (69,145,150,151).

B. Effector Cells

As macrophages are extensively distributed in the body, they can be obtained from every tissue (152,153). However, as the proportion of mononuclear phagocytes may vary considerably from one tissue to another, most experimental work has utilized conveniently available peritoneal cells as a source of effectors. A simple way to enrich mononuclear phagocytes is to take advantage of their distinctive capacity to quickly and tightly adhere to glass or plastic substratum. After removal of the nonadherent cells, contamination with other cells can be further diminished by prolonged culturing. Other methods of separating macrophages, in particular on gradients, tend to provide variable and mostly unsatisfactory results. When peritoneal cells from normal or induced rodents are incubated for 1-2 h, and the nonadherent cells then removed by repeated rinsing, a variable but mostly high proportion of the cells remaining on the culture vessel are phagocytic, show the morphologic and biochemical features of mononuclear phagocytes, and generally fail to synthesize DNA or to divide. Among the biochemical markers utilized for the identification of mononuclear phagocytes, lysozyme has proved particularly useful, as it is constantly produced and released from macrophages quite independently of their functional activity (154). Provided the tissue culture medium is replaced at appropriate intervals, the cells will survive for weeks but their cytostatic and lytic effector capacities are gradually diminished. The macrophage nature of this effector cell population is further assured by the observation that their effector capacities are effectively abolished by a variety of anti-macrophage agents.

1. Acquirement of Cytocidal Capacity. As mentioned previously, evidence continues to accumulate indicating that the descendants of mononuclear phagocytes present in the bone marrow pass sequentially at least two major steps before they express spontaneous cytotoxicity. The first stage involves proliferation and differentiation of a precursor cell into monocytes and/or macrophages, and is under the control of glycoprotein growth hormones such as CSA (cf. sect. III,A; 19,26,32, 41,42,105). The second stage involves activation, i.e. appropriate augmentation of metabolic activities in circulating monocytes and resting macrophages, requisite for expression of inherent cytolytic capacities. There is varied evidence for macrophage activation being a highly complex process which may be brought about by a variety of agents and through diverse biochemical routes. It seems nevertheless likely that other cell types and/or their products, in particular mediators derived from T lymphocytes, have a key role in the regulation of such macrophage effector capacities. In some experimental systems, homology at the I region between macrophages and T cells as well as the presence of macrophages bearing Ia molecules was required for the generation of cytocidal macrophages (93). The recent demonstration that colonies of pure macrophages were able to manifest tumoricidal activity upon exposure to serum enriched with the lymphocyte mediator MAF are particularly instructive (72). These findings suggest that the acquisition of the cytocidal potential by the progeny of colony-forming macrophages present in the peritoneal cavity of mice is primarily determined by environmental factors and is not restricted by a genetically limited functional heterogeneity. Incubation *in vitro* of macrophages with MAF has moreover been shown to considerably compress the time period required for the manifestation of target cell killing. It seems likely therefore that the lag phase required under the artificial *in vitro* conditions can be markedly shorter in the *in vivo* environment. The consistent observations that macrophages taken from nude mice manifest higher spontaneous cytotoxic activity than those from their normal congeners are a hint that, apart from T cell-derived lymphokines, other agents may effectively trigger the activation process (152,155-159). Adherent peritoneal cells obtained from normal rats and mice (resting resident macrophages) manifest limited but detectable spontaneous cytotoxicity (114,125,143,152). Although resting macrophages are effectively prepared to express tumoricidal ability upon exposure to MAF (93,160), *in vitro* interaction with agents such as BCG or *C. parvum*, widely utilized as effective activators *in vivo* (161-163), is not consistently associated with activation, possibly because other cell types and/or their products are critical. Other agents, such as endotoxin and double stranded RNA have been shown to be potent *in vitro*-inducers of spontaneous macrophage cytotoxicity (34, 68,69,158,164).

Various evidence suggests that the development of macrophage tumoricidal capacity which follows infection with *Mycobacteria*, *Toxoplasma*, *Listeria*, or interaction with lymphokines, is profoundly influenced by genetic factors (165,166). Thus, C3H/HeJ mice have been shown to carry a co-dominant mutation at the Lps locus that confers unresponsiveness to LPS and its derivatives (167,168) and also may lack the functional membrane component of B cells necessary for LPS triggering (169). It is interesting that C3H/HeJ mice have a high incidence of early appearing methylcholanthrene-induced tumors and are low responders to the prophylactic and therapeutic effects of BCG (170). However, under certain conditions, C3H/HeJ macrophages can be induced to pass the sequence of reactions necessary for the acquirement of tumoricidal capacity (70). Identification of nonresponder mouse strains (165) and analysis of the defects involved in intermediary reactions should provide useful information on the pathways of macrophage activation.

Local treatment with a variety of agents has been reported to increase the number and/or proportion of adherent effector cells and/or to promote their *in vitro* cytolytic potential (143,150,152,155,171-173). Among the stimulants utilized in our laboratory, proteose peptone induced an exudate consisting of at least 90% cells showing the characteristics of mononuclear phagocytes; however, these effectors expressed only intermediate cytolytic potential (21,50). In contrast, among the adherent cells harvested 5-10 days after intraperitoneal inoculation of heat-killed *C. parvum*, only approximately 70-75% were mononuclear phagocytes but these cells showed markedly increased capacity for cytotoxicity. These findings underline the crucial role of the agent used for macrophage stimulation and/or activation. The biochemical identity of the active principle in these products is gradually being clarified (174,175). Nevertheless, the biochemical processes involved in the acquirement of macrophage cytolytic capability still remain largely unknown.

In this context, the recent demonstration that peritoneal macrophages from 8 of 22 mouse strains failed to develop tumoricidal activity by 7 days after BCG infection, is of particular interest (165). Nonresponder mice could be divided into two broad categories: (1) mice of strains C3H/HeJ and C57B1/10ScCR with abnormal responsiveness to the lipid A region of LPS (157,167,168,176,177); (2) mice derived from the A strain with apparently normal lipid A responsiveness, exhibiting a profound defect in macrophage tumoricidal capacity to both *in vivo* and *in vitro* activation stimuli (71,178,179). These genetically determined defects in the tumoricidal capacity of macrophages could prove useful in analyzing the significance of this natural defense mechanism and of the effector mechanisms involved.

TABLE I. *Characteristics of Spontaneous Cell-Mediated Cytotoxicity Manifested by Rodent Macrophages*

Effector cell	Adherent, predominantly phagocytic, in culture stabile for 36-48 h.
Receptors	Fc, C3
Origin and distribution of effector cells	Bone marrow and limited local proliferation, monocyte-macrophage lineage; widely distributed in tissues, inducible by immunostimulants (BCG, **C. parvum**, etc.). Numerous in athymic mice.
Spontaneous cytotoxicity	**In vitro** expression after a lag phase of ~18 h. Effector:target cell ratio required for effective killing 5:1 to 10:1; enhanced by intercurrent infections; high in athymic mice.
Specificity	Affects a wide range of syngeneic, allogeneic and xenogeneic target cells from diverse tissues, with some selectivity for transformed cells; absence of immunologic memory.
Genetic differences between animal strains	None; defective in various mouse strains (cf. sect. IV,B,1).
Age dependence	In rats is fully developed a few days after birth, high in young animals, decreases progressively with increasing age.
Expression of cytotoxicity not affected by	X-irradiation, anti-Ig(anti-Fab), immune complexes, anti-Thy 1, anti-interferon, serum concentration, zymosan, trypsin, cytochalasin B.
Expression of cytotoxicity suppressed by	Lack of Ca^{++}, cycloheximide pretreatment, anti-macrophage sera, anti-macrophage agents, fetal liver cells, ^{89}Sr.

C. Characteristics of Natural Cytotoxicity

Expression of spontaneous cytotoxicity by macrophages is clearly dependent on the level of macrophage functional activity, the actual ratio of effectors to targets, and the inherent susceptibility of the target cell. Other variables, such as cell adhesion, spreading, and shape (180), the actual serum concentration (181) and, within a limited range, cell density (152), do not seem to play a critical role (cf. IV,C,3). The main features are summarized in Table I.

The difficulties in defining and reproducibly manipulating the functional activity of the mononuclear phagocyte has already been referred to. Whereas resident peritoneal macrophages from normal rodents manifest low spontaneous cytolytic activity, AM induced with microbial agents such as viable BCG or heat-killed *C. parvum* organisms, are effective in target cell killing. Under the artificial *in vitro* conditions, spontaneous cytotoxicity by AM requires 12-24 h interaction to be consistently detectable, and 24-36 h for its maximum expression (33). There is evidence, however, that under *in vivo* conditions, where lymphokines and other agents which stimulate macrophages are readily available, this lag phase is considerably compressed (96). Various other, indirect evidence suggests that close contact between effector and target cells is either required or at least greatly promotes the cytolytic potential (141,147,151,182-185).

A further characteristic of spontaneous macrophage-mediated cytotoxicity is its high lytic potential as manifested by the capacity to express cytolysis even at low effector to target cell ratios (10:1, 5:1 or even 1:1). The effector to target cell ratio which is effective in expressing cytotoxicity depends on the actual functional activity of effectors as well as on the type and susceptibility of the target cell.

1. Target Cell Susceptibility. The spectrum of target cells which are susceptible to macrophage killing is astonishingly extensive and clearly transgresses the narrow limits characteristic of immunospecific reactions (21,117,152). Thus, targets of syngeneic, allogeneic or xenogeneic origin, derived from epithelial and lymphoid tissue, and growing in monolayer and in suspension culture, are comparably susceptible to natural cytotoxicity manifested by macrophages. There are, however, considerable differences in degree of susceptibility from one target cell type to another. Although the particular properties which determine whether a target cell is susceptible or resistant to lysis still remains pretty much an enigma, it is obvious that for most tumor cell lines, such properties remain constant over prolonged periods and are thus a notable characteristic of that type of target. On the other hand, fully resistant primary explants of rat and mouse fibroblasts become more and more susceptible with progressive *in vitro* passaging (50,114,115,181). In all likelyhood, quantitative and perhaps even qualitative changes in target cell surface structures take place spontaneously during prolonged *in vitro* culture, determining the increased susceptibility to the lytic macrophage ability. In this context, observations indicating that tumor cell populations are able to adapt to the host environment, and in particular to the immune reactivity, by phenotypic alterations, are noteworthy (186-190).

2. *Target Cell Structure*. In view of the consistent findings that target cells of syngeneic, allogeneic or xenogeneic origin, derived from varied tissues are attacked similarly, classical immunological barriers are obviously irrelevant for the expression of natural macrophage cytotoxicity; thus, classical antigens are not involved in the recognition process. As tumor cells are generally amenable whereas fibroblasts are resistant, it had been assumed that spontaneous cytotoxicity might show some selectivity for transformed cells (23,115.125, 143,150,183,184,191-195). Results of further work showing no evident correlation between susceptibility of transformed cells and their degree of malignancy militate against such a simplistic view (20,47,114,117,155,171,181,196,197). It is remarkable, however, that the large majority of tumor cells is susceptible to spontaneous cytotoxicity by macrophages and that these cells retain their susceptibility over prolonged periods; this indicates that the derivation of macrophage-resistant variants is rare. Cells derived from normal tissues are mostly resistant.

The acquirement of cytocidal capacity in the course of the macrophage activation process is associated with the expression of a new, distinctive macrophage surface antigen (75). A similar association between a macrophage surface structure and its functional activity has recently been demonstrated for the Fc receptors (51,77). Other work indicates that after arming with a heat-labile component found in fresh human plasma, human mononuclear cells acquire nonspecific cytotoxicity towards xenogeneic red blood cells (198,199).

All in all these findings are in keeping with the concept that for the effective manifestation of natural cytotoxicity by macrophages, distinctive surface structures on both the effector and the target cell are required. Mononuclear phagocytes are entirely capable of discriminating not only between foreign and self components but also between self and alterations to self, as in effete or damaged tissue components or aberrant self constituents, such as tumor cells. The recognition abilities that underline this discriminatory capacity must have evolved in simple form with the emergence of primitive species and has since undergone further specialization in phylogeny, involving in vertebrates cooperation between components of the immune system. As mononuclear phagocytes appear to be able to recognize, to bind and to ingest foreign particulate material without the use of the more recently evolved Fc and C receptors, the more primitive forms of recognition are likely to have been retained. Indeed, the ability of phagocytes to adhere to various surfaces and to particulates in the absence of antibody or complement is well documented (200). This ability is regarded as immunologically nonspecific but the use of the term 'receptor' for the molecules involved in this reaction would seem justified. It is remarkable, however, given all the efforts expended, that the mechanisms underlying these highly important recognition abilities of phagocytes are still so poorly understood.

It seems likely, however, that integral membrane glycoproteins are the structures involved (201,202). Of particular interest are findings which suggest a role for the carbohydrates constituents of the bacterial cell wall in binding to the macrophage plasma membrane (201). Such interactions could conceivably be associated with the control of cell proliferation, tissue regeneration and tumor cell growth.

Another indication as to the nature of the structures recognized as non-self by mononuclear phagocytes has come from studies on fetal tissues. There is increasing appreciation that the growth of malignant tumors in experimental animals and in man can be accompanied by the renewed formation and exposure of fetal structures (203,204). It is interesting, therefore that the marked spontaneous cytotoxicity consistently manifested by AM against various targets is blocked in a dose-dependent manner by irradiated, syngeneic or allogeneic fetal liver cells but not by liver cells from adult donors (193). After birth, the property of fetal liver cells to compete with tumor targets is progressively and rapidly lost. The significance of these findings is further substantiated by *in vivo* studies (193); sect. V,D). However, much further work is required to understand the biochemical basis of the macrophage/target cell interaction. The results of several attempts in this direction recently performed in the author's laboratory are briefly summarized in following sections.

3. *Independence of Substratum Adhesiveness.* Cellular adhesiveness is a fundamental cell surface property known to play an important role in a variety of developmental, homoeostatic and pathological processes (205). As activation of macrophages by various interventions is paralleled by their spreading and increased adhesiveness to the substratum, it seemed conceivable that macrophage adherence could be a requirement for the expression of spontaneous cytotoxicity. Such a concept was also supported by findings indicating that following the addition of resistant fibroblasts to adherent macrophages, the macrophages were displaced from the substratum by the spreading and proliferating fibroblasts (115). Various recently introduced techniques were utilized as a discriminating means of assessing the role of substratum adhesiveness (180). Our finding that expression of spontaneous macrophage cytotoxicity against tumor targets growing in adherent or in suspension culture was similar, irrespective of whether interaction took place on plastic, on Teflon, or on plastic coated with varying concentrations of the polymer, poly(HEMA), indicated that in this *in vitro* system, target cell killing is quite independent of cell adhesion and cell shape (180). This is in agreement with earlier findings which have shown that agents, such as cytochalasin B or nocodazole, which interfere with the cytoskeleton and thus with directed movement and endocytosis were without effect on the expression of spontaneous cytotoxicity (152).

4. *Independence of Serum Concentration.* In utilizing the same effector and target cells, similar arrangement and population density but varying the actual serum concentration in the range between 1% and 50% fetal calf serum, it was sought to assess whether cytolysis expressed by macrophages was in any way dependent on the actual serum concentration. These experiments have shown that the killer effect of already activated macrophages against a given target was quite independent of the actual serum concentration (181). It should be noted,

however, that these findings were restricted to activated macrophages. Indeed, other work has demonstrated that the tumoricidal capacity of macrophages can be modulated by components of normal serum. Then too, particularly effective stimulation is evoked by agents such as MAF, interferon, or bacterial endotoxin, altogether indicating that the killer potential is markedly dependent on the local environment (34, 68,69,72,95,96,206).

5. *Suppression by Radioactive Strontium.* Radioactive strontium is taken up selectively by bone after parenteral administration and then continuously irradiates the marrow micro-environment; the marrow-dependent cells are eliminated without affecting mature T and B lymphocyte functions. Following such ^{89}Sr-treatment of mice, the capacity of resident macrophages from peritoneum and spleen to express spontaneous cytotoxicity against a variety of syngeneic, allogeneic and xenogeneic targets is abolished (47). Apparently, the effector cells which express spontaneous cytotoxicity pass a substantial part of their life in the bone marrow. In contrast, the capacity to mobilize mononuclear phagocytes and to enhance cytotoxicity in response to an appropriate stimulus were not impaired in ^{89}Sr-treated mice.

D. *Mechanisms of Natural Cytotoxicity*

It is now firmly established that fully activated macrophages manifest a considerable potential for killing a wide range of target cells *in vitro*. It is moreover possible to considerably compress the lag phase required for manifestation of the cytolytic capacity (96); it remains unresolved, however, whether the mechanisms involved in long-term and short-term cytotoxicity are indeed the same. Thus far, only a few kinds of nontoxic intervention have been found to consistently prevent cytolysis, namely suppression of protein synthesis in effector cells (33,152) and depletion of Ca^{++} in the medium (152).

The mechanisms underlying spontaneous macrophage-mediated cytotoxicity are still largely unknown. Although there is evidence to suggest that intimate cell-to-cell contact may favour cytolysis (22,147,151,182), macrophages and macrophage cell lines are known to release, under *in vitro* conditions, soluble lytic activity (207,208). Among the other mechanisms currently under consideration are (1) cell fusion between cytotoxic macrophages and target cells (183); (2) aberrant target cell division (209); (3) formation of cytotoxic oxidants by macrophages (H_2O_2; O_2^-; 158,210-212); (4) production of target cell membrane lesions by macrophage-derived proteases (68,152); (5) consequences of release of arginase by macrophages (213, 214); (6) synthesis and secretion of the third component of complement by macrophages, extracellular cleavage of C3 and generation of C3a which displays cytolytic capacity (84,101). Further possibilities are represented by an array of agents normally produced and secreted by macrophages; among these are interferon (84,215,216), prostaglandins (84), nucleosides (118, 119), and lysozyme. All these products, either alone or in combination, could well interfere with cell proliferation and/ or viability. Other soluble factors such as tumor necrosis factor (217-219) and heat-labile cytolytic factor (207), can be released from macrophages, but only under certain, still insufficiently defined conditions.

To establish that cytotoxicity is mediated by a particular agent, the following conditions should ideally be fulfilled: (1) under the culture conditions, in which macrophages express cytotoxicity, the purified agent should be able to mediate cytotoxicity equally well; (2) effector cells should release the agent(s) under the same assay conditions; (3) the amount and time course of release of the agent by macrophages should suffice fully to account for cytotoxicity; and (4) cytotoxicity should be prevented by more than one inhibitor of the release or the action of the agent. These criteria have been satisfied for some of the afore mentioned agents, but not for others. It is not intended to discuss in this context the various mechanisms in detail but rather brief mention of some of our recent findings which may be relevant for assessing the significance of some of the cytotoxic mechanisms.

1. *Role of Hydrogen Peroxide and Effects of Phorbol Esters.* Myeloperoxidase, hydrogen peroxide and halide ions which form a potent system for the intracellular killing of microbial pathogens (220), may also participate in the extracellular killing of eukaryotic cells. Hydrogen peroxide released by PMN's during phagocytosis (221-224) is able, together with myeloperoxidase and halide ions, to kill mammalian cells (225, 226). Upon triggering *in vitro,* activated peritoneal macrophages release almost comparable amounts of both superoxide anion and hydrogen peroxide (212,227). Exposure to the tumor promoter, PMA, a soluble membrane-active agent, triggers both H_2O_2 release and short-term (4 h) extracellular cytotoxicity by activated macrophages and by neutrophils; both H_2O_2 release and the manifestation of cytotoxicity were inhibited by

reduction in the actual glucose concentration and by catalase or ferricytochrome C (210,211). These findings strongly suggest that in analogy to the mechanisms operative in intracellular killing of microorganisms, toxic oxidants such as H_2O_2 could be involved in extracellular killing by AM as well as neutrophilic granulocytes. There is also evidence that PMN's have the potential to affect both the growth and viability of eukaryotic cells (22,228).

Studies in the author's laboratory indicate, however, that the situation may even be more complex. First, there are large differences among target cells in their susceptibility to lysis by H_2O_2 as well as by activated, PMA-triggered macrophages (210,211, Keller, unpublished). Probably only a selected number of target cell types, in particular P-388 cells, are susceptible to the amount of H_2O_2 released by PMN's or AM under such conditions. Secondly, under defined *in vitro* conditions, PMA in short-term assays not only triggers the release of H_2O_2 and other functions (210,211), but also markedly suppresses the expression of spontaneous short-term NK and of long-term macrophage cytotoxicity (229). These findings thus suggest that AM have the potential to release toxic oxidants such as H_2O_2, but the concentrations achieved *in vitro* are too low for killing the majority of target cells. The thesis that H_2O_2 is not involved in long-term spontaneous lysis by AM is further supported by the finding that catalase was without effect on its expression (229). This is in line with observations which indicated that the ionophore A 23187 which induces H_2O_2 production in PMN's had no major effects on the expression of natural cytotoxicity by AM (31,230).

2. Role of Prostaglandins. Prostaglandins, compounds synthesized by cyclo-oxigenation of unsaturated fatty acids, in particular arachidonic acid, are produced in substantial amounts by macrophages; their formation is stimulated by antigen-antibody complexes, zymosan, concanavalin A (84,231,232). Upon stimulation, the release of prostaglandins from macrophages continues for at least 24 h. Among the numerous inhibitory effects ascribed to prostaglandins are the suppression of primary *in vitro* antibody responses, and the inhibition of cellular responses to antigen or mitogens and of DNA synthesis (233-236).

On the basis of these findings, it has been postulated that cytolysis and in particular cytostasis manifested by AM might be mediated by prostaglandins. In order to verify the validity of such a hypothesis, the effect of two potent inhibitors of prostaglandin synthetase on the expression of macrophage

TABLE II. Expression of Spontaneous Cytotoxicity by C. parvum-*Induced Peritoneal Cells Is Not Affected by Inhibitors of Prostaglandin Synthetase*

Concentration of inhibitor (μg/ml)	*Inhibitor*	
	Indomethacin	*Diclofenac sodium*
none	*51 (±8)*	
5	*46 (±7)*	*48 (±8)*
10	*42 (±9)*	*44 (±8)*
25	*36 (±7)*	*45 (±7)*
50	*35 (±6)*[a]	*46 (±8)*
100	*35 (±7)*[a]	*55 (±10)*

Approximately $2x10^6$ *adherent, predominantly phagocytic DA rat peritoneal cells obtained 7 d after* C. parvum *i.p. were interacted for 36 h with* $2x20^5$ *polyoma virus-induced DA rat tumor cells (Py-12) which had been prelabeled with* ^{14}C*-thymidine (134). The values represent percent net thymidine release and are means (± s.d.) of at least 7 determinations, each performed in triplicate.*

[a]*Statistical significance (Student's* t*-test):* $p < 0.001$.

proliferative and cytolytic capacities has been examined. Neither promotion nor inhibition of target cell proliferation was in any way affected by the presence of the prostaglandin synthetase inhibitors, indomethacin or diclofenac sodium (237, 238). Moreover, nontoxic concentrations of these compounds (up to 50 μg/ml) did not significantly diminish natural cytotoxicity manifested by macrophages (Table II). These and other recent findings (239) thus point to absence of significant involvement of prostaglandins in the macrophage effects both on cellular proliferation and/or viability.

3. Role of Arginase. Recent work has indicated that several *in vitro* manifestations of macrophages might be due to arginase activity secreted by these cells (84,214,240). In particular, Ham stated that numerous suppressors of cell growth *in vitro* have later been identified as arginase (240). More recently, Currie (213) reported that activation of macrophages by zymosan or LPS induces the production and release of arginase, and suggested that the cytolytic activity of macrophages and/or their culture supernatants on target cells might be a consequence of arginine deprivation. This conclusion was corroborated by the finding that tumor cell killing was effectively prevented by the addition of arginine. It whould be borne in mind, however, that measurements of arginase activity have been complicated by unacceptably high background values (84); moreover, fetal calf sera often contain large amounts of arginase (241).

In utilizing a more objective, highly sensitive radiometric arginase assay, we have recently reevaluated the role of arginase. This study showed that fetal calf sera exhibit variable arginase activity whereas macrophages and serum-free supernatants from macrophage cultures consistently manifested low arginase activity (Tschopp and Keller, unpublished). These and other findings (173) do not support the thesis that arginase derived from macrophages and/or arginine deprivation of the medium are significantly involved in the mediation of natural cytotoxicity by macrophages.

4. *Role of Interferon.* Interferon, originally characterized as an antiviral agent produced by cells in response to virus infection (242), is now known to affect a variety of cellular functions quite unrelated to virus replication, suggesting a more general biologic role for this agent. Among the effects now ascribed to interferon are suppression of the proliferative response of lymphocytes to mitogens and antigen (243), inhibition of antibody formation (244-246), promotion of generation of cytotoxic lymphocytes (247-249), enhancement of phagocytosis and other capacities of mononuclear phagocytes (99,250-252), of natural short-term cytotoxicity expressed by NK cells (99,253-258) and of the excitability of cultured neurones (259), induction of varied modifications of the cell surface both *in vitro* (260-262) and *in vivo* (263), and pronounced antitumor effects (253,264). Various earlier work, recently reviewed by Allison (84), had indicated that interferon could be another product of macrophages with inherent regulatory potential. More recent findings have shown that upon stimulation by T cell-derived lymphokines, macrophages produce immune (type II) interferon (265,266). The possibility has therefore to be taken into account that some of the regulatory effects ascribed to macrophages are actually mediated by interferon.

Utilizing sheep anti-mouse interferon, a gift from Dr. I. Gresser, we have recently examined the thesis that cytolysis and/or cytostasis manifested by macrophages might be interferon-mediated. Interaction of *C. parvum*-induced adherent

TABLE III. α-Interferon Is Without Effect on the Expression of Spontaneous Cytotoxicity by AM

Initial ratio of AM to targets	*AM + targets*		*α-interferon + AM + targets*	
	P-815	*YAC-1*	*P-815*	*YAC-1*
25 : 1	63 (±8)	51 (±6)	64 (±9)	53 (±7)
10 : 1	39 (±6)	39 (±6)	43 (±8)	39 (±6)
5 : 1	25 (±5)	20 (±4)	25 (±6)	20 (±5)

$2.5x10^6$, $5x10^5$ or $2.5x10^5$ C. parvum-*induced adherent peritoneal effector cells (AM) from C57/Bl6 mice were interacted for 36 h with $5x10^4$ prelabeled target cells on Costar plates. Effects on viability were expressed as net percentage of ^{14}C-thymidine released (134). Values are means (±s.d.) of 10 determinations, each performed in triplicate. α-interferon globulin (267), a gift from Dr. I. Gresser, was present at a final dilution of 1:100. Within each line, no statistical difference (Student's* t-*test) between controls and α-interferon containing wells was detected.*

peritoneal effector cells from C57/B16 (Table III) or C3H/J mice with murine targets such as DBA/2 mastocytoma P-815 of A mouse Moloney leukemia YAC-1 cells, resulted in a similar spontaneous cytotoxicity irrespective of whether anti-interferon was present. These findings strongly suggest that macrophage-derived interferon is not necessarily involved in the lytic process itself. During the preparation of this review, Tagliabue *et al.* (125) reached similar conclusions. In additional, albeit limited experiments, the possible involvement of interferon in macrophage-mediated cytostasis has also been examined. The results in Table IV show that, particularly at low effector to target cell ratios, the presence of anti-interferon diminished slightly the expression of cytostasis. The possibility has thus to be considered that interferon might be involved in cytostasis manifested by macrophages.

Considering the aforegoing findings that anti-interferon is without effect on the expression of cytotoxicity by macrophages, it is worth recalling the results of recent work showing that anti-interferon sera not only completely blocked boosting by interferon of NK and K cell activities but even decreased the cytotoxic capacity of these effector cells to below unboosted levels, thus indicating a role for interferon

TABLE IV. Effect of α-Interferon on Cytostasis Mediated by AM

Initial ratio of AM to targets	*AM + targets*		*α-interferon + AM + targets*	
	P-815	*YAC-1*	*P-815*	*YAC-1*
25 : 1	28 (±6)	25 (±5)	28 (±7)	35 (±6)[a]
10 : 1	31 (±7)	33 (±6)	38 (±6)[a]	42 (±6)[a]
5 : 1	57 (±8)	59 (±8)	84 (±19)[a]	78 (±9)[a]

$2.5x10^5$, $5x10^5$ or $2.5x10^5$ C. parvum*-induced adherent peritoneal effector cells (AM) taken from C57/Bl6 mice were interacted for 4 h with $5x10^4$ target cells. Residual target cell proliferation was then assessed by exposing the cells for 60 min to 1 µCi ^{3}H-thymidine per well (22). Values which represent percent thymidine incorporation (controls in the absence of macrophages = 100%) are means (± s.d.) of 5 determinations, each performed in triplicate.*

[a]*Difference between controls and α-interferon-containing wells highly significant ($p < 0.001$; Studen's* t*-test).*

in normally maintaining these NK and K cell functions (254). Whereas spontaneous cytotoxicity of human blood lymphocytes against human lymphoblastoid cells was enhanced by interferon (249), it did not promote ADCC mediated by lymphocytes (256).

In summary, these findings make it unlikely that the putative effector molecules arginase, hydrogen peroxide, prostaglandins, and interferon play any major role in the expression of natural cytotoxicity by macrophages against a spectrum of target cell types. They are thus in keeping with recent evidence that the suppressive effect of alveolar macrophages on the *in vitro* immune response of rabbit lymphocytes to red blood cells could not be attributed to prostaglandins, arginase or thymidine (268). However, the mechanisms involved could differ depending on the functional activity of the effector cells (i.e. *C. parvum*-induced macrophages vs macrophages activated by LPS or MAF) and whether the kind of interaction is immunologically specific or not. It is moreover possible that the killer mechanism may depend on certain target cell characteristics. Thus, certain cell types, such as P-388 cells, are highly susceptible to hydrogen peroxide, whereas most other target cell types examined are rather resistant to this agent; EL-4 cells, on the other hand, are particularly susceptible to thymidine (83). It is conceivable that the mechanism by which macrophages kill targets is determined by the type of interaction (spontaneous vs immunospecific), the kind and extent of macrophage activity and the target cell characteristics.

V. MONONUCLEAR PHAGOCYTES IN NATURAL TUMOR RESISTANCE *IN VIVO*

The concept of the primacy of immunospecific mechanisms of host defense against neoplasia, which has dominated cancer research for more than a decade, is now increasingly confronted with evidence for the operation of a natural host defense system against tumors (1,2,11). The nude athymic mouse model, for example, originally thought to fulfill many of the predictions of the immune surveillance theory, has turned out to represent a natural model for the study of thymus-independent, spontaneous antitumor mechanisms (8,15,156). The relevance of T cell-independent surveillance mechanisms is further supported by the demonstration that the capacity to reject tumors is developed equally well in normal and in immunodeficient or immunosuppressed animals (269-271). It now seems likely that, in some analogy to resistance against microbial pathogens, the host disposes of a variety of natural and acquired cellular and humoral mechanisms capable of coping with tumors. The pattern of the defense responses elicited against a given tumor is likely to be determined by variables such as the type and primary localization of the tumor and the actual state of reactivity of the host. The important role of the tumor itself in determining the spectrum of host defense elicited is underlined by the general experience that immunospecific surveillance-like mechanisms are readily demonstrable and may become operative in viral oncogenesis (e.g. polyoma and other DNA viruses). In defense against various other tumors, amongst them spontaneous and carcinogen-induced tumors, T cell dependent antitumor reactivity has at best only a modest role (117, 231,270,272,273). It is moreover increasingly appreciated that the host-tumor relationship is not only decisively determined by the extent to which target cell surface structures recognized as non-self by the host are expressed but also on other target cell properties capable of profoundly affecting - either positively or negatively - distinctive host effector capacities (cf. sect. VI). The proportion and pattern of host cells which have infiltrated the tumor mass, parameters which vary considerably from one tumor to another but remain fairly constant for a given tumor, reflect in part the complex interaction between the tumor and the host (4,5,6). Thus, regression and/or progression of tumor growth and metastatic spread have been related to characteristic changes in the pattern of infiltrating host cells (18,274-277).

It is now more widely appreciated that a variety of cellular (16,22,278-283) and humoral mechanisms (12-14,208,219,284-286) may be involved in T independent, natural antitumor surveillance. Among the cellular components, a few types of lymphoreticular cells, namely mononuclear phagocytes (4,5,6,57, 125,131,145,173,194,198,199,269,275,277,287-289) and NK and/or K cells (7,8,15-17,289-297) have been most extensively investigated. In view of the variables and multifactorial nature of the host-tumor relationship and in the pattern of host defense mechanisms elicited against one tumor or another, it is indeed more realistic to limit this exposition to a single rat tumor model system which has been studied in some detail by various workers.

A. An In Vivo *Model System*

After injecting inbred female DA rats with DMBA, several tumors were obtained which were maintained by syngeneic *in vivo* passage (22). The DMBA-12 fibrosarcoma tumor which has been utilized most extensively, acquired the capacity to grow in ascites form (152,272,298). Upon s.c. or i.p. injection, this tumor grows locally; metastasis is observed only exceptionally. Inoculation into DA rats of 10^3 DMBA-12 cells consistently results in progressive tumor growth and death of the animal. Inoculation of smaller amounts of tumor cells is not always lethal.

The ascites tumor model, in which 10^3 DMBA-12 cells were inoculated i.p. as a standard challenge and the survival time taken as a measure of tumor growth, has turned out to be particularly convenient because of its simplicity and remarkable reproducibility. For the normal, untreated DA rat, the survival period is between 14 and 30 days (272). As DMBA-12 fibrosarcoma cells could also be cultured *in vitro* (in RPMI-1640 medium supplemented with 10% fetal calf serum), it was possible to examine the efficacy of various kinds of intervention on the growth of this particular tumor in parallel in the *in vivo* and *in vitro* model systems.

B. Natural Defense Mechanisms

For the induction of tumor growth, the inoculation of a minimal threshold number of tumor cells is required; this number is rather constant for a given host-tumor combination but varies over a wide range from one tumor to another. It has been argued that the threshold level could reflect the host's resistance to the particular tumor. The *in vitro*-demonstration of the existence of natural humoral and cell-mediated immunity in rodent and human systems has greatly promoted the concept that natural immune reactivity could involve a host surveillance mechanism against tumors.

In the present fibrosarcoma model system, no evidence for a major involvement of T cell-dependent immunity has been obtained thus far. In particular, concomitant immunity is only rarely detectable (33), and the course of a primary tumor challenge was not affected by previous repeated immunization with irradiated tumor cells (193). Rats surviving a first challenge given 7 d after *C. parvum* were generally as susceptible as untreated controls when rechallenged 2-3 m later. The findings that the capacity of adherent, predominantly phagocytic mononuclear cells to express cytotoxicity against diverse targets *in vitro* is already fully manifest a few days after birth (50) and that tumor resistance *in vivo* is highest in the youngest age group examined (299), are rather convincing evidence against any involvement of immunospecific mechanisms.

Work with the DMBA-12 tumor has shown that host resistance can be easily manipulated - enhanced or suppressed - by a variety of interventions in a clearly predictable manner. The most impressive message which has evolved from these experiments is that effects of both enhancing and suppressive agents is markedly dependent on the timing of their administration in relation to the tumor challenge (272). The consistent findings outlined below that the diverse interventions which result in suppression of host resistance against the tumor are only operative when administered locally shortly before or at the time of tumor cell challenge, attest to the central role of the very early phase of tumor growth and to readily available natural mechanisms as the likely effectors.

TABLE V. Spontaneous Cytotoxicity Manifested by Adherent Peritoneal Cells from Controls and at Various Intervals After C. parvum

Origin of peritoneal effector cells, days after C. parvum *(3 mg i.p.; 298)*	*Target cell type*		
	DMBA-12	*Polyoma-12*	*P-815*
Control	24 (±15)	40 (±12)	31 (±14)
d -3	26 (±17)	46 (±14)	32 (±12)
d -7	41 (±20)[a]	56 (±17)[a]	53 (±13)[a]
d -14	38 (±21)[b]	52 (±12)[a]	49 (±13)[a]
d -22	32 (±15)[c]	51 (±12)[a]	39 (±11)
d -30	23 (±9)	38 (±11)	16 (±13)

Approximately $2x10^6$ adherent, predominantly phagocytic peritoneal cells were interacted for 36 h with $2x10^5$ target cells which had been prelabeled with ^{14}C-thymidine (134). The values represent percent net thymidine release and are means of at least 10 determinations, each performed in triplicate.

Statistical significance (Student's t-*test): $^a p < 0.001$, $^b p < 0.005$, $^c p < 0.025$.*

C. Enhancement of Tumor Resistance

Numerous infectious agents such as BCG (161,300,301), *Corynebacteria* (162), *Listeria* (302), protozoa (303), or nematode parasites (304) as well as their products and still other stimulants have been shown to induce considerable antitumor activity in a variety of tumor implant models and in man (305). In the present model, *C. parvum* and BCG have a consistently demonstrable antitumor effect on both the solid subcutaneous tumor and the ascites form (298). Particularly relevant are the findings that in older animals the spontaneous antitumor resistance that diminishes with age can be effectively enhanced by *C. parvum* and BCG; this attests to the underlying persistence of the mechanisms expressing such resistance (299). The antitumor effect of these stimulants is most pronounced when administered 6-10 d prior to tumor challenge. In keeping with the time course of *in vivo* enhancement of antitumor resistance, the increase in *in vitro* cytolytic activity manifested by macrophage-like effectors was highest on day 7 after

TABLE VI. NK Activity of Spleen *cells in Controls and at Various Intervals After i.p.* C. parvum

Pretreatment with C. parvum *i.p. on day*	*Effector : target cell ratio (YAC, Cr^{51}, 4.5 h)*			
	100:1	*50:1*	*25:1*	*10:1*
None (controls)	*36 (±10)*	*20 (±8)*	*13 (±6)*	*4 (±3)*
d -3	*39 (±12)*	*24 (±20)*	*24 (±8)*	*6 (±5)*
d -7	*44 (±11)*	*29 (±12)[a]*	*14 (±8)*	*7 (±7)*
d -14	*41 (±11)*	*28 (±11)[a]*	*17 (±8)*	*9 (±5)*
d -22	*42 (±24)*	*28 (±12)[a]*	*16 (±8)*	*6 (±5)*
d -30	*36 (±12)*	*23 (±9)*	*12 (±6)*	*6 (±4)*
d -40	*38 (±12)*	*27 (±7)*	*17 (±4)*	*9 (±4)*

DA rat spleen cells were interacted for 4.5 h at the ratio indicated with YAC myeloma cells which had been prelabeled with ^{51}Cr (134). The values represent percent net chromium release and are means (±s.d.) of at least 12 determinations, each performed in triplicate.

[a]Statistical significance (Student's t*-test):* $p < 0.005$.

C. parvum, then gradually decreased and was no longer detectable after 4 weeks (Table V). Contrariwise, the spontaneous NK activity manifested by peritoneal and spleen cells (Table VI) remained unaffected by *C. parvum* pretreatment. The findings thus militate against a role for NK cells in stimulant-induced enhancement of resistance.

Resistance to progressively growing DMBA-12 tumor cells could also be enhanced by adoptive transfer of *C. parvum*-induced peritoneal cells (152,306). Remarkably enough, tumor growth was even diminished when the stimulated cells had previously been irradiated (2000 r) or were inoculated at a site remote from the tumor implant (306). Further studies ascertained that the adoptively transferred cells accumulated around the tumor mass (307,308). As rather large amounts of donor cells were required, it can, however, not be excluded that a minor, contamining cell population is responsible for the increase in spontaneous and the restoration of age-diminished host resistance to the tumor (152,272,299,306). The occasional finding that, under still poorly defined conditions, macrophages and/or their culture supernatants enhance tumor growth (272,306), are indicative of a critical balance between tumor suppressing and promoting mechanisms.

D. Suppression of Tumor Resistance

Experiments with various tumor model systems have shown that spontaneous resistance to the tumor is markedly reduced following local inoculation of agents as diverse as silica particles (193,306), carrageenan (306,309), dextran sulphate (272), polyvinyl sulphate (272), PMA (229,272), gold salts (310), or fetal tissues (193). Observations that these agents were either toxic or interfered with the *in vitro* expression of cytotoxicity by macrophages originally led to some optimism that they might provide a powerful means for a transient depletion or a functional blocking of the mononuclear phagocyte system. It is noteworthy, however, that such agents are by no means selective for macrophages as they directly affect other cellular and humoral systems. Moreover, they also give rise to a cascade of secondary cellular and humoral events which at various levels could interfere with host resistance and tumor growth (306,311).

In view of the complexity of the situation *in vivo*, the apparent uniformity with which these diverse agents affect host resistance against the tumor is rather unexpected. First, spontaneous resistance of the normal rat is markedly reduced after local administration of silica particles, carrageenan, dextran sulphate, polyvinyl sulphate, PMA or embryonal cells. Then too, enhanced tumor resistance, as induced by *C. parvum* or BCG, is totally abrogated by local treatment with the same agents (272, 298); frequently, the survival time of these animals is shortened considerably even below control levels. It is noteworthy that each of the diverse suppressive agents examined thus far in this respect, i.e. silica particles, carrageenan, dextran sulphate, polyvinyl sulphate, PMA and fetal tissue, was capable of markedly diminishing both spontaneous and induced tumor resistance only when inoculated briefly before or on the day of tumor cell implantation (193,229,272,298); beyond these narrow limits, their tumor-promoting effect is rapidly lost.

The fact that a series of quite unrelated agents share not only the capacity of suppressing host tumor resistance but also are collectively operative only in a narrow time span briefly before tumor challenge strongly supports the concept that the period immediately after introduction of tumor cells, at least in the present experimental model, determines the outcome of the host-tumor encounter. These observations suggest a role for natural resistance rather than acquired, immunospecific mechanisms.

The target mechanism(s) hampered by intervention with these varied agents is not easily assessed as they have been shown to affect various effector systems. Thus, both PMA and fetal tissue suppress spontaneous cytotoxicity mediated by mononuclear phagocytes and by NK cells. Among the various indications suggesting that macrophages are the critical target is the finding that silica particles, known to consistently effectively abrogate host tumor resistance *in vivo*, readily nullify spontaneous *in vitro* cytotoxicity expressed by macrophages without affecting NK activity. However, as the mononuclear phagocyte and the NK system share several attributes, much further investigation will be required to reliably identify the host defense mechanism(s) so readily modulated by these agents.

VI. COMPROMISE OF NATURAL TUMOR RESISTANCE BY TUMORS

The concept that the morphology and physiology of other tissues, and particularly the development and functional activity of macrophages, can be modified by tumor cells, or their products, is by no means novel (5,6,312-314). Although the mechanisms whereby small numbers of tumor cells modify macrophage development and activity are only poorly understood, there is convincing evidence that such factors can on occasions adversely affect macrophage development, motility and effector capacities, and thus put the host at a disadvantage (315,316). Utilizing the present DMBA-induced DA rat fibrosarcoma tumor, in which the percentage of macrophages is fairly constant during progressive growth of the tumor (level from 4-10%), Normann and his coworkers have developed evidence that in the tumor-bearing animal, macrophage accumulation to local stimuli in the peritoneal and pleural cavity, in subcutaneous tissues and within the tumor itself is impaired although the level in circulating monocytes was frequently increased (317-319). As the anti-inflammatory effect directed against macrophages was promptly corrected by tumor excision but recurred with metastasis, it was concluded that these alterations in the reactivity of mononuclear phagocytes are acquired and related to cancer progression. These findings are in keeping with observations in other animal models and in cancer patients (320-324).

It seems noteworthy, however, that, at least in the DMBA-induced DA rat fibrosarcoma model, these defects in the reactivity of mononuclear phagocytes are encountered only when the initial tumor burden was high, i.e. 10^6 to $2x10^6$ tumor cells. In particular, diminution of chemotaxis was only detectable after a rather sizeable tumor population had been achieved (33, 319,325). As outlined earlier, the outcome of the host-tumor encounter in the ascites tumor model is largely determined on the day of tumor cell challenge (10^3 tumor cells only). In this model system, reduction in the *in vitro* and *in vivo* reactivity of the mononuclear phagocyte system was detectable only in the terminal phase of tumor growth (33). As the methods available to assess these diverse parameters are still far from satisfactory, it would be premature to make any judgement regarding these complex tumor-host interactions.

VII. CODA

The evidence presently available suggests that, quite apart from their important intracellular capacities, mononuclear phagocytes manifest an array of basic extracellular functions. Among these physiological regulatory functions are promotion and/or inhibition of differentiation, clonal expansion and viability of other cell types. It now seems likely that it is these capacities which enable macrophages to profoundly influence tumor growth in diverse and at times oposing ways. Despite this newer knowledge, we are still far from being able to manipulate these macrophage functions in a qualitatively and quantitatively directed manner. The present work has focussed on tumor suppressive capacities, but it should be noted that macrophages can also enhance tumor growth.

The consequences of the interaction between macrophages and target cells *in vitro* are manifold and depend on numerous variables, notably the functional activity of effectors, the actual ratio of effectors to targets and attributes peculiar to the target cell. Macrophage cytotoxicity can be mediated via cellular and humoral mechanisms. But it is only the highly activated macrophage which is capable of expressing spontaneous extracellular cell-mediated cytotoxicity against a wide range of targets of syngeneic, allogeneic and xenogeneic origin. It is likely that this is the mechanism involved in the effects ascribed to macrophages during the earliest phase of tumor growth. In the later phase, when immunospecific antitumor reactivity has developed, macrophages armed with immunospecific structures derived from the lymphoid system or activated by soluble products of stimulated lymphocytes (lymphokines) are able to actively interfere with tumor growth.

Under *in vivo* conditions it has proved rather difficult to differentiate clearly between these diverse ways of macrophage/ target cell interaction but as well as between mononuclear phagocytes and other effector cells disposing of spontaneous tumoricidal potential, in particular NK cells. Moreover, evidence is increasing that the role of the various effector systems contributing to spontaneous antitumor resistance varies depending on the type of tumor cells and possibly still other variables. Despite these reservations and limitations, the central role of the mononuclear phagocyte in natural host resistance against diverse tumors now seems firmly established.

ACKNOWLEGMENTS

I thank Drs. Maurice Landy, and R. Gmür for reading the manuscript, and Miss R. Keist, Miss M. Marazzi and Miss U. Vogler for technical assistance.

REFERENCES

1. Möller, G. (ed.), "Immunological Surveillance Against Neoplasia", *Transplantation Rev. 7* (1971).
2. Möller, G. (ed.), "Experiments and the Concept of Immunological Surveillance", *Transplantation Rev. 28* (1976).
3. Prehn, R.T. *J. Natl. Cancer Inst. 59* 1043 (1977).
4. Nelson, D.S. (ed.) "Immunobiology of The Macrophage", Academic Press, New York, (1976).
5. Fink, M.A. (ed.) "The Macrophage in Neoplasia", Academic Press, New York, (1976).
6. James, K., McBride, W.H., and Stuart, A. (eds.) "The Macrophage and Cancer", Dept. of Surgery, University of Edinburgh, (1977).
7. Möller, G. (ed.) "Natural Killer Cells", *Immunological Rev. 44* (1979).
8. Kiessling, R., and Haller, O. *in* "Contemporary Topics in Immunobiology" vol. 8, chapt. 6 (N.L. Warner, and M.D. Cooper, eds.), p. 171. Plenum Press, New York, (1978).
9. Prehn, R.T., *Adv. Cancer Res. 23*, 203 (1976).
10. Hewitt, H.B., Blake, E.R., and Walder, A.S., *Br. J. Cancer 33*, 241 (1976).
11. Stutman, O., *Adv. Cancer Res. 22*, 261 (1975).
12. Martin, S.E., and Martin, W.J., *Int. J. Cancer 15*, 658 (1975).

13. Pierotti, M.A., and Colnaghi, M.I., *J. Natl. Cancer Inst. 55,* 945 (1975).
14. Rosenberg, S.A., *J. Natl. Cancer Inst. 58,* 1233 (1977).
15. Herberman, R.B., and Holden, H.T., *Adv. Cancer Res. 27,* 305 (1978).
16. Herberman, R.B., Holden, H.T., West, W.H., Bonnard, G.D. *et al., in* "Tumor Associated Antigens and Their Specific Immune Response" (F. Spreafico, and R. Arnon, eds.), Academic Press, New York, (1979).
17. Welsh, R.M., *J. Immunol. 121,* 1631 (1978).
18. Levy, M.H., and Wheelock, E.F., *Adv. Cancer Res. 20,* 131 (1974).
19. Keller, R., Proc. of the Internat. Meeting on Inflammation, Verona, 1979, *Supplement to Agents and Actions* (in press).
20. Keller, R., *Cellul. Immunol. 17,* 542 (1975).
21. Keller, R., *in* "Immunobiology of the Macrophage" (D.S. Nelson, ed.), p. 487. Academic Press, New York, (1976).
22. Keller, R., *J. exp. Med. 138,* 625 (1973).
23. Keller, R., *Br. J. Cancer 30,* 401 (1974).
24. Polverini, P.J., Cotran, R.S., Gimbrone, M.A., and Unanue, E.R., *Nature (Lond.) 269,* 804 (1977).
25. Möller, G. (ed.) "Role of Macrophages in the Immune Response", *Immunol. Rev. 40* (1978).
26. Chervenik, P.A., and LoBuglio, A.F., *Science 178,* 164 (1972).
27. Erb, P., Vogt, P., Meier, B., and Feldmann, M., *J. Immunol. 119,* 206 (1977).
28. Nelson, D.S., *in* "Immunobiology of the Macrophage" (D.S. Nelson, ed.), p. 235. Academic Press, New York, (1976).
29. Opitz, H.G., Lemke, H., and Hewlett, G., *Immunol. Rev. 40,* 53 (1978).
30. Persson, U., Hammarström, L., Möller, E., Möller, G. *et al., Immunol. Rev. 40,* 78 (1978).
31. Leibovich, S.J., *Exp. Cell Res. 113,* 47 (1978).
32. Gospodarowicz, D., and Moran, J.S., *Ann. Rev. Biochem. 45,* 531 (1976).
33. Keller, R., *in* "The Macrophage and Cancer" (K. James, W.H. McBride, and A.Stuart, eds.), p. 31. Dept. of Surgery, University of Edinburgh, (1977).
34. Alexander, P., and Evans, R., *Nature New Biol. 232,* 76 (1971).
35. Niederhuber, J.E., Allen, P., and Mayo, L., *J. Immunol. 122,* 1342 (1979).
36. Woodward, J.G., Fernandez, P.A., and Daynes, R.A., *J. Immunol. 122,* 1196 (1979).

37. Igarashi, T., Rodrigues, D., and Ting, C.-C., *J. Immunol. 122,* 1519 (1979).
38. Treves, A.J., *Immunol. Rev. 40,* 205 (1978).
39. van Furth, R., Langevoort, H.L., and Schaberg, A., *in* "Mononuclear Phagocytes in Immunity, Infection and Pathology" (R. van Furth, ed.), p. 1. Blackwell, Oxford, (1975).
40. van Oud Alblas, A.B., and van Furth, R., *J. exp. Med. 149,* 1504 (1979).
41. van der Meer, J.W.M., Beelen, R.H.J., Fluitsma, D.M., and van Furth, R., *J. exp. Med. 149,* 17 (1979).
42. Bainton, D.F., and Golde, D.W., *J. Clin Invest. 61,* 1555 (1978).
43. Buhles, W.C., *J. Reticuloendoth. Soc. 25,* 363 (1979).
44. Lohmann-Matthes, M.-L., Domzig, W., and Roder, J., *J. Immunol. 123,* 1883 (1979).
45. Spector, W.G., *in* "The Macrophage and Cancer" (K. James, W.H. McBride, and A. Stuart, eds.), p. 15. Dept. of Surgery, University of Edinburgh, (1977).
46. van Furth, R., Thompson, J., and Gassmann, A.E., *in* "Non-Specific Factors Influencing Host Resistance. A Reexamination" (W. Braun, and J. Ungar, eds.), p. 79. S. Karger, Basel, (1973).
47. Keller, R., *Immunology 37,* 333 (1979).
48. Territo, M., and Cline, M.J., *in* "Immunobiology of the Macrophage" (D.S. Nelson, ed.), p. 593. Academic Press, New York, (1976).
49. Berman, J.D., and Johnson, W.D., *Infect. and Immunity 19,* 898 (1978).
50. Keller, R., *Br. J. Cancer 37,* 742 (1978).
51. Rhodes, J., *J. Immunol. 114,* 976 (1975).
52. Lee, K.-C., and Berry, D., *J. Immunol. 118,* 1530 (1977).
53. Wing, E.J., Gardner, I.D., Ryning, F.W., and Remington, J.S., *Nature (Lond.) 268,* 642 (1977).
54. Walker, W.S., *in* "Immunobiology of the Macrophage" (D.S. Nelson, ed.), p. 91. Academic Press, New York, (1976).
55. Cowing, C., Schwartz, B.D., and Dickler, H.B., *J. Immunol. 120,* 378 (1978).
56. Stuart, A.E., *in* "The Macrophage and Cancer" (K. James, W.H. McBride, and A. Stuart, eds.), p. 1. Dept. of Surgery, University of Edinburgh, (1977).
57. Hibbs, J.B., Chapman, H.A., and Weinberg, J.B., *J. Reticuloendoth. Soc. 24,* 549 (1978).
58. Bodel, P.T., Nichols, B.A., and Bainton, D.F., *Am. J. Path. 91,* 107 (1978).

59. Norris, D.A., Morris, R.M., Sanderson, R.J., and Kohler, P.F., *J. Immunol. 123,* 166 (1979).
60. Davies, P., Bonney, R.J., Humes, J.L., and Kuehl, F.A., *in* "The Macrophage and Cancer" (K. James, W.H. McBride, and A. Stuart, eds.), p. 19. Dept. of Surgery, University of Edinburgh, (1977).
61. Unanue, E.R., *Am. J. Path. 83,* 396 (1976).
62. Karnovsky, M.L., and Lazdins, J.K., *J. Immunol. 121,* 809 (1978).
63. Mackaness, G.B., *in* "Mononuclear Phagocytes" (R. van Furth, ed.), p. 461. Blackwell, Oxford, (1970).
64. Allison, A.C., and Davies, P., *in* "Mononuclear Phagocytes in Immunity, Infection and Pathology" (R. van Furth, ed.), p. 487. Blackwell, Oxford, (1975).
65. North, R.J., *J. Immunol. 121,* 806 (1978).
66. Cohn, Z.A., *J. Immunol. 121,* 813 (1978).
67. Keller, R., Keist, R., and Ivatt, R.J., *Int. J. Cancer 14,* 678 (1974).
68. Hibbs, J.B., Taintor, R.R., Chapman, H.A., and Weinberg, J.B., *Science 197,* 279 (1977).
69. Russell, S.W., Doe, W.F., and McIntosh, A.T., *J. exp. Med. 146,* 1511 (1977).
70. Ruco, L.P., and Meltzer, M.S., *J. Immunol. 121,* 2035 (1978).
71. Boraschi, D., and Meltzer, M.S., *J. Immunol. 122,* 1592 (1979).
72. Stewart, C.C., Adles, C., and Hibbs, J.B., *J. Reticuloendoth. Soc. 24,* 107 (1978).
73. Lohmann-Matthes, M.-L., Domzig, W., and Taskov, H., *Eur. J. Immunol. 9,* 261 (1979).
74. Domzig, W., and Lohmann-Matthes, M.-L., *Eur. J. Immunol. 9,* 267 (1979).
75. Kaplan, A.M., Bear, H.D., Kirk, L., Cummins, C. *et al., J. Immunol. 120,* 2080 (1978).
76. Pearlstein, E., Dienstman, S.R., and Defendi, V., *J. Cell Biol. 79,* 263 (1978).
77. Kerbel, R.S., *Nature (Lond.) 259,* 226 (1976).
78. Montarroso, A.M., and Myrvik, Q.N., *J. Reticuloendoth. Soc. 24,* 93 (1978).
79. Walker, W.S., and Demus, A., *J. Immunol. 114,* 765 (1975).
80. Koren, H.S., Handwerger, B.S., and Wunderlich, J.R., *J. Immunol. 114,* 894 (1975).
81. Ralph, P., Moore, M.A.S., and Nilsson, K., *J. exp. Med. 143,* 1528 (1976).
82. Koren, H.S., Anderson, S.J., and Larrick, J.W., *Nature (Lond.) 279,* 328 (1979).

83. Unanue, E.R., *Immunol. Rev. 40*, 227 (1978).
84. Allison, A.C., *Immunol. Rev. 40*, 3 (1978).
85. Beller, D.I., and Unanue, E.R., *J. Immunol. 118*, 1780 (1977).
86. Yung, Y.P., and Cudkowicz, G., *J. Immunol. 121*, 1990 (1978).
87. de Weck, A.L. (ed.) "Biochemical Characterization of Lymphokines", Proc. 2nd Internat. Lymphokine Workshop, held at Ermatingen, Switzerland, 1979. Academic Press, New York (in press).
88. Mosier, D.E., *Science 158*, 1573 (1967).
89. Bloom, B.R., and Bennett, B., *Semin. Hematol. 7*, 215 (1970).
90. Guerry, D., Dusak, B.A., Schreiber, A.D., and Cooper, R. A., *J. Immunol. 121*, 2446 (1978).
91. McDougal, J.S., Shen, F.W., and Elster, P., *J. Immunol. 122*, 437 (1979).
92. Farr, A.G., Kiely, J.-M., and Unanue, E.R., *J. Immunol. 122*, 2395 (1979).
93. Farr, A.G., Wechter, W.J., Kiely, J.-M., and Unanue, E.R., *J. Immunol. 122*, 2405 (1979).
94. Lee, S.-T., and Paraskevas, F., *Cellul. Immunol. 40*, 141 (1978).
95. David, J.R., and Remold, H.G., *in* "Immunobiology of the Macrophage" (D.S. Nelson, ed.), p. 401. Academic Press, New York, (1976).
96. Sharma, S.D., and Piessens, W.F., *Cellul. Immunol. 37*, 20 (1978).
97. Hadden, J.W., Sadlik, J.R., and Hadden, E.M., *J. Immunol. 121*, 231 (1978).
98. Musson, R.A., and Henson, P.M., *J. Immunol. 122*, 2026 (1979).
99. Schellekens, H., Weimar, W., Cantell, K., and Stitz, L., *Nature (Lond.) 278*, 742 (1979).
100. Stebbing, N., Dawson, K.M., and Lindley, I.J.D., *Infect. and Immunity 19*, 5 (1978).
101. Ferluga, J., Schorlemmer, H.U., Baptista, L.C., and Allison, A.C., *Clin. exp. Immunol. 31*, 512 (1978).
102. Cruchaud, A., Montandon, N., and Welscher, H.D., *in* "Biochemical Characterization of Lymphokines", Proc. 2nd Internat. Lymphokine Workshop, held at Ermatingen, Switzerland, 1979, (A.L. de Weck, ed.). Academic Press, New York, (in press).
103. Hengartner, H., Luzzati, A.L., and Schreier, M., *in* "Lymphocyte Hybridomas" (F. Melchers, M. Potter, and N.L. Warner, eds.), p. 92. Springer, Berlin, (1979).

104. Schreier, M.H., and Nordin, A.A., *in* "B and T Cells in Immune Recognition" (F. Loor, and G.E. Roelants, eds.), p. 127. J. Wiley and Sons, Chichester, (1977).
105. Johnson, G.R., and Burgess, A.W., *J. Cell Biol. 77*, 35 (1978).
106. Cline, M.J., Rothman, B., and Golde, D.W., *J. Cell. Physiol. 84*, 193 (1974).
107. Cline, M.J., and Golde, D.W., *Nature (Lond.) 277*, 177 (1979).
108. Rinehart, J.J., Zanjani, E.D., Nomdedeu, B., Gormus, B.J. *et al.*, *J. Clin. Invest. 62*, 979 (1978).
109. Knapp, W., and Baumgartner, G., *J. Immunol. 121*, 1177 (1978).
110. Wood, D.D., *in* "Regulatory Mechanisms in Lymphocyte Activation", Proc. of the 11th Leukocyte Culture Conference, p. 117. Academic Press, New York, (1977).
111. Hoffmann, M.K., Koenig, S., Mittler, R.S., Dettgen, H.F. *et al.*, *J. Immunol. 122*, 497 (1979).
112. van der Zeijst, B.A.M., Stewart, C.C., and Schlesinger, S., *J. exp. Med. 147*, 1253 (1978).
113. de Vries, J.E., Caviles, A.P., Bont, W.S., and Mendelsohn, J., *J. Immunol. 122*, 1099 (1979).
114. Keller, R., *Br. J. Cancer 37*, 732 (1978).
115. Keller, R., Bregnard, A., Gehring, W.J., and Schroeder, H.E., *Exp. Cell Biol. 44*, 108 (1976).
116. Wahl, S.M., Wahl, L.M., McCarthy, J.B., Chedid, L. *et al.*, *J. Immunol. 122*, 2226 (1979).
117. Keller, R., *J. Natl. Cancer Inst. 56*, 369 (1976).
118. Stadecker, M.J., Calderon, J., Karnovsky, M.L., and Unanue, E.R., *J. Immunol. 119*, 1738 (1977).
119. Chan, T.-S., *Proc. Natl. Acad. Sci. USA 76*, 925 (1979).
120. Ansfield, M.J., Kaltreider, H.B., Caldwell, J.L. and Herskowitz, F.N., *J. Immunol. 122*, 542 (1979).
121. Goldman, R., and Hogg, N., *J. Immunol. 121*, 1657 (1978).
122. Pasternack, G.R., Johnson, R.J., and Shin, H.S., *J. Immunol. 120*, 1560 (1978).
123. Rice, L., Laughter, A.H., and Twomey, J.J., *J. Immunol. 122*, 991 (1979).
124. Kirchner, H., *Europ. J. Cancer 14*, 453 (1978).
125. Tagliabue, A., Mantovani, A., Kilgallen, M., Herberman, R.B. *et al.*, *J. Immunol. 122*, 2363 (1979).
126. Evans, R., and Alexander, P., *in* "Immunobiology of the Macrophage" (D.S. Nelson, ed.), p. 535. Academic Press, New York, (1976).

127. Lohmann-Matthes, M.-L., *in* "Immunobiology of the Macrophage" (D.S. Nelson, ed.), p. 463. Academic Press, New York, (1976).
128. McIvor, K.L., Piper, C.E., and Bell, R.B., *in* "The Macrophage in Neoplasia" (M.A. Fink, ed.), p. 135. Academic Press, New York, (1976).
129. Lohmann-Matthes, M.-L., and Fischer, H., *in* "Mononuclear Phagocytes in Immunity, Infection, and Pathology" (R. van Furth, ed.), p. 845. Blackwell, Oxford, (1975).
130. Galili, U., Rosenthal, L., Galili, N., and Klein, E., *J. Immunol. 122*, 878 (1979).
131. Pasternack, G.R., Johnson, R.J., and Shin, H.S., *J. Immunol. 120*, 1567 (1978).
132. Johnson, R.J., Siliciano, R.F., and Shin, H.S. *J. Immunol. 122*, 379 (1979).
133. Shaw, G.M., Levy, P.C., and LoBuglio, A.F., *J. Clin. Invest. 62*, 1172 (1978).
134. Keller, R., and Keist, R., *Br. J. Cancer 37*, 1078 (1978).
135. Oldham, R.K., Ortaldo, J.R., Holden, H.T., and Herberman, R.B., *J. Natl. Cancer Inst. 58*, 1061 (1977).
136. Ting, C.C., Park, J.Y., Nunn, M.E., and Herberman, R.B., *J. Natl. Cancer Inst. 58*, 232 (1977).
137. Fossati, G., Holden, H.T., and Herberman, R.B., *Cancer Res. 35*, 2600 (1975).
138. Hellström, I., and Hellström, K.E., *in* "In Vitro Methods of Cell-Mediated Immunity" (B.R. Bloom, and P.R. Glade, eds.), p. 409. Academic Press, New York, (1971).
139. Bean, M.A., Pees, H., Rosen, G., and Oettgen, H.F., *Natl. Cancer Inst. Monogr. 37*, 41 (1973).
140. Cerottini, J.-C., Engers, H.D., MacDonald, H.R., and Brunner, K.T., *J. exp. Med. 140*, 703 (1974).
141. Takasugi, M., and Klein, E., *Transplantation 9*, 219 (1970).
142. Sanderson, C.J., and Taylor, G.A., *Cell Tissue Kinet. 8*, 23 (1975).
143. Meltzer, M.S., Stevenson, M.M., Tucker, R.W., and Leonard, E., *in* "The Macrophage in Neoplasia" (M.A. Fink, ed.), p. 211. Academic Press, New York, (1976).
144. Brooks, C.G., *J. Immunol. Meth. 22*, 23 (1978).
145. Remington, J.S., Krahenbuhl, J.L., and Hibbs, J.B., *in* "Mononuclear Phagocytes in Immunity, Infection and Pathology" (R. van Furth, ed.), p. 869. Blackwell, Oxford, (1975).
146. Evans, R., and Alexander, P., *Nature (Lond.) 228*, 620 (1970).

147. Hanna, M.G., Bucana, C., Hobbs, B., and Fidler, I.J., *in* "The Macrophage in Neoplasia" (M.A. Fink, ed.), p. 113. Academic Press, New York, (1976).
148. Keller, R., *in* "Mononuclear Phagocytes in Immunity, Infection, and Pathology" (R. van Furth, ed.), p. 857. Blackwell, Oxford, (1975).
149. Stewart, C.C., Adles, C., and Hibbs, J.B., *in* "The Reticuloendothelial System in Health and Disease: Immunologic and Pathologic Aspects" (H. Friedman, M.R. Escobar, and S.M. Reichard, eds.), p. 423. Plenum Publishing Corp., New York, (1976).
150. Hibbs, J.B., Lambert, L.H., and Remington, J.S., *Nature New Biol. 235,* 48 (1972).
151. Hibbs, J.B., *in* "The Macrophage in Neoplasia" (M.A. Fink, ed.), p. 83. Academic Press, New York, (1976).
152. Keller, R., *in* "Current Trends in Tumor Immunology" (S. Ferrone, S. Gorini, R.B. Herberman, and R.A. Reisfeld, eds.), p. 121. Garland STPM Press, New York, (1979).
153. Vernon-Roberts, B. (ed.) "The Macrophage". Cambridge University Press, (1972).
154. Gordon, S., *in* "Mononuclear Phagocytes in Immunity, Infection and Pathology" (R. van Furth, ed.), p. 463. Blackwell, Oxford, (1975).
155. Kaplan, A.M., Morahan, P.S., and Regelson, W., *J. Natl. Cancer Inst. 52,* 1919 (1974).
156. Keller, R., *Immunology 27,* 285 (1974).
157. Ruco, L.P., Meltzer, M.S., and Rosenstreich, D.L. *J. Immunol. 121,* 543 (1978).
158. Nathan, C.F., Nogueira, N., Juangbhanich, C., Ellis, J. *et al., J. exp. Med. 149,* 1056 (1979).
159. Toh, K., Sato, N., and Kikuchi, K., *J. Reticuloendoth. Soc. 25,* 17 (1979).
160. Fidler, I.J., *J. Natl. Cancer Inst. 55,* 1159 (1975).
161. Laucius, J.F., Bodurtha, A.J., Mastrangelo, M.J., and Creech, R.M., *J. Reticuloendoth. Soc. 16,* 347 (1974).
162. Scott, M.T., *Semin. Oncology 1,* 367 (1974).
163. Woodruff, M.F.A., and Boak, J.L., *Br. J. Cancer 20,* 245 (1966).
164. Weinberg, J.B., Chapman, H.A., and Hibbs, J.B., *J. Immunol. 121,* 72 (1978).
165. Boraschi, D., and Meltzer, M.S., *Cell. Immunol. 45,* 188 (1979).
166. Ruco, L.P., and Meltzer, M.S., *J. Immunol. 120,* 329 (1978).
167. Coutinho, A., Gronowicz, E., and Sultzer, B.M., *Scand. J. Immunol. 4,* 139 (1975).

168. Skidmore, B.J., Morrison, D.C., Chiller, J.M., and Weigle, W.O., *J. exp. Med. 142*, 1488 (1975).
169. Watson, J., and Riblet, R., *J. Immunol. 114*, 1462 (1975).
170. Tokunaga, T., Yamamoto, S., Nakamura, R.M., Kurosawa, A. *et al., Japanese J. Med. Sci. Biol. 31*, 143 (1977).
171. Cleveland, R.P., Meltzer, M.S., and Zbar, B., *J. Natl. Cancer Inst. 52*, 1887 (1974).
172. Basić, I., Milas, L., Grdina, D.J., and Withers, H.R., *J. Natl. Cancer Inst. 52*, 1839 (1974).
173. Hopper, K.E., Harrison, J., and Nelson, D.S., *J. Reticuloendoth. Soc. 26*, 259 (1979).
174. Damais, C., Bona, C., Chedid, L., Fleck, J. *et al., J. Immunol. 115*, 268 (1975).
175. Fevrier, M., Birrien, J.L., Leclerc, C., Chedid, L. *et al., Eur. J. Immunol. 8*, 558 (1978).
176. Sultzer, B.M., *Nature (Lond.) 219*, 1253 (1968).
177. Coutinho, A., Forni, L., Melchers, F., and Watanabe, T., *Eur. J. Immunol. 7*, 325 (1977).
178. Heppner, G., and Weiss, D.W., *J. Bacteriol. 90*, 696 (1965).
179. Boraschi, D., and Meltzer, M.S., *J. Immunol. 122*, 1587 (1979).
180. Keller, R., *Exp. Cell Res. 124*, 121 (1979).
181. Keller, R., *Exp. Cell Biol. 47*, 269 (1979).
182. Piessens, W.F., *J. Immunol. 119*, 167 (1977).
183. Hibbs, J.B., *Science 184*, 468 (1974).
184. Hibbs, J.B., *J. Natl. Cancer Inst. 53*, 1487 (1974).
185. Piessens, W.F., *Cellul. Immunol. 35*, 303 (1978).
186. Weinhold, K.J., Miller, D.A., and Wheelock, E.F., *J. exp. Med. 149*, 745 (1979).
187. Fenyö, E.M., Klein, E., Klein, G., and Swiech, K., *J. Natl. Cancer Inst. 40*, 69 (1968).
188. Fidler, I.J., Gersten, D.M., and Budmen, M.B., *Cancer Res. 36*, 3160 (1976).
189. Biddison, W.E., and Palmer, J.C., *Proc. Natl. Acad. Sci. USA 74*, 329 (1977).
190. Pimm, M.V., and Baldwin, R.W., *Int. J. Cancer 20*, 37 (1977).
191. Holterman, O.A., Klein, E., and Casale, G.P., *Cellul. Immunol. 9*, 339 (1973).
192. Meltzer, M.S., Tucker, R.W., and Breuer, A.C., *Cellul. Immunol. 17*, 30 (1975).
193. Keller, R., *Br. J. Cancer 40*, 417 (1979).
194. Cameron, D.J., and Churchill, W.H., *J. Clin. Invest 63*, 977 (1979).

195. Somers, S.D., and Zwilling, B.S., *J. Immunol. 121,* 2453 (1978).
196. Gallily, R., *Cellul. Immunol. 15,* 419 (1975).
197. Jones, J.T., McBride, W.H., and Weir, D.M., *Cellul. Immunol. 18,* 375 (1975).
198. Muchmore, A.V., Decker, J.M., and Blaese, R.M., *J. Immunol. 122,* 1146 (1979).
199. Muchmore, A.V., Decker, J.M., and Blaese, R.M., *J. Immunol. 122,* 1152 (1979).
200. Stössel, T.P., *Semin. Hematol. 12,* 83 (1975).
201. Weir, D.M., and Ogmundsdóttir, H.M., *Clin. exp. Immunol. 30,* 323 (1977).
202. Sharon, N., and Lis, H., *Science 177,* 949 (1972).
203. Coggin, J.H., and Anderson, N.G., *Adv. Cancer Res. 19,* 105 (1974).
204. Medawar, P.B., and Hunt, R., *Nature (Lond.) 271,* 164 (1978).
205. Grinnell, F., *in* "Membranes and Neoplasia: New Approaches and Strategies", Progr. Clin. Biol. Res. vol. 9 (V.T. Marchesi, ed.), p. 227. Alan R. Liss, Inc., New York, (1976).
206. Schultz, R.M., and Chirigos, M.A., *Cancer Res. 38,* 1003 (1978).
207. Currie, G.A., and Basham, C., *J. exp. Med. 142,* 1600 (1975).
208. Askamit, R.R., and Kim, K.J., *J. Immunol. 122,* 1785 (1979).
209. Kaplan, A.M., Brown, J., Collins, J.M., Morahan, P.S. *et al., J. Immunol. 121,* 1781 (1978).
210. Nathan, C.F., Brukner, L.H., Silverstein, S.C., and Cohn, Z.A., *J. exp. Med. 149,* 84 (1979).
211. Nathan, C.F., Silverstein, S.C., Brukner, L.H., and Cohn, Z.A., *J. exp. Med. 149,* 100 (1979).
212. Johnston, R.B., Godzik, C.A., and Cohn, Z.A., *J. exp. Med. 148,* 115 (1978).
213. Currie, G.A., *Nature (Lond.) 273,* 758 (1978).
214. Kung, J.T., Brooks, S.B., Jakway, J.P., Leonard, L.L. *et al., J. exp. Med. 146,* 665 (1977).
215. Gresser, I., *in* "Advances in Cancer Research" (G. Klein, and S. Weinhouse, eds.), p. 97. Academic Press, New York, (1972).
216. de Maeyer, E., Fauve, R.M., and de Maeyer -Guignard, J., *Ann. Inst. Pasteur 120,* 438 (1971).
217. Carswell, E.A., Old, L.J., Kassel, R.L., Green, S., *et al., Proc. Natl. Acad. Sci. USA 72,* 3666 (1975).

218. Green, S., Dobrjansky, A., Carswell, E.A., Kassel, R.L. *et al.*, *Proc. Natl. Acad. Sci. USA 73*, 381 (1976).
219. Hoffmann, M.K., Oettgen, H.F., Old, L.J., Mittler, R.S. *et al.*, *J. Reticuloendoth. Soc. 23*, 307 (1978).
220. Klebanoff, S.J., *J. exp. Med. 126*, 1063 (1967).
221. Iyer, G.Y.N., Islam, D.M.F., and Quastel, J.H., *Nature (Lond.) 192*, 535 (1961).
222. Root, R.K., Metcalf, J., Oshino, N., and Chance, B., *J. Clin. Invest. 55*, 945 (1975).
223. Homann-Müller, J.W.T., Weening, R.S., and Roos, D., *J. Lab. Clin. Med. 85*, 198 (1975).
224. Goldstein, I.M., Cerqueira, M., Lind, S., and Kaplan, H.B. *J. Clin. Invest. 59*, 249 (1977).
225. Edelson, P.J., and Cohn, Z.A., *J. exp. Med. 138*, 318 (1973).
226. Clark, R.A., and Klebanoff, S.J., *J. exp. Med. 141*, 1442 (1975).
227. Nathan, C.F., and Root, R.K., *J. exp. Med. 146*, 1648 (1977).
228. Clark, R.A., and Klebanoff, S.J., *J. Immunol. 122*, 2605 (1979).
229. Keller, R., *Nature (Lond.) 282*, 729 (1979).
230. Root, R.K., and Metcalf, J., *Clin Res. 24*, 318 (1976).
231. Myatt, L., Bray, M.A., Gordon, D., and Morley, J., *Nature (Lond.) 257*, 227 (1975).
232. Humes, J.L., Bonney, R.J., Pelus, L., Dahlgren, M.E. *et al.*, *Nature (Lond.) 269*, 149 (1977).
233. Plescia, O.J., Smith, A.H., and Grinwich, K., *Proc. Natl. Acad. Sci. USA 72*, 1848 (1975).
234. Webb, D.R., and Nowowiejski, I., *Cellul. Immunol. 33*, 1 (1977).
235. Franks, D.J., Macmanus, J.P., and Whitfield, J.F., *Biochem. Biophys. Res. Comm. 44*, 1177 (1971).
236. Novogrodsky, A., Rubin, A.L., and Stenzel, K.H., *J. Immunol. 122*, 1 (1979).
237. Ku, E.C., Wasvary, J.M., and Cash, W.D., *Biochem. Pharmacol. 24*, 641 (1975).
238. Vane, J.R., *in* "Prostaglandin Synthetase Inhibitors" (H.J. Robinson, and J.R. Vane, eds.), p. 155. Raven Press, New York, (1974).
239. Shaw, J.O., Russell, S.W., Printz, M.P., and Skidgel, R.A. *J. Immunol. 123*, 50 (1979).
240. Ham, R.G., *In Vitro 10*, 119 (1974).
241. Kihara, H., and De la Flor, S.D., *Proc. Soc. Exp. Biol. Med. 129*, 303 (1968).

242. Isaacs, A., and Lindenmann, J., *Proc. Roy. Soc., Ser. B 147,* 258 (1957).
243. Lindahl-Magnusson, P., Leary, P., and Gresser, I., *Nature New Biol. 237,* 120 (1972).
244. Gisler, R.H., Lindahl, P., and Gresser, I., *J. Immunol. 113,* 438 (1974).
245. Braun, W., and Levy, H.B., *Proc. Soc. Exp. Biol. Med. 141,* 769 (1972).
246. Johnson, H.M., and Baron, S., *Cellul. Immunol. 25,* 106 (1976).
247. Lindahl, P., Leary, P., and Gresser, I., *Proc. Natl. Acad. Sci. USA 69,* 721 (1972).
248. Heron, I., Berg, K., and Cantell, K., *J. Immunol. 117,* 1370 (1976).
249. Skurkovich, S.V., Skorikova, A.S., and Eremkina, E.I., *J. Immunol. 121,* 1173 (1978).
250. Rabinovitch, M., and Hamburg, S.I., *in* "Functional Aspects of Mononuclear Phagocytes" (R. van Furth, and Z.A. Cohn, eds.). Martinus Nijhoff Publishers BV, The Hague, (1979, in press).
251. Donahoe, R.M., and Huang, K.-Y., *Infect. and Immunity 13,* 1250 (1976).
252. Schultz, R.M., Papamatheakis, J.D., and Chirigos, M.A., *Science 197,* 674 (1977).
253. Gidlund, M., Orn, A., Wigzell, H., Senik, A. *et al., Nature (Lond.) 273,* 759 (1978).
254. Herberman, R.B., Ortaldo, J.R., and Bonnard, G.D. *Nature (Lond.) 277,* 221 (1979).
255. Trinchieri, G., and Santoli, D., *J. exp. Med. 147,* 1314 (1978).
256. Trinchieri, G., Santoli, D., and Koprowski, H., *J. Immunol. 120,* 1849 (1978).
257. Djeu, J.Y., Heinbaugh, J.A., Holden, H.T., and Herberman, R.B., *J. Immunol. 122,* 175 (1979).
258. Djeu, J.Y., Heinbaugh, J.A., Holden, H.T., and Herberman, R.B., *J. Immunol. 122,* 182 (1979).
259. Calvet, M.-C., and Gresser, I., *Nature (Lond.) 278,* 558 (1979).
260. Lindahl, P., Leary, P., and Gresser, I., *Proc. Natl. Acad. Sci. USA 70,* 2785 (1973).
261. Huet, C., Gresser, I., Bandu, M.T., and Lindahl, P., *Proc. Soc. Exp. Biol. Med. 147,* 52 (1974).
262. Chang, E.H., Jay, F.T., and Friedman, R.M., *Proc. Natl. Acad. Sci. USA 75,* 1859 (1978).
263. Lindahl, P., Gresser, I., Leary, P., and Tovey, M., *Proc. Natl. Acad. Sci. USA 73,* 1284 (1976).

264. Gresser, I., *Texas Rep. Biol. Med. 35,* 394 (1977).
265. Neumann, C., and Sorg, C., *Europ. J. Immunol. 7,* 719 (1977).
266. Neumann, C., and Sorg, C., *Europ. J. Immunol. 8,* 582 (1978).
267. Gresser, I., Tovey, M.G., Bandu, M.-T., Maury, C. *et al., J. exp. Med. 144,* 1305 (1976).
268. Pennline, K.J., Conrad, R.E., Gerber, H.R., and Herscowitz, H.B., *J. Reticuloendoth. Soc. 25,* 495 (1979).
269. Chow, D.A., Greene, M.I., and Greenberg, A.H., *Int. J. Cancer 23,* 788 (1979).
270. Greenberg, A.H., and Greene, M., *Nature (Lond.) 264,* 356 (1976).
271. Dawson, P.J., Fieldsteel, A.H., and McCusker, J., *Br. J. Cancer 38,* 476 (1978).
272. Keller, R., *in* "Functional Aspects of Mononuclear Phagocytes" (R. van Furth, and Z.A. Cohn, eds.). Martinus Nijhoff Publishers BV, The Hague, (1979, in press).
273. Stutman, O., *in* "Mechanisms of Tumor Immunity" (I. Green, S. Cohen, and R.T. McCluskey, eds.), p. 27. John Wiley, New York, (1977).
274. Russell, S.W., and Cochrane, C.G., *Int. J. Cancer 13,* 54 (1974).
275. Russell, S.W., Doe, W.F., and Cochrane, C.G., *J. Immunol. 116,* 164 (1976).
276. Levy, R.B., Pierre, R.L.St., and Waksal, S.D., *Adv. Exp. Med. Biol. 73B,* 415 (1976).
277. Eccles, S.A., and Alexander, P., *Nature (Lond.) 250,* 667 (1974).
278. Fisher, B., and Saffer, E.A., *J. Natl. Cancer Inst. 60,* 687 (1978).
279. Stutman, O., Paige, C.J., and Figarella, E.F., *J. Immunol. 121,* 1819 (1978).
280. Paige, C.J., Figarella, E.F., Cuttito, M.J., Cahan, A. *et al., J. Immunol. 121,* 1827 (1978).
281. Perlmann, P., Troye, M., Pape, G.R., Harfast, D. *et al., in* "Natural and Induced Cell-Mediated Cytotoxicity. Effector and Regulatory Mechanisms" (G. Riethmüller, P. Wernet, and G. Cudkowitz, eds.). Academic Press, New York, (1979).
282. Nathan, C.F., Hill, V.M., and Terry, W.D., *Nature (Lond.) 260,* 146 (1976).
283. Perlmann, P., Perlmann, H., and Wigzell, H., *Transplantat. Rev. 13,* 91 (1972).
284. Wolosin, L.B., and Greenberg, A.H., *Int. J. Cancer 23,* 519 (1979).

285. Herberman, R.B., and Aoki, T., *J. exp. Med. 136,* 94 (1972).
286. Ménard, S., Colnaghi, M.I., and Della Porta, G., *Int. J. Cancer 19,* 267 (1977).
287. Schultz, R.M., Papamatheakis, J.D., and Chirigos, M.A., *in* "Immune Modulation and Control of Neoplasia by Adjuvant Therapy" (M.A. Chirigos, ed.), p. 459. Raven Press, New York, (1978).
288. Stutman, O., *Adv. Exp. Med. Biol. 73B,* 371 (1976).
289. Roder, J.C., Lohmann-Matthes, M.-L., Domzig, W., Kiessling, R. *et al., Europ. J. Immunol. 9,* 283 (1979).
290. Minato, N., Bloom, B.R., Jones, C., Holland, J. *et al., J. exp. Med. 149,* 1117 (1979).
291. Kasai, M., Leclerc, J.C., McVay-Boudreau, L., Shen, F.W. *et al., J. exp. Med. 149,* 1260 (1979).
292. Greenberg, A.H., and Playfair, J.H.L., *Clin. exp. Immunol. 16,* 99 (1974).
293. Shellam, G.R., *Int. J. Cancer 19,* 225 (1977).
294. Pape, G.R., Troye, M., Axelson, B., and Perlmann, P. *J. Immunol. 122,* 2251 (1979).
295. Kall, M.A., and Koren, H.S., *Cellul. Immunol. 40,* 58 (1978).
296. De Landazuri, M.O., Silva, A., Alvarez, J., and Herberman, R.B., *J. Immunol. 123,* 252 (1979).
297. Lotzová, E., and McCredie, K.B., *Cancer Immunol. Immunother. 4,* 215 (1978).
298. Keller, R., *J. Natl. Cancer Inst. 59,* 1751 (1977).
299. Keller, R., *Br. J. Cancer 38,* 557 (1978).
300. Bast, R., Zbar, B., Borsos, T., and Rapp, H.J., *New Engl. J. Med. 290,* 1413 (1974).
301. Pimm, M.V., Cook, A.J., Hopper, D.G., Dickinson, A.M. *et al., Int. J. Cancer 22,* 426 (1978).
302. Bast, R.C., Zbar, B., Mackaness, G.B., and Rapp, H.J., *J. Natl. Cancer Inst. 54,* 749 (1975).
303. Hibbs, J.B., Lambert, L.H., and Remington, J.S., *J. Infect. Dis. 124,* 587 (1971).
304. Keller, R., Ogilvie, B.M., and Simpson, E., *Lancet I,* 678 (1971).
305. Mathé, G., *Recent Results Cancer Res. 55,* 1 (1976).
306. Keller, R., *J. Natl. Cancer Inst. 57,* 1355 (1976).
307. Den Otter, W., Dullens, H.F.J., van Loveren, H., and Pels, E., *in* "The Macrophage and Cancer" (K. James, W.H. McBride, and A. Stuart, eds.), p. 119. Dept. of Surgery, University of Edinburgh, (1977).
308. Keller, R., and Hess, M.W., *Br. J. exp. Path. 53,* 570 (1972).

309. Thomson, A.W., and Fowler, E.F., *Transplantation 24*, 397 (1977).
310. McBride, W.H., Tuach, S., and Marmion, B.P., *Br. J. Cancer 32*, 558 (1975).
311. Catalona, W.J., Ratliff, T.L., and McCool, R.E., *Cellul. Immunol. 40*, 1 (1978).
312. Wong, A., Mankovitz, R., and Kennedy, J.C., *Int. J. Cancer 13*, 530 (1974).
313. Dvorak, H.F., Orenstein, N.S., Carvalho, A.C., Churchill, W.H. *et al.*, *J. Immunol. 122*, 166 (1979).
314. Fauve, R.M., Hevin, B., Jacob, H., Gaillard, J.A. *et al.*, *Proc. Natl. Acad. Sci. USA 71*, 4052 (1974).
315. James, K., *in* "The Macrophage and Cancer" (K. James, W.H. McBride, and A. Stuart, eds.), p. 225. Dept. of Surgery, University of Edinburgh, (1977).
316. Green, I., Cohen, S., and McCluskey, R.T. (eds.), "Mechanisms of Tumor Immunity". John Wiley, New York, (1977).
317. Normann, S.J., and Cornelius, J., *Cancer Res. 38*, 3453 (1978).
318. Normann, S.J., and Sorkin, E., *J. Natl. Cancer Inst. 57*, 135 (1976).
319. Normann, S.J., Schardt, M., and Sorkin, E., *in* "The Macrophage and Cancer" (K. James, W.H. McBride, and A. Stuart, eds.), p. 247. Dept. of Surgery, University of Edinburgh, (1977).
320. Boetcher, D.A., and Leonard, E.J., *J. Natl. Cancer Inst. 52*, 1091 (1974).
321. Eccles, S.A., *in* "The Macrophage and Cancer" (K. James, W.H. McBride, and A. Stuart, eds.), p. 308. Dept. of Surgery, University of Edinburgh, (1977).
322. Snyderman, R., Meadows, L., Holder, W., and Wells, S. *J. Natl. Cancer Inst. 60*, 737 (1978).
323. Snyderman, R., Pike, M.C., Blaylock, B.L., and Weinstein, P., *J. Immunol. 116*, 585 (1976).
324. Mantovani, A., *Int. J. Cancer 22*, 741 (1978).
325. Normann, S.J., Schardt, M., and Sorkin, E., *Int. J. Cancer 23*, 110 (1979).

NATURAL CYTOTOXICITY ON TUMOR CELLS OF HUMAN MONOCYTES AND MACROPHAGES[1]

Alberto Mantovani
Giuseppe Peri
Nadia Polentarutti
Paola Allavena

Istituto di Ricerche Farmacologiche
Mario Negri, Milan, Italy

Claudio Bordignon

Istituto di Patologia Medica 5[a]
University of Milan, Milan, Italy

Cristiana Sessa
Costantino Mangioni

I[a] Clinica Ostetrica e Ginecologica
University of Milan, Milan, Italy

I. INTRODUCTION

Cells of the monocyte-macrophage lineage can kill neoplastic cells by non-phagocytic mechanisms (reviewed by Evans and Alexander, 1976; Hibbs, 1976; Keller, 1976a). Studies have mainly focused on the tumoricidal capacity of murine macrophages exposed in vitro or in vivo to chemical or biological stimuli, but recent data indicate that unstimulated

[1]*This work was supported by C.N.R. (No. 79.00643.96, No. 79.02417.65 and No. 78.02166.04), by the Rotolo Fund and by Grant IROI CA 26824 from National Cancer Institute.*

ISBN 0-12-341350-8

cells of the monocyte-macrophage lineage can express significant levels of cytotoxicity (Keller, 1978a, b; Mantovani et al., 1979a,b and c; Mantovani et al., 1980a; Tagliabue et al., 1979; Horwitz et al., 1979).

Mononuclear phagocytes could act as a primitive surveillance mechanism against neoplasia (Hibbs, 1976; Evans and Alexander, 1976; Keller, 1976a) and could play a role in the control of established tumors and metastasis (Birbeck and Carter, 1972; Eccles and Alexander, 1974; Evans, 1972; 1976; Mantovani, 1978;Pross and Kerbel, 1976; Russell and McIntosh, 1977; Wood and Gillespie, 1975; Zarling and Tevethia, 1973). However the immunobiology of human monocytes and macrophages in relation to human neoplasia has been the object of limited investigation. Here we will summarize results on the tumoricidal activity of human mononuclear phagocytes and we will discuss issues of current interest in our laboratory.

II. EXPERIMENTAL PROCEDURES

The procedures used to isolate human macrophages and to test their *in vitro* tumoricidal capacity have been previously described in detail (Mantovani et al., 1979a,c; Mantovani et al., 1980a) and are only briefly summarized here.

Monocytes and macrophages were isolated by adherence on microexudate-coated plastic and exposure for 5-10 min to 1mM ethylene diamine tetraacetic acid (Ackerman and Douglas, 1978; Mantovani et al., 1979a,c and 1980a; Mantovani, 1980). Mononuclear phagocytes were isolated from the peripheral blood of adult donors or from cord blood (Mantovani et al., 1979a,c and 1980a); from peritoneal washings of patients undergoing surgery for non-malignant non-infectious gynecological diseases (Mantovani et al., 1980a); from the ascitic fluid of patients with liver cirrhosis and non-neoplastic, non-infectious gynecological diseases (Mantovani et al., 1980a); from the cystic fluid of benign ovarian cysts (Mantovani et al., 1980a); from pooled early lactation milk samples (Taylor-Papadimitriou et al., 1977; Mantovani et al., 1980a); from the bronchial washing of patients undergoing diagnostic bronchoscopy (Cantrell et al., 1973); from the peripheral blood and ascitic tumors of patients with ovarian carcinomatous ascites (Mantovani et al., 1979b).

Cytolytic activity of mononuclear phagocytes was measured as [^{3}H methyl] thymidine release from prelabelled tumor target cells after 48 h of interaction with effector cells (Mantovani et al., 1979a,c). Cytostatic activity was measured after 48-72 h of culture using a dye uptake test (Martin et al.,

1978; Mantovani *et al*., 1980a). Unless otherwise specified, the SV 40-transformed mKSA TU 5 (TU5) kidney line (Kit *et al*., 1969) was used in these studies.

III. NATURAL CYTOTOXICITY OF MONONUCLEAR PHAGOCYTES

Tables 1 and 2 show that human mononuclear phagocytes obtained from various anatomical sites (peripheral blood monocytes and monocyte-derived macrophages, milk foam cells and peritoneal macrophages) have significant cytolytic and cytostatic activity *in vitro* against TU5 target cells, cytotoxicity levels varying widely among different donors. Results presented in tables 1 and 2 were obtained using mononuclear phagocytes separated by adherence on microexudate-coated plastic and EDTA, but monocytes isolated by adherence and scraping (Mantovani *et al*., 1979a) or by lidocaine (unpublished data) had similar natural cytotoxicity levels. Moreover, adherent cells, belonging to the monocyte-macrophage lineage according to avid uptake of neutral red, non-specific esterase staining, phagocytosis of latex particles and binding and phagocytosis of sensitized red cells, were isolated from the cystic fluids of 4 patients with benign ovarian cysts. These adherent cells preparations had spontaneous cytotoxicity in the same range as the above mentioned mononuclear phagocyte populations. From the cystic fluids of 3 additional subjects with benign ovarian cysts, no adherent cells were separated. Unlike other mononuclear phagocyte populations, human alveolar macrophages had little or no cytolytic activity against TU5 tumor cells (table 1), but they did inhibit growth of these tumor cells as assessed by daily checking the cultures under an inverted microscope and by a dye uptake test (table 2). In agreement with these observations, rodent monocytes and macrophages were recently found to have appreciable levels of tumoricidal activity *in vitro* (Keller, 1978a, b; Tagliabue *et al*., 1979). Moreover, a similar spontaneous inhibition of tumor cell proliferation or cytolysis has been observed by other investigators working with human peripheral blood monocytes (Rinehart *et al*., 1978; Horwitz *et al*., 1979; Holtermann *et al*., 1974; Cameron and Churchill, 1979). Results presented in tables 1 and 2 were obtained with attacker to target (A:T) ratios ranging from 5:1 to 40:1. At low A:T ratios (5:1) stimulation of the proliferative capacity of some target cells was occasionally observed. This "feeding" effect of mononuclear phagocytes was better detected when A:T ratios of less than 5:1 were used. As shown in the typical experiment shown in table 3, peripheral blood monocytes enhanced the

TABLE 1. Natural Cytolytic Activity on TU5 Tumor Cells of Human Mononuclear Phagocytes Obtained from Various Anatomical Sites

Effector Cells	*% Specific Lysis* [a]			
	5:1 [b]	*10:1*	*20:1*	*40:1*
Peripheral blood monocytes (n=59)	*10.0 (2-30)*	*12.5 (5-42)*	*18.9 (7-50)*	*30.8 (8-66)*
In vitro matured monocyte-derived macrophages (n=6)	*18.9 (15-24)*	*23.4 (18-29)*	*28.8 (18-45)*	*-* [c]
Early lactation milk macrophages (n=3) [d]	*22.2 (20-45)*	*24.5 (24-27)*	*34.0 (33-35)*	*38.3*
Peritoneal exudate macrophages (n=18)	*13.0 (4-44)*	*20.0 (8-55)*	*25.0 (12-62)*	*37.0 (16-64)*
Ascitic macrophages (n=2) [e]	*19.5 (15-24)*	*24.0 (23-25)*	*34.1*	*49.1*
Benign ovarian cyst macrophages (n=4)	*10.3 (8-22)*	*12.9 (10-45)*	*14.4 (12-48)*	*25.3 (16-28)*
Alveolar macrophages (n=13)	*0 (0-0)*	*0 (0-0)*	*0 (0-9)*	*0 (0-0)*

[a] *Median with range shown in parenthesis*

[b] *A:T ratio*

[c] *Not tested*

[d] *Each early lactation milk sample was a pool of 5-10 donors*

[e] *Non-neoplastic ascites from two patients with liver cirrhosis and benign gynecological diseases*

proliferative capacity of TU5 cells at A:T ratios $\leq$ 1:1, had little effect between 2:1 and 5:1, and profoundly suppressed target cell proliferation at higher ratios. A stimulatory effect of mononuclear phagocytes on tumor cell proliferation has previously been reported with peritoneal (Keller, 1973, 1976a,b; Krahenbul et al., 1976; Namba and Hanaoka, 1972; Nathan and Terry, 1975; Olivotto and Bomford, 1974. Hewlett et al., 1977) or tumor-associated macrophages (Mantovani, 1978; Mantovani et al., 1979a,b) and was most easily observed with target cells poorly adapted to growth in culture and/or at

TABLE 2. Natural Cytostatic Activity on TU5 Tumor Cells of Human Mononuclear Phagocytes Obtained from Various Anatomical Sites.

Effector cells	% Growth inhibition[a]			
	5:1[b]	10:1	20:1	40:1
Peripheral blood monocytes (n=8)	0 (0-25)	41 (12-54)	56 (35-78)	82 (68-87)
Peritoneal exudate macrophage (n=1)	23		77	83
Alveolar macrophages (n=7)	26	40	72 (48-92)	–[c]

[a]Median with range shown in parenthesis

[b]A:T ratio

[c]Not tested

TABLE 3. Effect of Human Monocytes on the Proliferative Capacity of TU5 Target Cells.

Effector: Target cell ratio	% Growth inhibition (±S.D.)
0.2:1	-15 ± 2[#a]
0.5:1	-35 ± 1[##]
1:1	-28 ± 2[##]
2:1	-2 ± 2
5:1	11 ± 2
10:1	59 ± 1[##]
20:1	88 ± 1[##]

[a]Minus sign indicates stimulation of tumor growth

[#]Significantly different from tumor cells alone, $p < 0.05$

[##]Significantly different from tumor cells alone, $p < 0.01$

low effector to target cell ratios. Since the macrophage infiltration of poorly immunogenic metastasizing tumors tends to be low (Eccles and Alexander, 1974; Evans, 1976), it is possible to speculate that in these established advanced neoplasms the stimulatory capacity of macrophages may have some in vivo significance.

Under appropriate culture conditions, monocytes undergo a series of maturative steps which have been extensively investigated both morphologically and biochemically (Sutton, 1967). Table 4 shows that monocytes maintained in vitro for less than 10 days have cytotoxicity levels similar to fresh monocytes. In contrast, mononuclear phagocyte cultures beyond day 10, consisting primarily of epithelioid and multinucleated cells (Sutton, 1967), had little spontaneous cytocidal capacity (table 4) and failed to respond to lymphokines (Mantovani et al., 1980b).

Experiments summarized in tables 1-4 were performed with TU5 tumor cells as targets. When a series of human and murine tumor cell lines were tested for their susceptibility to human monocyte cytotoxicity, different target cells showed widely differing levels of lysis in the presence of effector cells. It is of interest that K 562 cells, highly susceptible to human NK cells, were not lysed (table 5) by unstimulated human peripheral blood monocytes nor was their growth inhibited (Mantovani et al., 1979a and b). When two pairs of untransformed or SV 40-transformed, early passage, human fibroblasts were tested (2303 and SV 40-2303; 2931 and SV 40-2931, table 5) natural human monocyte-mediated cytotoxicity was preferentially expressed on transformed, as compared to untransformed cells, although sparing of the latter was not absolute (Mantovani et al., 1979c).

Natural macrophage cytotoxicity is reportedly age-dependent in rats (Keller, 1978b) and, in a series of experiments, we studied the cytotoxic capacity of peripheral blood monocytes isolated from donors of different age (table 6). Adherent

TABLE 4. Cytolytic Activity of in vitro Cultivated Mononuclear Phagocytes on TU5 Target Cells.

Mononuclear phagocytes[a] cultivated in vitro for	*% Specific lysis (±S.D.)*
-	15.0 (0.5)[‡]
7 days	18.9 (0.7)[‡]
10 "	22.4 (4.9)[‡]
14 "	8.6 (0.4)[‡]
20 "	2.0 (0.6)

[a]Peripheral blood monocytes obtained from donor BD were cultivated in Neuman Tytell serumless medium supplemented with 40% autologous serum. Cytolytic activity against TU5 target cells was evaluted in a 72 h test at an A:T ratio of 20:1.

‡ Significantly above spontaneous release, $p < 0.05$

TABLE 5. *Susceptibility of Tumor Cell Lines to Human Monocyte-Mediated Cytotoxicity.*

	Target cells	%Specific lysis[a]
Murine lines	TU5 (SV_{40}-transformed) (n=59)	22.2 (7-45)
	1023 (Sarcoma) (n=6)	7.3 (6-39)
	TLX9 (Lymphoma) (n=10)	0 (0-8)
	RBL5 (Lymphoma) (n=3)	0 (0-4)
Human lines	Gll (breast ca) (n=4)	19.0 (18-34)
	CaLu (Lung ca) (n=4)	7.1 (6-10)
	E (Ovarian ca) (n=4)	10.0 (8-12)
Early passage human fibroblasts	2303 (n=5)	0
	SV_{40}-2303 (n=5)	28.0 (18-32)
	2931 (n=4)	0
	SV_{40}-2931 (n=4)	22.0 (17-33)

[a]*Median with range shown in parenthesis. The A:T ratio was 20:1.*

cell preparations from cord blood or from the peripheral blood of elderly (50-75 years of age) donors had cytolytic activity levels similar to young adult volunteers.

Experiments discussed so far, were performed in medium containing fetal bovine serum, but similar data were obtained when monocytes were separated and tested in the presence of autologous or pooled human serum (Mantovani et al., 1979a and unpublished data).

TABLE 6. Age-Dependency of Human Monocyte-Mediated Cytotoxicity.

Adherent cells obtained from	*Age[a] (years)*	*% Specific lysis[b]*			
		5:1[c]	*10:1*	*20:1*	*40:1*
Cord blood	-	*10.4*	*11.8*	*22.9*	*33.0*
	(n=7)	*(1-21)*	*(6-28)*	*(6-38)*	*(13-47)*
Adult volunteers	*32*	*10.0*	*12.5*	*18.9*	*30.8*
	(20-50,n=59)	*(2-30)*	*(5-42)*	*(7-50)*	*(8-66)*
	59	*13.0*	*19.2*	*24.5*	*26.5*
	(50-75,n=10)	*(4-28)*	*(12-31)*	*(18-50)*	*(16-47)*

[a]Median with range and number of subjects shown in parenthesis

[b]Median with range shown in parenthesis

[c]A:T ratio

IV. NATURE OF EFFECTOR CELLS

Several lines of evidence suggest that effector cells involved in natural cytotoxicity of human adherent cell preparations are not contaminating non-adherent NK cells and that they belong to the monocyte-macrophage series.

1) After thorough depletion of monocytes, non-adherent peripheral blood mononuclear cells rich in NK activity (Herberman et al., 1979) had essentially no cytotoxic activity against TU5, a target cell extremely susceptible to the natural cytolytic capacity of adherent cell preparations (Mantovani et al.,1979a). Conversely, adherent cells had little cytolytic and cytostatic capacity on K 562 target cells, a specific target for NK activity (Mantovani et al., 1979a,b). This latter finding differs from data from Horwitz et al. (1979) who observed lysis of K 562 by peripheral blood adherent cells.

2) Silica particles markedly inhibited monocyte or macrophage-mediated cytotoxicity. Conversely treatment with a potent and specific anti-T cell serum and complement, which inhibited NK activity, did not affect monocyte tumoricidal activity (Mantovani et al., 1979a).

3) Upon in vitro culture in medium with human serum, NK activity is greatly diminished (Ortaldo et al., 1977). In

contrast, human monocytes maintained in vitro under similar experimental conditions have cytotoxicity levels similar to or higher than fresh adherent effector cells (table 4; Mantovani et al., 1980a and b).

4) The organ distribution of NK and macrophage-mediated cytotoxicity is quite different. Table 7 shows that human peritoneal non-adherent mononuclear cells have NK activity extremely low when compared to peripheral blood lymphoid cells. Conversely, peritoneal adherent macrophages had natural cytotoxicity against TU5 similar or higher than peripheral blood monocytes.

V. PATHWAYS OF ACTIVATION

Lymphokines have been shown to regulate a number of functions of cells of the monocyte-macrophage lineage (reviewed by David, 1975) and, in rodents, to activate their cytotoxic capacity against tumor cells (Piessens et al., 1975; Churchill et al., 1975; Fidler, 1975; Fidler et al., 1976; Christie and Bomford, 1975; Ruco and Meltzer, 1977). It was therefore of interest to evaluate whether products of stimulated human lymphocytes could regulate the tumoricidal potential of human monocytes and macrophages (Mantovani et al., 1980a and b; Jett et al., 1980). As illustrated by the

TABLE 7. NK Activity and Natural Macrophage Cytotoxicity at Different Anatomical Sites

Target cells[a]	Effector cells		% Specific lysis
	Source	Adherence	
K 562	Peripheral Blood	Non-adherent	59
		Adherent	4
	Peritoneal Exudate	Non-adherent	6
		Adherent	4
TU5	Peripheral Blood	Non-adherent	6
		Adherent	35
	Peritoneal Exudate	Non-adherent	NT[b]
		Adherent	46

[a]Lysis was measured either as ^{5}Cr release (K 562) or as [^{3}H methyl] thymidine release (TU5) over 18 and 48 h of incubation, respectively. The A:T ratio was 20:1.

[b]Not tested

by the typical experiment presented in table 8, supernatants of lymphocyte cultures stimulated with mitogen (PHA, table 8) or specific antigen (PPD, Mantovani et al., 1980b) significantly increased the cytotoxic activity of human monocytes. Supernatants of stimulated lymphocytes contain Interferon (IF), an agent capable of increasing macrophage-mediated cytostasis in mice (Schultz et al., 1977). Moreover, as shown in table 9, IF can boost the tumoricidal activity of human peripheral blood monocytes and peritoneal macrophages (Mantovani et al., 1980a and b). In an effort to elucidate the possible role of IF, we took advantage of the biological properties of supernatants generated by coculture of human lymphocytes with Corynebacterium parvum (C.parvum) strain CN 6134 and CN 5888 (Sugiyama and Epstein, 1978; Epstein et al., 1979). C.parvum CN 6134 supernatants have relatively high concentrations of IF, whereas those elicited by strain CN 5888 contained little IF, but did inhibit the migration of human monocytes. Lymphokine supernatants elicited by both strains of anerobic coryneforms enhanced the tumoricidal activity of human monocytes, cytolysis levels being similar with the two stimuli. These observations strongly suggested

TABLE 8. Effect of Lymphokines on Monocyte-Mediated Cytotoxicity.

Supernatants from cultures with	A:T ratio	% Specific lysis (± S.D.)		
		1/3[c]	1/9	1/81
-	10:1	9.7(1.1)	10.9(2.1)	8.3(1.3)
PHA[a]	10:1	27.1(2.6)‡	20.1(0.7)‡	14.1(2.9)‡
-	20:1	13.2(0.8)	11.9(2.1)	10.3(0.1)
C.parvum CN 6134[b]	20:1	29.6(3.1)‡‡	21.8(3.0)‡‡	12.6(0.2)
C.parvum CN 5888	20:1	35.7(2.5)‡‡	24.4(0.8)‡‡	12.7(0.5)

[a]Lymphoid cells ($5x10^6$/ml) were cultured overnight with PHA (10 µg/ml) and washed thoroughly; supernatants were collected after further culture for 24 h.

[b]Supernatants of 6 days cultures with anaerobic coryneforms (140 µg/ml).

[c]Final dilution of the supernatants. Lymphokine supernatants, present throughout the cytolysis assay, did not affect the spontaneous release and proliferative capacity of TU5 tumor cells.

‡$p < 0.05$; ‡‡$p < 0.01$ versus control supernatants

TABLE 9. Effect of in vitro Preincubation with Interferon on Monocyte or Macrophage-Mediated Cytotoxicity

Effector cells[a]	*Interferon (units/ml)*			
	-	100	300	1000
Peritoneal macrophages	10.5(1.4)[b+]	12.6(0.8)[+]	16.3(0.6)[+≠]	27.4(2.1)[+≠]
Peripheral blood monocytes	8.2(0.9)[+]	7.8(1.8)[+]	15.9(1.2)[+≠]	28.6(1.9)[+≠]

[a]*Peripheral blood monocytes or peritoneal macrophages ($2x10^5$/well) were preincubated 20 h with Interferon (lot 45-10-9, HEM, Rockville, Md., USA) in 0.3 ml RPMI 1640 medium with 10% FBS. The wells were gently washed with 0.3 ml culture medium before adding 10^4 TU5 tumor cells.*

[b]*% specific lysis (± S.D.)*

[+]*Significantly above spontaneous release of tumor cells alone, $p < 0.05$*

[≠]*Significantly above specific lysis of effector cells alone, $p < 0.05$*

that lymphokines other than IF can play a role in the stimulation of the tumoricidal activity of human monocytes and macrophages. It was therefore proposed that activation of human monocyte-mediated cytotoxicity can involve at least two pathways, one involving IF and the other involving another still undefined lymphokine(s).

Further evidence for the existence of at least two pathway of stimulation of the tumoricidal activity of human mononuclear phagocytes came from studies on the responsiveness to lymphokines and IF of cells of the monocyte-macrophage series obtained from diverse anatomical sites. As shown in table 10, peripheral blood monocytes and peritoneal macrophages expressed enhanced cytotoxicity in the presence of IF or PHA-elicited lymphokine supernatants (Mantovani et al., 1980a and b; Jett et al., 1980). In contrast, alveolar macrophages did not have appreciable levels of natural cytotoxicity against TU5, nor did they show activation of cytotoxic activity in the presence of IF; however, in the presence of lymphokine supernatants, a significant though low stimulation of tumor cell cytolysis was observed. Moreover, enhanced citostasis was also observed Therefore, unlike peripheral blood monocytes and macrophages,

TABLE 10. *Effect of Interferon and Lymphokines on Alveolar Monophage Cytotoxicity.*

Effector cells	Stimulus	%specific lysis	%growth inhibition
Alveolar macrophages	-	0	70
	Interferon 1000 u/ml	4	68
	500 "	0	71
	250 "	0	75
	Lymphokine[a] 1/3	13[##]	95[##]
	1/6	3	73
	1/12	0	65
Blood monocytes	-	5	NT[b]
	Interferon 1000 u/ml	20[##]	NT
	Lymphokine 1/3	14[##]	NT

[a]Supernatant from PHA-stimulated lymphocites

[b]Not tested

[##]$p < 0.01$ compared to unstimulated effector cells

human alveolar macrophages do not show enhanced cytotoxicity when exposed to IF, but they do respond, weakly but significantly, to lymphokine supernatants. Thus data obtained with anaerobic coryneforms having different capacity to induce IF production, and with alveolar macrophages, showing defective natural cytotoxicity and defective responsiveness to IF, but capable of responding weakly to lymphokines, suggest the hypothesis that stimulation of human macrophage cytotoxicity by IF and by lymphokine supernatants involves two distinct biological pathways.

VI. TUMORICIDAL ACTIVITY OF MACROPHAGES FROM OVARIAN TUMORS

Ovarian carcinomas frequently spread in the peritoneal cavity and result in carcinomatous ascites. Human ascitic ovarian tumors are a source of relatively large amounts of tumor cells, tumor-associated macrophages and lymphocytes in suspension, and therefore we feel they provide unique opportunities to study the tumor-host relationship at an anatomical site directly involved by neoplasia. Macrophages can be isolated from ovarian carcinomatous ascites with relative ease by adherence in serum free medium (Mantovani et al., 1979b). More recently, we have been able to isolate highly purified, viable, lymphocytes and tumor cells by stepwise separation on discontinuous Ficoll-Hypaque gradients (Vose et al., 1977).

We previously observed that macrophages isolated from ascitic ovarian tumors can modulate tumor cell proliferative capacity in vitro, both stimulation and inhibition being detected depending on the A:T ratio, the incubation time and the target cell employed. Tumor-associated macrophages did not appear to express enhanced cytostasis when compared to normal peripheral blood monocytes (Mantovani et al., 1979b). Moreover macrophages isolated from carcinomatous ascites were capable of mediating antibody-dependent cytostasis on murine lymphoma cells (Mantovani et al., 1979b) as previously described for monocyte-derived macrophages (Mantovani et al., 1977). More recently, we studied the cytolytic activity against TU5 of tumor-associated macrophages and peripheral blood monocytes in patients with ascitic ovarian tumors (Mantovani et al., 1980c). As shown in Figure 1, tumor-associated

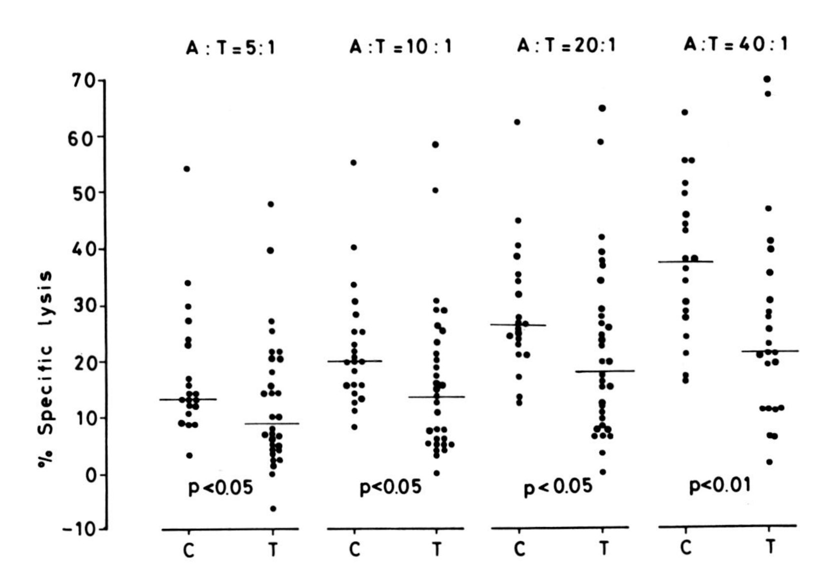

Fig. 1. Cytolytic activity on TU5 tumor cells of peritoneal macrophages from control subjects (C) undergoing surgery for non-malignant gynecological diseases and from ascitic ovarian tumors (T). Significance was assessed by Mann Whitney U test.

macrophages had significant cytolytic activity against TU5, cytotoxicity levels being significantly lower than control peritoneal macrophages from patients undergoing surgery for non-malignant non-infectious gynecological diseases (benign ovarian cysts, myomas, etc.). Similar results were obtained with peripheral blood monocytes (Mantovani et al., 1980c). Preliminary experiments indicate that tumor associated macrophages from ovarian cancer patients respond with increased tumoricidal capacity to in vitro exposure to IF or lymphokines and studies are in progress to compare their responsiveness to that of normal monocytes and macrophages.

TABLE 11. Effect of Chemotherapy on the Cytolytic Activity of Tumor-Associated Macrophages in Patients with Ascitic Ovarian Tumors.

Patient	Chemo-therapy cycles	Incubation time (h)	% specific lysis (± S.D.)		
			5:1[b]	10:1	20:1
B E	None	48	14.3(3.2)	18.6(3.6)	36.7(12.6)
		72	22.7(4.3)	23.1(1.6)	31.7(2.8)
	2 cycles	48	25.2(1.2)	34.2(2.1)	43.1(1.0)
		72	24.1(3.3)	36.3(2.9)	49.7(1.2)
C I	None	48	10.2(3.6)	10.8(3.1)	22.4(6.7)
	1 cycle	48	2.7(1.6)	9.5(3.7)	11.7(2.5)
D E	None	48	2.6(4.1)	3.8(3.7)	3.7(0.9)
		72	0.2(0.3)	4.6(8.9)	5.2(7.2)
	1 cycle	48	5.8(2.5)	0.6(3.8)	-2.7(2.2)
		72	7.8(4.5)	5.0(5.2)	4.6(1.4)
De V.	None	48	17.9(3.5)	25.0(2.7)	27.8(1.8)
	1 cycle	48	32.1(2.4)	36.2(10.6)	55.5(2.1)
T P	None	48	3.3(2.9)	3.2(0.8)	15.3(9.9)
		72	4.7(3.7)	4.4(1.5)	9.2(1.7)
	3 cycles	48	8.4(3.9)	6.5(1.5)	-[c]
		72	9.1(5.6)	15.7(2.9)	-

[a]*Ascitic fluid was obtained from ovarian cancer patients given chemotherapy cycles of Adriamycin (50 mg/m² i.v., day 1), cyclophosphamide (70 mg/m², orally, day 1-14) and cis Platinum (II)diamine dichloride (50 mg/m² i;v., day 1) or adriamycin, cylophosphamide and hexamethylmelamine (150 mg/m², orally, day 1-14).*
[b]*A:T ratio;* [c]*Not tested.*

In a limited number of untreated patients (5) the cytolytic activity of ascitic tumor-associated macrophages was tested both before and after the subjects were submitted to chemotherapy. No consistent inhibition of macrophage cytotoxicity was detected in this still limited series of experiments (table 11), whereas lymphoproliferative responses of peripheral blood lymphocytes to Phytohaemagglutinin and Pokweed mitogen were markedly suppressed in ovarian cancer patients given similar chemotherapeutic protocols (Mantovani et al., 1979d). A relative resistance of macrophage cytotoxicity to some chemotherapeutic agents, including Adriamycin and Cyclophosphamide used in these chemotherapy protocols (table 11), has previously been observed in mice (Mantovani, 1977 and unpublished data).

Different in vitro tumor cell lines differ significantly in their susceptibility to macrophage cytotoxicity (Mantovani et al., 1979a,b,c and Table 5). Thus, in an effort to elucidate further macrophage-tumor cell interactions in human ovarian carcinoma, the susceptibility of primary ovarian carcinoma cultures from 11 patients to macrophage cytotoxicity was investigated (Mantovani et al., 1980c).

TABLE 12. Susceptibility of Primary Ovarian Carcinoma Cultures to the Cytolytic Activity of Human Monocytes.

Primary culture	*Source*	*Histology*	*% Specific lysis (median)*[a]
AMA	*ascites*	*serous*	*22*
BE	*ascites*	*mucinous*	*12*
BM	*ascites*	*serous*	*8*
CI	*ascites*	*undifferentiated*	*0*
CP	*ascites*	*undifferentiated*	*0*
DeV	*ascites*	*serous*	*39*
FL	*solid*	*serous*	*0*
MA	*ascites*	*undifferentiated*	*-5*
MU	*ascites*	*serous*	*18*
	solid	*serous*	*13*
RI	*ascites*	*serous*	*6*
RS	*ascites*	*serous*	*13*

[a]*Median specific lysis with mononuclear phagocytes from 2-10 normal donors at an A:T ratio of 20:1.*

TABLE 13. *Susceptibility of Primary Ovarian Carcinoma Cultures to Human Mononuclear Phagocyte-Mediated Cytotoxicity*

Effector cells[a]		Target	% Specific lysis (± S.D.)			
Donor	Source		5:1	10:1	20:1	40:1
PG	Peripheral Blood	TU5	10.2(1.1)#	12.5(0.7)#	22.0(1.9)#	39.9(7.4)#
		BE[c]	0	11.0(0)#	11.8(1.4)#	23.8(2.3)#
LM	Tumor-associated macrophages	TU5	47.8(2.9)#	50.1(3.0)#	58.2(1.5)#	67.7(0)#
		FL[c]	–[f]	-6.5(2.0)[e]	-5.0(1.2)[e]	–
AMA	Tumor-associated macrophages	TU5	4.8(0.5)#	11.8(1.2)#	15.8(4.3)#	11.8(0.4)#
		AMA[c,d]	–	–	–	11.8(0)#
CI	Tumor-associated macrophages	TU5	10.2(3.6)#	10.8(2.1)#	22.4(6.7)#	22.3(5.2)#
		CI[c,d]	0	0	0	0
CP	Tumor-associated macrophages	TU5	6.2(0.5)#	7.1(2.9)#	14.6(1.4)#	20.4(1.1)#
		CP[c,d]	-6.7(9.5)[e]	-7.3(0.5)[e]	-4.3(1.4)[e]	0
		AMA[c]	–	25.3(3.3)#	26.9(8.6)#	–
DeV	Tumor-associated macrophages	TU5	17.9(3.5)#	20.5(2.7)#	27.8(2.8)#	46.7(7.0)#
		DeV[c,d]	18.3(9.5)#	33.4(2.1)#	29.7(2.2)#	16.8(9.6)#
		RI[c]	5.6(3.3)#	10.6(2.9)#	12.6(4.0)#	12.4(2.6)#

[a]Mononuclear phagocytes were obtained either from the peripheral blood of a normal adult healthy volunteer (PG) or from the ascitic tumors of ovarian carcinoma patients

[b]A:T ratio; [c]Primary ovarian carcinoma culture; [d]Autologous combination of ascitic tumor-associated macrophages and primary carcinoma culture; [e]Significantly below spontaneous release of tumor cells alone, $p < 0.05$; [f] Not tested

#Significantly above spontaneous release, $p < 0.05$

As shown in Table 12 where results with normal monocytes or macrophages at an A:T ratio of 20:1 are summarized, primary ovarian carcinoma cultures were heterogeneous in their susceptibility to the cytolytic activity of human mononuclear phagocytes. Ovarian cancer cells derived from 7 patients were consistently lysed by adherent effector cells whereas no consistent cytolytic effect was observed with the remaining 4 target cells (Tables 12 and 13). Similar results were obtained when tumor-associated macrophages were used as effectors (Table 13). In 4 experiments with the primary cultures AMA, CI, CP and DeV, lysis of tumor cells was tested using autologous tumor-associated macrophages. Autologous macrophages had no lytic activity or CI and CP target cells, but they did lyse susceptible heterologous tumor cells (TU5 and AMA). When ovarian tumor cells and macrophages from patient CP were tested, isotope release in the presence of autologous mononuclear phagocytes was significantly lower than baseline release of tumour cells alone. In contrast, macrophages isolated from the ascitic tumours of patients AMA and DeV had significant cytocidal activity against autologous neoplastic cells as shown fro instance by 33.4% specific lysis at an A:T ratio of 10:1 for DeV.

Cytotoxicity of mononuclear phagocytes against susceptible primary ovarian carcinoma cells was usually evident microscopically and, in a limited series of experiments (Table 14), the effect of mononuclear phagocytes on the proliferative activity of primary ovarian carcinoma cultures was quantitated spectrophotometrically (Martin et al., 1978. Mantovani et al., 1980a). Inhibition of tumour cell proliferative activity was detected with BE target cells, as expected on the basis of its significant susceptibility to lysis. In contrast, mononuclear phagocytes did not inhibit the proliferative capacity of CI and FL target cells, and in fact growth of these tumour cells was enhanced in the presence of effector cells.

TABLE 14. Effect of Mononuclear Phagocytes on the Proliferative Capacity of Primary Ovarian Carcinoma Cultures.

Ovarian target cells	*% Inhibition of tumor cell proliferation(±S.D.)*			
	5:1[a]	*10:1*	*20:1*	*40:1*
BE	*30 (2.2)*[‡]	*35 (11.8)*[‡]	*49 (9.8)*[‡]	*55 (8.8)*[‡]
Cl	*-6 (16)*[b]	*-6 (16)*	*-9 (21)*	*-19 (8.0)*[‡]
FL	*-*[c]	*-95 (8.4)*[‡]	*-54 (7.2)*[‡]	*-*

[a]*A:T ratio;* [b]*Minus sign indicates enhancement of tumor cell proliferative activity;* [c]*Not tested;* [‡]*$p < 0.05$*

VII. CONCLUSIONS AND SPECULATIONS

Human mononuclear phagocytes obtained from various anatomical sites (peripheral blood, peritoneal cavity, non-neoplastic ascites, benign ovarian cysts, and early lactation milk) have significant levels of spontaneous cytotoxicity against selected *in vitro* cell lines and primary ovarian carcinoma cultures. Moreover their cytocidal capacity can be enhanced by *in vitro* exposure to IF or lymphokines. In contrast, alveolar macrophages have no detectable spontaneous cytotoxic activity, no responsiveness to IF and weak, but significant, responsiveness to lymphokine supernatants. The heterogeneity of human mononuclear phagocyte populations in their tumoricidal capacity is hardly surprising. Alveolar macrophages differ from cells of the monocyte-macrophage series obtained from other anatomical sites in many respects, including metabolic characteristics, unresponsiveness to migration inhibition factor, effect of lymphocyte blastogenesis and prostaglandin (PG) production (Territo and Cline, 1976; Walker, 1976; Holt, 1979; Morley *et al*., 1979). The latter biological property, i.e. great capacity to produce PG compared to other mononuclear phagocytes (Morley *et al*., 1979), could play a role in the lack of enhanced cytotoxicity of these cells when exposed to IF, in as much as some PG of the E series have been reported to inhibit the stimulatory effect of IF on murine macrophage-mediated cytostasis (Schultz *et al*., 1978). Experiments to verify this possibility are in progress.

An alternative or complementary explanation for the defective tumoricidal capacity of alveolar macrophages stems from experiments with *in vitro* cultured monocytes. These cells undergo a series of maturative steps and, beyond day 10 in culture, lose their natural cytocidal capacity and their responsiveness to stimulation. It is therefore possible to speculate that, in the line of maturation of mononuclear phagocytes, macrophages removed by washing from lung alveoli, are beyond the stages which allow the expression of effective tumoricidal activity.

Exposure to chemical or biological stimuli can enhance the cytotoxic activity of rodent mononuclear phagocytes (Piessens *et al*., 1975; Fidler *et al*., 1976; Christie and Bomford, 1975; Ruco and Meltzer, 1977) and, similarly, IF or supernatants of antigen or mitogen-stimulated lymphocytes augment the tumoricidal capacity of human monocytes and macrophages. Supernatants of *C.parvum* CN 5888-stimulated lymphocytes have no detectable IF, but can effectively stimulate monocyte-mediated cytotoxicity. Conversely, human alveolar macrophages are totally unresponsive to IF, but show a weak, significant, stimulation of cytolysis and cytostasis in the presence of lymphokine supernatants. These two lines of evidence suggest that activation of the tumoricidal capacity of human mononuclear phagocytes can occur through two distinct pathways, one involving IF and the other lymphocyte products still not positively identified.

The *in vivo* relevance of human monocyte or macrophage-mediated cytotoxicity remains a matter of speculation. Cells of the monocyte-macrophage series are virtually ubiquitous in organs and tissues. Their natural tumoricidal capacity, preferentially expressed on transformed versus untrasformed target cells, could provide a mechanism of elimination of nascent tumor cells, not involving specific recognition by lymphocytes and subsequent activation of mononuclear phagocytes through specific release of mediators. Accordingly it is tempting to speculate that the protection against breast cancer conferred by early pregnancy may in part be related to an influex in the lactating mammary gland of macrophages with appreciable levels of spontaneous cytotoxicity against tumor cells.

The mechanisms through which mononuclear phagocytes acquire appreciable levels of spontaneous tumoricidal activity are unknown. It can be speculated that *in vivo* exposure to minute amounts of lymphokines released as a consequence of continuous exposure to environmental agents could account for the appreciable levels of spontaneous baseline cytotoxicity of monocytes and macrophages.

In established human and rodent neoplasms, macrophages can constitute a major component of the lymphoreticular infiltrate (Evans, 1976; Gauci and Alexander, 1975; Carr, 1977; Wood and Gollahon, 1977; Mantovani *et al*., 1979b). Macrophages isolated from ascitic ovarian tumors can modulate the *in vitro* growth of tumor cells and express cytolytic activity, cytotoxicity levels being similar or lower than those of peritoneal macrophages from control subjects. In considering the possible *in vivo* role of tumor-associated macrophages in the control of advanced human neoplasia, the susceptibility of tumor cells to attack by mononuclear phagocytes has to be taken into account. In fact we have observed that primary ovarian carcinoma cultures are considerably heterogeneous in their susceptibility to macrophage cytotoxicity. It is therefore conceivable that, provided tumor cells are susceptible to attack by mononuclear phagocytes, macrophages may act as a mechanism of restraint of ovarian tumor growth at least at this anatomical site (peritoneal cavity) where macrophage concentration relative to tumor cells is relatively high (Mantovani *et al*., 1979b). Conversely, in the presence of resistant ovarian tumor cells, it is unlikely that infiltrating mononuclear phagocytes, with cytotoxic capacity similar or lower than control, have any inhibitory effect on tumor cell proliferation, and neoplastic growth may actually be stimulated as observed in vitro.

Intraperitoneal administration of C.parvum can reportedly cause regression of ascitic ovarian tumors (Webb et al., 1978) and we have recently obtained similar results in a series of 6 patients unresponsive to chemotherapeutic agents.

Studies are currently in progress to elucidate the cellular basis of regression in these patients, in the hope that a better understanding of the tumor-host relationship at an anatomical site directly involved by this neoplasm may provide a rational for therapeutic attempts currently designed on an essentially empirical basis.

REFERENCES

Ackerman, S.K., and Douglas, S.D.(1978). *J.Immunol.* 120, 1372.

Birbeck, M.S.C., and Carter, R.L. (1972). *Int.J.Cancer* 9, 249.

Cameron, D.J., and Churchill, W.H.(1979). *J.Clin. Invest.* 63, 977.

Cantrell, E.T., Warr, G.A., Busbee, D.L., and Martin, R.R. (1973). *J.Clin.Invest.* 52, 1881.

Carr, I. (1977). *in* "The Macrophage and Cancer" (K.James, B. McBride, and A.Stuart,eds.), p.364. University of Edinburgh, Edinburgh .

Christie, G.H., and Bomford, R. (1975). *Cellular Immunology* 17, 141

Churchill, W.H.Jr., Piessens, W.F., Sulis, C.A., and David, J.R. (1975).*J.Immunol.* 115, 781.

David, J.R. (1975). *Fed.Proc.* 34, 1730.

Eccles, S.A., and Alexander, P. (1974). *Nature (London)* 250, 667.

Epstein, L.B., Dean, J.H., Herberman, R.B., Oppenheim, J.J., Rocklin, R.E., and Sugiyama, M. (1979). *in* "Proceedings of the 2nd.International Lymphokine Workshop", Abstract No. 64.

Evans, R. (1972). *Transplantation* 14, 468.

Evans, R. (1976). *in* "The Macrophage in Neoplasia" (M.A.Fink, ed.),p.27. Academic Press, New York.

Evans, R., and Alexander, P. (1976). *in*"Immunobiology of the Macrophage" (D.S.Nelson, ed.), p.535. Academic Press, New York.

Fidler, I.J. (1975). *J.Natl. Cancer Inst.* 55, 1159.

Fidler, I.J., Darnell, J.H., and Budmen, M.B. (1976). *Cancer Res.* 36, 3608.

Gauci, C.L., and Alexander, P. (1975). *Cancer Letters* 1, 29.

Herberman, R.B., Djeu, J.Y., Kay, H.D., Ortaldo, J.R., Riccardi, C., Bonnard, G.D., Holden, H.T., Fagnani, R., Santoni, A., and Puccetti, P. (1979). *Immunol. Reviews* 44, 43.

Hewlett, G., Opitz, H.-G., Schlumberger, H.D., and Lemke, H. (1977). *Eur.J.Immunol.* 7, 781.

Hibbs, J.B. (1976). *in* "The Macrophage in Neoplasia" (M.A. Fink, ed.), p. 83. Academic Press, New York.

Holt, P.G. (1979).*Immunology* 37, 429.

Holtermann, O.A., Djerassi, I., Lisafeld, B.A., Elias, E.G., Papermaster, B.W., and Klein, E. (1974). *Proc.Soc.Exp. Biol.Med.*147, 456.

Horwitz, D.A., Kight, N., Temple, A., and Allison, A.C. (1979). *Immunology* 36, 221.

Jett, J.R., Mantovani, A., and Herberman, R.B. (1980). Submitted to *Cellular Immunology*

Keller, R. (1973).*J.Exp.Med.*138, 625.

Keller, R. (1976a).*in* "Immunobiology of the Macrophage" (D.S.Nelson,ed.), p.487. Academic Press, New York.

Keller, R. (1976b). *J.Natl.Cancer Inst.*56, 369.

Keller, R. (1978a). *Br.J.Cancer* 37, 732.

Keller, R. (1978b). *Br.J.Cancer* 37, 742.

Kit, S., Kurimura, T., and Dubbs, D.R. (1969). *Int.J. Cancer* 4, 384.

Krahenbuhl, J.L., Lambert, L.H.Jr., and Remington, J.S. (1976). *Immunology* 31, 837.

Mantovani, A. (1977).*Cancer Res.* 37, 815.

Mantovani, A. (1978).*Int.J.Cancer* 22, 741.

Mantovani, A. (1980). *in* "Manual of Macrophage Methodology" (H.B.Herscowitz, H.T.Holden, J.A.Bellanti, A.Ghaffar, eds.), Marcel Dekker, New York, in press.

Mantovani, A., Bar Shavit, Z., Peri, G., Polentarutti, N., Bordignon, C., Sessa, C., and Mangioni, C. (1980a). *Clin. Exp.Immunol.* in press.

Mantovani, A., Caprioli, V., Gritti, P., and Spreafico, F. (1977). *Transplantation* 24, 291.

Mantovani, A., Dean, J.H., Jerrells, T.R., and Herberman, R.B. (1980b). Submitted to *J.Immunol.*

Mantovani, A., Jerrells, T.R., Dean, J.H., and Herberman, R.B. (1979a). *Int.J.Cancer* 23, 18.

Mantovani, A., Peri, G., Polentarutti, N., Bolis, G., Mangioni, C., and Spreafico, F. (1979b). *Int.J. Cancer* 23, 157.

Mantovani, A., Polentarutti, N., Gritti, P., Bolis, G., Maggioni, A., and Spreafico, F. (1979d). *Eur. J. Cancer* 15, 797.

Mantovani, A., Polentarutti, N., Peri, G., Bar Shavit, Z., Bolis, G., and Mangioni, C. (1980c). *J.Natl.Cancer Inst.* in press.

Mantovani, A., Tagliabue, A., Dean, J.H., Jerrells, T.R., Herberman, R.B. (1979c). *Int.J.Cancer* 23, 28.

Martin, F., Martin, M., Jeannin, J.-F., and Lagneau, A.(1978). *Eur.J. Immunol.* 8, 607.

Morley, J., Bray, M.A., Jones, R.W., Nugteren, D.H., and Van Dorp, D.A. (1979). *Prostaglandins* 17, 730.

Namba, Y., and Hanaoka, M. (1972). *J.Immunol.* 109, 1193.

Nathan, C.F., and Terry, W.D. (1975). *J.exp.Med.* 142, 887.

Olivotto, M., and Bomford, R. (1974). *Int.J.Cancer* 13, 478.

Ortaldo, J.R., Bonnard, G.D., and Herberman, R.B. (1977). *J. Immunol.* 119, 1351.

Piessens, W.F., Churchill,W.H,Jr., and David, J.R. (1975). *J. Immunol.* 114, 293.

Pross, H.F., and Kerbel, R.S. (1976). *J. Natl.Cancer Inst.* 57, 1157.

Rinehart, J.J., Lange, P., Gormus, B.J., and Kaplan, M.E. (1978). *Blood* 52, 211.

Ruco, L.P., and Meltzer, M.S. (1977). *J.Immunol.* 119, 889.

Russell, S.W., and McIntosh, A.T. (1977). *Nature(London)* 268, 69.

Schultz, R.M., Papamatheakis, J.D., and Chirigos, M.A. (1977). *Science* 197, 674.

Schultz, R.M., Pavlidis, N.A., Stylos, W.A., and Chirigos, M. A. (1978). *Science* 202, 320.

Sugiyama, M.,and Epstein, L.B. (1978). *Cancer Res.* 38, 4467.

Sutton, J.S. (1967). *Natl. Cancer Inst.Monogr.* 26, 71.

Tagliabue, A., Mantovani, A., Kilgallen, M., Herberman, R.B., McCoy, J.L. (1979). *J.Immunol.* 122, 2363.

Taylor-Papadimitriou, J., Shearer, M., and Tilly, R. (1977). *J. Natl. Cancer Inst.* 58, 1563.

Territo, M., and Cline, M.J. (1976). *in* "Immunobiology of the Macrophage" (D.S. Nelson, ed.), p. 593. Academic Press, New York.

Vose, B.M., Vánky, F., and Klein, E. (1977). *Int. J. Cancer* 20, 895.

Walker, W.S. (1976). *in* "Immunobiology of the Macrophage" (D.S. Nelson,ed.), p. 91. Academic Press, New York.

Webb, H.E., Oaten, S.W., and Pike, C.P. (1978). *Br.Med.J.* 1, 338.

Wood, G.W., and Gillespie,G.Y. (1975). *Int.J. Cancer* 16, 1022.

Wood, G.W., and Gollahon, K.A. (1977). *J. Natl.Cancer Inst.* 59, 1081.

Zarling, J.M., and Tevethia, S.S. (1973). *J. Natl. Cancer Inst.* 50, 149.

SUMMARY: NATURAL MACROPHAGE CYTOTOXICITY

Macrophages have been recognized for many years to play an important role in natural immunity. These effector cells, together with NK cells, appear to comprise the main components in natural resistance against tumor growth and other foreign invaders. There are proponents for the primacy of each effector mechanism in natural host defenses. However, the overall evidence does not permit such generalizations. It seems more likely that the presence of both of these celular systems is very beneficial to the host, since some tumors may be resistant to attack by one or the other but are less likely to evade the control of both.

The chapters in this section provide detailed reviews of natural macrophage cytotoxicity in rodents and in man. It would be redundant to try to summarize most of this information here. Rather, it seems most useful to indicate and discuss the similarities and differences in natural cytotoxicity by macrophages and NK cells. Some of the major points are listed in Table I.

I. SIMILARITIES AND POSITIVE ASSOCIATIONS BETWEEN MACROPHAGES AND NK CELLS

Most normal mice, rats and humans have been found to have appreciable levels of macrophage-mediated cytotoxicity, as well as NK reactivity. It is of interest that increased cytotoxic reactivity by macrophages, as well as NK cells has been observed in nude mice. Reactivity of both effector cells can be observed with a wide variety of target cells, including autologous, syngeneic, allogeneic and xenogeneic tumor cells. Although the activity of each is most apparent against transformed cells, effects may also be seen against some normal cells.

ISBN 0-12-341350-8

TABLE I. Similarities and Differences Between Macrophages and NK Cells, and Their Interrelationship

---

A. *Similarities and positive associations between macrophages and NK cells.*
   1. *Appreciable cytotoxic reactivity in most normal mice, rats and humans.*
   2. *Cytotoxicity against a wide range of target cells.*
   3. *Levels of reactivity augmented by variety of stimulating factors, with many having effects on both cell types.*
   4. *Some dependence on macrophages for reactivity of NK cells.*
   5. *Depressed function may be seen in tumor-bearing individuals.*
   6. *Evidence for in vivo role in resistance against tumor growth.*

B. *Differences and negative interactions between macrophages and NK cells.*
   1. *Distinctive cell surface and other characteristics.*
   2. *Different effects of various agents or treatments on activities (e.g. trypsin, protein synthesis inhibitors, lability in vitro.*
   3. *Cytolysis by macrophages usually requires longer period of time.*
   4. *Cytotoxic activity by macrophages appears earlier in life.*
   5. *Differences in susceptibility of some target cells to lysis by macrophages or NK cells.*
   6. *Differences in levels of activities in various organs and among mouse strains (e.g. beige, SJL, C3H/HeJ).*
   7. *Wider variety of known functions associated with macrophages.*
   8. *Suppression of NK activity by macrophages.*

The levels of reactivity of both macrophages and NK cells can be substantially augmented by a wide variety of stimulating factors. Interferon appears to be an important mediator of activation for macrophages as well as NK cells. However, in contrast to NK cells, other, apparently interferon-independent, mediators of boosting have been documented. Macrophage activating factor, a lymphokine produced by stimulated T cells, appears to play a centrol role in activation of cytotoxicity by macrophages. Endotoxins also have important stimulatory effects, apparently as interferon-independent triggers or accelerators of reactivity, on mouse macrophages.

Despite such differences in mechanisms of activation, it has been quite striking that most of the agents capable of boosting NK activity also have substantial effects on the activity of macrophages. Boosting of NK activity by some materials, e.g. poly I:C, has been found to be dependent on interferon production by macrophages. A further link between the two cell types has been the evidence that macrohages may play a similar role in the development and maintenance of spontaneous NK activity. Treatment of mice or rats with macrophage-toxic agents, silica or carrageenan, causes appreciable depression of NK activity. Other treatments, with ^{89}Sr or phorbol esters, also resulted in depression of cytotoxic activity by both macrophages and NK cells.

The parallel effects of many treatments on reactivity of macrophages and NK cells have led to difficulties in discriminating between their effects. Such problems have also arisen in *in vitro* studies because of some overlapping in the characteristics of these effector cells. Both cell types have Fc$_{\gamma}$ receptors and, as discussed earlier (sections IA and IC3), some NK cells, particularly after augmentation, can be adherent.

The levels of macrophage-mediated cytotoxicity in individuals bearing a variety of different tumors have not yet been extensively documented. However, in some tumor-bearers, cytotoxicity by macrophages, as well as NK activity, may be depressed.

II. DIFFERENCES AND NEGATIVE INTERACTIONS BETWEEN MACROPHAGES AND NK CELLS

Some of the major differences in the phenotype of NK cells and macrophages have been discussed in section IA. Some additional differences in their characteristics are worth pointing out here. Mouse NK cells tend to be quite labile *in vitro* at 37° and similarly, human NK cells lose much activity upon incubation overnight in medium containing human serum. In contrast, macrophages or monocytes appear to retain their natural cytotoxic reactivity for at least 1-2 days *in vitro*. Another feature of NK cells is their loss of activity upon treatment with trypsin (see earlier discussions,espicially in section IB). In contrast, the activity of macrophages appears to be trypsin-resistant (Keller). Also, as discussed in section IC4, treatment *in vivo* with estradiol selectively depresses NK activity. Conversely, the spontaneous cytotoxic activity of rodent macrophages, but not NK cells, is depressed or eliminated by treatment with inhibitors of protein synthesis.

Cytolysis of susceptible target cells by NK cells occurs very rapidly, being apparent in 4 hr assays, whereas substantially longer periods, usually 48-72 hrs, are required to detect spontaneous cytolytic reactivity by macrophages. Keller suggests that some of this longer period may be needed for activation of the macrophages and under some circumstances this can be circumvented.

Expression of cytotoxic reactivity by macrophages varies from that of NK cells in several respects. A major site for cytotoxic macrophages is the peritoneal cavity, where little spontaneous NK activity is found. Cytotoxic reactivity develops within a few days of birth in rats and mice, whereas NK activity first becomes detectable after 3-4 weeks. Some strains of mice have been found to have selective deficits in either NK or macrophage reactivity. For example, the low NK activity of beige or SJL mice is not accompanied by depressed macrophage-mediated cytotoxicity, and C3H/HeJ mice, that are deficient in spontaneous macrophge cytotoxicity, have high levels of NK activity.

The patterns of susceptibility of target cells to cytotoxicity by macrohages and NK cells vary considerably. Some targets that are very sensitive to lysis by NK cells are resistant to the effects of macrophages, and vice versa. For example, K562 is about the most sensitive target for human NK cells but is rather resistant to lysis by human monocytes, and while human NK cells don't show much activity against most mouse target cells, some of those lines are very sensitive to lysis by monocytes. As discussed in section ID, the cytotoxicity by NK cells appears to be dependent on recognition of a variety of antigens on target cells and there is evidence for subsets of effector cells that have restricted specificity. The general consensus is that macrophages are nonspecific in their action and do not recognize antigenic specificities. However, since they clearly do show selectivity towards certain target cells, and the pattern of reactivity by individual mouse macrophage cell lines varies somewhat from that of an unfractionated macrophage population (T. Taniyama and H.T. Holden, unpublished observations), it seems possible that macrophages may in fact have some heterogeneity and specificity in their cytotoxic reactivity.

As a class of cells, macrophages appear to be considerably more versatile in their range of functions than are NK cells. In addition to having cytolytic activity, macrophages also display various accessory and suppressor functions and have growth inhibitory or growth promoting activity against neoplastic and normal cells. The growth promoting activity seems to be primarily associated with target cells that are not rapidly proliferating *in vitro* and such stimulation of growth is usually referred to as "feeder effects." However, the mechanism of these growth promoting effects has not been elucidated and it is not clear whether macrophages can also cause acceleration of cell growth *in vivo*.

The other observed effect of macrophages that appears to run counter to host resistance is their suppressor activity. In addition to inhibiting lymphoproliferation, lymphokine production and generation of cytotoxic T lymphocytes, some activated macrophages appear to be able to suppress NK activity, perhaps due to their production of prostaglandins. As discussed earlier (section IC4) by Santoni *et al*, periods of macrophage activation are often accompanied by depression in NK activity.

It is yet clear whether the multiple functions associated with macrophages are possessed by the same cells. It is quite possible that there are subsets of macrophages, distinct from each other or at differnt stages of differentiation or activation, each having a more limited range of functions. Better markers and separation procedures are needed to resolve this important question.

III. RELATIVE *IN VIVO* ANTI-TUMOR ROLES OF MACROPHAGES AND NK CELLS

As discussed earlier, in section IF, there is considerable evidence for an *in vivo* role of NK cells in resistance against tumor growth. Keller points out that macrophages may also mediate natural resistance against growth of some tumors. The relative roles of each, and whether they usually act in concert or may interfere with each other, has not been well worked out. R. Evans has recently been reporting some instances in which macrophages actually appear to be interfering with effective resistance against tumor growth, but no similar situation has yet been found for NK cells.

It is important to note that, as with NK cells, there is almost no information regarding the effects of macrophages on growth of primary tumors. This is clearly an area that deserves more attention. Furthermore, it is often difficult to discriminate between the *in vivo* effects of NK cells and macrophages, and experiments need to be designed with this problem in mind. A potential example of such difficulty is that the effects on tumor growth of adoptively transferred macrophages could be mediated, not only by direct action of macrophages on tumor cells but also by the effects of these cells on NK cells, via interferon production on the one hand and suppression on the other. The use of experimental models or situations in which only the activity of NK cells or macrophages is depressed or augmented will be very important for better evaluating the *in vivo* roles of each. Some currently available possibilities for such studies are: a) for NK cells, beige or SJL mice or animals treated with estradiol; and b) for macrohages, C3H/HeJ mice.

THE ROLE OF GRANULOCYTES IN HOST DEFENSE AGAINST TUMORS

S. Korec

Laboratory of Immunodiagnosis
National Cancer Institute
Bethesda, Maryland

I. INTRODUCTION

In the past two decades much evidence has accumulated to indicate that the growth and development of neoplastic cells are subject to the influence of various factors of immune defense. Based on both *in vivo* and *in vitro* studies, antibodies (1, 2), lymphocytes (3, 4), and macrophages (5, 6) have been shown to be involved in host resistance to cancer. Granulocytes are the only major component of the immune apparatus that have been almost completely ignored by tumor immunologists. This is rather surprising since granulocytes are considered to be initially involved in almost all inflammatory reactions. They are known to operate under the influence of environmental signals but they are also known to secrete mediators regulating the activity of other cells participating in the reaction (7, 8, 9, 10). The inclusion of a chapter on granulocytes in this book on natural cell-mediated immunity against tumors is attributable to recent progress in our understanding of the biology of granulocytes and their possible role in tumor immunology.

II. NATURAL CYTOTOXICITY BY GRANULOCYTES

The first evidence on cytotoxicity by human granulocytes came from the work of Lundgren *et al*. (11). They reported damage (assessed by plaque formation) of human fibroblast monolayers by polymorphonuclear leukocytes (PMNs). Target cells were not killed, but detached from the surface of the

ISBN 0-12-341350-8

culture vessel into the medium and could be recultivated from the supernatant. Later Takasugi *et al.* (12) confirmed these results with adherent tumor target cell lines. They also observed detachment of targets by human granulocytes, without accompanying cell destruction, as measured by ^{51}Cr release. We have studied the cytolytic and cytostatic activity of human peripheral blood granulocytes against a variety of tumor-derived, virus-transformed and normal cell lines (13). In radioisotope release assays, we failed to detect lysis of any of the target cell lines tested, when examined for up to 72 hours, at the E/T (effector/target) cell ratios up to 100:1. In agreement with others we have seen disruption of target cell monolayers, by detachment of cells from the plastic. We have observed substantial growth-inhibitory activity of PMNs against adherent and non-adherent tumor cells, as measured by uptake of ^{3}H thymidine. Proliferation of normal fibroblast lines was inhibited to a lesser degree, and PHA-induced lymphoblasts were unaffected by the presence of PMNs in the culture.

Cytostasis of all but one target cell line was unaffected by addition of catalase to inhibit the peroxidase system (the fundamental granulocyte microbicidal mechanism) suggesting that other mechanisms are involved in the observed cytotoxicity (13).

When the activity of granulocytes from normals and patients was compared, cancer patients with clinically detectable disease showed lower levels of cytostasis (Fig. 1). In contrast, cancer patients without evidence of disease and patients with benign tumors had levels of cytostasis that were in the same range as those of normal adults.

The above results were obtained with granulocytes separated from blood by Plasmagel sedimentation of erythrocytes, followed by Ficoll-Hypaque centrifugation. However, with granulocytes obtained by a one-step method (separation of whole blood on discontinuous gradients formed by Ficoll-Hypaque and Percoll solutions of different densities) the reactivity of normals and cancer patients was the same, and in both groups was lower than seen with the previous method (Korec, S., Herberman, R. B., Cannon, G. B., Reid, J. and Braatz, J., in preparation). Addition of heat-inactivated normal pooled AB human serum increased the cytostatic activity of granulocytes of both normal donors and cancer patients usually to the same extent. In contrast, when autologous serum was added, the cytostatic activity of PMNs from cancer patients increased significantly less than that of normal individuals.

This suggested that the differences in cytostatic activity between cancer patients and normal donors might be due to serum factors. In support of this, when one-step

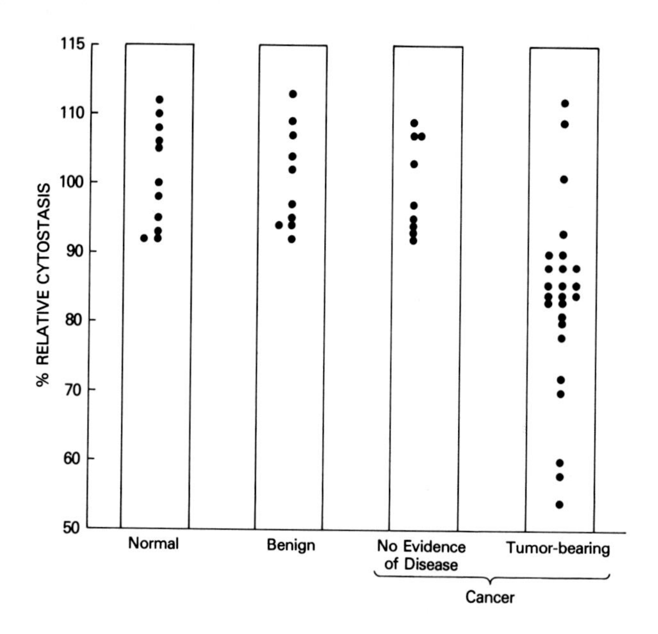

FIGURE 1. Cytostatic activity of granulocytes from patients and normal donors, tested against F265 lymphoblastoid cell line. Level of cytostasis of each individual calculated relative to mean % cytostasis of normal donors tested in same experiment.

separated granulocytes from normal donors were tested in the presence of sera from patients and controls, differences in reactivity were seen (Fig. 2), similar to those shown in Fig. 1. These experiments indicate that the decreased growth inhibitory activity of cancer patients' PMNs may be due mainly to some changes in serum factors, associated with tumor growth.

III. CYTOTOXICITY OF ACTIVATED GRANULOCYTES

A broad spectrum of agents is known to cause activation of granulocytes, with changes in their functional activity. Therefore it is important to make a distinction between results from experiments with resting and activated cells. Here we will discuss the function of granulocytes stimulated in the presence of other immune cells or humoral factors.

Rat peritoneal granulocytes induced by peptone-broth displayed substantial cytolytic activity against syngeneic

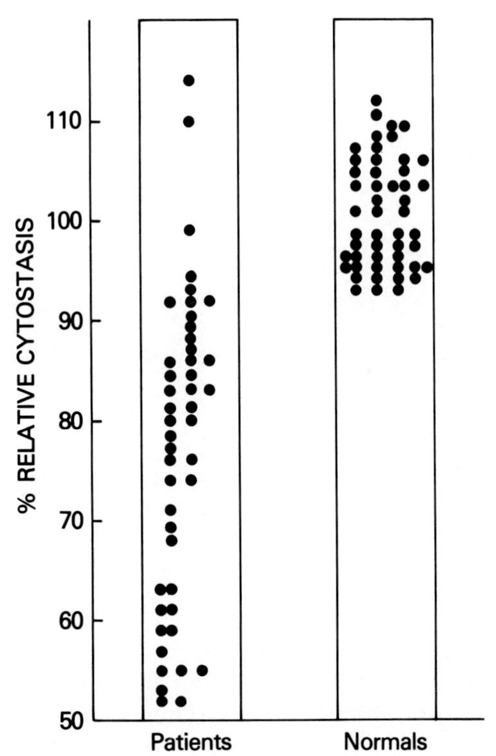

FIGURE 2. Cytostatic activity of one-step separated granulocytes of normal donors, tested in presence of sera from tumor-bearing patients or normal donors. Data expressed as in Figure 1.

ascitic tumor cells at E/T ratios as low as 2:1 (14). Dvorak *et al.* (15) observed destruction of mouse mammary adenocarcinoma cells 6 hours after intraperitoneal implantation. Tumor cells in contact with viable neutrophils displayed morphologic evidence of cell injury and death. The neutrophils remained fully granulated and nonphagocytic. In humans, granulocytes were found to form rosettes *in vivo* around ascitic lymphoma cells, in patients with an unusually prolonged course of disease (17). Involvement of antibodies in the attraction and binding of granulocytes to tumor cells was suspected.

The fact that granulocytes can function as effector cells in antibody-dependent cell-mediated cytotoxicity (ADCC) is well documented (17, 18, 19). An oxygen-dependent killing system has been implicated by most authors, but other mechanisms may also be involved (20). This ADCC activity is dependent on the presence of functional receptors for the Fc portion of IgG on the granulocyte cell membrane. Antibodies serve as a bridge keeping the granulocytes attached to the targets, and also as a stimulus for activating granulocyte metabolism. A similar mechanism seems to be involved in Concanavalin A-induced cytolysis by PMNs (21), where oxygen-dependent killing also has been suggested (22). Levels of cytolysis by activated granulocytes were comparable to those produced by lymphoid cells under similar conditions (19). Killing of tumor cells by phagocytosis-activated human granulocytes, as described by Clark *et al.* (23), seems to be mediated by the peroxidase system. Omission of phagocytosable particles, or addition of catalase, abolished cytotoxicity. The levels of cytolytic activity in these experiments were comparable to those seen in the above-mentioned studies with rat peritoneal granulocytes.

In mice, PMNs from tumor-bearing animals displayed significantly higher levels of cytotoxicity (detachment of adherent targets) against autologous tumor cells than against unrelated tumors (24). Since granulocytes do not appear capable of specific recognition, it is likely that this specificity was due to ADCC, with antibodies to the autologous tumor attached to the surface of PMNs.

Binding of complement-derived chemotactic factors (C3a, C5a or synthetic chemotactic factors) to the surface of PMNs results not only in chemotaxis but also in activation. The level of target killing by granulocytes activated with some of these factors varies from donor to donor, perhaps due to *in vivo* activation (25, 26), and also from target to target. In general, chemotactic factor-dependent cytolysis is of similar magnitude as ADCC.

IV. PARTICIPATION OF PMNS IN CYTOTOXICITY BY OTHER EFFECTOR CELLS

Bubenik *et al.* first reported higher levels of cytotoxicity by human peripheral blood mononuclear cells, when the effector cell population was contaminated by granulocytes (27). *In vivo* growth of tumors in rats was suppressed when tumor cells were transplanted subcutaneously with admixture of spleen cells and PMNs. Growth of tumor cells after mixture with spleen cells alone was similar to controls (28). In mice, local injection of the high molecular weight polysaccharide, levan, inhibited the growth of Lewis lung carcinoma (29). Histological studies showed that levan induced an intense polymorphonuclear reaction, followed by accumulation of macrophages. Destruction of tumor cells surrounded by PMNs and macrophages was observed. In humans, *in vitro* destruction of tumor cells by leukocytes from patients with gynecological tumors was observed (30). Participation of granulocytes was noted without further determination of their role.

CONCLUDING REMARKS

Polymorphonuclear leukocytes are an integral part of the immune system. In this short review, we have discussed situations in which PMNs have been shown to have cytotoxic reactivity against tumor cells. Reports in this field are still limited and inconclusive. The presence of granulocytes in proximity to tumor cells or indirect evidence on their possible antitumor activity are not convincing indications for a role of PMNs in resistance against tumors. However, the finding that normal granulocytes have *in vitro* cytostatic effects against a variety of tumor cells, and that upon activation cytolysis can result, raises the real possibility of an involvement of granulocytes in host defense against cancer. It would seem quite worthwile to vigorously pursue these leads and determine the *in vivo* role of granulocytes in tumor immunology.

REFERENCES

1. Fuller, T. C., Winn, H. J. (1975) *Transplantation Proc*, *5*, 585.
2. Johnson, R. Y., Pasternack, G. R., and Shin, H. S. (1977) *J. Immunol. 118*, 489.
3. Perlmann, P., Holm, G. (1969) *Adv. Immunol. 11*, 117.
4. Chu, E. H., Stjernsward, J., Clifford, P., Klein, G., (1967) *J. Nat. Canc. Inst. 39*,595.
5. Alexander, P., Evans, R. (1971) *Nature New Biol. 232*, 76.
6. Boyle, M., Ormerod, M. G. (1975) *J. Reticuloendoth. Soc. 17*, 73.
7. Nakamura, S., Yoshinaga, M., Hayashi, H. (1976) *J. Immunol. 117, 1*, 1.
8. Klostergaard, J., Lisafeld, B. H., Dunlop, B., Klein, E., Holterman, O. A. (1978) *Int. Arch. Allerg. Appl. Immun. 57*, 542.
9. Higuchi, Y., Ishida, M., Hayashi, H. (1979) *Cell. Immunol. 46*, 297.
10. Gordon, L. I., Douglas, S. D., Kay, N. E., Yamada, O., Osserman, E. F. (1979) *J. Clin. Invest. 69, 226.*

11. Lundgren, G., Zukoski, C. H. F., Moller, G. (1968) *Clin. Exp. Immunol. 3*, 817.
12. Takasugi, M., Akira, D., Kinoshita, K. (1975) *Cancer Res. 35*, 2169.
13. Korec, S., Herberman, R. B., Dean, J. H., Cannon, G. B. *Cell. Immunol.* (In press).
14. Pickaver, A. H., Ratcliffe, N. A., Williams, A. E., Smith, H. (1972). *Nature New Biology 235*, 186.
15. Dvorak, A. M., Connell, A. B., Proppe, K., Dvorak, H. F. (1978) *J. Immunol. 120, 4*, 1240.
16. Abelson, H. T., Stossel, T. P. (1978) *Lancet Jun. 1 (8075)*, 1217.
17. Hafeman, D. G., Lucas, Z. J. (1979) *J. Immunol. 123, 1*, 55.
18. Gale, R. P., Zighelboim, J., Ossorio, C., Fahey, J. C. (1974) *Clin. Res. 180, 22*, 180A.
19. Levy, P. C., Yhaw, G. M., Lo Buglio, A. (1979) *J. Immunol. 123, 2*, 594.
20. Clark, R. A., Klebanoff, S. J. (1977) *J. Immunol. 119*, 1413.
21. Simchowitz, L., Schur, P. H. (1976) *Immunology 31*, 303.
22. Clark, R. A., Klebanoff, S. J. (1979) *J. Immunol. 122*, 2605.
23. Clark, R. A., Klebanoff, S. J. (1975) *J. Exp. Med. 141*, 1442.
24. Fisher, B., Saffer, E. A. (1978) *J. Natl. Cancer Inst. 60, 3*, 687.
25. Saks, T., Moldow, C. F., Craddock, P. R., Bowers, T. K., Jacob, H. S. (1978) *J. Clin. Invest. 61, 5*, 1161.
26. Hunningheke, G., Gadek, J., Personal Communication.
27. Bubenik, J., Perlman, P., Helmstein, K., Moberger, G. (1970) *Int. J. Canc. 5*, 310.
28. Nakayama, M., Sendo, F., Miyake, J., Fuyama, S., Arai, S., Kobayashi, H. (1978) *J. Immunol. 120, 2*, 619.
29. Leibovici, J., Borit, A., Sandbank, V., Wolman, M. (1979) *Br. J. Cancer 40*, 597
30. Halbrecht, I., Komlos, L. (1974) *Obst. and Gyn. 43, 2*, 268.

SUMMARY: NATURAL GRANULOCYTE CYTOTOXICITY

Granulocytes are yet another class of effector cells that may play a significant role in natural resistance against tumors. While their activity against bacteria and fungi is well known, their anti-tumor effects have been largely neglected. From the limited data now available, it appears that they should be seriously considered, along with NK cells and macrophages. Granulocytes are well represented in the peripheral blood, spleen and at the site of growth of many tumors. As pointed out in the chapter by Becker (section IE), special efforts may be needed to separate them from other effector cells and to thereby adequately evaluate their role.

As with NK cells and macrophages, it is demonstrated here by Korec that human granulocytes from normal individuals have appreciable cytotoxic activity against a wide variety of target cells, especially transformed cells. In contrast to the other natural effector cells, unstimulated granulocytes appear to be only cytostatic and not cytolytic. However, as with NK cells and macrophages, granulocytes can become stimulated or activated and then have cytolytic activity. Interferon does not seem to be able to augment the reactivity of human granulocytes (S. Korec and R.B. Herberman, unpublished observations) and the factors which mediate their activation remain to be identified.

As another parallel with the other natural effector mechanisms, Korec has found that the cytostatic activity of human granulocytes is depressed in many patients bearing tumors. The observations of Becker that granulocytes are the main effector cells, that react against autologous tumor cells, within murine sarcoma virus-induced tumors of A strain mice are intriguing and much more work is needed to evaluate the possible *in vivo* role of granulocytes in resistance against tumor growth.

ISBN 0-12-341350-8

INDEX

A

D

E

F

G

H

I

J, K

L

M

N

O

T